KEY

Y compatible
N not compatible
P provisionally compatible; use within 15 minutes of preparation

? conflicting reports on compatibility; mixing not recommended
(A blank space indicates no available data on compatibility.)

	hydroxyzine	meperidine	morphine	nalbuphine	pentobarbital	phenobarbital	promethazine	scopolamine	secobarbital	sodium bicarbonate	thiopental
	P	Y	P	Y	P		Y	P		N	
	Y				N	N	Y	Y	N		N
	Y	Y	P		N	N	P	P	N	N	N
	P				N					N	
	N	N	N	N	N	N	N	N	N	N	N
	Y	Y	Y	Y	N		Y	Y	N	N	N
										N	N
	•	Y	P	Y	N	N	P	P		N	
	Y	•	N		N	N	Y	P		N	N
	P	N	•		?	N	?	P		N	N
	Y			•	N		?	Y			
	N	N	?	N	•		N	P		?	P
	N	N	N			•	N				Y
	P	Y	?	?	N	N	•	P			N
	P	P	P	Y	P		P	•	N	N	Y
								N	•		
	N	N	N		?			N		•	N
		N	N		P	Y	N	Y		N	•

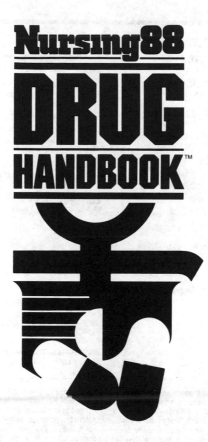

Nursing88 DRUG HANDBOOK™

NURSING88 BOOKS™
SPRINGHOUSE CORPORATION
SPRINGHOUSE, PENNSYLVANIA

NURSING88 DRUG HANDBOOK™

Staff for this volume

EDITORIAL DIRECTOR
Helen Klusek Hamilton

CLINICAL DIRECTOR
Barbara McVan, RN

ART DIRECTOR
John Hubbard

DRUG INFORMATION MANAGER
Larry Neil Gever, RPh, PharmD

CLINICAL EDITOR
Joanne Patzek DaCunha, RN, BS

ACQUISITIONS COORDINATOR
Margaret Belcher, RN, BSN

EDITORIAL SERVICES MANAGER
David Moreau

COPY EDITORS
Diane Labus, Doris Weinstock, Debra Young

PRODUCTION COORDINATOR
Susan Hopkins Rodzewich

ART PRODUCTION
Robert Perry (manager), Anna Brindisi, Don Knauss, Bob Wieder

TYPOGRAPHY
David C. Kosten (manager), Elizabeth DiCicco, Diane Paluba, Nancy Wirs

MANUFACTURING
Deborah C. Meiris (manager), T. Landis

EDITORIAL ASSISTANTS
Maree DeRosa, Denine Lichtfuss

Special thanks to Maryann Foley, RN, BSN.

The clinical procedures described and recommended in this publication are based on research and consultation with medical and nursing authorities. To the best of our knowledge, these procedures reflect currently accepted clinical practice; nevertheless, they can't be considered absolute and universal recommendations. For individual application, treatment recommendations must be considered in light of the patient's clinical condition and, before administration of new or infrequently used drugs, in light of latest package-insert information. The authors and the publisher disclaim responsibility for any adverse effects resulting directly or indirectly from the suggested procedures, from any undetected errors, or from the reader's misunderstanding of the text.

NURSING88 DRUG HANDBOOK
ISSN 0273-320X
ISBN 0-87434-126-4

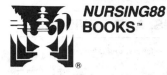

NURSING88 BOOKS™

NURSE'S REFERENCE LIBRARY®

Diseases	Practices
Diagnostics	Emergencies
Drugs	Signs & Symptoms
Assessment	Patient Teaching
Procedures	Treatments
Definitions	

NEW NURSING SKILLBOOK™ SERIES

Giving Emergency Care Competently
Monitoring Fluid and Electrolytes Precisely
Assessing Vital Functions Accurately
Coping with Neurologic Problems
   Proficiently
Reading EKGs Correctly
Combatting Cardiovascular Diseases
   Skillfully
Nursing Critically Ill Patients Confidently
Dealing with Death and Dying
Managing Diabetes Properly
Giving Cardiovascular Drugs Safely

NURSING PHOTOBOOK™ SERIES

Providing Respiratory Care
Managing I.V. Therapy
Dealing with Emergencies
Giving Medications
Assessing Your Patients
Using Monitors
Providing Early Mobility
Giving Cardiac Care
Performing GI Procedures
Implementing Urologic Procedures
Controlling Infection
Ensuring Intensive Care
Coping with Neurologic Disorders
Caring for Surgical Patients
Working with Orthopedic Patients
Nursing Pediatric Patients
Helping Geriatric Patients
Attending Ob/Gyn Patients
Aiding Ambulatory Patients
Carrying Out Special Procedures

NURSING NOW™ SERIES

Shock	Respiratory
Hypertension	Emergencies
Drug Interactions	Pain
Cardiac Crises	

NURSE'S CLINICAL LIBRARY®

Cardiovascular Disorders
Respiratory Disorders
Endocrine Disorders
Neurologic Disorders
Renal and Urologic Disorders
Gastrointestinal Disorders
Neoplastic Disorders
Immune Disorders

MEDIQUIK CARDS™

CLINICAL POCKET MANUAL™ SERIES

Diagnostic Tests	Neurologic Care
Emergency Care	Surgical Care
Fluids and	Medications and
Electrolytes	I.V.s
Signs and	Ob/Gyn Care
Symptoms	Pediatric Care
Cardiovascular	Assessment
Care	Drug Interactions
Respiratory Care	Documentation
Critical Care	

NURSE REVIEW™ SERIES

Cardiac Problems
Respiratory Problems
Gastrointestinal Problems
Neurologic Problems
Vascular Problems
Genitourinary Problems
Endocrine Problems
Musculoskeletal Problems
Metabolic Problems

NURSING YEARBOOK88
1987 Nursing Photobook Annual

CONSULTANTS, REVIEWERS, AND ADVISORS

At the time of publication, the clinical consultants, reviewers, and advisors held the following positions:

Clinical Consultants

Michael J. Booth, RN, CRNA, MA, Co-Director, Graduate Program of Nurse Anesthesia, and Assistant Professor, Department of Anesthesiology, Medical College of Pennsylvania and Hospital, Philadelphia

Karen E. Burgess, RN, MSN, Neuro/Ortho/Rehab Clinical Nurse Specialist, Huntington Memorial Hospital, Pasadena, Calif.

Charmaine J. Cummings, RN, MSN, Clinical Nurse Educator, Neurology, Eye, and Aging Research Nursing Service, Clinical Center Nursing Department, National Institutes of Health, Bethesda, Md.

Michele Donehower, RN, MSN, Clinical Nurse Specialist, The Johns Hopkins Oncology Center, Baltimore

Walter Carl Faubion, RN, MS, Manager, Parenteral and Enteral Nutrition Team; Clinical Assistant Professor, College of Pharmacy; and Adjunct Instructor, School of Nursing, University of Michigan Medical Center, Ann Arbor

Claire B. Forys, RN, BSN, Staff Nurse, Post Anesthesia Care Unit, Cooper Hospital–University Medical Center, Camden, N.J.

Deborah J. Henderson, RN, CIC, BSN, Special Assistant to the Director, NIAD, National Institutes of Health, Bethesda, Md.

Marcia Jo Hill, RN, MSN, Manager, Dermatologic Therapeutics, The Methodist Hospital, Houston

Karen Landis, RN, CCRN, MS, Pulmonary Clinical Nurse Specialist, Lehigh Valley Hospital Center, Allentown, Pa.

Chris Platt Moldovanyi, RN, CDE, MSN, Director of Nursing Education–Operating Room, and Endocrinology Clinical Nurse Specialist, Cleveland Clinic Foundation

Margaret A. Smellie-Belfield, RN, CCRN, BSN, Clinical Services Director, SICU/PACU, Veterans Administration Medical Center, San Diego

Nancy Baptie Walrath, RN, CGC, Director, Gastroenterology Department, Daniel Freeman Memorial and Marina Hospitals, Inglewood, Calif.

Special thanks to the following, who contributed to past editions: Jean Marie Amabile-Michiels, RN, MA, MSN; Wendy L. Baker, RN, MS, CCRN; Beverly A. Baldwin, RN, MA; Marjorie Davis Beck, RN; Therese E. Bowman, RN, BSN, MS; Heather Boyd-Monk, SRN, RN, BSN; Paula Brammer-Vetter, RN, BSN, CCRN; Nancy Burns, RN, PhD; Carla J. Burton, RN, BS; Priscilla A. Butts, RN, MSN; James J. Claffey, CRNA, BS; Maribel J. Clements, RN, MA; Elizabeth R. DiMeo, RN, MSN; Judy Donlen, RNC, MSN; Gail D'Onofrio, RN, MS; Jeanne Dupont, RN; DeAnn M. Englert, RN, MSN; Joel Glucroft, PhD; Margarethe Hawken, RN, MA, CNRN; Kathleen M. Hawkins, RN; Denise A. Hess, RN, BS; Tobie Hittle, RN, CCRN, BSN; Carolyn Holt, RN, BSEd; Maureen L. Metters, BSN; Kenneth J. Michalko, BSc Phm, PharmD; Margaret E. Miller, RN, MSN; John Nagelhout, CRNA, PhD; Brenda Marion Nevidson, RN, MSN; Elizabeth A. Phillips, RN, BA, BSN; Judith M. Rohde, RN, MS, CNP, CNRN; Dale Elizabeth Schreffler, RN, BSN; Roberta Seifer, RN, CNP, BS; Despina Seremelis, RN, BSN; Barbara Solomon, RN, MS; Robin Tourigian, RN, MSN; Carmen Brochu Wohrle, RN, MS; Patricia H. Worthington, RN, BSN

Pharmacy Reviewers

Steven R. Abel, RPh, PharmD, Assistant Director of Pharmacy, Clinical/Educational Services, Indiana University Hospitals, Indianapolis

Michael E. Burton, PharmD, Clinical Pharmacist, Veterans Administration Medical Center, Dallas

Robert B. Catalano, PharmD, Coordinator of Clinical Investigation, Fox Chase Cancer Center/American Oncologic Hospital, Philadelphia

Bruce D. Clayton, RPh, PharmD, Professor and Chairman, Department of Pharmacy Practice, College of Pharmacy, University of Arkansas for Medical Sciences, Little Rock

David W. Hawkins, PharmD, Associate Professor of Family Medicine, East Carolina University School of Medicine, Greenville, N.C.

CONTENTS

Autonomic Nervous System Drugs

Respiratory Tract Drugs

Gastrointestinal Tract Drugs

Hormonal Agents

Anesthetic Agents

Nutritional Agents

Miscellaneous Drug Categories

Index

FOREWORD

Nursing provides us with great opportunities to achieve professional fulfillment. However, with these opportunities come the obligatory responsibilities. One of the most difficult and complex of our responsibilities is that of administering and monitoring drug therapy.

The success or failure of a patient's treatment often depends on our first-hand knowledge of a drug's effects: the beneficial, or therapeutic, effects as well as the undesirable, or adverse, effects. How can we become so knowledgeable about the drugs our patients receive? Only with the help of a reliable drug reference. For almost a decade, the *Nursing Drug Handbook* has provided the reliable information we need to administer drug therapy with confidence.

Freshly reviewed for accuracy by both clinical nurse practitioners and clinical pharmacists, the *Nursing88 Drug Handbook* again offers all the drug information practicing nurses need. This year's edition, like preceding ones, has kept pace with current changes in the use of all the generic drugs (over 900) contained in it and adds 23 drugs newly approved during the past year. Also new in 1988, this volume offers information about a drug's potential effect on the fetus; it assigns a "pregnancy category" to every generic drug listed. With this knowledge, you'll be better able to counsel and advise patients who are pregnant or who expect to become pregnant.

You'll find new information as well as the familiar features that have made this handbook a leading drug reference—emphasis on clinical, not theoretical information; an easy-to-use format including mechanisms of action, indications and dosage, adverse reactions, interactions, and nursing considerations (which include contraindications, special precautions, and recommendations for easier administration, prevention of side effects, and safe storage)—all arranged for easy reference; and an easy-to-use index listing trade and generic names, combination products, and pharmacologic groups.

With the *Nursing88 Drug Handbook,* you can quickly and reliably validate any form of drug therapy. It is an indispensable source of accurate information you can use with confidence every day.

LUTHER CHRISTMAN, RN, PhD
Vice-President, Nursing Affairs, and Dean, College of Nursing
Rush–Presbyterian–St. Luke's Medical Center, Chicago

1

How to use Nursing88 Drug Handbook

Nursing88 Drug Handbook is meant to fill a very special need. It represents a joint effort by pharmacists and nurses to provide the nursing profession with drug information that focuses on what nurses need to know. With this in mind, it emphasizes clinical aspects and does not attempt to replace detailed pharmacology texts. For the same reason, the information is arranged in a format designed to make it readily accessible.

Introductory information
Following this chapter, Chapter 2 explains, in a general way, how drugs work. It also tells about side effects and adverse reactions and gives general guidelines about drug use in pregnancy and the presence of drugs in breast milk. Chapters 3 and 4 discuss the unique problems of administering drugs to children and the elderly and offer guidelines to minimize problems in these areas. In the remaining chapters, all drugs are classified according to their common, therapeutic uses.

Drug information
Each chapter begins with an alphabetically arranged list of the generic names of drugs described in that chapter. This is followed by a list of selected combination products in which these drugs are found. Specific information on each drug is arranged under six headings: *Name; Mechanism of Action; Indications and Dosage; Adverse Reactions; Interactions;* and *Nursing Considerations.*

Each drug's generic name is imme-

diately followed by an alphabetic list of its brand names. Brands available in both the United States and Canada are designated with a diamond (♦); those available *only* in Canada with a double diamond (♦♦). A brand name with no symbol after it is available only in the United States. If a drug is a controlled substance, that too is clearly indicated (example: Controlled Substance Schedule II). Products listed, although generally available, may not be approved by the Food and Drug Administration. The mention of a brand name in no way implies endorsement of that product or guarantees its legality.

The section titled *Mechanism of Action* succinctly describes *how* each specific drug provides its therapeutic effect. For example, although all antihypertensives lower blood pressure, they don't all do this by the same pharmacologic process.

The section titled *Indications and Dosage* lists general dosage information for adults (including recommended geriatric dosages, when available) and children, as applicable. Children's dosages are usually indicated in terms of mg/kg daily. Dosage instructions reflect current clinical trends in therapeutics and can't be considered as absolute and universal recommendations. For individual application, dosage instructions must be considered in light of the patient's clinical condition.

The section titled *Adverse Reactions* lists each drug's commonly observed adverse reactions (and selected rare ones if life-threatening). The most common and life-threatening adverse reactions are italicized for easy reference. An exception to this rule is an adverse reaction that, although normally considered hazardous, has been reported to be mild and reversible with the drug in question. For example, thrombocytopenia is considered a life-threatening adverse reaction of mithramycin (a chemotherapeutic drug), but the thrombocytopenia seen with methyldopa (Aldomet) is generally mild and reversible. Hence, thrombocytopenia listed as an adverse reaction to mithramycin is italicized, whereas the same reaction under methyldopa is not. Adverse reactions are grouped according to the body system in which they appear.

The next section, *Interactions,* lists each drug's confirmed, *clinically significant* interactions with other drugs, including additive effects, potentiated effects, and antagonistic effects. Also included are specific suggestions for dealing with dangerous drug interactions (for example, reducing doses or monitoring certain laboratory tests). Drug interactions are listed under the drug that is adversely affected. For example, magnesium trisilicate, an ingredient in antacids, interacts with tetracycline to cause decreased absorption of tetracycline. Therefore, this interaction is listed under tetracycline. To check on the possible effects of using two or more drugs simultaneously, refer to the interaction entry for *each* of the drugs in question.

The final section, *Nursing Considerations,* lists other useful information, starting with contraindications and precautions, followed by monitoring techniques and suggestions for prevention and treatment of adverse reactions. Also included are suggestions for patient comfort, for patient teaching, and for preparing, administering, and storing each drug.

FDA pregnancy categories

The Food and Drug Administration has established five pregnancy categories that indicate a drug's potential to cause birth defects. These categories, named A, B, C, D, and X, are listed below with an explanation of each. Drugs in Category A are considered generally safe to use in pregnancy; drugs in Category X are generally contraindicated.

• A: Adequate studies in pregnant women have failed to show a risk to the fetus in the first trimester of pregnancy—and there is no evidence of risk in later trimesters.

• B: Animal studies have not shown a risk to the fetus, but there are no adequate clinical studies in pregnant women.

• C: Animal studies *have* shown an adverse effect on the fetus, but there are no adequate studies in humans. The drug may be useful in pregnant women despite its potential risks.

• D: There is evidence of risk to the human fetus, but the potential benefits of use in pregnant women may be acceptable despite potential risks.

• X: Studies in animals or humans demonstrate fetal abnormalities, or adverse reaction reports indicate evidence of fetal risk. The risks involved clearly outweigh potential benefits.

• NR: No rating available.

Alcohol and tartrazine content

Many liquid drug preparations for oral use contain alcohol. Although the slight sedative effect that alcohol produces is not harmful in most patients—and can sometimes be beneficial—alcohol ingestion can be undesirable and even dangerous in some circumstances. So, alcohol-containing oral drugs should be given very cautiously, if at all, to patients who are:

• concomitantly taking potent CNS depressants, such as barbiturates.

• taking drugs that may produce a disulfiram-type reaction (such as chlorpropamide, metronidazole, and moxalactam).

• known alcoholics who are taking disulfiram (Antabuse) as part of a treatment program for their alcoholism. Patients taking disulfiram, upon ingestion of alcohol or alcohol-containing drugs, will exhibit severe symptoms that may include blurred vision, confusion, dyspnea, flushing, sweating, and tachycardia.

To help prevent inadvertent and potentially harmful exposure to alcohol, a single asterisk (*) follows the generic name of a drug if its liquid form contains alcohol. In many of the preparations so marked, the alcohol content is small. Nevertheless, in patients who are susceptible to developing adverse effects upon exposure to alcohol, these drugs should be avoided.

Tartrazine dye, also known as FD&C Yellow No. 5, is a common coloring agent used in some foods and drugs. Although usually harmless, it can provoke a severe allergic reaction in susceptible persons. For this reason, most drug manufacturers have begun to eliminate tartrazine from their products, but many drugs still contain it.

The incidence of tartrazine sensitivity is estimated at approximately 1 in 10,000 in the general population but somewhat higher in persons with asthma and/or sensitivity to aspirin. Why this is so is unknown. The most common symptoms of tartrazine sensitivity are urticaria, rhinorrhea, asthma (or exacerbation of existing asthma), and angioedema. Acutely sensitive persons may develop allergic vascular purpura, tachycardia, dyspnea, and chest pain. These allergic symptoms generally subside spontaneously upon discontinuation of the tartrazine-containing drug but occasionally require treatment with antihistamines or epinephrine.

Avoiding exposure to tartrazine is not simply a matter of avoiding yellow-colored drugs because this substance may be present in many other color blends, such as turquoise, green, and maroon. You can be sure to prevent exposure to tartrazine only by carefully checking the specific content of any drug preparation. To this end, this volume signals tartrazine content. The name of every brand of drug that may contain tartrazine will be followed by a double asterisk (**). If you suspect tartrazine sensitivity in a patient receiving such a drug, inform the doctor and contact the manufacturer to determine which dosage forms contain tartrazine.

A Guide to Abbreviations

b.i.d.	twice daily
CNS	central nervous system
CV	cardiovascular
EENT	eyes, ears, nose, throat
g	gram
G	gauge
GI	gastrointestinal
GU	genitourinary
I.M.	intramuscular
IU	international unit
I.V.	intravenous
kg	kilogram
L	liter
m²	square meter
MAO	monoamine oxidase
mcg	microgram
ml	milliliter
P.O.	by mouth
p.r.n.	as needed
q	every
q.i.d.	four times daily
S.C.	subcutaneous
t.i.d.	three times daily

Drug actions, reactions, and interactions explained

Administration of any drug provokes a series of physiochemical events within the body. The first event, when a drug combines with cell drug receptors, is known as the drug action. What follows as a result of this action of the drug is known as the drug effect. Depending on the number of different cellular drug receptors affected by a given drug, a drug effect can be local or systemic, or both. For example, the antipeptic ulcer drug cimetidine (Tagamet) acts solely by blocking histamine receptor cells in the parietal cells of the stomach. This is known as a local drug effect because the drug action is sharply limited to one area and does not spread to other parts of the body. On the other hand, diphenhydramine (Benadryl) produces a systemic effect in that it blocks histamine receptors in widespread areas of the body. In other words, local drug effects are specific to a limited number of organ systems, whereas systemic drug effects are generalized and affect different and diverse organ systems.

Three factors modify drug action
1. Absorption
Before a drug can act within the body, it must be absorbed into the bloodstream—usually after oral administration, the most frequently used route. Before a drug contained in a tablet or capsule can be absorbed, the dosage form must disintegrate, that is, break into smaller particles. Then, these smaller particles can dissolve in gastric juices. Only after so dissolving can a drug be absorbed into the bloodstream. Once absorbed and circulating in the bloodstream, it is said to be bioavailable, or ready to produce a drug effect. Of course, whether such absorption is complete or partial depends on several factors: the drug's physiochemical effects, its dosage form, its route of administration, its interactions with other substances in the gastrointestinal tract, and various patient characteristics. These same factors also determine the speed of absorption. Thus, oral solutions and elixirs, which bypass the need for disintegration and dissolution, are usually absorbed more rapidly. Drugs administered intramuscularly must first be absorbed through the muscle into the bloodstream. Rectal suppositories must dissolve to be absorbed through the rectal mucosa. Of course, drugs administered intravenously are placed directly into the circulation and are completely and immediately bioavailable.

2. Distribution
After absorption, a drug moves from the bloodstream into various fluids and tissues within the body; this is distribution. Individual patient variations can greatly alter the amount of drug that is distributed throughout the body. For example, in an edematous patient, a given dose must be distributed to a larger volume than in a nonedematous patient; the amount of drug must sometimes be increased to account for this. Remember, the dosage should be decreased when the edema is corrected. Conversely, in an

extremely dehydrated patient, the drug will be distributed to a much smaller volume, so the dose must then be decreased. The total area to which a drug is distributed is known as volume of distribution. Patients who are particularly obese may present another problem when considering drug distribution. Some drugs—such as digoxin, gentamicin, and tobramycin—are not well distributed to fatty tissue. Therefore, dosing based on actual body weight may lead to overdose and serious toxicity. In some cases, dosing must be based on lean body weight, which may be estimated from actuarial tables that give average weight range for height.

3. Metabolism and excretion (drug elimination)

Most drugs are metabolized in the liver and excreted by the kidneys. Hepatic diseases may affect one or more of the metabolic functions of the liver. Therefore, in patients with hepatic disease, the metabolism of a drug may be increased, decreased, or unchanged. Clearly, all patients with hepatic disease must be monitored closely for drug effect and toxicity. Some drugs (digoxin, gentamicin) are eliminated almost unchanged by the kidneys. For safe use of such drugs, renal function must be adequate or the drug will accumulate, producing toxic effects. Some drugs can alter the effect and excretion of other drugs. For example, they can stimulate hepatic metabolizing enzymes to speed up the rate of metabolism and change the drug effect. Or they can block or promote renal excretion of other drugs, causing them to accumulate and enhance their effects or causing them to be too rapidly excreted and so diminish their effects. Some slight elimination takes place by way of perspiration, saliva, breast milk, and so on. (Certain volatile anesthetics, however—halothane, for instance—are eliminated primarily by exhalation.)

The rate at which a drug is metabolized varies with the individual. In some patients, drugs are metabolized so quickly that their blood and tissue levels prove therapeutically inadequate. In others, the rate of metabolism is so slow that ordinary doses can produce toxic results.

Other modifying factors

An important factor that influences a drug's action and effect is its *binding to plasma proteins,* especially albumin, and other tissue components. Because only a free, unbound drug can act in the body, such binding greatly influences effectiveness and duration of effect.

The *patient's age* is another important factor. Elderly patients usually have decreased hepatic function, less muscle mass, and diminished renal function. Consequently, lower doses and sometimes longer dosage intervals are needed to avoid toxicity in the elderly. With similar consequences, neonates have underdeveloped metabolic enzyme systems and inadequate renal function. They need highly individualized dosage and careful monitoring.

Underlying disease can also markedly affect drug action and effect. For example, acidosis may cause insulin resistance. Genetic diseases, such as glucose-6-phosphate dehydrogenase (G6PD) deficiency and hepatic porphyria, may turn drugs into toxins with serious consequences. Patients with G6PD deficiency may develop hemolytic anemia when given sulfonamides or a number of other drugs. A genetically susceptible patient can develop an acute porphyria attack if given a barbiturate. Also, patients who have highly active hepatic enzyme systems (for example, rapid acetylators), when treated with isoniazid, can develop hepatitis from the rapid intrahepatic buildup of a toxic metabolite.

Things to consider about administration

1. Dosage forms do matter. Some tablets and capsules are too large to be readily swallowed by very ill patients. You may then request an oral solution or elixir of the same drug, but bear in mind that because a liquid is more easily and completely absorbed, it produces higher blood levels than a tablet. When a potentially toxic drug is given, the increased amount absorbed could cause toxicity. One example of this is digoxin tablets versus digoxin elixir. Sometimes a change in dosage form requires a change in dose.

2. Routes of administration are not therapeutically interchangeable. For example, phenytoin (Dilantin) is readily absorbed orally but is slowly and erratically absorbed intramuscularly. On the other hand, carbenicillin must be given parenterally because oral administration yields inadequate blood levels to treat systemic infections. However, it can be given orally to treat urinary tract infections because it concentrates in the urine.

3. The timing of drug administration can be important. Sometimes giving an oral drug during or shortly after mealtime decreases the amount of drug absorbed. This is not clinically significant with most drugs and may in fact be desirable with irritating drugs such as aspirin or phenylbutazone. But penicillins and tetracyclines should not be scheduled for administration at mealtimes because certain foods can inactivate them. If in doubt about the effect of food on a certain drug, check with the pharmacist.

4. Consider the patient's age, height, and weight. The doctor will need this information when calculating the dose for many drugs. It should be accurately recorded on the patient's chart. This chart should also include current laboratory data, especially kidney and liver function studies, so the doctor can consider them and adapt dosage as needed.

5. Watch for metabolic changes. Monitor for any physiologic change that might alter drug effect. Examples: depressed respiratory function and the development of acidosis or alkalosis.

6. Know the patient's history. Whenever possible, obtain a comprehensive family history from the patient or his family. Ask about past reactions to drugs, possible genetic traits that might alter drug response, and the current use of other drugs. Multiple drug therapy can dramatically change the effects of many drugs. These altered effects are known as drug interactions.

Drug interactions

When one drug administered in combination with or shortly after another drug alters the effect of one or both drugs, this is known as a drug interaction. Usually, the effect of one drug is increased or decreased. For instance, one drug may inhibit or stimulate the metabolism or excretion of the other; or it may release another from plasma protein-binding sites, freeing it for further action.

Combination therapy is based upon drug interaction. One drug, for example, may be given to potentiate another. Probenecid, which blocks the excretion of penicillin, is sometimes given with penicillin to maintain adequate blood levels of penicillin for a longer period. Often two drugs with similar action are given together precisely because of the additive effect that results. Aspirin and codeine, for instance, both analgesics, are often given in combination because together they provide greater relief from pain than either alone.

Drug interactions are sometimes used to prevent or antagonize certain side effects. Hydrochlorothiazide and spironolactone, both diuretics, are often administered in combination, because the former is potassium-depleting, while the latter is potassium-sparing.

But not all drug interactions are beneficial. Multiple drugs can interact to produce effects that are often undesirable and sometimes hazardous. Harmful drug interactions decrease efficacy or increase toxicity. A hypertensive patient well controlled with guanethidine may see his blood pressure rise to its former high level if he takes the antidepressant amitriptyline (Elavil) at the same time. Such a drug effect is known as antagonism. Drug combinations that produce these effects should be avoided if possible. Another kind of inhibiting effect occurs when a tetracycline drug is administered with calcium- or magnesium-containing drugs or foods (i.e., antacids or milk). These combine with tetracycline in the gastrointestinal tract and cause inadequate absorption of tetracycline.

Adverse reactions
Any drug effect other than what is therapeutically intended can be called an adverse reaction. It may be expected and benign, or unexpected and potentially harmful. Mild, but *predictable*, adverse reactions are sometimes called side effects. Drowsiness caused by antihistamines is an example of this. During hay fever season, a patient may have to contend with this drowsiness to get relief from hay fever symptoms. In such a case, the dose may be adjusted up or down to balance therapeutic effects with side effects.

An adverse reaction may be tolerated for a necessary therapeutic effect, or it may be hazardous and unacceptable and require discontinuation of the drug. Some adverse reactions subside with continued use. As an example, the drowsiness associated with methyldopa (Aldomet) and the orthostatic hypotension associated with

prazosin (Minipress) usually subside after several days, as the patient develops a tolerance to these effects. But many adverse reactions are dose-related and lessen or disappear only if dosage is reduced. Although most adverse reactions are not therapeutically desirable, an occasional one can be put to clinical use. An outstanding example of this is the drowsiness associated with diphenhydramine (Benadryl), which makes it clinically useful as a mild hypnotic.

Hypersensitivity, a term sometimes used interchangeably with drug allergy, is the result of an antigen-antibody immune reaction that occurs in the body when a drug is given to a susceptible patient. One of the most dangerous of all drug hypersensitivities is penicillin allergy. In its severest form, penicillin anaphylaxis can rapidly become fatal.

Rarely, idiosyncratic reactions occur. These are highly unpredictable, individual, and unusual. Probably the best known idiosyncratic drug reaction is the aplastic anemia caused by the antibiotic chloramphenicol (Chloromycetin). This reaction appears in only 1 out of 40,000 patients, but when it does, it is often fatal. A more common idiosyncratic reaction is extreme sensitivity to very low doses of a drug, or insensitivity to higher-than-normal doses.

To deal with adverse reactions correctly, you need to be alert to even minor changes in the patient's clinical status. Such minor changes may be an early warning of pending toxicity. Listen to the patient's complaints about his reactions to a drug, and consider each complaint objectively. You may be able to reduce adverse reactions in several ways. Obviously, dosage reduction often helps. But often so does a simple rescheduling of the same dose. For example, pseudoephedrine (Sudafed) may produce stimulation that will be no problem if it's given early in the day; similarly, the drowsiness that occurs with antihistamines or tranquilizers can be totally harmless if the dose is given at bedtime. Most important, your patient needs to be told what adverse reactions to expect so he won't become worried or even stop taking the drug on his own. Of course, the patient should report any unusual or unexpected adverse reactions to the doctor.

Recognizing drug allergies or serious idiosyncratic reactions can sometimes be lifesaving. Ask each patient about drugs he is taking or has taken in the past and what, if any, unusual effects he experienced from taking them. If a patient claims to be allergic to a drug, ask him to tell you exactly what happens when he takes it. He may be calling a harmless side effect such as upset stomach an allergic reaction, or he may have a true tendency to anaphylaxis. In either case, you and the doctor need to know this. Of course, you must record and report any clinical changes throughout the patient's hospital stay. If you suspect an adverse reaction, withhold the drug until you can check with the pharmacist and the doctor.

Toxic reactions
Chronic drug toxicities are generally due to the cumulative effect and resulting buildup of the drug in the body. These effects may be extensions of the desired therapeutic effect. For example, guanethidine-induced norepinephrine depletion produces a desired antihypertensive effect, but in larger doses, this same biochemical action often produces orthostatic hypotension.

Drug toxicities usually occur when drug blood levels rise due to impaired metabolism or excretion. For example, blood levels of theophylline rise when hepatic dysfunction impairs metabolism of the drug. Similarly, digoxin toxicity can follow impaired

renal function because digoxin is eliminated from the body almost exclusively by the kidneys (via glomerular filtration). Of course, toxic blood levels also follow excessive dosage. Aspirin tinnitus (ringing in ears) is usually a sign that the safe dose has been exceeded.

Most drug toxicity is predictable and dose-related; fortunately, most drug toxicity is also readily reversible upon dosage adjustment. So it's essential to monitor patients carefully for physiologic changes that might alter drug effect. Watch especially for impaired hepatic and renal function. Warn the patient about signs of pending toxicity, and tell him what to do if a toxic reaction occurs. Also, be sure to emphasize the importance of taking a drug exactly as prescribed. Warn the patient about serious problems that could arise if he changes the dose or the schedule for taking it.

Drugs and pregnancy
Ever since the thalidomide tragedy of the late 1950s—when thousands of malformed infants were born after their mothers used this mild sedative-hypnotic during pregnancy—use of drugs during pregnancy has been a source of serious medical concern and controversy. To identify drugs that may cause such teratogenic effects, preclinical drug studies always include tests on pregnant laboratory animals. These tests point out gross teratogenicity but do not clearly establish safety. Because different species react to drugs in different ways, animal studies do not rule out possible teratogenic effects in humans. For example, the preliminary studies on thalidomide gave no warning of teratogenic effects, and it was subsequently released for general use in Europe.

To prevent such tragedies, the Food and Drug Administration has established pregnancy categories (see Chapter 1).

What about the placental barrier? Once thought to protect the fetus from drug effects, the placenta isn't actually much of a barrier at all. Except for drugs with exceptionally large molecular structure, almost every drug administered to a pregnant woman crosses the placenta and enters the fetal circulation. An example of such large molecular size is heparin, the injectable anticoagulant. Theoretically, then, heparin could be used in a pregnant woman without fear of harming the fetus—but even heparin carries a warning for cautious use in pregnancy. Conversely, just because a drug crosses the placenta doesn't necessarily mean it's harmful to the fetus.

Actually, only one factor—stage of fetal development—seems clearly related to exaggerated risk during pregnancy. During two stages of pregnancy—the first and the third trimesters—the fetus is especially vulnerable to damage from maternal use of drugs. During these times, *all* drugs should be given with extreme caution.

The most sensitive period for drug-induced fetal malformation is the first trimester, when fetal organs are differentiating (organogenesis). During this time, *all* drugs should be withheld unless doing so would jeopardize the mother's health. Theoretically, during this sensitive time, even aspirin could harm the fetus. So, strongly advise your patient to avoid *all* self-prescribed drugs during early pregnancy.

The other time of special fetal sensitivity to drugs is the last trimester. The reason? At birth, when separated from his mother, the newborn must rely on his own metabolism to eliminate any remaining drug. Because his detoxifying systems are not fully developed, any residual drug may take a long time to be metabolized—and thus may induce prolonged toxic reactions. Consequently, drugs should be used only when absolutely necessary during the last 3 months of pregnancy.

Of course, in many circumstances, pregnant women must continue to take certain drugs. For example, an epileptic woman who is well controlled with an anticonvulsant should continue to take it even during pregnancy. Or a pregnant woman with a bacterial infection must receive antibiotics. In such cases, the potential risk to the fetus is overbalanced by the mother's need.

Following these general guidelines can prevent indiscriminate and potentially harmful use of drugs in pregnancy:

● Before a drug is prescribed for a woman of childbearing age, she should be asked the date of her last menstrual period and whether there is a possibility she is pregnant.

● Especially during the first and the third trimesters, a pregnant patient should avoid *all* drugs except those *essential* to maintain the pregnancy or maternal health.

● Topical drugs are not exempt from the warning against indiscriminate use during pregnancy. Many topically applied drugs can be absorbed in large enough amounts to be harmful to the fetus.

● When a pregnant patient needs *any* drug, the doctor should prescribe the *safest* possible drug in the *lowest* possible dose to minimize any harmful effect to the fetus.

● Every pregnant patient should check with her doctor before taking *any* drug.

Drugs and lactation

Most drugs a nursing mother takes appear in breast milk. Drug levels in breast milk tend to be high when blood levels are high—generally, shortly after taking each dose. Therefore, the mother should be advised to breast-feed *before* taking medication, not *after*.

Nevertheless, with very few excep-

tions, a mother who wishes to breast-feed may continue to do so with her doctor's permission. The exceptions: Breast-feeding should be temporarily interrupted and replaced with bottle-feeding when the mother must take:
• tetracyclines
• chloramphenicol
• sulfonamides (during first 2 weeks postpartum)
• oral anticoagulants
• iodine-containing drugs
• antineoplastics.

To protect her infant, a nursing mother should avoid taking drugs indiscriminately. If she needs to take a drug to maintain her own health, she should first check with her doctor to be sure of taking the safest drug at the safest dose.

Drug therapy in children

A child's absorption, distribution, metabolism, and excretion processes undergo profound changes that affect drug dosage. To ensure optimal drug effect and minimal toxicity, consider these factors when administering drugs to a child.

Absorption
Drug absorption in children depends on the form of the drug; its physical properties; other drugs or substances, such as food, taken simultaneously; physiologic changes; and concurrent disease.

• The pH of neonatal gastric fluid is neutral or slightly acidic and becomes more acidic as the infant matures. This affects drug absorption. For example, nafcillin and penicillin G, erratically absorbed or malabsorbed in an adult due to degradation by gastric acid, are better absorbed in an infant due to low gastric acidity.

• Various infant formulas or milk products may increase gastric pH and impede absorption of acidic drugs. So, if possible, give a child oral medications when his stomach is empty.

• Gastric emptying time and transit time through the small intestine—longer in children than in adults—can affect absorption. Also, intestinal hypermotility (as in diarrhea) can diminish the drug's absorption.

• A child's comparatively thin epidermis allows increased absorption of topical drugs.

Distribution
As with absorption, changes in body weight and physiology during childhood can significantly influence a drug's distribution and effects. In a premature infant, body fluid makes up about 85% of total body weight; in a full-term infant, 55% to 70%; and in an adult, 50% to 55%. Extracellular fluid (mostly blood) constitutes 40% of a neonate's body weight, compared with 20% in an adult. Intracellular fluid remains fairly constant throughout life and has little effect on drug dosage.

Since most drugs travel through extracellular fluid to reach their receptors, however, extracellular fluid volume influences a water-soluble drug's concentration and effect. Children have a larger proportion of fluid to solid body weight, so their distribution area is proportionately greater.

Because the proportion of fat to lean body mass increases with age, the distribution of fat-soluble drugs is more limited in children than adults. As a result, a drug's lipid- or water-solubility affects the dosage for a child.

Binding to plasma proteins
As the result of a decrease in either albumin concentration or intermolecular attraction between drug and plasma protein, many drugs are less bound to plasma proteins in infants than in adults.

Furthermore, preparations that bind plasma proteins may displace endogenous compounds, such as bilirubin or free fatty acids. Conversely, an endogenous compound may displace a weakly bound drug. For example, displacement of bound bilirubin can cause a rise in unbound bilirubin, which can lead to increased risk of kernicterus at normal bilirubin levels.

Since only an unbound, or free, drug has a pharmacologic effect, any alteration in ratio of a protein-bound to an unbound active drug can greatly influence effect.

Several diseases and disorders, such as nephrotic syndrome and malnutrition, can also decrease plasma protein and increase the concentration of an unbound drug, intensifying the drug's effect or producing toxicity.

Metabolism

A newborn's ability to metabolize a drug depends on the integrity of his hepatic enzyme system, his intrauterine exposure to the drug, and the nature of the drug itself.

Certain metabolic mechanisms are underdeveloped in neonates. Glucuronidation, the mechanism that neutralizes drugs, for example, is insufficiently developed to permit full pediatric doses until the infant is 1 month old. Because of this, the use of chloramphenicol in a newborn may cause gray baby syndrome, illustrating the newborn's inability to metabolize the drug. Use of chloramphenicol in neonates, therefore, requires decreased dosage (25 mg/kg/day) and monitoring of blood levels.

Conversely, intrauterine exposure to drugs may induce precocious development of hepatic enzyme mechanisms, increasing the infant's capacity to metabolize potentially harmful substances.

Older children can metabolize some drugs (theophylline, for example) more rapidly than adults. This ability may be due to their increased hepatic metabolic activity. Larger doses than those recommended for adults may be required.

Also, preparations given concurrently to a child may alter hepatic metabolism and induce release of hepatic enzymes. Phenobarbital, for example, can induce hepatic enzyme production and accelerate metabolism of drugs given concurrently.

Excretion

Renal excretion of a drug is the net effect of glomerular filtration, active tubular secretion, and passive tubular reabsorption. Because so many drugs are excreted in the urine, the degree of renal development or presence of renal disease can profoundly affect a child's dosage requirements.

If a child is unable to excrete a drug renally, drug accumulation and possible toxicity may result unless dosage is reduced.

Physiologically, an infant's kidneys differ from an adult's in that they have:
• high resistance to blood flow and subsequent decreased renal fraction of cardiac output
• incomplete glomerular and tubular development and short, incomplete loops of Henle (A child's glomerular filtration reaches adult values by age 2½ to 5 months; his tubular secretion may reach adult values by age 7 to 12 months.)
• low glomerular filtration rate (Penicillins are eliminated by this route.)
• decreased ability to concentrate urine or reabsorb various filtered compounds
• reduced ability by the proximal tubules to secrete organic acids.

Both children and adults have diurnal variations in urine pH that correlate with sleep-wake patterns.

Calculating and monitoring pediatric dosages

When calculating pediatric dosages, don't use formulas that modify adult dosages: a child is not a scaled-down version of an adult. Pediatric dosages should be calculated on the basis of either body weight (mg/kg) or body

surface area (mg/m^2).
• Reevaluate dosages at regular intervals to ensure necessary adjustments as the child develops.
• Although useful for adults and older children, don't use dosages based on body surface area in premature or full-term infants. Use the body weight method instead.
• Don't exceed the maximum adult dose when calculating amounts per kilogram of body weight (except with certain drugs, such as theophylline, if indicated).
• Obtain an accurate maternal drug history—prescription and nonprescription drugs, vitamins, and herbs or other health foods taken during pregnancy. In utero exposure may harm the neonate and hinder subsequent drug therapy.
• Drugs passed through breast milk can also have adverse effects on the nursing infant. Before a drug is prescribed for a breast-feeding mother, the potential effects on the infant should be investigated. For example, sulfa drugs given to a breast-feeding mother for a urinary tract infection appear in breast milk and may cause kernicterus at lower-than-normal levels of unconjugated bilirubin. Also, high concentrations of isoniazid appear in breast milk. Since this drug is metabolized by the liver, an infant's immature hepatic enzyme mechanisms cannot metabolize the drug, and the infant may suffer central nervous system (CNS) toxicity.

Oral medications
• *When giving oral medication to an infant,* administer it in liquid form if possible. For accuracy, measure and give the preparation by syringe; never use a vial or cup.
• Lift the patient's head to prevent aspiration of the medication, and press down on his chin to prevent choking.
• You may also place the drug in a nipple and allow the infant to suck the contents.
• *If the patient is a toddler,* explain how you're going to give him the medication. If possible, have the parents enlist the child's cooperation.
• Don't mix medication with food or call it "candy" even if it has a pleasant taste.
• Let the child drink liquid medication from a calibrated medication cup rather than from a spoon: it's easier and more accurate. If the preparation is available only in tablet form, crush it and mix it with a compatible syrup. (Check with the pharmacist to make sure the tablet can be crushed without losing its effectiveness.)
• *If the patient's an older child* who can swallow a tablet or capsule by himself, have him place the medication on the back of his tongue and swallow it with water or fruit juice. Remember, milk or milk products may interfere with drug absorption.

Intravenous infusions
When administering I.V. infusions to children, note the following special considerations.

Protecting the insertion site
In infants, use a peripheral vein or a scalp vein in the temporal region for I.V. infusions. The scalp vein is safest in that the needle is not likely to be dislodged; however, the head must be shaved around the site. Disfigurement may also result from the needle and infiltrated fluids. For these reasons, the scalp veins are not used as frequently today as they were in the past.
    The extremities are the most accessible insertion sites; however, since patients tend to move about, take these precautions:
• Protect the insertion site to prevent catheter or needle dislodgment.
• Use a padded arm board to minimize dislodgment.
• Place the clamp out of the child's reach; if extension tubing is used to

allow the child greater mobility, se-
curely tape the connection.
• Restrain the child only when necessary.
• To allay anxiety, give a simple explanation to the child who must be re-
strained while asleep.

*Maintaining flow rate and fluid bal-
ance*
While administering a continuous I.V.
infusion to a child, monitor flow rate
and check the patient's condition and
insertion site at least hourly—more
frequently when giving medication intermittently.

Adjust the flow rate only while the
patient is composed; crying and emotional upset can constrict blood vessels. Flow rate may be retarded if a
pump isn't used. Flow should be adequate because some drugs (calcium,
for example) can be very irritating at
low flow rates.

Making dilutions
Some drugs are hyperosmolar; in infants, these drugs must be diluted to
prevent radical changes in fluid that
might induce CNS hemorrhage. Sodium bicarbonate, for example, must
be diluted to half strength to lower osmolality and lessen the risk of CNS
bleeding.

In general, however, use the minimum amount of compatible fluid over
the shortest recommended period of
time. Remember also to check the total daily fluid intake and the amount
allotted to medication.

Intramuscular injections
Intramuscular injections are preferred
when the drug cannot be given by
other parenteral routes and rapid absorption is necessary.
• In children under 2 years, the vas-
tus lateralis muscle is the preferred
injection site; in older children, either
the ventrogluteal area or the gluteus
medius muscle can be used.

• To determine correct needle size,
consider the patient's age, muscle
mass, and nutritional status and the
drug's viscosity; record and rotate injection sites.
• Explain to the patient that the injection will hurt, but that the medication
will help him. Restrain him during the
injection, and comfort him afterward.

Dermatomucosal medications
• Use eardrops warmed to room
temperature; cold drops can cause
considerable pain and possibly vertigo.
• To administer drops, turn the patient on his side, with the affected
ear up. If he is younger than 3 years,
pull the pinna down and back; if he
is older than 3 years, pull the pinna
up and back.
• Avoid using inhalants in very
young children: obtaining their cooperation is difficult.
• Before attempting to administer
medication through a metered-dose
nebulizer to an older child, explain
the inhaler to him. Then have him
hold the nebulizer upside down and
close his lips around the mouthpiece. Have him exhale; pinch his
nostrils shut; and when he starts to
inhale, release one dose of medication into his mouth. Tell the patient
to continue inhaling until his lungs
feel full.
• Most inhaled agents are not useful
if taken orally; therefore, if you
doubt the patient's ability to use the
inhalant correctly, don't use it.

Parenteral nutrition
Intravenous nutrition is given to patients who can't or won't take adequate food orally and patients with
hypermetabolic conditions who need
I.V. supplementation. The latter
group includes premature infants
and children who have burns or
other major trauma, intractable
diarrhea, malabsorption syndromes,

gastrointestinal abnormalities, emotional disorders such as anorexia nervosa, and congenital abnormalities.

Before fat emulsions are administered to infants and children, however, potential benefits must be weighed against possible risks.

Fats—supplied as 10% or 20% emulsions—are administered both peripherally and centrally. Their use is limited by the child's ability to metabolize them. An infant or child with a diseased liver cannot efficiently metabolize fats, for example.

Some fats, however, must be supplied both to prevent essential fatty acid deficiency and to permit normal growth and development. A minimum of calories (2% to 4%) must be supplied as linoleic acid—an essential fatty acid found in lipids. In the infant, fats are essential for normal neurologic development.

Nevertheless, fat solutions may decrease oxygen perfusion and may adversely affect patients with pulmonary disease. This risk can be minimized by supplying only the minimum fat needed for essential fatty acid requirements and not the usual intake of 40% to 50% of the patient's total calories.

Fatty acids can also displace bilirubin bound to serum albumin, causing a rise in free, unconjugated bilirubin and an increased risk of kernicterus. However, fat solutions may interfere with some bilirubin assays and cause falsely elevated levels. To avoid this complication, a blood sample should be drawn 4 hours after infusion of the lipid emulsion; or if the emulsion is introduced over 24 hours, the blood sample should be centrifuged before the assay is performed.

Drug therapy in the elderly

If you're providing drug therapy for elderly patients, you'll want to understand physiologic and pharmacokinetic changes that may alter drug dosage, common adverse reactions, and compliance problems in the elderly.

Physiologic changes affecting drug action

As a person ages, gradual physiologic changes occur. Some of these age-related changes may alter the therapeutic and toxic effects of medications.

Body composition
Proportions of fat, lean tissue, and water in the body change with age. Total body mass and lean body mass tend to decrease; the proportion of body fat tends to increase.

Varying from person to person, these changes in body composition affect the relationship between a drug's concentration and solubility in the body.

For example, a *water-soluble* drug, such as gentamicin, is not distributed to fat. Since there's relatively less lean tissue in an elderly person, more drug remains in the blood.

Gastrointestinal function
In the elderly, decreases in gastric acid secretion and gastrointestinal motility slow emptying of stomach contents and movement of intestinal contents through the entire tract. Furthermore, although inconclusive, research shows the elderly may have more difficulty absorbing medica-

tions. This is a particularly significant problem with drugs having a narrow therapeutic range, such as digoxin, in which any change in absorption can be crucial.

Hepatic function
The liver's ability to metabolize certain drugs decreases with age. This is due to diminished blood flow to the liver, which results from the age-related decrease in cardiac output and from the diminished activity of certain liver enzymes. When an elderly patient takes certain sleep medications, such as secobarbital, his liver's reduced ability to metabolize the drug may produce a hangover effect the next morning.

Decreased hepatic function may cause:
• more intense drug effects due to higher blood levels
• longer-lasting drug effects due to prolonged blood concentrations
• greater incidence of drug toxicity.

Renal function
Although an elderly person's renal function is usually sufficient to eliminate excess body fluid and waste, his ability to eliminate some medications may be reduced by 50% or more.

Many medications commonly used by the elderly, such as digoxin, are excreted primarily through the kidneys. If the kidneys' ability to excrete the drug is decreased, high blood concentrations may result. Digoxin toxicity, therefore, is relatively common in elderly patients who are not receiving a reduced digoxin dosage to account for their decreased renal function.

Drug dosages can be modified to compensate for age-related decreases in renal function. Aided by laboratory tests, such as BUN and serum creatinine, clinical pharmacists and doctors can adjust medication dosages so the patient receives the expected therapeutic benefits without the risk of toxicity. Observe your patient for signs of toxicity. A patient taking digoxin, for example, may experience anorexia, nausea, vomiting, or confusion.

Adverse drug reactions

As compared with younger people, the elderly experience twice as many adverse drug reactions relating to greater drug consumption, poor compliance, and physiologic changes.

Signs and symptoms of adverse drug reactions—confusion, weakness, and lethargy—are often mistakenly attributed to senility or disease. If the adverse reaction isn't identified, the patient may continue to receive the drug. Furthermore, he may receive unnecessary additional medication to treat complications caused by the original medication. This can sometimes result in the pattern of inappropriate and excessive medication use referred to as "polypharmacy."

Although any medication can cause adverse reactions, most of the serious reactions in the elderly are caused by relatively few medications. Be particularly alert for toxicities resulting from diuretics, antihypertensives, digoxin, corticosteroids, sleep medications, and nonprescription drugs.

Diuretic toxicity
Because total body water content decreases with age, normal doses of potassium-wasting diuretics, such as hydrochlorothiazide and furosemide, may result in fluid loss and even dehydration in an elderly patient.

These diuretics may deplete serum potassium, causing weakness in the patient; and they may raise blood uric acid and glucose levels, complicating preexisting gout and diabetes mellitus.

Antihypertensive toxicity
Many elderly people experience lightheadedness or fainting when using antihypertensive medications. This is partially due to the fact that hypertension in the elderly is partly a response to such changes as atherosclerosis and decreased elasticity of the blood vessels. Antihypertensive drugs lower blood pressure too rapidly, resulting in a situation where insufficient blood flows to the brain. This may cause dizziness, fainting, or even stroke.

Consequently, dosages of antihypertensive drugs must be carefully individualized for each patient. In elderly people, overaggressive treatment of high blood pressure may clearly do more harm than good, so treatment goals should be reasonable. While it may be appropriate to bring blood pressure down to 120/85 mm Hg for a young hypertensive patient, a more reasonable goal for some (but not all) elderly hypertensive patients would be 150/95 mm Hg.

Digoxin toxicity
As the body's renal function and rate of excretion decline, digoxin concentrations in the blood may build to toxic levels, causing nausea, vomiting, diarrhea, and—most serious—cardiac dysrhythmias. Try to prevent severe toxicity by observing your patient for early signs such as appetite loss, confusion, or depression.

Corticosteroid toxicity
Elderly patients on corticosteroids may experience short-term effects, including fluid retention and psychological manifestations ranging from mild euphoria to acute psychotic reactions.

Long-term toxic effects, such as osteoporosis, can be especially severe in elderly patients who have been taking prednisone or related steroidal compounds for months or even years. To prevent serious toxicity, carefully monitor patients on long-term regimens. Observe them for subtle changes in appearance, mood, and mobility, as well as for signs of impaired healing and fluid and electrolyte disturbances.

Sleep medication toxicity
In some cases, sedatives or sleeping aids, such as flurazepam, cause excessive sedation or residual drowsiness.

Nonprescription drug toxicity
When aspirin and aspirin-containing analgesics are used in moderation, toxicity is minimal, but prolonged ingestion may cause gastrointestinal irritation and gradual blood loss resulting in severe anemia. Although anemia from chronic aspirin consumption can affect all age-groups, the elderly may be less able to compensate because of their already reduced iron stores.

Laxatives may cause diarrhea in elderly patients who are extremely sensitive to drugs such as bisacodyl. Chronic oral use of mineral oil as a lubricating laxative may result in lipid pneumonia due to aspiration of small residual oil droplets in the patient's mouth.

Patient noncompliance
Poor compliance is a problem with patients of all ages. However, in elderly patients, specific factors linked to aging—such as diminished visual acuity, hearing loss, forgetfulness, the common need for multiple drug therapy, and various socioeconomic factors—combine to make compliance a special problem. Approximately one third of the elderly fail to comply with

their prescribed drug therapy. They may fail to take prescribed doses or to follow the correct schedule; they may take medications prescribed for previous disorders, discontinue medications prematurely, or use p.r.n. medications indiscriminately.

Review your patient's medication regimen with him. Be sure he understands the medication amount and the time and frequency of doses. Also, explain how he should take each medication, that is, with food or water or by itself.

Give your patient whatever help you can to avoid drug therapy problems, and refer him to the doctor or pharmacist if he needs further information.

Amebicides and trichomonacides

carbarsone
chloroquine hydrochloride
   (See Chapter 8, ANTIMALARIALS.)
chloroquine phosphate
   (See Chapter 8, ANTIMALARIALS.)
emetine hydrochloride
iodoquinol (diiodohydroxyquin)
metronidazole
metronidazole hydrochloride
paromomycin sulfate

COMBINATION PRODUCTS
None.

carbarsone
Pregnancy Category: D

MECHANISM OF ACTION
An organic arsenic derivative with
amebicidal activity in the intestinal
lumen, possibly due to inhibition of
sulfhydryl enzymes.

INDICATIONS & DOSAGE
Intestinal amebiasis—
Adults: 250 mg P.O. b.i.d. or t.i.d.
for 10 days. Rectal (as retention
enema): 2 g dissolved in 200 ml warm
2% sodium bicarbonate solution, every other night for 5 doses. Discontinue oral therapy when enema is
given.
Children: average total dose is 75
mg/kg P.O. daily in 3 divided doses
over 10-day period. Recommended
total varies according to age—2 to 4
years, 2 g total; 5 to 8 years, 3 g total;
9 to 12 years, 4 g total; and over 12
years, 5 g total.

ADVERSE REACTIONS
Blood: *agranulocytosis.*
CNS: neuritis, convulsions, *hemorrhagic encephalitis.*
EENT: sore throat, retinal edema, visual disturbances.
GI: epigastric pain and burning, irritation, *nausea, vomiting,* diarrhea,
anorexia, constipation, increased motility, abdominal cramps.
GU: polyuria, albuminuria, kidney
damage.
Hepatic: hepatomegaly, jaundice,
hepatitis.
Skin: eruptions, *exfoliative dermatitis,* pruritus.
Other: edema of wrists, ankles, and
knees; weight loss; splenomegaly.

INTERACTIONS
None significant.

NURSING CONSIDERATIONS
• Contraindicated as initial treatment
in patients with hepatic or renal disease; in patients with contracted visual or color fields; and in patients
with known hypersensitivity or intolerance to any arsenical treatment.
• Don't exceed recommended dose;
toxicity may result. If second treatment is needed, allow at least 10 days
between courses.
• Divide carbarsone capsule to obtain
required dose. Give in ½ glass orange
juice or milk, in small amount of 1%
sodium bicarbonate solution, or in
jelly or other food.
• Discontinue upon first sign of intolerance or toxicity. Fatal exfoliative
dermatitis has been reported.

• Tell patient to report any unusual symptoms, even post-treatment.
• Liver function tests should precede therapy. Careful inspection of skin, vision testing, and palpation of liver and spleen should be repeated regularly.
• Monitor intake/output. Notify doctor of number, frequency, and character of stools.
• If ordered, give a cleansing enema before giving carbarsone enema.
• Deliver stool specimen to lab promptly; movements of parasites are seen only when stool is warm. Amebic cysts in stool indicate need for additional therapy. Stool specimen should be studied 1 week after stopping therapy and monthly for 1 year. To help prevent reinfestation, instruct patient in proper hygiene.

emetine hydrochloride
Pregnancy Category: X

MECHANISM OF ACTION
Kills *Entamoeba histolytica* by a mechanism related to the inhibition of protein synthesis.

INDICATIONS & DOSAGE
Acute fulminating amebic dysentery—
Adults: 1 mg/kg daily up to 60 mg daily (1 or 2 doses) deep S.C. or I.M. 3 to 5 days to control symptoms. Give another antiamebic drug simultaneously.
Children: 1 mg/kg daily in 2 doses I.M. for up to 5 days.
Amebic hepatitis and abscess—
Adults: 60 mg daily (1 or 2 doses) deep S.C. or I.M. for 10 days.

ADVERSE REACTIONS
CNS: dizziness, headache, mild sensory disturbances, central or peripheral nerve function changes, neuromuscular symptoms (weakness, aching, stiffness, tenderness, pain, tremors).

CV: *acute toxicity*—can occur at any dose (hypotension, tachycardia, precordial pain, dyspnea, *EKG abnormalities,* gallop rhythm, cardiac dilatation, severe acute degenerative myocarditis, pericarditis, congestive failure).
GI: *nausea, vomiting, diarrhea,* abdominal cramps, loss of sense of taste.
Metabolic: decreased serum potassium levels.
Skin: eczematous, urticarial purpuric lesions.
Local: skeletal muscle stiffness, aching, tenderness, *muscle weakness at injection site, cellulitis.*
Other: edema.

INTERACTIONS
None significant.

NURSING CONSIDERATIONS
• Contraindicated in patients with cardiac or renal disease, except those with amebic abscess or hepatitis not controlled by chloroquine or metronidazole; patients who have received a course of emetine less than 6 to 8 weeks previously; children, except for severe dysentery unresponsive to other amebicides; and in those with polyneuropathy or muscle disease. Use with caution in elderly or debilitated patients, patients with hypotension, or those about to undergo surgery.
• Record pulse rate and blood pressure 2 to 3 times daily. Discontinue use if drug produces tachycardia, precipitous fall in blood pressure, neuromuscular symptoms, marked gastrointestinal effects, or considerable weakness. Weakness and muscle symptoms usually precede more serious symptoms and serve as a guide for avoiding toxicity.
• Don't exceed recommended dose or extend therapy beyond 10 days. Patient confined to bed during treatment and for several days thereafter.

Italicized side effects are common or life-threatening.
*Liquid form contains alcohol.   **May contain tartrazine.

• Drug may alter EKG tracings for 6 weeks. EKG should be taken before therapy, after fifth dose, upon completion, and 1 week after therapy. Patterns can resemble those of myocardial infarction. First and most consistent change is T wave inversion.
• Deep S.C. administration is preferred; I.M. acceptable, but I.V. route is dangerous and contraindicated. Rotate sites and apply warm soaks.
• Record intake/output; odor and consistency of stools; and presence of mucus, blood, or other foreign matter. Send warm specimens to lab frequently. Repeat fecal examinations at 3-month intervals to assure elimination of amebae. Patients with acute amebic dysentery often become asymptomatic carriers. Check family members and suspected contacts.
• Suspect emetine-induced reaction if stools increase in number following initial relief of diarrhea.
• To help prevent reinfection, instruct patient in proper hygiene.
• Drug is very irritating. Avoid contact with eyes and mucous membranes.

iodoquinol (diiodohydroxyquin)
Diodoquin♦♦, Inserfem, Moebiquin, Yodoxin
Pregnancy Category: C

MECHANISM OF ACTION
An iodine derivative with amebicidal activity in the intestinal lumen. Its precise mechanism of action is unknown.

INDICATIONS & DOSAGE
Intestinal amebiasis—
Adults: 630 to 650 mg P.O. t.i.d. for 20 days. Total daily dose should not exceed 2 g.
Children: usual dose 30 to 40 mg/kg of body weight daily in 2 to 3 divided doses for 20 days.

Additional courses of iodoquinol therapy should not be repeated before a resting interval of 2 to 3 weeks.

ADVERSE REACTIONS
Blood: *agranulocytosis.*
CNS: neurotoxicity, dysesthesia, weakness, vertigo, malaise, headache, agitation, retrograde amnesia, ataxia, *peripheral neuropathy.*
EENT: *optic neuritis,* optic atrophy, loss of vision.
GI: anorexia, nausea, vomiting, abdominal cramps, diarrhea, increased motility, constipation, epigastric burning and pain, gastritis, anal irritation and itching.
Skin: pruritus, hives, papular and pustular eruptions, urticaria, discoloration of hair and nails.
Other: thyroid enlargement, fever, chills, generalized furunculosis, hair loss.

INTERACTIONS
None significant.

NURSING CONSIDERATIONS
• Contraindicated in patients with known hypersensitivity to 8-hydroxyquinoline derivatives or iodine-containing preparations. Diiodohydroxyquin causes hepatic damage in such patients. Also contraindicated in patients with hepatic or renal disease, or preexisting optic neuropathy.
• Patient should have periodic ophthalmologic examinations during treatment.
• Give after meals. Crush tablets and mix with applesauce or chocolate syrup.
• Record intake/output and color and amount of stool. Send warm specimens to lab frequently.
• Watch for diarrhea during the first 2 or 3 days of treatment. Notify doctor if it continues past 3 days.
• Advise patient not to discontinue the medication prematurely. Tell him to notify doctor if skin rash occurs.

• May interfere with thyroid function tests for up to 6 months after discontinuation of drug.

metronidazole
Apo-Metronidazole♦♦, Flagyl♦, Metryl, Neo-Tric♦♦, Novonidazol♦♦, PMS-Metronidazole♦♦, Satric, Trikacide♦♦

metronidazole hydrochloride
Flagyl I.V.♦, Flagyl I.V. R.T.U., Metro I.V.
Pregnancy Category: B

MECHANISM OF ACTION
A direct-acting trichomonacide and amebicide that works at both intestinal and extraintestinal sites.

INDICATIONS & DOSAGE
Amebic hepatic abscess—
Adults: 500 to 750 mg P.O. t.i.d. for 5 to 10 days.
Children: 35 to 50 mg/kg daily (in 3 doses) for 10 days.
Intestinal amebiasis—
Adults: 750 mg P.O. t.i.d. for 5 to 10 days.
Children: 35 to 50 mg/kg daily (in 3 doses) for 10 days. Follow this therapy with oral iodoquinol.
Trichomoniasis—
Adults (both male and female): 250 mg P.O. t.i.d. for 7 days or 2 g P.O. in single dose; 4 to 6 weeks should elapse between courses of therapy.
Refractory trichomoniasis—
Women: 250 mg P.O. b.i.d. for 10 days.
Treatment of bacterial infections caused by anaerobic microorganisms—
Adults: Loading dose is 15 mg/kg I.V. infused over 1 hour (approximately 1 g for a 70-kg adult). Maintenance dose is 7.5 mg/kg I.V. or P.O. q 6 hours (approximately 500 mg for a 70-kg adult). The first maintenance

dose should be administered 6 hours following the loading dose. Maximum dose not to exceed 4 g daily.
Giardiasis—
Adults: 250 mg P.O. t.i.d. for 5 days.
Children: 5 mg/kg P.O. t.i.d. for 5 days.
Prevention of postoperative infection in contaminated or potentially contaminated colorectal surgery—
Adults: 15 mg/kg infused over 30 to 60 minutes and completed approximately 1 hour before surgery. Then, 7.5 mg/kg infused over 30 to 60 minutes at 6 and 12 hours after the initial dose.

ADVERSE REACTIONS
Blood: transient leukopenia, neutropenia.
CNS: vertigo, headache, ataxia, incoordination, confusion, irritability, depression, restlessness, weakness, fatigue, drowsiness, insomnia, sensory neuropathy, paresthesias of extremities, psychic stimulation, neuromyopathy.
CV: EKG change (flattened T wave), edema (with I.V. R.T.U. preparation).
GI: abdominal cramping, stomatitis, *nausea, vomiting, anorexia,* diarrhea, constipation, proctitis, dry mouth.
GU: darkened urine, polyuria, dysuria, pyuria, incontinence, cystitis, decreased libido, dyspareunia, dryness of vagina and vulva, sense of pelvic pressure.
Skin: pruritus, flushing.
Local: *thrombophlebitis after I.V. infusion.*
Other: overgrowth of nonsusceptible organisms, especially *Candida* (glossitis, furry tongue), metallic taste, fever, gynecomastia.

INTERACTIONS
Alcohol: disulfiram-like reaction (nausea, vomiting, headache, cramps, flushing). Don't use together.
Disulfiram: acute psychoses and confusional states. Don't use together.

Italicized side effects are common or life-threatening.
*Liquid form contains alcohol.   **May contain tartrazine.

NURSING CONSIDERATIONS
Warning: This drug has been shown to be carcinogenic in mice and possibly rats. Unnecessary use should be avoided.
• If indicated during pregnancy for trichomoniasis, the 7-day regimen is preferred over the 2-g single-dose regimen.
• Use cautiously in patients with a history of blood dyscrasia or CNS disorder, and in patients with retinal or visual field changes. Use with caution in patients with hepatic disease or alcoholism; in conjunction with known hepatotoxic drugs.
• Tell patient to avoid alcohol or alcohol-containing medications for 48 hours after therapy is completed.
• Give with meals to minimize GI distress.
• Tell patient metallic taste and dark or red-brown urine are possible.
• Record number and character of stools when used in the treatment of amebiasis. Metronidazole should be used only after *Trichomonas vaginalis* has been confirmed by wet smear or culture or *Entamoeba histolytica* has been identified. Asymptomatic sexual partners of patients being treated for *T. vaginalis* infection should be treated simultaneously to avoid reinfection. Instruct patient in proper hygiene.
• The I.V. form should be administered by slow infusion only. Don't give I.V. push.
• Follow package instructions carefully when mixing the I.V. solution.
• Don't refrigerate Flagyl I.V. R.T.U.
• Flagyl I.V. R.T.U. may cause sodium retention. Observe carefully for edema, especially in patients also receiving corticosteroids.
• A 1% solution may be effective topically in treating decubitus ulcers.

paromomycin sulfate
Humatin
Pregnancy Category: C

MECHANISM OF ACTION
Acts as an amebicide in intestinal sites, effective in the presence or absence of bacteria. Its specific mechanism of action is unknown.

INDICATIONS & DOSAGE
Intestinal amebiasis, acute and chronic—
Adults and children: 25 to 35 mg/kg daily P.O. in 3 doses for 5 to 10 days after meals.
Tapeworms (fish, beef, pork, dog)—
Adults: 1 g P.O. q 15 minutes for 4 doses.
Children: 11 mg/kg P.O. q 15 minutes for 4 doses.

ADVERSE REACTIONS
Blood: eosinophilia.
CNS: headache, vertigo.
EENT: ototoxicity.
GI: anorexia, *nausea, vomiting, epigastric pain and burning, abdominal cramps,* diarrhea, constipation, increased motility, steatorrhea, pruritus ani, malabsorption syndrome.
GU: hematuria, nephrotoxicity.
Skin: rash, exanthema, pruritus.
Other: overgrowth of nonsusceptible organisms.

INTERACTIONS
None significant.

NURSING CONSIDERATIONS
• Contraindicated in patients with impaired renal function or intestinal obstruction. Use with caution in patients with ulcerative lesions of the bowel to avoid inadvertent absorption and resulting renal toxicity. Poorly absorbed orally, but will accumulate with renal impairment or ulcerative lesions.
• Ask about history of sensitivity to

drug before giving first dose.

• Administer after meals.

• Emphasize personal hygiene, particularly handwashing before eating and after defecation.

• Criterion of cure is absence of amebae in stools examined weekly for 6 weeks after treatment and thereafter at monthly intervals for 2 years. Examine feces of family members or suspected contacts.

• Avoid high doses or prolonged therapy.

• Watch for signs of superinfection (continued fever and other signs of new infections, especially monilial infections).

Anthelmintics

mebendazole
niclosamide
oxamniquine
piperazine adipate
piperazine citrate
praziquantel
pyrantel pamoate
pyrvinium pamoate
quinacrine hydrochloride
thiabendazole

COMBINATION PRODUCTS
None.

---

mebendazole
Vermox♦
Pregnancy Category: C

MECHANISM OF ACTION
Selectively and irreversibly inhibits uptake of glucose and other nutrients in susceptible helminths.

INDICATIONS & DOSAGE
Pinworm—
Adults and children over 2 years:
100 mg P.O. as a single dose. If infection persists 3 weeks later, repeat treatment.
Roundworm, whipworm, hookworm—
Adults and children over 2 years:
100 mg P.O. b.i.d. for 3 days. If infection persists 3 weeks later, repeat treatment.

ADVERSE REACTIONS
GI: occasional, transient abdominal pain and diarrhea in massive infection and expulsion of worms.

INTERACTIONS
None significant.

NURSING CONSIDERATIONS
• Tablets may be chewed, swallowed whole, or crushed and mixed with food.
• No dietary restrictions, laxatives, or enemas necessary.
• To avoid reinfection, wash perianal area daily. Change undergarments and bedclothes daily. Wash hands and clean fingernails after bowel movements and before meals. Treat all family members.

---

niclosamide
Niclocide
Pregnancy Category: B

MECHANISM OF ACTION
Inhibits the metabolic process of oxidative phosphorylation in tapeworms.

INDICATIONS & DOSAGE
Tapeworms (fish and beef)—
Adults: 4 tablets (2 g) chewed thoroughly as a single dose.
Children (more than 34 kg): 3 tablets (1.5 g) chewed thoroughly as a single dose.
Children (11 to 34 kg): 2 tablets (1 g) chewed thoroughly as a single dose.
Dwarf tapeworm—
Adults: 4 tablets chewed thoroughly as a single daily dose for 7 days.
Children (more than 34 kg): 3 tablets chewed thoroughly on the first day, then 2 tablets for the next 6 days.
Children (11 to 34 kg): 2 tablets

chewed thoroughly on the first day, then one tablet daily for the next 6 days.

ADVERSE REACTIONS
CNS: drowsiness, dizziness, headache.
EENT: oral irritation, bad taste in mouth.
GI: *nausea, vomiting, anorexia,* diarrhea.
Skin: rash, pruritus ani.

INTERACTIONS
None reported.

NURSING CONSIDERATIONS
• Instruct patient to chew tablets thoroughly and wash down with water; for smaller children, the tablets can be crushed and mixed with water or applesauce.
• Tablets should be taken as a single dose after breakfast.
• A mild laxative should be administered to cleanse the bowel prior to initiation of niclosamide therapy in patients who are constipated.
• When treating dwarf tapeworms, urge patient to drink fruit juices. This helps to eliminate the accumulated intestinal mucus under which they lodge.
• Patient is not considered cured until the stool has been negative for tapeworms for at least 3 months.

oxamniquine
Vansil
Pregnancy Category: C

MECHANISM OF ACTION
Reduces the egg load of *Schistosoma mansoni,* but its exact mechanism of action is unknown.

INDICATIONS & DOSAGE
Treatment of schistosomiasis caused by Schistosoma mansoni—
Adults and children: 12 to 15 mg/kg

given as a single oral dose.

ADVERSE REACTIONS
CNS: convulsions, *dizziness, drowsiness, headache.*
GI: nausea, vomiting, abdominal pain, anorexia.
Skin: urticaria.

INTERACTIONS
None significant.

NURSING CONSIDERATIONS
• There are no known contraindications.
• Use cautiously in patients with a history of convulsive conditions. Epileptiform convulsions have rarely been observed within the first few hours after ingestion. Patients with a history of convulsions should be kept under medical supervision.
• Instruct patient to avoid driving and other hazardous activities if he's dizzy or drowsy.
• Gastrointestinal tolerance is improved if you give the drug after meals.
• Although *S. mansoni* infection is rare in the United States and Canada, travelers or immigrants from such areas as Puerto Rico, Latin America, and Africa may have contracted the infection from contaminated water.

piperazine adipate
Entacyl♦♦

piperazine citrate
Antepar, Bryrel, Pin-Tega Tabs, Pipril, Ta-Verm, Veriga♦♦, Vermazine, Vermirex♦♦
Pregnancy Category: B

MECHANISM OF ACTION
Blocks neuromuscular action, paralyzing the worm and causing its expulsion by normal peristalsis.

INDICATIONS & DOSAGE
Pinworm—
Adults and children: 65 mg/kg P.O. daily 7 to 8 days. Maximum daily dose is 2.5 g.
Roundworm—
Adults: 3.5 g P.O. in single doses for 2 consecutive days.
Children: 75 mg/kg P.O. daily in single doses for 2 consecutive days. Maximum daily dose: 3.5 g.

ADVERSE REACTIONS
CNS: ataxia, tremors, choreiform movements, muscular weakness, myoclonus, hyporeflexia, paresthesias, convulsions, sense of detachment, EEG abnormalities, memory defect, *headache, vertigo*.
EENT: nystagmus, blurred vision, paralytic strabismus, cataracts with visual impairment, lacrimation, difficulty in focusing, rhinorrhea.
GI: *nausea, vomiting,* diarrhea, abdominal cramps.
Skin: urticaria, photodermatitis, *erythema multiforme,* purpura, eczematous skin reactions.
Other: arthralgia, fever, bronchospasm.

INTERACTIONS
Pyrantel pamoate: Possible pharmacologic antagonism. Don't administer together.

NURSING CONSIDERATIONS
• Contraindicated in patients with hepatic and/or renal impairment, or convulsive disorders. Use with caution in patients with severe malnutrition or anemia.
• Discontinue if CNS or significant GI reactions occur.
• Because of potential neurotoxicity, avoid prolonged or repeated treatment, especially in children.
• No dietary restrictions, laxatives, or enemas necessary.
• May be taken with food; but, for best absorption, tell patient to take on empty stomach.
• To avoid reinfection, wash perianal area daily. Change undergarments and bedclothes daily. Wash hands and clean fingernails before meals and after bowel movements. Treat all family members.
• Protect drug from air, light, and moisture.

praziquantel
Biltricide
Pregnancy Category: B

MECHANISM OF ACTION
Causes a contraction of schistosomes by a specific effect on the permeability of the cell membrane.

INDICATIONS & DOSAGE
Treatment of schistosomiasis caused by Schistosoma mekongi, S. japonicum, S. mansoni, *and* S. haematobium—
Adults and children 4 years and older: 20 mg/kg P.O. t.i.d. as a 1-day treatment. The interval between doses should be between 4 and 6 hours.

ADVERSE REACTIONS
CNS: *drowsiness, malaise,* headache, dizziness.
GI: abdominal discomfort, nausea.
Hepatic: minimal increase in liver enzymes.
Skin: urticaria.
Other: rise in body temperature.

INTERACTIONS
None significant.

NURSING CONSIDERATIONS
• Contraindicated in patients with ocular cysticercosis.
• May produce drowsiness. Tell patient to drive or operate machinery cautiously on the day of treatment and the day after treatment.
• Side effects may be more frequent or serious in patients with a heavy

worm burden.
- In the event of overdose, give a fast-acting laxative.
- Advise patient to take the tablet during meals and to wash down the unchewed tablet with a liquid.
- Tablets taste very bitter. Keeping them in the mouth may cause gagging or vomiting.
- Praziquantel is effective for several different species of *Schistosoma*.
- May also be effective against liver flukes.

pyrantel pamoate
Antiminth, Combantrin♦♦
Pregnancy Category: C

MECHANISM OF ACTION
Blocks neuromuscular action, paralyzing the worm and causing its expulsion by normal peristalsis.

INDICATIONS & DOSAGE
Roundworm and pinworm—
Adults and children over 2 years: single dose of 11 mg/kg P.O. Maximum dose 1 g. For pinworm, dose should be repeated in 2 weeks.

ADVERSE REACTIONS
CNS: headache, dizziness, drowsiness, insomnia.
GI: anorexia, nausea, vomiting, gastralgia, cramps, diarrhea, tenesmus.
Hepatic: transient elevation of SGOT.
Skin: rashes.
Other: fever, weakness.

INTERACTIONS
Piperazine salts: Possible pharmacologic antagonism. Don't administer together.

NURSING CONSIDERATIONS
- Use cautiously in severe malnutrition or anemia, or in hepatic dysfunction. Treat for anemia, dehydration, or malnutrition before giving drug.

- No dietary restrictions, laxatives, or enemas necessary.
- May be taken with food, milk, or fruit juices. Shake well before pouring.
- To avoid reinfection, wash perianal area daily. Change undergarments and bedclothes daily. Wash hands and clean fingernails before meals and after bowel movements. Treat all family members.
- Protect drug from light. Store below 30° C. (86° F.).
- Now available without a prescription. Urge patient to read the enclosed consumer information that tells how to identify and recognize pinworms.

pyrvinium pamoate
Pamovin♦♦, Povan, Vanquin♦♦
Pregnancy Category: C

MECHANISM OF ACTION
Appears to destroy parasites by preventing them from using exogenous carbohydrates.

INDICATIONS & DOSAGE
Pinworm—
Adults and children: 5 mg/kg P.O. single dose (maximum 350 mg). Repeat in 2 weeks if needed.

ADVERSE REACTIONS
GI: nausea, vomiting, cramping, diarrhea (vomiting more common with suspension than with tablets).
Hepatic: elevated enzymes.
Skin: photosensitivity, *erythema multiforme*.

INTERACTIONS
None significant.

NURSING CONSIDERATIONS
- Use cautiously in patients with pre-existing liver disease.
- Safe use in children who weigh less than 10 kg not established. Consult pediatrician.

Italicized side effects are common or life-threatening.
*Liquid form contains alcohol.   **May contain tartrazine.

- Swallow tablets whole to avoid staining teeth.
- Warn that drug stains fabrics, skin, teeth, vomitus, and stools bright red.
- No dietary restrictions, laxatives, or enemas necessary.
- To avoid reinfection, wash perianal area daily. Change undergarments and bedclothes daily. Wash hands and clean fingernails before meals and after bowel movements. Treat all family members.
- Protect drug from light.

quinacrine hydrochloride
Atabrine♦
Pregnancy Category: C

MECHANISM OF ACTION
Inhibits deoxyribonucleic acid metabolism.

INDICATIONS & DOSAGE
Treatment of giardiasis—
Adults: 300 mg P.O. in 3 divided doses for 5 to 7 days.
Children: 7 mg/kg/day P.O. given in 3 divided doses after meals for 5 days. Maximum 300 mg/day. If necessary, the dosage may be repeated in 2 weeks.
Tapeworms (beef, pork, and fish)—
Adults and children over 14 years: 4 doses of 200 mg given 10 minutes apart (800 mg total).
Children 11 to 14 years: 600 mg total dosage, administered in 3 or 4 divided doses, 10 minutes apart.
Children 5 to 10 years: 400 mg total dosage, administered in 3 or 4 divided doses, 10 minutes apart.

ADVERSE REACTIONS
CNS: *headache, dizziness, nervousness, vertigo, mood shifts, nightmares, seizures.*
GI: *diarrhea, anorexia, nausea, abdominal cramps,* vomiting.
Skin: pleomorphic skin eruptions.

INTERACTIONS
None significant.

NURSING CONSIDERATIONS
- Contraindicated if primaquine is being given concurrently since primaquine toxicity could be increased.
- Use with extreme caution in patients with porphyria or psoriasis; may exacerbate these conditions.
- Use with caution in patients with hepatic disease, alcoholism, severe renal or cardiac disease, psychosis, G-6-PD deficiency, and in those over 60 years or under 1 year.
- Give after meals with large glass of water, tea, or fruit juice to reduce GI irritation. Bitter taste may be disguised by jam or honey.
- Nausea and vomiting after large doses may be lessened by taking sodium bicarbonate with each dose.
- Administer a saline cathartic 1 to 2 hours after drug is given, to expel the worm.
- Collect all of stool after treatment. Don't put toilet paper in bedpan. Look for the scolex (attachment organ), which will be stained yellow from drug.
- Warn patient about temporary yellow color of skin and urine—it is not jaundice.
- Patient should be on a bland, nonfat, semisolid diet for 24 hours, and should fast after the evening meal before treatment.
- Induce emesis for overdose.

thiabendazole
Mintezol♦
Pregnancy Category: C

MECHANISM OF ACTION
Unknown.

INDICATIONS & DOSAGE
Systemic infection with pinworm, roundworm, threadworm, whipworm, cutaneous larva migrans, and trichi-

nosis—
Adults or children: 25 mg/kg P.O. in 2 doses daily for 2 successive days. Maximum dose is 3 g daily.
Cutaneous infestations with larva migrans (creeping eruption)—
Adults and children: 25 mg/kg P.O. b.i.d. for 2 to 5 days. Maximum 3 g daily. If lesions persist after 2 days, repeat course.
*Pinworm—*2 doses daily for 1 day; repeat in 7 days.
*Roundworm, threadworm, whipworm—*2 doses daily for 2 successive days.
*Trichinosis—*2 doses daily for 2 to 4 successive days.

ADVERSE REACTIONS
CNS: impaired mental alertness, impaired physical coordination, *drowsiness, giddiness,* headache, dizziness.
GI: *anorexia, nausea, vomiting,* diarrhea, epigastric distress.
Skin: rash, pruritus, *erythema multiforme.*
Other: lymphadenopathy, fever, flushing, chills.

INTERACTIONS
None significant.

NURSING CONSIDERATIONS
• Use with caution in patients with hepatic or renal dysfunction, severe malnutrition, anemia, and in patients who are vomiting. Supportive therapy indicated for anemic, dehydrated, or malnourished patients. In children under 15 kg, weigh benefits of therapy against risks.
• Warn that medication may cause drowsiness and dizziness.
• Give after meals. Shake suspension before measuring; chew tablets before swallowing.
• Laxatives, enemas, and diet restrictions not needed.
• To avoid reinfection, wash perianal area daily. Change undergarments and bedclothes daily. Wash hands and clean fingernails before meals and after bowel movements. Treat all family members.
• Disinfect toilet facilities daily.

7

Antifungals

amphotericin B
flucytosine (5-FC)
griseofulvin microsize
griseofulvin ultramicrosize
ketoconazole
miconazole
nystatin

COMBINATION PRODUCTS
MYSTECLIN-F CAPS: tetracycline HCl
250 mg and amphotericin B 50 mg
buffered with potassium metaphosphate.
MYSTECLIN-F CAPS: tetracycline HCl
125 mg and amphotericin B 25 mg
buffered with potassium metaphosphate.
MYSTECLIN-F SYRUP: tetracycline
HCl 125 mg and amphotericin B 25
mg per 5 ml buffered with potassium
metaphosphate.

---

amphotericin B
Fungizone♦
Pregnancy Category: B

MECHANISM OF ACTION
Probably acts by binding to sterols in
the fungal cell membrane, altering
cell permeability and allowing leakage of intracellular components.

INDICATIONS & DOSAGE
Systemic fungal infections (histoplasmosis, coccidioidomycosis, blastomycosis, cryptococcosis, disseminated moniliasis, aspergillosis, phycomycosis), meningitis—
Adults and children: initially, 1 mg
in 250 ml of dextrose 5% in water infused over 2 to 4 hours; or 0.25 mg/kg
daily by slow infusion over 6 hours.
Increase daily dose gradually as patient tolerance develops to maximum
1 mg/kg daily. Therapy must not exceed 1.5 mg/kg. If drug is discontinued for 1 week or more, administration must resume with initial dose and
again increase gradually.
Topical (3% cream, lotion, ointment):
apply liberally and rub well into affected area b.i.d. to q.i.d.
Intrathecal: 25 mcg/0.1 ml diluted
with 10 to 20 ml of cerebrospinal
fluid and administered by barbotage 2
or 3 times weekly. Initial dose should
not exceed 100 mcg.
Coccidioidal arthritis—
Adults: 5 to 15 mg into joint spaces.

ADVERSE REACTIONS
Blood: normochromic, normocytic
anemia.
CNS: headache, peripheral neuropathy; with intrathecal administration—
peripheral nerve pain, paresthesias.
GI: *anorexia, weight loss, nausea,*
vomiting, dyspepsia, diarrhea, epigastric cramps.
GU: abnormal renal function with *hypokalemia, azotemia, hyposthenuria,*
renal tubular acidosis, nephrocalcinosis; with large doses—permanent
renal impairment, anuria, oliguria.
Local: burning, stinging, irritation,
tissue damage with extravasation,
thrombophlebitis, pain at site of injection.
Other: arthralgia, myalgia, muscle
weakness secondary to hypokalemia,
fever, chills, malaise, generalized

---

pain.

INTERACTIONS
Other nephrotoxic antibiotics: may cause additive kidney toxicity. Administer very cautiously.

NURSING CONSIDERATIONS
• Use cautiously in patients with impaired renal function.
• Use parenterally only in hospitalized patients, under close supervision, when diagnosis of potentially fatal fungal infection has been confirmed.
• Monitor vital signs; fever may appear 1 to 2 hours after start of I.V. infusion and should subside within 4 hours of discontinuation.
• Monitor intake/output; report change in urine appearance or volume. Renal damage usually reversible if drug is stopped with first sign of dysfunction.
• Obtain liver and renal function studies weekly. If BUN exceeds 40 mg/100 ml, or if serum creatinine exceeds 3 mg/100 ml, doctor may reduce or stop drug until renal function improves. Monitor CBC weekly. Stop drug if Bromsulphalein, alkaline phosphatase, or bilirubin levels become elevated.
• Monitor potassium levels closely. Report any signs of hypokalemia. Check calcium and magnesium levels periodically.
• In the dry state, store at 2° to 8° C. (35.6° to 46.4° F.). Protect from light. Expires 2 years after date of manufacture. Reconstitute with 10 ml sterile water only. Mixing with solutions containing sodium chloride, other electrolytes, or bacteriostatic agents such as benzyl alcohol causes precipitation. Do not use if solution contains precipitate or foreign matter.
• Appears to be compatible with limited amounts of heparin sodium, hydrocortisone sodium succinate, and methylprednisolone sodium succinate.

• Reconstituted solution is stable for 1 week under refrigeration or 24 hours at room temperature. It has 24-hour stability in room light.
• An initial test dose may be prescribed: 1 mg is added to 50 to 150 ml of dextrose 5% in water and infused over 20 to 30 minutes.
• Severity of some side effects can be reduced by premedication with aspirin, antihistamines, antiemetics, or small doses of corticosteroids; addition of phosphate buffer and heparin to the solution; and alternate-day dose schedule. For severe reactions, drug may have to be stopped for varying periods.
• For I.V. infusion, an in-line membrane with mean pore diameter larger than 1 micron can be used. Infuse very slowly; rapid infusion may result in cardiovascular collapse. Warn patient of discomfort at infusion site and other potential side effects. Advise patient that several months of therapy may be needed to assure adequate response.
• Administer in distal veins. If veins become thrombosed, doctor can change to every-other-day regimen.
• Antibiotics should be given separately; don't mix or piggyback with amphotericin B.
• Topical preparations may stain clothing.

---

flucytosine (5-FC)
Ancobon, Ancotil♦♦
Pregnancy Category: C

MECHANISM OF ACTION
Appears to penetrate fungal cells, where it is converted to fluorouracil, a known metabolic antagonist. Causes defective protein synthesis.

INDICATIONS & DOSAGE
For severe fungal infections caused by susceptible strains of Candida *(including septicemia, endocarditis, urinary*

Italicized side effects are common or life-threatening.
*Liquid form contains alcohol.   **May contain tartrazine.

ANTIFUNGALS 33

tract and pulmonary infections) and
Cryptococcus *(meningitis, pulmonary
infection, and possible urinary tract
infections)—*
**Adults and children weighing more
than 50 kg:** 50 to 150 mg/kg daily q 6
hours P.O.
**Adults and children weighing less
than 50 kg:** 1.5 to 4.5 g/m²/day in 4
divided doses P.O.
Severe infections such as meningitis
may require doses up to 250 mg/kg.

ADVERSE REACTIONS
Blood: anemia, leukopenia, bone
marrow depression, thrombocyto-
penia.
CNS: dizziness, drowsiness, confu-
sion, headache, vertigo.
GI: *nausea, vomiting, diarrhea,* ab-
dominal bloating.
Hepatic: elevated SGOT, SGPT.
Metabolic: elevated serum alkaline
phosphatase, BUN, serum creatinine.
Skin: occasional rash.

INTERACTIONS
None significant.

NURSING CONSIDERATIONS
• Use with extreme caution in patients with impaired hepatic or renal
function, or bone marrow depression.
• Hematologic tests and renal and
liver function studies should precede
therapy and should be repeated at frequent intervals thereafter. Before
treatment, susceptibility tests should
establish that organism is flucytosine-
sensitive. Tests should be repeated
weekly to monitor drug resistance.
• Nausea, vomiting, and stomach upset are reduced if capsules are given
over a 15-minute period.
• Monitor intake and output; report
any marked change.
• If possible, blood level assays of
drug should be performed regularly to
maintain flucytosine at therapeutic
level (25 to 120 mcg/ml). Higher
blood levels may be toxic.

• Drug is always combined with amphotericin B; use may be synergistic.
• Store in light-resistant containers.
• Inform patient that adequate response may take weeks or months.

---

griseofulvin microsize
Fulvicin-U/F♦, Grifulvin V, Grisactin,
Grisovin-FP♦♦

griseofulvin ultramicrosize
Fulvicin P/G♦, Grisactin-Ultra, Gris-
PEG
Pregnancy Category: C

MECHANISM OF ACTION
Arrests fungal cell activity by disrupting its mitotic spindle structure.

INDICATIONS & DOSAGE
*Ringworm infections of skin, hair,
nails (tinea corporis, tinea pedis,
tinea capitis) when caused by* Tricho-
phyton, Microsporum, *or* Epidermo-
phyton—
Adults: 500 mg (microsize) P.O.
daily in single or divided doses. Severe infections may require up to 1 g
daily. Alternatively, may give 330 to
375 mg ultramicrosize in single or divided doses.
Tinea pedis and tinea unguium—
Adults: 0.75 to 1 g (microsize) P.O.
daily. Alternatively, may give 660 to
750 mg ultramicrosize P.O. daily.
Children: 11 mg/kg/day (microsize)
P.O. Alternatively, may give 7.3 mg/
kg/day of the ultramicrosize.

ADVERSE REACTIONS
Blood: leukopenia, *granulocytopenia*
(requires discontinuation of drug).
CNS: headaches (in early stages of
treatment), transient decrease in hearing, fatigue with large doses, occasional mental confusion, impaired
performance of routine activities,
psychotic symptoms.
GI: nausea, vomiting, excessive
thirst, flatulence, diarrhea.

Metabolic: porphyria.
Skin: rash, urticaria, photosensitive reactions (may aggravate lupus erythematosus).
Other: estrogen-like effects in children, oral thrush.

INTERACTIONS

Barbiturates: decreased griseofulvin absorption. Divide into 3 doses of griseofulvin per day.
Alcohol: may cause tachycardia, diaphoresis, and flushing. Avoid alcohol.

NURSING CONSIDERATIONS

• Contraindicated in patients with porphyria or hepatocellular failure. Since griseofulvin is a penicillin derivative, cross-sensitivity is possible. Use cautiously in penicillin-sensitive patients. Use only when topical treatment fails to arrest mycotic disease.
• CBC should be repeated regularly.
• Advise patient that prolonged treatment may be needed to control infection and prevent relapse, even if symptoms abate in first few days of therapy. Tell patient to keep skin clean and dry and to maintain good hygiene. Caution him to avoid intense sunlight.
• Most effectively absorbed and causes least GI distress when given after high-fat meal.
• Effective treatment of tinea pedis may require concomitant use of topical agent.
• Diagnosis of infecting organism should be verified in lab. Continue drug until clinical and laboratory examinations confirm complete eradication.
• Because griseofulvin ultramicrosize is dispersed in polyethylene glycol (PEG), it is absorbed more rapidly and completely than microsize preparations and is effective at one half to two thirds the usual griseofulvin dose.
• Advise patient to avoid alcoholic beverages.

ketoconazole

Nizoral♦
Pregnancy Category: C

MECHANISM OF ACTION

Inhibits purine transport and deoxyribonucleic acid, RNA, and protein synthesis; increases cell-wall permeability, making the fungus more susceptible to osmotic pressure.

INDICATIONS & DOSAGE

Treatment of systemic candidiasis, chronic mucocandidiasis, oral thrush, candiduria, coccidioidomycosis, histoplasmosis, chromomycosis, and paracoccidioidomycosis; severe cutaneous dermatophyte infections resistant to therapy with topical or oral griseofulvin—
Adults and children over 40 kg: initially, 200 mg P.O. daily single dose. Dosage may be increased to 400 mg once daily in patients who don't respond to lower dosage.
Children (less than 20 kg): 50 mg (¼ tablet) daily single dose.
Children (20 to 40 kg): 100 mg (½ tablet) daily single dose.

ADVERSE REACTIONS

CNS: headache, nervousness, dizziness.
GI: *nausea, vomiting,* abdominal pain, diarrhea, constipation.
Hepatic: elevated liver enzymes, *fatal hepatotoxicity.*
Skin: itching.
Other: gynecomastia with breast tenderness in males.

INTERACTIONS

Antacids, anticholinergics, H₂ blockers: decreased absorption of ketoconazole. Wait at least 2 hours after ketoconazole dose before administering these drugs.
Rifampin, isoniazid: increases ketoconazole metabolism. Monitor for decreased antifungal effect.

Italicized side effects are common or life-threatening.
*Liquid form contains alcohol.   **May contain tartrazine.

NURSING CONSIDERATIONS
• Ketoconazole is not effective in patients with achlorhydria. The drug requires acidity for dissolution and absorption. Instruct patient to dissolve each tablet in 4 ml aqueous solution of 0.2 N hydrochloric acid; and, to avoid contact with teeth, to sip the mixture through a straw (glass or plastic). Tell patient to follow with a glass of water.
• Make sure patient understands that treatment should be continued until all clinical and laboratory tests indicate that active fungal infection has subsided. If drug is discontinued too soon, infection will recur. Minimum treatment for candidiasis is 7 to 14 days. Minimum treatment for other systemic fungal infections is 6 months. Minimum treatment for resistant dermatophyte infections is at least 4 weeks.
• Reassure patient that, although nausea is common early in therapy, it will subside. To minimize nausea, you may, with doctor's permission, divide the daily dosage into 2 doses. Taking with meals also helps to decrease nausea.
• Also available as an oral suspension.
• Monitor for elevated liver enzymes and nausea that does not subside, as well as unusual fatigue, jaundice, dark urine or pale stools. May be sign of hepatotoxicity.
• Much larger doses (up to 800 mg/day) can be used to effectively treat fungal meningitis and intracerebral fungal lesions.
• Ketoconazole represents a major advance since it is the most effective oral antifungal drug available.
• Because of the potential of serious liver toxicity, ketoconazole should not be prescribed or used for such less serious conditions as fungus infections of the skin or nails.

miconazole
Monistat I.V.♦
Pregnancy Category: B

MECHANISM OF ACTION
Inhibits purine transport and deoxyribonucleic acid, RNA, and protein synthesis; increases cell-wall permeability, making the fungus more susceptible to osmotic pressure.

INDICATIONS & DOSAGE
Treatment of systemic fungal infections (coccidioidomycosis, candidiasis, cryptococcosis, paracoccidioidomycosis), chronic mucocutaneous candidiasis—
Adults: 200 to 3,600 mg per day. Doses may vary with diagnosis and with infective agent. May divide daily dose over 3 infusions, 200 to 1,200 mg per infusion. Dilute in at least 200 ml of 0.9% NaCl. Repeated courses may be needed due to relapse or reinfection.
Children: 20 to 40 mg/kg per day. Do not exceed 15 mg/kg per infusion.
Fungal meningitis—
Adults: 20 mg intrathecally as an adjunct to intravenous administration.

ADVERSE REACTIONS
Blood: transient decreases in hematocrit, thrombocytopenia.
CNS: dizziness, drowsiness.
GI: *nausea, vomiting,* diarrhea.
Metabolic: *transient decrease in serum sodium.*
Skin: *pruritic rash.*
Local: *phlebitis at injection site.*

INTERACTIONS
None significant.

NURSING CONSIDERATIONS
• Rapid injection of undiluted miconazole may produce arrhythmia. Dilute infusion with at least 200 ml of 0.9% NaCl and infuse over 30 to 60 minutes.

• Acute cardiorespiratory arrest has occurred with the first dose. A doctor should be present when the first dose is administered.
• Premedication with antiemetic may lessen nausea and vomiting.
• Avoid administration at mealtime in order to lessen GI adverse reactions.
• Lesser incidence and severity of adverse reactions with this drug may offer a significant advantage over other antifungals.
• Pruritic rash may persist for weeks after drug is discontinued. Pruritus may be controlled with oral or I.V. diphenhydramine.
• In treatment of fungal meningitis and urinary bladder infections, must be supplemented with intrathecal administration and bladder irrigation, respectively.
• Inform patient that adequate response may take weeks or months.
• Monitor levels of hemoglobin, hematocrit, electrolytes, and lipids regularly. Transient elevations in serum cholesterol and triglycerides may be due to castor oil vehicle.

---

nystatin
Mycostatin•, Nadostine••, Nilstat•, O-V Statin
Pregnancy Category: B

MECHANISM OF ACTION
Probably acts by binding to sterols in the fungal cell membrane, altering cell permeability and allowing leakage of intracellular components.

INDICATIONS & DOSAGE
Gastrointestinal infections—
Adults: 500,000 to 1,000,000 units as oral tablets, t.i.d.
Treatment of oral, vaginal, and intestinal infections caused by Candida albicans (Monilia) *and other* Candida *species—*
Adults: 400,000 to 600,000 units oral suspension q.i.d. for oral candidiasis.

Children and infants over 3 months: 250,000 to 500,000 units oral suspension q.i.d.
Newborn and premature infants: 100,000 units oral suspension q.i.d.
Vaginal infections—
Adults: 100,000 units, as vaginal tablets, inserted high into vagina, daily or b.i.d. for 14 days.

ADVERSE REACTIONS
GI: transient nausea, vomiting, diarrhea (usually with large oral dosage).

INTERACTIONS
None significant.

NURSING CONSIDERATIONS
• Nystatin is virtually nontoxic and nonsensitizing when used orally, vaginally, or topically, but advise patient to report redness, swelling, or irritation.
• Vaginal tablets can be used by pregnant women up to 6 weeks before term to prevent thrush in newborn. Continue therapy during menstruation. Instruct patient to wash applicator thoroughly after each use.
• Explain that use of antibiotics, oral contraceptives, and corticosteroids; diabetes; reinfection by sexual partner; and tight-fitting panty hose are predisposing factors of vaginal infection.
• For treatment of oral candidiasis (thrush): Be sure the mouth is clean of food debris before administering drug, then tell patient to hold suspension in mouth for several minutes before swallowing. When treating infants, swab medication on oral mucosa. Instruct patient in good oral hygiene techniques. Tell patient overuse of mouthwash or poorly fitting dentures, especially in older patients, may alter flora and promote infection.
• Advise patient to continue medication for 1 to 2 weeks after symptomatic improvement to ensure against reinfection. Consult doctor for exact

---

length of therapy.
- Immunosuppressed patients sometimes take vaginal tablets (100,000 units) by mouth as this provides prolonged contact with oral mucosa.
- Instruct patient in careful hygiene for affected areas.
- Store in tightly closed, light-resistant containers in cool place.
- Not effective against systemic infections.

Antimalarials

chloroquine hydrochloride
chloroquine phosphate
hydroxychloroquine sulfate
primaquine phosphate
pyrimethamine
quinine sulfate

COMBINATION PRODUCTS
ARALEN PHOSPHATE WITH PRIMA-
QUINE PHOSPHATE: chloroquine phosphate 500 mg (300 mg base) and primaquine phosphate 79 mg (45 mg
base).
FANSIDAR: sulfadoxine 500 mg and
pyrimethamine 25 mg.

---

chloroquine hydrochloride
Aralen HCl

chloroquine phosphate
Aralen Phosphate♦, Chlorocon,
Novochloroquine♦♦
Pregnancy Category: C

MECHANISM OF ACTION
As an antimalarial, may bind to and
alter the properties of DNA. As an
amebicide, mechanism of action is
unknown.

INDICATIONS & DOSAGE
*Suppressive prophylaxis and treatment
of acute attacks of malaria due to*
Plasmodium vivax, Plasmodium malariae, Plasmodium ovale, *and susceptible strains of* Plasmodium falciparum—
Adults: initially, 600 mg (base) P.O.,
then 300 mg P.O. at 6, 24, and 48
hours. Or 160 to 200 mg (base) I.M.
initially; repeat in 6 hours if needed.
Switch to oral therapy as soon as possible.
Children: initially, 10 mg (base)/kg
P.O., then 5 mg (base)/kg dose P.O. at
6, 24, and 48 hours (do not exceed
adult dose). Or 5 mg (base)/kg I.M.
initially; repeat in 6 hours if needed.
Switch to oral therapy as soon as possible.
Malaria suppressive treatment—
Adults and children: 5 mg (base)/kg
P.O. (not to exceed 300 mg) weekly
on same day of the week (begin 2
weeks before entering endemic area
and continue for 8 weeks after leaving). If treatment begins after exposure, double the initial dose (600 mg
for adults, 10 mg/kg for children) in 2
divided doses P.O. 6 hours apart.
Extraintestinal amebiasis—
Adults: 160 to 200 mg chloroquine
(hydrochloride) base I.M. daily for no
more than 12 days. As soon as possible, substitute 1 g (600 mg base)
chloroquine phosphate P.O. daily for
2 days; then 500 mg (300 mg base)
daily for at least 2 to 3 weeks. Treatment is usually combined with an effective intestinal amebicide.
Children: 10 mg/kg of chloroquine
(hydrochloride) base for 2 to 3 weeks.
Maximum 300 mg daily.
Rheumatoid arthritis—
250 mg chloroquine phosphate daily
with evening meal.

ADVERSE REACTIONS
Blood: *agranulocytosis,* hemolytic
anemia.
CNS: mild and transient headache,

Italicized side effects are common or life-threatening.
*Liquid form contains alcohol.   **May contain tartrazine.

neuromyopathy, psychic stimulation, fatigue, irritability, nightmares, convulsions, dizziness.
EENT: *visual disturbances* (blurred vision; difficulty in focusing; reversible corneal changes; generally irreversible, sometimes progressive or delayed, retinal changes, e.g., narrowing of arterioles; macular lesions; pallor of optic disk; optic atrophy; patchy retinal pigmentation, often leading to blindness); ototoxicity (nerve deafness, vertigo, tinnitus).
GI: anorexia, abdominal cramps, diarrhea, nausea, vomiting.
Skin: pruritus, lichen planus-like eruptions, skin and mucosal pigmentary changes, pleomorphic skin eruptions.

INTERACTIONS
Magnesium and aluminum salts, kaolin: Decreased GI absorption. Separate administration times.

NURSING CONSIDERATIONS
• Contraindicated in patients with retinal or visual field changes, porphyria. Use with extreme caution in presence of severe GI, neurologic, or blood disorders. Drug concentrates in liver; use cautiously in patients with hepatic disease or alcoholism. Use with caution in patients with G-6-PD deficiency or psoriasis; drug may exacerbate these conditions.
• Complete blood cell counts and liver function studies should be made periodically during prolonged therapy; if severe blood disorder appears that is not attributable to disease under treatment, drug may need to be discontinued.
• Overdosage can quickly lead to toxic symptoms: headache, drowsiness, visual disturbances, cardiovascular collapse and convulsions, followed by respiratory and cardiac arrest. Children are extremely susceptible to toxicity; avoid long-term treatment.

• Baseline and periodic ophthalmologic examinations needed. Report blurred vision, increased sensitivity to light, or muscle weakness. Check periodically for ocular muscle weakness after long-term use. Audiometric examinations recommended before, during, and after therapy, especially if long term.
• Give drug immediately before or after meals on same day each week.
• To avoid exacerbated drug-induced dermatoses, warn patient to avoid excessive exposure to sun.

---

hydroxychloroquine sulfate
Plaquenil Sulfate♦
Pregnancy Category: C

MECHANISM OF ACTION
May bind to and alter the properties of DNA.

INDICATIONS & DOSAGE
Suppressive prophylaxis of attacks of malaria due to Plasmodium vivax, Plasmodium malariae, Plasmodium ovale, *and susceptible strains of* Plasmodium falciparum—
Adults and children: for suppression: 5 mg (base)/kg body weight P.O. (not to exceed 310 mg) weekly on same day of the week (begin 2 weeks prior to entering and continue for 8 weeks after leaving endemic area). If not started prior to exposure, double initial dose (620 mg for adults, 10 mg/kg for children) in 2 divided doses P.O. 6 hours apart.
Treatment of acute malarial attacks—
Adults and children over 15 years: initially, 800 mg (sulfate) P.O., then 400 mg after 6 to 8 hours, then 400 mg daily for 2 days (total 2 g sulfate salt).
Children 11 to 15 years: 600 mg (sulfate) P.O. stat, then 200 mg 8 hours later, then 200 mg 24 hours later (total 1 g sulfate salt).
Children 6 to 10 years: 400 mg (sul-

fate) P.O. stat, then 2 doses of 200 mg
at 8-hour intervals (total 800 mg sulfate salt).
Children 2 to 5 years: 400 mg (sulfate) P.O. stat, then 200 mg 8 hours
later (total 600 mg sulfate salt).
Children under 1 year: 100 mg (sulfate) P.O. stat; then 3 doses of 100 mg
6 to 9 hours apart (total 400 mg sulfate salt).
Lupus erythematosus (chronic discoid
and systemic)—
Adults: 400 mg P.O. daily or b.i.d.,
continued for several weeks or
months, depending on response. Prolonged maintenance—200 to 400 mg
P.O. daily.
Rheumatoid arthritis—
Adults: initially, 400 to 600 mg P.O.
daily. When good response occurs
(usually in 4 to 12 weeks), cut dosage
in half.

ADVERSE REACTIONS
Blood: *agranulocytosis, leukopenia,*
thrombocytopenia, *aplastic anemia.*
CNS: irritability, nightmares, ataxia,
convulsions, psychic stimulation,
toxic psychosis, vertigo, tinnitus, nystagmus, lassitude, fatigue, dizziness,
hypoactive deep-tendon reflexes, skeletal muscle weakness.
EENT: visual disturbances (blurred
vision; difficulty in focusing; reversible corneal changes; generally irreversible, sometimes progressive or delayed, retinal changes, e.g., narrowing of arterioles; macular lesions; pallor of optic disk; optic atrophy; visual
field defects; patchy retinal pigmentation, often leading to blindness), ototoxicity (irreversible nerve deafness,
tinnitus, labyrinthitis).
GI: anorexia, abdominal cramps,
diarrhea, nausea, vomiting.
Skin: pruritus, lichen planus-like
eruptions, skin and mucosal pigmentary changes, pleomorphic skin eruptions.
Other: weight loss, bleaching of hair.

INTERACTIONS
Magnesium and aluminum salts, kaolin: Decreased GI absorption. Separate administration times.

NURSING CONSIDERATIONS
• Contraindicated in patients with
retinal or visual field changes, or porphyria. Use with extreme caution in
presence of severe GI, neurologic, or
blood disorders. Drug concentrates in
the liver; use cautiously in patients
with hepatic disease or alcoholism.
Use with caution in patients with G-6-PD deficiency or psoriasis; drug may
exacerbate these conditions.
• Complete blood cell counts and
liver function studies should be made
periodically during prolonged therapy; if severe blood disorder appears
that is not attributable to disease under treatment, consider discontinuing.
• Overdosage can quickly lead to
toxic symptoms: headache, drowsiness, visual disturbances, cardiovascular collapse and convulsions, followed by respiratory and cardiac arrest. Children are extremely susceptible to toxicity; avoid long-term treatment.
• Baseline and periodic ophthalmologic examinations needed. Report
blurred vision, increased sensitivity
to light, or muscle weakness. Check
periodically for ocular muscle weakness after long-term use. Audiometric
examinations recommended before,
during, and after therapy, especially if
long term.
• Give drug immediately before or after meals on same day of each week.

primaquine phosphate
Pregnancy Category: C

MECHANISM OF ACTION
A gametocidal drug that destroys exoerythrocytic forms and prevents delayed primary attack. Its precise
mechanism of action is unknown.

Italicized side effects are common or life-threatening.
*Liquid form contains alcohol.   **May contain tartrazine.

INDICATIONS & DOSAGE
Radical cure of relapsing vivax malaria, eliminating symptoms and infection completely; prevention of relapse—
Adults: 15 mg (base) P.O. daily for 14 days. (26.3 mg tablet = 15 mg of base).

ADVERSE REACTIONS
Blood: leukopenia, hemolytic anemia in G-6-PD deficiency, methemoglobinemia in NADH methemoglobin reductase deficiency, leukocytosis, mild anemia, *granulocytopenia, agranulocytosis.*
EENT: disturbances of visual accommodation.
GI: nausea, vomiting, epigastric distress, abdominal cramps.
Skin: urticaria.

INTERACTIONS
Magnesium and aluminum salts: Decreased gastrointestinal absorption. Separate administration times.

NURSING CONSIDERATIONS
• Contraindicated in patients with lupus erythematosus and rheumatoid arthritis; in patients taking bone marrow suppressants and potentially hemolytic drugs.
• Use with a fast-acting antimalarial, such as chloroquine. Use full dose to reduce possibility of drug-resistant strains.
• Light-skinned patients taking more than 30 mg daily, dark-skinned patients taking more than 15 mg (base) daily, and patients with severe anemia or suspected sensitivity should have frequent blood studies and urine examinations. Sudden fall in hemoglobin concentration, erythrocyte or leukocyte count, or marked darkening of the urine suggests impending hemolytic reactions.
• Observe closely for tolerance in patients with previous idiosyncrasy (manifested by hemolytic anemia,

methemoglobinemia, or leukopenia); family or personal history of favism; erythrocytic G-6-PD deficiency or NADH methemoglobin reductase deficiency.
• Administer drug with meals or with antacids.

---

pyrimethamine
Daraprim♦, Fansidar (with sulfadoxine)
Pregnancy Category: C

MECHANISM OF ACTION
Inhibits the enzyme dihydrofolate reductase, thereby impeding reduction of folic acid.

INDICATIONS & DOSAGE
Malaria prophylaxis and transmission control (pyrimethamine)—
Adults and children over 10 years: 25 mg P.O. weekly.
Children 4 to 10 years: 12.5 mg P.O. weekly.
Children under 4 years: 6.25 mg P.O. weekly.
Continue in all age groups at least 10 weeks after leaving endemic areas.
Acute attacks of malaria (Fansidar)—
Adults: 2 to 3 tablets as a single dose, either alone or in sequence with quinine or primaquine.
Children 9 to 14 years: 2 tablets.
Children 4 to 8 years: 1 tablet.
Children under 4 years: ½ tablet.
Malaria prophylaxis (Fansidar)—
Adults: 1 tablet weekly, or 2 tablets every 2 weeks.
Children 9 to 14 years: ¾ tablet weekly, or 1½ tablets every 2 weeks.
Children 4 to 8 years: ½ tablet weekly, or 1 tablet every 2 weeks.
Children under 4 years: ¼ tablet weekly, or ½ tablet every 2 weeks.
Acute attacks of malaria (pyrimethamine)—
Not recommended alone in nonimmune persons; use with faster-acting antimalarials, such as chloroquine,

---

for 2 days to initiate transmission control and suppressive cure.
Adults and children over 15 years: 25 mg P.O. daily for 2 days.
Children under 15 years: 12.5 mg P.O. daily for 2 days.
Toxoplasmosis (pyrimethamine)—
Adults: initially, 100 mg P.O., then 25 mg P.O. daily for 4 to 5 weeks; during same time give 1 g sulfadiazine P.O. q 6 hours.
Children: initially, 1 mg/kg P.O., then 0.25 mg/kg daily for 4 to 5 weeks, along with 100 mg sulfadiazine/kg P.O. daily, divided q 6 hours.

ADVERSE REACTIONS
Blood: *agranulocytosis, aplastic anemia,* megaloblastic anemia, bone marrow suppression, leukopenia, thrombocytopenia, pancytopenia.
CNS: stimulation and convulsions (acute toxicity).
GI: anorexia, vomiting, diarrhea, atrophic glossitis.
Skin: rashes, *erythema multiforme (Stevens-Johnson syndrome).*

INTERACTIONS
Folic acid and para-aminobenzoic acid: decreased antitoxoplasmic effects. May require dosage adjustment.

NURSING CONSIDERATIONS
• Sulfadoxine, an ingredient in Fansidar, is a sulfonamide; therefore, this combination is contraindicated in porphyria. Use cautiously in patients with impaired hepatic or renal function, severe allergy or bronchial asthma, or G-6-PD deficiency.
• Contraindicated in chloroquine-resistant malaria. Use cautiously in patients with convulsive disorders; smaller doses may be needed. Also use cautiously following treatment with chloroquine.
• Warn patient taking Fansidar to stop drug and notify doctor at first sign of skin rash.

• Dosages required to treat toxoplasmosis approach toxic levels. Twice-weekly blood counts, including platelets, are required. If signs of folic or folinic acid deficiency develop, dosage should be reduced or discontinued while patient receives parenteral folinic acid (leucovorin) until blood counts become normal.
• Give with meals to minimize GI distress.
• The first dose of Fansidar, when taken prophylactically, should be taken 1 to 2 days before traveling to an endemic area.
• Because of the possibility of severe skin reactions, Fansidar should be used only in regions where chloroquine-resistant malaria is prevalent and only when the traveler plans to stay in the region longer than 3 weeks.

quinine sulfate
Legatrin, Novoquine♦♦, Quinamm, Quintrol, Q-Vel, Strema
Pregnancy Category: X

MECHANISM OF ACTION
Mechanism of action is unknown, but the drug is often referred to as a generalized protoplasmic poison.

INDICATIONS & DOSAGE
Malaria due to Plasmodium falciparum *(chloroquine-resistant)—*
Adults: 650 mg P.O. q 8 hours for 10 days, with 25 mg pyrimethamine q 12 hours for 3 days, and with 500 mg sulfadiazine q.i.d. for 5 days.
Nocturnal leg cramps—
Adults: 260 to 300 mg P.O. at bedtime or after the evening meal.

ADVERSE REACTIONS
Blood: hemolytic anemia, thrombocytopenia, agranulocytosis, hypoprothrombinemia.
CNS: severe headache, apprehension, excitement, confusion, delirium, syncope, hypothermia, convulsions (with

toxic doses).

CV: hypotension, *cardiovascular collapse* with overdosage or rapid I.V. administration.

EENT: altered color perception, photophobia, blurred vision, night blindness, amblyopia, scotoma, diplopia, mydriasis, optic atrophy, tinnitus, impaired hearing.

GI: epigastric distress, diarrhea, nausea, vomiting.

GU: renal tubular damage, anuria.

Skin: rashes, pruritus.

Local: thrombosis at infusion site.

Other: asthma, flushing.

INTERACTIONS

Sodium bicarbonate: elevates quinine levels by decreasing quinine excretion. Use together cautiously.

NURSING CONSIDERATIONS

• Contraindicated in patients with G-6-PD deficiency. Use with caution in patients with cardiovascular conditions.

• Discontinue if any signs of idiosyncrasy or toxicity occur.

• Quinine is no longer used for acute attacks of malaria due to *Plasmodium vivax* or for suppression of malaria due to organism resistance.

• Administer after meals to minimize GI distress.

• When parenteral therapy is necessary or when oral therapy is not feasible, quinine dihydrochloride may be obtained from the CDC. Administer by slow infusion (over at least 1 hour).

Antituberculars and antileprotics

capreomycin sulfate
clofazimine
cycloserine
dapsone
ethambutol hydrochloride
ethionamide
isoniazid (INH)
para-aminosalicylate sodium
pyrazinamide
rifampin
streptomycin sulfate
   (See Chapter 10, AMINOGLYCOSIDES.)

COMBINATION PRODUCTS
P-I-N FORTE: isoniazid 100 mg and pyridoxine HCl 5 mg.
RIFAMATE: isoniazid 150 mg and rifampin 300 mg.
RIMACTANE/INH DUAL PACK: Thirty 300-mg isoniazid tablets and sixty 300-mg rifampin capsules.
TEEBACONIN AND VITAMIN B₆: isoniazid 100 mg and pyridoxine HCl 10 mg.

---

capreomycin sulfate
Capastat Sulfate♦
Pregnancy Category: C

MECHANISM OF ACTION
Unknown (bactericidal).

INDICATIONS & DOSAGE
Adjunctive treatment in pulmonary tuberculosis—
Adults: 15 mg/kg/day up to 1 g I.M. daily injected deeply into large muscle mass for 60 to 120 days; then 1 g 2 to 3 times weekly for a period of 18 to 24 months. Maximum dose should

not exceed 20 mg/kg daily. Must be given in conjunction with another antitubercular drug.

ADVERSE REACTIONS
Blood: eosinophilia, leukocytosis, leukopenia.
CNS: headache.
EENT: *ototoxicity* (tinnitus, vertigo, hearing loss).
GU: *nephrotoxicity* (elevated BUN and nonprotein nitrogen, proteinuria, casts, red blood cells, leukocytes; tubular necrosis, decreased creatinine clearance).
Local: pain, induration, excessive bleeding and sterile abscesses at injection site.
Metabolic: hypokalemia, alkalosis.

INTERACTIONS
None significant.

NURSING CONSIDERATIONS
• Contraindicated in patients receiving other ototoxic or nephrotoxic drugs. Use cautiously in patients with impaired renal function, history of allergies, or hearing impairment.
• Considered a "second-line" drug in the treatment of tuberculosis.
• Drug is never given I.V. Intravenous use may cause neuromuscular blockage. Administer deep into large muscle mass to minimize local reactions.
• Evaluate patient's hearing before and during therapy. Notify doctor if patient complains of tinnitus, vertigo, hearing impairment.
• Monitor renal function (output, specific gravity, urinalysis, BUN, serum

---

Italicized side effects are common or life-threatening.
*Liquid form contains alcohol.   **May contain tartrazine.

creatinine) before and during therapy; notify doctor of decreasing renal function. Dose must be reduced in renal impairment.
• Straw- or dark-colored solution does not indicate a loss in potency.

clofazimine
Lamprene
Pregnancy Category: C

MECHANISM OF ACTION
Inhibits mycobacterial growth by binding preferentially to mycobacterial DNA. Also has anti-inflammatory effects that suppress skin reactions of erythema nodosum leprosum.

INDICATIONS & DOSAGE
Treatment of dapsone-resistant leprosy—
Adults: 100 mg P.O. daily in combination with other antileprosy drugs for 3 years. Then, clofazimine *alone,* 100 mg daily.
Erythema nodosum leprosum—
Adults: 100 to 200 mg P.O. daily for up to 3 months. Taper dosage to 100 mg daily as soon as possible. Dosages above 200 mg daily are not recommended.

ADVERSE REACTIONS
EENT: conjunctival and corneal pigmentation.
GI: *epigastric pain, diarrhea, nausea, vomiting, gastrointestinal intolerance, bowel obstruction, GI bleeding.*
Skin: *Pink to brownish black pigmentation, ichthyosis and dryness,* rash, itching.
Other: *Splenic infarction,* discolored body fluids and excrement.

INTERACTIONS
None significant.

NURSING CONSIDERATIONS
• Use cautiously in patients with gastrointestinal problems, such as ab-

dominal pain and diarrhea.
• Advise patient to take the drug with meals.
• Doses that exceed 100 mg daily should be given for as short a period as possible and only under close medical supervision.
• If patient complains of colicky or burning abdominal pain or of any other gastrointestinal symptom, report this to the doctor, who may reduce the dose or increase the interval between doses.
• Warn patient that clofazimine may discolor skin, body fluids, and excrement. The color ranges from red to brownish black. Reassure patient that the unsightly skin discoloration is reversible but may not disappear until several months or years after drug treatment ends.
• Skin discoloration due to the drug may result in depression. Two suicides have been reported in patients taking clofazimine.
• Recommend application of skin oil or cream to help reverse skin dryness or ichthyosis.

cycloserine
Seromycin
Pregnancy Category: C

MECHANISM OF ACTION
Inhibits cell-wall biosynthesis by inhibiting the utilization of amino acids (bacteriostatic).

INDICATIONS & DOSAGE
Adjunctive treatment in pulmonary or extrapulmonary tuberculosis—
Adults: initially, 250 mg P.O. every 12 hours for 2 weeks; then, if blood levels are below 25 to 30 mcg/ml and there are no clinical signs of toxicity, dose is increased to 250 mg P.O. q 8 hours for 2 weeks. If optimum blood levels are still not achieved, and there are no signs of clinical toxicity, then dose is increased to 250 mg P.O. q 6

hours. Maximum dose is 1 g/day. If CNS toxicity occurs, drug is discontinued for 1 week, then resumed at 250 mg daily for 2 weeks. If no serious toxic effects occur, dose is increased by 250-mg increments every 10 days until blood level of 25 to 30 mcg/ml is obtained.

ADVERSE REACTIONS
CNS: drowsiness, headache, tremor, dysarthria, vertigo, confusion, loss of memory, *possible suicidal tendencies and other psychotic symptoms, nervousness, hallucinations, depression,* hyperirritability, paresthesias, paresis, hyperreflexia.
Other: hypersensitivity (allergic dermatitis).

INTERACTIONS
Isoniazid: monitor for CNS toxicity (dizziness or drowsiness).

NURSING CONSIDERATIONS
• Contraindicated in patients with seizure disorders, depression or severe anxiety, severe renal insufficiency, or chronic alcoholism. Use cautiously in patients with impaired renal function; reduced dosage required.
• Considered a "second-line" drug in the treatment of tuberculosis.
• Obtain specimen for culture and sensitivity tests before therapy begins and periodically thereafter to detect possible resistance.
• Serious neurologic effects can be precipitated by ingestion of alcohol; warn patient not to drink.
• Toxic reactions may occur with blood levels above 30 mcg/ml.
• Pyridoxine, anticonvulsants, tranquilizers, or sedatives may help to relieve adverse reactions.
• Observe for personality changes.
• Monitor hematologic tests and renal and liver function studies.
• Instruct patient to take drug exactly as prescribed; warn against discontin-uing use without doctor's consent.

---

dapsone
Avlosulfon♦♦
Pregnancy Category: A

MECHANISM OF ACTION
Inhibits folic acid biosynthesis (bactericidal).

INDICATIONS & DOSAGE
All forms of leprosy (Hansen's disease)—
Adults: 100 mg P.O. daily for indefinite period, plus rifampin 600 mg daily for 6 months.

ADVERSE REACTIONS
Blood: *aplastic anemia, agranulocytosis, hemolytic anemia;* methemoglobinemia; possible leukopenia.
CNS: psychosis, headache, dizziness, lethargy, severe malaise, paresthesias.
EENT: tinnitus, allergic rhinitis.
GI: anorexia, abdominal pain, nausea, vomiting.
Hepatic: hepatitis, cholestatic jaundice.
Skin: allergic dermatitis (generalized or fixed maculopapular rash).

INTERACTIONS
Probenecid: elevates levels of dapsone. Use together with extreme caution.

NURSING CONSIDERATIONS
• Use cautiously in chronic renal, hepatic, or cardiovascular disease or refractory types of anemia.
• Use cautiously in patients with G-6-PD deficiency.
• Therapy should be interrupted if generalized, diffuse dermatitis occurs.
• Dapsone dosage should be reduced or temporarily discontinued if hemoglobin falls below 9 g/dl; if leukocyte count falls below 5,000/mm³; if

---

Italicized side effects are common or life-threatening.
*Liquid form contains alcohol.   **May contain tartrazine.

erythrocyte count falls below 2.5 million/mm³ or remains low.

• Antihistamines may help to combat dapsone-induced allergic dermatitis.

• Erythema nodosum type of lepra reaction may occur during therapy as a result of *Mycobacterium leprae* bacilli (malaise, fever, painful inflammatory induration in the skin and mucosa, iritis, neuritis). In severe cases, therapy should be stopped and glucocorticoids given cautiously.

• Obtain CBC before treatment and monitor frequently throughout therapy (weekly for the first month, monthly for 6 months, and semiannually thereafter).

• Also used to treat relapsing polychondritis and as prophylaxis against malaria.

• Instruct nursing mothers to report cyanosis in infants, as this indicates high sulfone level.

---

ethambutol hydrochloride
Etibi♦♦, Myambutol♦
Pregnancy Category: B

MECHANISM OF ACTION
Interferes with the synthesis of RNA, thus inhibiting protein metabolism (bacteriostatic).

INDICATIONS & DOSAGE
Adjunctive treatment in pulmonary tuberculosis—
Adults and children over 13 years: initial treatment for patients who have not received previous antitubercular therapy 15 mg/kg P.O. daily single dose.
Re-treatment: 25 mg/kg P.O. daily single dose for 60 days with at least one other antitubercular drug; then decrease to 15 mg/kg P.O. daily single dose.

ADVERSE REACTIONS
CNS: headache, dizziness, mental confusion, possible hallucinations,

peripheral neuritis (numbness and tingling of extremities).
EENT: optic neuritis (vision loss and loss of color discrimination, especially red and green).
GI: anorexia, nausea, vomiting, abdominal pain.
Metabolic: *elevated uric acid.*
Other: anaphylactoid reactions, fever, malaise, bloody sputum.

INTERACTIONS
None significant.

NURSING CONSIDERATIONS
• Contraindicated in patients with optic neuritis and in children under 13 years. Use cautiously in patients with impaired renal function, cataracts, recurrent eye inflammations, gout, and diabetic retinopathy.

• Dose must be reduced in renal impairment.

• Perform visual acuity and color discrimination tests before and during therapy.

• Always monitor serum uric acid; observe patient for symptoms of gout.

• Reassure patient that visual disturbances will disappear several weeks to months after drug is stopped.

---

ethionamide
Trecator SC
Pregnancy Category: D

MECHANISM OF ACTION
Unknown (bacteriostatic).

INDICATIONS & DOSAGE
Adjunctive treatment in pulmonary or extrapulmonary tuberculosis (when primary therapy with streptomycin, isoniazid, and para-aminosalicylate sodium cannot be used or has failed)—
Adults: 500 mg to 1 g P.O. daily in divided doses. Concomitant administration of other effective antitubercular drugs and pyridoxine recom-

---

mended.
Children: 12 to 15 mg/kg P.O. daily in 3 to 4 doses. Maximum dose 750 mg.

ADVERSE REACTIONS
Blood: thrombocytopenia.
CNS: *peripheral neuritis,* psychic disturbances (especially mental depression).
CV: postural hypotension.
GI: *anorexia,* metallic taste in mouth, nausea, vomiting, sialorrhea, *epigastric distress,* diarrhea, stomatitis, weight loss.
Hepatic: jaundice, hepatitis, elevated SGOT and SGPT.
Skin: rash, *exfoliative dermatitis.*

INTERACTIONS
None significant.

NURSING CONSIDERATIONS
• Contraindicated in patients with severe hepatic damage. Use cautiously in patients with diabetes mellitus.
• Culture and sensitivity tests should be performed before starting therapy. Stop drug if skin rash occurs; may progress to exfoliative dermatitis.
• Monitor hepatic function every 2 to 4 weeks.
• Give with meals or antacids to minimize GI effects. Patient may require antiemetic.
• Pyridoxine may be ordered to prevent neuropathy.
• Instruct patient to take this drug exactly as prescribed; warn against discontinuing drug without doctor's consent.
• Warn patient to avoid excess alcohol ingestion because it may make him more vulnerable to liver damage.

isoniazid (INH)
Hyzyd, Isotamine♦♦, Laniazid, Nydrazid**, PMS-Isoniazid♦♦, Rimifon♦♦, Rolazid, Teebaconin
Pregnancy Category: C

MECHANISM OF ACTION
Inhibits cell-wall biosynthesis by interfering with lipid and DNA synthesis (bactericidal).

INDICATIONS & DOSAGE
Primary treatment against actively growing tubercle bacilli—
Adults: 5 mg/kg P.O. or I.M. daily single dose, up to 300 mg/day, continued for 9 months to 2 years.
Infants and children: 10 to 20 mg/kg P.O. or I.M. daily single dose, up to 300 to 500 mg/day, continued for 18 months to 2 years. Concomitant administration of at least one other effective antitubercular drug is recommended.
Preventive therapy against tubercle bacilli of those closely exposed or those with positive skin test whose chest X-rays and bacteriologic studies are consistent with nonprogressive tuberculous disease—
Adults: 300 mg P.O. daily single dose, continued for 1 year.
Infants and children: 10 mg/kg P.O. daily single dose, up to 300 mg/day, continued for 1 year.

ADVERSE REACTIONS
Blood: *agranulocytosis,* hemolytic anemia, *aplastic anemia,* eosinophilia, leukopenia, neutropenia, thrombocytopenia, methemoglobinemia, pyridoxine-responsive hypochromic anemia.
CNS: *peripheral neuropathy* (especially in the malnourished, alcoholics, diabetics, and slow acetylators), usually preceded by paresthesias of hands and feet, psychosis.
GI: nausea, vomiting, epigastric distress, constipation, dryness of the

---

Italicized side effects are common or life-threatening.
*Liquid form contains alcohol.   **May contain tartrazine.

mouth.
Hepatic: *hepatitis, occasionally severe and sometimes fatal, especially in the elderly.*
Metabolic: hyperglycemia, metabolic acidosis.
Local: irritation at injection site.
Other: rheumatic syndrome and systemic lupus erythematosus–like syndrome; hypersensitivity (fever, rash, lymphadenopathy, vasculitis).

INTERACTIONS
Aluminum-containing antacids and laxatives: may decrease the rate and amount of isoniazid absorbed. Give isoniazid at least 1 hour before antacid or laxative.
Disulfiram: neurologic symptoms, including changes in behavior and coordination, may develop with concomitant isoniazid use. Avoid concomitant use.
Carbamazepine: increased risk of isoniazid hepatotoxicity. Use together very cautiously.
Corticosteroids: may decrease therapeutic effectiveness. Monitor need for larger isoniazid dose.

NURSING CONSIDERATIONS
• Contraindicated in patients with acute hepatic disease, or isoniazid-associated hepatic damage. Use cautiously in patients with chronic non–isoniazid-associated hepatic disease, seizure disorder (especially those taking phenytoin), severe renal impairment, chronic alcoholism; in elderly patients; in slow acetylator phenotypes (approximately 50% of blacks and whites).
• Monitor hepatic function. Tell patient to notify doctor immediately if symptoms of hepatic impairment occur (loss of appetite, fatigue, malaise, jaundice, dark urine).
• Alcohol may be associated with increased incidence of isoniazid-related hepatitis. Discourage use.
• Pyridoxine should be given to pre-vent peripheral neuropathy, especially in malnourished patients.
• Instruct patient to take this drug exactly as prescribed; warn against discontinuing drug without doctor's consent.
• Encourage patient to fully comply with treatment, which may take months or years.
• Advise patient to take with food if GI irritation occurs.
• Reportedly effective when used investigationally to treat arthritis as well as action tremor in multiple sclerosis.

para-aminosalicylate sodium
Parasal Sodium, Pasdium♦
Pregnancy Category: C

MECHANISM OF ACTION
Inhibits the enzymes responsible for folic acid biosynthesis (bacteriostatic).

INDICATIONS & DOSAGE
Adjunctive treatment of tuberculosis—
Adults: 14 to 16 g P.O. daily, divided in 3 or 4 doses.
Children: 240 to 360 mg/kg P.O. daily, divided in 3 or 4 doses.

ADVERSE REACTIONS
Blood: *leukopenia, agranulocytosis,* eosinophilia, thrombocytopenia, hemolytic anemia.
CNS: encephalopathy.
CV: vasculitis.
GI: *nausea, vomiting,* diarrhea, *abdominal pain.*
GU: albuminuria, hematuria, crystalluria.
Hepatic: *jaundice, hepatitis.*
Metabolic: acidosis, hypokalemia.
Skin: rash.
Other: infectious mononucleosis–like syndrome, fever, lymphadenopathy.

INTERACTIONS

Ascorbic acid, ammonium chloride: acidify urine, increasing possibility of para-aminosalicylate sodium crystalluria. Avoid if possible.
Probenecid: may increase levels of para-aminosalicylate sodium. Use together cautiously.
Diphenhydramine: inhibits absorption of para-aminosalicylate sodium. Monitor for decreased para-aminosalicylate sodium effect.

NURSING CONSIDERATIONS

• Use cautiously in patients with impaired renal function, decreased hepatic function, and gastric ulcers.
• Para-aminosalicylate sodium should not be given to patients on sodium-restricted diets. A 15-g dose provides 1.6 g sodium.
• Give with meals or antacid to reduce gastrointestinal distress. Tell patient to swallow enteric-coated tablets whole and not with antacids.
• Monitor renal, hematopoietic, and hepatic functions and serum electrolytes.
• Tell patient to notify doctor at once if symptoms of hepatic impairment (loss of appetite, fatigue, malaise, jaundice, dark urine), fever, sore throat, or skin rash occurs.
• Instruct patient to take this drug exactly as prescribed; warn against discontinuing drug without doctor's consent.
• Protect from water, heat, and sun; don't use if drug turns brown or purple.
• Concomitant administration of at least one other effective antitubercular drug is recommended.

---

pyrazinamide
Tebrazid♦♦
Pregnancy Category: C

MECHANISM OF ACTION
Unknown (bactericidal).

INDICATIONS & DOSAGE

Adjunctive treatment of tuberculosis (when primary and secondary antitubercular drugs cannot be used or have failed)—
Adults: 20 to 35 mg/kg P.O. daily, divided in 3 to 4 doses. Maximum dose 3 g daily.

ADVERSE REACTIONS

Blood: sideroblastic anemia, possible bleeding tendency due to thrombocytopenia.
GI: anorexia, nausea, vomiting.
GU: dysuria.
Hepatic: hepatitis.
Metabolic: interference with control in diabetes mellitus, *hyperuricemia*.
Other: malaise, fever, arthralgia.

INTERACTIONS
None significant.

NURSING CONSIDERATIONS

• Contraindicated in patients with severe hepatic disease. Use cautiously in patients with diabetes mellitus or gout.
• Nearly 100% excreted in urine; reduced dose needed in patients with renal impairment.
• Perform liver function studies and examination for jaundice, liver tenderness, or enlargement before and frequently during therapy.
• Watch closely for signs of gout and of hepatic impairment (loss of appetite, fatigue, malaise, jaundice, dark urine, liver tenderness). Call doctor at once.
• Question doses that exceed 35 mg/kg, as they may cause liver damage.
• Monitor hematopoietic studies and serum uric acid levels.
• When used with surgical management of tuberculosis, start pyrazinamide 1 to 2 weeks before surgery and continue for 4 to 6 weeks postoperatively.

Italicized side effects are common or life-threatening.
*Liquid form contains alcohol.   **May contain tartrazine.

rifampin
Rifadin♦, Rimactane♦, Rofact♦♦
Pregnancy Category: C

MECHANISM OF ACTION
Inhibits DNA-dependent RNA polymerase, thus impairing ribonucleic acid synthesis (bactericidal).

INDICATIONS & DOSAGE
Primary treatment in pulmonary tuberculosis—
Adults: 600 mg P.O. daily single dose 1 hour before or 2 hours after meals.
Children over 5 years: 10 to 20 mg/kg P.O. daily single dose 1 hour before or 2 hours after meals. Maximum dose is 600 mg daily. Concomitant administration of other effective antitubercular drugs is recommended.
Meningococcal carriers—
Adults: 600 mg P.O. twice daily for 2 days.
Children over 5 years: 10 mg/kg twice daily P.O., not to exceed 600 mg/dose.

ADVERSE REACTIONS
Blood: thrombocytopenia, transient leukopenia, hemolytic anemia.
CNS: headache, fatigue, *drowsiness,* ataxia, dizziness, mental confusion, generalized numbness.
GI: epigastric distress, anorexia, nausea, vomiting, abdominal pain, diarrhea, flatulence, sore mouth and tongue.
Metabolic: hyperuricemia.
Hepatic: *serious hepatotoxicity as well as transient abnormalities in liver function tests.*
Skin: pruritus, urticaria, rash.
Other: flu-like syndrome.

INTERACTIONS
Para-aminosalicylate sodium, ketoconazole: may interfere with absorption of rifampin. Give these drugs 8 to 12 hours apart.
Probenecid: may increase rifampin levels. Use cautiously.

NURSING CONSIDERATIONS
• Contraindicated in patients with clinically active hepatitis.
• Use cautiously in patients with hepatic disease or in those receiving other hepatotoxic drugs.
• Monitor hepatic function, hematopoietic studies, and serum uric acid levels.
• Watch closely for signs of hepatic impairment (loss of appetite, fatigue, malaise, jaundice, dark urine, liver tenderness).
• Warn patient about drowsiness and the possibility of red-orange discoloration of urine, feces, saliva, sweat, sputum, and tears. Soft contact lenses may be permanently stained.
• Rifampin is not considered a teratogen. However, it may cause hemorrhaging in the newborns of rifampin-treated mothers.
• Advise patient to avoid alcoholic beverages while taking this drug. May increase risk of hepatotoxicity.
• Give 1 hour before or 2 hours after meals for optimal absorption; however, if GI irritation occurs, patient may take rifampin with meals.
• Increases enzyme activity of liver; may require increased doses of warfarin, corticosteroids, oral contraceptives, and oral hypoglycemics. See each drug entry for specific drug interactions.
• Concomitant treatment with at least one other antitubercular drug is recommended.

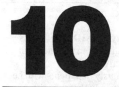

Aminoglycosides

amikacin sulfate
gentamicin sulfate
kanamycin sulfate
neomycin sulfate
netilmicin sulfate
streptomycin sulfate
tobramycin sulfate

COMBINATION PRODUCTS
NEOSPORIN G.U. IRRIGANT: 40 mg
neomycin sulfate and 200,000 units
polymixin B sulfate/ml.

---

amikacin sulfate
Amikin♦
Pregnancy Category: C

MECHANISM OF ACTION
Inhibits protein synthesis by binding
directly to the 30S ribosomal subunit.
Generally bactericidal.

INDICATIONS & DOSAGE
Serious infections caused by sensitive
Pseudomonas aeruginosa, Escherichia coli, Proteus, Klebsiella, Serratia, Enterobacter, Acinetobacter,
Providencia, Citrobacter, Staphylococcus—
**Adults and children with normal
renal function:** 15 mg/kg/day divided q 8 to 12 hours I.M. or I.V. infusion (in 100 to 200 ml dextrose 5%
in water run in over 30 to 60 minutes). May be given by direct I.V.
push if necessary.
**Neonates with normal renal func-
tion:** initially, 10 mg/kg I.M. or I.V.
infusion (in dextrose 5% in water run
in over 1 to 2 hours), then 7.5 mg/kg

q 12 hours I.M. or I.V. infusion.
Meningitis—
Adults: systemic therapy as above;
may also use up to 20 mg intrathecally or intraventricularly daily.
Children: systemic therapy as above;
may also use 1 to 2 mg intrathecally
daily.
*Uncomplicated urinary tract infec-
tions—*
Adults: 250 mg I.M. or I.V. b.i.d.
**Adults with impaired renal func-
tion:** initially, 7.5 mg/kg. Subsequent
doses and frequency determined by
blood amikacin levels and renal function studies.

ADVERSE REACTIONS
CNS: headache, lethargy, *neuromuscular blockade*.
EENT: *ototoxicity (tinnitus, vertigo,
hearing loss)*.
GU: *nephrotoxicity (cells or casts in
urine, oliguria, proteinuria, decreased creatinine clearance, increased BUN and serum creatinine
levels)*.

INTERACTIONS
I.V. loop diuretics (e.g. furosemide):
increase ototoxicity. Use cautiously.
Dimenhydrinate: may mask symp-
toms of ototoxicity. Use with caution.
Parenteral penicillins (e.g. carbenicil-
lin, ticarcillin): amikacin inactivation.
Don't mix together in I.V.
*Other aminoglycosides, amphotericin
B, cisplatin, methoxyflurane:* in-
creases nephrotoxicity. Use together
cautiously.
Cephalothin: increased nephrotoxic-

---

ity. Use together cautiously.

NURSING CONSIDERATIONS
• Use cautiously in patients with impaired renal function, in neonates and infants, and in elderly patients.
• Obtain specimen for culture and sensitivity before first dose. Therapy may begin pending test results.
• Weigh patient and obtain baseline renal function studies before therapy begins.
• Monitor renal function (output, specific gravity, urinalysis, BUN and creatinine levels, and creatinine clearance). Notify doctor of signs of decreasing renal function.
• Patient should be well hydrated while taking drug to minimize chemical irritation of the renal tubules.
• Evaluate patient's hearing before and during therapy. Notify doctor if patient complains of tinnitus, vertigo, or hearing loss.
• Watch for superinfection (continued fever and other signs of new infections, especially of upper respiratory tract).
• Usual duration of therapy is 7 to 10 days. If no response after 3 to 5 days, therapy should be stopped and new specimens obtained for culture and sensitivity.
• Peak blood levels that are above 35 mcg/ml and trough levels that are above 10 mcg/ml are associated with higher incidence of toxicity.
• After I.V. infusion, flush line with normal saline solution or 5% dextrose in water.
• Draw blood for peak amikacin level 1 hour after I.M. injection and 30 minutes to 1 hour after infusion ends; for trough levels, draw blood just before next dose.
• Don't collect blood in a heparinized tube.
• Potency of drug is not affected if solution turns light yellow.

gentamicin sulfate
Alcomicin♦♦, Cidomycin♦♦, Garamycin♦, Jenamicin
Pregnancy Category: C

MECHANISM OF ACTION
Inhibits protein synthesis by binding directly to the 30S ribosomal subunit. Generally bactericidal.

INDICATIONS & DOSAGE
Serious infections caused by sensitive Pseudomonas aeruginosa, Escherichia coli, Proteus, Klebsiella, Serratia, Enterobacter, Citrobacter, Staphylococcus—
Adults with normal renal function: 3 mg/kg daily in divided doses q 8 hours I.M. or I.V. infusion (in 50 to 200 ml of normal saline solution or dextrose 5% in water infused over 30 minutes to 2 hours). May be given by direct I.V. push if necessary. For life-threatening infections, patient may receive up to 5 mg/kg daily in 3 to 4 divided doses.
Children with normal renal function: 2 to 2.5 mg/kg I.M. or I.V. infusion q 8 hours.
Infants and neonates over 1 week with normal renal function: 2.5 mg/kg q 8 hours I.M. or I.V. infusion.
Neonates under 1 week: 2.5 mg/kg I.V. q 12 hours. For I.V. infusion, dilute in normal saline solution or dextrose 5% in water and infuse over 30 minutes to 2 hours.
Meningitis—
Adults: systemic therapy as above; may also use 4 to 8 mg intrathecally daily.
Children: systemic therapy as above; may also use 1 to 2 mg intrathecally daily.
Endocarditis prophylaxis for GI or GU procedure or surgery—
Adults: 1.5 mg/kg I.M. or I.V. 30 to 60 minutes before procedure or surgery and q 8 hours after, for 2 doses. Given with aqueous penicillin G or

ampicillin.

Children: 2.5 mg/kg I.M. or I.V. 30 to 60 minutes before procedure or surgery and q 8 hours after, for 2 doses. Given with aqueous penicillin G or ampicillin.

Patients with impaired renal function: initial dose is same as for those with normal renal function. Subsequent doses and frequency determined by renal function studies. *Posthemodialysis to maintain therapeutic blood levels—*
Adults: 1 to 1.7 mg/kg I.M. or I.V. infusion after each dialysis.
Children: 2 mg/kg I.M. or I.V. infusion after each dialysis.

ADVERSE REACTIONS
CNS: headache, lethargy, *neuromuscular blockade*.
EENT: *ototoxicity (tinnitus, vertigo, hearing loss).*
GU: *nephrotoxicity (cells or casts in the urine; oliguria; proteinuria; decreased creatinine clearance; increased BUN, nonprotein nitrogen, and serum creatinine levels).*

INTERACTIONS
I.V. loop diuretics (e.g. furosemide): increase ototoxicity. Use cautiously.
Dimenhydrinate: may mask symptoms of ototoxicity. Use with caution.
Parenteral penicillins (e.g. carbenicillin and ticarcillin): gentamicin inactivation. Don't mix together in I.V.
Cephalothin: increases nephrotoxicity. Use together cautiously.
Other aminoglycosides, methoxyflurane: increase ototoxicity and nephrotoxicity. Use together cautiously.

NURSING CONSIDERATIONS
• Use cautiously in patients with impaired renal function, and in neonates, infants, and elderly patients.
• Obtain specimen for culture and sensitivity before first dose. Therapy may begin pending test results.
• Weigh patient and obtain baseline

renal function studies before therapy begins.
• Monitor renal function (output, specific gravity, urinalysis, BUN and creatinine levels, and creatinine clearance). Notify doctor of signs of decreasing renal function.
• Patient should be well hydrated while taking drug to minimize chemical irritation of the renal tubules.
• After completing I.V. infusion, flush the line with normal saline solution or dextrose 5% in water.
• Evaluate patient's hearing before and during therapy. Notify doctor if patient complains of tinnitus, vertigo, or hearing loss.
• Watch for superinfection (continued fever and other signs of new infections, especially of upper respiratory tract).
• Usual duration of therapy is 7 to 10 days. If no response in 3 to 5 days, therapy should be stopped and new specimens obtained for culture and sensitivity.
• Peak blood levels above 12 mcg/ml and trough levels (those drawn just before next dose) above 2 mcg/ml are associated with higher incidence of toxicity.
• Draw blood for peak gentamicin level 1 hour after I.M. injection and 30 minutes to 1 hour after infusion ends; for trough levels, draw blood just before next dose.
• Don't collect blood in a heparinized tube.
• Hemodialysis (8 hours) removes up to 50% of drug from blood.
• Intrathecal form (without preservatives) should be used when intrathecal administration is indicated.

kanamycin sulfate
Anamid♦♦, Kantrex♦, Klebcil
Pregnancy Category: D

MECHANISM OF ACTION
Inhibits protein synthesis by binding

---

directly to the 30S ribosomal subunit. Generally bactericidal.

INDICATIONS & DOSAGE

Serious infections caused by sensitive Escherichia coli, Proteus, Enterobacter aerogenes, Klebsiella pneumoniae, Serratia marcescens, Acinetobacter—
Adults and children with normal renal function: 15 mg/kg daily divided q 8 to 12 hours deep I.M. into upper outer quadrant of buttocks or I.V. infusion (diluted 500 mg/200 ml of normal saline solution or dextrose 5% in water infused at 60 to 80 drops/minute). Maximum daily dose 1.5 g.
Neonates: 15 mg/kg daily I.M. or I.V. divided q 12 hours.
Adjunctive treatment in hepatic coma—
Adults: 8 to 12 g daily P.O. in divided doses.
Preoperative bowel sterilization—
Adults: 1 g P.O. q 1 hour for 4 doses, then q 4 hours for 4 doses; or 1 g P.O. q 1 hour for 4 doses, then q 6 hours for 36 to 72 hours.
Intraperitoneal irrigation—
500 mg in 20 ml sterile distilled water instilled via catheter into wound after patient fully recovered from anesthesia and neuromuscular blocking agent effects.
Wound irrigation—
Up to 2.5 mg/ml in normal saline irrigation solution.

ADVERSE REACTIONS

CNS: headache, lethargy, *neuromuscular blockade.*
EENT: *ototoxicity (tinnitus, vertigo, hearing loss).*
GU: *nephrotoxicity (cells or casts in the urine, oliguria, proteinuria, decreased creatinine clearance, increased BUN and serum creatinine levels).*

INTERACTIONS

I.V. loop diuretics (e.g. furosemide): increase ototoxicity. Use cautiously.

Dimenhydrinate: may mask symptoms of ototoxicity. Use with caution.
Parenteral penicillins (e.g. carbenicillin, ticarcillin): kanamycin inactivation. Don't mix together in I.V.
Cephalothin: increases nephrotoxicity. Use together cautiously.
Other aminoglycosides, amphotericin B, cisplatin, methoxyflurane: increases nephrotoxicity. Don't use together.

NURSING CONSIDERATIONS

• Oral use contraindicated in patients with intestinal obstruction and in treatment of systemic infection. Use cautiously in patients with impaired renal function and in the elderly.
• Obtain specimen for culture and sensitivity before first dose. Therapy may begin pending test results.
• Weigh patient and obtain baseline renal function studies before therapy begins.
• Monitor renal function (output, specific gravity, urinalysis, BUN, creatinine levels, and creatinine clearance). Notify doctor of signs of decreasing renal function.
• Patient should be well hydrated while taking drug to minimize chemical irritation of the renal tubules.
• Evaluate patient's hearing before and during therapy. Notify doctor if patient complains of tinnitus, vertigo, or hearing loss.
• Watch for superinfection (continued fever and other signs of new infection, especially of upper respiratory tract).
• If no response in 3 to 5 days, therapy should be stopped and new specimens obtained for culture and sensitivity.
• Peak blood levels over 30 mcg/ml and trough levels over 10 mcg/ml are associated with increased incidence of toxicity.

neomycin sulfate
Mycifradin Sulfate♦
Pregnancy Category: C

MECHANISM OF ACTION
Inhibits protein synthesis by binding directly to the 30S ribosomal subunit. Generally bactericidal.

INDICATIONS & DOSAGE
Infectious diarrhea caused by enteropathogenic Escherichia coli—
Adults: 50 mg/kg daily P.O. in 4 divided doses for 2 to 3 days.
Children: 50 to 100 mg/kg daily P.O. divided q 4 to 6 hours for 2 to 3 days.
Suppression of intestinal bacteria preoperatively—
Adults: 1 g P.O. q 1 hour for 4 doses, then 1 g q 4 hours for the balance of the 24 hours. A saline cathartic should precede therapy.
Children: 40 to 100 mg/kg daily P.O. divided q 4 to 6 hours. First dose should be preceded by saline cathartic.
Adjunctive treatment in hepatic coma—
Adults: 1 to 3 g P.O. q.i.d. for 5 to 6 days; or 200 ml of 1% or 100 ml of 2% solution as enema retained for 20 to 60 minutes q 6 hours.

ADVERSE REACTIONS
CNS: headache, lethargy.
EENT: *ototoxicity (tinnitus, vertigo, hearing loss).*
GI: nausea, vomiting.
GU: *nephrotoxicity (cells or casts in the urine, oliguria, proteinuria, decreased creatinine clearance, increased BUN and serum creatinine levels).*
Skin: rash, urticaria.

INTERACTIONS
I.V. loop diuretics (e.g. furosemide): increase ototoxicity. Use cautiously.
Dimenhydrinate: may mask symptoms of ototoxicity. Use with caution.

Cephalothin: Increases nephrotoxicity. Use together cautiously.
Other aminoglycosides, amphotericin B, cisplatin, methoxyflurane: increases nephrotoxicity. Use together cautiously.

NURSING CONSIDERATIONS
• Contraindicated in patients with intestinal obstruction. Use cautiously in patients with impaired renal function, ulcerative bowel lesions, and in elderly patients.
• Oral therapy not recommended for systemic infection; parenteral dosage form available for I.M. use but not recommended because of extreme ototoxicity and nephrotoxicity.
• Weigh patient and obtain baseline renal function studies before therapy begins.
• Monitor renal function (output, specific gravity, urinalysis, BUN and creatinine levels, and creatinine clearance). Notify doctor of signs of decreasing renal function.
• Patient should be well hydrated while taking drug to minimize chemical irritation of the renal tubules.
• Watch for respiratory depression in patients with renal disease, hypocalcemia, or neuromuscular diseases, such as myasthenia gravis.
• Evaluate hearing of patient with hepatic or renal disease before and during prolonged therapy. Notify doctor if patient complains of tinnitus, vertigo, or hearing loss. Onset of deafness may occur several weeks after drug is stopped.
• Sometimes used in the treatment of high blood cholesterol.
• Nonabsorbable at recommended dosage. However, more than 4 g of neomycin per day may be systemically absorbed and lead to nephrotoxicity.
• For preoperative disinfection, provide a low-residue diet and a cathartic immediately before oral administration of neomycin.
• Available in combination with poly-

Italicized side effects are common or life-threatening.
*Liquid form contains alcohol.   **May contain tartrazine.

myxin B as a urinary bladder irrigant.

netilmicin sulfate
Netromycin♦
Pregnancy Category: C

MECHANISM OF ACTION
Inhibits protein synthesis by binding directly to the 30S ribosomal subunit. Generally bactericidal.

INDICATIONS & DOSAGE
Serious infections caused by sensitive Pseudomonas aeruginosa, Escherichia coli, Proteus, Klebsiella, Serratia, Enterobacter, Citrobacter, Staphylococcus—
Adults and children over 12 years: 3 to 6.5 mg/kg/day by I.M. injection or I.V. infusion. May be given q 12 hours to treat serious urinary tract infections and q 8 to 12 hours to treat serious systemic infections.
Infants and children (6 weeks to 12 years): 5.5 to 8 mg/kg/day by I.M. injection or I.V. infusion given either as 1.8 to 2.7 mg/kg q 8 hours or as 2.7 to 4 mg/kg q 12 hours.
Neonates (under 6 weeks): 4 to 6.5 mg/kg/day by I.M. injection or I.V. infusion given as 2 to 3.25 mg/kg q 12 hours.

ADVERSE REACTIONS
CNS: headache, lethargy, *neuromuscular blockade.*
EENT: *ototoxicity (tinnitus, vertigo, hearing loss).*
GU: *nephrotoxicity (cells or casts in the urine; oliguria; proteinuria; decreased creatinine clearance; increased BUN, nonprotein nitrogen, and serum creatinine levels).*

INTERACTIONS
I.V. loop diuretics (e.g. furosemide): increase ototoxicity. Use cautiously.
Dimenhydrinate: may mask symptoms of ototoxicity. Use with caution.
Parenteral penicillins (e.g., carbenicillin, and ticarcillin): netilmicin inactivation. Don't mix together in I.V.
Cephalothin: increases nephrotoxicity. Use together cautiously.
Other aminoglycosides, amphotericin B, cisplatin, methoxyflurane: increases nephrotoxicity. Use together cautiously.

NURSING CONSIDERATIONS
• Use cautiously in patients with impaired renal function and in neonates, infants, and elderly patients.
• Obtain specimen for culture and sensitivity before first dose. Therapy may begin pending test results.
• Weigh patient and obtain baseline renal function studies before therapy begins.
• Monitor renal function (output, specific gravity, urinalysis, BUN and creatinine levels, and creatinine clearance). Notify doctor of signs of decreasing renal function.
• Patient should be well hydrated while taking drug to minimize chemical irritation of the renal tubules.
• After completing I.V. infusion, flush the line with normal saline solution or dextrose 5% in water.
• Evaluate patient's hearing before and during therapy. Notify doctor if patient complains of tinnitus, vertigo, or hearing loss.
• Watch for superinfection (continued fever and other signs of new infections, especially of upper respiratory tract).
• Usual duration of therapy is 7 to 10 days. If no response in 3 to 5 days, therapy should be stopped and new specimens obtained for culture and sensitivity.
• Peak blood levels above 16 mcg/ml and trough levels (those drawn just before next dose) above 4 mcg/ml are associated with higher incidence of toxicity.
• Draw blood for peak netilmicin level 1 hour after I.M. injection and 30 minutes to 1 hour after infusion

ends; for trough levels, draw blood just before next dose.
• Netromycin is the newest aminoglycoside. Some studies show that this drug is less nephrotoxic than other drugs in its class.

streptomycin sulfate
Pregnancy Category: D

MECHANISM OF ACTION
Inhibits protein synthesis by binding directly to the 30S ribosomal subunit. Generally bactericidal.

INDICATIONS & DOSAGE
Streptococcal endocarditis—
Adults: 10 mg/kg I.M. (maximum 0.5 g) q 12 hours for 2 weeks with penicillin.
Primary and adjunctive treatment in tuberculosis—
Adults: with normal renal function, 1 g I.M. daily for 2 to 3 months, then 1 g 2 or 3 times a week. Inject deeply into upper outer quadrant of buttocks.
Children: with normal renal function, 20 mg/kg daily in divided doses injected deeply into large muscle mass. Give concurrently with other antitubercular agents, but *not* with capreomycin, and continue until sputum specimen becomes negative.
Patients with impaired renal function: initial dose is same as for those with normal renal function. Subsequent doses and frequency determined by renal function study results.
Enterococcal endocarditis—
Adults: 1 g I.M. q 12 hours for 2 weeks, then 500 mg I.M. q 12 hours for 4 weeks with penicillin.
Tularemia—
Adults: 1 to 2 g I.M. daily in divided doses injected deep into upper outer quadrant of buttocks. Continue until patient is afebrile for 5 to 7 days.

ADVERSE REACTIONS
EENT: *ototoxicity (tinnitus, vertigo,*
hearing loss).
GU: some nephrotoxicity (not nearly as frequent as with other aminoglycosides).
Local: pain, irritation, and sterile abscesses at injection site.
Skin: *exfoliative dermatitis.*
Other: *hypersensitivity* (rash, fever, urticaria, and angioneurotic edema).

INTERACTIONS
Dimenhydrinate: may mask symptoms of streptomycin-induced ototoxicity. Use together cautiously.
I.V. Loop diuretics (e.g. furosemide): increase ototoxicity. Use cautiously.
Cephalothin: increases nephrotoxicity. Use together cautiously.

NURSING CONSIDERATIONS
• Contraindicated in labyrinthine disease. Use cautiously in patients with impaired renal function and in the elderly.
• Obtain specimen for culture and sensitivity before first dose except when treating tuberculosis. Therapy may begin pending test results.
• Patient should be well hydrated while taking drug to minimize chemical irritation of the renal tubules.
• Evaluate patient's hearing before, during, and 6 months after therapy. Notify doctor if patient complains of tinnitus, roaring noises, or fullness in ears.
• Watch for superinfection (continued fever and other signs of new infections).
• Protect hands when preparing. Drug is irritating.
• Endocarditis prophylaxis is recommended for all patients with rheumatic or congenital heart disease or with prosthetic heart valve. Patients should receive prophylactic antibiotics during GI or GU procedures or surgery.
• In primary treatment of tuberculosis, streptomycin is discontinued when sputum becomes negative.

tobramycin sulfate
Nebcin♦
Pregnancy Category: D

MECHANISM OF ACTION
Inhibits protein synthesis by binding directly to the 30S ribosomal subunit. Generally bactericidal.

INDICATIONS & DOSAGE
Serious infections caused by sensitive strains of Escherichia coli, Proteus, Klebsiella, Enterobacter, Serratia, Staphylococcus aureus, Pseudomonas, Citrobacter, Providencia—
Adults and children with normal renal function: 3 mg/kg I.M. or I.V. daily divided q 8 hours. Up to 5 mg/kg I.M. or I.V. daily divided q 6 to 8 hours for life-threatening infections.
Neonates under 1 week: up to 4 mg/kg I.M. or I.V. daily divided q 12 hours. For I.V. use, dilute in 50 to 100 ml normal saline solution or dextrose 5% in water for adults and in less volume for children. Infuse over 20 to 60 minutes.
Patients with impaired renal function: initial dose is same as for those with normal renal function. Subsequent doses and frequency determined by renal function study results.

ADVERSE REACTIONS
CNS: headache, lethargy, *neuromuscular blockade*.
EENT: *ototoxicity (tinnitus, vertigo, hearing loss)*.
GU: *nephrotoxicity (cells or casts in the urine, oliguria, proteinuria, decreased creatinine clearance, increased BUN and serum creatinine levels)*.

INTERACTIONS
I.V. loop diuretics (e.g. furosemide): increase ototoxicity. Use cautiously.
Dimenhydrinate: may mask symptoms of ototoxicity. Use with caution.
Parenteral penicillins (e.g., carbenicillin and ticarcillin): tobramycin inactivation. Don't mix together in I.V.
Cephalothin: increase nephrotoxicity. Use together cautiously.
Other aminoglycosides, amphotericin B, cisplatin, methoxyflurane: increases nephrotoxicity. Use together cautiously.

NURSING CONSIDERATIONS
• Use cautiously in patients with impaired renal function and in the elderly.
• Obtain specimen for culture and sensitivity before first dose. Therapy may begin pending test results.
• Weigh patient and obtain baseline renal function studies before starting therapy.
• Usual duration of therapy is 7 to 10 days.
• Monitor renal function (output, specific gravity, urinalysis, BUN and creatinine levels, and creatinine clearance). Notify doctor of signs of decreasing renal function.
• Patient should be well hydrated while taking drug to minimize chemical irritation of the renal tubules.
• Evaluate patient's hearing before and during therapy. Notify doctor if patient complains of tinnitus, vertigo, or hearing loss.
• Watch for superinfection (continued fever and other signs of new infections).
• Peak blood levels over 12 mcg/ml and trough levels above 2 mcg/ml are associated with increased incidence of toxicity.
• Draw blood for peak tobramycin level 1 hour after I.M. injection and 30 minutes to 1 hour after infusion ends; draw blood for trough level just before next dose. Don't collect blood in a heparinized tube.
• After I.V. infusion, flush line with normal saline solution or dextrose 5% in water.

11

Penicillins

amdinocillin
amoxicillin/potassium
  clavulanate
amoxicillin trihydrate
ampicillin
ampicillin sodium
ampicillin trihydrate
azlocillin sodium
bacampicillin hydrochloride
carbenicillin disodium
carbenicillin indanyl sodium
cloxacillin sodium
cyclacillin
dicloxacillin sodium
methicillin sodium
mezlocillin sodium
nafcillin sodium
oxacillin sodium
penicillin G benzathine
penicillin G potassium
penicillin G procaine
penicillin G sodium
penicillin V
penicillin V potassium
piperacillin sodium
ticarcillin disodium
ticarcillin disodium/clavulanate
  potassium

COMBINATION PRODUCTS
POLYCILLIN-PRB: ampicillin trihydrate 3.5g and probenecid 1g per bottle.
PRINCIPEN WITH PROBENECID: ampicillin trihydrate 3.5g and probenecid
1g per 9-capsule regimen.

amdinocillin
Coactin
Pregnancy Category: B

MECHANISM OF ACTION
Binds to a minor penicillin-binding
protein (PPB 2). This prevents bacterial cell from elongating. Generally
considered bacteriostatic.

INDICATIONS & DOSAGE
*Treatment of complicated and uncom-
plicated urinary tract infections due to
susceptible strains of* E. coli, Klebsiella, *and* Enterobacter—
Adults: 10 mg/kg I.M. or I.V. q 4 to 6
hours.

ADVERSE REACTIONS
Blood: *eosinophilia; thrombocytosis.*
CNS: dizziness.
GI: diarrhea, nausea, vomiting.
Local: thrombophlebitis.
Other: *hypersensitivity (erythematous
maculopapular rash, urticaria, ana-
phylaxis),* overgrowth of nonsuscepti-
ble organisms.

INTERACTIONS
Probenecid: increases blood levels of
penicillin.

NURSING CONSIDERATIONS
• Use cautiously in patients with
other drug allergies, especially to
cephalosporins (possible cross-allergenicity).
• Obtain cultures for sensitivity tests
before first dose. Unnecessary to wait
for results before beginning therapy.

Italicized side effects are common or life-threatening.
*Liquid form contains alcohol.   **May contain tartrazine.

• Before giving, ask patient about any allergic reactions to penicillin. However, a negative history doesn't rule out future penicillin allergy.
• Amdinocillin may act synergistically with other penicillins and cephalosporins and is frequently prescribed in combination with these drugs. May be a less toxic alternative to aminoglycosides.
• Dosage should be decreased in patients with moderate-to-severe renal failure.

---

amoxicillin/potassium clavulanate
Augmentin, Clavulin♦♦
Pregnancy Category: B

MECHANISM OF ACTION
Clavulanic acid increases amoxicillin effectiveness by inactivating beta lactamases, which destroy amoxicillin.

INDICATIONS & DOSAGE
Lower respiratory infections, otitis media, sinusitis, skin and skin structure infections, and urinary tract infections caused by susceptible strains of gram-positive and gram-negative organisms—
Adults: 250 mg (based on the amoxicillin component) P.O. q 8 hours. For more severe infections, 500 mg q 8 hours.
Children: 20 to 40 mg/kg/day (based on the amoxicillin component) given in divided doses q 8 hours.

ADVERSE REACTIONS
Blood: anemia, thrombocytopenia, thrombocytopenic purpura, eosinophilia, leukopenia.
GI: nausea, vomiting, *diarrhea*.
Other: *hypersensitivity (erythematous maculopapular rash, urticaria, anaphylaxis),* overgrowth of nonsusceptible organisms.

INTERACTIONS
Probenecid: increases blood levels of penicillin.

NURSING CONSIDERATIONS
• Use cautiously in patients with other drug allergies, especially to cephalosporins (possible cross-allergenicity), and in patients with mononucleosis (high incidence of maculopapular rash). Before giving, ask patient about any allergic reactions to penicillin. However, a negative history doesn't rule out future penicillin allergy.
• Obtain cultures for sensitivity tests before first dose. Unnecessary to wait for results before beginning therapy.
• Tell patient to take drug exactly as prescribed, even after he feels better. Patient should take entire quantity prescribed.
• Give with food to prevent GI distress.
• Incidence of diarrhea is greater than with amoxicillin alone.
• Large doses may cause increased yeast growth. Report symptoms to doctor.
• With prolonged therapy, bacterial and fungal superinfection may occur, especially in elderly, debilitated, or immunosuppressed patients. Close observation is essential.
• Both the "250" and "500" tablets contain the same amount of clavulanic acid (125 mg). Therefore, two "250" tablets are not equivalent to one "500" tablet.
• Particularly useful in clinical settings with high prevalence of amoxicillin-resistant organisms.
• Give penicillins at least 1 hour before bacteriostatic antibiotics.

---

amoxicillin trihydrate
Amoxican♦♦, Amoxil♦, Apo-
Amoxi,♦♦, Larotid, Polymox♦,
Robamox, Trimox, Utimox, Wymox
Pregnancy Category: B

MECHANISM OF ACTION
Bactericidal against microorganisms
by inhibiting cell-wall synthesis during active multiplication. Bacteria resist penicillin by producing penicillinases—enzymes that convert penicillin to inactive penicilloic acid.

INDICATIONS & DOSAGE
*Systemic infections, acute and chronic
urinary tract infections caused by susceptible strains of gram-positive and
gram-negative organisms—*
Adults: 750 mg to 1.5 g P.O. daily,
divided into doses given q 8 hours.
Children: 20 to 40 mg/kg P.O. daily,
divided into doses given q 8 hours.
Uncomplicated gonorrhea—
Adults: 3 g P.O. with 1 g probenecid
given as a single dose.
*Uncomplicated urinary tract infec-
tions due to susceptible organisms—*
Adults: 3 g P.O. given as a single
dose.

ADVERSE REACTIONS
Blood: anemia, thrombocytopenia,
thrombocytopenic purpura, eosinophilia, leukopenia.
GI: *nausea,* vomiting, *diarrhea.*
Other: *hypersensitivity (erythematous
maculopapular rash, urticaria, anaphylaxis),* overgrowth of nonsusceptible organisms.

INTERACTIONS
Probenecid: increases blood levels of
penicillin. Probenecid is often used
for this purpose.

NURSING CONSIDERATIONS
• Use cautiously in patients with
other drug allergies, especially to
cephalosporins (possible cross-allergenicity), and in patients with mononucleosis—high incidence of maculopapular rash in those receiving amoxicillin.
• Obtain cultures for sensitivity tests
before first dose. Unnecessary to wait
for results before beginning therapy.
• Before giving amoxicillin, ask patient if he's had any allergic reactions
to penicillin. However, a negative history of penicillin allergy is no guarantee against a future allergic reaction.
• Tell patient to take medication exactly as prescribed, even after he feels
better. Entire quantity prescribed
should be taken.
• Give with food to prevent GI distress.
• Large doses may cause increased
yeast growths. Report symptoms to
doctor.
• With prolonged therapy, bacterial
and fungal superinfection may occur,
especially in the elderly, debilitated,
or those with low resistance to infection due to immunosuppressives or irradiation. Close observation essential.
• Check expiration date. Warn patient
never to use leftover penicillin for a
new illness or to share penicillin with
family and friends.
• Trimox oral suspension may be
stored at room temperature for up to 2
weeks. Be sure to check individual
product labels for storage information.
• Tell patient to call the doctor if
rash, fever, or chills develop. A rash
is the most common allergic reaction.
The rash is most common if the patient is also taking allopurinol.
• Amoxicillin and ampicillin have
similar clinical applications.
• Urine glucose determinations may
be false-positive with copper sulfate
tests (Clinitest); glucose enzymatic
tests (Clinistix, Tes-Tape) are not affected.
• Give penicillins at least 1 hour before bacteriostatic antibiotics.

Italicized side effects are common or life-threatening.
*Liquid form contains alcohol.   **May contain tartrazine.

ampicillin
Amcap, Amcill, Ampicin♦♦,
Ampilean♦♦, D-Amp,
Novoampicillin♦♦, Penbritin♦♦,
Pfizerpen A, Principen,
Roampicillin

ampicillin sodium
Omnipen-N♦, Pen A/N, Polycillin-N,
Totacillin-N

ampicillin trihydrate
Omnipen
Pregnancy Category: B

MECHANISM OF ACTION
Bactericidal against microorganisms
by inhibiting cell-wall synthesis during active multiplication. Bacteria resist penicillin by producing penicillinases—enzymes that convert penicillin to inactive penicilloic acid.

INDICATIONS & DOSAGE
*Systemic infections, acute and chronic
urinary tract infections caused by susceptible strains of gram-positive and
gram-negative organisms—*
Adults: 1 to 4 g P.O. daily, divided
into doses given q 6 hours; 2 to 12 g
I.M. or I.V. daily, divided into doses
given q 4 to 6 hours.
Children: 50 to 100 mg/kg P.O.
daily, divided into doses given q 6
hours; or 100 to 200 mg/kg I.M. or
I.V. daily, divided into doses given q 6
hours.
Meningitis—
Adults: 8 to 14 g I.V. daily for 3 days,
then I.M. divided q 3 to 4 hours.
Children: up to 300 mg/kg I.V. daily
for 3 days, then I.M. divided q 4
hours.
Uncomplicated gonorrhea—
Adults: 3.5 g P.O. with 1 g probenecid given as a single dose.

ADVERSE REACTIONS
Blood: anemia, thrombocytopenia,
thrombocytopenic purpura, eosinophilia, leukopenia.
GI: *nausea,* vomiting, *diarrhea,* glossitis, stomatitis.
Local: pain at injection site, vein irritation, thrombophlebitis.
Other: *hypersensitivity (erythematous
maculopapular rash, urticaria, anaphylaxis), overgrowth of nonsusceptible organisms.*

INTERACTIONS
Probenecid: increases blood levels of
penicillin. Probenecid is often used
for this purpose.

NURSING CONSIDERATIONS
• Use cautiously in patients with
other drug allergies, especially to
cephalosporins (possible cross-allergenicity), and in patients with mononucleosis—high incidence of maculopapular rash in those receiving ampicillin.
• Obtain cultures for sensitivity tests
before first dose. Unnecessary to wait
for results before beginning therapy.
• Before giving ampicillin, ask patient if he's had any allergic reactions
to penicillin. However, a negative history of penicillin allergy is no guarantee against a future allergic reaction.
• Tell patient to take medication exactly as prescribed, even after he feels
better. Entire quantity prescribed
should be taken.
• Tell the patient to call the doctor if
rash, fever, or chills develop. A rash
is the most common allergic reaction.
Rash is most common if the patient is
also taking allopurinol.
• When given orally, drug may cause
GI disturbances. Food may interfere
with absorption, so give 1 to 2 hours
before meals or 2 to 3 hours after.
• Don't give I.M. or I.V. unless infection is severe or patient can't take oral
dose.
• Dosage should be altered in patients
with impaired renal functions.
• When giving I.V., mix with dextrose 5% in water or a saline solution.

Don't mix with other drugs or solutions: they might be incompatible.
• Give I.V. intermittently to prevent vein irritation. Change site every 48 hours.
• Large doses may cause increased yeast growths. Report symptoms to doctor.
• With prolonged therapy, bacterial or fungal superinfection may occur, especially in the elderly, debilitated, or those with low resistance to infection due to immunosuppressives or irradiation. Close observation is essential.
• Check expiration date. Warn patient never to use leftover penicillin for a new illness or to share penicillin with family and friends.
• Initial dilution in vial is stable for 1 hour. Follow manufacturer's direction for stability data when ampicillin is further diluted for I.V. infusion.
• In pediatric meningitis, may be given concurrently with parenteral chloramphenicol for 24 hours pending cultures.
• Urine glucose determinations may be false-positive with copper sulfate tests (Clinitest); glucose enzymatic tests (Clinistix, Tes-Tape) are not affected.
• Give penicillins at least 1 hour before bacteriostatic antibiotics.

azlocillin sodium
Azlin
Pregnancy Category: B

MECHANISM OF ACTION
Bactericidal against microorganisms by inhibiting cell-wall synthesis during active multiplication. Bacteria resist penicillin by producing penicillinases—enzymes that convert penicillin to inactive penicilloic acid.

INDICATIONS & DOSAGE
Serious infections caused by susceptible strains of Pseudomonas aeruginosa—
Adults: 200 to 350 mg/kg daily I.V. given in 4 to 6 divided doses. Usual dose is 3 g q 4 hours (18 g daily). Maximum daily dosage is 24 g. May be administered by I.V. intermittent infusion or by direct slow I.V. injection.
Children with acute exacerbation of cystic fibrosis: 75 mg/kg q 4 hours (450 mg/kg daily). Maximum daily dosage is 24 g.
Azlocillin shouldn't be used in neonates.

ADVERSE REACTIONS
Blood: *bleeding with high doses,* neutropenia, eosinophilia, leukopenia, *thrombocytopenia.*
CNS: neuromuscular irritability, headache, dizziness.
GI: nausea, diarrhea.
Local: pain at injection site, vein irritation, phlebitis.
Metabolic: *hypokalemia.*
Other: *hypersensitivity (edema, fever, chills, rash, pruritus, urticaria, anaphylaxis), overgrowth of nonsusceptible organisms.*

INTERACTIONS
Aminoglycoside antibiotics (e.g., gentamicin, tobramycin): chemically incompatible. Don't mix together in I.V. solution.

NURSING CONSIDERATIONS
• Use cautiously in patients hypersensitive to drugs, especially to cephalosporins (possible cross-allergenicity), and in those with bleeding tendencies, uremia, or hypokalemia.
• Obtain cultures for sensitivity tests before starting therapy. Unnecessary to wait for results before starting therapy.
• Before giving azlocillin, ask patient if he's had allergic reactions to penicillin. A negative history of penicillin allergy, however, is no guarantee against future allergic reactions.

Italicized side effects are common or life-threatening.
*Liquid form contains alcohol.   **May contain tartrazine.

- Dosage should be altered in patients with impaired renal functions.
- Check CBC frequently. Drug may cause thrombocytopenia.
- Monitor serum potassium level.
- Patient with high serum level of this drug may have convulsions. Take seizure precautions.
- When giving I.V., mix with dextrose 5% in water or other suitable I.V. fluids.
- Give I.V. intermittently to prevent vein irritation. Change site every 48 hours.
- Rapid administration may cause chest discomfort. Don't infuse over a period of less than 5 minutes.
- Almost always used with another antibiotic, such as gentamicin.
- With prolonged therapy, superinfections may occur, especially in the elderly or debilitated, or in those patients with low resistance to infection due to immunosuppressors or irradiation. Monitor patient closely.
- Check drug expiration date.
- Azlocillin is less likely to cause hypokalemia than similar antibiotics, such as carbenicillin and ticarcillin.
- Drug may be better suited to patients on salt-free diets than carbenicillin and ticarcillin (contains 2.17 mEq Na⁺/g of azlocillin).
- Give penicillins at least 1 hour before bacteriostatic antibiotics.

bacampicillin hydrochloride
Penglobe♦♦, Spectrobid
Pregnancy Category: B

MECHANISM OF ACTION
Bactericidal against microorganisms by inhibiting cell-wall synthesis during active multiplication. Bacteria resist penicillin by producing penicillinases—enzymes that convert penicillin to inactive penicilloic acid.

INDICATIONS & DOSAGE
Upper and lower respiratory tract infections due to streptococci, pneumococci, staphylococci, and Hemophilus influenzae; *urinary tract infections due to* Escherichia coli, Proteus mirabilis, *and* Streptococcus faecalis; *skin infections due to streptococci and susceptible staphylococci—*
Adults and children weighing more than 25 kg: 400 to 800 mg P.O. q 12 hours.
Gonorrhea—
Usual dosage is 1.6 g plus 1 g probenecid given as a single dose.
Not recommended for children under 25 kg.

ADVERSE REACTIONS
Blood: anemia, thrombocytopenia, thrombocytopenic purpura, eosinophilia, leukopenia.
GI: *nausea,* vomiting, *diarrhea,* glossitis, stomatitis.
Other: *hypersensitivity (erythematous maculopapular rash, urticaria, anaphylaxis),* overgrowth of nonsusceptible organisms.

INTERACTIONS
Probenecid: increases blood levels of bacampicillin or other penicillins. Probenecid is often used for this purpose.

NURSING CONSIDERATIONS
- Use cautiously in patients with other drug allergies, especially to cephalosporins (possible cross-allergenicity), and in patients with mononucleosis. This drug, like ampicillin, is linked to a high incidence of maculopapular rash.
- Obtain cultures for sensitivity tests before first dose. Unnecessary to wait for results before beginning therapy.
- Before giving bacampicillin, ask patient if he's had any previous allergic reactions to penicillin. However, a negative history of penicillin allergy is no guarantee against a future allergic reaction.
- Bacampicillin is especially formu-

lated to produce high blood levels of antibiotic when administered twice daily.

• Diarrhea may occur less frequently with bacampicillin than with ampicillin.

• Tell patient to take medication even after he feels better. Entire quantity prescribed should be taken.

• Tell patient to call the doctor if rash, fever, or chills develop. A rash is the most common allergic reaction.

• With prolonged therapy, bacterial or fungal superinfection may occur, especially in the elderly or the debilitated, and in those with low resistance to infection due to immunosuppressors or irradiation. Close observation is essential.

• Check expiration date. Warn patient never to use leftover penicillin products for a new illness or to share penicillin with family and friends.

• Unlike ampicillin, bacampicillin tablets may be taken with meals without fear of diminished drug absorption. Give with food to prevent GI distress. However, bacampicillin suspension should be taken on an empty stomach.

• Administer penicillins at least 1 hour before bacteriostatic antibiotics.

---

carbenicillin disodium
Geopen♦, Pyopen♦
Pregnancy Category: B

MECHANISM OF ACTION
Bactericidal against microorganisms by inhibiting cell-wall synthesis during active multiplication. Bacteria resist penicillin by producing penicillinases—enzymes that convert penicillin to inactive penicilloic acid.

INDICATIONS & DOSAGE
Systemic infections caused by susceptible strains of gram-positive and especially gram-negative organisms (Proteus, Pseudomonas aeruginosa)—

Adults: 30 to 40 g daily I.V. infusion, divided into doses given q 4 to 6 hours.
Children: 300 to 500 mg/kg daily I.V. infusion, divided into doses given q 4 to 6 hours.
Urinary tract infections—
Adults: 200 mg/kg daily I.M. or I.V. infusion, divided into doses given q 4 to 6 hours.
Children: 50 to 200 mg/kg daily I.M. or I.V. infusion, divided into doses given q 4 to 6 hours.

ADVERSE REACTIONS
Blood: *bleeding with high doses,* neutropenia, eosinophilia, leukopenia, *thrombocytopenia.*
CNS: neuromuscular irritability.
GI: nausea.
Local: pain at injection site, vein irritation, phlebitis.
Metabolic: *hypokalemia.*
Other: *hypersensitivity (edema, fever, chills, rash, pruritus, urticaria, anaphylaxis),* overgrowth of nonsusceptible organisms.

INTERACTIONS
Probenecid: increases blood levels of penicillin. Probenecid is often used for this purpose.
Aminoglycoside antibiotics (e.g., gentamicin, tobramycin): chemically incompatible. Don't mix together in I.V.

NURSING CONSIDERATIONS
• Use cautiously in patients with other drug allergies, especially to cephalosporins (possible cross-allergenicity), and in those with bleeding tendencies, uremia, hypokalemia. Use cautiously in patients on sodium-restricted diets; contains 4.7 mEq sodium/g.

• Obtain cultures for sensitivity tests before first dose. Unnecessary to wait for test results before beginning therapy.

• Before giving carbenicillin, ask patient if he's had any allergic reactions

---

Italicized side effects are common or life-threatening.
*Liquid form contains alcohol.   **May contain tartrazine.

to penicillin. However, a negative history of penicillin allergy is no guarantee against a future allergic reaction.
• Dosage should be altered in patients with impaired renal function. Patients with impaired renal function are susceptible to nephrotoxicity. Monitor intake and output.
• Check CBC frequently. Drug may cause thrombocytopenia.
• Monitor serum potassium. Patients may develop hypokalemia due to large amount of sodium in the preparation.
• If patient has high blood level of this drug, he may have convulsions. Be prepared by keeping side rails up on bed.
• When giving I.V., mix with dextrose 5% in water or other suitable I.V. fluids.
• Give I.V. intermittently to prevent vein irritation. Change site every 48 hours.
• Almost always used with another antibiotic, such as gentamicin.
• Large doses may cause increased yeast growths. Report symptoms to doctor.
• With prolonged therapy, other superinfections may occur, especially in the elderly, debilitated, or those with low resistance to infection due to immunosuppressives or irradiation. Close observation is essential.
• Check expiration date; do not use any penicillin that is outdated.
• Give penicillins at least 1 hour before bacteriostatic antibiotics.

---

carbenicillin indanyl sodium
Geocillin, Geopen Oral♦♦
Pregnancy Category: B

MECHANISM OF ACTION
Bactericidal against microorganisms by inhibiting cell-wall synthesis during active multiplication. Bacteria resist penicillin by producing penicillinases—enzymes that convert penicil-

lin to inactive penicilloic acid.

INDICATIONS & DOSAGE
Urinary tract infection and prostatitis caused by susceptible strains of gram-negative organisms—
Adults: 382 to 764 mg P.O. q.i.d. Not recommended for children.

ADVERSE REACTIONS
Blood: leukopenia, neutropenia, eosinophilia, anemia, thrombocytopenia.
GI: *nausea,* vomiting, *diarrhea, flatulence, abdominal cramps, unpleasant taste.*
Other: *hypersensitivity (rash, chills, fever, urticaria, pruritus, anaphylaxis),* overgrowth of nonsusceptible organisms.

INTERACTIONS
None significant.

NURSING CONSIDERATIONS
• Use cautiously in patients with other drug allergies, especially to cephalosporins (possible cross-allergenicity).
• Obtain cultures for sensitivity tests before first dose. Unnecessary to wait for test results before starting therapy.
• Before giving carbenicillin, ask patient if he's had any allergic reactions to penicillin. However, a negative history of penicillin allergy is no guarantee against a future allergic reaction.
• Tell patient to take medication exactly as prescribed, even after he feels better. Entire quantity prescribed should be taken.
• Tell patient to call the doctor if he develops rash, fever, or chills. A rash is the most common allergic reaction.
• When given orally, drug may cause GI disturbances. Food may interfere with absorption, so give 1 to 2 hours before meals or 2 to 3 hours after.
• Large doses may cause increased yeast growths. Report symptoms to doctor.

• With prolonged therapy, other superinfections may occur, especially in the elderly, debilitated, or those with low resistance to infection due to immunosuppressives or irradiation. Close observation is essential.

• Check expiration date. Warn patient never to use leftover penicillin for a new illness or to share penicillin with family and friends.

• Use only in patients whose creatinine clearance is 10 ml/minute or more.

• Excellent treatment for *Pseudomonas* urinary tract infections in ambulatory patients.

• May be useful in treatment of cystitis, but not pyelonephritis.

• Not effective for any systemic infection because blood levels are nil.

---

cloxacillin sodium
Apo Cloxi♦♦, Bactopen♦♦,
Cloxapen, Novocloxin♦♦,
Orbenin♦♦, Tegopen♦
Pregnancy Category: B

MECHANISM OF ACTION
Bactericidal against microorganisms by inhibiting cell-wall synthesis during active multiplication. Bacteria resist penicillin by producing penicillinases—enzymes that convert penicillin to inactive penicilloic acid. Cloxacillin resists these enzymes.

INDICATIONS & DOSAGE
Systemic infections caused by penicillinase-producing staphylococci—
Adults: 2 to 4 g P.O. daily, divided into doses given q 6 hours.
Children: 50 to 100 mg/kg P.O. daily, divided into doses given q 6 hours.

ADVERSE REACTIONS
Blood: eosinophilia.
GI: *nausea,* vomiting, *epigastric distress, diarrhea.*
Other: *hypersensitivity (rash, urti-*caria, chills, fever, sneezing, wheezing, anaphylaxis),* overgrowth of nonsusceptible organisms.

INTERACTIONS
Probenecid: increases blood levels of penicillin. Probenecid is often used for this purpose.

NURSING CONSIDERATIONS
• Use with caution in patients with other drug allergies, especially to cephalosporins (possible cross-allergenicity).

• Obtain cultures for sensitivity tests before first dose. Unnecessary to wait for test results before starting therapy.

• Before giving cloxacillin, ask patient if he's had any allergic reactions to penicillin. However, a negative history of penicillin allergy is no guarantee against a future allergic reaction.

• Tell patient to take medication exactly as prescribed, even if he feels better. Entire quantity prescribed should be taken.

• Tell patient to call the doctor if rash, fever, or chills develop. A rash is the most common allergic reaction.

• When given orally, drug may cause GI disturbances. Food may interfere with absorption, so give 1 to 2 hours before meals or 2 to 3 hours after.

• Patient should take each dose with a full glass of water, not fruit juice or carbonated beverage, because acid will inactivate the drug.

• With prolonged therapy, other superinfections may occur, especially in the elderly, debilitated, or those with low resistance to infection due to immunosuppressives or irradiation. Close observation is essential.

• Check expiration date. Warn patient never to use leftover penicillin for a new illness or to share penicillin with family and friends.

• Give penicillins at least 1 hour before bacteriostatic antibiotics.

Italicized side effects are common or life-threatening.
*Liquid form contains alcohol.   **May contain tartrazine.

cyclacillin
Cyclapen-W
Pregnancy Category: B

MECHANISM OF ACTION
Bactericidal against microorganisms by inhibiting cell-wall synthesis during active multiplication. Bacteria resist penicillin by producing penicillinases—enzymes that convert penicillin to inactive penicilloic acid.

INDICATIONS & DOSAGE
Systemic and urinary tract infections caused by susceptible strains of gram-positive and gram-negative organisms—
Adults: 250 to 500 mg P.O. q.i.d. in equally spaced doses.
Children: 50 to 100 mg/kg daily t.i.d. in equally divided doses.

ADVERSE REACTIONS
Blood: anemia, thrombocytopenia, thrombocytopenic purpura, leukopenia, neutropenia, eosinophilia.
GI: *nausea*, vomiting, diarrhea.
Other: *hypersensitivity (edema, fever, chills, rash, pruritus, urticaria, anaphylaxis)*, overgrowth of nonsusceptible organisms.

INTERACTIONS
Probenecid: increases blood levels of penicillin. Probenecid is often used for this purpose.

NURSING CONSIDERATIONS
• Contraindicated in patients allergic to other penicillins.
• Obtain cultures for sensitivity tests before first dose. Unnecessary to wait for test results before starting therapy.
• Before giving cyclacillin, ask patient if he's had any allergic reactions to penicillin. However, a negative history of penicillin allergy is no guarantee against a future allergic reaction.
• Tell patient he must take all medication exactly as prescribed, for as long as ordered, even after he feels better.
• Patients with renal insufficiency should receive less drug in accordance with their creatinine clearance level.
• Large doses of penicillin may cause increased yeast growths. Watch for signs and symptoms, and report to doctor.
• With prolonged therapy, bacterial and fungal superinfection may occur, especially in the elderly, debilitated, or those with low resistance to infection due to immunosuppressives or irradiation. Close observation is essential.
• Check expiration date before giving this drug. Warn patient never to use leftover penicillin for a new illness or to share his penicillin with family and friends.
• Tell patient to call the doctor if he develops rash, fever, or chills. A rash is the most common allergic reaction.
• Studies show that cyclacillin is as effective as amoxicillin in treating acute otitis media and causes less diarrhea.
• Give penicillins at least 1 hour before bacteriostatic antibiotics.

dicloxacillin sodium
Dycill, Dynapen♦, Pathocil
Pregnancy Category: B

MECHANISM OF ACTION
Bactericidal against microorganisms by inhibiting cell-wall synthesis during active multiplication. Bacteria resist penicillin by producing penicillinases—enzymes that convert penicillin to inactive penicilloic acid. Dicloxacillin resists these enzymes.

INDICATIONS & DOSAGE
Systemic infections caused by penicillinase-producing staphylococci—
Adults: 1 to 2 g daily P.O., divided into doses given q 6 hours.
Children: 25 to 50 mg/kg P.O. daily, divided into doses given q 6 hours.

ADVERSE REACTIONS
Blood: eosinophilia.
GI: *nausea,* vomiting, *epigastric distress,* flatulence, *diarrhea.*
Other: *hypersensitivity (pruritus, urticaria, rash, anaphylaxis),* overgrowth of nonsusceptible organisms.

INTERACTIONS
Probenecid: increases blood levels of penicillin. Probenecid is often used for this purpose.

NURSING CONSIDERATIONS
• Use cautiously in patients allergic to cephalosporins (possible cross-allergenicity).
• Obtain cultures for sensitivity tests before first dose. Unnecessary to wait for test results before starting therapy.
• Before giving dicloxacillin, ask patient if he's had any allergic reactions to penicillin. However, a negative history of penicillin allergy is no guarantee against a future allergic reaction.
• Tell patient to take medication exactly as prescribed, even if he feels better. Entire quantity prescribed should be taken.
• Tell patient to call the doctor if rash, fever, or chills develop. A rash is the most common allergic reaction.
• Drug may cause GI disturbances. Food may interfere with absorption, so give 1 to 2 hours before meals or 2 to 3 hours after.
• With prolonged therapy, other superinfections may occur, especially in the elderly, debilitated, or those with low resistance to infection due to immunosuppressives or irradiation. Close observation is essential.
• Periodic assessments of renal, hepatic, and hematopoietic function should be made when therapy is prolonged.
• Check expiration date. Warn patient never to use leftover penicillin for a new illness or to share penicillin with family and friends.
• Give penicillins at least 1 hour be-

fore bacteriostatic antibiotics.

---

methicillin sodium
Staphcillin♦
Pregnancy Category: B

MECHANISM OF ACTION
Bactericidal against microorganisms by inhibiting cell-wall synthesis during active multiplication. Bacteria resist penicillin by producing penicillinases—enzymes that convert penicillin to inactive penicilloic acid. Methicillin resists these enzymes.

INDICATIONS & DOSAGE
Systemic infections caused by penicillinase-producing staphylococci—
Adults: 4 to 12 g I.M. or I.V. daily, divided into doses given q 4 to 6 hours.
Children: 100 to 200 mg/kg I.M. or I.V. daily, divided into doses given q 4 to 6 hours.

ADVERSE REACTIONS
Blood: *eosinophilia,* hemolytic anemia, transient neutropenia.
CNS: neuropathy, convulsions with high doses.
GI: glossitis, stomatitis.
GU: interstitial nephritis.
Local: *vein irritation, thrombophlebitis.*
Other: *hypersensitivity (chills, fever, edema, rash, urticaria, anaphylaxis),* overgrowth of nonsusceptible organisms.

INTERACTIONS
Probenecid: increases blood levels of penicillin. Probenecid is often used for this purpose.

NURSING CONSIDERATIONS
• Use cautiously in patients with other drug allergies, especially to cephalosporins (possible cross-allergenicity), and in infants.
• Obtain cultures for sensitivity tests

before first dose. Unnecessary to wait for test results before starting therapy. Methicillin-resistant strains of Staphylococci should be treated with vancomycin.

• Before giving methicillin, ask patient if he's had any allergic reactions to penicillin. However, a negative history of penicillin allergy is no guarantee against a future allergic reaction.

• If ordered 4 times a day, be sure to give every 6 hours—even during the night.

• Urinalysis should be done frequently to monitor renal function.

• If patient has high blood level of this drug, he may have convulsions. Be prepared by keeping side rails up on bed.

• When giving I.V., mix with a normal saline solution. Don't mix with others because methicillin may be inactivated. Initial dilution must be made with sterile water for injection.

• Give I.V. intermittently to prevent vein irritation. Change site every 48 hours.

• With prolonged therapy, other superinfections may occur, especially in the elderly, debilitated, or those with low resistance to infection due to immunosuppressives or irradiation. Close observation is essential.

• Periodic assessment of hepatic, renal, and hematopoietic function is required during prolonged therapy.

• Check expiration date.

• Give penicillins at least 1 hour before bacteriostatic antibiotics.

mezlocillin sodium
Mezlin
Pregnancy Category: B

MECHANISM OF ACTION
Bactericidal against microorganisms by inhibiting cell-wall synthesis during active multiplication. Bacteria resist penicillin by producing penicillinases—enzymes that convert penicil-

lin to inactive penicilloic acid.

INDICATIONS & DOSAGE
Systemic infections caused by susceptible strains of gram-positive and especially gram-negative organisms (Proteus, Pseudomonas aeruginosa)—
Adults: 200 to 300 mg/kg daily I.V. or I.M. given in 4 to 6 divided doses. Usual dose is 3 g q 4 hours or 4 g q 6 hours. For very serious infections, up to 24 g daily may be administered.
Children to age 12: 50 mg/kg q 4 hours by I.V. infusion or direct I.V. injection.

ADVERSE REACTIONS
Blood: *bleeding with high doses,* neutropenia, eosinophilia, leukopenia, *thrombocytopenia.*
CNS: neuromuscular irritability.
GI: nausea, diarrhea.
Local: pain at injection site, vein irritation, phlebitis.
Metabolic: *hypokalemia.*
Other: *hypersensitivity (edema, fever, chills, rash, pruritus, urticaria, anaphylaxis), overgrowth of nonsusceptible organisms.*

INTERACTIONS
Aminoglycoside antibiotics (e.g., gentamicin, tobramycin): chemically incompatible. Don't mix together in I.V. solution. Give 1 hour apart, especially in patients with renal insufficiency.

NURSING CONSIDERATIONS
• Use cautiously in patients hypersensitive to drugs, especially to cephalosporins (possible cross-hypersensitivity), and those with bleeding tendencies, uremia, hypokalemia.

• Obtain cultures for sensitivity tests before starting therapy. Unnecessary to wait for culture and sensitivity results before starting therapy.

• Before giving mezlocillin, ask patient if he's had allergic reactions to penicillin. A negative history of penicillin allergy, however, is no guaran-

tee against future allergic reaction.
• Dosage should be altered in patients with impaired renal function.
• Check CBC frequently. Drug may cause thrombocytopenia.
• Monitor serum potassium level.
• Patient with high serum level of this drug may have convulsions. Take seizure precautions.
• When giving I.V., mix with dextrose 5% in water or other suitable I.V. fluids.
• Give I.V. intermittently to prevent vein irritation. Change site every 48 hours.
• Almost always used with another antibiotic, such as gentamicin.
• With prolonged therapy, superinfections may occur, especially in the elderly or debilitated, or those with low resistance to infection due to immunosuppressors or irradiation. Monitor patient closely.
• Check drug expiration date.
• Compared with similar antibiotics such as carbenicillin and ticarcillin, mezlocillin is less likely to cause hypokalemia.
• Drug may be better suited to patients on salt-free diets than carbenicillin and ticarcillin (contains 1.85 mEq Na/g of mezlocillin).
• Give penicillins at least 1 hour before bacteriostatic antibiotics.

nafcillin sodium
Nafcil, Nallpen, Unipen♦
Pregnancy Category: B

MECHANISM OF ACTION
Bactericidal against microorganisms by inhibiting cell-wall synthesis during active multiplication. Bacteria resist penicillin by producing penicillinases—enzymes that convert penicillin to inactive penicilloic acid.

INDICATIONS & DOSAGE
Systemic infections caused by penicillinase-producing staphylococci—

Adults: 2 to 4 g P.O. daily, divided into doses given q 6 hours; 2 to 12 g I.M. or I.V. daily, divided into doses given q 4 to 6 hours.
Children: 50 to 100 mg/kg P.O. daily, divided into doses given q 4 to 6 hours; or 100 to 200 mg/kg I.M. or I.V. daily, divided into doses given q 4 to 6 hours.

ADVERSE REACTIONS
Blood: transient leukopenia, neutropenia, granulocytopenia, thrombocytopenia with high doses.
GI: *nausea,* vomiting, diarrhea.
Local: *vein irritation, thrombophlebitis.*
Other: *hypersensitivity (chills, fever, rash, pruritus, urticaria, anaphylaxis).*

INTERACTIONS
Probenecid: increases blood levels of penicillin. Probenecid is often used for this purpose.

NURSING CONSIDERATIONS
• Use cautiously in patients with other drug allergies, especially to cephalosporins (possible cross-allergenicity), and in those with gastrointestinal distress.
• Obtain cultures for sensitivity tests before first dose. Unnecessary to wait for test results before starting therapy.
• Before giving nafcillin, ask patient if he's had any allergic reactions to penicillin. However, a negative history of penicillin allergy is no guarantee against a future allergic reaction.
• Tell patient to take medication exactly as prescribed, even if he feels better. Entire quantity prescribed should be taken.
• Tell patient to call the doctor if rash, fever, or chills develop. A rash is the most common allergic reaction.
• When given orally, drug may cause GI disturbances. Food may interfere with absorption, so give 1 to 2 hours before meals or 2 to 3 hours after.

- When giving I.V., mix with dextrose 5% in water or a saline solution.
- Give I.V. intermittently to prevent vein irritation. Change site every 48 hours.
- With prolonged therapy, other superinfections may occur, especially in the elderly, debilitated, or those with low resistance to infection due to immunosuppressives or irradiation. Close observation is essential.
- Check expiration date.
- Give penicillins at least 1 hour before bacteriostatic antibiotics.

oxacillin sodium
Bactocill, Prostaphlin♦
Pregnancy Category: B

MECHANISM OF ACTION
Bactericidal against microorganisms by inhibiting cell-wall synthesis during active multiplication. Bacteria resist penicillin by producing penicillinases—enzymes that convert penicillin to inactive penicilloic acid. Oxacillin resists these enzymes.

INDICATIONS & DOSAGE
Systemic infections caused by penicillinase-producing staphylococci—
Adults: 2 to 4 g P.O. daily, divided into doses given q 6 hours; 2 to 12 g I.M. or I.V. daily, divided into doses given q 4 to 6 hours.
Children: 50 to 100 mg/kg P.O. daily, divided into doses given q 6 hours; 100 to 200 mg/kg I.M. or I.V. daily, divided into doses given q 4 to 6 hours.

ADVERSE REACTIONS
Blood: granulocytopenia, thrombocytopenia, eosinophilia, hemolytic anemia, transient neutropenia.
CNS: neuropathy.
GI: oral lesions.
GU: interstitial nephritis, transient hematuria, proteinuria.
Hepatic: hepatitis, elevated enzymes.

Local: *thrombophlebitis.*
Other: *hypersensitivity (fever, chills, rash, urticaria, anaphylaxis),* overgrowth of nonsusceptible organisms.

INTERACTIONS
Probenecid: increases blood levels of penicillin. Probenecid is often used for this purpose.

NURSING CONSIDERATIONS
- Use cautiously in patients with other drug allergies, especially to cephalosporins (possible cross-allergenicity), in premature newborns, and in infants.
- Obtain cultures for sensitivity tests before first dose. Unnecessary to wait for test results before starting therapy.
- Before giving oxacillin, ask patient if he's had any allergic reactions to penicillin. However, a negative history of penicillin allergy is no guarantee against a future allergic reaction.
- Tell the patient to take medication exactly as prescribed, even if he feels better. The entire quantity prescribed should be taken.
- Tell patient to call the doctor if rash, fever, or chills develop. A rash is the most common allergic reaction.
- When given orally, drug may cause GI disturbances. Food may interfere with absorption, so give 1 to 2 hours before meals or 2 to 3 hours after.
- Don't give I.M. or I.V. unless infection is severe or patient can't take oral dose.
- Periodic liver function studies are indicated; watch for elevated SGOT and SGPT.
- When giving I.V., mix with dextrose 5% in water or a saline solution.
- Give I.V. intermittently to prevent vein irritation. Change site every 48 hours.
- With prolonged therapy, other superinfections may occur, especially in the elderly, debilitated, or those with low resistance to infection due to immunosuppressives or irradiation.

Close observation is essential.
- Check expiration date.
- Give penicillins at least 1 hour before bacteriostatic antibiotics.

penicillin G benzathine
Bicillin L-A♦, Megacillin
Suspension♦, Permapen
Pregnancy Category: B

MECHANISM OF ACTION
Bactericidal against microorganisms by inhibiting cell-wall synthesis during active multiplication. Bacteria resist penicillin by producing penicillinases—enzymes that convert penicillin to inactive penicilloic acid.

INDICATIONS & DOSAGE
Congenital syphilis—
Children under age 2: 50,000 units/kg I.M. as a single dose.
Group A streptococcal upper respiratory infections—
Adults: 1.2 million units I.M. in a single injection.
Children over 27 kg: 900,000 units I.M. in a single injection.
Children under 27 kg: 300,000 to 600,000 units I.M. in a single injection.
Prophylaxis of poststreptococcal rheumatic fever—
Adults and children: 1.2 million units I.M. once a month or 600,000 units twice a month.
Syphilis of less than 1 year's duration—
Adults: 2.4 million units I.M. in a single dose.
Syphilis of more than 1 year's duration—
Adults: 2.4 million units I.M. weekly for 3 successive weeks.

ADVERSE REACTIONS
Blood: eosinophilia, hemolytic anemia, thrombocytopenia, leukopenia.
CNS: neuropathy, convulsions with high doses.

Local: pain and sterile abscess at injection site.
Other: *hypersensitivity (maculopapular and exfoliative dermatitis, chills, fever, edema, anaphylaxis).*

INTERACTIONS
Probenecid: increases blood levels of penicillin. Probenecid is often used for this purpose.

NURSING CONSIDERATIONS
- Use cautiously in patients with other drug allergies, especially to cephalosporins (possible cross-allergenicity).
- Obtain cultures for sensitivity tests before first dose. Unnecessary to wait for test results before beginning therapy.
- Before giving penicillin, ask patient if he's had any allergic reactions to this drug. However, a negative history of penicillin allergy is no guarantee against a future allergic reaction.
- Tell patient to call the doctor if rash, fever, or chills develop. Fever and eosinophilia are the most common allergic reactions.
- Shake medication well before injection.
- Never give I.V.—inadvertent I.V. administration has caused cardiac arrest and death.
- Very slow absorption time makes allergic reactions difficult to treat.
- Inject deeply into upper outer quadrant of buttocks in adults; in midlateral thigh in infants and small children.
- Check expiration date.
- Give penicillins at least 1 hour before bacteriostatic antibiotics.

Italicized side effects are common or life-threatening.
*Liquid form contains alcohol.   **May contain tartrazine.

penicillin G potassium

Biotic-T, Cryspen, Deltapen,
Falapen♦♦, Lanacillin,
Megacillin♦♦, P-50♦♦, Parcillin,
Pensorb, Pentids**, Pfizerpen
Pregnancy Category: B

MECHANISM OF ACTION

Bactericidal against microorganisms by inhibiting cell-wall synthesis during active multiplication. Bacteria resist penicillin by producing penicillinases—enzymes that convert penicillin to inactive penicilloic acid.

INDICATIONS & DOSAGE

Moderate to severe systemic infections—
Adults: 1.6 to 3.2 million units P.O. daily, divided into doses given q 6 hours (1 mg = 1,600 units); 1.2 to 24 million units I.M. or I.V. daily, divided into doses given q 4 hours.
Children: 25,000 to 100,000 units/kg P.O. daily, divided into doses given q 6 hours; or 25,000 to 300,000 units/kg I.M. or I.V. daily, divided into doses given q 4 hours.

ADVERSE REACTIONS

Blood: hemolytic anemia, leukopenia, thrombocytopenia.
CNS: neuropathy, convulsions with high doses.
Metabolic: possible severe potassium poisoning with high doses (hyperreflexia, convulsions, coma).
Local: *thrombophlebitis, pain at injection site.*
Other: *hypersensitivity (rash, urticaria, maculopapular eruptions, exfoliative dermatitis, chills, fever, edema, anaphylaxis),* overgrowth of nonsusceptible organisms.

INTERACTIONS

Probenecid: increases blood levels of penicillin. Probenecid is often used for this purpose.

NURSING CONSIDERATIONS

• Use cautiously in patients with other drug allergies, especially to cephalosporins (possible cross-allergenicity).
• Obtain cultures for sensitivity tests before first dose. Unnecessary to wait for results before beginning therapy.
• Before giving penicillin, ask patient if he's had any allergic reactions to this drug. However, a negative history of penicillin allergy is no guarantee against a future allergic reaction.
• Tell patient to take medication exactly as prescribed, even if he feels better.
• Tell patient to call the doctor if rash, fever, or chills develop. A rash is the most common allergic reaction.
• When given orally, drug may cause GI disturbances. Food may interfere with absorption, so give 1 to 2 hours before meals or 2 to 3 hours after.
• Extremely painful when given I.M. Inject deep into large muscle.
• Patients with poor renal function are predisposed to high blood levels. Monitor renal function closely.
• If patient has high blood level of this drug, he may have convulsions. Be prepared by keeping side rails up on bed.
• When giving I.V., mix with dextrose 5% in water or a saline solution.
• Give I.V. intermittently to prevent vein irritation. Change site every 48 hours.
• With prolonged therapy, other superinfections may occur, especially in the elderly, debilitated, or those with low resistance to infection due to immunosuppressives or irradiation. Close observation is essential.
• Check expiration date. Warn patient never to use leftover penicillin for a new illness or to share penicillin with family and friends.
• Give penicillins at least 1 hour before bacteriostatic antibiotics.

Unmarked trade names available in the United States only.
♦ Also available in Canada.   ♦♦ Available in Canada only.

penicillin G procaine
Ayercillin♦♦, Crysticillin A.S.,
Duracillin A.S., Pfizerpen A.S.,
Wycillin♦
Pregnancy Category: B

MECHANISM OF ACTION
Bactericidal against microorganisms
by inhibiting cell-wall synthesis during active multiplication. Bacteria resist penicillin by producing penicillinases—enzymes that convert penicillin to inactive penicilloic acid.

INDICATIONS & DOSAGE
*Moderate to severe systemic infec-
tions—*
Adults: 600,000 to 1.2 million units
I.M. daily given as a single dose.
Children: 300,000 units I.M. daily
given as a single dose.
Uncomplicated gonorrhea—
Adults and children over 12 years:
give 1 g probenecid; then 30 minutes
later give 4.8 million units of penicillin G procaine I.M., divided into two
injection sites.
Pneumococcal pneumonia—
Adults and children over 12 years:
300,000 to 600,000 units I.M. daily q
6 to 12 hours.

ADVERSE REACTIONS
Blood: thrombocytopenia, hemolytic
anemia, leukopenia.
CNS: arthralgia, convulsions.
Other: *hypersensitivity (rash, urticaria, chills, fever, edema, prostra-
tion, anaphylaxis),* overgrowth of
nonsusceptible organisms.

INTERACTIONS
Probenecid: increases blood levels of
penicillin. Probenecid is often used
for this purpose.

NURSING CONSIDERATIONS
• Contraindicated in patients with hypersensitivity to procaine. Use cautiously in patients with other drug allergies, especially to cephalosporins
(possible cross-allergenicity).
• Obtain cultures for sensitivity tests
before first dose. Unnecessary to wait
for test results before beginning therapy.
• Before giving penicillin, ask patient
if he's had any allergic reactions to
this drug. However, a negative history
of penicillin allergy is no guarantee
against a future allergic reaction.
• Tell patient to call doctor if rash, fever, or chills develop. A rash is the
most common allergic reaction.
• Give deep I.M. in upper outer
quadrant of buttocks in adults; in midlateral thigh in small children. Do not
give subcutaneously. Don't massage
injection site.
• Never give I.V.—inadvertent I.V.
administration has caused death, due
to CNS toxicity from procaine.
• Due to slow absorption rate, allergic reactions are hard to treat.
• With prolonged therapy, other superinfections may occur, especially in
the elderly, debilitated, or those with
low resistance to infection due to immunosuppressives or irradiation.
Close observation is essential.
• Periodic evaluations of renal and
hematopoietic function are recommended.
• Check expiration date.
• Give penicillins at least 1 hour before bacteriostatic antibiotics.

penicillin G sodium
Crystapen♦♦
Pregnancy Category: B

MECHANISM OF ACTION
Bactericidal against microorganisms
by inhibiting cell-wall synthesis during active multiplication. Bacteria resist penicillin by producing penicillinases—enzymes that convert penicillin to inactive penicilloic acid.

INDICATIONS & DOSAGE

Moderate to severe systemic infections—
Adults: 1.2 to 24 million units daily I.M. or I.V., divided into doses given q 4 hours.
Children: 25,000 to 300,000 units/kg daily I.M. or I.V., divided into doses given q 4 hours.
Endocarditis prophylaxis for dental surgery—
Adults: 2 million units I.V. or I.M. 30 to 60 minutes before procedure, then 1 million units 6 hours later.

ADVERSE REACTIONS

Blood: hemolytic anemia, leukopenia, thrombocytopenia.
CNS: arthralgia, neuropathy, convulsions.
CV: *congestive heart failure with high doses.*
Local: *vein irritation, pain at injection site, thrombophlebitis.*
Other: *hypersensitivity (chills, fever, edema, maculopapular rash, exfoliative dermatitis, urticaria, anaphylaxis),* overgrowth of nonsusceptible organisms.

INTERACTIONS

Probenecid: increases blood levels of penicillin. Probenecid is often used for this purpose.

NURSING CONSIDERATIONS

• Contraindicated in patients on sodium restriction. Use cautiously in patients with other drug allergies, especially to cephalosporins (possible cross-allergenicity).
• Obtain cultures for sensitivity tests before first dose. Unnecessary to wait for test results before beginning therapy.
• Before giving penicillin, ask patient if he's had any allergic reactions to this drug. However, a negative history of penicillin allergy is no guarantee against a future allergic reaction.
• If patient has high blood level of

this drug, he may have convulsions. Be prepared by keeping side rails up on bed.
• Give I.V. intermittently to prevent vein irritation. Change site every 48 hours.
• With prolonged therapy, other superinfections may occur, especially in the elderly, debilitated, or those with low resistance to infection due to immunosuppressives or irradiation.
• Give penicillins at least 1 hour before bacteriostatic antibiotics.

---

penicillin V

penicillin V potassium

Betapen VK, Biotic-V-Powder, Bopen V-K, Cocillin V-K, Lanacillin VK, Ledercillin VK♦, LV, Nadopen-V♦♦, Novopen VK♦♦, Penapar VK, Penbec-V♦♦, Pen-Vee-K♦, Pfizerpen VK, PVF K♦♦, Robicillin-VK, SK-Penicillin VK, Uticillin VK, V-Cillin K♦, Veetids**
Pregnancy Category: B

MECHANISM OF ACTION

Bactericidal against microorganisms by inhibiting cell-wall synthesis during active multiplication. Bacteria resist penicillin by producing penicillinases—enzymes that convert penicillin to inactive penicilloic acid.

INDICATIONS & DOSAGE

Mild to moderate systemic infections—
Adults: 250 to 500 mg (400,000 to 800,000 units) P.O. q 6 hours.
Children: 15 to 50 mg/kg (25,000 to 90,000 units/kg) P.O. daily, divided into doses given q 6 to 8 hours.
Endocarditis prophylaxis for dental surgery—
Adults: 2 g P.O. 30 to 60 minutes before procedure, then 500 mg P.O. q 6 hours for 8 doses.
Children under 30 kg: ½ of the adult dose.

ADVERSE REACTIONS
Blood: eosinophilia, hemolytic anemia, leukopenia, thrombocytopenia.
CNS: neuropathy.
GI: *epigastric distress,* vomiting, diarrhea, *nausea.*
Other: *hypersensitivity (rash, urticaria, chills, fever, edema, anaphylaxis),* overgrowth of nonsusceptible organisms.

INTERACTIONS
Neomycin: decreases absorption of penicillin. Give penicillin by injection.
Probenecid: increases blood levels of penicillin. Probenecid is often used for this purpose.

NURSING CONSIDERATIONS
• Use cautiously in patients with other drug allergies, especially to cephalosporins (possible cross-allergenicity) and GI disturbances.
• Obtain cultures for sensitivity tests before first dose. Unnecessary to wait for test results before beginning therapy.
• Before giving penicillin, ask patient if he's had any allergic reactions to this drug. However, a negative history of penicillin allergy is no guarantee against a future allergic reaction.
• Tell patient to take medication exactly as prescribed, even if he feels better. Entire quantity prescribed should be taken.
• Tell patient to call the doctor if rash, fever, or chills develop. A rash is the most common allergic reaction.
• May cause GI disturbances. Food may interfere with absorption, so give 1 to 2 hours before meals or 2 to 3 hours after.
• Patient should take each dose with a full glass of water, not fruit juice or a carbonated beverage, because acid will inactivate the drug.
• Patients being treated for streptococcal infections should take the drug until the full 10-day course is completed.
• With prolonged therapy, other superinfections may occur, especially in the elderly, debilitated, or those with low resistance to infection due to immunosuppressives or irradiation. Close observation is essential.
• Periodic renal and hematopoietic function studies are recommended in patients receiving prolonged therapy.
• Check expiration date. Warn patient never to use leftover penicillin for a new illness or to share penicillin with family and friends.
• Give penicillins at least 1 hour before bacteriostatic antibiotics.

piperacillin sodium
Pipracil♦
Pregnancy Category: B

MECHANISM OF ACTION
Bactericidal against microorganisms by inhibiting cell-wall synthesis during active multiplication. Bacteria resist penicillin by producing penicillinases—enzymes that convert penicillin to inactive penicilloic acid.

INDICATIONS & DOSAGE
*Systemic infections caused by susceptible strains of gram-positive and especially gram-negative organisms (*Proteus, Pseudomonas aeruginosa*)—*
Adults and children over 12 years: 100 to 300 mg/kg daily divided q 4 to 6 hours I.V. or I.M. Doses for children under 12 years not established.
Prophylaxis of surgical infections—
Adults: 2 g I.V., given 30 to 60 minutes before surgery. Depending on type of surgery, dose may be repeated during surgery, and once or twice more after surgery.

ADVERSE REACTIONS
Blood: *bleeding with high doses,* neutropenia, eosinophilia, leukopenia, *thrombocytopenia.*
CNS: neuromuscular irritability,

headache, dizziness.
GI: nausea, diarrhea.
Local: pain at injection site, vein irritation, phlebitis.
Metabolic: *hypokalemia*.
Other: *hypersensitivity (edema, fever, chills, rash, pruritus, urticaria, anaphylaxis)*, overgrowth of nonsusceptible organisms.

INTERACTIONS
Aminoglycoside antibiotics (e.g., gentamicin, tobramycin): chemically incompatible.

NURSING CONSIDERATIONS
• Use cautiously in patients hypersensitive to drugs, especially to cephalosporins (possible cross-hypersensitivity), and those with bleeding tendencies, uremia, hypokalemia.
• Cystic fibrosis patients tend to be most susceptible to fever or rash.
• Obtain cultures for sensitivity tests before starting therapy. Unnecessary to wait for culture and sensitivity results before starting therapy.
• Before giving piperacillin, ask patient if he's had allergic reactions to penicillin. A negative history of penicillin allergy, however, is no guarantee against future allergic reaction.
• Dosage should be altered in patients with impaired renal function.
• Check CBC frequently. Drug may cause thrombocytopenia.
• Monitor serum potassium level.
• Patient with high serum level of this drug may have convulsions. Take seizure precautions.
• Give I.V. intermittently to prevent vein irritation. Change site every 48 hours.
• Almost always used with another antibiotic, such as gentamicin.
• With prolonged therapy, superinfections may occur, especially in the elderly or debilitated, or those with low resistance to infection due to immunosuppressors or irradiation. Monitor patient closely.

• Drug may be better suited to patients on salt-free diets than carbenicillin and ticarcillin (contains 1.98 mEq Na/g of piperacillin).
• Piperacillin has shown greater activity against *Pseudomonas aeruginosa* than carbenicillin, ticarcillin, or mezlocillin.
• Give penicillins at least 1 hour before bacteriostatic antibiotics.

ticarcillin disodium
Ticar♦
Pregnancy Category: B

MECHANISM OF ACTION
Bactericidal against microorganisms by inhibiting cell-wall synthesis during active multiplication. Bacteria resist penicillin by producing penicillinases—enzymes that convert penicillin to inactive penicilloic acid.

INDICATIONS & DOSAGE
Severe systemic infections caused by susceptible strains of gram-positive and especially gram-negative organisms (Pseudomonas, Proteus)—
Adults: 18 g I.V. or I.M. daily, divided into doses given q 4 to 6 hours.
Children: 200 to 300 mg/kg I.V. or I.M. daily, divided into doses given q 4 to 6 hours.

ADVERSE REACTIONS
Blood: leukopenia, neutropenia, eosinophilia, *thrombocytopenia,* hemolytic anemia.
CNS: convulsions, neuromuscular excitability.
GI: nausea, diarrhea.
Metabolic: *hypokalemia*.
Local: pain at injection site, vein irritation, phlebitis.
Other: *hypersensitivity (rash, pruritus, urticaria, chills, fever, edema, anaphylaxis)*, overgrowth of nonsusceptible organisms.

Unmarked trade names available in the United States only.
♦Also available in Canada.   ♦♦Available in Canada only.

INTERACTIONS
Probenecid: increases blood levels of penicillin. Probenecid is often used for this purpose.
Aminoglycoside antibiotics (e.g., gentamicin, tobramycin): chemically incompatible. Don't mix together in I.V.

NURSING CONSIDERATIONS
• Use cautiously in patients with other drug allergies, especially to cephalosporins (possible cross-allergenicity), and in patients with impaired renal function, hemorrhagic conditions, hypokalemia, or sodium restrictions (contains 5.2 mEq Na/g).
• Obtain cultures for sensitivity tests before first dose. Unnecessary to wait for test results before beginning therapy.
• Before giving ticarcillin, ask patient if he's had any allergic reactions to penicillin. However, a negative history of penicillin allergy is no guarantee against a future allergic reaction.
• Dosage should be decreased in patients with impaired renal functions.
• Check CBC frequently. Drug may cause thrombocytopenia.
• If patient has high blood level of this drug, he may develop convulsions. Be prepared by keeping side rails up on bed.
• When giving I.V., mix with dextrose 5% in water or other suitable I.V. fluids.
• Give I.V. intermittently to prevent vein irritation. Change site every 48 hours.
• Administer deep I.M. into large muscle.
• Almost always used with another antibiotic, such as gentamicin.
• With prolonged therapy, other superinfections may occur, especially in the elderly, debilitated, or those with low resistance to infection due to immunosuppressives or irradiation. Close observation is essential.
• Monitor serum potassium.
• Check expiration date.

• Give penicillins at least 1 hour before bacteriostatic antibiotics.

---

ticarcillin disodium/ clavulanate potassium
Timentin
Pregnancy Category: B

MECHANISM OF ACTION
Clavulanic acid increases ticarcillin's effectiveness by inactivating beta lactamases, which destroy ticarcillin.

INDICATIONS & DOSAGE
Treatment of infections of the lower respiratory tract, urinary tract, bones and joints, skin and skin structure, and septicemia when caused by beta-lactamase–producing strains of bacteria or by ticarcillin-susceptible organisms—
Adults: 3.1-g vial (contains ticarcillin 3 g and clavulanate potassium 0.1 g) administered by I.V. infusion q 4 to 6 hours.

ADVERSE REACTIONS
Blood: leukopenia, neutropenia, cosinophilia, *thrombocytopenia,* hemolytic anemia.
CNS: convulsions, neuromuscular excitability.
GI: nausea, diarrhea.
Metabolic: *hypokalemia.*
Local: pain at injection site, vein irritation, phlebitis.
Other: *hypersensitivity (rash, pruritus, urticaria, chills, fever, edema, anaphylaxis),* overgrowth of nonsusceptible organisms.

INTERACTIONS
Probenecid: increases blood levels of penicillin.
Aminoglycoside antibiotics (e.g., gentamicin, tobramycin): chemically incompatible. Don't mix together in I.V.

NURSING CONSIDERATIONS
• Use cautiously in patients with

Italicized side effects are common or life-threatening.
*Liquid form contains alcohol.   **May contain tartrazine.

other drug allergies, especially to cephalosporins (possible cross-allergenicity), and in patients with impaired renal function, hemorrhagic conditions, hypokalemia, or sodium restrictions.

• Before giving Timentin, ask patient if he's had any allergic reactions to penicillin. However, a negative history of penicillin allergy is no guarantee against a future allergic reaction.

• Dosage should be decreased in patients with impaired renal functions.

• Check CBC frequently. Drug may cause thrombocytopenia.

• Monitor serum potassium.

• Administer by I.V. infusion over 30 minutes. Don't give by I.V. push or I.M.

• Particularly useful in clinical settings with a high prevalence of ticarcillin-resistant organisms.

• Give penicillins at least 1 hour before bacteriostatic antibiotics.

12

Cephalosporins

cefaclor
cefadroxil monohydrate
cefamandole nafate
cefazolin sodium
cefonicid sodium
cefoperazone sodium
ceforanide
cefotaxime sodium
cefotetan disodium
cefoxitin sodium
ceftazidime
ceftizoxime sodium
ceftriaxone sodium
cefuroxime sodium
cephalexin monohydrate
cephalothin sodium
cephapirin sodium
cephradine
moxalactam disodium

COMBINATION PRODUCTS
None.

---

cefaclor
Ceclor◆
Pregnancy Category: B

MECHANISM OF ACTION
Inhibits cell-wall synthesis, promoting osmotic instability. Usually bactericidal.

INDICATIONS & DOSAGE
Treatment of infections of respiratory or urinary tracts, skin, and soft tissue; and otitis media due to Hemophilus influenzae, Streptococcus pneumoniae, Streptococcus pyogenes, Escherichia coli, Proteus mirabilis, Klebsiella *species, and staphylo-*

cocci—
Adults: 250 to 500 mg P.O. q 8 hours. Total daily dose should not exceed 4 g.
Children: 20 mg/kg daily P.O. in divided doses q 8 hours. In more serious infections, 40 mg/kg daily are recommended, not to exceed 1 g per day.

ADVERSE REACTIONS
Blood: transient leukopenia, lymphocytosis, anemia, eosinophilia.
CNS: dizziness, headache, somnolence.
GI: *nausea,* vomiting, *diarrhea,* anorexia, *pseudomembranous colitis.*
GU: red and white cells in urine, vaginal moniliasis, vaginitis.
Skin: *maculopapular rash,* dermatitis.
Other: hypersensitivity, fever.

INTERACTIONS
Probenecid: may inhibit excretion and increase blood levels of cefaclor.

NURSING CONSIDERATIONS
• Contraindicated in hypersensitivity to other cephalosporins. Use cautiously in patients with impaired renal status and in those with history of sensitivity to penicillin. Ask patient if he's had any reaction to previous cephalosporin or penicillin therapy before administering first dose.
• Prolonged use may result in overgrowth of nonsusceptible organisms. Careful observation of patient for superinfection is essential.
• Obtain cultures for sensitivity tests before first dose, but therapy may be-

Italicized side effects are common or life-threatening.
*Liquid form contains alcohol.   **May contain tartrazine.

gin pending test results.
- Major clinical use appears to be in treating otitis media caused by *H. influenzae* when resistant to ampicillin or amoxicillin. Drug is a second-generation cephalosporin.
- Tell patient to take medication exactly as prescribed, even after he feels better.
- Call doctor if skin rash develops.
- Store reconstituted suspension in refrigerator. Stable for 14 days if refrigerated. Shake well before using.
- Drug may be taken with meals.
- Cefaclor is a relatively expensive antibiotic and should be used only when the organism is resistant to other agents.
- If ordered, total daily dose of cefaclor may be administered twice daily rather than 3 times daily with similar therapeutic results.
- Urine glucose determinations may be false-positive with copper sulfate tests (Clinitest); glucose-enzymatic tests (Clinistix, Tes-Tape) are not affected.

---

cefadroxil monohydrate
Duricef♦, Ultracef
Pregnancy Category: B

MECHANISM OF ACTION
Inhibits cell-wall synthesis, promoting osmotic instability. Usually bactericidal.

INDICATIONS & DOSAGE
Treatment of urinary tract infections caused by Escherichia coli, Proteus mirabilis, *and* Klebsiella *species; infections of skin and soft tissue; and streptococcal pharyngitis*—
Adults: 500 mg to 2 g P.O. per day, depending on the infection being treated. Usually given in once-daily or b.i.d. dosage.
Children: 30 mg/kg daily in 2 divided doses.

ADVERSE REACTIONS
Blood: transient neutropenia, eosinophilia, leukopenia, anemia.
CNS: dizziness, headache, malaise, paresthesias.
GI: *pseudomembranous colitis, nausea,* anorexia, vomiting, *diarrhea,* glossitis, *dyspepsia,* abdominal cramps, anal pruritus, tenesmus, oral candidiasis (thrush).
GU: genital pruritus, moniliasis.
Skin: *maculopapular and erythematous rashes.*
Other: dyspnea.

INTERACTIONS
Probenecid: may inhibit excretion and increase blood levels of cefadroxil.

NURSING CONSIDERATIONS
- Contraindicated in hypersensitivity to other cephalosporins. Use cautiously in patients with impaired renal status and in those with history of sensitivity to penicillin. Ask patient if he's had any reaction to previous cephalosporin or penicillin therapy before administering first dose.
- Prolonged use may result in overgrowth of nonsusceptible organisms. Careful observation of patient for superinfection is essential.
- Obtain cultures for sensitivity tests before first dose, but therapy may begin pending test results.
- If creatinine clearance is below 50 ml/minute, dosage interval should be lengthened so drug doesn't accumulate.
- Tell patient to take medication exactly as prescribed, even after he feels better.
- Call doctor if skin rash develops.
- Since absorption not delayed by presence of food, tell the patient to take with food or milk to lessen GI discomfort.
- Longer half-life permits once- or twice-daily dosing.
- Urine glucose determinations may be false-positive with copper sulfate tests

---

(Clinitest); glucose-enzymatic tests (Clinistix, Tes-Tape) are not affected.

cefamandole nafate
Mandol♦
Pregnancy Category: B

MECHANISM OF ACTION
Inhibits cell-wall synthesis, promoting osmotic instability. Usually bactericidal.

INDICATIONS & DOSAGE
Treatment of serious infections of respiratory and genitourinary tracts, skin and soft-tissue infections, bone and joint infections, septicemia, and peritonitis due to Escherichia coli *and other coliform bacteria,* Staphylococcus aureus *(penicillinase- and nonpenicillinase-producing),* Staphyloccus epidermidis, *group A beta-hemolytic streptococci,* Klebsiella, Hemophilus influenzae, Proteus mirabilis, *and* Enterobacter *species*—
Adults: 500 mg to 1 g q 4 to 8 hours. In life-threatening infections, up to 2 g q 4 hours may be needed.
Infants and children: 50 to 100 mg/kg daily in equally divided doses q 4 to 8 hours. May be increased to total daily dose of 150 mg/kg (not to exceed maximum adult dose) for severe infections.
Total daily dosage is same for I.M. or I.V. administration and depends on susceptibility of organism and severity of infection. In patients with impaired renal function, doses or frequency of administration must be modified according to degree of renal impairment, severity of infection, and susceptibility of organism. Should be injected deep I.M. into a large muscle mass, such as gluteus or lateral aspect of thigh.

ADVERSE REACTIONS
Blood: transient neutropenia, eosinophilia, hemolytic anemia, *hypopro-*

thrombinemia, bleeding.
CNS: headache, malaise, paresthesias, dizziness.
GI: *pseudomembranous colitis,* nausea, anorexia, vomiting, *diarrhea,* glossitis, dyspepsia, abdominal cramps, tenesmus, anal pruritus, oral candidiasis (thrush).
GU: genital pruritus and moniliasis.
Skin: *maculopapular and erythematous rashes,* urticaria.
Local: *at injection site—pain, induration, sterile abscesses,* temperature elevation, tissue sloughing; *phlebitis and thrombophlebitis with I.V. injection.*
Other: *hypersensitivity,* dyspnea.

INTERACTIONS
Ethyl alcohol: may cause a disulfiramlike reaction. Warn patients not to drink alcohol for several days after discontinuing cefamandole.
Probenecid: may inhibit excretion and increase blood levels of cefamandole.

NURSING CONSIDERATIONS
• Contraindicated in hypersensitivity to other cephalosporins. Use cautiously in patients with impaired renal status and in those with history of sensitivity to penicillin. Ask patient if he's had any reaction to previous cephalosporin or penicillin therapy before administering first dose.
• Prolonged use may result in overgrowth of nonsusceptible organisms. Careful observation of patient for superinfection is essential.
• Obtain cultures for sensitivity tests before first dose, but therapy may begin pending test results.
• Not as effective as cefoxitin in treating anaerobic infections.
• For most cephalosporin-sensitive organisms, cefamandole offers little advantage over previously available agents.
• For I.V. use, reconstitute 1 g with 10 ml of sterile water for injection, dextrose 5% or 0.9% sodium chloride

---

Italicized side effects are common or life-threatening.
*Liquid form contains alcohol.   **May contain tartrazine.

for injection.
• Don't mix with I.V. infusions containing magnesium or calcium ions; chemically incompatible.
• I.M. cefamandole is not as painful as cefoxitin. Does not require addition of lidocaine.
• After reconstitution, remains stable for 24 hours at room temperature or 96 hours under refrigeration.
• The chemical structure of this drug includes the methylthiotetrazole (MTT) side chain that has been associated with bleeding disorders. If bleeding occurs, it can be promptly reversed with administration of vitamin K.
• Urine glucose determinations may be false-positive with copper sulfate tests (Clinitest); glucose-enzymatic tests (Clinistix, Tes-Tape) are not affected.

cefazolin sodium
Ancef♦, Kefzol♦
Pregnancy Category: B

MECHANISM OF ACTION
Inhibits cell-wall synthesis, promoting osmotic instability. Usually bactericidal.

INDICATIONS & DOSAGE
Treatment of serious infections of respiratory and genitourinary tracts, skin and soft-tissue infections, bone and joint infections, septicemia, and endocarditis due to Escherichia coli, *Enterobacteriaceae, gonococci,* Hemophilus influenzae, Klebsiella, Proteus mirabilis, Staphylococcus aureus, Streptococcus pneumoniae, *and group A beta-hemolytic streptococci; and perioperative prophylaxis—*
Adults: 250 mg I.M. or I.V. q 8 hours to 1 g q 6 hours. Maximun 12g/day in life-threatening situations.
Children over 1 month: 8 to 16 mg/kg I.M. or I.V. q 8 hours, or 6 to 12 mg/kg q 6 hours.

Total daily dosage is same for I.M. or I.V. administration and depends on susceptibility of organism and severity of infection. In patients with impaired renal function, doses or frequency of administration must be modified according to degree of renal impairment, severity of infection, and susceptibility of organism. Should be injected deep I.M. into a large muscle mass, such as gluteus or lateral aspect of thigh.

ADVERSE REACTIONS
Blood: transient neutropenia, leukopenia, eosinophilia, anemia.
CNS: dizziness, headache, malaise, paresthesias.
GI: *pseudomembranous colitis,* nausea, anorexia, vomiting, *diarrhea,* glossitis, dyspepsia, abdominal cramps, anal pruritus, tenesmus, oral candidiasis (thrush).
GU: genital pruritus and moniliasis, vaginitis.
Skin: *maculopapular and erythematous rashes, urticaria.*
Local: *at injection site—pain, induration, sterile abscesses, tissue sloughing; phlebitis and thrombophlebitis with I.V. injection.*
Other: *hypersensitivity,* dyspnea.

INTERACTIONS
Probenecid: may inhibit excretion and increase blood levels of cefazolin.

NURSING CONSIDERATIONS
• Use cautiously in patients with impaired renal status and in those with history of sensitivity to penicillin. Ask patient if he's ever had any reaction to cephalosporin or penicillin therapy before administering first dose.
• Avoid doses greater than 4 g daily in patients with severe renal impairment.
• Prolonged use may result in overgrowth of nonsusceptible organisms. Watch carefully for superinfection.

- Obtain cultures for sensitivity tests before first dose, but therapy may begin pending test results.
- Because of long duration of effect, most infections can be treated with a single dose q 8 hours.
- For I.M. administration, reconstitute with sterile water, bacteriostatic water, or 0.9% sodium chloride solution as follows: 2 ml to 250-mg vial; 2 ml to 500-mg vial; 2.5 ml to 1-g vial. Shake well until dissolved. Resultant concentration: 125 mg/ml, 225 mg/ml, 330 mg/ml, respectively.
- Not as painful as other cephalosporins when given I.M.
- Alternate injection sites if I.V. therapy lasts longer than 3 days. Use of small I.V. needles in the larger available veins may be preferable.
- Reconstituted cefazolin sodium is stable for 24 hours at room temperature, for 96 hours under refrigeration.
- About 40% to 75% of patients receiving cephalosporins show a false-positive direct Coombs' test; only a few of these indicate hemolytic anemia.
- Considered the first-generation cephalosporin of choice by most authorities.
- Urine glucose determinations may be false-positive with copper sulfate tests (Clinitest); glucose-enzymatic tests (Clinistix, Tes-Tape) are not affected.

---

cefonicid sodium
Monocid
Pregnancy Category: B

MECHANISM OF ACTION
Inhibits cell-wall synthesis, promoting osmotic instability. Usually bactericidal.

INDICATIONS & DOSAGE
Treatment of serious infections of the lower respiratory and urinary tract; skin and skin structure infections;
septicemia; and bone and joint infections. Susceptible microorganisms include Streptococcus pneumoniae, Klebsiella pneumoniae, E. coli, Hemophilus influenzae, Proteus mirabilis, Staphyloccus aureus and epidermidis, and Streptococcus pyogenes—
Adults: Usual dosage is 1 g I.V. or I.M. q 24 hours. In life-threatening infections, 2 g q 24 hours.

Total daily dosage is same for I.M. or I.V. administration and depends on susceptibility of organism and severity of infection. In patients with impaired renal function, doses or frequency of administration must be modified according to degree of renal impairment, severity of infection, and susceptibility of organism. Should be injected deep I.M. into a large muscle mass, such as gluteus or lateral aspect of thigh.

ADVERSE REACTIONS
Blood: transient neutropenia, leukopenia, eosinophilia, anemia.
CNS: dizziness, headache, malaise, paresthesias.
GI: *pseudomembranous colitis,* nausea, anorexia, vomiting, diarrhea, glossitis, dyspepsia, abdominal cramps, anal pruritus, tenesmus, oral candidiasis (thrush).
GU: genital pruritus and moniliasis, vaginitis.
Skin: *maculopapular and erythematous rashes, urticaria.*
Local: *at injection site—pain, induration, sterile abscesses, tissue sloughing; phlebitis and thrombophlebitis with I.V. injection.*
Other: hypersensitivity, dyspnea.

INTERACTIONS
Probenecid: may inhibit excretion and increase blood levels of cefonicid.

NURSING CONSIDERATIONS
- Contraindicated in hypersensitivity to other cephalosporins. Use cautiously in patients with impaired renal

---

Italicized side effects are common or life-threatening.
*Liquid form contains alcohol.   **May contain tartrazine.

function and in those with history of sensitivity to penicillin. Ask patient if he's had any reaction to previous cephalosporin or penicillin therapy before administering first dose.

• Prolonged use may result in overgrowth of nonsusceptible organisms. Observe patient carefully for superinfection.

• Obtain cultures for sensitivity tests before therapy, but therapy may begin pending results of cultures and sensitivity tests.

• When administering 2 g I.M. doses once daily, one-half the dose should be administered in different large muscle masses.

• Has been promoted as a cost-effective agent for surgical prophylaxis.

cefoperazone sodium
Cefobid♦
Pregnancy Category: B

MECHANISM OF ACTION
Inhibits cell-wall synthesis, promoting osmotic instability. Usually bactericidal.

INDICATIONS & DOSAGE
Treatment of serious infections of the respiratory tract; intraabdominal, gynecologic, and skin infections; bacteremia, septicemia. Susceptible microorganisms include Streptococcus pneumoniae *and* Streptococcus pyogenes; Staphylococcus aureus *(penicillinase and nonpenicillinase-producing);* Staphylococcus epidermidis; *enterococcus;* Escherichia coli; Klebsiella; Hemophilus influenzae; Enterobacter; Citrobacter; Proteus; *some* Pseudomonas *species including* Pseudomonas aeruginosa; *and* Bacteroides fragilis—
Adults: Usual dosage is 1 to 2 g q 12 hours I.M. or I.V. In severe infections, or infections caused by less sensitive organisms, the total daily dosage or frequency may be increased up

to 16 g/day in certain situations. No dosage adjustment is usually necessary in patients with renal impairment. However, doses of 4 g/day should be given very cautiously in patients with hepatic disease. Should be injected deep I.M. into a large muscle mass, such as gluteus or lateral aspect of the thigh.

ADVERSE REACTIONS
Blood: transient neutropenia, eosinophilia, hemolytic anemia, *hypoprothrombinemia, bleeding*.
CNS: headache, malaise, paresthesias, dizziness.
GI: *pseudomembranous colitis,* nausea, anorexia, vomiting, *diarrhea,* glossitis, dyspepsia, abdominal cramps, tenesmus, anal pruritus, oral candidiasis (thrush).
Hepatic: mildly elevated liver enzymes.
GU: genital pruritus and moniliasis.
Skin: *maculopapular and erythematous rashes, urticaria.*
Local: *at injection site—pain, induration, sterile abscesses, temperature elevation, tissue slough; phlebitis and thrombophlebitis with I.V. injection.*
Other: hypersensitivity, dyspnea.

INTERACTIONS
Probenecid: may inhibit excretion and increase blood levels of cefoparazone.
Ethyl alcohol: may cause a disulfiram-like reaction. Warn patients not to drink alcohol for several days after discontinuing cefoperazone.

NURSING CONSIDERATIONS
• Contraindicated in hypersensitivity to other cephalosporins. Use cautiously in patients with impaired renal function and in those with history of sensitivity to penicillin. Ask patient if he's had any reaction to previous cephalosporin or penicillin therapy before administering first dose.
• Prolonged use may result in overgrowth of nonsusceptible organisms.

Careful observation of patient for superinfection is essential.

• Obtain cultures for sensitivity tests before therapy, but therapy may begin pending results of cultures and sensitivity tests.

• Cefoperazone is one of the third-generation cephalosporins. It has increased activity over the first-generation cephalosporins against gram-negative organisms, yet it is the least active of the third-generation cephalosporins currently available.

• Because of high degree of biliary excretion, may cause more diarrhea than other cephalosporins.

• The chemical structure of this drug includes the methylthiotetrazole (MTT) side chain that has been associated with bleeding disorders. If bleeding occurs, it can be promptly reversed with administration of vitamin K. Monitor prothrombin time regularly.

• Urine glucose determinations may be false-positive with copper sulfate tests (Clinitest); glucose enzymatic tests (Clinistix, Tes-Tape) are not affected.

ceforanide
Precef
Pregnancy Category: B

MECHANISM OF ACTION
Inhibits cell-wall synthesis, promoting osmotic instability. Usually bactericidal.

INDICATIONS & DOSAGE
Treatment of serious infections of the lower respiratory and urinary tract; skin and skin structure infections; endocarditis; septicemia; and bone and joint infections. Susceptible microorganisms include Streptococcus pneumoniae, Klebsiella pneumoniae, E. coli, Hemophilus influenzae, Proteus mirabilis, Staphylococcus aureus *and* epidermidis, *and* Streptococcus pyogenes—

Adults: 0.5 to 1 g I.V. or I.M. q 12 hours.

Children: 20 to 40 mg/kg/day in equally divided doses q 12 hours.
Prophylaxis of surgical infections—
0.5 to 1 g I.M. or I.V. 1 hour prior to surgery.
Total daily dosage is same for I.M. or I.V. administration and depends on susceptibility of organism and severity of infection. In patients with impaired renal function, doses or frequency of administration must be modified according to degree of renal impairment, severity of infection, and susceptibility of organism. Should be injected deep I.M. into a large muscle mass, such as gluteus or lateral aspect of thigh.

ADVERSE REACTIONS
Blood: transient neutropenia, leukopenia, eosinophilia, thrombocytopenia.
CNS: confusion, headache, lethargy.
GI: *pseudomembranous colitis,* nausea, anorexia, vomiting, diarrhea, glossitis, dyspepsia, abdominal cramps, oral candidiasis (thrush).
GU: genital pruritus and moniliasis, vaginitis.
Hepatic: transient elevation in liver enzymes.
Skin: *maculopapular and erythematous rashes, urticaria.*
Local: *at injection site—pain, induration, sterile abscesses, tissue sloughing; phlebitis and thrombophlebitis with I.V. injection.*
Other: hypersensitivity, dyspnea.

INTERACTIONS
Probenecid: may inhibit excretion and increase blood levels of ceforanide.

NURSING CONSIDERATIONS
• Contraindicated in hypersensitivity to other cephalosporins. Use cautiously in patients with impaired renal function and in those with history of

---

Italicized side effects are common or life-threatening.
*Liquid form contains alcohol.   **May contain tartrazine.

sensitivity to penicillin. Ask patient if he's had a previous reaction to cephalosporin or penicillin therapy before administering first dose.

• Obtain cultures for sensitivity tests before therapy; but therapy may begin pending results of cultures and sensitivity tests.

• Upon reconstitution, ceforanide injection may appear cloudy. Let stand briefly to allow solution to deaerate and clarify.

• Prolonged use may result in overgrowth of nonsusceptible organisms. Observe patient carefully for superinfection.

• Ceforanide is a second-generation cephalosporin which may be administered twice daily.

---

cefotaxime sodium
Claforan♦
Pregnancy Category: B

MECHANISM OF ACTION
Inhibits cell-wall synthesis, promoting osmotic instability. Usually bactericidal.

INDICATIONS & DOSAGE
Treatment of serious infections of the lower respiratory and urinary tracts, CNS infections, gynecological infections, bacteremia, septicemia, and skin infections. Among susceptible microorganisms are streptococci, in-cluding Streptococcus pneumoniae *and* pyogenes; Staphylococcus aureus *(penicillinase- and nonpenicillinase-producing);* Staphylococcus epidermidis; Escherichia coli; Klebsiella *species;* Hemophilus influenzae; Enterobacter *species;* Proteus *species; and* Peptostreptococcus *species*—
Adults: usual dose is 1 g I.V. or I.M. q 6 to 8 hours. Up to 12 g daily can be administered in life-threatening infections.
Total daily dosage is same for I.M. or I.V. administration and depends on

susceptibility of organism and severity of infection. In patients with impaired renal function, doses or frequency of administration must be modified according to degree of renal impairment, severity of infection, and susceptibility of organism. Should be injected deep I.M. into a large muscle mass, such as gluteus or lateral aspect of thigh.

ADVERSE REACTIONS
Blood: transient neutropenia, eosinophilia, hemolytic anemia.
CNS: headache, malaise, paresthesias, dizziness.
GI: *pseudomembranous colitis,* nausea, anorexia, vomiting, *diarrhea,* glossitis, dyspepsia, abdominal cramps, tenesmus, anal pruritus, oral candidiasis (thrush).
GU: genital pruritus and moniliasis.
Skin: *maculopapular and erythematous rashes, urticaria.*
Local: *at injection site—pain, induration, sterile abscesses, temperature elevation, tissue slough; phlebitis and thrombophlebitis with I.V. injection.*
Other: hypersensitivity, dyspnea.

INTERACTIONS
Probenecid: may inhibit excretion and increase blood levels of cefotaxime. Use together cautiously.

NURSING CONSIDERATIONS
• Contraindicated in hypersensitivity to other cephalosporins. Use cautiously in patients with impaired renal function and in those with history of sensitivity to penicillin. Ask patient if he's had any reaction to previous cephalosporin or penicillin therapy before administering first dose.

• Prolonged use may result in overgrowth of nonsusceptible organisms. Careful observation of patient for superinfection is essential.

• Obtain cultures for sensitivity tests before therapy, but therapy may begin pending results of cultures and sensi-

---

tivity tests.
• Cefotaxime was the first of the so-called third-generation cephalosporins. It has increased antibacterial activity against gram-negative microorganisms.
• Some doctors may prescribe cefotaxime in clinical situations in which they formerly prescribed aminoglycosides. However, this drug is not effective against infections caused by *Pseudomonas* organisms.
• Urine glucose determinations may be false-positive with copper sulfate tests (Clinitest); glucose enzymatic tests (Clinistix, Tes-Tape) are not affected.

---

cefotetan disodium
Cefotan♦
Pregnancy Category: B

MECHANISM OF ACTION
Inhibits cell-wall synthesis, promoting osmotic instability. Usually bactericidal.

INDICATIONS & DOSAGE
Treatment of serious infections of the urinary and lower respiratory tracts, gynecologic, skin and skin structure, intraabdominal, and bone and joint infections. Among susceptible microorganisms are streptococci, Staphylococcus aureus *(penicillinase- and nonpenicillinase-producing),* Staphylococcus epidermidis, Escherichia coli, Klebsiella *species,* Enterobacter *species,* Proteus *species,* Hemophilus influenzae, Neisseria gonorrhoeae, *and* Bacteroides *species, including* B. fragilis.
Adults: 1 to 2 g I.V. or I.M. q 12 hours for 5 to 10 days. Up to 6 g daily in life-threatening infections. Total daily dosage is same for I.M. or I.V. administration and depends on susceptibility of organism and severity of infection. In patients with impaired renal function, doses or frequency of

administration must be modified according to degree of renal impairment, severity of infection, and susceptibility of organism. Should be injected deep I.M. into a large muscle mass, such as gluteus or lateral aspect of thigh.

ADVERSE REACTIONS
Blood: transient neutropenia, eosinophilia, hemolytic anemia.
CNS: headache, malaise, paresthesias, dizziness.
GI: *pseudomembranous colitis,* nausea, anorexia, vomiting, *diarrhea,* glossitis, dyspepsia, abdominal cramps, tenesmus, anal pruritus.
GU: genital pruritus and moniliasis.
Skin: *maculopapular and erythematous rashes, urticaria.*
Local: *at injection site—pain, induration, sterile abscesses, tissue sloughing; phlebitis and thrombophlebitis with I.V. injection.*
Other: *hypersensitivity,* dyspnea, elevated temperature.

INTERACTIONS
Probenecid: may inhibit excretion and increase blood levels of cefotetan.
Ethyl alcohol: may cause a disulfiram-like reaction. Warn patients not to drink alcohol for several days after discontinuing cefotetan.

NURSING CONSIDERATIONS
• Contraindicated in hypersensitivity to other cephalosporins. Use cautiously in patients with impaired renal status and in those with history of sensitivity to penicillin. Ask patient if he's had any reaction to previous cephalosporin or penicillin therapy before administering first dose.
• Prolonged use may result in overgrowth of nonsusceptible organisms. Observe patient for superinfection.
• Obtain cultures for sensitivity tests before first dose, but therapy may begin pending test results.
• For I.V. use, reconstitute with ster-

Italicized side effects are common or life-threatening.
*Liquid form contains alcohol.   **May contain tartrazine.

ile water for injection. Then, may be mixed with 50 to 100 ml of dextrose 5% in water or 0.9% sodium chloride solution.
• I.M. injection may be reconstituted with sterile water or bacteriostatic water for injection, normal saline, 0.5% or 1% lidocaine hydrochloride. Shake to dissolve and let stand until clear.
• Reconstituted solution remains stable for 24 hours at room temperature or for 96 hours when refrigerated.
• The chemical structure of this drug includes the methylthiotetrazole (MTT) side chain that has been associated with bleeding disorders. However, such bleeding has not been reported with this drug.
• Cefotetan is similar to cefoxitin in that it's particularly useful in intraabdominal and gynecologic infection (highly active against *B.fragilis*).

cefoxitin sodium
Mefoxin♦
Pregnancy Category: B

MECHANISM OF ACTION
Inhibits cell-wall synthesis, promoting osmotic instability. Usually bactericidal.

INDICATIONS & DOSAGE
Treatment of serious infection of respiratory and genitourinary tracts, skin and soft-tissue infections, bone and joint infections, bloodstream and intra-abdominal infections due to Escherichia coli *and other coliform bacteria,* Staphylococcus aureus *(penicillinase- and nonpenicillinase-producing),* Staphylococcus epidermidis, *streptococci,* Klebsiella, Hemophilus influenzae, *and* Bacteroides *species, including* B. fragilis—
Adults: 1 to 2 g q 6 to 8 hours for uncomplicated forms of infection. Up to 12 g daily in life-threatening infections.

Children: 80 to 160 mg/kg daily given in 4 to 6 equally divided doses. Total daily dosage is same for I.M. or I.V. administration and depends on susceptibility of organism and severity of infection. In patients with impaired renal function, doses or frequency of administration must be modified according to degree of renal impairment, severity of infection, and susceptibility of organism. Should be injected deep I.M. into a large muscle mass, such as gluteus or lateral aspect of thigh.

ADVERSE REACTIONS
Blood: transient neutropenia, eosinophilia, hemolytic anemia.
CNS: headache, malaise, paresthesias, dizziness.
GI: *pseudomembranous colitis,* nausea, anorexia, vomiting, *diarrhea,* glossitis, dyspepsia, abdominal cramps, tenesmus, anal pruritus, oral candidiasis (thrush).
GU: genital pruritus and moniliasis.
Skin: *maculopapular and erythematous rashes, urticaria.*
Local: *at injection site—pain, induration, sterile abscesses, tissue sloughing; phlebitis and thrombophlebitis with I.V. injection.*
Other: *hypersensitivity,* dyspnea, elevated temperature.

INTERACTIONS
Probenecid: may inhibit excretion and increase blood levels of cefoxitin.

NURSING CONSIDERATIONS
• Contraindicated in hypersensitivity to other cephalosporins. Use cautiously in patients with impaired renal status and in those with history of sensitivity to penicillin. Ask patient if he's had any reaction to previous cephalosporin or penicillin therapy before administering first dose.
• Prolonged use may result in overgrowth of nonsusceptible organisms. Observe patient for superinfection.

• Obtain cultures for sensitivity tests before first dose, but therapy may begin pending test results.

• A very useful cephalosporin when anaerobic or mixed aerobic-anaerobic infection is suspected, especially *B. fragilis.*

• Associated with development of thrombophlebitis. Assess I.V. site frequently.

• For I.V. use, reconstitute 1 g with at least 10 ml of sterile water for injection, and 2 g with 10 to 20 ml. Solutions of dextrose 5% and 0.9% sodium chloride for injection can also be used.

• I.M. injection can be reconstituted with 0.5% or 1% lidocaine HCl (without epinephrine) to minimize pain.

• After reconstitution, remains stable for 24 hours at room temperature or 1 week under refrigeration.

• Urine glucose determinations may be false-positive with copper sulfate tests (Clinitest); glucose-enzymatic tests (Clinistix, Tes-Tape) are not affected.

ceftazidime
Fortaz, Tazicef, Tazidime♦
Pregnancy Category: B

MECHANISM OF ACTION
Inhibits cell-wall synthesis, promoting osmotic instability. Usually bactericidal.

INDICATIONS & DOSAGE
Treatment of serious infections of the lower respiratory and urinary tracts, gynecologic infections, bacteremia, septicemia, intraabdominal infections, CNS infections, and skin infections. Among susceptible microorganisms are streptococci, including Streptococcus pneumoniae *and* S. pyogenes; Staphylococcus aureus *(penicillinase- and nonpenicillinase-producing);* Escherichia coli; Klebsiella

species; Proteus *species;* Enterobacter *species;* Hemophilus influenzae; Pseudomonas *species, and some strains of* Bacteroides *species.*

Adults: 1 g I.V. or I.M. q 8 to 12 hours; up to 6 g daily in life-threatening infections.

Children 1 month to 12 years: 30 to 50 mg/kg I.V. q 8 hours.

Neonates 0 to 4 weeks: 30 mg/kg I.V. q 12 hours.

Total daily dosage is same for I.M. or I.V. administration and depends on susceptibility of organism and severity of infection. In patients with impaired renal function, doses or frequency of administration must be modified according to degree of renal impairment, severity of infection, and susceptibility of organism. Should be injected deep I.M. into a large muscle mass, such as gluteus or lateral aspect of thigh.

ADVERSE REACTIONS
Blood: *eosinophilia; thrombocytosis,* leukopenia.

CNS: headache, dizziness.

GI: *pseudomembranous enterocolitis,* nausea, vomiting, diarrhea, dysgeusia, abdominal cramps.

GU: genital pruritus and moniliasis.

Hepatic: transient elevation in liver enzymes.

Skin: *maculopapular and erythematous rashes, urticaria.*

Local: *at injection site—pain, induration, sterile abscesses, tissue sloughing; phlebitis and thrombophlebitis with I.V. injection.*

Other: *hypersensitivity,* dyspnea, elevated temperature.

INTERACTIONS
Sodium bicarbonate–containing solutions: make ceftazidime unstable. Don't mix together.

NURSING CONSIDERATIONS
• Contraindicated in hypersensitivity to other cephalosporins. Use cau-

tiously in patients with history of sensitivity to penicillin. Ask patient if he's had any previous reaction to cephalosporin or penicillin therapy before administering first dose.
• Obtain cultures for sensitivity tests before first dose, but therapy may begin pending test results.
• Prolonged use may result in overgrowth of nonsusceptible organisms. Watch carefully for superinfection.
• The vials of ceftazidime are supplied under reduced pressure. When the antibiotic is dissolved, carbon dioxide is released and a positive pressure develops. Each brand of ceftazidime includes specific instructions for reconstitution. Read and follow these instructions carefully.
• This third-generation cephalosporin has excellent activity against infections caused by *Pseudomonas aeruginosa*. May be prescribed for these infections, especially when aminoglycosides are potentially too dangerous.

ceftizoxime sodium
Cefizox
Pregnancy Category: B

MECHANISM OF ACTION
Inhibits cell-wall synthesis, promoting osmotic instability. Usually bactericidal.

INDICATIONS & DOSAGE
Treatment of serious infections of the lower respiratory and urinary tracts, gynecological infections, bacteremia, septicemia, meningitis, intraabdominal infections, bone and joint infections, and skin infections. Among susceptible microorganisms are streptococci, including Streptococcus pneumoniae and pyogenes; Staphylococcus aureus (penicillinase- and nonpenicillinase-producing); Staphylococcus epidermidis; Escherichia coli; Klebsiella species; Hemophilus influenzae; Enterobacter species; Proteus species;
some Pseudomonas *species, and* Peptostreptococcus *species*—
Adults: Usual dosage is 1 to 2 g I.V. or I.M. q 8 to 12 hours. In life-threatening infections, up to 2 g q 4 hours. Total daily dosage is same for I.M. or I.V. administration and depends on susceptibility of organism and severity of infection. In patients with impaired renal function, doses or frequency of administration must be modified according to degree of renal impairment, severity of infection, and susceptibility of organism. Should be injected deep I.M. into a large muscle mass, such as gluteus or lateral aspect of thigh.

ADVERSE REACTIONS
Blood: transient neutropenia, eosinophilia, hemolytic anemia.
CNS: headache, malaise, paresthesias, dizziness.
GI: *pseudomembranous colitis,* nausea, anorexia, vomiting, *diarrhea,* glossitis, dyspepsia, abdominal cramps, tenesmus, anal pruritus.
GU: genital pruritus and moniliasis.
Skin: *maculopapular and erythematous rashes, urticaria.*
Local: *at injection site—pain, induration, sterile abscesses, tissue sloughing; phlebitis and thrombophlebitis with I.V. injection.*
Other: *hypersensitivity, dyspnea, elevated temperature.*

INTERACTIONS
Probenecid: may inhibit excretion and increase blood levels of ceftizoxime.

NURSING CONSIDERATIONS
• Contraindicated in hypersensitivity to other cephalosporins. Use cautiously in patients with impaired renal function and in those with history of sensitivity to penicillin. Ask patient if he's had any reaction to previous cephalosporin or penicillin therapy before administering first dose.
• Prolonged use may result in over-

Unmarked trade names available in the United States only.
♦ Also available in Canada.   ♦♦ Available in Canada only.

growth of nonsusceptible organisms. Watch carefully for superinfection.
• Obtain cultures for sensitivity tests before first dose, but therapy may begin pending test results.
• Ceftizoxime is a third-generation cephalosporin, which is comparable in activity to cefotaxime, moxalactam, ceftriaxone and cefoperazone. No significant degree of bleeding or disulfiram-type reaction has been reported with its use.

ceftriaxone sodium
Rocephin
Pregnancy Category: B

MECHANISM OF ACTION
Inhibits cell-wall synthesis, promoting osmotic instability. Usually bactericidal.

INDICATIONS & DOSAGE
Treatment of serious infections of the lower respiratory and urinary tracts, gynecological infections, bacteremia, septicemia, intraabdominal infections, and skin infections. Susceptible microorganisms are streptococci, in-cluding Streptococcus pneumoniae *and* pyogenes; Staphylococcus aureus *(penicillinase- and nonpenicillinase-producing);* Staphylococcus epidermidis; Escherichia coli; Klebsiella *species;* Hemophilus influenzae; Enterobacter *species;* Proteus *species;* Pseudomonas *species; and* Peptostreptococcus *species—*
Adults: 1 to 2 g I.M. or I.V. once daily or in equally divided doses twice daily. Total daily dose should not exceed 4 g.
Children: 50 to 75 mg/kg, given in divided doses q 12 hours.
Treatment of meningitis—
Adults and children: 100 mg/kg given in divided doses q 12 hours. May give loading dose of 75 mg/kg. Total daily dose is same for I.M. or I.V. administration and depends on

susceptibility of organism and severity of infection. Should be injected deep I.M. into a large muscle mass, such as gluteus or lateral aspect of thigh.

ADVERSE REACTIONS
Blood: *eosinophilia; thrombocytosis,* leukopenia.
CNS: headache, dizziness.
GI: *pseudomembranous enterocolitis,* nausea, vomiting, diarrhea, dysgeusia, abdominal cramps.
GU: genital pruritus and moniliasis.
Hepatic: transient elevation in liver enzymes.
Skin: *maculopapular and erythematous rashes, urticaria.*
Local: *at injection site—pain, induration, sterile abscesses, tissue sloughing; phlebitis and thrombophlebitis with I.V. injection.*
Other: hypersensitivity, dyspnea, elevated temperature.

INTERACTIONS
Probenecid: may inhibit excretion and increase blood levels of ceftriaxone.

NURSING CONSIDERATIONS
• Contraindicated in hypersensitivity to other cephalosporins. Use cautiously in patients with history of sensitivity to penicillin. Ask patient if he's had any previous reaction to cephalosporin or penicillin therapy before administering first dose.
• Obtain cultures for sensitivity tests before first dose, but therapy may begin pending test results.
• Prolonged use may result in overgrowth of nonsusceptible organisms. Watch carefully for superinfection.
• A third-generation cephalosporin with the longest half-life of any available cephalosporin. Allows once-daily dose regimen.
• Dosage adjustment generally not needed in patients with renal insufficiency.
• Commonly used in home antibiotic

Italicized side effects are common or life-threatening.
*Liquid form contains alcohol.   **May contain tartrazine.

programs for outpatient treatment of serious infections, such as osteomyelitis.

cefuroxime sodium
Zinacef♦
Pregnancy Category: B

MECHANISM OF ACTION
Inhibits cell-wall synthesis, promoting osmotic instability. Usually bactericidal.

INDICATIONS & DOSAGE
Treatment of serious infections of the lower respiratory and urinary tract; skin and skin structure infections; septicemia, meningitis, and gonorrhea. Among susceptible organisms are Streptococcus pneumoniae, Hemophilus influenzae, Klebsiella *species,* Staphylococcus aureus, Streptococcus pyogenes, E. coli, Enterobacter, *and* Neisseria gonorrhoeae—
Adults: Usual dosage is 750 mg to 1.5 g I.M. or I.V. q 8 hours, usually for 5 to 10 days. For life-threatening infections and infections caused by less susceptible organisms, 1.5 g I.M. or I.V. q 6 hours; for bacterial meningitis, up to 3 g I.V. q 6 hours.
Children and infants over 3 months: 50 to 100 mg/kg/day I.M. or I.V. Higher doses are administered when treating meningitis.
Total daily dosage is same for I.M. or I.V. administration and depends on susceptibility of organism and severity of infection. In patients with impaired renal function, doses or frequency of administration must be modified according to degree of renal impairment, severity of infection, and susceptibility of organism. Should be injected deep I.M. into a large muscle mass, such as gluteus or lateral aspect of thigh.

ADVERSE REACTIONS
Blood: transient neutropenia, eosino-

philia, hemolytic anemia, decrease in hemoglobin and hematocrit.
CNS: headache, malaise, paresthesias, dizziness.
GI: *pseudomembranous colitis,* nausea, anorexia, vomiting, *diarrhea,* glossitis, dyspepsia, abdominal cramps, tenesmus, anal pruritus.
GU: genital pruritus and moniliasis.
Skin: *maculopapular and erythematous rashes, urticaria.*
Local: *at injection site—pain, induration, sterile abscesses, temperature elevation, tissue sloughing; phlebitis and thrombophlebitis with I.V. injection.*
Other: hypersensitivity, dyspnea.

INTERACTIONS
Probenecid: may inhibit excretion and increase blood levels of cefuroxime.

NURSING CONSIDERATIONS
• Contraindicated in hypersensitivity to other cephalosporins. Use cautiously in patients with impaired renal function and in those with history of sensitivity to penicillin. Ask patient if he's had any reaction to previous cephalosporin or penicillin therapy before administering first dose.
• Prolonged use may result in overgrowth of nonsusceptible organisms. Watch patient carefully for superinfection.
• Obtain cultures for sensitivity tests before therapy, but therapy may begin pending results of cultures and sensitivity tests.
• Cefuroxime is a second-generation cephalosporin similar to cefamandole. However, cefuroxime has not been associated with prothrombin deficiency and bleeding as are some of the other cephalosporins. Advantage over some other cephalosporins is that cefuroxime is useful in treating meningitis.

cephalexin monohydrate
Ceporex♦♦, Keflex♦, Novolexin♦♦
Pregnancy Category: B

MECHANISM OF ACTION
Inhibits cell-wall synthesis, promoting osmotic instability. Usually bactericidal.

INDICATIONS & DOSAGE
Treatment of infections of respiratory or genitourinary tract, skin and soft-tissue infections, bone and joint infections, and otitis media due to Escherichia coli *and other coliform bacteria, group A beta-hemolytic streptococci,* Hemophilus influenzae, Klebsiella, Proteus mirabilis, Streptococcus pneumoniae, *and staphylococci*—
Adults: 250 mg to 1 g P.O. q 6 hours.
Children: 6 to 12 mg/kg P.O. q 6 hours. Maximum 25 mg/kg q 6 hours.

ADVERSE REACTIONS
Blood: transient neutropenia, eosinophilia, anemia.
CNS: dizziness, headache, malaise, paresthesias.
GI: *pseudomembranous colitis, nausea, anorexia,* vomiting, *diarrhea,* glossitis, dyspepsia, abdominal cramps, anal pruritus, tenesmus, oral candidiasis (thrush).
GU: genital pruritus and moniliasis, vaginitis.
Skin: *maculopapular and erythematous rashes, urticaria*.
Other: *hypersensitivity*, dyspnea.

INTERACTIONS
Probenecid: may increase blood levels of cephalosporins.

NURSING CONSIDERATIONS
• Use cautiously in patients with impaired renal status and in those with history of sensitivity to penicillin. Ask patient if he's had any reaction to previous cephalosporin or penicillin therapy before administering first dose.
• Prolonged use may result in overgrowth of nonsusceptible organisms. Watch closely for superinfection.
• Obtain cultures for sensitivity tests before first dose, but therapy may begin pending test results.
• Tell patient to take medication exactly as prescribed, even after he feels better. Group A beta-hemolytic streptococcal infections should be treated for a minimum of 10 days.
• Tell patient to take with food or milk to lessen GI discomfort.
• Call doctor if skin rash develops.
• Preparation of oral suspension: add required amount of water to powder in two portions. Shake well after each addition. After mixing, store in refrigerator. Stable for 14 days without significant loss of potency. Keep tightly closed and shake well before using.
• About 40% to 75% of patients receiving cephalosporins show a false-positive direct Coombs' test, but only a few of these indicate hemolytic anemia.
• Urine glucose determinations may be false-positive with copper sulfate tests (Clinitest); glucose-enzymatic tests (Clinistix, Tes-Tape) are not affected.

cephalothin sodium
Ceporacin♦♦,Keflin♦, Seffin
Pregnancy Category: B

MECHANISM OF ACTION
Inhibits cell-wall synthesis, promoting osmotic instability. Usually bactericidal.

INDICATIONS & DOSAGE
Treatment of serious infections of respiratory, genitourinary, or gastrointestinal tract; skin and soft-tissue infections (including peritonitis); bone and joint infections; septicemia; endocarditis; and meningitis due to Esche-

richia coli *and other coliform bacteria, Enterobacteriaceae, enterococci, gonococci, group A beta-hemolytic streptococci,* Hemophilus influenzae, Klebsiella, Proteus mirabilis, Salmonella, Staphylococcus aureus, Shigella, Streptococcus pneumoniae, *staphylococci, and* Streptococcus viridans—

Adults: 500 mg to 1 g I.M. or I.V. (or intraperitoneally) q 4 to 6 hours; in life-threatening infections, up to 2 g q 4 hours.

Children: 14 to 27 mg/kg I.V. q 4 hours, or 20 to 40 mg/kg q 6 hours; dose should be proportionately less in accordance with age, weight, and severity of infection.

Dosage schedule is determined by degree of renal impairment, severity of infection, and susceptibility of causative organism. Should be injected deep I.M. into a large muscle mass, such as gluteus or lateral aspect of thigh. I.V. route is preferable in severe or life-threatening infections.

ADVERSE REACTIONS

Blood: transient neutropenia, eosinophilia, hemolytic anemia.
CNS: headache, malaise, paresthesias, dizziness.
GI: *pseudomembranous colitis,* nausea, anorexia, vomiting, *diarrhea,* glossitis, dyspepsia, abdominal cramps, tenesmus, anal pruritus, oral candidiasis (thrush).
GU: *nephrotoxicity,* genital pruritus and moniliasis.
Skin: *maculopapular and erythematous rashes, urticaria.*
Local: *at injection site—pain, induration, sterile abscesses, tissue sloughing; phlebitis and thrombophlebitis with I.V. injection.*
Other: *hypersensitivity,* dyspnea, temperature elevation.

INTERACTIONS

Probenecid: may increase blood levels of cephalosporins. Use together cau-

tiously.
Aminoglycosides: increased nephrotoxicity. Monitor kidney function tests carefully.

NURSING CONSIDERATIONS

• Use cautiously in patients with impaired renal function and in those with history of sensitivity to penicillin. Ask patient if he's had any reaction to previous cephalosporin or penicillin therapy before administering first dose.
• Obtain cultures for sensitivity tests before first dose, but therapy may begin pending test results.
• Prolonged use may result in overgrowth of nonsusceptible organisms. Watch for superinfection.
• Drug causes severe pain when administered I.M.; avoid this route if possible.
• When giving this drug I.V., check frequently for vein irritation and phlebitis. Alternate injection sites if I.V. therapy lasts longer than 3 days. Use of small I.V. needle in the larger available veins may be preferable. Addition of a small concentration of heparin (100 units) or hydrocortisone (10 to 25 mg) may reduce incidence of phlebitis.
• For I.M. administration, reconstitute each gram of cephalothin sodium with 4 ml of sterile water for injection, providing 500 mg in each 2.2 ml. If vial contents do not dissolve completely, add an additional 0.2 to 0.4 ml diluent, and warm contents slightly.
• For I.V. administration, dilute contents of 4-g vial with at least 20 ml of sterile water for injection, dextrose 5% injection, or 0.9% sodium chloride injection and add to one of following I.V. solutions: acetated Ringer's injection, dextrose 5% injection, dextrose 5% in lactated Ringer's injection, Ionosol B in dextrose 5% in water, lactated Ringer's injection, Normosol-N in dextrose 5% in water,

Plasma-Lyte injection, Plasma-Lyte-N injection in dextrose 5%, Ringer's injection, or 0.9% sodium chloride injection. Choose solution and fluid volume according to patient's fluid and electrolyte status.

• About 40% to 75% of patients receiving cephalosporins show a false-positive direct Coombs' test; only a few of these indicate hemolytic anemia.

• Urine glucose determinations may be false-positive with copper sulfate tests (Clinitest); glucose-enzymatic tests (Clinistix, Tes-Tape) are not affected.

---

cephapirin sodium
Cefadyl♦
Pregnancy Category: B

MECHANISM OF ACTION
Inhibits cell-wall synthesis, promoting osmotic instability. Usually bactericidal.

INDICATIONS & DOSAGE
Serious infections of respiratory, genitourinary, or gastrointestinal tract; skin and soft-tissue infections; bone and joint infections (including osteomyelitis); septicemia; endocarditis due to Streptococcus pneumoniae, Escherichia coli, *group A beta-hemolytic streptococci,* Hemophilus influenzae, Klebsiella, Proteus mirabilis, Staphylococcus aureus, *and* Streptococcus viridans—
Adults: 500 mg to 1 g I.V. or I.M. q 4 to 6 hours up to 12 g daily.
Children over 3 months: 10 to 20 mg/kg I.V. or I.M. q 6 hours; dose depends on age, weight, and severity of infection.
Should be injected deep I.M. into a large muscle mass, such as gluteus or lateral aspect of thigh. Depending on causative organism and severity of infection, patients with reduced renal function may be treated adequately with a lower dose (7.5 to 15 mg/kg q 12 hours). Patients with severely reduced renal function and who are to be dialyzed should receive same dose just before dialysis and q 12 hours thereafter.

ADVERSE REACTIONS
Blood: transient neutropenia, eosinophilia, anemia.
CNS: dizziness, headache, malaise, paresthesias.
GI: *pseudomembranous colitis,* nausea, anorexia, vomiting, *diarrhea,* glossitis, dyspepsia, abdominal cramps, tenesmus, anal pruritus, oral candidiasis (thrush).
GU: genital pruritus and moniliasis, vaginitis.
Skin: *maculopapular and erythematous rashes, urticaria.*
Local: *at injection site—pain, induration, sterile abscesses, tissue sloughing; phlebitis and thrombophlebitis with I.V. injection.*
Other: *hypersensitivity,* dyspnea.

INTERACTIONS
Probenecid: may increase blood levels of cephalosporins.

NURSING CONSIDERATIONS
• Use cautiously in patients with impaired renal function and in those with a history of sensitivity to penicillin. Ask patient if he's had any reaction to previous cephalosporin or penicillin therapy before administering first dose.
• Prolonged use may result in overgrowth of nonsusceptible organisms. Watch for superinfection.
• Obtain cultures for sensitivity tests before first dose, but therapy may begin pending test results.
• For I.M. administration, reconstitute 1-g vial with 2 ml sterile water for injection or bacteriostatic water for injection so that 1.2 ml contains 500 mg of cephapirin. I.M. injection is painful; prepare patient for this.

Italicized side effects are common or life-threatening.
*Liquid form contains alcohol.   **May contain tartrazine.

• When giving this drug I.V., check frequently for vein irritation and phlebitis. Alternate injection sites if I.V. therapy lasts longer than 3 days. Use of small I.V. needles in the larger available veins may be preferable.

• Prepare I.V. infusion using dextrose injection, sodium chloride injection, or bacteriostatic water for injection as diluent: 20 ml yields 1 g per 10 ml; 50 ml yields 1 g per 25 ml; 100 ml yields 1 g per 50 ml.

• I.V. infusion with Y-tubing: during infusion of cephapirin solution, it is desirable to stop other solution. Check volume of cephapirin solution carefully so that calculated dose is infused. When Y-tubing is used, dilute 4-g vial with 40 ml of diluent.

• Reconstituted cephapirin is stable and compatible for 10 days under refrigeration and for 24 hours at room temperature.

• About 40% to 75% of patients receiving cephalosporins show a false-positive direct Coombs' test, but only a few indicate hemolytic anemia.

• Urine glucose determinations may be false-positive with copper sulfate tests (Clinitest); glucose-enzymatic tests (Clinistix, Tes-Tape) are not affected.

cephradine
Anspor, Velosef♦**
Pregnancy Category: B

MECHANISM OF ACTION
Inhibits cell-wall synthesis, promoting osmotic instability. Usually bactericidal.

INDICATIONS & DOSAGE
Serious infection of respiratory, genitourinary, or gastrointestinal tract; skin and soft-tissue infections; bone and joint infections; septicemia; endocarditis; and otitis media due to Escherichia coli *and other coliform bacteria, group A beta-hemolytic strepto-cocci,* Hemophilus influenzae, Klebsiella, Proteus mirabilis, Staphylococcus aureus, Streptococcus pneumoniae, *staphylococci, and* Streptococcus viridans—
Adults: 500 mg to 1 g I.M. or I.V. 2 to 4 times daily; do not exceed 8 g daily. Or 250 to 500 mg P.O. q 6 hours. Severe or chronic infections may require larger and/or more frequent doses (up to 1 g P.O. q 6 hours).
Children over 1 year: 6 to 12 mg/kg P.O. q 6 hours. 12 to 25 mg/kg I.M. or I.V. q 6 hours.
Otitis media—19 to 25 mg/kg P.O. q 6 hours. Do not exceed 4 g daily.
All patients, regardless of age and weight: larger doses (up to 1 g q.i.d.) may be given for severe or chronic infections. Parenteral therapy may be followed by oral. Injections should be given deep I.M. into a large muscle mass, such as gluteus or lateral aspect of thigh.

ADVERSE REACTIONS
Blood: transient neutropenia, eosinophilia.
CNS: dizziness, headache, malaise, paresthesias.
GI: *pseudomembranous colitis, nausea, anorexia,* vomiting, heartburn, glossitis, dyspepsia, abdominal cramping, *diarrhea,* tenesmus, anal pruritus, oral candidiasis (thrush).
GU: genital pruritus and moniliasis, vaginitis.
Skin: *maculopapular and erythematous rashes, urticaria.*
Local: *at injection site—pain, induration, sterile abscesses, tissue sloughing; phlebitis and thrombophlebitis with I.V. injection.*
Other: *hypersensitivity,* dyspnea.

INTERACTIONS
Probenecid: may increase blood levels of cephalosporins.

NURSING CONSIDERATIONS
• Contraindicated in hypersensitivity

to other cephalosporins.
• Use cautiously in patients with impaired renal function and in those with a history of sensitivity to penicillin. Ask patient if he's had any reaction to previous cephalosporin or penicillin therapy before administering first dose.
• Obtain cultures for sensitivity tests before first dose, but therapy may begin pending test results.
• Prolonged use may result in overgrowth of nonsusceptible organisms. Watch for superinfection.
• When giving this drug I.V., check frequently for vein irritation and phlebitis. Alternate injection sites if I.V. therapy lasts longer than 3 days. Use of small I.V. needle in the larger available veins may be preferable.
• Tell patient to take medication exactly as prescribed, even after he feels better. Group A beta-hemolytic streptococcal infections should be treated for a minimum of 10 days.
• Tell patient to take the oral dosage form with food or milk to lessen GI discomfort.
• I.M. injection is painful.
• For I.M. administration, reconstitute with sterile water for injection or with bacteriostatic water for injection as follows: 1.2 ml to 250-mg vial; 2 ml to 500-mg vial; 4 ml to 1-g vial. I.M. solutions must be used within 2 hours if kept at room temperature and within 24 hours if refrigerated. Solutions may vary in color from light straw to yellow without affecting potency.
• When preparing cephradine for intravenous administration, when available, use preparation specifically supplied for infusion. Follow specific product directions carefully when reconstituting.
• About 40% to 75% of patients receiving cephalosporins show a false-positive direct Coombs' test, but only a few indicate hemolytic anemia.
• Urine glucose determinations may

be false-positive with copper sulfate tests (Clinitest); glucose-enzymatic tests (Clinistix, Tes-Tape) are not affected.
• Cephradine is the only cephalosporin available in both oral and injectable forms.

moxalactam disodium
Moxam♦
Pregnancy Category: C

MECHANISM OF ACTION
Inhibits cell-wall synthesis, promoting osmotic instability. Usually bactericidal.

INDICATIONS & DOSAGE
Treatment of serious infections of lower respiratory and urinary tract, CNS infections, intraabdominal infections, gynecologic infections, bacteremia, septicemia, and skin infections. Susceptible microorganisms include Streptococcus pneumoniae *and* pyogenes; Staphylococcus aureus *(penicillinase- and nonpenicillinase-producing);* Staphylococcus epidermidis; Escherichia coli; Klebsiella; Hemophilus influenzae; Enterobacter; Proteus; *some* Pseudomonas *species; and* Peptostreptococcus—
Adults: Usual daily dose is 2 to 6 g I.M. or I.V. administered in divided doses q 8 hours for 5 to 10 days, or up to 14 days. Up to 12 g daily may be needed in life-threatening infections or in infections due to less susceptible organisms.
Children: 50 mg/kg I.M. or I.V. q 6 to 8 hours.
Neonates: 50 mg/kg I.M. or I.V. q 8 to 12 hours.
Total daily dosage is same for I.M. or I.V. administration and depends on susceptibility of organism and severity of infection. In patients with impaired renal function, doses or frequency of administration must be modified according to degree of im-

pairment, severity of infection, and susceptibility of organism. Should be injected deep I.M. into the gluteus or lateral aspect of thigh.

ADVERSE REACTIONS
Blood: transient neutropenia, eosinophilia, hemolytic anemia, *hypoprothrombinemia, bleeding*.
CNS: headache, malaise, paresthesias, dizziness.
GI: *pseudomembranous colitis,* nausea, anorexia, vomiting, *diarrhea,* glossitis, dyspepsia, abdominal cramps, tenesmus, pruritus ani, oral candidiasis (thrush).
GU: genital moniliasis.
Skin: *maculopapular and erythematous rashes, urticaria.*
Local: *pain at injection site, induration, sterile abscesses, tissue sloughing; phlebitis and thrombophlebitis with I.V. injection.*
Other: *hypersensitivity,* dyspnea, elevated temperature.

INTERACTIONS
Ethyl alcohol: may cause a disulfiram-like reaction. Warn patients not to drink alcohol for several days after discontinuing moxalactam.

NURSING CONSIDERATIONS
• Contraindicated in hypersensitivity to other cephalosporins. Use cautiously in patients with impaired renal function and in those with history of sensitivity to penicillin. Before administering first dose, ask patient if he's had any reaction to cephalosporin or penicillin.
• Prolonged use may result in overgrowth of nonsusceptible organisms. Monitor closely for superinfection.
• Obtain cultures for sensitivity tests before therapy. Unnecessary to wait for culture and sensitivity results before starting therapy.
• Moxalactam is one of the third-generation cephalosporins.
• For direct intermittent I.V. administration, add 10 ml of sterile water for injection, dextrose 5% injection, or 0.9% NaCl injection/g of moxalactam.
• Bleeding associated with hypoprothrombinemia can be prevented with vitamin K. Doctor may order 10 mg vitamin K per week to be given prophylactically.
• The chemical structure of this drug includes the methylthiotetrazole (MTT) side chain that has been associated with bleeding disorders. If bleeding occurs, it can be promptly reversed with the administration of vitamin K. Monitor prothrombin times regularly.
• Moxalactam does not interefere with urine glucose determinations.

13

Tetracyclines

demeclocycline hydrochloride
doxycycline hyclate
minocycline hydrochloride
oxytetracycline hydrochloride
tetracycline hydrochloride

COMBINATION PRODUCTS
MYSTECLIN-F CAPS: tetracycline HCl 250 mg and amphotericin B 50 mg buffered with potassium metaphosphate.
MYSTECLIN-F SYRUP: tetracycline HCl 125 mg and amphotericin B 25 mg per 5 ml, buffered with potassium metaphosphate.
For additional combinations, see Chapter 15, URINARY TRACT ANTISEPTICS.

---

demeclocycline hydrochloride
Declomycin♦, Ledermycin
Pregnancy Category: D

MECHANISM OF ACTION
Exerts bacteriostatic effect by binding to the 30S ribosomal subunit of microorganisms, thus inhibiting protein synthesis.

INDICATIONS & DOSAGE
Infections caused by susceptible gram-negative and gram-positive organisms, trachoma, rickettsiae—
Adults: 150 mg P.O. q 6 hours or 300 mg P.O. q 12 hours.
Children over 8 years: 6 to 12 mg/kg P.O. daily, divided q 6 to 12 hours.
Gonorrhea—
Adults: 600 mg P.O. initially, then 300 mg P.O. q 12 hours for 4 days (total 3 g).
Uncomplicated urethral, endocervical, or rectal infection caused by Chlamydia trachomatis—
Adults: 300 mg P.O. q.i.d. for at least 7 days.
Syndrome of inappropriate ADH (a hyposmolar state)—
Adults: 600 to 1,200 mg P.O. daily in divided doses.

ADVERSE REACTIONS
Blood: neutropenia, eosinophilia.
CV: pericarditis.
EENT: dysphagia, glossitis.
GI: anorexia, *nausea, vomiting, diarrhea,* enterocolitis, anogenital inflammation.
Metabolic: *increased BUN,* diabetes insipidus syndrome (polyuria, polydipsia, weakness).
Skin: *maculopapular and erythematous rashes, photosensitivity, increased pigmentation, urticaria.*
Other: hypersensitivity.

INTERACTIONS
Antacids (including NaHCO₃) and laxatives containing aluminum, magnesium, or calcium; food, milk, or other dairy products: decrease antibiotic absorption. Give antibiotic 1 hour before or 2 hours after any of the above.
Ferrous sulfate and other iron products, zinc: decrease antibiotic absorption. Give demeclocycline 3 hours after or 2 hours before iron administration.
Methoxyflurane: may cause nephro-

---

toxicity with tetracyclines. Monitor carefully.

NURSING CONSIDERATIONS

• Use with extreme caution in impaired renal or hepatic function. Use of these drugs during last half of pregnancy and in children younger than 8 years may cause permanent discoloration of teeth, enamel defects, and retardation of bone growth.

• Obtain cultures before starting therapy.

• Check expiration date. Outdated or deteriorated demeclocycline may cause nephrotoxicity.

• Do not expose these drugs to light or heat; store in tight container.

• Watch for overgrowth of nonsusceptible organisms. Check patient's tongue for signs of monilia infection. Stress good oral hygiene. If superinfection occurs, drug should be discontinued.

• Observe patient for diarrhea, which may result from local irritation or superinfection.

• Warn patient to avoid direct sunlight and ultraviolet light. A sunscreen may help prevent photosensitivity reactions. Photosensitivity persists for some time after discontinuation of drug.

• Effectiveness is reduced when taken with milk or other dairy products, food, antacids, or iron products. Explain this to patient. Tell patient to take each dose with a full glass of water on an empty stomach, at least 1 hour before meals or 2 hours afterward. Give at least 1 hour before bedtime to prevent esophagitis.

• Instruct patient to take medication for as long as prescribed, exactly as prescribed, even after he feels better.

• May cause false-negative reading of Clinistix or Tes-Tape.

doxycycline hyclate
Doxy-100, Doxy-200, Doxy-Caps, Doxychel, Doxy-Lemmon, Doxy-Tabs, Vibramycin♦, Vibra Tabs
Pregnancy Category: D

MECHANISM OF ACTION
Exerts bacteriostatic effect by binding to the 30S ribosomal subunit of microorganisms, thus inhibiting protein synthesis.

INDICATIONS & DOSAGE
Infections caused by sensitive gram-negative and gram-positive organisms, trachoma, rickettsiae, Mycoplasma, and Chlamydia—
Adults: 100 mg P.O. q 12 hours on first day, then 100 mg P.O. daily; or 200 mg I.V. on first day in 1 or 2 infusions, then 100 to 200 mg I.V. daily.
Children over 8 years (under 45 kg): 4.4 mg/kg P.O. or I.V. daily, divided q 12 hours first day, then 2.2 to 4.4 mg/kg daily. Over 45 kg, same as adults.

Give I.V. infusion slowly (minimum 1 hour). Infusion must be completed within 12 hours (within 6 hours in lactated Ringer's solution or dextrose 5% in lactated Ringer's solution).
Gonorrhea in patients allergic to penicillin—
Adults: 200 mg P.O. initially, followed by 100 mg P.O. at bedtime, and 100 mg P.O. b.i.d. for 3 days; or 300 mg P.O. initially and repeat dose in 1 hour.
Primary or secondary syphilis in patients allergic to penicillin—
Adults: 300 mg P.O. daily in divided doses for 10 days.
Uncomplicated urethral, endocervical or rectal infections caused by Chlamydia trachomatis *or* Ureaplasma urealyticum—
Adults: 100 mg P.O. b.i.d. for at least 7 days.
To prevent "Traveler's Diarrhea" commonly caused by enterotoxigenic E.

coli—
Adults: 100 mg P.O. daily.

ADVERSE REACTIONS
Blood: neutropenia, eosinophilia.
CNS: intracranial hypertension.
CV: pericarditis.
EENT: sore throat, glossitis, dysphagia.
GI: anorexia, *epigastric distress, nausea*, vomiting, *diarrhea*, enterocolitis, anogenital inflammation.
Skin: *maculopapular and erythematous rashes, photosensitivity, increased pigmentation, urticaria.*
Local: thrombophlebitis.
Other: hypersensitivity.

INTERACTIONS
Antacids (including NaHCO₃) and laxatives containing aluminum, magnesium, or calcium: decrease antibiotic absorption. Give antibiotic 1 hour before or 2 hours after any of the above.
Ferrous sulfate and other iron products, zinc: decrease antibiotic absorption. Give doxycycline 3 hours after or 2 hours before iron administration.
Phenobarbital, carbamazepine, alcohol: decrease antibiotic effect. Avoid if possible.

NURSING CONSIDERATIONS
• Use of these drugs during last half of pregnancy and in children younger than 8 years may cause permanent discoloration of teeth, enamel defects, and retardation of bone growth.
• Patient may develop thrombophlebitis with I.V. administration.
• Obtain cultures before starting therapy.
• Check expiration date.
• Don't expose drug to light or heat. Protect from sunlight during infusion.
• Watch for overgrowth of nonsusceptible organisms. Check patient's tongue for signs of monilia infection. Stress good oral hygiene. If superinfection occurs, drug should be discon-

tinued.
• Observe patient for diarrhea, which may result from local irritation or superinfection.
• May be taken with milk or food if GI side effects develop.
• Do not give with antacids.
• Tell patient to take medication exactly as prescribed, even after he feels better.
• Reconstitute powder for injection with sterile water for injection. Use 10 ml in 100-mg vial and 20 ml in 200-mg vial. Dilute solution to 100 to 1,000 ml for I.V. infusion. Do not infuse solutions more concentrated than 1 mg/ml.
• Reconstituted solution is stable for 72 hours refrigerated.
• Doxycycline may be used in patients with renal impairment; does not accumulate or cause a significant rise in BUN.
• Parenteral form may cause false-positive reading of Clinitest. All forms may cause false-negative reading of Clinistix or Tes-Tape.
• Should not be taken within 1 hour of bedtime because of increased incidence of dysphagia.

minocycline hydrochloride
Minocin♦*, Vectrin*
Pregnancy Category: D

MECHANISM OF ACTION
Exerts bacteriostatic effect by binding to the 30S ribosomal subunit of microorganisms, thus inhibiting protein synthesis.

INDICATIONS & DOSAGE
Infections caused by sensitive gram-negative and gram-positive organisms, trachoma, amebiasis—
Adults: initially, 200 mg P.O., I.V.; then 100 mg q 12 hours or 50 mg P.O. q 6 hours.
Children over 8 years: initially, 4 mg/kg P.O., I.V.; then 4 mg/kg P.O.

Italicized side effects are common or life-threatening.
*Liquid form contains alcohol.   **May contain tartrazine.

daily, divided q 12 hours. Give I.V. in 500 to 1,000 ml solution without calcium, over 6 hours.
Gonorrhea in patients sensitive to penicillin—
Adults: initially, 200 mg, then 100 mg q 12 hours for 4 days.
Syphilis in patients sensitive to penicillin—
Adults: initially, 200 mg, then 100 mg q 12 hours for 10 to 15 days.
Meningococcal carrier state—
100 mg P.O. q 12 hours for 5 days.
Uncomplicated urethral, endocervical, or rectal infection caused by Chlamydia trachomatis *or* Ureaplasma urealyticam—
Adults: 100 mg b.i.d. for at least 7 days.
Uncomplicated gonoccocal urethritis in men—
Adults: 100 mg b.i.d. for 5 days.

ADVERSE REACTIONS
Blood: neutropenia, eosinophilia.
CNS: *light-headedness, dizziness from vestibular toxicity.*
CV: pericarditis.
EENT: dysphagia, glossitis.
GI: *anorexia,* epigastric distress, *nausea,* vomiting, *diarrhea,* enterocolitis, inflammatory lesions in anogenital region.
Metabolic: increased BUN.
Skin: *maculopapular and erythematous rashes, photosensitivity, increased pigmentation, urticaria.*
Local: *thrombophlebitis.*
Other: hypersensitivity.

INTERACTIONS
Antacids (including NaHCO₃) and laxatives containing aluminum, magnesium, or calcium: decrease antibiotic absorption. Give antibiotic 1 hour before or 2 hours after any of the above.
Ferrous sulfate and other iron products, zinc: decrease antibiotic absorption. Tetracyclines should be given 3 hours after or 2 hours before iron administration.
Methoxyflurane: may cause severe nephrotoxicity with tetracyclines. Monitor carefully.

NURSING CONSIDERATIONS
• Use with extreme caution in patients with impaired renal or hepatic function. Use during last half of pregnancy and in children younger than 8 years may cause permanent discoloration of teeth, enamel defects, and retardation of bone growth.
• Patient may develop thrombophlebitis with I.V. administration of this drug. Avoid extravasation.
• Obtain cultures before starting therapy.
• Check expiration date.
• Do not expose these drugs to light or heat. Keep cap tightly closed.
• Watch for overgrowth of nonsusceptible organisms. Check patient's tongue for signs of monilia infection. Stress good oral hygiene. If superinfection occurs, drug should be discontinued.
• Observe patient for diarrhea, which may result from local irritation or superinfection.
• May be taken with food. Tell patient to take medication exactly as prescribed, even after he feels better.
• May cause tooth discoloration in young adults. Observe for brown pigmentation and inform doctor if it occurs.
• Reconstitute 100 mg powder with 5 ml sterile water for injection, with further dilution of 500 to 1,000 ml for I.V. infusion. Stable for 24 hours at room temperature.
• Parenteral form may cause false-positive reading of Clinitest. All forms may cause false-negative reading of Clinistix or Tes-Tape.

oxytetracycline hydrochloride

Dalimycin, E.P. Mycin, Oxlopar, Oxy-Kesso-Tetra, Oxytetraclor, Terramycin♦, Uri-tet
Pregnancy Category: D

MECHANISM OF ACTION

Exerts bacteriostatic effect by binding to the 30S ribosomal subunit of microorganisms, thus inhibiting protein synthesis.

INDICATIONS & DOSAGE

Infections caused by sensitive gram-negative and gram-positive organisms, trachoma, rickettsiae—
Adults: 250 mg P.O. q 6 hours; 100 mg I.M. q 8 to 12 hours; 250 mg I.M. as a single dose.
Children over 8 years: 25 to 50 mg/kg P.O. daily, divided q 6 hours; 15 to 25 mg/kg I.M. daily, divided q 8 to 12 hours; or 10 to 20 mg/kg I.V. daily, divided q 12 hours.
Brucellosis—
Adults: 500 mg P.O. q.i.d. for 3 weeks with streptomycin 1 g I.M. q 12 hours first week, once daily second week.
Syphilis in patients sensitive to penicillin—
Adults: 30 to 40 g total dose P.O., divided equally over 10 to 15 days.
Gonorrhea in patients sensitive to penicillin—
Adults: initially, 1.5 g P.O. followed by 0.5 g q.i.d. for a total of 9 g.

ADVERSE REACTIONS

Blood: neutropenia, eosinophilia.
CNS: intracranial hypertension.
CV: pericarditis.
EENT: dysphagia, glossitis.
GI: *anorexia, nausea,* vomiting, *diarrhea,* enterocolitis, anogenital inflammation.
Metabolic: *increased BUN.*
Skin: *maculopapular and erythematous rashes, urticaria, photosensitivity, increased pigmentation.*
Local: *irritation after I.M. injection, thrombophlebitis.*
Other: hypersensitivity.

INTERACTIONS

Antacids (including NaHCO$_3$) and laxatives containing aluminum, magnesium, or calcium; food, milk, or other dairy products: decrease antibiotic absorption. Give antibiotic 1 hour before or 2 hours after.
Ferrous sulfate and other iron products, zinc: decrease antibiotic absorption. Give tetracyclines 3 hours after or 2 hours before iron administration.
Methoxyflurane: may cause severe nephrotoxicity with tetracyclines.

NURSING CONSIDERATIONS

• Use with extreme caution in patients with impaired renal or hepatic function. Use during last half of pregnancy and in children younger than 8 years may cause permanent discoloration of teeth, enamel defects, and retardation of bone growth.
• Patient may develop thrombophlebitis with I.V. administration. Avoid extravasation.
• Obtain cultures before starting therapy.
• Check expiration date. Outdated or deteriorated oxytetracycline may cause nephrotoxicity.
• Do not expose these drugs to light or heat.
• Inject I.M. dose deeply. Warn that it may be painful. Rotate sites. I.M. preparations contain a local anesthetic; ask patient about hypersensitivity to local anesthetics.
• Watch for overgrowth of nonsusceptible organisms. Check patient's tongue for signs of monilia infection. Stress good oral hygiene. If superinfection occurs, drug should be discontinued.
• Observe patient for diarrhea, which may result from local irritation or superinfection.

Italicized side effects are common or life-threatening.
*Liquid form contains alcohol.   **May contain tartrazine.

- Warn patient to avoid direct sunlight and ultraviolet light. A sunscreen may help prevent photosensitivity reactions. Photosensitivity persists for considerable time after discontinuation of drug.
- Effectiveness is reduced when taken with milk or other dairy products, food, antacids, or iron products. Explain this to patient. Tell patient to take each dose with a full glass of water on an empty stomach, at least 1 hour before meals or 2 hours afterward. Give at least 1 hour before bedtime to prevent esophagitis.
- Tell patient to take medication exactly as prescribed, even after he feels better.
- For I.V. use, reconstitute 250 mg and 500 mg powder for injection with 10 ml sterile water.
- Dilute to at least 100 ml in dextrose 5% in water, normal saline solution, or Ringer's solution. Do not mix with any other drug.
- Store reconstituted solutions in refrigerator. Stable for 48 hours.
- Parenteral form may cause false-positive reading of Clinitest. All forms may cause false-negative reading of Clinistix or Tes-Tape.

---

tetracycline hydrochloride
Achromycin♦, Achromycin V♦, Amer-Tet, Bicycline, Cefracycline♦♦, Centet-250, Cyclopar, Maso-Cycline, Medicycline♦♦, Neo-Tetrine♦♦, Nor-Tet 500, Novotetra♦♦, Panmycin**, Robitet, Sarocycline, Scotrex, SK-Tetracycline*, Sumycin, Tet-Cy, Tetra-C, Tetraclor, Tetra-Co, Tetracyn♦, Tetralan, Tetralean♦♦, Tetram, Tetramax, Tetram S, Trexin
Pregnancy Category: D

MECHANISM OF ACTION
Exerts bacteriostatic effect by binding to the 30S ribosomal subunit of microorganisms, thus inhibiting protein synthesis.

INDICATIONS & DOSAGE
Infections caused by sensitive gram-negative and gram-positive organisms, trachoma, rickettsiae, Mycoplasma, *and* Chlamydia—
Adults: 250 to 500 mg P.O. q 6 hours; 250 mg I.M. daily or 150 mg I.M. q 12 hours; or 250 to 500 mg I.V. q 8 to 12 hours (I.M. and I.V. hydrochloride salt only).
Children over 8 years: 25 to 50 mg/kg P.O. daily, divided q 6 hours; 15 to 25 mg/kg daily (maximum 250 mg) I.M. single dose or divided q 8 to 12 hours; or 10 to 20 mg/kg I.V. daily, divided q 12 hours.
Uncomplicated urethral, endocervical, or rectal infection caused by Chlamydia trachomatis—
Adults: 500 mg P.O. q.i.d. for at least 7 days.
Brucellosis—
Adults: 500 mg P.O. q 6 hours for 3 weeks with streptomycin 1 g I.M. q 12 hours week 1 and daily week 2.
Gonorrhea in patients sensitive to penicillin—
Adults: initially, 1.5 g P.O., then 500 mg q 6 hours for 7 days.
Syphilis in patients sensitive to penicillin—
Adults: 30 to 40 g total in equally divided doses over 10 to 15 days.
Acne—
Adults and adolescents: initially, 250 mg P.O. q 6 hours, then 125 to 500 mg P.O. daily or every other day.
Shigellosis—
Adults: 2.5 g P.O. in 1 dose.

ADVERSE REACTIONS
Blood: neutropenia, eosinophilia.
CNS: dizziness, headache, intracranial hypertension.
CV: pericarditis.
EENT: sore throat, glossitis, dysphagia.
GI: anorexia, *epigastric distress, nausea,* vomiting, *diarrhea,* stomatitis,

enterocolitis, inflammatory lesions in anogenital region.
Hepatic: hepatotoxicity with large doses given I.V.
Metabolic: *increased BUN.*
Skin: *maculopapular and erythematous rashes, urticaria, photosensitivity, increased pigmentation.*
Local: *irritation after I.M. injection, thrombophlebitis.*

INTERACTIONS
Antacids (including NaHCO₃) and laxatives containing aluminum, magnesium, or calcium; food, milk, or other dairy products: decrease antibiotic absorption. Give antibiotic 1 hour before or 2 hours after any of the above.
Ferrous sulfate and other iron products, zinc: decrease antibiotic absorption. Give tetracyclines 3 hours after or 2 hours before iron administration.
Methoxyflurane: may cause severe nephrotoxicity with tetracyclines.

NURSING CONSIDERATIONS
• Use with extreme caution in patients with impaired renal or hepatic function. Use during last half of pregnancy and in children younger than 8 years may cause permanent discoloration of teeth, enamel defects, and retardation of bone growth.
• Obtain cultures before starting therapy.
• Effectiveness reduced when taken with milk or other dairy products, food, antacids, or iron products. Explain this to patient. Tell patient to take each dose with a full glass of water on an empty stomach, at least 1 hour before meals or 2 hours afterward. Give at least 1 hour before bedtime to prevent esophagitis.
• Patient may develop thrombophlebitis with I.V. administration. Avoid extravasation.
• Check expiration date. Outdated or deteriorated tetracycline may cause nephrotoxicity.

• Discard I.M. solutions after 24 hours because they deteriorate. Exception: discard Achromycin solution in 12 hours.
• Do not expose to light or heat.
• Inject I.M. dose deeply. Warn patient that it may be painful. Rotate sites. I.M. preparations often contain a local anesthetic; ask patient about hypersensitivity to local anesthetics.
• Watch for overgrowth of nonsusceptible organisms. Check patient's tongue for signs of monilia infection. Stress good oral hygiene. Stop drug if superinfection occurs.
• Observe patient for diarrhea, which may result from local irritation or superinfection.
• Warn patient to avoid direct sunlight and ultraviolet light. A sunscreen may help prevent photosensitivity reactions. Photosensitivity persists after discontinuation of drug.
• Tell patient to take drug exactly as prescribed, even after he feels better.
• For I.V. use, reconstitute 100 mg and 250 mg powder for injection with 5 ml sterile water; with 10 ml for 500 mg. Further dilute in 100 to 1,000 ml volume of dextrose 5% in 0.9% saline solution. Refrigerate diluted solution for I.V. use and use within 24 hours. Exception: use Achromycin solution immediately.
• Do not mix tetracycline solution with any other I.V. additive.
• For I.M. use, reconstitute 100 mg powder for injection with 2 ml sterile water for injection. Concentration will be 50 mg/ml. Amount of diluent for 250-mg injection varies according to brand. Check with pharmacy or follow manufacturer's instructions.
• Parenteral form may cause false-positive reading of Clinitest. All forms may cause false-negative reading of Clinistix or Tes-Tape.
• Tetracycline may be used as a pleural sclerosing agent in malignant pleural effusions. Instilled through chest tube.

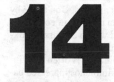

14

Sulfonamides

co-trimoxazole
sulfadiazine
sulfamethoxazole
sulfasalazine
sulfisoxazole

COMBINATION PRODUCTS
AZO GANTANOL: sulfamethoxazole 500 mg and phenazopyridine hydrochloride 100 mg.
AZO GANTRISIN: sulfisoxazole 500 mg and phenazopyridine hydrochloride 50 mg.
NEOTRIZINE: sulfadiazine 167 mg, sulfamerazine 167 mg, and sulfamethazine 167 mg.
SULFALOID: sulfadiazine 167 mg, sulfamerazine 167 mg, and sulfamethazine 167 mg.
TERFONYL: sulfadiazine 167 mg, sulfamerazine 167 mg, and sulfamethazine 167 mg.
THIOSULFIL-A: sulfamethizole 250 mg and phenazopyridine hydrochloride 50 mg.
TRIPLE SULFA: sulfadiazine 167 mg, sulfamerazine 167 mg, and sulfamethazine 167 mg.
UROBIOTIC-250: sulfamethizole 250 mg, oxytetracycline (as the hydrochloride) 250 mg, and phenazopyridine hydrochloride 50 mg.

co-trimoxazole
(sulfamethoxazole-trimethoprim)
Apo-Sulfatrim♦♦, Bactrim♦*,
Bactrim DS, Bactrim I.V. Infusion,
Cotrim, Cotrim D.S., Septra♦*,
Septra DS, Septra I.V. Infusion
Pregnancy Category: C (D if near term)

MECHANISM OF ACTION
The sulfamethoxazole component inhibits the formation of dihydrofolic acid from para-aminobenzoic acid (PABA). The trimethoprim component inhibits dihydrofolate reductase. Both decrease bacterial folic acid synthesis.

INDICATIONS & DOSAGE
Urinary tract infections and shigellosis—
Adults: 160 mg trimethoprim/800 mg sulfa (double-strength tablet) q 12 hours for 10 to 14 days in urinary tract infections and for 5 days in shigellosis. For simple cystitis or acute urethral syndrome, may give one to three double-strength tablets as a single dose.
Children: 8 mg/kg trimethoprim/40 mg/kg sulfa per 24 hours, in 2 divided doses q 12 hours (10 days for urinary tract infections; for 5 days in shigellosis).
Otitis media—
Children: 8 mg/kg trimethoprim/40 mg/kg sulfa per 24 hours, in 2 divided doses q 12 hours for 10 days.
Pneumocystis carinii pneumonitis—
Adults and children: 20 mg/kg tri-

methoprim/ 100 mg/kg sulfa per 24 hours, in equally divided doses q 6 hours for 14 days.
Chronic bronchitis—
Adults: 160 mg trimethoprim/800 mg sulfa q 12 hours for 10 to 14 days. Not recommended for infants less than 2 months old.

ADVERSE REACTIONS
Blood: *agranulocytosis, aplastic anemia,* megaloblastic anemia, thrombocytopenia, leukopenia, hemolytic anemia.
CNS: headache, mental depression, convulsions, hallucinations.
GI: *nausea, vomiting, diarrhea,* abdominal pain, anorexia, stomatitis.
GU: toxic nephrosis with oliguria and anuria, crystalluria, hematuria.
Hepatic: jaundice.
Skin: *erythema multiforme (Stevens-Johnson syndrome), generalized skin eruption, epidermal necrolysis, exfoliative dermatitis,* photosensitivity, urticaria, pruritus.
Other: *hypersensitivity, serum sickness, drug fever, anaphylaxis.*

INTERACTIONS
Ammonium chloride, ascorbic acid: doses sufficient to acidify urine may cause precipitation of sulfonamide and crystalluria. Don't use together.

NURSING CONSIDERATIONS
• Contraindicated in patients with porphyria. Use cautiously and in reduced dosages in patients with impaired hepatic or renal function and in those with severe allergy or bronchial asthma, G-6-PD deficiency, blood dyscrasias.
• Adverse reactions, especially hypersensitivity reactions, occur much more frequently in AIDS patients.
• I.V. infusion must be diluted in dextrose 5% in water prior to administration. Don't mix with other drugs or solutions.
• I.V. infusion must be infused slowly

over 60 to 90 minutes. Don't give by rapid infusion or bolus injection. Must be used within 2 hours of mixing. Do not refrigerate.
• This combination is often used in extremely ill immunosuppressed patients when prescribed for treatment of *Pneumocystis* pneumonia.
• Oral suspension available.
• Note that the "DS" product means "double strength."
• Promptly report skin rash, sore throat, fever, or mouth sores—early signs of blood dyscrasias.
• Used effectively for treatment of chronic bacterial prostatitis.
• Used prophylactically for recurrent urinary tract infections in women and for "Traveler's diarrhea."

---

sulfadiazine
Microsulfon
Pregnancy Category: B (D if near term)

MECHANISM OF ACTION
Inhibits formation of dihydrofolic acid from para-aminobenzoic acid (PABA), decreasing bacterial folic acid synthesis.

INDICATIONS & DOSAGE
Urinary tract infection—
Adults: initially, 2 to 4 g P.O., then 500 mg to 1 g P.O. q 6 hours.
Children: initially, 75 mg/kg or 2 g/m^2 P.O., then 150 mg/kg or 4 g/m^2 P.O. in 4 to 6 divided doses daily. Maximum daily dose 6 g.
Rheumatic fever prophylaxis, as an alternative to penicillin—
Children over 30 kg: 1 g P.O. daily.
Children under 30 kg: 500 mg P.O. daily.
Adjunctive treatment in toxoplasmosis—
Adults: 4 g P.O. in divided doses q 6 hours for 3 to 4 weeks, discontinued for 1 week; given with pyrimethamine 25 mg P.O. daily for 3 to 4 weeks.

Italicized side effects are common or life-threatening.
*Liquid form contains alcohol.   **May contain tartrazine.

Children: 100 mg/kg P.O. in divided doses q 6 hours for 3 to 4 weeks; given with pyrimethamine 2 mg/kg daily for 3 days, then 1 mg/kg daily for 3 to 4 weeks.

ADVERSE REACTIONS

Blood: *agranulocytosis, aplastic anemia,* megaloblastic anemia, thrombocytopenia, leukopenia, hemolytic anemia.
CNS: headache, mental depression, convulsions, hallucinations.
GI: *nausea, vomiting, diarrhea,* abdominal pain, anorexia, stomatitis.
GU: toxic nephrosis with oliguria and anuria, crystalluria, hematuria.
Hepatic: jaundice.
Skin: *erythema multiforme (Stevens-Johnson syndrome), generalized skin eruption, epidermal necrolysis, exfoliative dermatitis,* photosensitivity, urticaria, pruritus.
Local: irritation, extravasation.
Other: *hypersensitivity, serum sickness, drug fever, anaphylaxis.*

INTERACTIONS

Ammonium chloride, ascorbic acid: doses sufficient to acidify urine may cause precipitation of sulfonamide and crystalluria. Don't use together.
PABA-containing drugs: inhibit antibacterial action. Don't use together.

NURSING CONSIDERATIONS

• Contraindicated in patients with porphyria or in infants younger than 2 months (except in congenital toxoplasmosis). Use cautiously in reduced doses in patients with impaired hepatic or renal function, bronchial asthma, history of multiple allergies, G-6-PD deficiency, blood dyscrasias.
• Tell patient to drink a full glass of water with each dose and to drink plenty of water throughout the day to prevent crystalluria. Monitor fluid intake and urinary output. Intake should be sufficient to produce output of 1,500 ml daily (between 3,000 and 4,000 ml daily for adults). To aid in prevention of crystalluria, sodium bicarbonate may be administered to alkalinize urine. Monitor urine pH daily.
• Tell patient to take medication for as long as prescribed, even if he feels better. Warn patient to avoid direct sunlight and ultraviolet light to prevent photosensitivity reaction.
• Give drug on schedule to maintain constant blood level.
• Watch for signs of blood dyscrasias (purpura, ecchymosis, sore throat, fever, pallor). Report them immediately.
• Monitor urine cultures, CBCs, and urinalyses before and during therapy.
• Folic or folinic acid may be used during rest periods in toxoplasmosis therapy to reverse hematopoietic depression and/or anemia associated with pyrimethamine and sulfadiazine.
• Protect drug from light.

---

sulfamethoxazole
Gantanol♦, Urobak
Pregnancy Category: B (D if near term)

MECHANISM OF ACTION
Inhibits formation of dihydrofolic acid from para-aminobenzoic acid (PABA), decreasing bacterial folic acid synthesis.

INDICATIONS & DOSAGE
Urinary tract and systemic infections—
Adults: initially, 2 g P.O., then 1 g P.O. b.i.d. up to t.i.d. for severe infections.
Children and infants over 2 months: initially, 50 to 60 mg/kg P.O., then 25 to 30 mg/kg b.i.d. Maximum dose should not exceed 75 mg/kg daily.
Lymphogranuloma venereum (genital, inguinal, or anorectal infection)—
Adults: 1 g daily for at least 2 weeks.

ADVERSE REACTIONS
Blood: *agranulocytosis, aplastic anemia,* megaloblastic anemia, thrombocytopenia, leukopenia, hemolytic anemia.
CNS: headache, mental depression, convulsions, hallucinations.
GI: *nausea, vomiting, diarrhea,* abdominal pain, anorexia, stomatitis.
GU: toxic nephrosis with oliguria and anuria, crystalluria, hematuria.
Hepatic: jaundice.
Skin: *erythema multiforme (Stevens-Johnson syndrome), generalized skin eruption, epidermal necrolysis, exfoliative dermatitis,* photosensitivity, urticaria, pruritus.
Other: *hypersensitivity, serum sickness, drug fever, anaphylaxis.*

INTERACTIONS
Ammonium chloride, ascorbic acid: doses sufficient to acidify urine may cause precipitation of sulfonamide and crystalluria. Don't use together.
PABA-containing drugs: inhibit antibacterial action. Don't use together.

NURSING CONSIDERATIONS
• Contraindicated in patients with porphyria or in infants younger than 2 months (except in congenital toxoplasmosis). Use cautiously and in reduced dosages in patients with impaired hepatic or renal function and in those with severe allergy or bronchial asthma, G-6-PD deficiency, blood dyscrasias.
• Tell patient to drink a full glass of water with each dose and to drink plenty of water during the day to prevent crystalluria. Monitor fluid intake/urinary output. Intake should be sufficient to produce output of 1,500 ml daily (between 3,000 and 4,000 ml daily for adults). To aid in prevention of crystalluria, sodium bicarbonate may be administered to alkalinize urine. Monitor urine pH daily.
• Tell patient to take medication for as long as prescribed, even after he

feels better. Warn patient to avoid direct sunlight and ultraviolet light to prevent photosensitivity reaction.
• Monitor urine cultures, CBCs, and urinalyses before and during therapy.
• Sulfamethoxazole is also used in adjunctive therapy for treatment of toxoplasmosis.
• Instruct patient to report early signs of blood dyscrasias (sore throat, fever, pallor) to doctor immediately.

---

sulfasalazine
Azulfidine, Azulfidine En-Tabs, Salazopyrin♦♦, SAS-500♦
Pregnancy Category: B (D if near term)

MECHANISM OF ACTION
Inhibits formation of dihydrofolic acid from para-aminobenzoic acid (PABA), decreasing bacterial folic acid synthesis.

INDICATIONS & DOSAGE
Mild to moderate ulcerative colitis, adjunctive therapy in severe ulcerative colitis—
Adults: initially, 3 to 4 g P.O. daily in evenly divided doses; usual maintenance dose is 1.5 to 2 g P.O. daily in divided doses q 6 hours. May need to start with 1 to 2 g initially, with a gradual increase in dose to minimize adverse reactions.
Children over 2 years: initially, 40 to 60 mg/kg P.O. daily, divided into 3 to 6 doses; then 30 mg/kg daily in 4 doses. May need to start at lower dose if gastrointestinal intolerance occurs.

ADVERSE REACTIONS
Blood: *agranulocytosis, aplastic anemia,* megaloblastic anemia, thrombocytopenia, leukopenia, hemolytic anemia.
CNS: headache, mental depression, convulsions, hallucinations.
GI: *nausea, vomiting, diarrhea,* abdominal pain, anorexia, stomatitis.

Italicized side effects are common or life-threatening.
*Liquid form contains alcohol.   **May contain tartrazine.

GU: toxic nephrosis with oliguria and anuria, crystalluria, hematuria.
Hepatic: jaundice, hepatoxicity.
Skin: *erythema multiforme (Stevens-Johnson syndrome), generalized skin eruption, epidermal necrolysis, exfoliative dermatitis,* photosensitivity, urticaria, pruritus.
Other: *hypersensitivity, serum sickness, drug fever, anaphylaxis,* oligospermia, infertility.

INTERACTIONS
None significant.

NURSING CONSIDERATIONS
• Contraindicated in porphyria. Use cautiously and in reduced dosages in patients with impaired hepatic or renal function and in those with severe allergy or bronchial asthma, G-6-PD deficiency. Also contraindicated in patients with intestinal and urinary obstruction, and in patients allergic to salicylates.
• Instruct patient to take medication for as long as prescribed, even after he feels better. Warn patient to avoid direct sunlight and ultraviolet light to prevent photosensitivity reaction.
• Colors alkaline urine orange-yellow.
• Adverse reactions are usually those affecting GI tract. Minimize symptoms by spacing doses evenly and administering after food intake.
• Also available as an oral suspension.

---

sulfisoxazole
Barazole, Gantrisin♦, G-Sox, J-Sul, Lipo Gantrisin, Novosoxazole♦♦, Rosoxol, Sosol, Soxa, Soxomide, Sulfagan, Urisoxin, Urizole, Velmatrol
Pregnancy Category: B (D if near term)

MECHANISM OF ACTION
Inhibits formation of dihydrofolic

acid from para-aminobenzoic acid (PABA), decreasing bacterial folic acid synthesis.

INDICATIONS & DOSAGE
Urinary tract and systemic infections—
Adults: initially, 2 to 4 g P.O., then 1 to 2 g P.O. q.i.d.; extended-release suspension 4 to 5 g P.O. q 12 hours.
Children over 2 months: initially, 75 mg/kg P.O. daily or 2 g/m² P.O. daily in divided doses q 6 hours, then 150 mg/kg or 4 g/m² P.O. daily in divided doses q 6 hours; extended-release suspension 60 to 70 mg/kg P.O. q 12 hours.

ADVERSE REACTIONS
Blood: *agranulocytosis, aplastic anemia,* megaloblastic anemia, thrombocytopenia, leukopenia, hemolytic anemia.
CNS: headache, mental depression, convulsions, hallucinations.
GI: *nausea, vomiting, diarrhea,* abdominal pain, anorexia, stomatitis.
GU: toxic nephrosis with oliguria and anuria, crystalluria, hematuria.
Hepatic: jaundice.
Skin: *erythema multiforme (Stevens-Johnson syndrome), generalized skin eruption, epidermal necrolysis, exfoliative dermatitis,* photosensitivity, urticaria, pruritus.
Other: *hypersensitivity, serum sickness, drug fever, anaphylaxis.*

INTERACTIONS
PABA-containing drugs: inhibit antibacterial action. Don't use together.
Ammonium chloride, ascorbic acid: doses sufficient to acidify urine may cause crystalluria and precipitation of sulfonamide. Don't use together.

NURSING CONSIDERATIONS
• Contraindicated in patients with porphyria and in infants younger than 2 months (except in congenital toxoplasmosis). Use cautiously in patients

with impaired hepatic or renal function, severe allergy or bronchial asthma, G-6-PD deficiency.

• Tell patient to drink a full glass of water with each dose and to drink plenty of water throughout the day to prevent crystalluria. Monitor fluid intake and urinary output. Intake should be sufficient to produce output of 1,500 ml daily (between 3,000 and 4,000 ml daily for adults). To aid in prevention of crystalluria, sodium bicarbonate may be administered to alkalinize urine. Monitor urine pH daily.

• Tell patient to take medication for as long as prescribed, even after he feels better. Warn patient to avoid direct sunlight and ultraviolet light to prevent photosensitivity reaction.

• Monitor urine cultures, CBCs, prothrombin time, and urinalyses before and during therapy.

• Gantrisin suspension and Lipo Gantrisin suspension cannot be interchanged, since the latter is an extended-release preparation.

• Sulfisoxazole/pyrimethamine combination is used to treat toxoplasmosis.

• Tell patient to report early signs of blood dyscrasias (sore throat, fever, pallor) immediately to doctor.

• When given preoperatively, the patient should receive a low-residue diet and a minimal number of enemas and cathartics.

• Although often given, initial loading dose is not pharmacologically necessary.

Italicized side effects are common or life-threatening.
*Liquid form contains alcohol.   **May contain tartrazine.

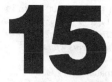

Urinary tract antiseptics

cinoxacin
methenamine hippurate
methenamine mandelate
methylene blue
nalidixic acid
nitrofurantoin
nitrofurantoin macrocrystals
norfloxacin

COMBINATION PRODUCTS
AZO GANTANOL: sulfamethoxazole 500 mg and phenazopyridine HCl 100 mg.
AZO GANTRISIN: sulfisoxazole 500 mg and phenazopyridine HCl 50 mg.
AZO-MANDELAMINE: methenamine mandelate 500 mg and phenazopyridine HCl 50 mg.
CYSTEX: methenamine 165 mg, salicylamide 65 mg, sodium salicylate 97 mg, and benzoic acid 32 mg.
CYSTISED (IMPROVED): methenamine 40.8 mg, phenyl salicylate 18.1 mg, atropine sulfate 0.03 mg, hyoscyamine 0.03 mg, benzoic acid 4.5 mg, methylene blue 5.4 mg, and gelsemium 6.1 mg.
HEXALOL: methenamine 40.8 mg, phenyl salicylate 18.1 mg, atropine sulfate 0.03 mg, hyoscyamine 0.03 mg, benzoic acid 4.5 mg, and methylene blue 5.4 mg.
PROSED: methylene blue 5.4 mg, methenamine 40.8 mg, phenyl salicylate 18.1 mg, atropine sulfate 0.03 mg, hyoscyamine 0.03 mg, and benzoic acid 4.5 mg.
THIOSULFIL-A: sulfamethizole 250 mg and phenazopyridine HCl 50 mg.
URO-PHOSPHATE: methenamine 300 mg and sodium acid phosphate 500

mg. Sugar coated.
UROQUID-ACID: methenamine mandelate 350 mg and sodium acid phosphate 200 mg.
UROQUID-ACID NO. 2: methenamine mandelate 500 mg and sodium acid phosphate 500 mg.

cinoxacin
Cinobac
Pregnancy Category: B

MECHANISM OF ACTION
Inhibits microbial DNA synthesis.

INDICATIONS & DOSAGE
Treatment of initial and recurrent urinary tract infections caused by susceptible strains of Escherichia coli, Klebsiella, Enterobacter, Proteus mirabilis, Proteus vulgaris, *and* Proteus morgani, Serratia, *and* Citrobacter—
Adults and children 12 years or older: 1 g daily, in two to four divided doses for 7 to 14 days.
Not recommended for children under age 12.

ADVERSE REACTIONS
CNS: *dizziness, headache,* drowsiness, insomnia, convulsions.
EENT: sensitivity to light.
GI: *nausea, vomiting, abdominal pain,* diarrhea.
Skin: rash, urticaria, pruritus, photosensitivity.

INTERACTIONS
Probenecid: may decrease urinary

levels of cinoxacin by inhibiting renal tubular secretion. Monitor for increased toxicity and reduced antibacterial effectiveness.

NURSING CONSIDERATIONS
• Contraindicated in patients who are hypersensitive to nalidixic acid. Use cautiously in patients with impaired renal and hepatic function.
• Not effective against *Pseudomonas,* enterococci, or staphylococci.
• Obtain clean-catch urine specimen for culture and sensitivity before starting therapy and repeat p.r.n.
• High urine levels permit twice-daily dosing.
• Report CNS side effects to doctor immediately. They indicate serious toxicity and usually mean that administration of drug should be stopped.
• Cinoxacin should be taken with meals to help decrease GI side effects.
• Warn patient about photophobic effects of drug, and advise him to avoid very bright sunlight.

---

methenamine hippurate
Hiprex**, Hip-Rex♦♦, Urex

methenamine mandelate
Mandelamine♦, Sterine♦♦
Pregnancy Category: C

MECHANISM OF ACTION
In acid urine, methenamines are hydrolyzed to ammonia and to formaldehyde, which is responsible for antibacterial action against gram-positive and gram-negative organisms. Mandelic and hippuric acids, with which methenamines are combined, are also antibacterial by unknown mechanisms.

INDICATIONS & DOSAGE
Long-term prophylaxis or suppression of chronic urinary tract infections—
Adults and children over 12 years: 1 g (hippurate) P.O. q 12 hours.

Children 6 to 12 years: 500 mg to 1 g (hippurate) P.O. q 12 hours.
Urinary tract infections, infected residual urine in patients with neurogenic bladder—
Adults: 1 g (mandelate) P.O. q.i.d. after meals.
Children 6 to 12 years: 500 mg (mandelate) P.O. q.i.d. after meals.
Children under 6 years: 50 mg/kg (mandelate) divided in 4 doses after meals.

ADVERSE REACTIONS
GI: nausea, vomiting, diarrhea.
GU: with high doses, urinary tract irritation, dysuria, frequency, albuminuria, hematuria.
Hepatic: elevated liver enzymes.
Skin: rashes.

INTERACTIONS
Alkalinizing agents: inhibit methenamine action. Don't use together.
Acetazolamide: antagonizes methenamine effect. Use together cautiously.

NURSING CONSIDERATIONS
• Contraindicated in patients with renal insufficiency, severe hepatic disease, or severe dehydration.
• Ineffective against *Candida* infection.
• Oral suspension contains vegetable oil. Administer cautiously to elderly or debilitated patients, because aspiration could cause lipid pneumonia.
• Monitor intake and output. Intake should be at least 1,500 to 2,000 ml daily.
• Obtain a clean-catch urine specimen for culture and sensitivity tests before starting therapy, and repeat p.r.n.
• Limit intake of alkaline foods, such as vegetables, milk, and peanuts. May drink cranberry, plum, and prune juices. These juices or ascorbic acid may be used to acidify urine.
• Warn patient not to take antacids, including Alka-Seltzer and sodium bi-

---

Italicized side effects are common or life-threatening.
*Liquid form contains alcohol.   **May contain tartrazine.

carbonate.
• For best results, maintain urine pH at 5.5 or less. Use Nitrazine paper to check pH. Large doses of ascorbic acid (12 g/day) may be necessary to effectively acidify urine.
• *Proteus* and *Pseudomonas* tend to raise urine pH; urinary acidifiers are usually necessary when treating these infections.
• Obtain liver function studies periodically during long-term therapy.
• Administer after meals to minimize GI upset.
• If rash appears, hold dose and contact doctor.

methylene blue
MG-Blue, Urolene Blue, Wright's Stain
Pregnancy Category: C (D if injected intra-amniotically)

MECHANISM OF ACTION
Methylene blue is a mildly antiseptic dye. High concentrations convert the ferrous iron of reduced hemoglobin to ferric iron to form methemoglobin. This mechanism is the basis for its use as an antidote in cyanide poisoning. Low concentrations of methylene blue can hasten conversion of methemoglobin to hemoglobin.

INDICATIONS & DOSAGE
Cystitis, urethritis—
Adults: 65 mg P.O. b.i.d. or t.i.d. after meals with glass of water.
Methemoglobinemia and cyanide poisoning—
Adults and children: 1 to 2 mg/kg of 1% sterile solution slow I.V.

ADVERSE REACTIONS
Blood: anemia (long-term use).
GI: nausea, vomiting, diarrhea.
GU: dysuria, bladder irritation.
Other: fever (large doses).

INTERACTIONS
None significant.

NURSING CONSIDERATIONS
• Contraindicated in patients with renal insufficiency.
• Monitor intake and output carefully. Intake should be at least 2,000 ml daily.
• Monitor hemoglobin; possibility of anemia from accelerated destruction of erythrocytes.
• Turns urine and stool blue-green.
• Seldom used as urinary tract antiseptic.
• I.V. form has been used to treat nitrite intoxication.

nalidixic acid
NegGram♦
Pregnancy Category: B

MECHANISM OF ACTION
Inhibits microbial DNA synthesis.

INDICATIONS & DOSAGE
Acute and chronic urinary tract infections caused by susceptible gram-negative organisms (Proteus, Klebsiella, Enterobacter, *and* Escherichia coli)—
Adults: 1 g P.O. q.i.d. for 7 to 14 days; 2 g daily for long-term use.
Children over 3 months: 55 mg/kg P.O. daily divided q.i.d. for 7 to 14 days; 33 mg/kg daily for long-term use.

ADVERSE REACTIONS
Blood: eosinophilia.
CNS: drowsiness, weakness, headache, dizziness, vertigo, convulsions in epileptics, confusion, hallucinations.
EENT: sensitivity to light, change in color perception, diplopia, blurred vision.
GI: *abdominal pain, nausea, vomiting,* diarrhea.
Skin: pruritus, photosensitivity, urti-

caria, rash.
Other: angioedema, fever, chills, increased intracranial pressure and bulging fontanelles in infants and children.

INTERACTIONS
None significant.

NURSING CONSIDERATIONS
• Contraindicated in patients with convulsive disorders. Use with caution in impaired hepatic or renal function, or severe cerebral arteriosclerosis. Should be used very cautiously in prepubertal children; erosion of cartilage of immature animals has been reported.
• Not effective against *Pseudomonas* or if infection's found outside of the urinary tract.
• Tell the patient to report visual disturbances; these usually disappear with reduced dose.
• Obtain culture and sensitivity tests before starting therapy and repeat p.r.n.
• Obtain CBC, renal and liver function studies during long-term therapy.
• Resistant bacteria may emerge within the first 48 hours of therapy.
• May cause a false-positive Clinitest reaction. Use Clinistix or Tes-Tape to monitor urine glucose. Also gives false elevations in urine vanillylmandelic acid (VMA) and 17-ketosteroids. Repeat tests after therapy is completed.
• Avoid undue exposure to sunlight due to photosensitivity. Patient may continue to be photosensitive for as long as 3 months after drug is discontinued.

nitrofurantoin
Furadantin, Furalan, Furantoin, J-Dantin, Nephronex♦♦, Nitrex, Novofuran♦♦, Sarodant

nitrofurantoin macrocrystals
Macrodantin♦
Pregnancy Category: B

MECHANISM OF ACTION
Bacteriostatic in low concentration and possibly bactericidal in high concentration. Interferes with bacterial enzyme systems.

INDICATIONS & DOSAGE
Pyelonephritis, pyelitis, and cystitis due to susceptible Escherichia coli, Staphylococcus aureus, *enterococci; certain strains of* Klebsiella, Proteus, *and* Enterobacter—
Adults and children over 12 years: 50 to 100 mg P.O. q.i.d. with meals. Or, 180 mg I.V. b.i.d. in patients over 54 kg; 6.6 mg/kg daily I.V. in patients under 54 kg.
Children 1 month to 12 years: 5 to 7 mg/kg P.O. daily, divided q.i.d.
Long-term suppression therapy—
Adults: 50 to 100 mg P.O. daily at bedtime.

ADVERSE REACTIONS
Blood: hemolysis in patients with G-6-PD deficiency (reversed after stopping drug), *agranulocytosis,* thrombocytopenia.
CNS: peripheral neuropathy, headache, dizziness, drowsiness, *ascending polyneuropathy with high doses or renal impairment.*
GI: *anorexia, nausea, vomiting,* abdominal pain, *diarrhea.*
Hepatic: hepatitis.
Skin: maculopapular, erythematous, or eczematous eruption; pruritus; urticaria; *exfoliative dermatitis; Stevens-Johnson syndrome.*
Other: asthmatic attacks in patients

Italicized side effects are common or life-threatening.
*Liquid form contains alcohol.   **May contain tartrazine.

with history of asthma; *anaphylaxis;* hypersensitivity; transient alopecia; drug fever; overgrowth of nonsusceptible organisms in the urinary tract; *pulmonary sensitivity reactions (cough, chest pains, fever, chills, dyspnea).*

INTERACTIONS
Magnesium-containing antacids: decreased nitrofurantoin absorption. Separate administration times by 1 hour.
Probenecid, sulfinpyrazone: increased blood levels and decreased urine levels. May result in increased toxicity and lack of therapeutic effect. Don't use together.

NURSING CONSIDERATIONS
• Contraindicated in patients with moderate-to-severe renal impairment, anuria, oliguria, creatinine clearance under 40 ml/minute; use cautiously in patients with G-6-PD deficiency.
• Hypersensitivity may develop when used for long-term therapy.
• Obtain culture and sensitivity tests before starting therapy and repeat p.r.n.
• Monitor CBC regularly.
• Give with food or milk to minimize GI distress.
• I.M. route painful and should not be used for more than 5 days.
• Dilute I.V. nitrofurantoin to 500 ml of suitable I.V. solution before administering. Constitute in sterile water without preservatives.
• Monitor intake/output carefully. May turn urine brown or darker.
• Store in amber container. Keep away from metals other than stainless steel or aluminum to avoid precipitate formation. Warn patients not to use pillboxes made of these materials.
• Continue treatment for 3 days after sterile urine specimens have been obtained.
• Monitor pulmonary status.
• Has no effect in blood or tissue outside the urinary tract.
• Use of nitrofurantoin may result in growth of nonsusceptible organisms, especially *Pseudomonas.*
• May cause false-positive results with urine sugar test using copper sulfate reduction method (Clinitest) but not with glucose oxidase tests (Tes-Tape, Diastix, Clinistix).

norfloxacin
Noroxin
Pregnancy Category: C

MECHANISM OF ACTION
Inhibits bacterial DNA synthesis, mainly by inhibiting DNA gyrase. Bactericidal.

INDICATIONS & DOSAGE
Treatment of complicated or uncomplicated urinary tract infections caused by susceptible strains of Escherichia coli, Klebsiella, Enterobacter, Proteus, Pseudomonas aeruginosa, Citrobacter, Staphylococcus aureus *(and* epidermidis*), and group D streptococci—*
Adults: For uncomplicated infections, 400 mg P.O. b.i.d. for 7 to 10 days. For complicated infections, 400 mg b.i.d. for 10 to 21 days.

ADVERSE REACTIONS
CNS: fatigue, somnolence, headache, dizziness.
GI: nausea, constipation, flatulence, heartburn.
Hepatic: transient elevations of SGOT and SGPT.
Skin: rash.

INTERACTIONS
Nitrofurantoin: decreases norfloxacin's effectiveness. Don't use together.
Antacids: may hinder absorption.

NURSING CONSIDERATIONS
• Contraindicated in patients allergic to nalidixic acid and cinoxacin.

• Warn patients not to exceed the recommended dosages. Advise them to drink several glasses of water throughout the day to maintain hydration and adequate urinary output.

• Advise patients to take the drug 1 hour before or 2 hours after meals since the presence of food may hinder absorption.

• Because norfloxacin may cause dizziness, patients should avoid hazardous activities that require alertness and good coordination until their response to this drug has been established.

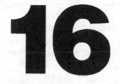

Antivirals

acyclovir sodium
amantadine hydrochloride
ribavirin
vidarabine monohydrate
zidovudine (formerly
  azidothymidine, AZT)

COMBINATION PRODUCTS
None.

---

acyclovir sodium
Zovirax♦
Pregnancy Category: C

MECHANISM OF ACTION
Becomes incorporated into viral deoxyribonucleic acid and inhibits viral multiplication.

INDICATIONS & DOSAGE
Treatment of initial and recurrent episodes of mucocutaneous herpes simplex virus (HSV-1 and HSV-2) infections in immunocompromised patients; severe initial episodes of herpes genitalis in patients who are not immunocompromised—
Adults and children over 11 years: 5 mg/kg, given at a constant rate over a period of 1 hour by I.V. infusion q 8 hours for 7 days (5 days for herpes genitalis).
Children under 12 years: 250 mg/m², given at a constant rate over a period of 1 hour by I.V. infusion q 8 hours for 7 days (5 days for herpes genitalis).
Treatment of initial genital herpes—
Adults: 200 mg P.O. q 4 hours while awake (a total of 5 capsules daily).

Treatment should continue for 10 days.
Intermittent therapy for recurrent genital herpes—
Adults: 200 mg P.O. q 4 hours while awake (a total of 5 capsules daily). Treatment should continue for 5 days. Initiate therapy at the first sign of recurrence.
Chronic suppressive therapy for recurrent genital herpes—
Adults: 200 mg P.O. t.i.d. for up to 6 months.

ADVERSE REACTIONS
CNS: (associated with I.V. dosage): *headache, encephalopathic changes (lethargy, obtundation, tremors, confusion, hallucinations, agitation, seizures, coma).*
CV: hypotension.
GI: (associated with P.O. dosage): *nausea, vomiting,* diarrhea.
GU: *transient elevations of serum creatinine,* hematuria.
Local: *inflammation, vesicular eruptions and phlebitis at injection site.*
Skin: rash, itching.

INTERACTIONS
Probenecid: increased acyclovir blood levels. Monitor for possible toxicity.

NURSING CONSIDERATIONS
For I.V. form:
• Don't administer topically, intramuscularly, orally, subcutaneously, or ophthalmically.
• Don't give by bolus injection.
• Infusion must be administered over at least 1 hour to prevent renal tubular

---

damage. Bolus injection, dehydration, preexisting renal disease, and the concomitant use of other nephrotoxic drugs increases the risk of renal toxicity.
• Notify doctor if serum creatinine level does not return to normal within a few days. He may increase hydration, adjust dose, or discontinue acyclovir.
• Encephalopathic changes are more likely in patients with neurologic disorders or in those who have had neurologic reactions to cytotoxic drugs.
• Patient must be adequately hydrated during acyclovir infusion.
For P.O. form:
• Teach patient that drug is effective in managing the disease but does not eliminate or cure it.
• Instruct patient that acyclovir will not prevent spread of infection to others.
• Urge patient to recognize the early symptoms of infection (such as tingling, itching, or pain) so he can take acyclovir before the infection fully develops.

---

amantadine hydrochloride
Symmetrel♦
Pregnancy Category: C

MECHANISM OF ACTION
Interferes with influenza A virus penetration into susceptible cells. Its action in the treatment of parkinsonism is unknown.

INDICATIONS & DOSAGE
Prophylaxis or symptomatic treatment of influenza type A virus, respiratory tract illnesses—
Adults to age 64 and children age 10 and over: 200 mg P.O. daily in a single dose or divided b.i.d.
Children 1 to 9 years: 4.4 to 8.8 mg/kg P.O. daily, divided b.i.d. or t.i.d. Don't exceed 150 mg daily.
Adults over age 64: 100 mg P.O. once daily.
Treatment should continue for 24 to 48 hours after symptoms disappear. Prophylaxis should start as soon as possible after initial exposure and continue for at least 10 days after exposure. May continue prophylactic treatment up to 90 days for repeated or suspected exposures if influenza vaccine unavailable. If used with influenza vaccine, continue dose for 2 to 3 weeks until protection from vaccine develops.
To treat drug-induced extrapyramidal reactions—
Adults: 100 mg P.O. b.i.d., up to 300 mg daily in divided doses. Patient may benefit from as much as 400 mg daily, but doses over 200 mg must be closely supervised.
To treat idiopathic parkinsonism, parkinsonian syndrome—
Adults: 100 mg P.O. b.i.d.; in patients who are seriously ill or receiving other antiparkinsonism drugs, 100 mg daily for at least 1 week, then 100 mg b.i.d., p.r.n.

ADVERSE REACTIONS
CNS: depression, fatigue, confusion, dizziness, psychosis, hallucinations, anxiety, *irritability*, ataxia, *insomnia*, weakness, headache, light-headedness, difficulty in concentrating.
CV: peripheral edema, orthostatic hypotension, congestive heart failure.
GI: anorexia, nausea, constipation, vomiting, dry mouth.
GU: urinary retention.
Skin: *livedo reticularis* (with prolonged use).

INTERACTIONS
None significant.

NURSING CONSIDERATIONS
• Use cautiously in patients with history of epilepsy, congestive heart failure, peripheral edema, hepatic disease, mental illness, eczematoid rash, renal impairment, orthostatic

---

hypotension, cardiovascular disease, and in elderly patients.
• For best absorption, drug should be taken after meals.
• Instruct patient to report side effects to the doctor, especially dizziness, depression, anxiety, nausea, and urinary retention.
• Elderly are more susceptible to neurological adverse reactions. Taking the drug in two daily doses rather than single dose may reduce their incidence.
• If orthostatic hypotension occurs, instruct patient not to stand or change positions too quickly.
• If insomnia occurs, dose should be taken several hours before bedtime.
• When prescribed for parkinsonism, warn patient against discontinuing drug abruptly since this might precipitate a parkinsonian crisis.

ribavirin
Virazole
Pregnancy Category: X

MECHANISM OF ACTION
Inhibits viral activity by an unknown mechanism. Thought to inhibit RNA and DNA synthesis by depleting intracellular nucleotide pools.

INDICATIONS & DOSAGE
Treatment of hospitalized infants and young children infected by respiratory syncytial virus (RSV)—
Infants and young children: Solution in concentration of 20 mg/ml delivered via the Viratek Small Particle Aerosol Generator (SPAG-2). Treatment is carried out for 12 to 18 hours/day for at least 3, and no more than 7, days.

ADVERSE REACTIONS
Blood: anemia, reticulocytosis.
CV: *cardiac arrest,* hypotension.
Local: *worsening of respiratory status, bacterial pneumonia, pneumo-*

thorax, apnea, ventilator dependence.

INTERACTIONS
None significant.

NURSING CONSIDERATIONS
• Contraindicated in females who are or may become pregnant during treatment with drug.
• Ribavirin aerosol is indicated only for severe lower respiratory tract infection due to respiratory syncytial virus (RSV). Although treatment may be started while awaiting diagnostic test results, existence of RSV infection must be eventually documented.
• Most infants and children with RSV infection don't require treatment because the disease is often mild and self-limiting. Infants with underlying conditions, such as prematurity or cardiopulmonary disease get RSV in its severest form, and benefit most from treatment with ribavirin aerosol.
• This treatment must be accompanied by, and does not replace, supportive respiratory and fluid management.
• Ribavirin aerosol *must* be administered by the Viratek Small Particle Aerosol Generator (SPAG-2). Don't use any other aerosol generating device.
• The water used to reconstitute this drug must not contain any antimicrobial agent. Use sterile USP water for injection, *not* bacteriostatic water.
• Discard solutions placed in the SPAG-2 unit at least every 24 hours before adding newly reconstituted solution.
• Store reconstituted solutions at room temperature for 24 hours.

vidarabine monohydrate
Vira-A♦
Pregnancy Category: C

MECHANISM OF ACTION
Becomes incorporated into viral de-

oxyribonucleic acid and inhibits viral multiplication.

INDICATIONS & DOSAGE
Herpes simplex virus encephalitis—
Adults and children (including neonates): 15 mg/kg daily for 10 days. Slowly infuse the total daily dose by I.V. infusion at a constant rate over 12-to 24-hour period. Avoid rapid or bolus injection.

ADVERSE REACTIONS
Blood: anemia, neutropenia, thrombocytopenia.
CNS: tremor, dizziness, hallucinations, confusion, psychosis, ataxia.
GI: *anorexia, nausea,* vomiting, diarrhea.
Hepatic: elevated SGOT, bilirubin.
Skin: pruritus, rash.
Local: pain at injection site.
Other: weight loss.

INTERACTIONS
Allopurinol: concurrent therapy increases risk of CNS adverse reactions.

NURSING CONSIDERATIONS
• Will reduce mortality caused by herpes simplex virus encephalitis from 70% to 28%. No evidence that vidarabine is effective in encephalitis due to other viruses.
• Don't give I.M. or subcutaneously because of low solubility and poor absorption.
• Monitor hematologic tests, such as hemoglobin, hematocrit, WBC, and platelets during therapy. Also monitor renal and liver function studies.
• Patient with impaired renal function may need dosage adjustment.
• Once in solution, vidarabine is stable at room temperature for at least 2 weeks.
• Use with an I.V. filter of 0.45 μm or smaller.
• Must be diluted to a concentration of less than 0.5 mg/ml.
• Any intravenous solution is suitable

as a diluent.

zidovudine (AZT)
Retrovir
Pregnancy Category: C

MECHANISM OF ACTION
Prevents replication of the human immunodeficiency virus (HIV) by inhibiting the enzyme reverse transcriptase.

INDICATIONS & DOSAGE
Patients with AIDS or advanced AIDS-related complex who have confirmed Pneumocystis carinii *pneumonia or a* T_4 *lymphocyte count below 200—*
Adults: 200 mg P.O. q 4 hours around the clock.

ADVERSE REACTIONS
Blood: *Severe bone marrow depression (resulting in anemia), granulocytopenia, thrombocytopenia.*
CNS: *headache,* agitation, restlessness, insomnia, confusion, anxiety.
Skin: rash, itching.

INTERACTIONS
Co-trimoxazole, acetaminophen: may impair hepatic metabolism of zidovudine, increasing the drug's toxicity.
Other cytotoxic drugs: additive adverse effects on the bone marrow.
Acyclovir: possible lethargy and fatigue. Use together cautiously.

NURSING CONSIDERATIONS
• Zidovudine frequently causes a low red blood cell count by depressing the bone marrow. Advise patients that they may need blood transfusions during treatment with zidovudine.
• The drug is in short supply and cannot be prescribed by the doctor and dispensed by the pharmacist except to patients who are declared eligible to receive zidovudine by the Burroughs-Wellcome Retrovir Center. Eligible patients are assigned unique enrollment numbers that must accompany

---

Italicized side effects are common or life-threatening.
*Liquid form contains alcohol.   **May contain tartrazine.

all prescriptions.

• Remind patients that they *must* comply with the every-4-hour dosage schedule. Suggest ways to avoid missing doses, such as the use of alarm clocks.

• Warn patients not to take any other drugs for AIDS (especially from the "street") unless their doctors have approved them. Some purported AIDS "cures" may interfere with zidovudine's effectiveness.

• The drug has been shown to temporarily decrease morbidity and mortality in certain patients with AIDS or AIDS-related complex.

• The optimum duration of treatment, as well as the dosage for optimum effectiveness and minimum toxicity, is not yet known.

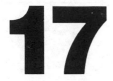

Miscellaneous anti-infectives

aztreonam
bacitracin
chloramphenicol
chloramphenicol palmitate
chloramphenicol sodium
    succinate
clindamycin hydrochloride
clindamycin palmitate
    hydrochloride
clindamycin phosphate
erythromycin base
erythromycin estolate
erythromycin ethylsuccinate
erythromycin gluceptate
erythromycin lactobionate
erythromycin stearate
imipenem/cilastatin sodium
lincomycin hydrochloride
pentamidine isethionate
polymyxin B sulfate
spectinomycin dihydrochloride
trimethoprim
vancomycin hydrochloride

COMBINATION PRODUCTS
None.

---

aztreonam
Azactam
Pregnancy Category: B

MECHANISM OF ACTION
Inhibits bacterial cell wall synthesis,
ultimately causing cell wall destruction. Bactericidal.

INDICATIONS & DOSAGE
*Treatment of urinary tract infections,
lower respiratory tract infections, septicemia, skin and skin-structure infec-*
*tions, intraabdominal infections, and
gynecologic infections caused by various gram-negative organisms—*
Adults: 500 mg to 2 g I.V. or I.M. q 8
to 12 hours. For severe systemic or
life-threatening infections, 2 g q 6 to
8 hours may be given. Maximum dose
is 8 g daily.

ADVERSE REACTIONS
GI: diarrhea, nausea, vomiting.
Hepatic: transient elevations of
SGOT and SGPT.
Local: thrombophlebitis at I.V. site,
discomfort and swelling at I.M. injec-
tion site.

INTERACTIONS
None significant.

NURSING CONSIDERATIONS
• Use cautiously in elderly patients
and in those with diminished renal
function.
• Aztreonam is a narrow-spectrum
antibiotic, effective solely against
gram-negative organisms. Because it
is ineffective against gram-positive
and anaerobic organisms, aztreonam
must be used with other antibiotics
for immediate treatment of life-
threatening illnesses.
• Patients who are allergic to penicillins or cephalosporins may not be allergic to aztreonam since there is no
cross-allergenicity.
• To administer a bolus of aztreonam,
inject it slowly (over 3 to 5 minutes)
directly into a vein or I.V. tubing.
• Intramuscular injections should be
given deep into a large muscle mass,

Italicized side effects are common or life-threatening.
*Liquid form contains alcohol.   **May contain tartrazine.

such as the upper outer quadrant of the gluteus maximus or the lateral part of the thigh.

• Aztreonam is the first commercially available member of a new antibiotic family, the monobactams. Its effectiveness against gram-negative organisms is comparable to that of the aminoglycoside antibiotics, without the ototoxicity or nephrotoxicity usually associated with the aminoglycosides.

---

bacitracin
Pregnancy Category: C

MECHANISM OF ACTION
Hinders bacterial cell-wall synthesis, damaging the bacterial plasma membrane and making the cell more vulnerable to osmotic pressure.

INDICATIONS & DOSAGE
Pneumonia or empyema caused by susceptible staphylococci—
Infants over 2.5 kg: 1,000 units/kg I.M. daily, divided q 8 to 12 hours.
Infants under 2.5 kg: 900 units/kg I.M. daily, divided q 8 to 12 hours. Although the FDA approves the use of bacitracin in infants only, adults with susceptible staphylococcal infections may receive 10,000 to 25,000 units I.M. q 6 hours (maximum 25,000 units/dose, 100,000 units daily).

ADVERSE REACTIONS
Blood: blood dyscrasias, eosinophilia.
GI: nausea, vomiting, anorexia, diarrhea, rectal itching or burning.
GU: *nephrotoxicity (albuminuria,* cylindruria, oliguria, anuria, increased BUN, tubular and glomerular necrosis).
Skin: urticaria, rash.
Local: *pain at injection site.*
Other: superinfection, fever, *anaphylaxis,* neuromuscular blockade.

INTERACTIONS
None significant.

NURSING CONSIDERATIONS
• Contraindicated in patients with impaired renal function. Use cautiously in myasthenia gravis or neuromuscular disease.
• Culture and sensitivity test should be done before starting treatment.
• For I.M. administration only. Give deep I.M.; injection may be painful; dilute in solution containing sodium chloride and 2% procaine hydrochloride (if hospital policy permits). Do not give if patient is sensitive to procaine or PABA derivatives.
• Maintain adequate fluid intake, and monitor urinary output closely. If intake or output decreases, notify the doctor.
• Obtain baseline renal function studies before starting therapy. Monitor daily during therapy. Notify doctor of any change.
• Concentration of bacitracin should be between 5,000 and 10,000 units/ml. Store in refrigerator. Drug is inactivated at room temperature.
• Report side effects to the doctor immediately.
• May be used with neomycin as a bowel prep, or in solution as a wound irrigating agent.
• Urine pH should be kept above 6.0.
• Prolonged therapy may result in overgrowth of nonsusceptible organisms, especially *Candida albicans.*
• Don't administer by I.V. route; drug is irritating to vein and predisposes to severe thrombophlebitis.

chloramphenicol

chloramphenicol palmitate

chloramphenicol sodium succinate

Chloromycetin♦, Mychel,
Novochlorocap♦♦
Pregnancy Category: C

MECHANISM OF ACTION
Inhibits bacterial protein synthesis by binding to the 50S subunit of the ribosome.

INDICATIONS & DOSAGE
Hemophilus influenzae *meningitis, acute* Salmonella typhi *infection, severe infections caused by sensitive* Salmonella *species,* Rickettsia, *lymphogranuloma, psittacosis, various sensitive gram-negative organisms causing meningitis, bacteremia, or other serious infections*—
Adults and children: 50 to 100 mg/ kg P.O. or I.V. daily, divided q 6 hours. Maximum dose is 100 mg/kg daily.
Premature infants and neonates (2 weeks or younger): 25 mg/kg P.O. or I.V. daily, divided q 6 hours. I.V. route must be used to treat meningitis.

ADVERSE REACTIONS
Blood: *aplastic anemia,* hypoplastic anemia, *granulocytopenia,* thrombocytopenia.
CNS: headache, mild depression, confusion, delirium, peripheral neuropathy with prolonged therapy.
CV: *cardiovascular collapse in newborns ("gray syndrome").*
EENT: optic neuritis (in patients with cystic fibrosis), glossitis, decreased visual acuity.
GI: nausea, vomiting, stomatitis, diarrhea, enterocolitis.
Other: infections by nonsusceptible organisms, hypersensitivity reaction (fever, rash, urticaria, *anaphylaxis*), *gray baby syndrome in premature and newborn infants (abdominal distention, gray cyanosis, vasomotor collapse, respiratory distress, death within a few hours of onset of symptoms).*

INTERACTIONS
Acetaminophen: elevates chloramphenicol levels. Monitor for chloramphenicol toxicity.

NURSING CONSIDERATIONS
• Use cautiously in patients with impaired hepatic or renal function, and with other drugs causing bone marrow depression or blood disorders. *Don't use for infections caused by organisms susceptible to other agents or for trivial infections; use only when clearly indicated for severe infection.*
• Culture and sensitivity test may be done concurrently with first dose and p.r.n.
• Monitor CBC, platelets, serum iron, and reticulocytes before and every 2 days during therapy. Stop drug immediately if anemia, reticulocytopenia, leukopenia, or thrombocytopenia develops.
• Instruct patient to report adverse reactions to the doctor, especially nausea, vomiting, diarrhea, fever, confusion, sore throat, or mouth sores.
• Tell patient to take medication for as long as prescribed, exactly as directed, even after he feels better.
• Give I.V. slowly over 1 minute. Check injection site daily for phlebitis and irritation.
• Reconstitute 1-g vial of powder for injection with 10 ml sterile water for injection. Concentration will be 100 mg/ml. Stable for 30 days at room temperature, but refrigeration recommended. Do not use cloudy solutions.
• Watch for evidence of superinfection by nonsusceptible organisms.

Italicized side effects are common or life-threatening.
*Liquid form contains alcohol.   **May contain tartrazine.

clindamycin hydrochloride

clindamycin palmitate hydrochloride

clindamycin phosphate

Cleocin, Dalacin C♦♦
Pregnancy Category: B

MECHANISM OF ACTION

Inhibits bacterial protein synthesis by binding to the 50S subunit of the ribosome.

INDICATIONS & DOSAGE

Infections caused by sensitive staphylococci, streptococci, pneumococci, Bacteroides, Fusobacterium, Clostridium perfringens, *and other sensitive aerobic and anaerobic organisms—*
Adults: 150 to 450 mg P.O. q 6 hours; or 300 mg I.M. or I.V. q 6, 8, or 12 hours. Up to 2,700 mg I.M. or I.V. daily, divided q 6, 8, or 12 hours. May be used for severe infections.
Children over 1 month: 8 to 25 mg/ kg P.O. daily, divided q 6 to 8 hours; or 15 to 40 mg/kg I.M. or I.V. daily, divided q 6 hours.

ADVERSE REACTIONS

Blood: transient leukopenia, eosinophilia, thrombocytopenia.
GI: *nausea,* vomiting, abdominal pain, *diarrhea, pseudomembranous enterocolitis,* esophagitis, flatulence, anorexia, *bloody or tarry stools, dysphagia.*
Hepatic: elevated SGOT, alkaline phosphatase, bilirubin.
Skin: maculopapular rash, urticaria.
Local: *pain,* induration, *sterile abscess with I.M. injection;* thrombophlebitis, erythema, and pain after I.V. administration.
Other: unpleasant or bitter taste, *anaphylaxis.*

INTERACTIONS

Erythromycin: antagonist that may block access of clindamycin to its site of action; don't use together.

NURSING CONSIDERATIONS

• Contraindicated in patients with known hypersensitivity to the antibiotic congener lincomycin; also in patients with history of GI disease, especially colitis. Use cautiously in newborns and patients with renal or hepatic disease, asthma, or significant allergies.
• Monitor renal, hepatic, and hematopoietic functions during prolonged therapy.
• Culture and sensitivity test should be performed before starting treatment and p.r.n.
• Don't use in meningitis. Drug does not penetrate CSF.
• Don't refrigerate reconstituted oral solution, as it will thicken. Drug is stable for 2 weeks at room temperature.
• Instruct patient to report side effects to the doctor, especially diarrhea. Warn patient not to treat such diarrhea himself.
• Advise patients taking the capsule form to take with a full glass of water to prevent dysphagia.
• Don't give diphenoxylate compound (Lomotil) to treat drug-induced diarrhea. May prolong and worsen diarrhea.
• Give deep I.M. Rotate sites. Warn that I.M. injection may be painful. Doses greater than 600 mg per injection are not recommended.
• When giving I.V., check site daily for phlebitis and irritation. For I.V. infusion, dilute each 300 mg in 50 ml solution, and give no faster than 30 mg/minute.
• I.M. injection may cause CPK levels to rise due to muscle irritation.
• Topical form available to treat acne.

erythromycin base
E-Mycin♦, Eryc, Ery-Tab, Erythromid♦♦, Ethril 500, Ilotycin♦, Novorythro♦♦, Robimycin, Staticin PCE

erythromycin estolate
Ilosone♦, Novorythro♦♦

erythromycin ethylsuccinate
E.E.S., Erythrocin♦, Pediamycin, Wyamycin Liquid

erythromycin glucepate
Ilotycin♦

erythromycin lactobionate
Erythrocin♦

erythromycin stearate
E-Biotic, Erypar, Erythrocin♦, Ethril**, Novorythro♦♦, SK-Erythromycin, Wintrocin, Wyamycin
Pregnancy Category: B

MECHANISM OF ACTION
Inhibits bacterial protein synthesis by binding to the 50S subunit of the ribosome.

INDICATIONS & DOSAGE
Acute pelvic inflammatory disease caused by Neisseria gonorrhoeae—
Women: 500 mg I.V. (erythromycin glucepate, lactobionate) q 6 hours for 3 days, then 250 mg (erythromycin base, estolate, stearate) or 400 mg (erythromycin ethylsuccinate) P.O. q 6 hours for 7 days.
Endocarditis prophylaxis for dental procedures in patients allergic to penicillin—
Adults: 1 g (erythromycin base, estolate, stearate) P.O. 1 hour before procedure, then 500 mg P.O. 6 hours later.
Intestinal amebiasis—
Adults: 250 mg (erythromycin base, estolate, stearate) P.O. q 6 hours for

10 to 14 days.
Children: 30 to 50 mg/kg (erythromycin base, estolate, stearate) P.O. daily, divided q 6 hours for 10 to 14 days.
Mild-to-moderately severe respiratory tract, skin, and soft-tissue infections caused by sensitive group A beta-hemolytic streptococci, Diplococcus pneumoniae, Mycoplasma pneumoniae, Corynebacterium diphtheriae, Bordetella pertussis, Listeria monocytogenes—
Adults: 250 to 500 mg (erythromycin base, estolate, stearate) P.O. q 6 hours; or 400 to 800 mg (erythromycin ethylsuccinate) P.O. q 6 hours; or 15 to 20 mg/kg I.V. daily, as continuous infusion or divided q 6 hours.
Children: 30 mg/kg to 50 mg/kg (oral erythromycin salts) P.O. daily, divided q 6 hours; or 15 to 20 mg/kg I.V. daily, divided q 4 to 6 hours.
Syphilis—
Adults: 500 mg (erythromycin base, estolate, stearate) P.O. q.i.d. for 15 days.
Legionnaire's Disease—
Adults: 500 mg to 1 g I.V. or P.O. q 6 hours for 21 days.
Uncomplicated urethral, endocervical, or rectal infections where tetracyclines are contraindicated—
Adults: 500 mg P.O. q.i.d. for at least 7 days.
Urogenital Chlamydia trachomatis *infections during pregnancy—*
Adults: 500 mg P.O. q.i.d. for at least 7 days or 250 mg P.O. q.i.d. for at least 14 days.
Conjunctivitis caused by Chlamydia trachomatis *in newborns—*
Newborns: 50 mg/kg/day in 4 divided doses for at least 2 weeks.
Pneumonia of infancy due to Chlamydia trachomatis—
Infants: 50 mg/kg/day in 4 divided doses for at least 3 weeks.

ADVERSE REACTIONS
EENT: hearing loss with high intra-

Italicized side effects are common or life-threatening.
*Liquid form contains alcohol. ** May contain tartrazine.

venous doses.
GI: *abdominal pain and cramping,*
nausea, vomiting, diarrhea.
Hepatic: cholestatic jaundice (with
erythromycin estolate).
Skin: urticaria, rashes.
Local: *venous irritation, thrombo-*
phlebitis following I.V. injection.
Other: overgrowth of nonsusceptible
bacteria or fungi; *anaphylaxis;* fever.

INTERACTIONS

Clindamycin, lincomycin: may be antagonistic. Don't use together.
Theophylline: decreased erythromycin
blood levels and increased theophylline toxicity. Use together cautiously.

NURSING CONSIDERATIONS

• Erythromycin estolate contraindicated in hepatic disease. Use other
erythromycin salts cautiously in patients with impaired hepatic function.
• Culture and sensitivity test should
be performed before starting treatment and p.r.n.
• For best absorption, instruct patient
to take oral form of drug with a full
glass of water 1 hour before or 2
hours after meals. If tablets are
coated, they may be taken with meals.
Tell patient not to drink fruit juice
with medication. Chewable erythromycin tablets should not be swallowed
whole.
• Coated forms of erythromycin are
associated with lower incidence of
gastrointestinal problems. May be
more tolerable in patients who cannot
easily tolerate erythromycin.
• When administering suspension, be
sure to note the concentration.
• May cause overgrowth of nonsusceptible bacteria or fungi. Watch for
signs and symptoms of superinfection.
• Tell patient to take medication for
as long as prescribed, exactly as directed, even after he feels better.
Treat streptococcal infections for 10
days.

• Report adverse reactions, especially
nausea, abdominal pain, or fever.
• Erythromycin estolate may cause
serious hepatotoxicity in adults (reversible cholestatic jaundice). Monitor hepatic function (increased levels
of bilirubin, SGOT, SGPT, alkaline
phosphatase may occur). Other erythromycin salts cause hepatotoxicity to
a lesser degree. Patients who develop
hepatotoxicity from estolate may react
similarly to treatment with any erythromycin preparation.
• I.V. dose should be administered
over 60 minutes. Reconstitute according to manufacturer's directions and
dilute each 250 mg in at least 100 ml
0.9% normal saline solution.
• Erythromycin lactobionate should
not be administered with other drugs.
• Topical form available to treat acne.

imipenem/cilastatin sodium
Primaxin
Pregnancy Category: C

MECHANISM OF ACTION
Imipenem is bactericidal and inhibits
bacterial cell wall synthesis. Cilasta-
tin inhibits the enzymatic breakdown
of imipenem in the kidney, making it
effective in the urinary tract.

INDICATIONS & DOSAGE
Treatment of serious infections of the
lower respiratory and urinary tracts,
intraabdominal and gynecologic in-
fections, bacterial septicemia, bone
and joint infections, skin and soft tis-
sue infections, and endocarditis. Most
known microorganisms susceptible:
Staphylococcus *and* Streptococcus
species, Escherichia coli, Klebsiella,
Proteus, Enterobacter *species,* Pseudomonas aeruginosa, *and* Bacteroides
species including B. fragilis—
Adults: 250 mg to 1 g by I.V. infusion
q 6 to 8 hours. Maximum daily dosage
is 50 mg/kg/day or 4 g/day, whichever
is less.

ADVERSE REACTIONS
CNS: *seizures,* dizziness.
CV: hypotension.
GI: nausea, vomiting, diarrhea, *pseudomembranous colitis.*
Skin: rash, urticaria, pruritus.
Local: *thrombophlebitis, pain at injection site.*
Other: *hypersensitivity.*

INTERACTIONS
None significant.

NURSING CONSIDERATIONS
• Use cautiously in patients allergic to penicillins or cephalosporins because this drug is chemically similar. Ask patient if he's had a hypersensitivity reaction to either of these drugs before administering first dose of imipenem.
• Use cautiously in patients who have a history of seizure disorders, especially if they also have compromised renal function. If patient develops seizures that persist despite anticonvulsant therapy, notify doctor. The drug should then be discontinued.
• Don't administer by direct I.V. bolus injection. Each 250- or 500-mg dose should be given by intravenous infusion over 20 to 30 minutes. Each 1-g dose should be infused over 40 to 60 minutes. If nausea occurs, the infusion may be slowed.
• When reconstituting powder, shake until the solution is clear. Solutions may range from colorless to yellow and variations of color within this range don't affect the drug's potency. After reconstitution, solution is stable for 10 hours at room temperature and for 48 hours when refrigerated.
• Imipenem/cilastatin has the broadest antibacterial spectrum of any available antibiotic. The drug is most valuable for empiric treatment of infections and for mixed infections that would otherwise require a combination of antibiotics, often including an aminoglycoside.

lincomycin hydrochloride
Lincocin♦
Pregnancy Category: B

MECHANISM OF ACTION
Inhibits bacterial protein synthesis by binding to the 50S subunit of the ribosome.

INDICATIONS & DOSAGE
Respiratory tract, skin and soft-tissue, and urinary tract infections; osteomyelitis, septicemia caused by sensitive group A beta-hemolytic streptococci, pneumococci, and staphylococci—
Adults: 500 mg P.O. q 6 to 8 hours (not to exceed 8 g daily); or 600 mg I.M. daily or q 12 hours; or 600 mg to 1 g I.V. q 8 to 12 hours (not to exceed 8 g daily).
Children over 1 month: 30 to 60 mg/kg P.O. daily, divided q 6 to 8 hours; or 10 mg/kg I.M. daily or divided q 12 hours; or 10 to 20 mg/kg I.V. daily, divided q 6 to 8 hours. For I.V. infusion, dilute to 100 ml; infuse over 1 hour to avoid hypotension.

ADVERSE REACTIONS
Blood: *neutropenia, leukopenia,* thrombocytopenia, purpura.
CNS: dizziness, headache.
CV: hypotension with rapid I.V. infusion.
EENT: glossitis, tinnitus.
GI: nausea, vomiting, *pseudomembranous colitis, persistent diarrhea,* abdominal cramps, stomatitis, pruritus ani.
GU: vaginitis.
Hepatic: cholestatic jaundice.
Skin: rashes, urticaria.
Local: pain at injection site.
Other: hypersensitivity, angioedema.

INTERACTIONS
Antidiarrheal medication (kaolin, pectin, attapulgite): reduce oral absorption of lincomycin by as much as 90%. Antidiarrheals should be

MISCELLANEOUS ANTI-INFECTIVES   133

avoided or given at least 2 hours before lincomycin.

NURSING CONSIDERATIONS
• Contraindicated in known hypersensitivity to clindamycin. Use cautiously in patients with history of GI disorders (especially colitis); asthma or significant allergies; hepatic or renal disease; and endocrine or metabolic disorders.
• Culture and sensitivity tests should be done before starting treatment and p.r.n.
• For best absorption, instruct patient to take drug with a full glass of water 1 hour before or 2 hours after meals.
• Tell patient to take medication exactly as directed, even after he feels better.
• Tell patient to report side effects to doctor, especially diarrhea. Warn him not to treat diarrhea himself. Watch for signs of superinfection, especially when therapy exceeds 10 days.
• Never treat drug-induced diarrhea with diphenoxylate compound (Lomotil); it may prolong or worsen diarrhea.
• Give deep I.M. Rotate sites. Warn that I.M. injection may be painful.
• When giving I.V., check site daily for phlebitis and irritation. Rotate infusion sites regularly.
• Rapid I.V. infusion may cause hypotension and syncope.
• Monitor blood pressure in patients receiving the drug parenterally.
• Monitor hepatic function (increased levels of alkaline phosphatase, SGOT, SGPT, bilirubin may occur).
• Monitor CBC and platelets. Stop drug immediately if neutropenia, leukopenia, or other blood disorders develop.

pentamidine isethionate
Pentam 300
Pregnancy Category: C

MECHANISM OF ACTION
Interferes with biosynthesis of DNA, RNA, phospholipids, and proteins.

INDICATIONS & DOSAGE
Treatment of pneumonia due to Pneumocystis carinii—
Adults and children: 4 mg/kg I.V. or I.M. once a day for 14 days.

ADVERSE REACTIONS
Blood: *leukopenia,* thrombocytopenia, anemia.
CNS: confusion, hallucinations.
CV: *hypotension,* tachycardia.
Endocrine: *hypoglycemia,* hypocalcemia.
GI: nausea, anorexia, metallic taste.
GU: *elevated serum creatinine,* renal toxicity.
Hepatic: elevated liver enzymes.
Local: *sterile abscess, pain or induration at injection site.*
Skin: rash, facial flushing, pruritus.
Other: fever.

INTERACTIONS
None significant.

NURSING CONSIDERATIONS
• Once the diagnosis of *Pneumocystis carinii* has been firmly established, there are no absolute contraindications to pentamidine therapy.
• Use cautiously in patients with hypertension, hypotension, hypoglycemia, hypocalcemia, leukopenia, thrombocytopenia, anemia, and hepatic or renal dysfunction.
• Patient should be lying down when receiving the drug because sudden, severe hypotension may develop. Monitor blood pressure during administration and several times thereafter until blood pressure is stable.
• When administering I.V., infuse

over 60 minutes to minimize risk of hypotension.
• Monitor blood glucose levels, serum creatinine, and BUN daily.
• Pain and induration occur universally with I.M. injection. Administer by deep I.M. injection.
• In patients with AIDS, pentamidine produces less severe adverse reactions than does the alternative treatment trimethoprim-sulfamethoxazole. Therefore, in AIDS patients, pentamidine is considered the treatment of choice.

polymyxin B sulfate
Aerosporin♦
Pregnancy Category: B

MECHANISM OF ACTION
Hinders bacterial cell-wall synthesis, damaging the bacterial plasma membrane and making the cell more vulnerable to osmotic pressure.

INDICATIONS & DOSAGE
Acute urinary tract infections or septicemia caused by sensitive Pseudomonas aeruginosa, *or when other antibiotics are ineffective or contraindicated; bacteremia caused by sensitive* Enterobacter aerogenes *and* Klebsiella pneumoniae, *or acute urinary tract infections caused by* Escherichia coli—
Adults and children: 15,000 to 25,000 units/kg daily I.V. infusion, divided q 12 hours; or 25,000 to 30,000 units/kg daily, divided q 4 to 8 hours. I.M. not advised due to severe pain at injection site.
Meningitis caused by sensitive P. aeruginosa *or* Hemophilus influenzae *when other antibiotics ineffective or contraindicated—*
Adults and children over 2 years: 50,000 units intrathecally once daily for 3 to 4 days, then 50,000 units every other day for at least 2 weeks after cerebrospinal fluid tests are negative

and cerebrospinal fluid sugar is normal.
Children under 2 years: 20,000 units intrathecally once daily for 3 to 4 days, then 25,000 units every other day for at least 2 weeks after cerebrospinal fluid tests are negative and cerebrospinal fluid sugar is normal.

ADVERSE REACTIONS
CNS: irritability, drowsiness, facial flushing, weakness, ataxia, respiratory paralysis, headache and meningeal irritation with intrathecal administration, peripheral and perioral paresthesias, convulsions, *coma*.
EENT: blurred vision.
GU: *nephrotoxicity* (albuminuria, cylindruria, hematuria, proteinuria, decreased urine output, increased BUN).
Skin: urticaria.
Local: *pain at I.M. injection site*.
Other: hypersensitivity reactions with fever, *anaphylaxis*.

INTERACTIONS
None significant.

NURSING CONSIDERATIONS
• Use cautiously in patients with impaired renal function or myasthenia gravis.
• Give only to hospitalized patients under constant medical supervision.
• For meningitis, must give intrathecally to achieve adequate cerebrospinal fluid levels.
• Give deep I.M. Warn that injection may be painful. If patient isn't allergic to procaine, use 1% procaine (if hospital policy permits) as diluent to decrease pain. Rotate sites.
• Don't give solution containing local anesthetics I.V. or intrathecally.
• When giving I.V., check site daily for phlebitis and irritation. Dilute each 500,000 units in 300 to 500 ml dextrose 5% in water; infuse over 60 to 90 minutes. Rotate I.V. sites regularly.

Italicized side effects are common or life-threatening.
*Liquid form contains alcohol.   **May contain tartrazine.

- Parenteral solutions should be refrigerated and used within 72 hours.
- Monitor renal function (BUN, serum creatinine, creatinine clearance, urinary output) before and during therapy. Intake should be sufficient to maintain output at 1,500 ml/day (between 3,000 and 4,000 ml/day for adults).
- Discontinue therapy if BUN increases and urinary output decreases.
- Notify doctor immediately if patient develops fever, CNS adverse reactions, rash, or symptoms of nephrotoxicity.
- If patient is scheduled for surgery, notify anesthesiologist of preoperative treatment with this drug since neuromuscular blockade can occur.

spectinomycin dihydrochloride
Trobicin◆
Pregnancy Category: B

MECHANISM OF ACTION
Inhibits protein synthesis by binding to the 30S subunit of the ribosome.

INDICATIONS & DOSAGE
Gonorrhea—
Adults: 2 to 4 g I.M. single dose injected deeply into the upper outer quadrant of the buttock.

ADVERSE REACTIONS
CNS: insomnia, dizziness.
GI: nausea.
GU: decreased urine output.
Skin: urticaria.
Local: pain at injection site.
Other: fever, chills (may mask or delay symptoms of incubating syphilis).

INTERACTIONS
None significant.

NURSING CONSIDERATIONS
- Not effective in the treatment of syphilis.

- Serologic test for syphilis should be done before treatment dose and 3 months after.
- Use 20G needle to administer drug. The 4-g dose (10 ml) should be divided into two 5-ml injections—one in each buttock.
- Shake vial vigorously after reconstitution and before withdrawing dose. Store at room temperature after reconstitution and use within 24 hours.
- Should be reserved for penicillin-resistant strains of gonorrhea.

trimethoprim
Proloprim◆, Trimpex
Pregnancy Category: C

MECHANISM OF ACTION
Interferes with the action of dihydrofolate reductase, inhibiting bacterial synthesis of folic acid.

INDICATIONS & DOSAGE
Treatment of uncomplicated urinary tract infections caused by susceptible strains of Escherichia coli, Proteus mirabilis, Klebsiella, *and* Enterobacter *species—*
Adults: 100 mg P.O. every 12 hours for 10 days.
Not recommended for children under 12 years.

ADVERSE REACTIONS
Blood: thrombocytopenia, leukopenia, megaloblastic anemia, methemoglobinemia.
GI: *epigastric distress, nausea, vomiting,* glossitis.
Skin: *rash, pruritus, exfoliative dermatitis.*
Other: fever.

INTERACTIONS
None significant.

NURSING CONSIDERATIONS
- Contraindicated in documented

megaloblastic anemia due to folate deficiency.
• Clinical signs such as sore throat, fever, pallor, or purpura may be early indications of serious blood disorders. Complete blood counts should be done routinely. Prolonged use of trimethoprim at high doses may cause bone marrow depression.
• Dose should be decreased in patients with severely impaired renal function. Give cautiously to patients with impaired hepatic function.
• To be of benefit, full course of therapy must be completed.

vancomycin hydrochloride
Vancocin•
Pregnancy Category: C

MECHANISM OF ACTION
Hinders bacterial cell-wall synthesis, damaging the bacterial plasma membrane and making the cell more vulnerable to osmotic pressure.

INDICATIONS & DOSAGE
Severe staphylococcal infections when other antibiotics ineffective or contraindicated—
Adults: 500 mg I.V. q 6 hours, or 1 g q 12 hours.
Children: 44 mg/kg I.V. daily, divided q 6 hours.
Neonates: 10 mg/kg I.V. daily, divided q 6 to 12 hours.
Antibiotic-associated pseudomembranous and staphylococcal enterocolitis—
Adults: 125 to 500 mg P.O. q 6 hours for 7 to 10 days.
Children: 44 mg/kg P.O. daily, divided q 6 hours.
Endocarditis prophylaxis for dental procedures—
Adults: 1 g I.V. slowly over 1 hour, starting 1 hour before procedure. No repeat dose is necessary.

ADVERSE REACTIONS
Blood: transient eosinophilia, leukopenia.
EENT: tinnitus, ototoxicity (deafness).
GI: nausea.
Skin: "red-neck" syndrome (maculopapular rash on face, neck, trunk, and extremities).
Local: *pain or thrombophlebitis with I.V. administration, necrosis.*
Other: chills, fever, *anaphylaxis,* overgrowth of nonsusceptible organisms.

INTERACTIONS
None significant.

NURSING CONSIDERATIONS
• Use cautiously in patients receiving other neurotoxic, nephrotoxic, or ototoxic drugs. Use cautiously in patients with impaired hepatic or renal function; also in those with preexisting hearing loss; in patients over 60 years; and in patients with allergies to other antibiotics.
• Tell patient to take medication exactly as directed, even after he feels better. Treat staphylococcal endocarditis for at least 4 weeks.
• Patients should receive auditory function tests before and during therapy.
• Tell patient to report adverse reactions at once, especially fullness or ringing in ears. Stop drug immediately if these occur.
• Do not give drug I.M.
• For I.V. infusion, dilute in 200 ml sodium chloride injection or 5% glucose solution and infuse over 60 minutes. Check site daily for phlebitis and irritation. Report pain at infusion site. Avoid extravasation. Severe irritation and necrosis can result.
• Monitor patient carefully for "red-neck syndrome." Stop infusion and notify doctor promptly if you see this reaction.
• Refrigerate I.V. solution after re-

constitution and use within 96 hours.
• Monitor renal function (BUN,
serum creatinine, urinalysis, creatinine clearance, urinary output) before
and during therapy. Watch for signs of
superinfection.
• Oral preparation stable for 2 weeks
if refrigerated.

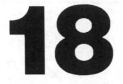

Cardiac glycosides, glycoside neutralizer, and amrinone

amrinone lactate
deslanoside
digitoxin
digoxin
digoxin immune FAB

COMBINATION PRODUCTS
None.

---

amrinone lactate
Inocor
Pregnancy Category: C

MECHANISM OF ACTION
Produces inotropic action by increasing cellular levels of cAMP. Produces vasodilation through a direct relaxant effect on vascular smooth muscle.

INDICATIONS & DOSAGE
Short-term management of congestive heart failure—
Adults: initially, 0.75 mg/kg I.V. bolus over 2 to 3 minutes. Then begin maintenance infusion of 5 to 10 mcg/kg/minute. Additional bolus of 0.75 mg/kg may be given 30 minutes after start of therapy. Total daily dose should not exceed 10 mg/kg.

ADVERSE REACTIONS
Blood: *thrombocytopenia.*
CV: *arrhythmias,* hypotension.
GI: nausea, vomiting, cramps, dyspepsia, diarrhea.
Hepatic: enzyme elevation, possible hepatotoxicity.
Local: burning at site of injection.

Other: *hypersensitivity.*

INTERACTIONS
Disopyramide: excessive hypotension. Don't administer concurrently.
Furosemide: will form precipitate. Don't mix together.

NURSING CONSIDERATIONS
• Don't use in patients with severe aortic or pulmonic valvular disease. Use cautiously in patients with hypertrophic subaortic stenosis.
• Dosage should be based on clinical response, including assessment of pulmonary artery pressures and cardiac output.
• Amrinone should be administered solely via an intravenous pump.
• Monitor blood pressure and heart rate throughout the infusion. Slow or stop infusion, and notify doctor if patient's blood pressure falls.
• Monitor platelet count. Platelet count below 150,000 mm³ usually requires a decreased dosage.
• Administer amrinone as supplied, or dilute in normal or half-normal saline solution to a concentration of 1 mg/ml to 3 mg/ml. Use diluted solution within 24 hours.
• Don't dilute the drug with solutions containing dextrose because a slow chemical reaction occurs over 24 hours. However, amrinone can be injected into running dextrose infusions through a Y-connector or directly into the tubing.
• Amrinone is primarily prescribed

Italicized side effects are common or life-threatening.
*Liquid form contains alcohol. **May contain tartrazine.

for patients who have not responded to therapy with digitalis, diuretics, and vasodilators.

deslanoside
Cedilanid♦♦, Cedilanid-D
Pregnancy Category: C

MECHANISM OF ACTION
Promotes movement of calcium from extracellular to intracellular cytoplasm and inhibits adenosine triphosphatase (ATPase). These actions strengthen myocardial contraction.

INDICATIONS & DOSAGE
Congestive heart failure, paroxysmal atrial tachycardia, atrial fibrillation and flutter—
Adults: loading dose 1.2 to 1.6 mg I.M. or I.V. in 2 divided doses over 24 hours; for maintenance, use another glycoside. Not recommended for children.

ADVERSE REACTIONS
The following are signs of toxicity that may occur with all cardiac glycosides:
CNS: *fatigue, generalized muscle weakness, agitation,* hallucinations, headache, malaise, dizziness, vertigo, stupor, paresthesias.
CV: *increased severity of congestive heart failure, arrhythmias (most commonly conduction disturbances with or without AV block, premature ventricular contractions, and supraventricular arrhythmias),* hypotension.
Toxic effects on heart may be life-threatening and require immediate attention.
EENT: *yellow-green halos around visual images, blurred vision,* light flashes, photophobia, diplopia.
GI: *anorexia, nausea,* vomiting, diarrhea.

INTERACTIONS
Amphotericin B, carbenicillin, ticarcillin, corticosteroids, and diuretics

(including loop diuretics, chlorthalidone, metolazone, and thiazides): hypokalemia, predisposing patient to digitalis toxicity. Monitor serum potassium.
Parenteral calcium, thiazides: hypercalcemia and hypomagnesemia, predisposing patient to digitalis toxicity. Monitor serum calcium and serum magnesium.

NURSING CONSIDERATIONS
• Contraindicated in presence of any digitalis-induced toxicity; ventricular fibrillation; ventricular tachycardia unless caused by congestive heart failure. Administering calcium salts to digitalized patient is contraindicated. Calcium affects cardiac contractility and excitability in much the same way that glycosides do and may lead to serious arrhythmias in digitalized patient. Use with extreme caution in the elderly, and in patients with acute myocardial infarction, incomplete AV block, chronic constrictive pericarditis, idiopathic hypertrophic subaortic stenosis, renal insufficiency, severe pulmonary disease, or hypothyroidism.
• Hypothyroid patients are very sensitive to glycosides; hyperthyroid patients may need larger doses.
• Obtain baseline data (heart rate and rhythm, blood pressure, electrolytes) before giving first dose.
• Question patient about recent use of cardiac glycosides (within the previous 2 to 3 weeks) before administering a loading dose. Always divide loading dose over first 24 hours unless clinical situation indicates otherwise.
• Use only for rapid digitalization, not maintenance.
• Dose is adjusted to patient's clinical condition and is monitored by serum levels of cardiac glycoside, calcium, potassium, magnesium, and by EKG.
• Take apical-radial pulse for a full minute. Record and report to doctor any significant changes (sudden in-

crease or decrease in rate, pulse deficit, irregular beats, and particularly regularization of a previously irregular rhythm). Check blood pressure and obtain 12-lead EKG with these changes.
• Excessive slowing of the pulse rate (60 beats/minute or less) may be a sign of digitalis toxicity. Hold drug and notify doctor.
• Observe eating patterns. Ask patient about nausea, vomiting, anorexia, visual disturbances, and other symptoms of toxicity.
• I.M. injection is painful; give I.V. if possible.
• Monitor serum potassium carefully. Take corrective action *before* hypokalemia occurs.

---

digitoxin
Crystodigin
Pregnancy Category: C

MECHANISM OF ACTION
Promotes movement of calcium from extracellular to intracellular cytoplasm and inhibits adenosine triphosphatase (ATPase). These actions strengthen myocardial contraction.

INDICATIONS & DOSAGE
Congestive heart failure, paroxysmal atrial tachycardia, atrial fibrillation and flutter—
Adults: loading dose 1.2 to 1.6 mg I.V. or P.O. in divided doses over 24 hours; maintenance 0.1 mg daily.
Children 2 to 12 years: loading dose 0.03 mg/kg or 0.75 mg/m^2 I.M., I.V., or P.O. in divided doses over 24 hours; maintenance $1/_{10}$ loading dose or 0.003 mg/kg or 0.075 mg/m^2 daily. Monitor closely for toxicity.
Children 1 to 2 years: loading dose 0.04 mg/kg over 24 hours in divided doses; maintenance 0.004 mg/kg daily. Monitor closely for toxicity.
Children 2 weeks to 1 year: loading dose 0.045 mg/kg I.M., I.V., or P.O.

in divided doses over 24 hours; maintenance 0.0045 mg/kg daily. Monitor closely for toxicity.
Premature infants, neonates, severely ill older infants: loading dose 0.022 mg/kg I.M., I.V., or P.O. in divided doses over 24 hours; maintenance 0.0022 mg/kg daily. Monitor closely for toxicity.

ADVERSE REACTIONS
The following are signs of toxicity that may occur with all cardiac glycosides:
CNS: *fatigue, generalized muscle weakness, agitation, hallucinations,* headache, malaise, dizziness, vertigo, stupor, paresthesias.
CV: *increased severity of congestive heart failure, arrhythmias (most commonly conduction disturbances with or without AV block, premature ventricular contractions, and supraventricular arrhythmias),* hypotension.
Toxic effects on heart may be life-threatening and require immediate attention.
EENT: *yellow-green halos around visual images, blurred vision,* light flashes, photophobia, diplopia.
GI: *anorexia, nausea,* vomiting, diarrhea.

INTERACTIONS
Antacids, kaolin-pectin: decreased absorption of oral digitoxin. Schedule doses as far as possible from oral digitoxin administration.
Cholestyramine, colestipol, metoclopramide: decreased absorption of oral digitoxin. Monitor for decreased effect and low blood levels. Dosage may have to be increased.
Amphotericin B, carbenicillin, ticarcillin, corticosteroids, and diuretics (including loop diuretics, chlorthalidone, metolazone, and thiazides): hypokalemia, predisposing patient to digitalis toxicity. Monitor serum potassium.
Parenteral calcium, thiazides: hypercalcemia and hypomagnesemia, pre-

---

Italicized side effects are common or life-threatening.
*Liquid form contains alcohol.   **May contain tartrazine.

disposing patient to digitalis toxicity. Monitor serum calcium and serum magnesium.

Phenylbutazone, phenobarbital, phenytoin, rifampin: faster metabolism and shorter duration of digitoxin. Observe for underdigitalization.

Cimetidine: decreased digitoxin metabolism. Monitor for digitoxin toxicity.

NURSING CONSIDERATIONS

• Contraindicated in presence of any digitalis-induced toxicity; ventricular fibrillation; ventricular tachycardia unless caused by congestive heart failure. Administering calcium salts to digitalized patient is contraindicated. Calcium affects cardiac contractility and excitability in much the same way that glycosides do and may lead to serious arrhythmias in digitalized patient. Use with extreme caution in patients with acute myocardial infarction, incomplete AV block, chronic constrictive pericarditis, idiopathic hypertrophic subaortic stenosis, severe pulmonary disease, hypothyroidism, and in the elderly.

• Hypothyroid patients are very sensitive to glycosides; hyperthyroid patients may need larger doses.

• Obtain baseline data (heart rate and rhythm, blood pressure, electrolytes) before giving first dose.

• Question patient about recent use of cardiac glycosides (within the previous 2 to 3 weeks) before administering a loading dose. Always divide loading dose over first 24 hours unless clinical situation indicates otherwise.

• Dose is adjusted to patient's clinical condition and is monitored by serum levels of cardiac glycoside, calcium, potassium, magnesium, and by EKG.

• Take apical-radial pulse for a full minute. Record and report to doctor any significant changes (sudden increase or decrease in rate, pulse deficit, irregular beats, and particularly regularization of a previously irregu-

lar rhythm). Check blood pressure and obtain 12-lead EKG with these changes.

• Excessive slowing of the pulse rate (60 beats/minute or less) may be a sign of digitalis toxicity. Hold drug and notify doctor.

• Observe eating patterns. Ask patient about nausea, vomiting, anorexia, visual disturbances, and other symptoms of toxicity.

• Watch closely for signs of toxicity, especially in children and the elderly.

• Monitor serum potassium carefully. Take corrective action *before* hypokalemia occurs.

• I.M. injection is painful and poorly absorbed; give I.V. if parenteral route is necessary.

• Digitoxin is a long-acting drug; watch for cumulative effects.

• Protect solution from light.

• Instruct patient and responsible family member about drug action, dosage regimen, how to take pulse, reportable signs, and follow-up plans.

• Don't substitute one brand for another.

• Therapeutic blood levels of digitoxin range from 25 to 35 ng/ml.

---

digoxin
Lanoxicaps, Lanoxin♦*
Pregnancy Category: C

MECHANISM OF ACTION
Promotes movement of calcium from extracellular to intracellular cytoplasm and inhibits adenosine triphosphatase (ATPase). These actions strengthen myocardial contraction.

INDICATIONS & DOSAGE
Congestive heart failure, atrial fibrillation and flutter, paroxysmal atrial tachycardia—
Adults: loading dose 0.5 to 1 mg I.V. or P.O. in divided doses over 24 hours; maintenance 0.125 to 0.5 mg I.V. or P.O. daily (average 0.25 mg).

Larger doses are often needed for treatment of arrhythmias, depending on patient response.

Adults over 65: 0.125 mg P.O. daily as maintenance dose. Frail or very small elderly patients may require only 0.0625 mg daily or 0.125 mg every other day.

Children over 2 years: loading dose 0.02 to 0.04 mg/kg P.O. divided q 8 hours over 24 hours; I.V. loading dose 0.015 to 0.035 mg/kg; maintenance 0.012 mg/kg P.O. daily divided q 12 hours.

Children 1 month to 2 years: loading dose 0.035 to 0.060 mg/kg P.O. divided into three doses over 24 hours; I.V. loading dose 0.03 to 0.05 mg/kg; maintenance 0.01 to 0.02 mg/kg P.O. daily divided q 12 hours.

Neonates under 1 month: loading dose 0.035 mg/kg P.O. divided q 8 hours over 24 hours; I.V. loading dose 0.02 to 0.03 mg/kg; maintenance 0.01 mg/kg P.O. daily divided q 12 hours.

Premature infants: loading dose 0.025 mg/kg I.V. divided into 3 doses over 24 hours; maintenance 0.01 mg/kg I.V. daily divided q 12 hours.

ADVERSE REACTIONS

The following are signs of toxicity that may occur with all cardiac glycosides:
CNS: *fatigue, generalized muscle weakness, agitation, hallucinations,* headache, malaise, dizziness, vertigo, stupor, paresthesias.
CV: *increased severity of congestive heart failure, arrhythmias (most commonly conduction disturbances with or without AV block, premature ventricular contractions, and supraventricular arrhythmias),* hypotension.
Toxic effects on heart may be life-threatening and require immediate attention.
EENT: *yellow-green halos around visual images, blurred vision,* light flashes, photophobia, diplopia.
GI: *anorexia, nausea,* vomiting, diarrhea.

INTERACTIONS

Antacids, kaolin-pectin: decreased absorption of oral digoxin. Schedule doses as far as possible from oral digoxin administration.
Cholestyramine, colestipol, metoclopramide: decreased absorption of oral digoxin. Monitor for decreased effect and low blood levels. Dosage may have to be increased.
Quinidine, diltiazem, amiodarone, nifedipine, and verapamil: increased digoxin blood levels. Monitor for toxicity.
Amphotericin B, carbenicillin, ticarcillin, corticosteroids, and diuretics (including loop diuretics, chlorthalidone, metolazone, and thiazides): hypokalemia, predisposing patient to digitalis toxicity. Monitor serum potassium.
Parenteral calcium, thiazides: hypercalcemia and hypomagnesemia, predisposing patient to digitalis toxicity. Monitor serum calcium and serum magnesium.
Anticholinergics: may increase digoxin absorption of oral tablets. Monitor blood levels and observe for toxicity.
Amiloride: inhibits and increases digoxin excretion. Monitor for altered digoxin effect.

NURSING CONSIDERATIONS

• Contraindicated in presence of any digitalis-induced toxicity; ventricular fibrillation; ventricular tachycardia unless caused by congestive heart failure. Administering calcium salts to digitalized patient is contraindicated. Calcium affects cardiac contractility and excitability in much the same way that glycosides do and may lead to serious arrhythmias in digitalized patient. Use with extreme caution in the elderly, and in patients with acute myocardial infarction, incomplete AV block, chronic constrictive pericardi-

tis, idiopathic hypertrophic subaortic stenosis, renal insufficiency, severe pulmonary disease, or hypothyroidism. Dose must be reduced in renal impairment.
• Infuse intravenous dose slowly over at least 5 minutes.
• Hypothyroid patients are very sensitive to glycosides; hyperthyroid patients may need larger doses.
• Obtain baseline data (heart rate and rhythm, blood pressure, electrolytes) before giving first dose.
• Question patient about recent use of cardiac glycosides (within the previous 2 to 3 weeks) before administering a loading dose. Always divide loading dose over first 24 hours unless clinical situation indicates otherwise.
• Dose is adjusted to patient's clinical condition and is monitored by serum levels of cardiac glycoside, calcium, potassium, magnesium, and by EKG.
• Take apical-radial pulse for a full minute. Record and report to doctor any significant changes (sudden increase or decrease in rate, pulse deficit, irregular beats, and particularly regularization of a previously irregular rhythm). Check blood pressure and obtain 12-lead EKG with these changes.
• Excessive slowing of the pulse rate (60 beats/minute or less) may be a sign of digitalis toxicity. Hold drug and notify doctor.
• Observe eating patterns. Ask patient about nausea, vomiting, anorexia, visual disturbances, and other symptoms of toxicity.
• Monitor serum potassium carefully. Take corrective action *before* hypokalemia occurs.
• Withhold for 1 to 2 days before elective electrocardioversion. Adjust dose after cardioversion.
• Instruct patient and responsible family member about drug action, dosage regimen, how to take pulse, reportable signs, and follow-up plans.
• Don't substitute one brand for another.
• Digoxin solution enclosed in a recently available soft capsule (Lanoxicaps). Because absorption is better than for tablets, the dose is usually slightly smaller.
• Therapeutic blood levels of digoxin range from 0.5 to 2.5 ng/ml.

digoxin immune FAB (ovine)
Digibind
Pregnancy Category: C

MECHANISM OF ACTION
Binds molecules of digoxin and digitoxin, making them unavailable for binding at their site of action on cells in the body.

INDICATIONS & DOSAGE
Treatment of potentially life-threatening digoxin or digitoxin intoxication—
Adults and children: administered I.V. over 30 minutes or as a bolus if cardiac arrest is imminent. The dosage varies according to the amount of digoxin or digitoxin to be neutralized. Average dose is 10 vials (400 mg). However, if the toxicity resulted from acute digoxin ingestion, and neither a serum digoxin level nor an estimated ingestion amount is known, 20 vials (800 mg) should be administered. See package insert for complete, specific dosage instructions.

ADVERSE REACTIONS
CV: congestive heart failure, rapid ventricular rate (both due to reversal of the cardiac glycoside's therapeutic effects).
Metabolic: hypokalemia.
Other: *hypersensitivity.*

INTERACTIONS
None reported.

NURSING CONSIDERATIONS
• Since digoxin immune FAB is derived from digoxin-specific antibody fragments obtained from immunized sheep, use cautiously in persons known to be allergic to ovine proteins. In these high-risk patients, skin testing is recommended. A limited supply of this drug is available at major medical centers or from the manufacturer (1-800-334-4828 or, in North Carolina, 1-800-672-7223).
• This antidote should be used only for life-threatening overdosage in patients in shock or cardiac arrest; for ventricular arrhythmias, such as ventricular tachycardia or fibrillation; for progressive bradyarrhythmias, such as severe sinus bradycardia; or for second- or third-degree AV block not responsive to atropine.
• Monitor potassium levels closely during treatment.
• In most patients, signs of digitalis toxicity disappear within a few hours.
• Best to infuse this drug through a 0.22-μm membrane filter. However, give by bolus injection if cardiac arrest is considered imminent.
• Reconstituted product must be used within 24 hours. Store in refrigerator.

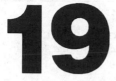

Antiarrhythmics

amiodarone hydrochloride
atropine sulfate
bretylium tosylate
disopyramide
disopyramide phosphate
encainide hydrochloride
esmolol hydrochloride
flecainide acetate
lidocaine hydrochloride
mexiletine hydrochloride
phenytoin
(See Chapter 29, ANTICONVULSANTS.)
phenytoin sodium
(See Chapter 29, ANTICONVULSANTS.)
procainamide hydrochloride
propranolol hydrochloride
(See Chapter 20, ANTIANGINALS.)
quinidine gluconate
quinidine polygalacturonate
quinidine sulfate
tocainide hydrochloride

COMBINATION PRODUCTS
None.

amiodarone hydrochloride
Cordarone
Pregnancy Category: C

MECHANISM OF ACTION
A Group III antiarrhythmic that prolongs the refractory period and repolarization.

INDICATIONS & DOSAGE
Ventricular and supraventricular arrhythmias, including recurrent supraventricular tachycardia (WPW syndrome), atrial fibrillation and flutter, and ventricular tachycardia—

Adults: loading dose is 5 to 10 mg/kg by I.V. infusion via central line, followed by I.V. infusion of 10 mg/kg per day for 3 to 5 days. Or, give loading dose of 800 to 1600 mg P.O. daily for 1 to 3 weeks until initial therapeutic response occurs. Maintenance dose: 200 to 600 mg P.O. daily. (Note: Intravenous use of amiodarone is investigational.)

ADVERSE REACTIONS
CNS: peripheral neuropathy and extrapyramidal symptoms, headache, *malaise, fatigue.*
CV: bradycardia, hypotension.
EENT: *corneal microdeposits,* visual disturbances.
Endocrine: hypothyroidism, hyperthyroidism, gynecomastia.
GI: *nausea, vomiting,* constipation.
Hepatic: *altered liver enzymes,* hepatic dysfunction.
Respiratory: *severe pulmonary toxicity (pneumonitis/alveolitis).*
Skin: *photosensitivity,* blue-gray skin pigmentation.
Other: muscle weakness.

INTERACTIONS
None significant.

NURSING CONSIDERATIONS
• Use cautiously in patients with preexisting bradycardia or sinus node disease; conduction disturbances; severely depressed ventricular function; and marked cardiomegaly.
• Amiodarone is often effective for treatment of arrhythmias resistant to other drug therapy. However, large in-

cidence of side effects limits its use.
• Most patients treated show corneal microdeposits upon slit-lamp ophthalmologic examination. Onset of this effect from 1 to 4 months after beginning amiodarone therapy. However, only 2% to 3% have actual visual disturbances. To minimize this complication, recommend instillation of methylcellulose ophthalmic solution during amiodarone therapy.
• Monitor carefully for pulmonary toxicity, which may be fatal. Incidence increases in patients receiving more than 400 mg per day.
• Monitor blood pressure, heart rate and rhythm frequently. Notify doctor of any significant change.
• Monitor hepatic function tests; thyroid function tests.
• Monitor for symptoms of pneumonitis—exertional dyspnea, nonproductive cough, and pleuritic chest pain. Monitor pulmonary function tests and chest X-ray.
• Divide oral loading dose into three equal doses and give with meals to decrease GI intolerance. Maintenance dose may be given once daily, but may be divided into two doses taken with meals if GI intolerance occurs.
• Advise patient to use a sunscreen to prevent photosensitivity. Monitor for burn or tingling skin followed by erythema and possible skin blistering.
• Amiodarone's side effects are more prevalent at high doses but are generally reversible when drug therapy is stopped. Resolution of side effects may take up to 4 months.

---

atropine sulfate
Pregnancy Category: C

MECHANISM OF ACTION
An anticholinergic, it inhibits acetylcholine at the parasympathetic neuroeffector junction, blocking vagal effects on the SA node; this enhances conduction through the AV node and speeds heart rate.

INDICATIONS & DOSAGE
Symptomatic bradycardia, bradyarrhythmia (junctional or escape rhythm)—
Adults: usually 0.5 to 1 mg I.V. push; repeat q 5 minutes, to maximum 2 mg. Lower doses (less than 0.5 mg) can cause bradycardia.
Children: 0.01 mg/kg dose up to maximum 0.4 mg; or 0.3 mg/m² dose; may repeat q 4 to 6 hours.
Antidote for anticholinesterase insecticide poisoning—
Adults and children: 2 mg I.M. or I.V. repeated at hourly intervals until muscarinic symptoms disappear. Severe cases may require up to 6 mg I.M. or I.V. q 1 hour.
Preoperatively for diminishing secretions and blocking cardiac vagal reflexes—
Adults: 0.4 to 0.6 mg I.M. 45 to 60 minutes before anesthesia.
Children: 0.01 mg/kg I.M. up to a maximum dose of 0.4 mg 45 to 60 minutes before anesthesia.

ADVERSE REACTIONS
Blood: leukocytosis.
CNS: *headache, restlessness,* ataxia, disorientation, hallucinations, delirium, coma, *insomnia, dizziness;* excitement, agitation, and confusion (especially in elderly).
CV: *1 to 2 mg—tachycardia, palpitations; greater than 2 mg—extreme tachycardia, angina.*
EENT: *1 mg—slight mydriasis,* photophobia; *2 mg—blurred vision, mydriasis.*
GI: *dry mouth (common even at low doses),* thirst, *constipation,* nausea, vomiting.
GU: *urinary retention.*
Skin: hot, flushed skin.

INTERACTIONS
Methotrimeprazine: may produce extrapyramidal symptoms. Monitor pa-

---

Italicized side effects are common or life-threatening.
*Liquid form contains alcohol.   **May contain tartrazine.

tient carefully.

NURSING CONSIDERATIONS
• Contraindicated in narrow-angle glaucoma, obstructive uropathy, obstructive disease of GI tract, myasthenia gravis, paralytic ileus, intestinal atony, unstable cardiovascular status in acute hemorrhage, and toxic megacolon.
• Adverse reactions vary considerably with dose. Most common is dry mouth.
• Many of the adverse effects (such as dry mouth and constipation) are an extension of the drug's pharmacologic activity and may be expected.
• Watch for tachycardia in cardiac patients.
• Antidote for atropine overdose is physostigmine salicylate.
• Other anticholinergic drugs may increase vagal blockage.
• When given I.V., may cause paradoxical initial bradycardia. Usually disappears within 2 minutes.
• Monitor intake/output. Drug causes urinary retention and hesitancy; have patient void before receiving the drug.
• Monitor closely for urinary retention in elderly males with benign prostatic hypertrophy (BPH).

bretylium tosylate
Bretylate♦♦, Bretylol
Pregnancy Category: C

MECHANISM OF ACTION
A Group III antiarrhythmic that initially exerts transient adrenergic stimulation through release of norepinephrine. Subsequent depletion of norepinephrine causes adrenergic blocking actions to predominate. Repolarization is prolonged.

INDICATIONS & DOSAGE
Ventricular fibrillation—
Adults: 5 mg/kg by rapid I.V. injection. If necessary, increase dose to 10

mg/kg and repeat q 15 to 30 minutes until 30 mg/kg have been given.
Other ventricular arrhythmias—
Adults: initially, 500 mg diluted to 50 ml with dextrose 5% in water or normal saline solution and infused I.V. over more than 8 minutes at 5 to 10 mg/kg. Dose may be repeated in 1 to 2 hours. Thereafter, dose q 6 to 8 hours.
I.V. maintenance—
Adults: infused in diluted solution of 500 ml dextrose 5% in water or normal saline solution at 1 to 2 mg/minute.
I.M. injection—
Adults: 5 to 10 mg/kg undiluted. Repeat in 1 to 2 hours if needed. Thereafter, repeat q 6 to 8 hours.
Not recommended for children.

ADVERSE REACTIONS
CNS: *vertigo, dizziness, light-headedness, syncope* (usually secondary to hypotension).
CV: *severe hypotension (especially orthostatic), bradycardia,* anginal pain.
GI: severe nausea, vomiting (with rapid infusion).

INTERACTIONS
All antihypertensives: may potentiate hypotension. Monitor blood pressure.

NURSING CONSIDERATIONS
• Contraindicated in digitalis-induced arrhythmias. Use cautiously in patients with fixed cardiac output, aortic stenosis, and pulmonary hypertension to avoid severe and sudden drop in blood pressure.
• Monitor blood pressure, heart rate and rhythm frequently. Notify doctor immediately of any significant change. If supine systolic blood pressure falls below 75 mm Hg, notify doctor; he may order norepinephrine or dopamine, or volume expansion to raise blood pressure.
• Keep patient in the supine position until tolerance to hypotension devel-

ops.
• Avoid sudden postural changes due to postural hypotension.
• Follow dosage directions carefully to avoid nausea and vomiting.
• Give I.V. injections for ventricular fibrillation as rapidly as possible. Do not dilute.
• Rotate I.M. injection sites to prevent tissue damage, and don't exceed 5-ml volume in any one site.
• To be used with other cardiopulmonary-resuscitative measures such as CPR, countershock, epinephrine, sodium bicarbonate, and lidocaine.
• Avoid subtherapeutic doses (less than 5 mg/kg), since such doses may cause hypotension.
• Ventricular tachycardia and other ventricular arrhythmias respond less rapidly to treatment than ventricular fibrillation does.
• Dosage should be decreased in renal impairment.
• Monitor carefully if pressor amines (sympathomimetics) are given to correct hypotension, as bretylium potentiates pressor amines.
• Ineffective treatment for atrial arrhythmias.
• Has been used investigationally to treat hypertension.
• Observe for increased anginal pain in susceptible patients.
• Observe patient for side effects and notify doctor if any occur.

---

disopyramide
Rythmodan♦

disopyramide phosphate
Norpace♦, Norpace CR♦
Pregnancy Category: C

MECHANISM OF ACTION
A Class Ia antiarrhythmic that depresses phase O. It prolongs the action potential. All Class I drugs have membrane stabilizing effects.

INDICATIONS & DOSAGE
Premature ventricular contractions (unifocal, multifocal, or coupled); ventricular tachycardia not severe enough to require electrocardioversion—

Adults: Usual maintenance dose 150 to 200 mg P.O. q 6 hours; for patients who weigh less than 50 kg or those with renal, hepatic, or cardiac impairment—100 mg P.O. q 6 hours. May give sustained-release capsule q 12 hours. Recommended doses in advanced renal insufficiency: Creatinine clearance 15 to 40 ml/minute: 100 mg q 10 hours; creatinine clearance 5 to 15 ml/minute: 100 mg q 20 hours; creatinine clearance 1 to 5 ml/minute: 100 mg q 30 hours.
Children 12 to 18 years: 6 to 15 mg/kg daily.
Children 4 to 12 years: 10 to 15 mg/kg daily.
Children 1 to 4 years: 10 to 20 mg/kg daily.
Children less than 1 year: 10 to 30 mg/kg daily.
All children's doses should be divided into equal amounts and given every 6 hours.

ADVERSE REACTIONS
CNS: dizziness, agitation, depression, fatigue, muscle weakness, syncope.
CV: *hypotension, congestive heart failure, heart block, edema, weight gain.*
EENT: *blurred vision, dry eyes, dry nose.*
GI: nausea, vomiting, anorexia, bloating, abdominal pain, *constipation, dry mouth.*
GU: *urinary retention and hesitancy.*
Hepatic: cholestatic jaundice.
Metabolic: hypoglycemia.
Skin: rash in 1% to 3% of patients.

INTERACTIONS
Phenytoin: increases disopyramide's metabolism. Monitor for decreased

---

Italicized side effects are common or life-threatening.
*Liquid form contains alcohol.   **May contain tartrazine.

antiarrhythmic effect.

NURSING CONSIDERATIONS
• Contraindicated in cardiogenic shock or second- or third-degree heart block with no pacemaker. Use very cautiously, and avoid, if possible, in congestive heart failure. Use cautiously in underlying conduction abnormalities, urinary tract diseases (especially prostatic hypertrophy), hepatic or renal impairment, myasthenia gravis, narrow-angle glaucoma. Adjust dosage in renal insufficiency.
• Don't give sustained-release capsule for rapid control of ventricular arrhythmias; when therapeutic blood levels must be rapidly attained; in patients with cardiomyopathy or possible cardiac decompensation; or in patients with severe renal impairment.
• When transferring your patient from immediate-release to sustained-release capsules, advise him to begin a sustained-release capsule 6 hours after the last immediate-release capsule was taken.
• Discontinue if heart block develops, if QRS complex widens by more than 25%, or if Q-T interval lengthens by more than 25% above baseline.
• Correct any underlying electrolyte abnormalities before use.
• Watch for recurrence of arrhythmias; check for side effects; notify doctor.
• Check apical pulse before administering drug. Notify doctor if pulse rate is slower than 60 beats per minute (bpm) or faster than 120 bpm.
• Teach patient the importance of taking drug on time, exactly as prescribed. To do this, he may have to use an alarm clock for night doses.
• Relieve discomfort of dry mouth by chewing gum or hard candy.
• Manage constipation with proper diet or bulk laxatives.
• Use of disopyramide with other antiarrhythmics may cause further myo-

cardial depression.
• Most doctors prefer to prescribe disopyramide for patients not in heart failure who can't tolerate quinidine or procainamide.
• Pharmacist may prepare disopyramide suspension. 100-mg capsules are used to prepare suspension with cherry syrup. May be best for young children.

---

encainide hydrochloride
Enkaid
Pregnancy Category: C

MECHANISM OF ACTION
A Class Ic antiarrhythmic that depresses phase O. Unlike Class Ia and Ib agents, it does not prolong or shorten the action potential. All Class I drugs have membrane-stabilizing effects.

INDICATIONS & DOSAGE
Treatment of documented life-threatening arrhythmias, nonsustained ventricular tachycardia, and frequent PVCs—
Adults: initially, 25 mg P.O. t.i.d. at approximately 8-hour intervals. After 3 to 5 days, dosage may be increased to 35 mg t.i.d. if necessary. After an additional 3 to 5 days, dosage may be increased to 50 mg t.i.d. Maximum daily dose is 75 mg q.i.d.

ADVERSE REACTIONS
CNS: *dizziness, blurred vision, insomnia, headache.*
CV: *arrhythmias, palpitations,* edema, *chest pains.*
GI: dry mouth, constipation, nausea, vomiting.
Other: *dyspnea, weakness.*

INTERACTIONS
Cimetidine: may increase encainide blood levels. Use together cautiously.

NURSING CONSIDERATIONS
• Contraindicated in patients with preexisting second- or third-degree AV block or with right bundle branch block when associated with a left hemiblock, unless a pacemaker is present; contraindicated in cardiogenic shock.
• Use cautiously in patients with preexisting congestive heart failure, cardiomyopathy, or sick sinus syndrome.
• Patients who receive encainide dosage of 200 mg per day or more should be hospitalized.
• Monitor for possible new or worsened arrhythmias. Encainide may increase frequency of PVCs and possibly severe ventricular tachycardia. These "proarrhythmic events" usually occur during the 1st week of therapy and are much more common when dosage exceeds 200 mg per day.
• Allowing at least 3 days to adjust to the dose before increasing it significantly reduces the risk of proarrhythmia. Warn patient of the risk of increasing his own encainide dose.
• Some patients who are well controlled on 50 mg t.i.d. or less may be treated as effectively with a 12-hour dosage schedule to ease compliance. Discuss this possibility with the doctor.

---

esmolol hydrochloride
Brevibloc
Pregnancy Category: C

MECHANISM OF ACTION
Blocks response to beta stimulation. Decreases heart rate and blood pressure.

INDICATIONS & DOSAGE
Supraventricular tachycardia—
Adults: as a loading dose, 500 mcg/kg/minute by I.V. infusion over 1 minute, followed by a 4-minute maintenance infusion of 50 mcg/kg/minute. If adequate response does not occur

within 5 minutes, repeat the loading dose followed by a maintenance infusion of 100 mcg/kg/minute. Maximum maintenance infusion is 200 mcg/kg/minute.

ADVERSE REACTIONS
CNS: dizziness, somnolence, headache, agitation, fatigue.
CV: *hypotension* (sometimes with diaphoresis).
GI: *nausea,* vomiting.
Local: *inflammation and induration at infusion site.*
Other: bronchospasm.

INTERACTIONS
Morphine: may increase esmolol blood levels. Avoid using together.

NURSING CONSIDERATIONS
• Contraindicated in patients with sinus bradycardia, heart block greater than first degree, cardiogenic shock, or overt heart failure.
• Use cautiously in patients with impaired renal function, diabetes, or bronchospasm.
• Up to 50% of all patients treated with esmolol develop hypotension. Monitor closely, especially if patient's pretreatment blood pressure was low.
• Hypotension can usually be reversed within 30 minutes by decreasing the dose or, if necessary, by stopping the infusion.
• Esmolol is recommended only for short-term use, no longer than 48 hours.
• If a local reaction develops at the infusion site, change to another site. Avoid butterfly needles.
• Don't give esmolol by direct I.V. injection. Drug must be diluted before infusion.
• When patient's heart rate becomes stable, esmolol will be replaced by alternative (longer-acting) antiarrhythmics, such as propranolol, digoxin, or verapamil. As the replacement drug is started, the esmolol infusion should

be gradually reduced over 1 hour.
• Esmolol has an ultrashort duration of action and can be accurately titrated. Therefore, it has advantages over other beta blockers in treating cardiac arrhythmias.

flecainide acetate
Tambocor
Pregnancy Category: C

MECHANISM OF ACTION
A Class Ic antiarrhythmic that depresses phase O. Unlike Class Ia and Ib agents, however, it does not prolong or shorten the action potential. All Class I drugs have membrane stabilizing effects.

INDICATIONS & DOSAGE
Treatment of symptomatic ventricular tachycardia and premature ventricular contractions—
Adults: 100 mg P.O. q 12 hours. May be increased in increments of 50 mg b.i.d. every 4 days until efficacy is achieved. Maximum dose is 400 mg daily for most patients.

ADVERSE REACTIONS
CNS: *dizziness, headache,* fatigue, tremor.
CV: *arrhythmias,* chest pain.
EENT: *blurred vision and other visual disturbances.*
GI: nausea, constipation, abdominal pain.
Other: *dyspnea,* edema.

INTERACTIONS
None significant.

NURSING CONSIDERATIONS
• Contraindicated in patients with preexisting second- or third-degree AV block or with right bundle branch block when associated with a left hemiblock, unless a pacemaker is present; contraindicated in cardiogenic shock.

• Therapy with flecainide should usually begin in a hospital setting because of risk of arrhythmias ("proarrhythmic events").
• Use cautiously in patients with preexisting congestive heart failure or cardiomyopathy and in patients with sick sinus syndrome.
• Hypokalemia or hyperkalemia may alter the effect of flecainide and should be corrected before this drug is given.
• Incidence of adverse effects increases when trough blood levels exceed 1 mcg/ml. Periodically monitor blood levels, especially in patients with renal failure or congestive heart failure.
• Most patients can be adequately maintained on an every-12-hour dosage schedule, but some need to receive flecainide every 8 hours.
• Full therapeutic effect of flecainide may take 3 to 5 days. The doctor may order I.V. lidocaine while awaiting full effect.
• Loading doses may aggravate arrhythmias and are therefore not recommended.
• Flecainide is the first of the Ic class of antiarrhythmics. This class of drugs appears to be highly efficacious and has a relatively low incidence of adverse effects.
• Twice-daily dosing for flecainide aids patient compliance.

lidocaine hydrochloride
Lido Pen Auto-Injector, Xylocaine♦
Pregnancy Category: B

MECHANISM OF ACTION
A Class Ib antiarrhythmic that depresses phase O. It shortens the action potential. All Class I drugs have membrane stabilizing effects.

INDICATIONS & DOSAGE
Ventricular arrhythmias from myocardial infarction, cardiac manipulation,

or cardiac glycosides; ventricular tachycardia—

Adults: 50 to 100 mg (1 to 1.5 mg/kg) I.V. bolus at 25 to 50 mg/minute. Give half this amount to elderly or lightweight patients, and to those with congestive heart failure or hepatic disease. Repeat bolus q 3 to 5 minutes until arrhythmias subside or side effects develop. Don't exceed 300-mg total bolus during a 1-hour period. Simultaneously, begin constant infusion: 1 to 4 mg/minute. Use lower dose in elderly patients, those with congestive heart failure or hepatic disease, or patients who weigh less than 50 kg. If single bolus has been given, repeat smaller bolus 15 to 20 minutes after start of infusion to maintain therapeutic serum level. After 24 hours of continuous infusion, decrease rate by half.
I.M. administration: 200 to 300 mg in deltoid muscle only.
Children: 1 mg/kg by I.V. bolus, followed by infusion of 30 mcg/kg/minute.

ADVERSE REACTIONS
CNS: *confusion, tremors,* lethargy, somnolence, *stupor, restlessness,* slurred speech, euphoria, depression, *light-headedness,* paresthesias, muscle twitching, *convulsions.*
CV: *hypotension,* bradycardia, further arrhythmias.
EENT: *tinnitus, blurred or double vision.*
Other: *anaphylaxis,* soreness at injection site, sensations of cold, diaphoresis.

INTERACTIONS
Cimetidine, beta blockers: decreased metabolism of lidocaine. Monitor for toxicity.
Phenytoin: additive cardiac depressant effects. Monitor carefully.

NURSING CONSIDERATIONS
• Contraindicated if allergic to re-

lated local anesthetics of the amide type, such as Nupercaine.
• Use cautiously in complete or second-degree heart block. Use of lidocaine with epinephrine (for local anesthesia) to treat arrhythmias contraindicated. Use with caution in elderly patients, those with congestive heart failure, renal or hepatic disease, or patients who weigh less than 50 kg. Such patients will need a reduced dose.
• In many severely ill patients, convulsions may be the first clinically apparent sign of toxicity. However, severe reactions usually are preceded by somnolence, confusion, and paresthesias.
• If toxic signs (dizziness) occur, stop drug at once and notify doctor. Continued infusion could lead to convulsions and coma. Give oxygen via nasal cannula, if not contraindicated. Keep oxygen and CPR equipment handy.
• Patients receiving infusions must be *attended at all times,* and be on a cardiac monitor. Use an infusion pump or a microdrip system and timer for monitoring infusion precisely. Never exceed an infusion rate of 4 mg/minute, if possible. A faster rate greatly increases risk of toxicity.
• Monitor patient's response, especially blood pressure, serum electrolytes, BUN, and creatinine. Notify doctor promptly if abnormalities develop.
• A bolus dose not followed by infusion will have a short-lived effect.
• A patient who has received lidocaine I.M. will show a sevenfold increase in serum CPK level. Such CPK originates in the skeletal muscle, not the heart. Test isoenzymes if using I.M. route.
• Used investigationally to treat refractory status epilepticus.
• Therapeutic serum levels are 2 to 5 mcg/ml.

mexiletine hydrochloride
Mexitil
Pregnancy Category: C

MECHANISM OF ACTION
A Class Ib antiarrhythmic that depresses phase O. It shortens the action potential. All Group I drugs have membrane stabilizing effects.

INDICATIONS & DOSAGE
Treatment of refractory ventricular dysrhythmias, including ventricular tachycardia and premature ventricular contractions—
Adults: 200-400 mg P.O. followed by 200 mg q 8 hours. May increase dose to 400 mg q 8 hours if satisfactory control is not obtained. Some patients may respond well to an every-12-hour schedule. May give up to 450 mg q 12 hours.

ADVERSE REACTIONS
CNS: *tremor, dizziness,* blurred vision, ataxia, diplopia, confusion, nystagmus, nervousness, headache.
CV: hypotension, bradycardia, widened QRS complex.
GI: *nausea, vomiting.*
Skin: rash.

INTERACTIONS
Phenytoin, rifampin, phenobarbital: decreased mexiletine blood levels. Monitor carefully.
Cimetidine: increased mexiletine blood levels. Monitor carefully.

NURSING CONSIDERATIONS
• Contraindicated in patients with cardiogenic shock or preexisting second- or third-degree AV block (if pacemaker is not present).
• Early sign of mexiletine toxicity is tremor, usually a fine tremor of the hands. This progresses to dizziness and later to ataxia and nystagmus as the drug's blood level increases. Question your patient about these symptoms.
• When changing from lidocaine to mexiletine, stop the infusion when the first mexiletine dose is given. Keep the infusion line open, however, until the arrhythmia appears to be satisfactorily controlled.
• May administer oral dose with meals.
• Therapeutic levels range from 0.75 to 2 mcg/ml.
• Monitor blood pressure, heart rate and rhythm frequently. Notify doctor of any significant change.
• Patients who respond well to mexiletine can often be maintained on a q 12 hour schedule. Notify doctor if you feel the patient is a good candidate for q 12 hour therapy. Twice-a-day dosage eases compliance.

procainamide hydrochloride
Procan SR, Promine, Pronestyl♦**, Pronestyl-SR, Sub-Quin
Pregnancy Category: C

MECHANISM OF ACTION
A Class Ia antiarrhythmic that depresses phase O. It prolongs the action potential. All Class I drugs have membrane stabilizing effects.

INDICATIONS & DOSAGE
Premature ventricular contractions, ventricular tachycardia, atrial arrhythmias unresponsive to quinidine, paroxysmal atrial tachycardia—
Adults: 100 mg q 5 minutes slow I.V. push, no faster than 25 to 50 mg/minute until arrhythmias disappear, side effects develop, or 1 g has been given. When arrhythmias disappear, give continuous infusion of 2 to 6 mg/minute. Usual effective dose 500 to 600 mg. If arrhythmias recur, repeat bolus as above and increase infusion rate; 0.5 to 1 g I.M. q 4 to 8 hours until oral therapy begins.
Loading dose for atrial fibrillation or

paroxysmal atrial tachycardia—
Adults: 1 to 1.25 g P.O. If arrhythmias persist after 1 hour, give additional 750 mg. If no change occurs, give 500 mg to 1 g q 2 hours until arrhythmias disappear or side effects occur.
Loading dose for ventricular tachycardia—
Adults: 1 g P.O. Maintenance 50 mg/kg daily given at 3-hour intervals; average 250 to 500 mg q 3 hours.
Note: Sustained-release tablet may be used for maintenance dosing when treating ventricular tachycardia, atrial fibrillation, and paroxysmal atrial tachycardia. Dose is 500 mg to 1 g q 6 hours.

ADVERSE REACTIONS
Blood: thrombocytopenia, *neutropenia* (especially with sustained-release forms), *agranulocytosis,* hemolytic anemia, *increased ANA titer.*
CNS: hallucinations, confusion, convulsions, depression.
CV: *severe hypotension, bradycardia,* AV block, ventricular fibrillation (after parenteral use).
GI: *nausea, vomiting, anorexia, diarrhea, bitter taste.*
Skin: *maculopapular rash.*
Other: *fever, lupus erythematosus syndrome (especially after prolonged administration),* myalgia.

INTERACTIONS
Cimetidine: may increase procainamide blood levels. Monitor for toxicity.
Amiodarone: increased procainamide levels and possible drug toxicity.

NURSING CONSIDERATIONS
• Contraindicated in patients with hypersensitivity to procaine and related drugs; with complete, second-, or third-degree heart block unassisted by electrical pacemaker; or with myasthenia gravis. Use with caution in congestive heart failure or other conduction disturbances, such as bundle branch block or cardiac glycoside intoxication, or with hepatic or renal insufficiency.
• Patients receiving infusions must be *attended at all times.* Use an infusion pump or a microdrip system and timer to monitor the infusion precisely.
• Monitor blood pressure and EKG continuously during I.V. administration. Watch for prolonged Q-T and QRS intervals, heart block, or increased arrhythmias. If these occur, withhold drug, obtain rhythm strip, and notify doctor immediately.
• Keep patient supine for I.V. administration if hypotension occurs.
• If procainamide is administered too rapidly, I.V. hypotension can occur. Watch closely for side effects and notify doctor if they occur. Instruct patient to report fever, rash, muscle pain, diarrhea, bleeding, bruises, or pleuritic chest pain.
• Procainamide solution for injection may become discolored. If so, check with pharmacy and prepare to discard.
• Monitor CBC frequently during first 3 months of therapy, particularly in patients taking sustained-release dosage forms.
• Decrease dose in hepatic and renal dysfunction, and give over 6 hours. Half-life of procainamide is increased as much as threefold in these states.
• N-acetylprocainamide (NAPA), an active metabolite, may accumulate when renal function is decreased. This may add to toxicity.
• Patient with congestive heart failure has a lower volume of distribution and can be treated with lower doses.
• Positive antinuclear antibody titer common in about 60% of patients who don't have symptoms of lupus erythematosus syndrome. This response seems related to prolonged use, not dosage.
• After long-standing atrial fibrillation, restoration of normal rhythm may result in thromboembolism, due

---

Italicized side effects are common or life-threatening.
*Liquid form contains alcohol.   **May contain tartrazine.

to dislodgment of thrombi from atrial wall. Anticoagulation usually advised before restoration of normal sinus rhythm.
• Stress importance of taking drug exactly as prescribed. Patient may have to set an alarm clock for night doses.
• Geriatric patients may be more likely to develop hypotension. Monitor BP carefully.

quinidine gluconate
(62% quinidine base)
Duraquin, Quinaglute Dura-Tabs♦, Quinate♦♦, Quinatime, Quin-Release

quinidine polygalacturonate
(60.5% quinidine base)
Cardioquin♦

quinidine sulfate
(83% quinidine base)
CinQuin, Novoquindin♦♦, Quine, Quinidex Extentabs♦, Quinora, SK-Quinidine Sulfate
Pregnancy Category: C

MECHANISM OF ACTION
A Class Ia antiarrhythmic that depresses phase O. It prolongs the action potential. All Class I drugs have membrane stabilizing effects.

INDICATIONS & DOSAGE
Atrial flutter or fibrillation—
Adults: 200 mg quinidine sulfate or equivalent base P.O. q 2 to 3 hours for 5 to 8 doses with subsequent daily increases until sinus rhythm is restored or toxic effects develop. Administer quinidine only after digitalization to avoid increasing AV conduction. Maximum 3 to 4 g daily.
Paroxysmal supraventricular tachycardia—
Adults: 400 to 600 mg I.M. gluconate q 2 to 3 hours until toxic side effects develop or arrhythmia subsides.

Premature atrial and ventricular contractions; paroxysmal atrioventricular junctional rhythm; paroxysmal atrial tachycardia; paroxysmal ventricular tachycardia; maintenance after cardioversion of atrial fibrillation or flutter—
Adults: test dose 50 to 200 mg P.O., then monitor vital signs before beginning therapy. Quinidine sulfate or equivalent base 200 to 400 mg P.O. q 4 to 6 hours; or initially, quinidine gluconate 600 mg I.M., then up to 400 mg q 2 hours, p.r.n.; or quinidine gluconate 800 mg I.V. diluted in 40 ml dextrose 5% in water, infused at 16 mg (1 ml)/minute.
Children: test dose 2 mg/kg; 3 to 6 mg/kg q 2 to 3 hours for 5 doses P.O. daily.

ADVERSE REACTIONS
Blood: *hemolytic anemia, thrombocytopenia, agranulocytosis.*
CNS: *vertigo, headache, lightheadedness,* confusion, restlessness, cold sweat, pallor, fainting, dementia.
CV: *premature ventricular contractions; severe hypotension; SA and AV block; ventricular fibrillation, tachycardia; aggravated congestive heart failure; EKG changes (particularly widening of QRS complex, notched P waves, widened Q-T interval, ST segment depression).*
EENT: *tinnitus,* excessive salivation, blurred vision.
GI: *diarrhea, nausea, vomiting,* anorexia, abdominal pains.
Hepatic: hepatotoxicity including granulomatous hepatitis.
Skin: rash, petechial hemorrhage of buccal mucosa, pruritus.
Other: angioedema, acute asthmatic attack, respiratory arrest, *fever, cinchonism.*

INTERACTIONS
Acetazolamide, antacids, sodium bicarbonate: may increase quinidine blood levels due to alkaline urine.

Monitor for increased effect.
Barbiturates, phenytoin, rifampin:
may antagonize quinidine activity.
Monitor for decreased quinidine effect.
Verapamil: May result in hypotension.
Monitor blood pressure.
Nifedipine: may decrease quinidine
blood levels. Monitor carefully.

NURSING CONSIDERATIONS
• Contraindicated in cardiac glycoside toxicity when AV conduction is
grossly impaired; complete AV block
with AV nodal or idioventricular
pacemaker. Use with caution in myasthenia gravis. Anticholinesterase drug
doses may have to be increased.
• May increase toxicity of digitalis
derivatives. Use with caution in patients previously digitalized. Monitor
digoxin levels.
• Monitor liver function tests during
the first 4 to 8 weeks of therapy.
• The I.V. route should only be used
to treat acute arrhythmias. For maintenance, give only by oral or I.M.
route.
• Dosage varies—some patients may
require drug q 4 hours, others q 6
hours. Titrate dose by both clinical response and blood levels.
• When changing route of administration, alter dosage to compensate for
variations in quinidine base content.
• Dose should be decreased in congestive heart failure and hepatic disease.
• Check apical pulse rate and blood
pressure before starting therapy. If
you detect extremes in pulse rate,
withhold drug and notify doctor at
once.
• Lidocaine may be effective in treating quinidine-induced arrhythmias,
since it increases AV conduction.
• GI side effects, especially diarrhea,
are signs of toxicity. Notify doctor.
Check quinidine blood levels, which
are toxic when greater than 8 mcg/ml.
GI symptoms may be decreased by

giving with meals. Monitor drug response carefully.
• Instruct patient to notify doctor if
skin rash, fever, unusual bleeding,
bruising, ringing in ears, or visual
disturbance occurs.
• After long-standing atrial fibrillation, restoration of normal sinus
rhythm may result in thromboembolism due to dislodgment of thrombi
from atrial wall. Anticoagulation often advised before restoration of normal atrial rhythm.
• Never use discolored (brownish)
quinidine solution.
• Store away from heat and direct
light.

tocainide hydrochloride
Tonocard
Pregnancy Category: C

MECHANISM OF ACTION
A Class Ib antiarrhythmic that depresses phase O. It shortens the action
potential. All Class I drugs have
membrane stabilizing effects.

INDICATIONS & DOSAGE
*Suppression of symptomatic ventricular arrhythmias, including frequent
premature ventricular contractions
and ventricular tachycardia—*
Adults: initially, 400 mg P.O. q 8
hours. Usual dosage is between 1,200
and 1,800 mg per day, divided into 3
doses.

ADVERSE REACTIONS
Blood: *aplastic anemia.*
CNS: *light-headedness, tremors,* restlessness, paresthesias, confusion, dizziness.
CV: hypotension.
EENT: blurred vision.
GI: *nausea, vomiting, epigastric
pain,* constipation, diarrhea, anorexia.
Hepatic: hepatitis.
Skin: skin rash.

INTERACTIONS
None significant.

NURSING CONSIDERATIONS
• Contraindicated in patients who are hypersensitive to lidocaine or other amide-type local anesthetics and in patients with second- or third-degree atrioventricular block in the absence of a ventricular pacemaker.
• Use cautiously in patients with congestive heart failure or diminished cardiac reserve.
• Administer cautiously to patients with hepatic or renal impairment. These patients may often be treated effectively with a lower dose.
• Therapeutic blood levels range from 4 to 10 mcg/ml.
• Adverse reactions are generally mild, transient, and reversible by reducing dosage. Gastrointestinal reactions can be minimized by taking the drug with food.
• Dizziness and falling are more likely to occur in the elderly.
• Monitor patient for tremor. This may indicate the approaching of maximum dose.
• Considered by cardiologists as an "oral lidocaine." May ease transition from intravenous lidocaine to oral antiarrhythmic therapy. Monitor patient carefully during this transition period.

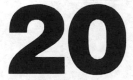

Antianginals

diltiazem hydrochloride
erythrityl tetranitrate
isosorbide dinitrate
nadolol
nifedipine
nitroglycerin
pentaerythritol tetranitrate
propranolol hydrochloride
verapamil hydrochloride

COMBINATION PRODUCTS
CARTRAX-10: pentaerythritol tetranitrate 10 mg and hydroxyzine HCl 10 mg.
CARTRAX-20: pentaerythritol tetranitrate 20 mg and hydroxyzine HCl 10 mg.
COROVAS TYMCAPS: pentaerythritol tetranitrate 30 mg and secobarbital 50 mg.
MILTRATE-10: pentaerythritol tetranitrate 10 mg and meprobamate 200 mg.
MILTRATE-20**: pentaerythritol tetranitrate 20 mg and meprobamate 200 mg.

diltiazem hydrochloride
Cardizem♦
Pregnancy Category: C

MECHANISM OF ACTION
Reduces cardiac oxygen demand by inhibiting the influx of calcium through the muscle cell. This dilates the coronary arteries and decreases systemic vascular resistance (afterload).

INDICATIONS & DOSAGE
Management of vasospastic (also called Prinzmetal's or variant) angina and classic chronic stable angina pectoris—
Adults: 30 mg P.O. q.i.d., before meals and at bedtime. Dosage may be gradually increased to 240 mg/day, in divided doses.

ADVERSE REACTIONS
CNS: *headache, fatigue, drowsiness,* dizziness, nervousness, depression, insomnia, confusion.
CV: *edema, arrhythmia,* flushing, bradycardia, hypotension, conduction abnormalities.
GI: *nausea,* vomiting, diarrhea.
GU: nocturia, polyuria.
Hepatic: transient elevation of liver enzymes.
Skin: *rash,* pruritus.
Other: photosensitivity.

INTERACTIONS
Propranolol (and other beta blockers): may prolong cardiac conduction time. Use together cautiously.

NURSING CONSIDERATIONS
• Contraindicated in sick sinus syndrome, unless a functioning ventricular pacemaker is present; in hypotension when systolic blood pressure is less than 90 mm Hg; and second- or third-degree AV block.
• Use cautiously in elderly because duration of action may be prolonged.
• Use cautiously in patients with impaired ventricular function or conduction abnormalities.

Italicized side effects are common or life-threatening.
*Liquid form contains alcohol.   **May contain tartrazine.

• Use cautiously in patients with impaired liver or kidney function.
• Assist patients with ambulation during initiation of diltiazem therapy because dizziness may occur.
• If nitrate therapy is prescribed during titration of diltiazem dosage, urge patient to continue compliance. Sublingual nitroglycerin, especially, may be taken concomitantly as needed when anginal symptoms are acute.
• Of the available calcium antagonists, diltiazem may offer the lowest risk of side effects.
• Diltiazem is being prescribed in some centers as a treatment for mild to moderate hypertension.
• Used investigationally to treat supraventricular tachycardia.
• May be useful as migraine prophylaxis in some patients. However, diltiazem itself may cause headaches.

---

erythrityl tetranitrate
Cardilate♦
Pregnancy Category: C

MECHANISM OF ACTION
Reduces cardiac oxygen demand by decreasing left ventricular end-diastolic pressure (preload) and systemic vascular resistance (afterload). Also increases blood flow through the collateral coronary vessels.

INDICATIONS & DOSAGE
Prophylaxis and long-term management of frequent or recurrent anginal pain, reduced exercise tolerance associated with angina pectoris—
Adults: 5 mg orally, sublingually, or buccally t.i.d., increasing in 2 to 3 days if needed.

ADVERSE REACTIONS
CNS: *headache, sometimes with throbbing; dizziness;* weakness.
CV: *orthostatic hypotension, tachycardia, flushing, palpitations,* fainting.

GI: nausea, vomiting.
Local: sublingual burning.
Skin: cutaneous vasodilation.
Other: hypersensitivity reactions.

INTERACTIONS
None significant.

NURSING CONSIDERATIONS
• Contraindicated in hypersensitivity to nitrites, head trauma, cerebral hemorrhage, severe anemia. Use with caution in hypotension.
• Monitor blood pressure, and intensity and duration of response to drug.
• May cause headaches, especially at first. Treat headache with aspirin or acetaminophen. Dosage may need to be reduced temporarily, but tolerance usually develops.
• Tell patient to take medication regularly, even long-term, if ordered, and to keep it easily accessible at all times. Physiologically necessary but not habit-forming.
• Additional dose may be taken before anticipated stress or at bedtime if angina is nocturnal.
• Advise patient to avoid alcoholic beverages; they may produce increased hypotension.
• May cause orthostatic hypotension. To minimize it, patient should change to upright position slowly. He should go up and down stairs carefully, and lie down at the first sign of dizziness.
• Tell patient to wet the sublingual tablet with saliva, place it under the tongue until completely absorbed, and sit down and rest. If patient complains of tingling sensation with drug placed sublingually, he may try holding tablet in buccal pouch.
• Teach patient to take oral tablet on empty stomach, either ½ hour before or 1 to 2 hours after meals, and to swallow oral tablets whole.
• Drug should not be discontinued abruptly—coronary vasospasm may occur.
• Store medication in cool place, in

---

tightly closed container, away from light. To assure freshness, replace supply every 3 months. Remove cotton from container, since it absorbs drug.

isosorbide dinitrate
Coronex♦♦, Dilatrate-SR, Iso-Bid, Iso-D, Isordil♦, Isosorb, Sorate, Sorbitrate
Pregnancy Category: C

MECHANISM OF ACTION
Reduces cardiac oxygen demand by decreasing left ventricular end-diastolic pressure (preload) and systemic vascular resistance (afterload). Also increases blood flow through the collateral coronary vessels.

INDICATIONS & DOSAGE
Treatment of acute anginal attacks (sublingual and chewable only); prophylaxis in situations likely to cause attacks; treatment of chronic ischemic heart disease (by preload reduction)—
Adults:
Sublingual form—2.5 to 10 mg under the tongue for prompt relief of anginal pain, repeated q 2 to 3 hours during acute phase, or q 4 to 6 hours for prophylaxis.
Chewable form—5 to 10 mg, p.r.n., for acute attack or q 2 to 3 hours for prophylaxis but only after initial test dose of 5 mg to determine risk of severe hypotension.
Oral form—5 to 30 mg P.O. q.i.d. for prophylaxis only (use smallest effective dose); sustained-release forms 40 mg P.O. q 6 to 12 hours.
Adjunct with other vasodilators, such as hydralazine and prazosin, in treatment of severe chronic congestive heart failure—
Adults:
Oral or chewable form—20 to 40 mg q 4 hours.

ADVERSE REACTIONS
CNS: *headache, sometimes with throbbing; dizziness;* weakness.
CV: *orthostatic hypotension, tachycardia, palpitations, ankle edema,* fainting.
GI: nausea, vomiting.
Local: sublingual burning.
Skin: cutaneous vasodilation, *flushing*.
Other: hypersensitivity reactions.

INTERACTIONS
None significant.

NURSING CONSIDERATIONS
• Contraindicated in hypersensitivity to nitrites, head trauma, cerebral hemorrhage, severe anemia. Use with caution in hypotension.
• Monitor blood pressure, and intensity and duration of response to drug.
• May cause headaches, especially at first. Treat headache with aspirin or acetaminophen. Dosage may need to be reduced temporarily, but tolerance usually develops.
• Tell patient to take medication regularly, even long-term, if ordered, and to keep it easily accessible at all times. Physiologically necessary but not habit-forming.
• Additional dose may be taken before anticipated stress or at bedtime if angina is nocturnal.
• Advise patient to avoid alcoholic beverages; they may produce increased hypotension.
• May cause orthostatic hypotension. To minimize it, patient should change to upright position slowly. He should go up and down stairs carefully, and lie down at the first sign of dizziness.
• Teach patient to take sublingual tablet at first sign of attack. He should wet the tablet with saliva, place it under the tongue until completely absorbed, and sit down and rest. Burning sensation indicates potency. Dose may be repeated every 10 to 15 minutes for a maximum of three doses. If

no relief, patient should call doctor or go to hospital emergency room. If patient complains of tingling sensation with drug placed sublingually, he may try holding tablet in buccal pouch.
• Warn patient not to confuse sublingual with oral form.
• Teach patient to take oral tablet on empty stomach, either ½ hour before or 1 to 2 hours after meals; to swallow oral tablets whole; and to chew chewable tablets thoroughly before swallowing.
• Drug should not be discontinued abruptly—coronary vasospasm may occur.
• Store in cool place, in tightly closed container, away from light.
• Has been used investigationally in treatment of congestive heart failure and diffuse esophageal spasms.

nadolol
Corgard♦
Pregnancy Category: C

MECHANISM OF ACTION
A beta-adrenergic blocker that reduces cardiac oxygen demand by blocking catecholamine-induced increases in heart rate, blood pressure, and force of myocardial contraction. Depresses renin secretion.

INDICATIONS & DOSAGE
Management of angina pectoris—
Adults: 40 mg P.O. once daily, initially. Dosage may be increased in 40- to 80-mg increments until optimum response occurs. Usual maintenance dosage range: 80 to 240 mg once daily.
Treatment of hypertension—
Adults: 40 mg P.O. once daily, initially. Dosage may be increased in 40- to 80-mg increments until optimum response occurs. Usual maintenance dosage: 80 to 320 mg once daily. Doses of 640 mg may be necessary in rare cases.

ADVERSE REACTIONS
CNS: fatigue, lethargy.
CV: *bradycardia, hypotension, congestive heart failure,* peripheral vascular disease.
GI: nausea, vomiting, diarrhea.
Metabolic: hypoglycemia without tachycardia.
Skin: rash.
Other: *increased airway resistance,* fever.

INTERACTIONS
Insulin, hypoglycemic drugs (oral): can alter dosage requirements in previously stabilized diabetics. Observe patient carefully.
Cardiac glycosides: excessive bradycardia and increased depressant effect on myocardium. Use together cautiously.
Epinephrine: severe vasoconstriction. Monitor blood pressure and observe patient carefully.
Indomethacin: decreased antihypertensive effect. Monitor blood pressure and adjust dosage.

NURSING CONSIDERATIONS
• Contraindicated in patients with bronchial asthma, sinus bradycardia and greater than first-degree conduction block, and cardiogenic shock.
• Elderly may experience enhanced adverse reactions. Dose may need to be adjusted.
• Use cautiously in patients with heart failure, chronic bronchitis, renal or hepatic insufficiency, or emphysema.
• Always check patient's apical pulse before giving this drug. If slower than 60 beats per minute, hold drug and call doctor.
• Monitor blood pressure frequently. If patient develops severe hypotension, administer a vasopressor as ordered.
• Don't discontinue abruptly: can exacerbate angina and MI.
• Teach patient about his disease and

therapy. Explain why it's important to take this drug, even when he's feeling well. Tell outpatient not to discontinue drug suddenly, but to call doctor if unpleasant side effects develop.
• Has been used in a limited number of patients with atrial flutter or fibrillation. Also has been used for a few patients in the treatment of migraine headaches.
• This drug masks common signs of shock, hyperthyroidism, and hypoglycemia.
• May be given without regard to meals.

nifedipine
Adalat♦♦, Procardia
Pregnancy Category: C

MECHANISM OF ACTION
Reduces cardiac oxygen demand by inhibiting the influx of calcium through the muscle cell. This dilates the coronary arteries and decreases systemic vascular resistance (afterload).

INDICATIONS & DOSAGE
Management of vasospastic (also called Prinzmetal's or variant) angina and classic chronic stable angina pectoris; treatment of hypertension and Raynaud's syndrome—
Adults: Starting dose is 10 mg P.O. t.i.d.
Usual effective dose range is 10 to 20 mg t.i.d. Some patients may require up to 30 mg q.i.d. Maximum daily dose is 180 mg.

ADVERSE REACTIONS
CNS: *dizziness, light-headedness, flushing, headache,* weakness, syncope.
CV: peripheral edema, hypotension, palpitations.
EENT: nasal congestion.
GI: *nausea, heartburn,* diarrhea.
Metabolic: hypokalemia.

Other: muscle cramps, dyspnea.

INTERACTIONS
Propranolol (and other beta blockers): may cause hypotension and heart failure. Use together cautiously.

NURSING CONSIDERATIONS
• Use cautiously in patients with congestive heart failure or hypotension.
• Monitor blood pressure regularly, especially of patients who are also taking beta blockers or antihypertensives.
• Use cautiously in elderly because duration of action may be prolonged.
• Monitor serum potassium levels regularly.
• Patient may briefly develop anginal exacerbation when beginning drug therapy or at times of dosage increase. Reassure him that this symptom is temporary.
• Although rebound effect hasn't been observed when drug is stopped, dosage should still be reduced slowly under doctor's supervision.
• If patient is kept on nitrate therapy while drug dosage is being titrated, urge him to continue his compliance. Sublingual nitroglycerin, especially, may be taken as needed when anginal symptoms are acute.
• Instruct patient to swallow the capsule whole without breaking, crushing, or chewing.
• There's no sublingual form of nifedipine available. However, the liquid in the oral capsule can be withdrawn by puncturing the capsule with a needle. Instill the drug into the buccal pouch.
• Protect capsules from direct light and store at room temperature.
• Store capsules at room temperature, away from light and moisture.

Italicized side effects are common or life-threatening.
*Liquid form contains alcohol.   **May contain tartrazine.

nitroglycerin

Cardabid, Corobid, Deponit, Glyceryl Trinitrate, Gly-Trate, Nitro-Bid♦, Nitro-Bid I.V., Nitrocap, Nitrocels, Nitro-Dial, Nitrodisc, Nitro-Dur, Nitro-Dur II, Nitrogard, Nitroglyn, Nitrol♦, Nitrol TSAR, Nitrolingual, Nitro-Lyn, Nitrong♦, Nitrospan, Nitrostabilin♦♦, Nitrostat♦, Nitrostat I.V.♦, NTS, Nyglycon, Transderm-Nitro, Trates**, Tridil♦
Pregnancy Category: C

MECHANISM OF ACTION
Reduces cardiac oxygen demand by decreasing left ventricular end-diastolic pressure (preload) and systemic vascular resistance (afterload). Also increases blood flow through the collateral coronary vessels.

INDICATIONS & DOSAGE
Prophylaxis against chronic anginal attacks—
Adults: 1 sustained-release capsule q 8 to 12 hours; or 2% ointment: Start with ½″ ointment, increasing with ½″ increments until headache occurs, then decreasing to previous dose. Range of dosage with ointment 2″ to 5″. Usual dose 1″ to 2″. Alternatively, transdermal disc or pad (Nitrodisc, Nitro-Dur, or Transderm-Nitro) may be applied to hairless site once daily.
Relief of acute angina pectoris, prophylaxis to prevent or minimize anginal attacks when taken immediately prior to stressful events—
Adults: 1 sublingual tablet (gr ¼₀₀, ¹⁄₂₀₀, ¹⁄₁₅₀, ¹⁄₁₀₀) dissolved under the tongue or in the buccal pouch immediately upon indication of anginal attack. May repeat q 5 minutes for 15 minutes. Or, using Nitrolingual spray, spray one or two doses into mouth, preferably onto or under the tongue. May repeat every 3 to 5 minutes to a maximum of 3 doses within a 15 minute period. Or, transmucosally, 1 to 3

mg every 3 to 5 hours during waking hours.
To control hypertension associated with surgery; to treat congestive heart failure associated with myocardial infarction; to relieve angina pectoris in acute situations; to produce controlled hypotension during surgery (by I.V. infusion)—
Adults: Initial infusion rate is 5 mcg/minute. May be increased by 5 mcg/minute q 3 to 5 minutes until a response is noted. If a 20 mcg/minute rate doesn't produce a response, dosage may be increased by as much as 20 mcg/minute q 3 to 5 minutes.

ADVERSE REACTIONS
CNS: *headache, sometimes with throbbing; dizziness;* weakness.
CV: *orthostatic hypotension, tachycardia, flushing, palpitations,* fainting.
GI: nausea, vomiting.
Skin: cutaneous vasodilation.
Local: sublingual burning.
Other: hypersensitivity reactions.

INTERACTIONS
None significant.

NURSING CONSIDERATIONS
• Contraindicated in hypersensitivity to nitrites, head trauma, cerebral hemorrhage, severe anemia. Use with caution in hypotension.
• Monitor blood pressure, and intensity and duration of response to drug.
• May cause headaches, especially at first. Treat headache with aspirin or acetaminophen. Dosage may need to be reduced temporarily, but tolerance usually develops.
• Tell patient to take medication regularly, even long-term, if ordered, and to keep it easily accessible at all times. Physiologically necessary but not habit-forming.
• Additional dose may be taken before anticipated stress or at bedtime if angina is nocturnal.

• Advise patient to avoid alcoholic beverages; they may produce increased hypotension.

• May cause orthostatic hypotension. To minimize it, patient should change to upright position slowly. He should go up and down stairs carefully, and lie down at the first sign of dizziness.

• Teach patient to take sublingual tablet at first sign of attack. He should wet the tablet with saliva, place it under the tongue until completely absorbed, and sit down and rest. If no relief, patient should call doctor or go to hospital emergency room. If patient complains of tingling sensation with drug placed sublingually, he may try holding tablet in buccal pouch.

• Although a burning sensation used to be an indication of tablet potency, today many brands don't produce this sensation.

• Store in cool, dark place, in tightly closed container. To assure freshness, replace supply of sublingual tablets every 3 months. Remove cotton from container, since it absorbs drug.

• Tell patient to store nitroglycerin sublingual tablets in original container or other container specifically approved for this use.

• Advise patient not to carry bottle close to body. He should carry it in jacket pocket or purse.

• Teach patient to take oral tablet on empty stomach, either ½ hour before or 1 to 2 hours after meals; to swallow oral tablets whole; and to chew chewable tablets thoroughly before swallowing.

• To apply ointment, spread in uniform, thin layer on any nonhairy area. Do not rub in. Cover with plastic film to aid absorption and to protect clothing. If using Tape-Surrounded Appli-Ruler (TSAR) system, keep the TSAR on skin to protect patient's clothing and to ensure that ointment remains in place.

• Be sure to remove all excess ointment from previous site before applying next dose.

• Avoid getting ointment on fingers.

• Transdermal dosage forms can be applied to any hairless part of the skin except distal parts of the arms or legs, because absorption will not be maximal at these sites.

• Be sure to remove transdermal patch before defibrillation. Because of its aluminum backing, the electric current may cause the patch to explode.

• When terminating transdermal treatment of angina, gradually reduce the dosage and frequency of application over 4 to 6 weeks.

• Instruct patient to use caution when wearing transdermal patch near microwave oven. Leaking radiation may heat patch's metallic backing and cause burns.

• The various brands of transdermal nitroglycerin products can be interchanged to achieve the prescribed dose. Now, standardized labels specify the amount of nitroglycerin released over 24 hours.

• If nitroglycerin lingual aerosol (Nitrolingual) has been prescribed for patient, instruct him how to use this device correctly. Remind him he should *not* inhale the spray, but should release the spray onto or under the tongue. Also tell him not to swallow immediately after administering the spray—wait about 10 seconds or so before swallowing.

• The transmucosal dosage form may be used to provide relief from an acute anginal attack as well as for prophylaxis.

• Tell patient to place the transmucosal tablet between lip and gum above the incisors, or between cheek and gum. Tell him not to swallow or chew tablet; this will make it ineffective.

• When administering as an intravenous infusion, be sure to use the special nonabsorbing tubing supplied by the manufacturer, because up to 80%

Italicized side effects are common or life-threatening.
*Liquid form contains alcohol.   **May contain tartrazine.

of the drug can be absorbed by regular plastic tubing. Also, be sure to prepare in a glass bottle or container.
• Closely monitor vital signs during infusion.

---

pentaerythritol tetranitrate
Angijen Green, Arcotrate Nos. 1 & 2, Baritrate, Desatrate 30, Desatrate 50, Dilar, Duotrate, Maso-Trol, Nitrin, Penta-Cap-No. 1, Penta-E., Penta-E. S.A., Pentaforte-T, Penta-Tal No. 1 & 2, Pentrate T.D., Pentritol, Pent-T-80, Peritrate♦, PETN, Petro-20 mg, P-T-T, Quintrate, Rate, Vasolate, Vasolate-80
Pregnancy Category: C

MECHANISM OF ACTION
Reduces cardiac oxygen demand by decreasing left ventricular end-diastolic pressure (preload) and systemic vascular resistance (afterload). Also increases blood flow through the collateral coronary vessels.

INDICATIONS & DOSAGE
Prophylaxis against angina pectoris—
Adults: 10 to 20 mg P.O. q.i.d.; may be titrated upward to 40 mg P.O. q.i.d. ½ hour before or 1 hour after meals and h.s.; 80 mg sustained-release preparations P.O. b.i.d.

ADVERSE REACTIONS
CNS: *headache, sometimes with throbbing; dizziness;* weakness.
CV: *orthostatic hypotension, tachycardia, flushing, palpitations,* fainting.
GI: nausea, vomiting.
Skin: cutaneous vasodilation.
Other: hypersensitivity reactions.

INTERACTIONS
None significant.

NURSING CONSIDERATIONS
• Contraindicated in head trauma, cerebral hemorrhage, severe anemia. Use with caution in hypotension and glaucoma.
• Monitor blood pressure, and intensity and duration of response to drug.
• Medication may cause headaches, especially at first. Treat with aspirin or acetaminophen. Dosage may need to be reduced temporarily, but tolerance usually develops.
• Medication should be taken regularly, even long-term, if ordered. Physiologically necessary but not habit-forming.
• Additional doses may be taken before anticipated stress or at bedtime for nocturnal angina.
• Not to be used for relief of acute anginal attacks.
• Medication may cause orthostatic hypotension. To minimize it, patient should change to upright position slowly. He should go up and down stairs carefully, and lie down at the first sign of dizziness.
• Advise patient to avoid alcoholic beverages, which may exacerbate hypotension.
• Drug should not be discontinued abruptly—coronary vasospasm may occur.
• Store medication in cool place in tightly covered, light-resistant container.

---

propranolol hydrochloride
Inderal♦, Inderal LA♦
Pregnancy Category: C

MECHANISM OF ACTION
A beta-adrenergic blocker that reduces cardiac oxygen demand by blocking catecholamine-induced increases in heart rate, blood pressure, and force of myocardial contraction. Depresses renin secretion. Also prevents vasodilation of the cerebral arteries.

INDICATIONS & DOSAGE

Management of angina pectoris—
Adults: 10 to 20 mg t.i.d. or q.i.d.
Or, one 80-mg sustained-release capsule daily. Dosage may be increased at 7- to 10-day intervals. The average optimum dose is 160 mg daily.

To reduce mortality following myocardial infarction—
Adults: 180 to 240 mg P.O. daily in divided doses. Usually administered 3 to 4 times daily.

Supraventricular, ventricular, and atrial arrhythmias; tachyarrhythmias due to excessive catecholamine action during anesthesia, hyperthyroidism, and pheochromocytoma—
Adults: 1 to 3 mg I.V. diluted in 50 ml dextrose 5% in water or normal saline solution infused slowly, not to exceed 1 mg/minute. After 3 mg have been infused, another dose may be given in 2 minutes; subsequent doses no sooner than q 4 hours. Usual maintenance 10 to 80 mg P.O. t.i.d. or q.i.d.

Hypertension—
Adults: initial treatment of hypertension: 80 mg P.O. daily in 2 to 4 divided doses or the sustained-release form once daily. Increase at 3- to 7-day intervals to maximum daily dose of 640 mg. Usual maintenance dose for hypertension: 160 to 480 mg daily.

Prevention of frequent, severe, uncontrollable, or disabling migraine or vascular headache—
Adults: initially, 80 mg daily in divided doses or one sustained-release capsule once daily. Usual maintenance dose: 160 to 240 mg daily, divided t.i.d. or q.i.d.

ADVERSE REACTIONS

CNS: *fatigue, lethargy,* vivid dreams, hallucinations.
CV: *bradycardia, hypotension, congestive heart failure,* peripheral vascular disease.
GI: nausea, vomiting, diarrhea.
Metabolic: hypoglycemia without

tachycardia.
Skin: rash.
Other: *increased airway resistance,* fever, arthralgia.

INTERACTIONS

Insulin, hypoglycemic drugs (oral): can alter requirements for these drugs in previously stabilized diabetics. Monitor for hypoglycemia.
Cardiac glycosides: excessive bradycardia and increased depressant effect on myocardium. Use together cautiously.
Aminophylline: antagonized beta-blocking effects of propranolol. Use together cautiously.
Isoproterenol, glucagon: antagonized propranolol effect. May be used therapeutically and in emergencies.
Cimetidine: inhibits propranolol's metabolism. Monitor for greater beta-blocking effect.
Epinephrine: severe vasoconstriction. Monitor blood pressure and observe patient carefully.

NURSING CONSIDERATIONS

• Contraindicated in diabetes mellitus, asthma, allergic rhinitis; during ethyl ether anesthesia; in sinus bradycardia and in heart block greater than first degree; in cardiogenic shock; in right ventricular failure secondary to pulmonary hypertension. Use with caution in patients with congestive heart failure or respiratory disease, and in patients taking other antihypertensive drugs.
• Elderly may experience enhanced adverse reactions. Dose may need to be adjusted.
• Always check patient's apical pulse rate before giving this drug. If you detect extremes in pulse rates, hold medication and call the doctor immediately.
• Monitor blood pressure, EKG, and heart rate and rhythm frequently, especially during I.V. administration. If patient develops severe hypotension,

Italicized side effects are common or life-threatening.
*Liquid form contains alcohol.   **May contain tartrazine.

notify doctor. He may prescribe a vasopressor.
• After prolonged atrial fibrillation, restoration of normal sinus rhythm may result in thromboembolism due to dislodgment of thrombi from atrial wall. Anticoagulation often advised before restoration of normal atrial rhythm.
• Teach patient about his disease and therapy. Explain why it's important to take this drug exactly as prescribed, even when he's feeling well. Tell outpatient not to discontinue his drug suddenly; abrupt discontinuation can exacerbate angina and MI. Tell patient to call doctor if unpleasant side effects develop.
• This drug masks common signs of shock and hypoglycemia.
• Food may increase the absorption of propranolol. Give consistently with meals.
• Now available in 90-mg (light purple) tablet strength.
• Compliance may be improved by administering this drug twice daily, or by sustained-release capsule. Check with doctor.
• Has also been used to treat aggression and rage, stage fright, recurrent GI bleeding, and menopausal symptoms.
• *Don't discontinue before surgery for pheochromocytoma.* Before any surgical procedure, notify anesthesiologist that patient is receiving propranolol.
• Double-check dose and route. I.V. doses much smaller than P.O.
• Glucagon may be prescribed to reverse propranolol overdose.

---

verapamil hydrochloride
Calan, Calan SR, Isoptin♦, Isoptin SR
Pregnancy Category: C

MECHANISM OF ACTION
Reduces cardiac oxygen demand by inhibiting the influx of calcium through the muscle cell. This dilates the coronary arteries and decreases systemic vascular resistance (afterload). Also depresses SA and AV nodal conduction.

INDICATIONS & DOSAGE
Management of vasospastic (also called Prinzmetal's or variant) angina and classic chronic, stable angina pectoris—
Adults: starting dose is 80 mg P.O. t.i.d. or q.i.d. Dosage may be increased at weekly intervals. Some patients may require up to 480 mg daily.
Treatment of atrial arrhythmias—
Adults: 0.075 to 0.15 mg/kg (5 to 10 mg) I.V. push over 2 minutes with EKG and blood pressure monitoring. Repeat dose in 30 minutes if no response. Follow bolus injection with maintenance infusion of 0.005 mg/kg/minute.
Children 1 to 15 years: 0.1 to 0.3 mg/kg and I.V. bolus over 2 minutes.
Children less than 1 year: 0.1 to 0.2 mg/kg as I.V. bolus over 2 minutes under continuous EKG monitoring. Dose can be repeated in 30 minutes if no response.
Migraine headache prophylaxis—
Adults: 80 mg P.O. q.i.d.
Treatment of hypertension—
Adults: 240-mg sustained-release tablet once daily in the morning. If response is not adequate, may give an additional half tablet in the evening or one tablet every 12 hours. Alternatively, may give 80-mg immediate-release tablet t.i.d. or q.i.d.

ADVERSE REACTIONS
CNS: dizziness, headache, fatigue.
CV: *transient hypotension, heart failure,* bradycardia, AV block, ventricular asystole, peripheral edema.
GI: *constipation,* nausea (primarily from oral form).
Hepatic: elevated liver enzymes.

INTERACTIONS
Propranolol (and other beta blockers), *disopyramide:* may cause heart failure. Use together cautiously.
Quinidine: may result in hypotension. Monitor blood pressure.

NURSING CONSIDERATIONS
• Contraindicated in patients with advanced heart failure, AV block, severe left ventricular dysfunction, cardiogenic shock, sinus node disease, and severe hypotension.
• Use cautiously in elderly because duration of action may be prolonged.
• Use cautiously in patients with myocardial infarction followed by coronary occlusion, sick sinus syndrome, impaired AV conduction, or heart failure with atrial tachyarrhythmia; and in patients with hepatic or renal disease.
• All patients receiving I.V. verapamil should be monitored electrocardiographically. Monitor the R-R interval.
• Liver function tests should be done periodically.
• Patients with severely compromised cardiac function or those receiving beta blockers should receive lower doses of verapamil. Monitor these patients very closely.
• In older patients, I.V. doses should be administered over at least 3 minutes to minimize the risk of adverse effects.
• Notify doctor if such signs of congestive heart failure as swelling of hands and feet or shortness of breath occur.
• If patient is kept on nitrate therapy while drug dosage of oral verapamil is being titrated, urge him to continue his compliance. Sublingual nitroglycerin, especially, may be taken as needed when anginal symptoms are acute.
• Preliminary studies show verapamil to be highly effective in the prophylaxis of migraine headache.

Italicized side effects are common or life-threatening.
*Liquid form contains alcohol.   **May contain tartrazine.

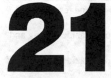

Antihypertensives

acebutolol
atenolol
captopril
clonidine hydrochloride
diazoxide
enalapril maleate
guanabenz acetate
guanadrel sulfate
guanethidine sulfate
guanfacine hydrochloride
hydralazine hydrochloride
labetalol
methyldopa
metoprolol tartrate
metyrosine
minoxidil
nadolol
(See Chapter 20, ANTIANGINALS.)
nitroprusside sodium
pargyline hydrochloride
phenoxybenzamine
   hydrochloride
phentolamine mesylate
pindolol
prazosin hydrochloride
propranolol hydrochloride
(See Chapter 20, ANTIANGINALS.)
rauwolfia serpentina
rescinnamine
reserpine
timolol maleate
trimethaphan camsylate

COMBINATION PRODUCTS

ALDOCLOR-150: chlorothiazide 150 mg and methyldopa 250 mg.
ALDOCLOR-250: chlorothiazide 250 mg and methyldopa 250 mg.
ALDORIL-15♦: hydrochlorothiazide 15 mg and methyldopa 250 mg.
ALDORIL-25♦: hydrochlorothiazide 25 mg and methyldopa 250 mg.
ALDORIL D30: hydrochlorothiazide 30 mg and methyldopa 500 mg.
ALDORIL D50: hydrochlorothiazide 50 mg and methyldopa 500 mg.
APRESAZIDE 25/25: hydrochlorothiazide 25 mg and hydralazine HCl 25 mg.
APRESAZIDE 50/50: hydrochlorothiazide 50 mg and hydralazine HCl 50 mg.
APRESAZIDE 100/50: hydrochlorothiazide 50 mg and hydralazine HCl 100 mg.
APRESODEX: hydrochlorothiazide 15 mg and hydralazine HCl 25 mg.
APRESOLINE-ESIDRIX: hydrochlorothiazide 15 mg and hydralazine HCl 25 mg.
CAM-AP-ES: hydrochlorothiazide 15 mg, hydralazine HCl 25 mg, and reserpine 0.1 mg.
COMBIPRES 0.1♦: chlorthalidone 15 mg and clonidine HCl 0.1 mg.
COMBIPRES 0.2: chlorthalidone 15 mg and clonidine HCl 0.2 mg.
CORZIDE: nadolol 40 mg or 80 mg and bendroflumethiazide 5 mg.
DEMI-REGROTON: chlorthalidone 25 mg and reserpine 0.125 mg.
DIUPRES-250: chlorothiazide 250 mg and reserpine 0.125 mg.
DIUPRES-500: chlorothiazide 500 mg and reserpine 0.125 mg.
DIURESE-R: trichlormethiazide 4 mg and reserpine 0.1 mg.
DIUTENSEN: methyclothiazide 2.5 mg and cryptenamine 2 mg (as tannate).
DIUTENSEN-R: methyclothiazide 2.5 mg and reserpine 0.1 mg.
ENDURONYL: methyclothiazide 5 mg

and deserpidine 0.25 mg.

ENDURONYL-FORTE: methyclothiazide 5 mg and deserpidine 0.5 mg.

ESIMIL: hydrochlorothiazide 25 mg
and guanethidine monosulfate 10 mg.

EUTRON FILMTABS: methyclothiazide
5 mg and pargyline HCl 25 mg.

EXNA-R TABLETS: benzthiazide 50
mg and reserpine 0.125 mg.

HYDRAL 25/25: hydrochlorothiazide
25 mg and hydralazine HCl 25 mg.

HYDRAL 50/50: hydrochlorothiazide
50 mg and hydralazine HCl 50 mg.

HYDROMOX-R: quinethazone 50 mg
and reserpine 0.125 mg.

HYDRO PLUS: hydrochlorothiazide 50
mg and reserpine 0.125 mg.

HYDROPRES-25♦: hydrochlorothiazide 25 mg and reserpine 0.125 mg.

HYDROPRES-50♦: hydrochlorothiazide 50 mg and reserpine 0.125 mg.

HYDRO-RESERP: hydrochlorothiazide
50 mg and reserpine 0.125 mg.

HYDROSERP: hydrochlorothiazide 50
mg and reserpine 0.125 mg.

HYDROSERPINE: hydrochlorothiazide
50 mg and reserpine 0.125 mg.

HYDROTENSIN-25 TABLETS: hydrochlorothiazide 25 mg and reserpine
0.125 mg.

HYDROTENSIN-50: hydrochlorothiazide 50 mg and reserpine 0.125 mg.

HYSERP: hydrochlorothiazide 15 mg,
hydralazine HCl 25 mg, and reserpine
0.1 mg.

INDERIDE 40/25: propranolol HCl 40
mg and hydrochlorothiazide 25 mg.

INDERIDE 80/25: propranolol HCl 80
mg and hydrochlorothiazide 25 mg.

INDERIDE LA 80/50: propranolol HCl
80 mg and hydrochlorothiazide 50
mg.

LOPRESSOR HCT 50/25: metoprolol
tartrate 50 mg and hydrochlorothiazide 25 mg.

LOPRESSOR HCT 100/25: metoprolol
tartrate 100 mg and hydrochlorothiazide 25 mg.

MAXZIDE: triamterene 75 mg and hydrochlorothiazide 50 mg.

METATENSIN TABLETS: trichlorme-

thiazide 2 or 4 mg and reserpine 0.1
mg.

MINIZIDE 1: polythiazide 0.5 mg and
prazosin 1 mg.

MINIZIDE 2: polythiazide 0.5 mg and
prazosin 2 mg.

MINIZIDE 5: polythiazide 0.5 mg and
prazosin 5 mg.

NAQUIVAL: trichlormethiazide 4 mg
and reserpine 0.1 mg.

NATURETIN W/K 2.5 mg♦: bendroflumethiazide 2.5 mg and potassium
chloride 500 mg.

NATURETIN W/K 5 mg♦: bendroflumethiazide 5 mg and potassium chloride 500 mg.

ORETICYL 25: hydrochlorothiazide 25
mg and deserpidine 0.125 mg.

ORETICYL 50: hydrochlorothiazide 50
mg and deserpidine 0.125 mg.

ORETICYL FORTE: hydrochlorothiazide 25 mg and deserpidine 0.25 mg.

RAUTRAX**: flumethiazide 400 mg,
potassium chloride 400 mg, and powdered rauwolfia serpentina 50 mg.

RAUTRAX-N**: bendroflumethiazide
4 mg, powdered rauwolfia serpentina
50 mg, and potassium chloride 400
mg.

RAUZIDE**: bendroflumethiazide 4
mg and powdered rauwolfia serpentina 50 mg.

REGROTON: chlorthalidone 50 mg and
reserpine 0.25 mg.

RENESE-R: polythiazide 2 mg and reserpine 0.25 mg.

REZIDE: hydrochlorothiazide 15 mg,
hydralazine HCl 25 mg, and reserpine
0.1 mg.

R-HCTZ-H: hydrochlorothiazide 15
mg, hydralazine HCl 25 mg, and reserpine 0.1 mg.

SALUTENSIN♦: hydroflumethiazide 50
mg and reserpine 0.125 mg.

SALUTENSIN DEMI: hydroflumethiazide 25 mg and reserpine 0.125 mg.

SER-A-GEN: hydrochlorothiazide 15
mg, hydralazine HCl 25 mg, and reserpine 0.1 mg.

SERALAZIDE: hydrochlorothiazide 15
mg, hydralazine HCl 25 mg, and re-

Italicized side effects are common or life-threatening.
♦ ~uid form contains alcohol.   **May contain tartrazine.

serpine 0.1 mg.

SER-AP-ES♦: hydrochlorothiazide 15 mg, reserpine 0.1 mg, and hydralazine HCl 25 mg.

SERPASIL-APRESOLINE #1**: reserpine 0.1 mg and hydralazine HCl 25 mg.

SERPASIL-APRESOLINE #2♦: reserpine 0.2 mg and hydralazine HCl 50 mg.

SERPASIL-ESIDRIX #1♦: hydrochlorothiazide 25 mg and reserpine 0.1 mg (called Serpasil-Esidrix 25 in Canada).

TENORETIC 50: atenolol 50 mg and chlorthalidone 25 mg.

TENORETIC 100: atenolol 100 mg and chlorthalidone 25 mg.

TIMOLIDE 10/25: timolol maleate 10 mg and hydrochlorothiazide 25 mg.

TRI-HYDROSERPINE: hydrochlorothiazide 15 mg, hydralazine HCl 25 mg, and reserpine 0.1 mg.

UNIPRES: hydrochlorothiazide 15 mg, reserpine 0.1 mg, and hydralazine HCl 25 mg.

VASERETIC: enalapril maleate 10 mg and hydrochlorothiazide 25 mg.

---

acebutolol
Sectral
Pregnancy Category: B

MECHANISM OF ACTION
Blocks response to beta stimulation and depresses renin secretion.

INDICATIONS & DOSAGE
Treatment of hypertension—
Adults: 400 mg P.O. either as a single daily dose or divided b.i.d. Patients may receive as much as 1,200 mg daily.
Ventricular arrhythmias—
Adults: 400 mg P.O. daily divided b.i.d. Dose is then increased to provide an adequate clinical response. Usual dose is 600 to 1,200 mg per day.

ADVERSE REACTIONS
CNS: *fatigue,* headache, dizziness, insomnia.
CV: chest pain, edema, bradycardia, congestive heart failure, *hypotension.*
GI: nausea, constipation, diarrhea, dyspepsia.
Metabolic: hypoglycemia without tachycardia.
Skin: rash.
Other: fever.

INTERACTIONS
Insulin, hypoglycemic drugs (oral): can alter dosage requirements in previously stabilized diabetics. Observe patient carefully.
Cardiac glycosides: excessive bradycardia and increased depressant effect on myocardium. Use together cautiously.
Indomethacin: decreased antihypertensive effect. Monitor blood pressure and adjust dosage.

NURSING CONSIDERATIONS
• Contraindicated in persistently severe bradycardia, second- and third-degree heart block, overt cardiac failure, and cardiogenic shock.
• Use cautiously in patients with cardiac failure.
• Similar to metoprolol, acebutolol is a cardioselective beta blocker. This drug should be used with caution in patients with bronchospastic diseases such as asthma and emphysema.
• Dosage should be reduced in patients with decreased renal function.
• Geriatric patients may require lower acebutolol doses. For such patients, dosage should not exceed 800 mg per day.
• Always check patient's apical pulse before giving this drug; if slower than 60 beats per minute, hold drug and call doctor.
• Before surgery, notify anesthesiologist if patient's receiving this drug.
• Do not discontinue abruptly; can exacerbate angina and MI.

• Teach patient about his disease and therapy. Explain the importance of taking this drug as prescribed, even when he's feeling well. Tell patient not to discontinue drug suddenly, but to call doctor if unpleasant adverse effects develop.

---

atenolol
Tenormin♦
Pregnancy Category: C

MECHANISM OF ACTION
Blocks response to beta stimulation and depresses renin secretion.

INDICATIONS & DOSAGE
Treatment of hypertension—
Adults: initially, 50 mg P.O. daily single dose. Dosage may be increased to 100 mg once daily after 7 to 14 days. Dosages greater than 100 mg are unlikely to produce further benefit. Dosage adjustment is necessary in patients with creatinine clearance below 35 ml/minute.
Angina pectoris—
Adults: 50 mg P.O. once daily. May increase to 100 mg daily after 7 days for optimal effect. May give as much as 200 mg daily.

ADVERSE REACTIONS
CNS: fatigue, lethargy.
CV: *bradycardia, hypotension, congestive heart failure,* peripheral vascular disease.
GI: nausea, vomiting, diarrhea.
Skin: rash.
Other: fever.

INTERACTIONS
Insulin, hypoglycemic drugs (oral): can alter dosage requirements in previously stabilized diabetics. Observe patient carefully.
Cardiac glycosides: excessive bradycardia and increased depressant effect on myocardium. Use together cautiously.

Indomethacin: decrease in antihypertensive effect. Monitor blood pressure and adjust dosage.

NURSING CONSIDERATIONS
• Contraindicated in sinus bradycardia and greater than first degree conduction block, and cardiogenic shock.
• Use cautiously in patients with cardiac failure.
• Similar to metoprolol, atenolol is a cardioselective beta blocker. Although atenolol can be used in patients with bronchospastic diseases such as asthma and emphysema, the drug should still be used cautiously in such patients—especially when 100 mg are given.
• Dosage should be reduced if patient has renal insufficiency.
• Once-a-day dosage encourages patient compliance. Counsel your patient to take the drug at a regular time every day. Drug can be dispensed in a 28-day calendar pack.
• Always check patient's apical pulse before giving this drug; if slower than 60 beats per minute, hold drug and call doctor.
• Monitor blood pressure frequently.
• Don't discontinue abruptly; can exacerbate angina and MI.
• Teach patient about his disease and therapy. Explain the importance of taking this drug, even when he's feeling well. Tell patient not to discontinue drug suddenly, but to call doctor if unpleasant side effects develop.
• This drug masks common signs of shock and hypoglycemia. However, atenolol doesn't potentiate insulin-induced hypoglycemia or delay recovery of blood glucose to normal levels.
• Has been prescribed effectively in the treatment of angina pectoris and in patients with alcohol withdrawal syndrome.
• Atenolol, as well as other beta blockers, is being prescribed to decrease mortality following myocardial infarction.

Italicized side effects are common or life-threatening.
*Liquid form contains alcohol.   **May contain tartrazine.

captopril
Capoten♦
Pregnancy Category: C

MECHANISM OF ACTION
By inhibiting angiotensin-converting enzyme, prevents pulmonary conversion of angiotensin I to angiotensin II.

INDICATIONS & DOSAGE
Hypertension—
Adults: 25 mg P.O. b.i.d. or t.i.d. initially. If blood pressure isn't satisfactorily controlled in 1 to 2 weeks, dose may be increased to 50 mg t.i.d. If not satisfactorily controlled after another 1 to 2 weeks, a diuretic should be added to regimen. If further blood pressure reduction is necessary, dose may be raised to as high as 150 mg t.i.d. while continuing the diuretic. Maximum dose is 450 mg daily. Daily dose may also be administered b.i.d.
Heart failure—
Adults: 25 mg P.O. t.i.d. initially. May be increased to 50 mg t.i.d. Maximum dose 450 mg daily. In patients also taking diuretics, initial dose is 6.25 to 12.5 mg t.i.d.

ADVERSE REACTIONS
Blood: *leukopenia, agranulocytosis, pancytopenia.*
CNS: dizziness, fainting.
CV: *tachycardia, hypotension,* angina pectoris, congestive heart failure, pericarditis.
EENT: *loss of taste (dysgeusia).*
GU: *proteinuria, nephrotic syndrome, membranous glomerulopathy, renal failure,* urinary frequency.
GI: anorexia.
Metabolic: hyperkalemia.
Skin: *urticarial rash, maculopapular rash,* pruritus.
Other: fever, angioedema of face and extremities, transient increases in liver enzymes.

INTERACTIONS
Nonsteroidal anti-inflammatory drugs including aspirin: may reduce antihypertensive effect. Monitor blood pressure.
Potassium supplements: increased risk of hyperkalemia. Avoid these supplements unless hypokalemic blood levels are confirmed.
Antacids: decreased captopril effect. Separate administration times.

NURSING CONSIDERATIONS
• Use cautiously in patients with impaired renal function or serious autoimmune disease (particularly systemic lupus erythematosus), or those who have been exposed to other drugs known to affect white cell counts or immune response.
• Proteinuria and nephrotic syndrome may occur in patients who are on captopril therapy. Those who develop persistent proteinuria or proteinuria that exceeds 1 g daily should have their captopril therapy reevaluated.
• Monitor patient's blood pressure and pulse rate frequently.
• Perform WBC and differential counts before starting treatment, every 2 weeks for the first 3 months of therapy, and periodically thereafter.
• Advise patients to report any sign of infection (sore throat, fever).
• Although captopril can be used alone, its beneficial effects are increased when a thiazide diuretic is added.
• May cause dizziness or fainting; advise patient to avoid sudden postural changes.
• Elderly patients may be more sensitive to the hypotensive effects.
• Question patient about impaired taste sensation.
• Should be taken 1 hour before meals since food in the GI tract may reduce absorption.
• Has been prescribed to treat rheumatoid arthritis.

Unmarked trade names available in the United States only.
♦Also available in Canada.   ♦♦Available in Canada only.

clonidine hydrochloride

Catapres ♦, Catapres-TTS,
Dixarit♦♦
Pregnancy Category: C

MECHANISM OF ACTION

Inhibits the central vasomotor centers, thereby decreasing sympathetic outflow.

INDICATIONS & DOSAGE

Essential, renal, and malignant hypertension—
Adults: initially, 0.1 mg P.O. b.i.d. Then increase by 0.1 to 0.2 mg daily on a weekly basis. Usual dose range: 0.2 to 0.8 mg daily in divided doses. Infrequently, doses as high as 2.4 mg daily. No dosing recommendations for children.

Or, apply transdermal patch to a hairless area of intact skin on the upper arm or torso, once every 7 days.
To suppress abstinence symptoms during narcotics withdrawal—
Adults: 0.1 mg P.O. t.i.d.

ADVERSE REACTIONS

CNS: *drowsiness,* dizziness, fatigue, sedation, nervousness, headache.
CV: orthostatic hypotension, bradycardia, *severe rebound hypertension.*
EENT: *mouth dryness.*
GI: *constipation.*
GU: urinary retention.
Metabolic: glucose intolerance.
Skin: *pruritus, dermatitis* (from transdermal patch).
Other: impotence.

INTERACTIONS

Tricyclic antidepressants and MAO inhibitors: may decrease antihypertensive effect. Use together cautiously.
Propranolol and other beta blockers: paradoxical hypertensive response. Monitor carefully.

NURSING CONSIDERATIONS

• Use cautiously in patients with severe coronary insufficiency, diabetes, myocardial infarction, cerebral vascular disease, chronic renal failure, or history of depression, or in those taking other antihypertensives.
• Monitor blood pressure and pulse rate frequently. Dosage is usually adjusted to patient's blood pressure and tolerance.
• May be given to rapidly lower blood pressure in some hypertensive emergency situations.
• Reduce dose gradually over 2 to 4 days. If discontinued abruptly, this drug may cause severe hypertension.
• Teach patient about his disease and therapy. Explain why it's important to take this drug exactly as prescribed, even when he's feeling well. Tell outpatient not to discontinue this drug suddenly, but to call the doctor if unpleasant side effects develop. Severe rebound hypertension will occur if patient discontinues the drug suddenly. Warn that this drug can cause drowsiness, but that tolerance to this side effect will develop.
• Observe for tolerance to the drug's therapeutic effects that may require an increased dosage.
• Inform patient that orthostatic hypotension can be minimized by rising slowly and avoiding sudden position changes.
• Elderly patients may be more sensitive to hypotensive effects.
• Last dose should be taken immediately before retiring.
• Transdermal patch provides antihypertensive activity for up to 7 days. Available in three strengths: TTS-1 contains 2.5 mg; TTS-2 contains 5 mg; TTS contains 7.5 mg of clonidine.
• Transdermal patch usually adheres despite showering and other routine daily activities. An adhesive "overlay" is available to provide additional skin adherence if necessary.
• Has been used investigationally for migraine headache prophylaxis and

---

Italicized side effects are common or life-threatening.
*Liquid form contains alcohol.   **May contain tartrazine.

treatment of dysmenorrhea. May also suppress craving for nicotine in nicotine addiction.

diazoxide
Hyperstat♦ (I.V. only)
Pregnancy Category: C

MECHANISM OF ACTION
Directly relaxes arteriolar smooth muscle.

INDICATIONS & DOSAGE
Hypertensive crisis—
Adults: 300 mg I.V. bolus push, administered in 30 seconds or less into peripheral vein. Repeat at intervals of 4 to 24 hours, p.r.n. Mini-boluses of 1 to 3 mg/kg repeated at intervals of 5 to 15 minutes or infusions of 15 mg/minute are equally effective. Switch to therapy with oral antihypertensives as soon as possible.
Children: 5 mg/kg I.V. rapid bolus push.

ADVERSE REACTIONS
CNS: *headaches,* dizziness, lightheadedness, euphoria.
CV: *sodium and water retention, orthostatic hypotension,* sweating, flushing, warmth, angina, myocardial ischemia, arrhythmias, EKG changes.
GI: *nausea, vomiting,* abdominal discomfort.
Metabolic: *hyperglycemia,* hyperuricemia.
Local: inflammation and pain from extravasation.

INTERACTIONS
Hydralazine: may cause severe hypotension. Use together cautiously.
Thiazide diuretics: may increase the effects of diazoxide. Use together cautiously.

NURSING CONSIDERATIONS
• Use cautiously in patients with impaired cerebral or cardiac function,

diabetes, or uremia, or in those taking other antihypertensives.
• Check patient's standing blood pressure before discontinuing close monitoring for hypotension.
• Monitor blood pressure frequently. Notify doctor immediately if severe hypotension develops. Keep norepinephrine available.
• Monitor patient's intake and output carefully. If fluid or sodium retention develops, doctor may want to order diuretics.
• Take care to avoid extravasation.
• This drug may alter requirements for insulin, diet, or oral hypoglycemic drugs in previously controlled diabetics. Monitor blood glucose daily.
• Weigh patient daily. Notify doctor of any weight increase.
• Watch diabetics closely for signs of severe hyperglycemia or hyperosmolar nonketotic coma. Insulin may be needed.
• Check patient's uric acid levels frequently. Report abnormalities to doctor.
• Inform patient that orthostatic hypotension can be minimized by rising slowly and avoiding sudden position changes. Instruct patient to remain supine for 30 minutes after injection.
• Infusion of diazoxide has been shown to be as effective as a bolus in some patients.

enalapril maleate
Vasotec
Pregnancy Category: C

MECHANISM OF ACTION
By inhibiting angiotensin-converting enzyme, prevents pulmonary conversion of angiotensin I to angiotensin II.

INDICATIONS & DOSAGE
Treatment of hypertension—
Adults: Initially, 5 mg P.O. once daily, then adjust according to response. Usual dosage range is 10 to 40

mg daily as a single dose or two divided doses.

ADVERSE REACTIONS
Blood: neutropenia, *agranulocytosis.*
CNS: *headache, dizziness, fatigue,* insomnia.
CV: *hypotension.*
GI: diarrhea, nausea.
Skin: rash.
Other: cough, *angioedema.*

INTERACTIONS
None significant.

NURSING CONSIDERATIONS
• Use cautiously in patients with pre-existing renal impairment or collagen vascular disease.
• If patient is taking a diuretic, it should be discontinued 2 to 3 days before beginning enalapril therapy. This will reduce the risk of hypotension. Then, if enalapril does not control blood pressure, diuretic therapy may be added.
• Angioedema (including laryngeal edema) may occur, especially after the first enalapril dose. Advise patient to report any signs or symptoms such as swelling of face, eyes, lips, tongue, or breathing difficulty.
• Advise patient to report light-headedness, especially during the first few days of therapy, when it's most likely to occur.
• Advise patient to report any sign of infection.
• Enalapril is similar to captopril, the other angiotensin-converting enzyme inhibitor, but has a longer duration of action. Many patients may get satisfactory therapeutic results by taking enalapril once daily.

guanabenz acetate
Wytensin
Pregnancy Category: C

MECHANISM OF ACTION
An alpha-adrenergic stimulator that alters sympathetic outflow.

INDICATIONS & DOSAGE
Treatment of hypertension—
Adults: initially, 4 mg P.O. b.i.d. Dosage may be increased in increments of 4 to 8 mg/day every 1 to 2 weeks. Maximum dose is 32 mg b.i.d.

ADVERSE REACTIONS
CNS: *drowsiness, sedation, dizziness, weakness,* headache, ataxia, depression.
CV: *severe rebound hypertension.*
EENT: *dry mouth.*
GU: sexual dysfunction.

INTERACTIONS
CNS depressants: may cause increased sedation. Use together cautiously.

NURSING CONSIDERATIONS
• Use cautiously in patients with vascular insufficiency, coronary insufficiency, recent MI, cerebrovascular disease, or severe hepatic or renal failure.
• Don't stop guanabenz therapy abruptly. Rebound hypertension may occur.
• Advise your patient to drive a car or operate machinery very cautiously until the CNS effects of the drug are determined.
• Elderly patients may be more sensitive to hypotensive effects.
• Warn your patient that his tolerance to alcohol or other CNS depressants may be diminished.
• Guanabenz can be used alone or in combination with a thiazide diuretic.
• Teach patient about his disease and

Italicized side effects are common or life-threatening.
*Liquid form contains alcohol.   **May contain tartrazine.

therapy. Explain why it's important to take this drug exactly as prescribed, even when he's feeling well.
• To relieve dry mouth, tell patient to chew sugarless gum or dissolve ice chips in the mouth.

guanadrel sulfate
Hylorel
Pregnancy Category: B

MECHANISM OF ACTION
Acts peripherally, inhibiting norepinephrine release and depleting norepinephrine stores in adrenergic nerve endings.

INDICATIONS & DOSAGE
Treatment of hypertension—
Adults: initially, 5 mg P.O. b.i.d. Dosage can be adjusted until blood pressure is controlled. Most patients require doses of 20 to 75 mg/day, usually given b.i.d.

ADVERSE REACTIONS
CNS: *fatigue, dizziness,* drowsiness, faintness.
CV: *orthostatic hypotension,* edema.
GI: diarrhea.
Other: impotence, ejaculation disturbances.

INTERACTIONS
MAO inhibitors, ephedrine, norepinephrine, methylphenidate, tricyclic antidepressants, amphetamines, phenothiazines: may inhibit the antihypertensive effect of guanadrel. Adjust dose accordingly.

NURSING CONSIDERATIONS
• Contraindicated in patients with known or suspected pheochromocytoma or frank congestive heart failure.
• Use cautiously in patients with known regional vascular disease, asthmatic patients, and patients with history of peptic ulcer disease.

• Guanadrel should be discontinued 48 to 72 hours before surgery to minimize the risk of vascular collapse during anesthesia.
• Don't give concurrently or within 1 week of therapy with an MAO inhibitor.
• Patient response varies widely with this drug and dosage must be individualized. Monitor both supine and standing blood pressure, especially during the period of dosage adjustment.
• Teach patient about his disease and therapy. Explain why it's important to take this drug exactly as prescribed, even when he's feeling well. Tell patient not to discontinue this drug suddenly but to call the doctor if unpleasant side effects develop.
• Tell outpatient to avoid strenuous exercise, and warn that hot showers may cause hypotensive reaction.
• Inform patient that orthostatic hypotension can be minimized by rising slowly from a supine position and avoiding sudden position changes.
• Elderly patients may be more sensitive to hypotensive effects.

guanethidine sulfate
Ismelin♦
Pregnancy Category: C

MECHANISM OF ACTION
Acts peripherally, inhibiting norepinephrine release and depleting norepinephrine stores in adrenergic nerve endings.

INDICATIONS & DOSAGE
For moderate to severe hypertension; usually used in combination with other antihypertensives—
Adults: initially, 10 mg P.O. daily. Increase by 10 mg at weekly to monthly intervals, p.r.n. Usual dose is 25 to 50 mg daily. Some patients may require up to 300 mg.
Children: initially, 200 mcg/kg P.O.

daily. Increase gradually every 1 to 3 weeks to maximum of 8 times initial dose.

ADVERSE REACTIONS
CNS: *dizziness, weakness, syncope*.
CV: *orthostatic hypotension, bradycardia*, congestive heart failure, arrhythmias.
EENT: *nasal stuffiness*, mouth dryness.
GI: *diarrhea*.
Other: *edema, weight gain, inhibition of ejaculation*.

INTERACTIONS
Levodopa, alcohol: may increase hypotensive effect of guanethidine. Use together cautiously.
MAO inhibitors, ephedrine, norepinephrine, methylphenidate, tricyclic antidepressants, amphetamines, phenothiazines: may inhibit the antihypertensive effect of guanethidine. Adjust dose accordingly.

NURSING CONSIDERATIONS
• Contraindicated in patients with pheochromocytoma. Use cautiously in patients with severe cardiac disease, recent MI, cerebrovascular disease, peptic ulcer, impaired renal function, or bronchial asthma, or in those taking other antihypertensives.
• Discontinue drug 2 to 3 weeks before elective surgery to reduce the possibility of vascular collapse and cardiac arrest during anesthesia.
• Teach patient about his disease and therapy. Explain why it's important to take this drug exactly as prescribed, even when he's feeling well. Tell patient not to discontinue this drug suddenly, but to call the doctor if unpleasant side effects develop.
• Tell outpatient to avoid strenuous exercise, and warn that hot showers may cause hypotensive reaction.
• Patient should receive instruction on low-sodium diet. Monitor for possible weight gain and edema.

• A hot environment may also potentiate the hypotensive effects of guanethidine.
• Inform patient that orthostatic hypotension can be minimized by rising slowly and avoiding sudden position changes. Mouth dryness can be relieved with sugarless chewing gum, sour hard candy, or ice chips.
• Elderly patients may be more sensitive to hypotensive effects.
• If patient develops diarrhea, doctor may prescribe atropine or paregoric.

guanfacine hydrochloride
Tenex
Pregnancy Category: B

MECHANISM OF ACTION
Inhibits the central vasomotor center, thereby decreasing sympathetic outflow.

INDICATIONS & DOSAGE
Treatment of mild to moderate hypertension—
Adults: initially, 0.5 to 1 mg P.O. daily, at bedtime. Average dose is 1 to 3 mg daily.

ADVERSE REACTIONS
CNS: *drowsiness, dizziness*, fatigue, headache, insomnia.
CV: bradycardia, orthostatic hypotension, rebound hypertension.
GI: *constipation, dry mouth*, diarrhea, nausea.
Skin: dermatitis, pruritus.

INTERACTIONS
None significant.

NURSING CONSIDERATIONS
• Use cautiously in patients with severe coronary insufficiency, recent MI, cerebrovascular disease, or chronic renal or hepatic insufficiency.
• Warn patients not to discontinue therapy abruptly. Rebound hypertension is less common than with similar

---

Italicized side effects are common or life-threatening.
*Liquid form contains alcohol.   **May contain tartrazine.

drugs, such as clonidine, but may occur.
• Guanfacine reportedly has no adverse effect on blood lipids.
• May be used alone or with a diuretic.
• The incidence and severity of adverse reactions increase with higher dosages.
• Because guanfacine causes drowsiness, advise patient to avoid activities that require alertness until response to the drug is established.
• Guanfacine appears to be as effective as methyldopa and clonidine; long half-life permits once-daily dosing.

hydralazine hydrochloride
Apresoline♦**, Hydralyn, Rolazine
Pregnancy Category: C

MECHANISM OF ACTION
Directly relaxes arteriolar smooth muscle.

INDICATIONS & DOSAGE
Essential hypertension (oral, alone or in combination with other antihypertensives); to reduce afterload in severe congestive heart failure (with nitrates); and severe essential hypertension (parenteral to lower blood pressure quickly)—
Adults: initially, 10 mg P.O. q.i.d.; gradually increased to 50 mg q.i.d. Maximum recommended dosage is 200 mg daily, but some patients may require 300 to 400 mg daily.
I.V.—20 to 40 mg given slowly and repeated as necessary, generally q 4 to 6 hours. Switch to oral antihypertensives as soon as possible.
I.M.—20 to 40 mg repeated as necessary, generally q 4 to 6 hours. Switch to oral antihypertensives as soon as possible.
Children: initially, 0.75 mg/kg P.O. daily in 4 divided doses (25 mg/m² daily). May increase gradually to 10

times this dose, if necessary.
I.V.—give slowly 1.7 to 3.5 mg/kg daily or 50 to 100 mg/m² daily in 4 to 6 divided doses.
I.M.—1.7 to 3.5 mg/kg daily or 50 to 100 mg/m² daily in 4 to 6 divided doses.

ADVERSE REACTIONS
Blood: neutropenia, leukopenia.
CNS: peripheral neuritis, *headache,* dizziness.
CV: orthostatic hypotension, *tachycardia,* arrhythmias, *angina, palpitations, sodium retention.*
GI: *nausea, vomiting, diarrhea, anorexia.*
Skin: rash.
Other: *lupus erythematosus-like syndrome, weight gain.*

INTERACTIONS
Diazoxide: may cause severe hypotension. Use together cautiously.

NURSING CONSIDERATIONS
• Use cautiously in patients with cardiac disease or in those taking other antihypertensives.
• Monitor patient's blood pressure and pulse rate frequently.
• Watch patient closely for signs of lupus erythematosus-like syndrome (sore throat, fever, muscle and joint aches, skin rash). Call doctor immediately if any of these develop.
• Teach patient about his disease and therapy. Explain why it's important to take this drug exactly as prescribed, even when he's feeling well. Tell outpatient not to discontinue this drug suddenly, but to call the doctor if unpleasant side effects develop.
• Inform patient that orthostatic hypotension can be minimized by rising slowly and avoiding sudden position changes.
• Elderly patients may be more sensitive to hypotensive effects.
• Give this drug with meals to increase absorption.

• Compliance may be improved by administering this drug b.i.d. Check with doctor.
• Complete blood count, LE cell preparation, and antinuclear antibody titer determinations should be done before therapy and periodically during long-term therapy.
• Has been prescribed during pregnancy for treatment of eclampsia. Administered I.V.

labetalol
Normodyne, Trandate
Pregnancy Category: C

MECHANISM OF ACTION
Blocks response to alpha and beta stimulation and depresses renin secretion.

INDICATIONS & DOSAGE
Treatment of hypertension—
Adults: 100 mg P.O. b.i.d. with or without a diuretic. Dose may be increased to 200 mg b.i.d. after 2 days. Further dose increases may be made every 1 to 3 days until optimum response is reached. Usual maintenance dose is 200 to 400 mg b.i.d.
For severe hypertension and hypertensive emergencies—
Adults: Dilute 200 mg to 200 ml with 5% dextrose in water. Infuse at 2 mg per minute until satisfactory response is obtained. Then stop the infusion. may repeat q 6 to 8 hours.
Alternatively, administer by repeated I.V. injection: Initially, give 20 mg I.V. slowly over 2 minutes. May repeat injections of 40 to 80 mg q 10 minutes until maximum dose of 300 mg is reached.

ADVERSE REACTIONS
CNS: vivid dreams, fatigue, headache.
CV: *orthostatic hypotension and dizziness,* peripheral vascular disease, bradycardia.

EENT: nasal stuffiness.
Endocrine: hypoglycemia without tachycardia.
GI: nausea, vomiting, diarrhea.
GU: sexual dysfunction, urinary retention.
Skin: rash.
Other: increased airway resistance, transient scalp tingling.

INTERACTIONS
Insulin, hypoglycemic drugs (oral): can alter dosage requirements in previously stabilized diabetics. Observe patient carefully.
Cimetidine: may enhance labetalol's effect. Give together cautiously.

NURSING CONSIDERATIONS
• Contraindicated in patients with bronchial asthma.
• Use cautiously in congestive heart failure, chronic bronchitis, emphysema, preexisting peripheral vascular disease, and pheochromocytoma.
• Monitor blood pressure frequently.
• Teach patient about his disease and therapy. Explain why it's important to take this drug exactly as prescribed, even when he's feeling well. Tell outpatient not to discontinue this drug suddenly; abrupt discontinuation can exacerbate angina and MI. Tell patient to call doctor if unpleasant side effects develop.
• This drug masks common signs of shock and hypoglycemia.
• Labetalol is a beta-adrenergic blocker which also has unique alpha-adrenergic blocking effects.
• Unlike other beta blockers, labetalol does not decrease heart rate or cardiac output.
• Dizziness is the most troublesome side effect and tends to occur in early stages of treatment, in patients also receiving diuretics, and in patients receiving higher dosages. Inform patient that this can be minimized by rising slowly and avoiding sudden position changes. Taking a dose at bed-

---

Italicized side effects are common or life-threatening.
*Liquid form contains alcohol.   **May contain tartrazine.

time will also help minimize this adverse reaction.
• Transient scalp tingling occurs occasionally at the beginning of labetalol therapy. This usually subsides quickly.
• When administered I.V. for hypertensive emergencies, labetalol produces a rapid, predictable fall in blood pressure within 5 to 10 minutes. Patient should remain supine for 3 hours after infusion.

methyldopa
Aldomet♦, Dopamet♦♦, Medimet-250♦♦, Novomedopa♦♦
Pregnancy Category: C

MECHANISM OF ACTION
An alpha-adrenergic stimulator that alters sympathetic outflow.

INDICATIONS & DOSAGE
For sustained mild to severe hypertension; should not be used for acute treatment of hypertensive emergencies—
Adults: initially, 250 mg P.O. b.i.d. to t.i.d. in first 48 hours. Then increase as needed every 2 days. May give entire daily dose in the evening or at bedtime. Dosages may need adjustment if other antihypertensive drugs are added to or deleted from therapy.
Maintenance dosages—500 mg to 2 g daily in 2 to 4 divided doses. Maximum recommended daily dose is 3 g.
I.V.—500 mg to 1 g q 6 hours, diluted in dextrose 5% in water, and administered over 30 to 60 minutes. Switch to oral antihypertensives as soon as possible.
Children: initially, 10 mg/kg daily P.O. in 2 to 3 divided doses; or 20 to 40 mg/kg daily I.V. in 4 divided doses. Increase dose daily until desired response occurs. Maximum daily dose 65 mg/kg.

ADVERSE REACTIONS
Blood: *hemolytic anemia,* reversible granulocytopenia, thrombocytopenia.
CNS: *sedation,* headache, asthenia, weakness, dizziness, *decreased mental acuity,* involuntary choreoathetotic movements, psychic disturbances, depression, nightmares.
CV: bradycardia, *orthostatic hypotension,* aggravated angina, myocarditis, *edema, and weight gain.*
EENT: *dry mouth, nasal stuffiness.*
GI: diarrhea, pancreatitis.
Hepatic: *hepatic necrosis.*
Other: gynecomastia, lactation, skin rash, *drug-induced fever,* impotence.

INTERACTIONS
Norepinephrine, phenothiazines, tricyclic antidepressants, amphetamines: possible hypertensive effects. Monitor carefully.

NURSING CONSIDERATIONS
• Use cautiously in patients receiving other antihypertensives or MAO inhibitors and in patients with impaired hepatic function. Monitor blood pressure and pulse rate frequently.
• Observe for involuntary choreoathetoid movements. Report to doctor; he may discontinue drug.
• Observe patient for side effects, particularly unexplained fever. Report side effects to doctor.
• After dialysis, monitor patient for hypertension. Patient may need an extra dose of methyldopa.
• If patient requires blood transfusion, make sure he gets direct and indirect Coombs' tests to avoid cross-matching problems.
• Monitor blood studies (complete blood count) before and during therapy.
• If patient has been on this drug for several months, positive reaction to direct Coombs' test indicates hemolytic anemia.
• Weigh patient daily. Notify doctor of any weight increase. Salt and water

retention may occur but can be relieved with diuretics.

• Tell patient that urine may turn dark in toilet bowls treated with bleach.

• Teach patient about his disease and therapy. Explain why it's important to take this drug exactly as prescribed, even when he's feeling well. Tell outpatient not to stop this drug suddenly, but to call the doctor if unpleasant side effects develop. Once-daily dosage administered at bedtime will minimize drowsiness during daytime. Check with doctor.

• Inform patient that orthostatic hypotension can be minimized by rising slowly and avoiding sudden position changes. Mouth dryness can be relieved with sugarless chewing gum, sour hard candy, or ice chips.

• Elderly patients are more likely to experience sedation and hypotension.

---

metoprolol tartrate
Betaloc♦♦, Lopresor♦♦, Lopressor
Pregnancy Category: B

MECHANISM OF ACTION
Blocks response to beta stimulation and depresses renin secretion.

INDICATIONS & DOSAGE
For hypertension; may be used alone or in combination with other antihypertensives—
Adults: 50 mg b.i.d. or 100 mg once daily P.O. initially. Up to 200 to 400 mg daily in 2 to 3 divided doses. No dosage recommendations for children.
Early intervention in acute myocardial infarction—
Adults: Three injections of 5-mg I.V. boluses q 2 minutes. Then, 15 minutes after last dose, administer 50 mg P.O. q 6 hours for 48 hours. Maintenance dose is 100 mg P.O. b.i.d.

ADVERSE REACTIONS
CNS: fatigue, lethargy.
CV: *bradycardia, hypotension, con-*

gestive heart failure, peripheral vascular disease.
GI: nausea, vomiting, diarrhea.
Skin: rash.
Other: fever, arthralgias.

INTERACTIONS
Insulin, hypoglycemic drugs (oral): can alter dosage requirements in previously stabilized diabetics. Observe patient carefully.
Cardiac glycosides: excessive bradycardia and increased depressant effect on myocardium. Use together cautiously.
Barbiturates, rifampin: increased metabolism of metoprolol. Monitor for decreased effect.
Chlorpromazine, cimetidine: inhibits metoprolol's metabolism. Monitor for greater beta-blocking effect.
Indomethacin: decrease in antihypertensive effect. Monitor blood pressure and adjust dosage.

NURSING CONSIDERATIONS
• Use cautiously in patients with heart failure, diabetes, or respiratory disease, or in those taking other antihypertensives. Always check patient's apical pulse rate before giving this drug. If it's slower than 60 beats per minute, hold drug and call doctor immediately.

• Although most patients with asthma and bronchitis can take this drug without fear of worsening their condition, doses over 100 mg daily should be used cautiously in those patients.

• Monitor blood pressure frequently.

• Teach patient about his disease and therapy. Explain why it's important to take this drug, even when he's feeling well. Tell outpatient not to discontinue this drug suddenly; abrupt discontinuation can exacerbate angina and MI. Instruct patient to call doctor if unpleasant side effects develop.

• This drug masks common signs of shock and hypoglycemia. However,

---

Italicized side effects are common or life-threatening.
*Liquid form contains alcohol.   **May contain tartrazine.

metoprolol doesn't potentiate insulin-induced hypoglycemia or delay recovery of blood glucose to normal levels.
• Food may increase absorption of metoprolol. Give consistently with meals.

metyrosine
Demser
Pregnancy Category: C

MECHANISM OF ACTION
Inhibits the enzyme tyrosine hydroxylase.

INDICATIONS & DOSAGE
Preoperative preparation of patients with pheochromocytoma; management of such patients when surgery is contraindicated; to control or prevent hypertension before or during pheochromocytomectomy—
Adults and children over 12 years: 250 mg P.O. q.i.d. May be increased by 250 to 500 mg q day to a maximum of 4 g daily in divided doses. When used for preoperative preparation, optimally effective dosage should be given for at least 5 to 7 days.

ADVERSE REACTIONS
CNS: *sedation,* extrapyramidal symptoms, such as speech difficulty and tremors, disorientation.
GI: *diarrhea,* nausea, vomiting, abdominal pain.
GU: *crystalluria,* hematuria.
Other: impotence, hypersensitivity.

INTERACTIONS
Phenothiazines and haloperidol: increased inhibition of catecholamine synthesis may result in extrapyramidal symptoms. Use cautiously.

NURSING CONSIDERATIONS
• During surgery, monitor blood pressure and EKG continuously. If a serious arrhythmia occurs during anesthesia and surgery, treatment with a beta-blocking drug or lidocaine may be necessary.
• Warn patient that sedation almost always occurs in those treated with metyrosine. Sedation usually subsides after several days' treatment.
• Instruct patient to increase daily fluid intake to prevent crystalluria. Daily urine volume should be 2,000 ml or more.
• Tell patient to notify doctor if any of the listed side effects occur.
• Insomnia may occur when metyrosine is stopped.
• If patient's hypertension is not adequately controlled by metyrosine, an alpha-adrenergic blocking agent, such as phenoxybenzamine, should be added to the regimen.
• Available as 250-mg capsules.

minoxidil
Loniten♦
Pregnancy Category: C

MECHANISM OF ACTION
Produces direct arteriolar vasodilation.

INDICATIONS & DOSAGE
Treatment of severe hypertension—
Adults: 5 mg P.O. initially as a single dose. Effective dosage range is usually 10 to 40 mg daily. Maximum dose 100 mg daily.
Children under 12 years: 0.2 mg/kg as a single daily dose. Effective dosage range usually 0.25 to 1 mg/kg daily. Maximum dose is 50 mg.

ADVERSE REACTIONS
CV: *edema, tachycardia, pericardial effusion and tamponade, congestive heart failure,* EKG changes.
Skin: rash, *Stevens-Johnson syndrome.*
Other: *hypertrichosis* (elongation, thickening, and enhanced pigmentation of fine body hair), breast tenderness.

INTERACTIONS
Guanethidine: severe orthostatic hypotension. Advise patient to stand up slowly.

NURSING CONSIDERATIONS
• Contraindicated in patients with pheochromocytoma.
• A potent vasodilator: Use only when other antihypertensives have failed.
• Instruct patient to take his own pulse. Patient should report an increase greater than 20 beats per minute to the doctor.
• Closely monitor blood pressure and pulse at beginning of therapy.
• Monitor intake and output; check for weight gain and edema.
• Elderly patients may be more sensitive to hypotensive effects.
• About 8 out of 10 patients will experience hypertrichosis within 3 to 6 weeks of beginning treatment. Unwanted hair can be controlled with a depilatory or shaving. Assure patient that extra hair will disappear within 1 to 6 months of stopping minoxidil. Advise patient, however, not to discontinue drug without doctor's consent.
• Drug is usually prescribed with a beta-blocking drug to control tachycardia and a diuretic to counteract fluid retention. Make sure patient complies with total treatment regimen.
• A patient package insert (PPI) has been prepared by the manufacturer of minoxidil, describing in layman's terms the drug and its side effects. Be sure your patient receives this insert and reads it thoroughly. Provide an oral explanation also.
• Prescribed in various topical forms for treatment of some types of male alopecia.

nitroprusside sodium
Nipride♦, Nitropress
Pregnancy Category: C

MECHANISM OF ACTION
Relaxes both arteriolar and venous smooth muscle.

INDICATIONS & DOSAGE
To lower blood pressure quickly in hypertensive emergencies; to control hypotension during anesthesia; to reduce preload and afterload in cardiac pump failure or cardiogenic shock; may be used with or without dopamine—
Adults: 50-mg vial diluted with 2 to 3 ml of dextrose 5% in water I.V. and then added to 250, 500, or 1,000 ml dextrose 5% in water. Infuse at 0.5 to 10 mcg/kg/minute.
Average dose: 3 mcg/kg/minute.
Maximum infusion rate: 10 mcg/kg/minute.
Patients taking other antihypertensive drugs along with nitroprusside are very sensitive to this drug. Adjust dosage accordingly.

ADVERSE REACTIONS
The following side effects generally indicate overdosage:
CNS: *headache, dizziness,* ataxia, loss of consciousness, coma, weak pulse, absent reflexes, widely dilated pupils, *restlessness, muscle twitching, diaphoresis.*
CV: distant heart sounds, palpitations, dyspnea, shallow breathing.
GI: *vomiting, nausea, abdominal pain.*
Metabolic: acidosis.
Skin: pink color.

INTERACTIONS
None significant.

NURSING CONSIDERATIONS
• Use cautiously in patients with hypothyroidism or hepatic or renal disease, or in those receiving other anti-

---

Italicized side effects are common or life-threatening.
*Liquid form contains alcohol.   **May contain tartrazine.

hypertensives.
• Due to light sensitivity, wrap I.V. solution in foil. It's not necessary to wrap the tubing in foil. Fresh solution should have faint brownish tint. Discard after 24 hours.
• Obtain baseline vital signs before giving this drug, and find out what parameters the doctor wants to achieve.
• Check blood pressure every 5 minutes at start of infusion and every 15 minutes thereafter. If severe hypotension occurs, turn off I.V. nitroprusside—effects of drug quickly reversed. Notify doctor. If possible, an arterial pressure line should be started. Regulate drug flow to specified level.
• Don't use bacteriostatic water for injection or sterile saline solution for reconstitution.
• Infuse with automatic infusion pump.
• This drug is best run piggyback through a peripheral line with no other medication. Don't adjust rate of main I.V. line while drug is running. Even small bolus of nitroprusside can cause severe hypotension.
• This drug can cause cyanide toxicity, so check serum thiocyanate levels every 72 hours. Thiocyanate levels of greater than 100 mcg/ml are associated with toxicity. Watch for signs of thiocyanate toxicity: profound hypotension, metabolic acidosis, dyspnea, headache, loss of consciousness, ataxia, vomiting. If these occur, discontinue drug immediately and notify doctor.

pargyline hydrochloride
Eutonyl
Pregnancy Category: C

MECHANISM OF ACTION
Inhibits the enzyme monoamine oxidase (MAO).

INDICATIONS & DOSAGE
For moderate to severe hypertension, usually given in combination with other drugs—
Adults: initially, 25 to 50 mg P.O. once daily, if not receiving any other antihypertensive drugs. Then increase dosage by 10 mg daily at weekly intervals. Maximum daily dosage 200 mg. Usual daily dose for patients over 65 years or those who've had sympathectomy: 10 to 25 mg. When used in combination with other drugs, total daily dose of pargyline should not exceed 25 mg. No dosage recommendations for children.

ADVERSE REACTIONS
CNS: *tremors,* convulsions, choreiform movements, psychic changes, *nightmares, hyperexcitability, sweating,* dizziness, fainting, drowsiness.
CV: palpitations, *orthostatic hypotension,* fluid retention.
EENT: *mouth dryness,* optic damage.
GI: *nausea, vomiting, increased appetite, constipation.*
Other: impotence.

INTERACTIONS
Amphetamines, ephedrine, levodopa, metaraminol, methotrimeprazine, methylphenidate, phenylephrine, phenylpropanolamine, pseudoephedrine: enhanced pressor effects. Use together cautiously.
Alcohol, barbiturates, and other sedatives; tranquilizers; narcotics; dextromethorphan; tricyclic antidepressants: unpredictable interactions. Should be used with caution and in reduced dosage.

NURSING CONSIDERATIONS
• Contraindicated in patients with advanced renal failure, pheochromocytoma, hyperthyroidism, or Parkinson's disease; in patients who are hyperactive and hyperexcitable. Use cautiously in patients who are receiving other antihypertensives or who

have hepatic disease.
• Discontinue this drug at least 2 weeks before elective surgery.
• Hypotensive effects of this drug are increased by high temperatures, fever, stress, or severe illness. If patient develops severe hypotension, counteract with ephedrine or phenylephrine.
• Monitor blood pressure and pulse rate frequently. Take blood pressure while patient is standing.
• Patient should have periodic ophthalmic evaluations during therapy.
• If patient is scheduled for surgery and has been taking this drug, be sure narcotic dosages are reduced.
• This drug may require up to several weeks to reach optimal effect.
• Advise patient to take drug in the morning to avoid insomnia.
• Warn patient not to take any other medications, including over-the-counter cold remedies, without first asking doctor.
• This drug is an MAO inhibitor. Tell patient not to eat foods with high tyramine content: for example, aged cheese, chianti wine, sour cream, canned figs, raisins, chicken livers, yeast extract, pickled herring.
• Teach patient about his disease and therapy. Explain why it's important to take this drug exactly as prescribed, even when he's feeling well. Tell outpatient not to discontinue this drug suddenly, but to call the doctor if unpleasant side effects develop.
• Inform patient that orthostatic hypotension can be minimized by rising slowly and avoiding sudden position changes. Mouth dryness can be relieved with sugarless chewing gum, sour hard candy, or ice chips.

phenoxybenzamine hydrochloride
Dibenzyline
Pregnancy Category: C

MECHANISM OF ACTION
An alpha-adrenergic blocker that noncompetitively blocks the effect of catecholamines on alpha-adrenergic receptors.

INDICATIONS & DOSAGE
To control hypertension and sweating secondary to pheochromocytoma; may be used in combination with propranolol to control excessive tachycardia—
Adults: initially, 10 mg P.O. daily. Increase by 10 mg daily every 4 days. Maintenance dose: 20 to 60 mg daily.
Children: initially, 0.2 mg/kg or 6 mg/m² P.O. daily in a single dose. Maintenance dose: 12 to 36 mg/m² daily as a single dose or in divided doses.
To control Raynaud's syndrome, frostbite, acrocyanosis—
Adults: initially, 10 mg P.O., then increase by 10 mg q 4 days to a maximum of 60 mg daily.

ADVERSE REACTIONS
CNS: lethargy, drowsiness.
CV: *orthostatic hypotension, tachycardia,* shock.
EENT: *nasal stuffiness, dry mouth, miosis.*
GI: vomiting, abdominal distress.
Other: *impotence, inhibition of ejaculation.*

INTERACTIONS
None significant.

NURSING CONSIDERATIONS
• Use cautiously in patients with cerebrovascular or coronary insufficiency, advanced renal disease, respiratory disease.
• Watch patient closely for side effects, and call doctor promptly if they

occur. If severe hypotension develops, patient may require norepinephrine to counteract effect.

• Nasal congestion, inhibition of ejaculation, and impotence usually decrease with continued therapy.

• Patient with tachycardia may require concurrent propranolol therapy.

• Monitor patient's heart rate and blood pressure frequently.

• This drug may take several weeks to achieve optimal effect.

• Monitor respiratory status carefully. This drug may aggravate symptoms of pneumonia and asthma.

• Teach patient about his disease and therapy. Explain why it's important to take this drug exactly as prescribed, even when he's feeling well. Tell outpatient not to discontinue this drug suddenly, but to call the doctor if unpleasant side effects develop.

• Inform patient that orthostatic hypotension can be minimized by rising slowly and avoiding sudden position changes. Mouth dryness can be relieved with sugarless chewing gum, sour hard candy, or ice chips.

• Used investigationally to treat chronic urinary retention.

• Small initial doses are increased gradually until desired effect is obtained. Patient should be observed at each dose for at least 4 days.

---

phentolamine mesylate
Regitine, Rogitine♦♦
Pregnancy Category: C

MECHANISM OF ACTION
An alpha-adrenergic blocker that competitively blocks the effects of catecholamines on alpha-adrenergic receptors.

INDICATIONS & DOSAGE
To aid in diagnosis of pheochromocytoma; to control or prevent hypertension before or during pheochromocytomectomy—

Adults:
I.V. diagnostic dose: 5 mg, with close monitoring of blood pressure.
Before surgical removal of tumor, give 2 to 5 mg I.M. or I.V. During surgery, patient may need small I.V. doses (1 mg) or small I.M. doses (3 mg).

Children:
I.V. diagnostic dose: 0.1 mg/kg or 3 mg/m² as single dose, with close monitoring of blood pressure.
Before surgical removal of tumor give 1 mg I.V. or 3 mg I.M.
During surgery, patient may need small I.V. doses (1 mg).
To treat extravasation—infiltrate area with 5 to 10 mg phentolamine in 10 ml normal saline solution. Must be done within 12 hours.

ADVERSE REACTIONS
CNS: *dizziness, weakness, flushing.*
CV: *hypotension*, shock, *arrhythmias*, palpitations, *tachycardia*, angina pectoris.
GI: *diarrhea*, abdominal pain, *nausea, vomiting*, hyperperistalsis.
Other: *nasal stuffiness*, hypoglycemia.

INTERACTIONS
None significant.

NURSING CONSIDERATIONS
• Contraindicated in patients with angina, coronary artery disease, and history of MI. Use cautiously in patients with gastritis or peptic ulcer and in those receiving other antihypertensives.

• Don't administer epinephrine to treat phentolamine-induced hypotension. May cause additional fall in blood pressure.

• When this drug is given for diagnostic test, check patient's blood pressure first. Make frequent blood pressure checks during administration.

• Diagnosis positive for pheochromocytoma if severe hypotension results

---

from I.V. test dose.
- Administer norepinephrine to counteract severe hypotensive effect of this drug. Don't administer epinephrine to raise blood pressure, as this may cause further drop.
- Don't give sedatives or narcotics 24 hours before diagnostic test. Rauwolfia alkaloids should be withdrawn at least 4 weeks before testing.

pindolol
Visken♦
Pregnancy Category: B

MECHANISM OF ACTION
Blocks response to beta stimulation and depresses renin secretion.

INDICATIONS & DOSAGE
Treatment of hypertension—
Adults: initially, 5 mg P.O. b.i.d. Dosage may be increased by 10 mg/day every 2 to 3 weeks up to a maximum of 60 mg/day.

ADVERSE REACTIONS
CNS: *insomnia, fatigue, dizziness, nervousness,* vivid dreams, hallucinations, lethargy.
CV: *edema,* bradycardia, congestive heart failure, peripheral vascular disease, hypotension.
EENT: visual disturbances.
GI: *nausea,* vomiting, diarrhea.
Metabolic: hypoglycemia without tachycardia.
Skin: rash.
Other: *increased airway resistance, muscle pain, joint pain,* chest pain.

INTERACTIONS
Insulin, hypoglycemic drugs (oral): can alter requirements for these drugs in previously stabilized diabetics. Monitor for hypoglycemia.
Cardiac glycosides: excessive bradycardia and increased depressant effect on myocardium. Use together cau-

tiously.
Cimetidine: inhibits pindolol metabolism. Monitor for greater beta-blocking effect.
Epinephrine: severe vasoconstriction. Monitor blood pressure and observe patient carefully.
Indomethacin: decreased antihypertensive affect. Monitor blood pressure and adjust dosage.

NURSING CONSIDERATIONS
- Contraindicated in diabetes mellitus, asthma, allergic rhinitis; during ethyl ether anesthesia; in sinus bradycardia and heart block greater than first degree; in cardiogenic shock; in right ventricular failure secondary to pulmonary hypertension. Use with caution in patients with congestive heart failure or respiratory disease, and in patients taking other antihypertensive drugs.
- Always check patient's apical pulse rate before giving this drug. If you detect extremes in pulse rates, hold medication and call the doctor immediately.
- Monitor blood pressure frequently. If patient develops severe hypotension, notify doctor. He may prescribe a vasopressor.
- Teach patient about his disease and therapy. Explain why it's important to take this drug exactly as prescribed, even when he's feeling well. Tell outpatient not to discontinue this drug suddenly; abrupt discontinuation can exacerbate angina and MI. Tell patient to call doctor if unpleasant side effects develop.
- This drug masks common signs of shock and hypoglycemia.
- Pindolol may be taken without any special regard for meals.
- Many patients respond favorably to a dose of 5 mg t.i.d.
- The first commercially available beta-blocker with partial beta-*agonist* activity. In other words, pindolol also *stimulates* beta-adrenergic receptors

as well as blocks them. Therefore, it decreases cardiac output less than other beta-adrenergic blockers.
• May be advantageous for patients who develop bradycardia with other beta blockers.

prazosin hydrochloride
Minipress♦
Pregnancy Category: C

MECHANISM OF ACTION
Relaxes both arteriolar and venous smooth muscle.

INDICATIONS & DOSAGE
For mild to moderate hypertension; used alone or in combination with a diuretic or other antihypertensive drugs; also used to decrease afterload in severe chronic congestive heart failure—
Adults: P.O. test dose: 1 mg given before bedtime to prevent "first-dose syncope." Initial dose: 1 mg t.i.d. Increase dosage slowly. Maximum daily dose 20 mg. Maintenance dose: 3 to 20 mg daily in 3 divided doses. A few patients have required dosages larger than this (up to 40 mg daily). If other antihypertensive drugs or diuretics are added to this drug, decrease prazosin dosage to 1 to 2 mg t.i.d. and retitrate.

ADVERSE REACTIONS
CNS: *dizziness*, headache, drowsiness, weakness, *"first-dose syncope,"* depression.
CV: orthostatic hypotension, *palpitations.*
EENT: blurred vision, dry mouth.
GI: vomiting, diarrhea, abdominal cramps, constipation, *nausea.*
GU: priapism, impotence.

INTERACTIONS
Propranolol and other beta blockers: syncope with loss of consciousness may occur more frequently. Advise

patient to sit or lie down if he feels dizzy.

NURSING CONSIDERATIONS
• Use cautiously in patients receiving other antihypertensive drugs.
• Monitor patient's blood pressure and pulse rate frequently.
• If initial dose is greater than 1 mg, patient may develop severe syncope with loss of consciousness (first-dose syncope). Increase dosage slowly. Instruct patient to sit or lie down if he experiences dizziness.
• Elderly patients may be more sensitive to hypotensive effects.
• Teach patient about his disease and therapy. Explain why it's important to take this drug exactly as prescribed, even when he's feeling well. Tell outpatient not to discontinue this drug suddenly, but to call the doctor if unpleasant side effects develop.
• Inform patient that orthostatic hypotension can be minimized by rising slowly and avoiding sudden position changes. Mouth dryness can be relieved with sugarless chewing gum, sour hard candy, or ice chips.
• Compliance *may* be improved by giving this drug once a day. Check with doctor.
• Has been used to treat Raynaud's vasospasm.

rauwolfia serpentina
HBP, Hiwolfia, Hyper-Rauw, Rau, Raudixin♦**, Rauja, Raumason, Rauneed, Raupoid, Rausertina, Rauval, Rauwoldin, Rawfola, Serfia, T-Rau
Pregnancy Category: D

MECHANISM OF ACTION
Acts peripherally, inhibiting norepinephrine release and depleting norepinephrine stores in adrenergic nerve endings.

INDICATIONS & DOSAGE

Mild to moderate hypertension—
Adults: initially and for 1 to 3 weeks thereafter, 200 to 400 mg P.O. daily as a single dose or in 2 divided doses. Maintenance dose: 50 to 300 mg daily.
No dosing recommendations for children.

ADVERSE REACTIONS

CNS: mental confusion, *depression, drowsiness, nervousness, paradoxical anxiety,* nightmares, sedation, headache, extrapyramidal symptoms.
CV: *orthostatic hypotension, bradycardia, syncope.*
EENT: *mouth dryness, nasal stuffiness,* glaucoma.
GI: *hypersecretion of gastric acid, nausea, vomiting,* gastrointestinal bleeding.
Skin: pruritus, rash.
Other: *impotence, weight gain.*

INTERACTIONS

MAO inhibitors: may cause excitability and hypertension. Use together cautiously.

NURSING CONSIDERATIONS

• Contraindicated in patients with depression. Use cautiously in patients with severe cardiac or cerebrovascular disease, impaired renal function, peptic ulcer, ulcerative colitis, gallstones; in those undergoing surgery; and in those taking other antihypertensives or tricyclic antidepressants.
• Monitor patient's blood pressure and pulse rate frequently.
• Teach patient about his disease and therapy. Explain why it's important to take this drug exactly as prescribed, even when he's feeling well. Tell outpatient not to discontinue this drug suddenly, but to call the doctor if unpleasant side effects develop. Warn that this drug can cause drowsiness.
• Watch patient closely for signs of mental depression. Warn him to no-

tify doctor promptly if he starts having nightmares.
• Inform patient that orthostatic hypotension can be minimized by rising slowly and avoiding sudden position changes. Mouth dryness can be relieved with sugarless chewing gum, sour hard candy, or ice chips. Tell patient to contact doctor if relief is needed for nasal stuffiness.
• Give this drug with meals.
• Patient should weigh himself daily and notify doctor of any weight gain.
• Effects of this drug may last for 10 days after it's discontinued.

rescinnamine
Anaprel, Moderil
Pregnancy Category: D

MECHANISM OF ACTION

Acts peripherally, inhibiting norepinephrine release and depleting norepinephrine stores in adrenergic nerve endings.

INDICATIONS & DOSAGE

For mild to moderate hypertension; may be used alone or in combination with other antihypertensives—
Adults: initially, 0.5 mg b.i.d. Maintenance dose: 0.25 to 0.5 mg daily. No dosing recommendations for children.

ADVERSE REACTIONS

CNS: mental confusion, *depression, drowsiness, nervousness, anxiety, nightmares,* sedation, parkinsonism.
CV: *orthostatic hypotension, bradycardia, syncope.*
EENT: *mouth dryness, nasal stuffiness,* glaucoma.
GI: *hypersecretion of gastric acid, nausea, vomiting,* gastrointestinal bleeding.
Skin: pruritus, rash.
Other: *impotence, weight gain.*

Italicized side effects are common or life-threatening.
*Liquid form contains alcohol.   **May contain tartrazine.

INTERACTIONS
MAO inhibitors: may cause excitability and hypertension. Use together cautiously.

NURSING CONSIDERATIONS
• Contraindicated in patients with depression. Use cautiously in patients with severe cardiac or cerebrovascular disease, peptic ulcer, ulcerative colitis, gallstones, or in those undergoing surgery. Also use cautiously in patients taking other antihypertensives.
• Monitor patient's blood pressure and pulse rate frequently.
• Teach patient about his disease and therapy. Explain why it's important to take this drug exactly as prescribed, even when he's feeling well. Tell outpatient not to discontinue this drug suddenly, but to call the doctor if unpleasant side effects develop. Warn that this drug can cause drowsiness.
• Watch patient closely for signs of mental depression. Warn him to notify doctor promptly if he starts having nightmares.
• Inform patient that orthostatic hypotension can be minimized by rising slowly and avoiding sudden position changes. Mouth dryness can be relieved with sugarless chewing gum, sour hard candy, or ice chips. Tell patient to contact doctor if relief is needed for nasal stuffiness.
• Give this drug with meals.
• Patient should weigh himself daily and notify doctor of any weight gain.
• Effects of this drug may last for 10 days after it's discontinued.

reserpine
Arcum R-S, Broserpine, De Serpa, Elserpine, Hyperine, Rau-Sed, Releserp-5, Reserfia♦♦, Reserpaneed, Rolserp, Serp, Serpalan, Serpanray, Serpasil♦*, Serpate, Serpena, Sertabs, Sertina, Tensin, T-Serp, Zepine
Pregnancy Category: D

MECHANISM OF ACTION
Acts peripherally, inhibiting norepinephrine release and depleting norepinephrine stores in adrenergic nerve endings.

INDICATIONS & DOSAGE
Mild to moderate essential hypertension (oral); hypertensive emergencies (parenteral)—
Adults: initially, 0.5 mg P.O. daily for 1 to 2 weeks. Maintenance dose: 0.1 to 0.5 mg daily.
Children: 0.07 mg/kg or 2 mg/m² with hydralazine I.M. every 12 to 24 hours.

ADVERSE REACTIONS
CNS: mental confusion, *depression, drowsiness, nervousness, paradoxical anxiety, nightmares,* extrapyramidal symptoms, sedation.
CV: *orthostatic hypotension, bradycardia, syncope.*
EENT: *mouth dryness, nasal stuffiness,* glaucoma.
GI: *hyperacidity, nausea, vomiting,* gastrointestinal bleeding.
Skin: pruritus, rash.
Other: *impotence, weight gain.*

INTERACTIONS
MAO inhibitors: may cause excitability and hypertension. Use together cautiously.

NURSING CONSIDERATIONS
• Contraindicated in patients with depression. Use cautiously in patients with severe cardiac or cerebrovascu-

lar disease, peptic ulcer, ulcerative colitis, gallstones, mental depressive disorders; in those undergoing surgery; and in those taking other antihypertensive drugs.
• Monitor patient's blood pressure and pulse rate frequently.
• Teach patient about his disease and therapy. Explain why it's important to take this drug exactly as prescribed, even when he's feeling well. Tell outpatient not to discontinue this drug suddenly, but to call doctor if unpleasant side effects develop. Warn that this drug can cause drowsiness.
• Warn female patient to notify doctor if she becomes pregnant.
• Watch patient closely for signs of mental depression. Warn him to notify doctor promptly if he starts having nightmares.
• Inform patient that orthostatic hypotension can be minimized by rising slowly and avoiding sudden position changes. Mouth dryness can be relieved with sugarless chewing gum, sour hard candy, or ice chips. Tell patient to contact doctor if relief is needed for nasal stuffiness.
• Give this drug with meals.
• Patient should weigh himself daily and notify doctor of any weight gain.
• Effects of this drug may last for 10 days after it's discontinued.
• To calculate m² for dosage, use a nomogram.

---

timolol maleate
Blocadren♦
Pregnancy Category: C

MECHANISM OF ACTION
Blocks response to beta stimulation and depresses renin secretion.

INDICATIONS & DOSAGE
Hypertension—
Adults: Initial dosage is 10 mg P.O. b.i.d. Usual daily maintenance dosage is 20 to 40 mg. Maximum daily

dosage is 60 mg. Drug is used either alone or in combination with diuretics.
Myocardial infarction (long-term prophylaxis in patients who have survived acute phase)—
Adults: Recommended dosage for long-term prophylaxis in survivors of acute myocardial infarction (MI) is 10 mg P.O. b.i.d.

ADVERSE REACTIONS
CNS: fatigue, lethargy, vivid dreams.
CV: *bradycardia, hypotension, congestive heart failure (CHF),* peripheral vascular disease.
GI: nausea, vomiting, diarrhea.
Metabolic: hypoglycemia without tachycardia.
Skin: rash.
Other: *increased airway resistance,* fever.

INTERACTIONS
Insulin, hypoglycemic drugs (oral): can alter requirements for these drugs in previously stabilized diabetics. Monitor for hypoglycemia.
Cardiac glycosides: excessive bradycardia and increased depressant effect on myocardium. Use together cautiously.
Indomethacin: decrease in antihypertensive effect. Monitor blood pressure and adjust dosage.

NURSING CONSIDERATIONS
• Contraindicated in diabetes mellitus, asthma, allergic rhinitis; during ethyl ether anesthesia; in sinus bradycardia and heart block greater than first degree; in cardiogenic shock; in right ventricular failure secondary to pulmonary hypertension. Use with caution in CHF and respiratory disease, and in patients taking other antihypertensives.
• Always check patient's apical pulse rate before giving this drug. If you detect extremes in pulse rates, withhold medication and call the doctor imme-

diately.
- Monitor blood pressure frequently.
- Instruct patient about the disease and therapy. Explain the importance of taking drug exactly as prescribed, even when he's feeling well. Tell patient not to discontinue drug suddenly: abrupt discontinuation can exacerbate angina and MI. Tell patient to call doctor if unpleasant side effects develop.
- This drug masks common signs of shock and hypoglycemia.
- If patient is taking the drug for hypertension, warn him not to increase the dosage without first consulting his doctor. At least 7 days should intervene between increases in dosage.
- Do not discontinue therapy abruptly. Reduce dosage gradually over 1 to 2 weeks.
- Timolol is the first beta blocker approved for use in post-MI patients. Like other beta blockers, it prolongs survival of MI patients.

trimethaphan camsylate
Arfonad♦
Pregnancy Category: C

MECHANISM OF ACTION
A ganglionic blocker that stabilizes postsynaptic membranes.

INDICATIONS & DOSAGE
To lower blood pressure quickly in hypertensive emergencies; for controlled hypotension during surgery—
Adults: 500 mg (10 ml) diluted in 500 ml dextrose 5% in water to yield concentration of 1 mg/ml I.V. Start I.V. drip at 1 to 2 mg/minute and titrate to achieve desired hypotensive response. Range: 0.3 mg to 6 mg/minute.

ADVERSE REACTIONS
CNS: dilated pupils, *extreme weakness.*
CV: *severe orthostatic hypotension,*

tachycardia.
GI: anorexia, *nausea, vomiting, dry mouth.*
GU: *urinary retention.*
Other: respiratory depression.

INTERACTIONS
None significant.

NURSING CONSIDERATIONS
- Contraindicated in patients with anemia, respiratory insufficiency. Use cautiously in patients with arteriosclerosis; cardiac, hepatic, or renal disease; degenerative CNS disorders; Addison's disease; diabetes. Also use cautiously in patients receiving glucocorticoids; or in those receiving other antihypertensives.
- Monitor patient's blood pressure and vital signs frequently.
- May require elevation of the head of the bed for maximal effect to avoid cerebral anoxia. Do not elevate bed more than 30°.
- Large doses have caused apnea and respiratory arrest.
- If extreme hypotension occurs, discontinue drug and call doctor. Use phenylephrine or mephentermine to counteract hypotension.
- Watch closely for respiratory distress, especially if large doses are used.
- Patient should receive oxygen therapy during use of this agent.
- Use infusion pump to administer this drug slowly and precisely.
- Discontinue drug before wound closure in surgery to allow blood pressure to return to normal.

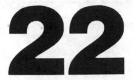

Vasodilators

amyl nitrite
cyclandelate
dipyridamole
ethaverine hydrochloride
isoxsuprine hydrochloride
nylidrin hydrochloride
papaverine hydrochloride

COMBINATION PRODUCTS
DEAPRIL-ST: dihydroergocornine mesylate 0.167 mg, dihydroergocristine mesylate 0.167 mg, and dihydroergocryptine mesylate 0.167 mg.
HYDERGINE: dihydroergocornine mesylate 0.167 mg, dihydroergocristine mesylate 0.167 mg, and dihydroergocryptine mesylate 0.167 mg.

amyl nitrite
Pregnancy Category: C

MECHANISM OF ACTION
Reduces cardiac oxygen demand by decreasing left ventricular end-diastolic pressure (preload) and systemic vascular resistance (afterload). Also increases blood flow through the collateral coronary vessels. Converts hemoglobin to methemoglobin in the treatment of cyanide poisoning.

INDICATIONS & DOSAGE
Relief of angina pectoris, bronchospasm, biliary spasm—
Adults and children: 0.2 to 0.3 ml by inhalation (one glass ampul inhaler), p.r.n.
Antidote for cyanide poisoning—
0.2 or 0.3 ml by inhalation for 30 to 60 seconds q 5 minutes until conscious.

ADVERSE REACTIONS
Blood: methemoglobinemia.
CNS: *headache, sometimes with throbbing;* dizziness; weakness.
CV: *orthostatic hypotension, tachycardia,* flushing, palpitations, fainting.
GI: nausea, vomiting.
Skin: cutaneous vasodilation.
Other: hypersensitivity reactions.

INTERACTIONS
None significant.

NURSING CONSIDERATIONS
• Contraindicated in hypersensitivity to nitrites. Use with caution in cerebral hemorrhage, hypotension, head injury, and glaucoma.
• Watch for orthostatic hypotension. Have patient sit down and avoid rapid position changes while inhaling drug.
• Extinguish all cigarettes before use, or ampul may ignite.
• Wrap ampul in cloth and crush. Hold near patient's nose and mouth so vapor is inhaled.
• Effective within 30 seconds but has a short duration of action (4 to 8 minutes).
• Keeping the head low, deep breathing, and movement of extremities may help relieve dizziness, syncope, or weakness from postural hypotension.
• Drug is often abused. Claimed to have aphrodisiac benefits. Sometimes called "Amy."
• Seldom, if ever, used for treatment of angina because it is expensive, in-

convenient, and frequently causes adverse reactions.

cyclandelate
Cyclospasmol♦
Pregnancy Category: C

MECHANISM OF ACTION
Directly relaxes smooth muscle due to the inhibition of phosphodiesterase, resulting in increased concentrations of cyclic adenosine monophosphate.

INDICATIONS & DOSAGE
Adjunct in intermittent claudication, arteriosclerosis obliterans, vasospasm and muscular ischemia associated with thrombophlebitis, nocturnal leg cramps, Raynaud's phenomenon, selected cases of ischemic cerebral vascular disease—
Adults: initially, 200 mg P.O. q.i.d. (before meals and h.s.); maximum 400 mg P.O. q.i.d. When clinical response is noted, decrease dosage gradually until maintenance dosage is reached. Maintenance dose 400 to 800 mg daily in divided doses.

ADVERSE REACTIONS
CNS: *headache, tingling of the extremities, dizziness.*
CV: *mild flushing,* tachycardia.
GI: pyrosis, eructation, nausea, heartburn.
Other: *sweating.*

INTERACTIONS
None significant.

NURSING CONSIDERATIONS
• Use with extreme caution in severe obliterative coronary artery or cerebrovascular disease, since circulation to these diseased areas may be compromised by vasodilatory effects of the drug elsewhere (coronary steal syndrome). Use with caution in patients with glaucoma, hypotension.
• Give with food or antacids to lessen GI distress.
• Use in conjunction with, not as a substitute for, appropriate medical or surgical therapy for peripheral or cerebrovascular disease.
• Short-term therapy of little benefit. Instruct patient to expect long-term treatment and to continue to take medication.
• Side effects usually disappear after several weeks of therapy.

dipyridamole
Persantine♦**
Pregnancy Category: C

MECHANISM OF ACTION
Inhibits platelet adhesion in patients with prosthetic heart valves. Also inhibits the enzymes adenosine deaminase and phosphodiesterase.

INDICATIONS & DOSAGE
Prevention of recurrent transient ischemic attack—
Adults: 50 mg P.O. t.i.d. at least 1 hour before meals, to maximum of 400 mg daily.
Inhibition of platelet adhesion in patients with prosthetic heart valves, in combination with warfarin or aspirin—
Adults: 100 to 400 mg P.O. daily.
Transient ischemic attack—
Adults: 400 to 800 mg P.O. daily in divided doses.

ADVERSE REACTIONS
CNS: *headache, dizziness,* weakness.
CV: flushing, fainting, *hypotension.*
GI: *nausea,* vomiting, diarrhea.
Skin: rash.

INTERACTIONS
None significant.

NURSING CONSIDERATIONS
• Use with caution in hypotension, anticoagulant therapy.
• Observe for side effects, especially

with large doses. Monitor blood pressure.
• Administer 1 hour before meals. May administer with meals if patient develops gastrointestinal distress.
• Watch for signs of bleeding, prolonged bleeding time (large doses, long-term).
• Dipyridamole is no longer approved or recommended for the treatment of angina pectoris.

ethaverine hydrochloride
Circubid, Etalent, Ethaquin, Ethatab, Ethavex, Isovex, Pavaspan, Spasodil
Pregnancy Category: C

MECHANISM OF ACTION
Directly relaxes smooth muscle due to the inhibition of phosphodiesterase, resulting in increased concentrations of cyclic adenosine monophosphate.

INDICATIONS & DOSAGE
Long-term treatment of peripheral and cerebrovascular insufficiency associated with arterial spasm; spastic conditions of gastrointestinal and genitourinary tracts—
Adults: 100 to 200 mg P.O. t.i.d. or 150 mg of sustained-release preparation P.O. q 12 hours.

ADVERSE REACTIONS
CNS: *headache,* drowsiness.
CV: *hypotension, flushing,* sweating, vertigo, cardiac depression, arrhythmias.
GI: *nausea, anorexia, abdominal distress, dryness of throat,* constipation, diarrhea.
Hepatic: jaundice, altered liver function tests.
Skin: rash.
Other: respiratory depression, malaise, lassitude.

INTERACTIONS
None significant.

NURSING CONSIDERATIONS
• Contraindicated in complete AV dissociation and in severe hepatic disease. Use with caution in women who are pregnant or of childbearing age, and in patients with glaucoma or pulmonary embolus; may precipitate arrhythmias.
• Hold dose and call doctor if signs of hepatic hypersensitivity develop (gastrointestinal symptoms, altered liver function tests, jaundice, eosinophilia).
• Monitor and record vital signs during therapy.
• FDA has announced this drug may not be effective for disease states indicated.

isoxsuprine hydrochloride
Rolisox, Vasodilan♦, Vasoprine
Pregnancy Category: C

MECHANISM OF ACTION
Stimulates beta receptors and may also be a direct-acting peripheral vasodilator.

INDICATIONS & DOSAGE
Adjunct for relief of symptoms associated with cerebrovascular insufficiency, peripheral vascular diseases (such as arteriosclerosis obliterans, thromboangiitis obliterans, Raynaud's disease)—
Adults: 10 to 20 mg P.O. t.i.d. or q.i.d.

ADVERSE REACTIONS
GI: vomiting, abdominal distress, intestinal distention.
Skin: severe rash.

INTERACTIONS
None significant.

NURSING CONSIDERATIONS
• Contraindicated in immediate postpartum period and arterial bleeding.
• Safe use in pregnancy and lactation

Italicized side effects are common or life-threatening.
*Liquid form contains alcohol.   **May contain tartrazine.

not established, although drug has been used to inhibit contractions in premature labor.
• Discontinue if rash develops.

nylidrin hydrochloride
Arlidin♦, Rolidrin
Pregnancy Category: C

MECHANISM OF ACTION
Stimulates beta receptors and may directly relax vascular smooth muscle.

INDICATIONS & DOSAGE
To increase blood supply in vasospastic disorders (arteriosclerosis obliterans, thromboangiitis obliterans, diabetic vascular disease, night leg cramps, Raynaud's phenomenon and disease, ischemic ulcer, frostbite, acrocyanosis, acroparesthesia, sequelae of thrombophlebitis); and in circulatory disturbances of the middle ear (primary cochlear ischemia, cochlear striae, vascular ischemia, macular or ampullar ischemia); other disturbances due to labyrinth artery spasm or obstruction—
Adults: 3 to 12 mg P.O. t.i.d. or q.i.d.

ADVERSE REACTIONS
CNS: trembling, *nervousness,* weakness, *dizziness (not associated with labyrinth artery insufficiency).*
CV: *palpitations, hypotension,* flushing.
GI: *nausea, vomiting.*

INTERACTIONS
None significant.

NURSING CONSIDERATIONS
• Contraindicated in acute myocardial infarction, paroxysmal tachycardia, angina pectoris, thyrotoxicosis. Use with caution in uncompensated heart disease or peptic ulcer.

papaverine hydrochloride
BP-Papaverine, Cerebid, Cerespan, Cirbed, Delapav, Lapav*, Myobid, Papacon, PapKaps-150, P-A-V, Pavabid, Pavacap, Pavacen, Pavaclor, Pavacron, Pavadel, Pavadur, Pavadyl, Pava-lyn, Pava-Par, Pava-Rx, Pavasule, Pavatime, Pava-Wol, Paverolan, Pavex, Ro-Papav, Vasal, Vazosan
Pregnancy Category: C

MECHANISM OF ACTION
Directly relaxes smooth muscle due to the inhibition of phosphodiesterase, resulting in increased concentrations of cyclic adenosine monophosphate.

INDICATIONS & DOSAGE
Relief of cerebral and peripheral ischemia associated with arterial spasm and myocardial ischemia; treatment of smooth-muscle spasm (coronary occlusion, angina pectoris, sequelae of peripheral and pulmonary embolism, certain cerebral angiospastic states); and visceral spasms (biliary, ureteral, or gastrointestinal colic)—
Adults: 60 to 300 mg P.O. 1 to 5 times daily, or 150 to 300 mg sustained-release preparations q 8 to 12 hours; 30 to 120 mg I.M. or I.V. q 3 hours, as indicated.

ADVERSE REACTIONS
CNS: *headache.*
CV: *increased heart rate, increased blood pressure* (with parenteral use), depressed AV and intraventricular conduction, arrhythmias.
GI: constipation, *nausea.*
Other: *sweating, flushing,* malaise, increased depth of respiration.

INTERACTIONS
None significant.

NURSING CONSIDERATIONS
• Contraindicated for I.V. use in com-

plete AV block. Use with caution in glaucoma.

• Monitor blood pressure, heart rate and rhythm, especially in cardiac disease. Hold dose and notify doctor immediately if changes occur.

• Not often used parenterally, except when immediate effect is desired.

• Give I.V. slowly (over 1 to 2 minutes) to avoid serious side effects.

• Most effective when given early in the course of a disorder.

• Tell patient to take medication regularly; long-term therapy is required.

• Do not add lactated Ringer's injection to the injectable form; will precipitate.

• FDA has announced this drug may not be effective for disease states indicated.

Italicized side effects are common or life-threatening.
*Liquid form contains alcohol.   **May contain tartrazine.

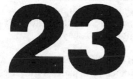

Antilipemics

cholestyramine
clofibrate
colestipol hydrochloride
dextrothyroxine sodium
gemfibrozil
niacin
   (See Chapter 98, VITAMINS AND MINERALS.)
probucol

COMBINATION PRODUCTS
None.

cholestyramine
Questran♦**
Pregnancy Category: C

MECHANISM OF ACTION
Combines with bile acid to form an insoluble compound that is excreted.

INDICATIONS & DOSAGE
Primary hyperlipidemia, pruritus, and diarrhea due to excess bile acid; as adjunctive therapy for the reduction of elevated serum cholesterol in patients with primary hypercholesterolemia, and to reduce the risks of atherosclerotic coronary artery disease and myocardial infarction—
Adults: 4 g before meals and h.s., not to exceed 32 g daily. Each scoop or packet of Questran contains 4 g cholestyramine.
Children: 240 mg/kg daily P.O. in 3 divided doses with beverage or food. Safe dosage not established for children under 6 years.

ADVERSE REACTIONS
GI: *constipation*, fecal impaction, hemorrhoids, *abdominal discomfort,* flatulence, *nausea*, vomiting, steatorrhea.
Skin: *rashes*, irritation of skin, tongue, and perianal area.
Other: *vitamin A, D, and K deficiency from decreased absorption;* hyperchloremic acidosis with long-term use or very high dosage.

INTERACTIONS
None significant.

NURSING CONSIDERATIONS
• Patients who are taking this drug to reduce the risks of atherosclerotic heart disease should be encouraged to be aware of other cardiac disease risk factors. Recommend weight-control and stop-smoking programs.
• Monitor serum cholesterol and triglyceride levels regularly during cholestyramine therapy.
• To mix, sprinkle powder on surface of preferred beverage or wet food. Let stand a few minutes, then stir to obtain uniform suspension.
• Mixing with carbonated beverages may result in excess foaming. To avoid, use large glass, and mix slowly.
• Administer all other medications at least 1 hour before or 4 to 6 hours after cholestyramine to avoid blocking their absorption.
• Observe bowel habits; treat constipation as needed. Encourage a diet high in roughage and fluids. If severe constipation develops, decrease dosage, add a stool softener, or discontinue drug.

• Monitor cardiac glycoside levels in patients receiving both medications concurrently. Should cholestyramine therapy be discontinued, cardiac glycoside toxicity may result unless dosage is adjusted.

• Watch for signs of vitamin A, D, and K deficiency.

• May cause decreased absorption of many drugs due to binding. Check drug interaction list of individual drugs.

clofibrate
Atromid-S♦, Claripex♦♦
Pregnancy Category: C

MECHANISM OF ACTION
Seems to inhibit biosynthesis of cholesterol at an early stage, but the exact mechanism is unknown.

INDICATIONS & DOSAGE
Hyperlipidemia and xanthoma tuberosum; Type III hyperlipidemia that does not respond adequately to diet—
Adults: 2 g P.O. daily in 4 divided doses. Some patients may respond to lower doses as assessed by serum lipid monitoring.
Should not be used in children.

ADVERSE REACTIONS
Blood: leukopenia.
CNS: fatigue, weakness.
GI: *nausea, diarrhea, vomiting,* stomatitis, *dyspepsia,* flatulence.
GU: decreased libido.
Hepatic: gallstones, *transient and reversible elevations of liver function tests.*
Skin: rashes, urticaria, pruritus, dry skin and hair.
Other: *myalgias and arthralgias,* resembling a flu-like syndrome; *weight gain; polyphagia;* fever.

INTERACTIONS
Oral contraceptives, rifampin: may antagonize clofibrate's lipid-lowering

effect. Monitor blood lipid level.
Probenecid: increased clofibrate effect. Monitor for toxicity.

NURSING CONSIDERATIONS
• Contraindicated in patients with severe renal or hepatic disease.

• Warn patient to report flu-like symptoms to doctor immediately.

• Monitor renal and hepatic function, blood counts, serum electrolyte and blood sugar levels. If liver function tests show steady rise, clofibrate should be discontinued.

• Should not be used indiscriminately. May pose increased risk of gallstones, heart disease, and cancer.

• Monitor serum cholesterol and triglyceride levels regularly during clofibrate therapy.

• If significant lipid lowering is not achieved within 3 months, drug should be discontinued.

colestipol hydrochloride
Colestid
Pregnancy Category: C

MECHANISM OF ACTION
Combines with bile acid to form an insoluble compound that is excreted.

INDICATIONS & DOSAGE
Primary hypercholesterolemia and xanthomas—
Adults: 15 to 30 g P.O. daily in 2 to 4 divided doses.

ADVERSE REACTIONS
GI: *constipation (common, may require decreasing the dosage),* fecal impaction, hemorrhoids, abdominal discomfort, flatulence, nausea, vomiting, steatorrhea.
Skin: rashes, irritation of skin, tongue, and perianal area.
Other: vitamin A, D, and K deficiency from decreased absorption; hyperchloremic acidosis with long-term use or very high dosage.

Italicized side effects are common or life-threatening.
*Liquid form contains alcohol.   **May contain tartrazine.

INTERACTIONS
Oral hypoglycemics: may antagonize response to colestipol. Monitor blood lipid level.

NURSING CONSIDERATIONS
• Administer all other medications at least 1 hour before or 4 to 6 hours after colestipol to avoid blocking their absorption.
• Monitor cardiac glycoside levels in patients receiving both medications concurrently. Should colestipol therapy be discontinued, cardiac glycoside toxicity may result unless dosage is adjusted.
• Watch for signs of vitamin A, D, and K deficiency.
• Lowering dosage or adding stool softener may relieve constipation.
• May cause decreased absorption of many drugs due to binding. Check drug interaction list of individual drugs.
• Administer this drug in at least 3 oz (90 ml) of juice, milk, or water. After drinking this preparation, patient should swirl a small additional amount of liquid in the same glass and then drink it to ensure ingestion of the entire dose.

dextrothyroxine sodium
Choloxin♦**
Pregnancy Category: C

MECHANISM OF ACTION
Accelerates hepatic catabolism of cholesterol and increases bile secretion to lower cholesterol levels.

INDICATIONS & DOSAGE
Hyperlipidemia in euthyroid patients, especially when cholesterol and triglyceride levels are elevated—
Adults: initial dose 1 to 2 mg daily, increased by 1 to 2 mg daily at monthly intervals to a total of 4 to 8 mg daily.
Children: initial dose 0.05 mg/kg

daily, increased by 0.05 mg/kg daily at monthly intervals to a total of 4 mg daily.

ADVERSE REACTIONS
CV: palpitations, angina pectoris, arrhythmias, ischemic myocardial changes on EKG, *myocardial infarction.*
EENT: visual disturbances, ptosis.
GI: nausea, vomiting, diarrhea, constipation, decreased appetite.
Metabolic: *insomnia, weight loss, sweating,* flushing, hyperthermia, hair loss, menstrual irregularities.

INTERACTIONS
None significant.

NURSING CONSIDERATIONS
• Contraindicated in patients with hepatic or renal disease, or iodism. Patients with history of cardiac disease, including arrhythmias, hypertension, or angina pectoris, should receive very small doses.
• May increase need for insulin, diet therapy, or oral hypoglycemics in patients with diabetes.
• If the use of anticoagulants is being considered, discontinue drug 2 weeks before surgery to avoid possible potentiation of anticoagulant effect.
• Observe patient for signs of hyperthyroidism, such as nervousness, insomnia, weight loss. If these occur, dosage should be decreased or drug discontinued.

gemfibrozil
Lopid♦
Pregnancy Category: B

MECHANISM OF ACTION
Inhibits peripheral lipolysis and also reduces triglyceride synthesis in the liver.

INDICATIONS & DOSAGE
Treatment of type IV hyperlipidemia

(hypertriglyceridemia) and severe hypercholesterolemia unresponsive to diet and other drugs—
Adults: 1,200 mg P.O. administered in two divided doses. Usual dosage range 900 to 1,500 mg daily.

ADVERSE REACTIONS
Blood: anemia, leukopenia.
CNS: blurred vision, headache, dizziness.
GI: *abdominal and epigastric pain, diarrhea, nausea,* vomiting, flatulence.
Hepatic: elevated enzymes.
Skin: rash, dermatitis, pruritus.
Other: painful extremities.

INTERACTIONS
None significant.

NURSING CONSIDERATIONS
• Contraindicated in hepatic or severe renal dysfunction—including primary biliary cirrhosis—and in preexisting gallbladder disease.
• CBC and liver function tests should be done periodically during the first 12 months of therapy.
• Gemfibrozil is very closely related to clofibrate both chemically and pharmacologically.
• Instruct patient to take drugs ½ hour before breakfast and dinner.
• Should not be used indiscriminately. May pose risk of gallstones, heart disease, and cancer.
• Patient should adhere strictly to prescribed diet, avoiding saturated fats, cholesterol, and sugars.
• Because of possible dizziness and blurred vision, patient should avoid driving or other hazardous activities until CNS response to drug is determined.

probucol
Lorelco♦
Pregnancy Category: C

MECHANISM OF ACTION
Inhibits cholesterol transport from the intestine and may also decrease cholesterol synthesis. Appears to be more effective in patients with mild cholesterol elevations than in those with severe hypercholesterolemia.

INDICATIONS & DOSAGE
Primary hypercholesterolemia—
Adults: 2 tablets (500 mg total) P.O. b.i.d. with morning and evening meals. Not recommended in children.

ADVERSE REACTIONS
GI: *diarrhea, flatulence, abdominal pain, nausea, vomiting.*
Other: *hyperhidrosis,* fetid sweat, angioneurotic edema.

INTERACTIONS
None significant.

NURSING CONSIDERATIONS
• Drug's effect is enhanced when taken with food.
• Contraindicated in patients with arrhythmias. Drug should be stopped in any patient whose EKG shows prolonged Q-T interval.

Italicized side effects are common or life-threatening.
*Liquid form contains alcohol.   **May contain tartrazine.

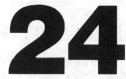

Nonnarcotic analgesics and antipyretics

Salicylates
aspirin
choline magnesium trisalicylate
choline salicylate
magnesium salicylate
salsalate
sodium salicylate
sodium thiosalicylate

Urinary tract analgesic
phenazopyridine hydrochloride

Miscellaneous
acetaminophen
diflunisal
methotrimeprazine
  (See Chapter 28, SEDATIVE-HYPNOTICS.)

COMBINATION PRODUCTS
AMAPHEN: acetaminophen 325 mg, caffeine 40 mg, and butalbital 50 mg.
ANACIN: aspirin 400 mg and caffeine 32 mg.
ANOQUAN: acetaminophen 325 mg, caffeine 40 mg, and butalbital 50 mg.
ARTHRALGEN: acetaminophen 250 mg and salicylamide 250 mg.
AXOTAL: aspirin 650 mg and butalbital 50 mg.
BC POWDER: aspirin 650 mg, salicylamide 195 mg, and caffeine 32 mg.
BC TABLETS: aspirin 325 mg, salicylamide 95 mg, and caffeine 16 mg.
BUTAL: aspirin 325 mg, caffeine 40 mg, and butalbital 50 mg.
CAMA, ARTHRITIS STRENGTH: aspirin 500 mg, magnesium oxide 150 mg, and aluminum hydroxide 150 mg.
COPE: aspirin 421 mg, caffeine 32 mg, magnesium hydroxide 50 mg, and aluminum hydroxide 25 mg.

DURADYNE: acetaminophen 180 mg, aspirin 230 mg, and caffeine 15 mg.
ESGIC: acetaminophen 325 mg, caffeine 40 mg, and butalbital 50 mg.
EXCEDRIN P.M.: acetaminophen 500 mg and diphenhydramine citrate 38 mg.
EXCEDRIN TABLETS: aspirin 250 mg, acetaminophen 250 mg, caffeine 65 mg.
FEMCAPS: acetaminophen 324 mg, caffeine 32 mg, ephedrine sulfate 8 mg, and atropine sulfate 0.0325 mg.
FIORICET: acetaminophen 325 mg, butalbital 50 mg, and caffeine 40 mg
FIORINAL: aspirin 325 mg, caffeine 40 mg, and butalbital 50 mg.
G-1: acetaminophen 500 mg, caffeine 40 mg, and butalbital 50 mg.
GEMNISYN: aspirin 325 mg and acetaminophen 325 mg.
ISOLLYL: aspirin 325 mg, caffeine 40 mg, and butalbital 50 mg.
MIDOL: aspirin 454 mg, caffeine 32.4 mg, and cinnemedrine HCl 14.9 mg.
PAC NEW REVISED FORMULA: aspirin 400 mg and caffeine 32 mg.
PHRENILIN: acetaminophen 325 mg and butalbital 50 mg.
PHRENILIN FORTE: acetaminophen 650 mg and butalbital 50 mg.
SINUTAB: acetaminophen 325 mg, chlorpheniramine 2 mg, and pseudoephedrine HCl 30 mg.
SINUTAB II MAXIMUM STRENGTH: acetaminophen 500 mg and pseudoephedrine HCl 30 mg.
SYNALGOS: aspirin 356.4 mg and caffeine 30 mg.
TRIGESIC: acetaminophen 125 mg, aspirin 230 mg, and caffeine 30 mg.

TRILISATE: choline salicylate 293 mg and magnesium salicylate 362 mg.
VANQUISH: aspirin 227 mg, acetaminophen 194 mg, caffeine 33 mg, aluminum hydroxide 25 mg, and magnesium hydroxide 50 mg.

acetaminophen
Acephen, Atasol♦♦, Campain♦♦, Datril-500, Dolanex, Halenol, Liquiprin, Panadol♦♦, Phendex, Robigesic♦♦, Rounox♦♦, Tapar*, Tempra♦*, Tylenol♦* **, Valadol*
Pregnancy Category: B

MECHANISM OF ACTION
Produces analgesia by blocking generation of pain impulses. This action is probably due to inhibition of prostaglandin synthesis; it may also be due to inhibition of the synthesis or action of other substances that sensitize pain receptors to mechanical or chemical stimulation. It relieves fever by central action in the hypothalamic heat-regulating center.

INDICATIONS & DOSAGE
Mild pain or fever—
Adults and children over 11 years: 325 to 650 mg P.O. or rectally q 4 hours, p.r.n. Maximum dose shouldn't exceed 4 g daily. Dosage for long-term therapy shouldn't exceed 2.6 g daily.
Children 11 years: 480 mg/dose.
Children 9 to 10 years: 400 mg/dose.
Children 6 to 8 years: 320 mg/dose.
Children 4 to 5 years: 240 mg/dose.
Children 2 to 3 years: 160 mg/dose.
Children 12 to 23 months: 120 mg/dose.
Children 4 to 11 months: 80 mg/dose.
Children up to 3 months: 40 mg/dose.

ADVERSE REACTIONS
Hepatic: *severe liver damage with toxic doses.*

Skin: rash, urticaria.

INTERACTIONS
Diflunisal: increases acetaminophen blood levels. Don't use together.
Cholestyramine: inhibits acetaminophen's absorption. Avoid concurrent administration.

NURSING CONSIDERATIONS
• Repeated use is contraindicated in patients with anemia, or renal or hepatic disease.
• Has no significant anti-inflammatory effect.
• Warn patient that high doses or unsupervised chronic use can cause hepatic damage. Excessive ingestion of alcoholic beverages may increase the risk of hepatotoxicity.
• Don't use for self-medication of marked fever (greater than 103.1° F., or 39.5° C.), fever persisting longer than 3 days, or recurrent fever unless directed by doctor.
• May increase the hypoprothrombinemic activity of warfarin when taken chronically for pain.
• Many nonprescription products contain acetaminophen. Be aware of this when calculating total daily dosages.
• Recommend the liquid form for children and for all patients who have difficulty swallowing.

aspirin
Ancasal♦♦, A.S.A., Aspergum, Aspirin♦♦, Aspirjen Jr., Bayer Timed-Release♦, Buffinol, Easprin, Ecotrin♦, Empirin, Entrophen♦♦, Measurin, Novasen♦♦, Sal-Adult♦♦, Sal-Infant♦♦, Supasa♦♦, Zorprin
Pregnancy Category: C (D in 3rd trimester)

MECHANISM OF ACTION
• Produces analgesia by an ill-defined effect on the hypothalamus (central action) and by blocking gen-

---

Italicized side effects are common or life-threatening.
*Liquid form contains alcohol.   **May contain tartrazine.

eration of pain impulses (peripheral action). The peripheral action may involve inhibition of prostaglandin synthesis.
• Exerts its anti-inflammatory effect by inhibiting prostaglandin synthesis; may also inhibit the synthesis or action of other mediators of the inflammatory response.
• Relieves fever by acting on the hypothalamic heat-regulating center to produce peripheral vasodilation. This increases peripheral blood supply and promotes sweating, which leads to loss of heat and to cooling by evaporation.
• Also appears to impede clotting by blocking prostaglandin synthetase action, which prevents formation of the platelet-aggregating substance thromboxane A_2.

INDICATIONS & DOSAGE
Adults:
Arthritis—2.6 to 5.2 g P.O. daily in divided doses.
Mild pain or fever—325 to 650 mg P.O. or rectally q 4 hours, p.r.n.
Thromboembolic disorders—325 to 650 mg P.O. daily or b.i.d.
Transient ischemic attacks in men—650 mg P.O. b.i.d. or 325 mg q.i.d.
To reduce the risk of heart attack in patients with previous myocardial infarction or unstable angina—325 mg P.O. once daily.
Children:
Arthritis—90 to 130 mg/kg P.O. daily divided q 4 to 6 hours.
Fever—40 to 80 mg/kg P.O. or rectally daily divided q 6 hours, p.r.n.
Mild pain—65 to 100 mg/kg P.O. or rectally daily divided q 4 to 6 hours, p.r.n.

ADVERSE REACTIONS
Blood: *prolonged bleeding time.*
EENT: *tinnitus and hearing loss*
GI: *nausea, vomiting, GI distress, occult bleeding.*
Hepatic: abnormal liver function

studies, hepatitis.
Skin: *rash,* bruising.
Other: *hypersensitivity manifested by anaphylaxis and/or asthma.*

INTERACTIONS
Ammonium chloride (and other urine acidifiers): increased blood levels of aspirin products. Monitor for aspirin toxicity.
Antacids in high doses (and other urine alkalinizers): decreased levels of aspirin products. Monitor for decreased aspirin effect.
Corticosteroids: enhance salicylate elimination. Monitor for decreased salicylate effect.
Oral anticoagulants and heparin: increase risk of bleeding. Avoid using together if possible.

NURSING CONSIDERATIONS
• Contraindicated in GI ulcer, GI bleeding, aspirin hypersensitivity. Use cautiously in patients with hypoprothrombinemia, vitamin K deficiency, bleeding disorders, and in asthmatics with nasal polyps (may cause severe bronchospasm).
• Because of epidemiologic association with Reye's syndrome, the Centers for Disease Control recommends that children or teenagers with chicken pox or influenza-like illness should not be given salicylates.
• Febrile, dehydrated children can develop toxicity rapidly.
• Elderly patients may be more susceptible to aspirin's toxic effects.
• Give with food, milk, antacid, or large glass of water to reduce GI side effects.
• Because of the many possible drug interactions involving aspirin, warn patients taking prescription drugs to check with doctor or pharmacist before taking over-the-counter combinations containing aspirin.
• Therapeutic blood salicylate level in arthritis is 20 to 30 mg/100 ml.
• Alcohol may increase risk of gas-

trointestinal bleeding.
• May cause increase in serum levels of SGOT, SGPT, alkaline phosphatase, and bilirubin.
• Keep out of reach of children—aspirin is one of the leading causes of poisoning in children. Encourage use of child-resistant containers.
• Advise patients receiving large doses of aspirin for an extended period of time to watch for petechiae, bleeding gums, signs of GI bleeding, and to maintain adequate fluid intake. Obtain hemoglobin and prothrombin tests periodically.
• Enteric-coated products are slowly absorbed and are not suitable for acute effects. They do cause less GI bleeding and may be more suited for long-term therapy, such as arthritis therapy.
• There's no evidence that aspirin is effective in reducing the incidence of transient ischemic attacks in women.
• Recent research shows that aspirin can prevent sunburn and treat sunburn pain by preventing cells from manufacturing prostaglandins.
• If possible, stop aspirin dosage 1 week before elective surgery.
• For patients with swallowing difficulties, aspirin can be crushed and combined with soft food or dissolved in liquid. After mixing it with a liquid, administer it immediately, because the drug doesn't stay in solution.

---

choline magnesium trisalicylate

Trilisate♦
Pregnancy Category: C

MECHANISM OF ACTION
• Produces analgesia by an ill-defined effect on the hypothalamus (central action) and by blocking generation of pain impulses (peripheral action). The peripheral action may involve inhibition of prostaglandin syn-

thesis.
• Exerts its anti-inflammatory effect by inhibiting prostaglandin synthesis; may also inhibit the synthesis or action of other mediators of the inflammatory response.
• Relieves fever by acting on the hypothalamic heat-regulating center to produce peripheral vasodilation. This increases peripheral blood supply and promotes sweating, which leads to loss of heat and to cooling by evaporation.

INDICATIONS & DOSAGE
Arthritis, mild—
Adults: 1 to 2 teaspoonfuls or tablets b.i.d. Total daily dose can also be given at one time.
Rheumatoid arthritis and osteoarthritis—
Adults: 2 to 3 teaspoonfuls or tablets b.i.d. Total daily dose can also be given at one time.
Each '500' tablet or teaspoonful is equal in salicylate content to 650 mg aspirin.
Juvenile rheumatoid arthritis—
Children (12-37 kg): 50 mg/kg/day P.O. in divided doses.
Children (more than 37 kg): 2,250 mg given in divided doses.
Mild-to-moderate pain and fever—
Adults: 2 to 3 g P.O. daily in divided doses.
Children (12-37 kg): 50 mg/kg/day in divided doses.

ADVERSE REACTIONS
EENT: *tinnitus and hearing loss.*
GI: *nausea, vomiting, GI distress, occult bleeding.*
Hepatic: abnormal liver function studies, hepatitis.
Skin: *rash,* bruising.
Other: *hypersensitivity manifested by anaphylaxis, and/or asthma.*

INTERACTIONS
Ammonium chloride (and other urine acidifiers): increased blood levels of

---

Italicized side effects are common or life-threatening.
*Liquid form contains alcohol.   **May contain tartrazine.

salicylates. Monitor for salicylate toxicity.

Antacids in high doses (and other urine alkalinizers): decreased levels of salicylates. Monitor for decreased salicylate effect.

Corticosteroids: enhance salicylate elimination. Monitor for decreased salicylate effect.

Oral anticoagulants and heparin: increase risk of bleeding. Avoid using together if possible.

NURSING CONSIDERATIONS
• Contraindicated in GI ulcer, GI bleeding, aspirin hypersensitivity. Use cautiously in patients with hypoprothrombinemia, vitamin K deficiency, bleeding disorders, and in asthmatics with nasal polyps (may cause severe bronchospasm).
• Because of epidemiologic association with Reye's syndrome, the Centers for Disease Control recommends that children or teenagers with chicken pox or influenza-like illness should not be given salicylates.
• May cause less GI distress than aspirin. If antacid is needed, give it 2 hours after meals and give choline magnesium trisalicylate before meals.
• Tell patient to take tablets with food or a full glass of water.
• Febrile, dehydrated children can develop toxicity rapidly.
• Therapeutic blood salicylate level in arthritis is 20 to 30 mg/100 ml.
• Alcohol may increase risk of gastrointestinal bleeding.
• May cause an increase in serum levels of SGOT, SGPT, alkaline phosphatase, and bilirubin.
• Obtain hemoglobin and prothrombin tests periodically in patients receiving large doses over an extended period of time.

choline salicylate
Arthropan♦
Pregnancy Category: C

MECHANISM OF ACTION
• Produces analgesia by an ill-defined effect on the hypothalamus (central action) and by blocking generation of pain impulses (peripheral action). The peripheral action may involve inhibition of prostaglandin synthesis.
• Exerts its anti-inflammatory effect by inhibiting prostaglandin synthesis; may also inhibit the synthesis or action of other mediators of the inflammatory response.
• Relieves fever by acting on the hypothalamic heat-regulating center to produce peripheral vasodilation. This increases peripheral blood supply and promotes sweating, which leads to loss of heat and to cooling by evaporation.

INDICATIONS & DOSAGE
Arthritis—
Adults: 5 to 10 ml P.O. q.i.d.
Minor pain or fever—
Adults: 870 mg (5 ml) P.O. q 3 to 4 hours, p.r.n.
Children 3 to 6 years: 105 to 210 mg P.O. q 4 hours, p.r.n.
Each 870 mg (5 ml) equals 650 mg aspirin.

ADVERSE REACTIONS
EENT: *tinnitus and hearing loss (first signs of toxicity).*
GI: *nausea, vomiting, GI distress, occult bleeding.*
Hepatic: abnormal liver function studies, hepatitis.
Skin: *rash,* bruising.
Other: *hypersensitivity manifested by anaphylaxis and/or asthma.*

INTERACTIONS
Ammonium chloride (and other urine acidifiers): increased blood levels of

salicylates. Monitor for salicylate toxicity.
Antacids in high doses (and other urine alkalinizers): decreased levels of salicylates. Monitor for decreased salicylate effect.
Corticosteroids: enhance salicylate elimination. Monitor for decreased salicylate effect.
Oral anticoagulants: increase risk of bleeding. Avoid using together if possible.

NURSING CONSIDERATIONS
• Contraindicated in GI ulcer, GI bleeding, aspirin hypersensitivity. Use cautiously in patients with hypoprothrombinemia, vitamin K deficiency, bleeding disorders, and in asthmatics with nasal polyps (may cause severe bronchospasm).
• Because of epidemiologic association with Reye's syndrome, the Centers for Disease Control recommends that children or teenagers with chicken pox or influenza-like illness should not be given salicylates.
• May cause less GI distress than aspirin. If antacid is needed, give it 2 hours after meals and give choline salicylate before meals.
• May mix drug with water, fruit juice, or carbonated drinks.
• Febrile, dehydrated children can develop toxicity rapidly.
• Therapeutic blood salicylate level in arthritis is 20 to 30 mg/100 ml.
• Alcohol may increase risk of gastrointestinal bleeding.
• May cause an increase in serum levels of SGOT, SGPT, alkaline phosphatase, and bilirubin.
• Obtain hemoglobin and prothrombin tests periodically in patients receiving large doses over an extended period of time.

diflunisal
Dolobid♦
Pregnancy Category: C

MECHANISM OF ACTION
Mechanism of action is unknown, but it is probably related to inhibition of prostaglandin synthesis.

INDICATIONS & DOSAGE
Mild to moderate pain and osteoarthritis—
Adults: 500 to 1,000 mg daily in two divided doses, usually q 12 hours. Maximum dosage 1,500 mg daily.
Adults over 65: Start with one-half the usual adult dose.

ADVERSE REACTIONS
CNS: *dizziness, somnolence, insomnia, headache.*
EENT: *tinnitus.*
GI: *nausea, dyspepsia, gastrointestinal pain, diarrhea,* vomiting, constipation, flatulence.
Skin: *rash,* pruritus, sweating, dry mucous membranes, stomatitis.

INTERACTIONS
Aspirin, antacids: decreased diflunisal blood levels. Monitor for possible decreased therapeutic effect.

NURSING CONSIDERATIONS
• Contraindicated for patients in whom acute asthmatic attacks, urticaria, or rhinitis are precipitated by aspirin or other nonsteroidal anti-inflammatory drugs.
• Use cautiously in patients with active gastrointestinal bleeding or history of peptic ulcer disease; renal impairment; compromised cardiac function; or those taking anticoagulants.
• Similar to aspirin, diflunisal is a salicylic acid derivative but is metabolized differently.
• May be administered with water, milk, or meals.

Italicized side effects are common or life-threatening.
*Liquid form contains alcohol.   **May contain tartrazine.

magnesium salicylate
Analate, Arthrin, Efficin, Magan, Mobidin
Pregnancy Category: C

MECHANISM OF ACTION
• Produces analgesia by an ill-defined effect on the hypothalamus (central action) and by blocking generation of pain impulses (peripheral action). The peripheral action may involve inhibition of prostaglandin synthesis.
• Exerts its anti-inflammatory effect by inhibiting prostaglandin synthesis; may also inhibit the synthesis or action of other mediators of the inflammatory response.
• Relieves fever by acting on the hypothalamic heat-regulating center to produce peripheral vasodilation. This increases peripheral blood supply and promotes sweating, which leads to loss of heat and to cooling by evaporation.

INDICATIONS & DOSAGE
Arthritis—
Adults: up to 9.6 g daily in divided doses.
Mild pain or fever—
Adults: 600 mg P.O. t.i.d. or q.i.d.

ADVERSE REACTIONS
EENT: *tinnitus and hearing loss.*
GI: *nausea, vomiting, GI distress, occult bleeding.*
Hepatic: abnormal liver function studies, hepatitis.
Skin: *rash,* bruising.
Other: *hypersensitivity manifested by anaphylaxis and/or asthma.*

INTERACTIONS
Ammonium chloride (and other urine acidifiers): increased blood levels of salicylates. Monitor for salicylate toxicity.
Antacids in high doses (and other urine alkalinizers): decreased levels of salicylates. Monitor for decreased salicylate effect.
Corticosteroids: enhance salicylate elimination. Monitor for decreased salicylate effect.
Oral anticoagulants and heparin: increase risk of bleeding. Avoid using together if possible.

NURSING CONSIDERATIONS
• Contraindicated in severe chronic renal insufficiency because of risk of magnesium toxicity; GI ulcer; GI bleeding; aspirin hypersensitivity. Use cautiously in hypoprothrombinemia, vitamin K deficiency and bleeding disorders.
• Because of epidemiologic association with Reye's syndrome, the Centers for Disease Control recommends that children or teenagers with chicken pox or influenza-like illness should not be given salicylates.
• Febrile, dehydrated children can develop toxicity rapidly.
• Give with food, milk, antacid, or large glass of water to reduce GI side effects.
• Therapeutic blood salicylate level in arthritis is 20 to 30 mg/100 ml.
• Alcohol may increase risk of gastrointestinal bleeding.
• May cause an increase in serum levels of SGOT, SGPT, alkaline phosphatase, and bilirubin.
• Obtain hemoglobin and prothrombin tests periodically in patients receiving large doses over an extended period of time.

phenazopyridine hydrochloride
Azogesic, Azo-Pyridon, Azo-Standard, Baridium, Di-Azo, Diridone, Phenazo♦♦, Phen-Azo, Phenazodine, Pyridiate, Pyridium♦, Urodine
Pregnancy Category: B

MECHANISM OF ACTION
Exerts local anesthetic action on urinary mucosa through unknown mechanism.

INDICATIONS & DOSAGE
Pain with urinary tract irritation or infection—
Adults: 100 to 200 mg P.O. t.i.d.
Children: 100 mg P.O. t.i.d.

ADVERSE REACTIONS
CNS: headache, vertigo.
GI: nausea.

INTERACTIONS
None significant.

NURSING CONSIDERATIONS
• Contraindicated in renal and hepatic insufficiency.
• Colors urine red or orange. May stain fabrics.
• Use only as analgesic. Use with antibiotic to treat urinary tract infection.
• Drug may be stopped in 3 days if pain is relieved.
• May alter Clinistix or Tes-Tape results. Use Clinitest for accurate urine glucose test results.
• Stop drug if skin or sclera becomes yellow-tinged. May indicate accumulation due to impaired renal excretion.

salsalate
Disalcid, Mono-Gesic
Pregnancy Category: C

MECHANISM OF ACTION
• Produces analgesia by an ill-de-fined effect on the hypothalamus (central action) and by blocking generation of pain impulses (peripheral action). The peripheral action may involve inhibition of prostaglandin synthesis.
• Exerts its anti-inflammatory effect by inhibiting prostaglandin synthesis; may also inhibit the synthesis or action of other mediators of the inflammatory response.
• Relieves fever by acting on the hypothalamic heat-regulating center to produce peripheral vasodilation. This increases peripheral blood supply and promotes sweating, which leads to loss of heat and to cooling by evaporation.

INDICATIONS & DOSAGE
Minor pain or fever, arthritis—
Adults: 1 g P.O. b.i.d., t.i.d., or q.i.d., p.r.n.

ADVERSE REACTIONS
EENT: *tinnitus and hearing loss.*
GI: *nausea, vomiting, GI distress, occult bleeding.*
Hepatic: abnormal liver function studies, hepatitis.
Skin: *rash,* bruising.
Other: *hypersensitivity manifested by anaphylaxis and/or asthma.*

INTERACTIONS
Ammonium chloride (and other urine acidifiers): increased blood levels of salicylates. Monitor for salicylate toxicity.
Antacids in high doses (and other urine alkalinizers): decreased levels of salicylates. Monitor for decreased salicylate effect.
Corticosteroids: enhance salicylate elimination. Monitor for decreased salicylate effect.
Oral anticoagulants and heparin: increase risk of bleeding. Avoid using together if possible.

Italicized side effects are common or life-threatening.
*Liquid form contains alcohol.   **May contain tartrazine.

NURSING CONSIDERATIONS
• Contraindicated in GI bleeding, aspirin hypersensitivity. Use cautiously in hypoprothrombinemia, vitamin K deficiency and bleeding disorders.
• Because of epidemiologic association with Reye's syndrome, the Centers for Disease Control recommends that children or teenagers with chicken pox or influenza-like illness should not be given salicylates.
• Give with food, milk, antacid, or large glass of water to reduce GI side effects.
• Therapeutic blood salicylate level in arthritis is 20 to 30 mg/100 ml.
• Alcohol may increase risk of gastrointestinal bleeding.
• May increase serum alkaline phosphatase, bilirubin, SGOT, and SGPT levels.
• Advise patients receiving large doses for extended period of time to watch for petechiae, bleeding gums, and signs of GI bleeding, and to maintain adequate fluid intake. Obtain hemoglobin and prothrombin tests periodically.

sodium salicylate
Uracel
Pregnancy Category: C

MECHANISM OF ACTION
• Produces analgesia by an ill-defined effect on the hypothalamus (central action) and by blocking generation of pain impulses (peripheral action). The peripheral action may involve inhibition of prostaglandin synthesis.
• Exerts its anti-inflammatory effect by inhibiting prostaglandin synthesis; may also inhibit the synthesis or action of other mediators of the inflammatory response.
• Relieves fever by acting on the hypothalamic heat-regulating center to produce peripheral vasodilation. This increases peripheral blood supply and promotes sweating, which leads to loss of heat and to cooling by evaporation.

INDICATIONS & DOSAGE
Minor pain or fever—
Adults: 325 to 650 mg P.O. q 4 to 6 hours, p.r.n., or 500 mg slow I.V. infusion over 4 to 8 hours. Maximum dose 1 g daily.

ADVERSE REACTIONS
EENT: *tinnitus and hearing loss (first signs of toxicity).*
GI: *nausea, vomiting, GI distress, occult bleeding.*
Hepatic: abnormal liver function studies, hepatitis.
Skin: *rash,* bruising.
Other: *hypersensitivity manifested by anaphylaxis and/or asthma.*
Local: thrombophlebitis (from I.V.).

INTERACTIONS
Ammonium chloride (and other urine acidifiers): increased blood levels of salicylates. Monitor for salicylate toxicity.
Antacids in large doses (and other urine alkalinizers): decreased levels of salicylates. Monitor for decreased salicylate effect.
Corticosteroids: enhance salicylate elimination. Monitor for decreased salicylate effect.
Oral anticoagulants and heparin: increase risk of bleeding. Avoid using together if possible.

NURSING CONSIDERATIONS
• Contraindicated in GI ulcer, GI bleeding, aspirin hypersensitivity. Use cautiously in hypoprothrombinemia, vitamin K deficiency, bleeding disorders, asthma with nasal polyps (may cause severe bronchospasm).
• Use cautiously in congestive heart failure and hypertension, because of increased sodium load.
• Because of epidemiologic association with Reye's syndrome, the Cen-

ters for Disease Control recommends that children or teenagers with chicken pox or influenza-like illness should not be given salicylates.
• Febrile, dehydrated children can develop toxicity rapidly.
• Give with food, milk, antacid, or large glass of water to reduce GI side effects.
• Therapeutic salicylate level in arthritis is 20 to 30 mg/100 ml.
• Alcohol may increase risk of gastrointestinal bleeding.
• May increase serum alkaline phosphatase, bilirubin, SGOT, and SGPT levels.
• Advise patients receiving large doses for extended period of time to watch for petechiae, bleeding gums, and signs of GI bleeding, and to maintain adequate fluid intake. Obtain hemoglobin and prothrombin tests periodically.

sodium thiosalicylate
Arthrolate, Osteolate, Thiodyne, Thiolate, Thiosal
Pregnancy Category: C

MECHANISM OF ACTION
• Produces analgesia by an ill-defined effect on the hypothalamus (central action) and by blocking generation of pain impulses (peripheral action). The peripheral action may involve inhibition of prostaglandin synthesis.
• Exerts its anti-inflammatory effect by inhibiting prostaglandin synthesis; may also inhibit the synthesis or action of other mediators of the inflammatory response.
• Relieves fever by acting on the hypothalamic heat-regulating center to produce peripheral vasodilation. This increases peripheral blood supply and promotes sweating, which leads to loss of heat and to cooling by evaporation.

INDICATIONS & DOSAGE
Mild pain—
Adults: 50 to 100 mg I.M. daily or every other day.
Arthritis—
Adults: 100 mg I.M. daily.
Rheumatic fever—
Adults: 100 to 150 mg I.M. b.i.d. until asymptomatic.

ADVERSE REACTIONS
EENT: *tinnitus and hearing loss.*
GI: *nausea, vomiting, GI distress, occult bleeding.*
Hepatic: abnormal liver function studies, hepatitis.
Skin: *rash,* bruising.
Other: *hypersensitivity manifested by anaphylaxis.*

INTERACTIONS
Ammonium chloride (and other urine acidifiers): increased blood levels of salicylates. Monitor for salicylate toxicity.
Antacids in large doses (and other urine alkalinizers): decreased levels of salicylates. Monitor for decreased salicylate effect.
Corticosteriods: enhance salicylate elimination. Monitor for decreased salicylate effects.
Oral anticoagulants and heparin: increase risk of bleeding. Avoid using together if possible.

NURSING CONSIDERATIONS
• Contraindicated in GI ulcer, GI bleeding, aspirin hypersensitivity. Use cautiously in hypoprothrombinemia, vitamin K deficiency, bleeding disorders and asthma with nasal polyps (may cause severe bronchospasm).
• Because of epidemiologic association with Reye's syndrome, the Centers for Disease Control recommends that children or teenagers with chicken pox or influenza-like illness should not be given salicylates.
• Tinnitus, headache, dizziness, confusion, fever, sweating, thirst, drowsi-

ness, dim vision, hyperventilation, and tachycardia are signs of mild toxicity.
• Alcohol may increase risk of gastrointestinal bleeding.
• May increase serum alkaline phosphatase, bilirubin, SGOT, and SGPT levels.
• Advise patients receiving large doses for extended period of time to watch for petechiae, bleeding gums, and signs of GI bleeding, and to maintain adequate fluid intake. Obtain hemoglobin and prothrombin tests periodically.

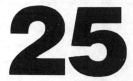

Nonsteroidal anti-inflammatory agents

fenoprofen calcium
ibuprofen
indomethacin
indomethacin sodium trihydrate
ketoprofen
meclofenamate
mefenamic acid
naproxen
naproxen sodium
oxyphenbutazone
phenylbutazone
piroxicam
sulindac
suprofen
tolmetin sodium

COMBINATION PRODUCTS
None.

fenoprofen calcium
Nalfon♦
Pregnancy Category: B (D in 3rd trimester)

MECHANISM OF ACTION
Produces anti-inflammatory, analgesic, and antipyretic effects, possibly through inhibition of prostaglandin synthesis.

INDICATIONS & DOSAGE
Rheumatoid arthritis and osteoarthritis—
Adults: 300 to 600 mg P.O. q.i.d. Maximum 3.2 g daily.
Mild to moderate pain—
Adults: 200 mg P.O. q 4 to 6 hours, p.r.n.

ADVERSE REACTIONS
Blood: prolonged bleeding time, anemia.
CNS: headache, drowsiness, dizziness.
CV: peripheral edema.
GI: *epigastric distress, nausea, occult blood loss,* constipation, anorexia.
GU: reversible renal failure.
Hepatic: elevated enzymes.
Skin: pruritus, rash, urticaria.

INTERACTIONS
None significant.

NURSING CONSIDERATIONS
• Contraindicated in asthmatics with nasal polyps and in patients with hypersensitivity to aspirin. Use cautiously in patients with GI disorders, angioedema, cardiovascular disease, or hypersensitivity to other noncorticosteroid anti-inflammatory drugs.
• Use cautiously in patients with history of peptic ulcer disease.
• Tell patient that full therapeutic effect may be delayed for 2 to 4 weeks.
• Check renal, hepatic, and auditory function periodically in long-term therapy. Stop drug if abnormalities occur.
• Give dose 30 minutes before or 2 hours after meals. If GI side effects occur, give with milk or meals.
• Prothrombin time may be prolonged in patients receiving coumarin-type anticoagulants. Fenoprofen decreases platelet aggregation and may prolong bleeding time.

---

ibuprofen
Amersol♦♦, Haltran, Ibuprin,
Medipren, Midol 200, Motrin♦,
Rufen, Trendar
Pregnancy Category: B (D in 3rd
trimester)

MECHANISM OF ACTION
Produces anti-inflammatory, analgesic, and antipyretic effects, possibly
through inhibition of prostaglandin
synthesis.

INDICATIONS & DOSAGE
*Arthritis, primary dysmenorrhea,
gout, postextraction dental pain—*
Adults: 200 to 600 mg P.O. q.i.d.

ADVERSE REACTIONS
Blood: prolonged bleeding time.
CNS: headache, drowsiness, dizziness, aseptic meningitis.
CV: peripheral edema.
EENT: visual disturbances, tinnitus.
GI: *epigastric distress, nausea, occult blood loss.*
GU: reversible renal failure.
Hepatic: elevated enzymes.
Skin: pruritus, rash, urticaria.
Other: bronchospasm, edema.

INTERACTIONS
None significant.

NURSING CONSIDERATIONS
• Contraindicated in asthmatics with
nasal polyps. Use cautiously in GI
disorders, angioedema, hypersensitivity to other noncorticosteroid anti-inflammatory drugs including aspirin,
hepatic or renal disease, cardiac decompensation, or known intrinsic coagulation defects.
• Use cautiously in patients with history of peptic ulcer disease.
• Tell patient that full therapeutic effect may be delayed for 2 to 4 weeks.
• Check renal and hepatic function
periodically in long-term therapy.
Stop drug if abnormalities occur.

• Tell patient to report to doctor immediately any GI symptoms or signs
of bleeding, visual disturbances, skin
rashes, weight gain, or edema.
• Give with meals or milk to reduce
GI side effects.
• Available as several brands without
prescription in the 200-mg tablet
strength.

indomethacin
Indocid♦♦, Indocin, Indocin SR,
Indo-Lemmon, Indomed

indomethacin sodium trihydrate
Indocin I.V.
Pregnancy Category: B (D in 3rd
trimester)

MECHANISM OF ACTION
Produces anti-inflammatory, analgesic, and antipyretic effects, possibly
through inhibition of prostaglandin
synthesis.

INDICATIONS & DOSAGE
Moderate to severe arthritis, ankylosing spondylitis—
Adults: 25 mg P.O. or per rectum
b.i.d. or t.i.d. with food or antacids;
may increase dose by 25 mg daily q 7
days up to 200 mg daily. Alternatively, sustained-release capsules (75
mg) may be given: 75 mg to start, in
the morning or at bedtime, followed,
if necessary, by 75 mg b.i.d.
Acute gouty arthritis—
50 mg t.i.d. Reduce dose as soon as
possible, then stop. Sustained-release
capsules shouldn't be used for this
condition.
To close a hemodynamically significant patent ductus arteriosus in premature infants (I.V. form only)—
Age less than 48 hours: 0.2 mg/kg
I.V. followed by 2 doses of 0.1 mg/kg
at 12- to 24-hour intervals.
Age 2-7 days: 0.2 mg/kg I.V. followed by 2 doses of 0.2 mg/kg at 12-

to 24-hour intervals.
Over 7 days: 0.2 mg/kg I.V. followed by 2 doses of 0.25 mg/kg at 12- to 24-hour intervals.

ADVERSE REACTIONS
Oral form:
Blood: *hemolytic anemia, aplastic anemia, agranulocytosis,* leukopenia, *thrombocytopenic purpura,* iron deficiency anemia.
CNS: *headache, dizziness,* depression, drowsiness, confusion, peripheral neuropathy, convulsions, psychic disturbances, syncope, *vertigo.*
CV: hypertension, *edema.*
EENT: *blurred vision, corneal and retinal damage,* hearing loss, tinnitus.
GI: *nausea, vomiting,* anorexia, *diarrhea, severe GI bleeding.*
GU: hematuria, hyperkalemia, acute renal failure.
Hepatic: elevated enzymes.
Skin: pruritus, urticaria, *Stevens-Johnson syndrome.*
Other: hypersensitivity (shocklike symptoms, rash, respiratory distress, angioedema).
I.V. form:
Blood: decreased platelet aggregation.
GI: *bleeding,* vomiting.
GU: *renal dysfunction.*
Metabolic: *hyponatremia, hyperkalemia,* hypoglycemia.

INTERACTIONS
Diflunisal, Probenecid: decreases indomethacin excretion; watch for increased incidence of indomethacin side effects.
Furosemide: impaired response to both drugs. Avoid if possible.
Triamterene: possible nephrotoxicity. Don't use together.

NURSING CONSIDERATIONS
Oral form:
• Contraindicated in aspirin hypersensitivity and GI disorders. Use cautiously in patients with epilepsy, par-

kinsonism, hepatic or renal disease, cardiovascular disease, infection, history of mental illness, and in elderly patients.
• Severe headache may occur. Decrease dose if headache persists.
• Has an antipyretic effect.
• Tell patient to notify doctor immediately if any visual or hearing changes occur. Patients taking drug long-term should have regular eye examinations and hearing tests.
• Very irritating to GI tract. Give with meals. Advise patient to notify doctor of any GI side effects.
• CNS side effects are more common and serious in elderly patients.
• Monitor for bleeding in patients receiving anticoagulants.
• Causes sodium retention; monitor for increased blood pressure in patients with hypertension.
• Used investigationally as prophylaxis for gout when colchicine is not well tolerated.
• Patients taking drug long-term should receive periodic testing of CBC, renal function, and eye examinations.
• Due to high incidence of side effects when used chronically, indomethacin should not be used routinely as an analgesic or antipyretic.
I.V. form:
• Contraindicated in infants with untreated infection; active bleeding; coagulation defects or thrombocytopenia; necrotizing enterocolitis; or impaired renal function.
• Don't administer second or third scheduled dose if anuria or marked oliguria is evident.
• If ductus arteriosus reopens, a second course of one to three doses may be given. If ineffective, surgery may be necessary.
• Monitor carefully for bleeding and for reduced urine output. Stop drug and notify doctor if either occurs.

Italicized side effects are common or life-threatening.
*Liquid form contains alcohol.   **May contain tartrazine.

ketoprofen
Orudis
Pregnancy Category: B (D in 3rd trimester)

MECHANISM OF ACTION
Produces anti-inflammatory, analgesic, and antipyretic effects, possibly through inhibition of prostaglandin synthesis.

INDICATIONS & DOSAGE
Rheumatoid arthritis and osteoarthritis—
Adults: 150 to 300 mg P.O. divided into three or four doses. Usual dose is 75 mg t.i.d. Maximum 300 mg/day.

ADVERSE REACTIONS
Blood: prolonged bleeding time.
CNS: *headache,* dizziness, *CNS inhibition or excitation.*
EENT: tinnitus, visual disturbances.
GI: *nausea, abdominal pain, diarrhea, constipation, flatulence,* anorexia, vomiting, stomatitis.
GU: nephrotoxicity, *increased BUN.*
Hepatic: elevated enzymes.
Skin: rash.

INTERACTIONS
None significant.

NURSING CONSIDERATIONS
• Contraindicated in patients who are hypersensitive to aspirin or other nonsteroidal anti-inflammatory drugs.
• Use cautiously in patients with history of peptic ulcer disease or renal dysfunction.
• Tell patient that full therapeutic effect may be delayed for 2 to 4 weeks.
• Check renal and hepatic function periodically during long-term therapy.
• Give dose 30 minutes before or 2 hours after meals. If GI side effects occur, give with milk or meals.

meclofenamate
Meclomen
Pregnancy Category: B (D in 3rd trimester)

MECHANISM OF ACTION
Produces anti-inflammatory, analgesic, and antipyretic effects, possibly through inhibition of prostaglandin synthesis.

INDICATIONS & DOSAGE
Rheumatoid arthritis and osteoarthritis—
Adults: 200 to 400 mg/day P.O. in 3 or 4 equally divided doses.

ADVERSE REACTIONS
Blood: leukopenia, thrombocytopenia, *agranulocytosis, aplastic anemia.*
CNS: *drowsiness, dizziness,* nervousness, headache.
CV: edema
EENT: blurred vision, eye irritation.
GI: nausea, vomiting, *diarrhea,* hemorrhage.
GU: dysuria, hematuria, nephrotoxicity.
Hepatic: hepatotoxicity.
Skin: rash, urticaria.

INTERACTIONS
None significant.

NURSING CONSIDERATIONS
• Contraindicated in GI ulceration or inflammation. Use cautiously in patients with hepatic or renal disease, cardiovascular disease, blood dyscrasias, diabetes mellitus, and in asthmatics with nasal polyps.
• Use cautiously in patients with history of peptic ulcer disease. Also use cautiously in the elderly, who are more likely to experience adverse reactions.
• Warn patient against activities that require alertness until CNS response to drug is determined.

Unmarked trade names available in the United States only.
♦ Also available in Canada.   ♦♦ Available in Canada only.

• Stop drug if rash or diarrhea develops.
• Administer with food to minimize GI side effects.
• Almost identical in chemical structure to mefenamic acid.
• False-positive reactions for urine bilirubin using the diazo tablet test have been reported.
• Patients taking drug long-term should receive periodic testing of CBC, renal and hepatic function.

mefenamic acid
Ponstan♦♦, Ponstel
Pregnancy Category: C

MECHANISM OF ACTION
Produces anti-inflammatory, analgesic, and antipyretic effects, possibly through inhibition of prostaglandin synthesis.

INDICATIONS & DOSAGE
Mild to moderate pain, dysmenorrhea—
Adults and children over 14 years: 500 mg P.O. initially, then 250 mg q 4 hours, p.r.n.
Maximum therapy 1 week.

ADVERSE REACTIONS
Blood: leukopenia, thrombocytopenia, *agranulocytosis, aplastic anemia.*
CNS: drowsiness, dizziness, nervousness, headache.
CV: edema.
EENT: blurred vision, eye irritation.
GI: nausea, vomiting, *diarrhea,* hemorrhage.
GU: dysuria, hematuria, nephrotoxicity.
Hepatic: hepatotoxicity.
Skin: rash, urticaria.

INTERACTIONS
None significant.

NURSING CONSIDERATIONS
• Contraindicated in GI ulceration or inflammation. Use cautiously in patients with hepatic or renal disease, cardiovascular disease, blood dyscrasias, diabetes mellitus, and in asthmatics with nasal polyps.
• Use cautiously in patients with history of peptic ulcer disease.
• Warn patient against activities that require alertness until CNS response to drug is determined.
• Severe hemolytic anemia may occur with prolonged use.
• Stop drug if rash or diarrhea develops.
• Should not be administered for more than 1 week at a time, because incidence of toxicity increases.
• Administer with food to minimize GI side effects.
• False-positive reactions for urine bilirubin using the diazo tablet test have been reported.

naproxen
Naprosyn♦

naproxen sodium
Anaprox♦
Pregnancy Category: B (D in 3rd trimester)

MECHANISM OF ACTION
Produces anti-inflammatory, analgesic, and antipyretic effects, possibly through inhibition of prostaglandin synthesis.

INDICATIONS & DOSAGE
Arthritis, primary dysmenorrhea (free base)—
Adults: 250 to 500 mg P.O. b.i.d. Maximum 1,000 mg daily.
Mild to moderate pain and for treatment of primary dysmenorrhea (naproxen sodium)—
Adults: 2 tablets (275 mg each tablet) to start, followed by 275 mg q 6 to 8 hours as needed. Maximum daily

---

Italicized side effects are common or life-threatening.
*Liquid form contains alcohol.   **May contain tartrazine.

dose should not exceed 1,375 mg.

ADVERSE REACTIONS
Blood: prolonged bleeding time, *agranulocytosis*, neutropenia.
CNS: headache, drowsiness, dizziness.
CV: peripheral edema.
EENT: visual disturbances.
GI: *epigastric distress, occult blood loss, nausea.*
GU: nephrotoxicity.
Hepatic: elevated enzymes.
Skin: pruritus, rash, urticaria.

INTERACTIONS
None significant.

NURSING CONSIDERATIONS
• Contraindicated in asthmatics with nasal polyps.
• Use cautiously in patients with renal disease, cardiovascular disease, GI disorders, angioedema, and in those allergic to noncorticosteroid anti-inflammatory agents, including aspirin.
• Use cautiously in patients with history of peptic ulcer disease.
• Monitor CBC periodically.
• Tell patient taking naproxen that full therapeutic effect may be delayed 2 to 4 weeks.
• Warn patient against taking both naproxen and naproxen sodium at the same time because both circulate in the blood as the naproxen anion.
• 275 mg naproxen sodium is equivalent to 250 mg naproxen free base.
• Check renal and hepatic function periodically in long-term therapy. Stop drug if abnormalities occur.
• Advise periodic eye examinations during long term therapy.
• Monitor hemoglobin and bleeding time periodically.

oxyphenbutazone
Pregnancy Category: D

MECHANISM OF ACTION
Produces anti-inflammatory, analgesic, and antipyretic effects, possibly through inhibition of prostaglandin synthesis.

INDICATIONS & DOSAGE
Pain, inflammation in arthritis, bursitis, superficial venous thrombosis—
Adults: 100 to 200 mg P.O. with food or milk t.i.d. or q.i.d.
Acute gouty arthritis—
Adults: 400 mg initially as single dose, then 100 mg q 4 hours for 4 days or until relief is obtained.

ADVERSE REACTIONS
Blood: *bone-marrow depression (fatal aplastic anemia, agranulocytosis, thrombocytopenia),* hemolytic anemia, leukopenia.
CNS: restlessness, confusion, lethargy.
CV: hypertension, pericarditis, myocarditis, *cardiac decompensation.*
EENT: optic neuritis, blurred vision, retinal hemorrhage or detachment, hearing loss.
GI: *nausea, vomiting, diarrhea,* ulceration, occult blood loss.
GU: proteinuria, hematuria, glomerulonephritis, nephrotic syndrome, *renal failure.*
Hepatic: *hepatitis.*
Metabolic: toxic and nontoxic goiter, respiratory alkalosis, and metabolic acidosis.
Skin: petechiae, pruritus, purpura, various dermatoses from rash to *toxic necrotizing epidermolysis.*

INTERACTIONS
None significant.

NURSING CONSIDERATIONS
• Contraindicated in children under 14 years; in patients with senility; GI

ulcer; blood dyscrasias; renal, hepatic, cardiac, and thyroid disease. Should not be used in patients receiving long-term anticoagulant therapy.
• Tell patient to stop drug and notify doctor immediately if fever, sore throat, mouth ulcers, GI discomfort, black or tarry stools, bleeding, bruising, rash, or weight gain occurs.
• Give with food, milk, or antacids.
• Complete physical examination and laboratory evaluation are recommended before therapy. Warn patient to remain under close medical supervision and to keep all doctor and laboratory appointments.
• Monitor CBC every 2 weeks or weekly in elderly patients. Report any abnormality to doctor immediately.
• Record patient's weight, intake, and output daily. May cause sodium retention and edema.
• Response should be seen in 2 or 3 days. Drug should be stopped if no response seen within 1 week.
• Patients over age 60 should not receive drug for longer than 1 week. Younger patients, too, should only receive it for short periods.
• Has antipyretic effect.

phenylbutazone
Algoverine♦♦, Azolid, Butagesic♦♦, Butazolidin♦, Intrabutazone♦♦, Malgesic♦♦, Neo-Zoline♦♦
Pregnancy Category: D

MECHANISM OF ACTION
Produces anti-inflammatory, analgesic, and antipyretic effects, possibly through inhibition of prostaglandin synthesis.

INDICATIONS & DOSAGE
Pain, inflammation in arthritis, bursitis, acute superficial thrombophlebitis—
Adults: initially, 100 to 200 mg P.O. t.i.d. or q.i.d. Maximum dose 600 mg per day. When improvement is ob-

tained, decrease dose to 100 mg t.i.d. or q.i.d.
Acute, gouty arthritis—
Adults: 400 mg initially as single dose, then 100 mg q 4 hours for 4 days or until relief is obtained.

ADVERSE REACTIONS
Blood: *bone-marrow depression (fatal aplastic anemia, agranulocytosis,* thrombocytopenia), hemolytic anemia, leukopenia.
CNS: agitation, confusion, lethargy.
CV: hypertension, edema, pericarditis, myocarditis, *cardiac decompensation.*
EENT: optic neuritis, blurred vision, retinal hemorrhage or detachment, hearing loss.
GI: *nausea, vomiting, diarrhea,* ulceration, occult blood loss.
GU: proteinuria, hematuria, glomerulonephritis, nephrotic syndrome, *renal failure.*
Hepatic: *hepatitis.*
Metabolic: hyperglycemia, toxic and nontoxic goiter, respiratory alkalosis, and metabolic acidosis.
Skin: petechiae, pruritus, purpura, various dermatoses from rash to *toxic necrotizing epidermolysis.*

INTERACTIONS
Cholestyramine: may alter phenylbutazone absorption. Give 1 hour before cholestyramine.

NURSING CONSIDERATIONS
• Contraindicated in children under 14 years; in patients with senility; GI ulcer; blood dyscrasias; renal, hepatic, cardiac, and thyroid disease. Should not be used in patients receiving long-term anticoagulant therapy.
• Warn patient to stop drug and notify doctor immediately if fever, sore throat, mouth ulcers, GI discomfort, black or tarry stools, bleeding, bruising, rash, or weight gain occurs.
• Give with food, milk, or antacids.
• Complete physical examination and

Italicized side effects are common or life-threatening.
*Liquid form contains alcohol.   **May contain tartrazine.

NONSTEROIDAL ANTI-INFLAMMATORY AGENTS   221

laboratory evaluation are recommended before therapy. Patient should remain under close medical supervision and keep all doctor and laboratory appointments.
• Monitor CBC every 2 weeks or weekly in elderly patients. Report any abnormalities to doctor right away.
• Record patient's weight, intake, and output daily. May cause sodium retention and edema.
• Response should be seen in 3 to 4 days. Stop drug if no response within 1 week.
• Patients over age 60 should not receive drug for longer than 1 week. Younger patients, too, should only receive it for short periods.
• This drug has limited use because it produces adverse reactions in up to 45% of patients.

piroxicam
Feldene♦
Pregnancy Category: C

MECHANISM OF ACTION
Produces anti-inflammatory, analgesic, and antipyretic effects, possibly through inhibition of prostaglandin synthesis.

INDICATIONS & DOSAGE
Osteoarthritis and rheumatoid arthritis—
Adults: 20 mg P.O. once daily. If desired, the dose may be divided.

ADVERSE REACTIONS
Blood: prolonged bleeding time, anemia.
CNS: headache, drowsiness, dizziness.
CV: peripheral edema.
GI: *epigastric distress, nausea, occult blood loss, severe gastrointestinal bleeding.*
GU: nephrotoxicity.
Hepatic: elevated enzymes.
Skin: pruritus, rash, urticaria, *photo-*

sensitivity.

INTERACTIONS
None significant.

NURSING CONSIDERATIONS
• Contraindicated in asthmatics with nasal polyps. Use cautiously in patients with angioedema, GI disorders, cardiac disease, or hypersensitivity to other nonsteroidal anti-inflammatory drugs.
• Use cautiously in patients with history of peptic ulcer disease.
• Tell patient full therapeutic effect may be delayed for 2 to 4 weeks.
• Causes adverse skin reactions more often than other drugs in its class. Photosensitivity reactions are the most common.
• Check renal, hepatic, and auditory function periodically during prolonged therapy. Drug should be discontinued if abnormalities occur.
• If GI side effects occur, give with milk or meals.
• Prothrombin time may be prolonged in patients receiving coumarin-type anticoagulants. Piroxicam decreases platelet aggregation and may prolong bleeding time.
• The first nonsteroidal anti-inflammatory drug approved by the FDA for once-daily administration. Has a longer half-life and, hence, a longer duration of action than other similar drugs.

sulindac
Clinoril♦
Pregnancy Category: B (D in 3rd trimester)

MECHANISM OF ACTION
Produces anti-inflammatory, analgesic, and antipyretic effects, possibly through inhibition of prostaglandin synthesis.

INDICATIONS & DOSAGE

Osteoarthritis, rheumatoid arthritis, ankylosing spondylitis—
Adults: 150 mg P.O. b.i.d. initially; may increase to 200 mg P.O. b.i.d.
Acute subacromial bursitis or supraspinatus tendinitis, acute gouty arthritis—
Adults: 200 mg P.O. b.i.d. for 7 to 14 days. Dose may be reduced as symptoms subside.

ADVERSE REACTIONS

Blood: prolonged bleeding time, *aplastic anemia.*
CNS: dizziness, headache, nervousness.
EENT: tinnitus, transient visual disturbances.
GI: *epigastric distress, occult blood loss, nausea.*
Hepatic: elevated enzymes.
Skin: rash, pruritus.
Other: edema.

INTERACTIONS

None significant.

NURSING CONSIDERATIONS

• Contraindicated in acute asthmatics whose conditions are precipitated by aspirin or other nonsteroidal anti-inflammatory agents; in patients who have active ulcers and GI bleeding. Use cautiously in patients with a history of ulcers and GI bleeding, renal dysfunction, compromised cardiac function, hypertension; or in those receiving oral anticoagulants or oral hypoglycemic agents.
• To reduce GI side effects, give with food, milk, or antacids.
• Patient should notify doctor and have complete visual examination if any visual disturbances occur.
• Tell patient to notify doctor immediately if prolonged bleeding occurs.
• Drug causes sodium retention. Patient should report edema and have blood pressure checked periodically.
• Of all the nonsteroidal anti-inflam-

matory drugs, sulindac is the safest to use when mild renal impairment exists. Less likely to cause further renal toxicity.

suprofen
Suprol
Pregnancy Category: B (D in 3rd trimester)

MECHANISM OF ACTION

Produces anti-inflammatory, analgesic, and antipyretic effects, possibly through inhibition of prostaglandin synthesis.

INDICATIONS & DOSAGE

Mild to moderate pain and treatment of primary dysmenorrhea—
Adults: 200 mg q 4 to 6 hours p.r.n. Doses exceeding 800 mg daily are not recommended.

ADVERSE REACTIONS

Blood: thrombocytopenia, leukopenia.
CNS: headache, dizziness, sedation, mood changes, sleep disturbances.
CV: edema.
GI: *nausea, dyspepsia, diarrhea,* abdominal pain, vomiting, flatulence, constipation, gastrointestinal bleeding.
GU: *flank pain, nephrotoxicity.*
Hepatic: elevated enzymes.
Skin: dermatitis, pruritus, rash.
Other: muscle cramps, upper respiratory congestion.

INTERACTIONS

None significant.

NURSING CONSIDERATIONS

• Contraindicated in patients with hypersensitivity to aspirin or other nonsteroidal anti-inflammatory drugs.
• Substantial uricosuria may occur within 1 or more hours after the first suprofen dose. Therefore, patients should be well hydrated when they first take this drug.

• Use cautiously in patients with fluid retention, heart failure or hypertension. Assess for peripheral edema.

• Use cautiously in patients with history of peptic ulcer disease or kidney disease.

• Advise patient to take suprofen on an empty stomach if possible. However, if gastrointestinal upset occurs, tell him to take the drug with a small amount of milk or antacid.

• Tell patient to report to doctor immediately any flank pain, GI symptoms or signs of bleeding, visual disturbances, skin rashes, weight gain, or edema.

• Tell patient that suprofen is for the relief of acute pain only. It is not recommended for chronic, prolonged use.

• Because this drug may cause serious nephrotoxicity, the FDA has warned against using it as an initial treatment.

---

tolmetin sodium
Tolectin♦, Tolectin DS♦**
Pregnancy Category: B (D in 3rd trimester)

MECHANISM OF ACTION
Produces anti-inflammatory, analgesic, and antipyretic effects, possibly through inhibition of prostaglandin synthesis.

INDICATIONS & DOSAGE
Rheumatoid arthritis and osteoarthritis, gout, dysmenorrhea, juvenile rheumatoid arthritis—
Adults: 400 mg P.O. t.i.d. or q.i.d. Maximum 2 g daily.
Children 2 years or older: 15 to 30 mg/kg daily in divided doses.

ADVERSE REACTIONS
Blood: prolonged bleeding time.
CNS: headache, dizziness, drowsiness.
GI: *epigastric distress, occult blood loss, nausea.*
GU: nephrotoxicity, pseudoproteinuria.
Skin: rash, urticaria, pruritus.
Other: sodium retention, edema.

INTERACTIONS
None significant.

NURSING CONSIDERATIONS
• Contraindicated in asthmatics with nasal polyps. Use cautiously in cardiac and renal disease, and GI bleeding.

• Use cautiously in patients with history of peptic ulcer disease.

• Give with food, milk, or antacids to reduce GI side effects.

• Tell patient therapeutic effect should begin within 1 week, but full therapeutic effect may be delayed 2 to 4 weeks.

• Double-strength capsule (400 mg) is available.

• Extended therapy should be accompanied by periodic eye examinations and renal function studies.

• Only nonsteroidal antiinflammatory reported to falsely elevate urinary protein causing pseudoproteinuria.

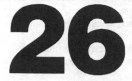

Narcotic and opioid analgesics

alfentanil hydrochloride
buprenorphine hydrochloride
butorphanol tartrate
codeine phosphate
codeine sulfate
fentanyl citrate
hydromorphone hydrochloride
levorphanol tartrate
meperidine hydrochloride
methadone hydrochloride
morphine sulfate
nalbuphine hydrochloride
oxycodone hydrochloride
oxymorphone hydrochloride
pentazocine hydrochloride
pentazocine lactate
propoxyphene hydrochloride
propoxyphene napsylate
sufentanil citrate

COMBINATION PRODUCTS

AMACODONE: hydrocodone bitartrate 5 mg and acetaminophen 500 mg.
BANCAP HC: hydrocodone bitartrate 5 mg and acetaminophen 500 mg.
BUFF-A-COMP NO. 3: codeine phosphate 30 mg, aspirin 325 mg, caffeine 40 mg, and butalbital 50 mg.
CAPITAL WITH CODEINE: codeine phosphate 30 mg and acetaminophen 325 mg.
DARVOCET-N 50: propoxyphene napsylate 50 mg and acetaminophen 325 mg.
DARVOCET-N 100: propoxyphene napsylate 100 mg and acetaminophen 650 mg.
DARVON COMPOUND: propoxyphene HCl 32 mg, aspirin 389 mg, and caffeine 32.4 mg.
DARVON COMPOUND-65: propoxy-phene HCl 65 mg, aspirin 389 mg, and caffeine 32.4 mg.
DARVON-N WITH ASA: propoxyphene napsylate 100 mg and aspirin 325 mg.
DARVON WITH ASA: propoxyphene HCl 65 mg and aspirin 325 mg.
DEMEROL APAP: meperidine HCl 50 mg and acetaminophen 300 mg.
DOLACET: propoxyphene HCl 65 mg and acetaminophen 650 mg.
DOLENE AP-65: propoxyphene HCl 65 mg and acetaminophen 650 mg.
DOLENE COMPOUND-65: propoxy-phene HCl 65 mg, aspirin 389 mg, and caffeine 32.4 mg.
DOXAPHENE COMPOUND: propoxy-phene HCl 65 mg, aspirin 389 mg, and caffeine 32.4 mg.
DURADYNE DHC: hydrocodone bitar-trate 5 mg and acetaminophen 500 mg.
EMPIRIN WITH CODEINE NO. 2: aspirin 325 mg and codeine phosphate 15 mg.
EMPIRIN WITH CODEINE NO. 3: aspirin 325 mg and codeine phosphate 30 mg.
EMPIRIN WITH CODEINE NO. 4: aspirin 325 mg and codeine phosphate 60 mg.
EMPRACET WITH CODEINE NO. 3: co-deine phosphate 30 mg and acetamin-ophen 300 mg.
EMPRACET WITH CODEINE NO. 4: co-deine phosphate 60 mg and acetamin-ophen 300 mg.
FIORINAL WITH CODEINE NO. 1: co-deine phosphate 7.5 mg, aspirin 325 mg, caffeine 40 mg, and butalbital 50 mg.
FIORINAL WITH CODEINE NO. 2♦: co-

deine phosphate 15 mg, aspirin 325 mg, caffeine 40 mg, and butalbital 50 mg.
FIORINAL WITH CODEINE NO. 3♦: codeine phosphate 30 mg, aspirin 325 mg, caffeine 40 mg, and butalbital 50 mg.
HYCODAPHEN: hydrocodone bitartrate 5 mg and acetaminophen 500 mg.
INNOVAR (INJECTION)♦: fentanyl (as the citrate) 0.05 mg and droperidol 2.5 mg per ml.
ISOLLYL WITH CODEINE: codeine phosphate 30 mg, aspirin 325 mg, caffeine 40 mg, and butalbital 50 mg.
PANTOPON♦: hydrochlorides of opium alkaloids. 20 mg is therapeutically equivalent to 15 mg morphine.
PERCOCET-5: acetaminophen 325 mg and oxycodone hydrochloride 5 mg.
PERCODAN♦: oxycodone hydrochloride 4.5 mg, oxycodone terephthalate 0.38 mg, and aspirin 325 mg.
PERCODAN-DEMI♦: oxycodone hydrochloride 2.25 mg, oxycodone terephthalate 0.19 mg, and aspirin 325 mg.
PHENAPHEN-650 WITH CODEINE: codeine phosphate 30 mg and acetaminophen 650 mg.
PHENAPHEN WITH CODEINE NO. 3: codeine phosphate 30 mg and acetaminophen 325 mg.
PHENAPHEN WITH CODEINE NO. 4: codeine phosphate 60 mg and acetaminophen 325 mg.
PHRENILIN WITH CODEINE NO. 3: codeine phosphate 30 mg, acetaminophen 325 mg, and butalbital 50 mg.
PROVAL NO. 3: codeine phosphate 30 mg and acetaminophen 325 mg.
TALACEN: pentazocine hydrochloride 25 mg and acetaminophen 650 mg.
TALWIN COMPOUND: pentazocine HCl 12.5 mg and aspirin 325 mg.
TYLENOL WITH CODEINE NO 1: acetaminophen 300 mg and codeine phosphate 7.5 mg.
TYLENOL WITH CODEINE NO. 2: acetaminophen 300 mg and codeine phosphate 15 mg.

TYLENOL WITH CODEINE NO. 3: acetaminophen 300 mg and codeine phosphate 30 mg.
TYLENOL WITH CODEINE NO. 4: acetaminophen 300 mg and codeine phosphate 60 mg.
TYLOX: acetaminophen 500 mg and oxycodone hydrochloride 5 mg.
VICODIN: hydrocodone bitartrate 5 mg and acetaminophen 500 mg.
WYGESIC: propoxyphene HCl 65 mg and acetaminophen 650 mg.
ZYDONE: hydrocodone bitartrate 5 mg and acetaminophen 500 mg.

---

alfentanil hydrochloride
Alfenta
Controlled Substance Schedule II
Pregnancy Category: B (D for prolonged use or use of high doses at term)

MECHANISM OF ACTION
Binds with opiate receptors at many sites in the central nervous system (brain, brain stem, and spinal cord), altering both perception of and emotional response to pain through an unknown mechanism.

INDICATIONS & DOSAGE
Adjunct to general anesthetic—
Adults: initially, 8 to 50 mcg/kg I.V., then give increments of 3 to 15 mcg/kg I.V.
As a primary anesthetic—
Adults: initially, 130 to 245 mcg/kg I.V., then give 0.5 to 1.5 mcg/kg/minute I.V.

ADVERSE REACTIONS
CV: hypotension, hypertension, bradycardia, tachycardia.
GI: nausea, vomiting.
Skin: itching.
Other: chest wall rigidity, intraoperative muscle movement, *respiratory depression*.

INTERACTIONS
Alcohol, CNS depressants: additive effects. Use together cautiously.

NURSING CONSIDERATIONS
• Use cautiously in patients with pulmonary disease or decreased respiratory reserve.
• Should be administered only by persons specifically trained in the use of intravenous anesthetics.
• As a primary anesthetic, alfentanil may be prescribed for induction of anesthesia for general surgery requiring endotracheal intubation and medical ventilation.
• Discontinue infusion at least 10 to 15 minutes before the end of surgery.
• To administer small volumes of alfentanil accurately, use a tuberculin syringe.
• Keep narcotic antagonist (naloxone) and resuscitative equipment available when giving drug.
• Dose should be reduced in elderly and debilitated patients.
• Monitor vital signs routinely.

---

buprenorphine hydrochloride
Controlled Substance Schedule V
Buprenex
Pregnancy Category: C (D for prolonged use or use of high doses at term)

MECHANISM OF ACTION
Binds with opiate receptors at many sites in the central nervous system (brain, brain stem, and spinal cord), altering both perception of and emotional response to pain through an unknown mechanism.

INDICATIONS & DOSAGE
Moderate to severe pain—
Adults: 0.3 mg I.M. or slow I.V. q 6 hours, p.r.n. or around the clock. May administer up to 0.6 mg per dose if necessary.

ADVERSE REACTIONS
CNS: *dizziness, sedation, headache,* confusion, nervousness, euphoria.
CV: hypotension.
GI: *nausea,* vomiting, constipation.
Skin: pruritus.
Other: *respiratory depression,* hypoventilation.

INTERACTIONS
Alcohol, CNS depressants: additive effects. Use together cautiously.
Narcotic analgesics: avoid concomitant use. Possible decreased analgesic effect.

NURSING CONSIDERATIONS
• Use cautiously in patients with head injury and increased intracranial pressure, severe liver and kidney impairment, CNS depression, thyroid irregularities, and prostatic hypertrophy.
• Naloxone will not completely reverse the respiratory depression provided by buprenorphine. Therefore, an overdose may necessitate mechanical ventilation. Larger than customary doses of naloxone (more than 0.4 mg) and doxapram may also be ordered.
• Psychological and physical addiction may occur.
• If dependence occurs, withdrawal symptoms may appear up to 14 days after drug is stopped.
• Possesses narcotic antagonist properties. May precipitate abstinence syndrome in narcotic-dependent patients.
• Subcutaneous administration not recommended.
• Buprenorphine 0.3 mg is equal to 10 mg morphine and 75 mg meperidine in analgesic potency. Has a longer duration of action than morphine or meperidine.

Italicized side effects are common or life-threatening.
*Liquid form contains alcohol.   **May contain tartrazine.

butorphanol tartrate

Stadol♦
Pregnancy Category: B (D for
prolonged use or use of high doses
at term)

MECHANISM OF ACTION

Binds with opiate receptors at many
sites in the central nervous system
(brain, brain stem, and spinal cord),
altering both perception of and emotional response to pain through an unknown mechanism.

INDICATIONS & DOSAGE

Moderate to severe pain—
Adults: 1 to 4 mg I.M. q 3 to 4 hours,
p.r.n. or around the clock; or 0.5 to 2
mg I.V. q 3 to 4 hours, p.r.n. or
around the clock.

ADVERSE REACTIONS

CNS: *sedation, headache, vertigo,
floating sensation,* lethargy, confusion, nervousness, unusual dreams,
agitation, euphoria, hallucinations,
flushing.
CV: palpitations, fluctuation in blood
pressure.
EENT: diplopia, blurred vision.
GI: *nausea,* vomiting, dry mouth,
constipation.
Skin: rash, hives, *clamminess, excessive sweating.*
Other: *respiratory depression.*

INTERACTIONS

Alcohol, CNS depressants: additive
effects. Use together cautiously.
Narcotic analgesics: avoid concomitant use. Possible decreased analgesic
effect.

NURSING CONSIDERATIONS

• Contraindicated in narcotic addiction; may precipitate narcotic abstinence syndrome. Use cautiously in
head injury, increased intracranial
pressure, acute MI, ventricular dysfunction, coronary insufficiency, respiratory disease or depression, renal
or hepatic dysfunction.
• Psychological and physical addiction may occur.
• Possesses narcotic antagonist properties. May precipitate abstinence
syndrome in narcotic-dependent patients.
• Respiratory depression apparently
does not increase with increased dosage.
• Subcutaneous route not recommended.
• Also approved for use as a preoperative medication, as the analgesic
component of balanced anesthesia,
and for relief of postpartum pain.

codeine phosphate

codeine sulfate

Controlled Substance Schedule II
Pregnancy Category: C (D for
prolonged use or use of high doses
at term)

MECHANISM OF ACTION

Binds with opiate receptors at many
sites in the central nervous system
(brain, brain stem, and spinal cord),
altering both perception of and emo
tional response to pain through an unknown mechanism. Also supresses
the cough reflex by a direct central action in the medulla.

INDICATIONS & DOSAGE

Mild to moderate pain—
Adults: 15 to 60 mg P.O. or 15 to 60
mg (phosphate) S.C. or I.M. q 4
hours, p.r.n. or around the clock.
Children: 3 mg/kg daily divided q 4
hours, p.r.n. or around the clock.
Nonproductive cough—
Adults: 8 to 20 mg P.O. q 4 to 6
hours. Maximum 120 mg/24 hours.
Children: 1 to 1.5 mg/kg P.O. daily
in 4 divided doses. Maximum 60 mg/
24 hours.

ADVERSE REACTIONS
CNS: *sedation, clouded sensorium, euphoria,* convulsions with large doses, dizziness.
CV: *hypotension,* bradycardia.
GI: *nausea, vomiting, constipation, dry mouth,* ileus.
GU: *urinary retention.*
Skin: pruritus, flushing.
Other: *respiratory depression,* physical dependence.

INTERACTIONS
Alcohol, CNS depressants: additive effects. Use together cautiously.

NURSING CONSIDERATIONS
• Use with extreme caution in patients with head injury, increased intracranial pressure, increased cerebrospinal fluid pressure, hepatic or renal disease, hypothyroidism, Addison's disease, acute alcoholism, seizures, severe CNS depression, bronchial asthma, COPD, respiratory depression, shock, and in elderly or debilitated patients.
• Warn ambulatory patient to avoid activities that require alertness.
• Monitor respiratory and circulatory status and bowel function.
• For full analgesic effect, give before patient has intense pain.
• Codeine and aspirin or acetaminophen are often prescribed together to provide enhanced pain relief.
• Do not administer discolored injection solution.
• If used with general anesthetics, other narcotic analgesics, tranquilizers, sedatives, hypnotics, alcohol, tricyclic antidepressants, or MAO inhibitors, CNS depression is increased. Use together with extreme caution. Monitor patient's response.
• An antitussive; don't use when cough is a valuable diagnostic sign or beneficial (as after thoracic surgery).
• Monitor cough type and frequency.
• Constipating effect makes codeine useful in the treatment of diarrhea.

• The abuse potential is much less than that of morphine.

fentanyl citrate
Controlled Substance Schedule II
Sublimaze♦
Pregnancy Category: B (D for prolonged use or use of high doses at term)

MECHANISM OF ACTION
Binds with opiate receptors at many sites in the central nervous system (brain, brain stem, and spinal cord), altering both perception of and emotional response to pain through an unknown mechanism.

INDICATIONS & DOSAGE
Adjunct to general anesthetic—
Adults: 0.05 to 0.1 mg I.V. repeated q 2 to 3 minutes, p.r.n. Dose should be reduced in elderly and poor-risk patients.
Postoperatively—
Adults: 0.05 to 0.1 mg I.M. q 1 to 2 hours, p.r.n.
Children 2 to 12 years: 0.02 to 0.03 mg per 9 kg.
Preoperatively—
Adults: 0.05 to 0.1 mg I.M. 30 to 60 minutes before surgery.

ADVERSE REACTIONS
CNS: *sedation, somnolence, clouded sensorium, euphoria,* convulsions with large doses.
CV: *hypotension,* bradycardia.
GI: nausea, vomiting, *constipation,* ileus.
GU: *urinary retention.*
Other: *respiratory depression,* muscle rigidity, physical dependence.

INTERACTIONS
Alcohol, CNS depressants: additive effects. Use together cautiously.

NURSING CONSIDERATIONS
• Contraindicated in patients who

Italicized side effects are common or life-threatening.
*Liquid form contains alcohol.   **May contain tartrazine.

have received MAO inhibitors within 14 days and who have myasthenia gravis. Use cautiously in patients with head injury, increased cerebrospinal fluid pressure, asthma, COPD, respiratory depression, seizures, hepatic or renal disease, hypothyroidism, Addison's disease, alcoholism, increased intracranial pressure, CNS depression, shock, and in elderly or debilitated patients.
• Keep narcotic antagonist (naloxone) and resuscitative equipment available when giving drug I.V.
• Monitor respirations of newborns exposed to drug during labor.
• Use as postoperative analgesic only in recovery room. Make sure another analgesic is ordered for later use.
• Often used with droperidol (Innovar) to produce neuroleptanalgesia.
• Monitor circulatory and respiratory status carefully.
• Respiratory depression, hypotension, profound sedation, and coma may result if used with other narcotic analgesics, general anesthetics, tranquilizers, alcohol, sedatives, hypnotics, tricyclic antidepressants, or MAO inhibitors. Fentanyl citrate dose should be reduced by ¼ to ⅓. Also give above drugs in reduced dosages.
• For better analgesic effect, give before patient has intense pain.
• When used postoperatively, encourage turning, coughing, and deep breathing to avoid atelectasis.
• Epidural injection or infusion has been used for postoperative analgesia, chronic pain management, or postpartum pain control.
• When administered by epidural injection, monitor the patient closely for respiratory depression. Immediately report a respiratory rate below 12.
• High doses can produce muscle rigidity. This effect can be reversed by administration of neuromuscular blocking agents.

hydromorphone hydrochloride
Controlled Substance Schedule II
Dilaudid♦**, Dilaudid HP, Dilaudid Cough Syrup*
Pregnancy Category: B (D for prolonged use or use of high doses at term)

MECHANISM OF ACTION
Binds with opiate receptors at many sites in the central nervous system (brain, brain stem, and spinal cord), altering both perception of and emotional response to pain through an unknown mechanism. Also suppresses the cough reflex by direct action on the cough center in the medulla.

INDICATIONS & DOSAGE
Moderate to severe pain—
Adults: 1 to 6 mg P.O. q 4 to 6 hours, p.r.n. or around the clock; or 2 to 4 mg I.M., S.C., or I.V. q 4 to 6 hours, p.r.n. or around the clock (I.V. dose should be given over 3 to 5 minutes); or 3 mg rectal suppository at bedtime, p.r.n. or around the clock.
Cough—
Adults: 1 mg P.O. q 3 to 4 hours, p.r.n.
Children 6 to 12 years: 0.5 mg P.O. q 3 to 4 hours, p.r.n.

ADVERSE REACTIONS
CNS: *sedation, somnolence, clouded sensorium, euphoria,* convulsions with large doses.
CV: *hypotension,* bradycardia.
GI: *nausea, vomiting, constipation,* ileus.
GU: *urinary retention.*
Local: induration with repeated S.C. injection.
Other: *respiratory depression,* physical dependence.

INTERACTIONS
Alcohol, CNS depressants: additive effects. Use together cautiously.

NURSING CONSIDERATIONS

• Contraindicated in increased intracranial pressure and status asthmaticus. Use with extreme caution in patients with increased cerebrospinal fluid pressure, respiratory depression, hepatic or renal disease, hypothyroidism, shock, Addison's disease, acute alcoholism, seizures, head injury, severe CNS depression, brain tumor, bronchial asthma, COPD, and in elderly or debilitated patients.

• Warn ambulatory patient to avoid activities that require alertness.

• Monitor respiratory and circulatory status and bowel function.

• Keep narcotic antagonist (naloxone) available.

• Respiratory depression and hypotension can occur with I.V. administration. Give very slowly and monitor constantly.

• Rotate injection sites to avoid induration with subcutaneous injection.

• Commonly abused narcotic.

• If used with general anesthetics, other narcotic analgesics, tranquilizers, sedatives, hypnotics, alcohol, tricyclic antidepressants, or MAO inhibitors, CNS depression is increased. Hydromorphone dose should be reduced. Use together with extreme caution. Monitor patient's response.

• Oral dosage form is particularly convenient for patients with chronic pain because tablets are available in 1 mg, 2 mg, 3 mg, and 4 mg. This enables these patients to titrate their own dose.

• For better analgesic effect, give before patient has intense pain.

• When used postoperatively, encourage turning, coughing, and deep breathing to avoid atelectasis.

• May worsen or mask gallbladder pain.

• Dilaudid HP, a highly concentrated form (10 mg/ml), may be administered in smaller volumes, preventing the discomfort associated with large-volume I.M. or S.C. injections.

levorphanol tartrate
Controlled Substance Schedule II
Levo-Dromoran♦
Pregnancy Category: B (D for prolonged use or use of high doses at term)

MECHANISM OF ACTION
Binds with opiate receptors at many sites in the central nervous system (brain, brain stem, and spinal cord), altering both perception of and emotional response to pain through an unknown mechanism.

INDICATIONS & DOSAGE
Moderate to severe pain—
Adults: 2 to 3 mg P.O. or S.C. q 6 to 8 hours, p.r.n. or around the clock.

ADVERSE REACTIONS
CNS: *sedation, somnolence, clouded sensorium, euphoria,* convulsions with large doses.
CV: *hypotension,* bradycardia.
GI: *nausea, vomiting, constipation,* ileus.
GU: *urinary retention.*
Other: *respiratory depression,* physical dependence.

INTERACTIONS
Alcohol, CNS depressants: additive effects. Use together cautiously.

NURSING CONSIDERATIONS
• Contraindicated in patients with acute alcoholism, bronchial asthma, increased intracranial pressure, respiratory depression, and anoxia. Use with extreme caution in patients with hepatic or renal disease, hypothyroidism, Addison's disease, seizures, head injury, severe CNS depression, brain tumor, COPD, shock, and in elderly or debilitated patients.

• Warn ambulatory patient to avoid activities that require alertness.

• Monitor circulatory and respiratory status and bowel function.

Italicized side effects are common or life-threatening.
*Liquid form contains alcohol.   **May contain tartrazine.

- Warn patient drug has bitter taste.
- Protect from light.
- Keep narcotic antagonist (naloxone) available.
- If used with general anesthetics, other narcotic analgesics, tranquilizers, sedatives, hypnotics, alcohol, tricyclic antidepressants, or MAO inhibitors, CNS depression is increased. Reduce levorphanol dose. Use together with extreme caution. Monitor patient's response.
- For better analgesic effect, give before patient has intense pain.
- When used postoperatively, encourage turning, coughing, and deep breathing to avoid atelectasis.

meperidine hydrochloride
Controlled Substance Schedule II
Demer-Idine♦♦, Demerol♦
Pregnancy Category: B (D for prolonged use or use of high doses at term)

MECHANISM OF ACTION
Binds with opiate receptors at many sites in the central nervous system (brain, brain stem, and spinal cord), altering both perception of and emotional response to pain through an unknown mechanism.

INDICATIONS & DOSAGE
Moderate to severe pain—
Adults: 50 to 150 mg P.O., I.M., or S.C. q 3 to 4 hours, p.r.n. or around the clock.
Children: 1 mg/kg P.O., I.M., or S.C. q 4 to 6 hours. Maximum—100 mg q 4 hours, p.r.n. or around the clock.
Preoperatively—
Adults: 50 to 100 mg I.M. or S.C. 30 to 90 minutes before surgery.
Children: 1 to 2.2 mg/kg I.M. or S.C. 30 to 90 minutes before surgery.

ADVERSE REACTIONS
CNS: *sedation, somnolence, clouded*
sensorium, euphoria, paradoxical excitement, tremors, convulsions with large doses.
CV: *hypotension,* bradycardia, tachycardia.
GI: *nausea, vomiting, constipation,* ileus.
GU: *urinary retention.*
Local: pain at injection site, local tissue irritation and induration after S.C. injection; phlebitis after I.V. injection.
Other: *respiratory depression,* physical dependence, muscle twitching.

INTERACTIONS
MAO inhibitors, barbiturates, isoniazid: increased CNS excitation or depression can be severe or fatal. Don't use together.
Alcohol, CNS depressants: additive effects. Use together cautiously.
Phenytoin: decreased blood levels of meperidine. Monitor for decreased analgesia.

NURSING CONSIDERATIONS
- Contraindicated if patient has used MAO inhibitors within 14 days. Use with extreme caution in patients with increased intracranial pressure, increased cerebrospinal fluid pressure, shock, CNS depression, head injury, asthma, COPD, respiratory depression, supraventricular tachycardias, seizures, acute abdominal conditions, hepatic or renal disease, hypothyroidism, Addison's disease, urethral stricture, prostatic hypertrophy, alcoholism, in children under 12 years, and in elderly or debilitated patients.
- May be used in some patients allergic to morphine.
- Meperidine and active metabolite normeperidine accumulate. Monitor for increased toxic effect, especially in patients with poor renal function.
- Because meperidine toxicity often appears after several days of treatment, this drug is not recommended for treatment of chronic pain.

• Meperidine may be given slow I.V., preferably as a diluted solution. S.C. injection very painful.

• Keep narcotic antagonist (naloxone) available when giving this drug I.V.

• Warn ambulatory patient to avoid activities that require alertness.

• Monitor respirations of newborns exposed to drug during labor. Have resuscitation equipment available.

• P.O. dose less than half as effective as parenteral dose. Give I.M. if possible. When changing from parenteral to P.O. route, dose should be increased.

• Syrup has local anesthetic effect. Give with full glass of water.

• Chemically incompatible with barbiturates. Don't mix together.

• Monitor respiratory and cardiovascular status carefully. Don't give if respirations are below 12/minute or if change in pupils is noted.

• Watch for withdrawal symptoms if stopped abruptly after long-term use.

• If used with other narcotic analgesics, general anesthetics, phenothiazines, sedatives, hypnotics, tricyclic antidepressants, or alcohol, respiratory depression, hypotension, profound sedation, or coma may occur. Reduce meperidine dose. Use together with extreme caution.

• For better analgesic effect, give before patient has intense pain. Initially, administration on a fixed schedule may result in better pain control with a smaller daily dose by reducing patient anxiety. Once good pain control has been achieved, adjust scheduling per individual requirements.

• Alternating centrally active narcotic with a more peripherally active nonnarcotic analgesic (ASA, acetaminophen, NSAIDs) may improve pain control while requiring lower narcotic doses.

• When used postoperatively, encourage turning, coughing, and deep breathing to avoid atelectasis.

methadone hydrochloride
Controlled Substance Schedule II
Dolophine, Methadone HCl Oral Solution
Pregnancy Category: B (D for prolonged use or use of high doses at term)

MECHANISM OF ACTION
Binds with opiate receptors at many sites in the central nervous system (brain, brain stem, and spinal cord), altering both perception of and emotional response to pain through an unknown mechanism.

INDICATIONS & DOSAGE
Severe pain—
Adults: 2.5 to 10 mg P.O., I.M., or S.C. q 4 to 12 hours, p.r.n. or around the clock.
Narcotic abstinence syndrome—
Adults: 15 to 40 mg P.O. daily (highly individualized).
Maintenance: 20 to 120 mg P.O. daily. Adjust dose as needed. Daily doses greater than 120 mg require special state and federal approval.

ADVERSE REACTIONS
CNS: *sedation, somnolence, clouded sensorium, euphoria,* convulsions with large doses.
CV: *hypotension,* bradycardia.
GI: *nausea, vomiting, constipation,* ileus.
GU: *urinary retention.*
Local: pain at injection site, tissue irritation, induration following S.C. injection.
Other: *respiratory depression,* physical dependence.

INTERACTIONS
Rifampin: withdrawal symptoms; reduced blood levels of methadone. Use together cautiously.
Ammonium chloride and other urine acidifiers, phenytoin: may reduce methadone effect. Monitor for de-

creased pain control.

Alcohol, CNS depressants: additive effects. Use together cautiously.

NURSING CONSIDERATIONS
• Give with extreme caution in elderly or debilitated patients, or in patients with acute abdominal conditions, severe hepatic or renal impairment, hypothyroidism, Addison's disease, prostatic hypertrophy, urethral stricture, head injury, increased intracranial pressure, asthma, COPD, respiratory depression, CNS depression.
• Safe use in adolescent addicts as maintenance drug not established.
• One daily dose adequate for maintenance. No advantage to divided doses.
• Oral liquid form legally required in maintenance programs.
• Oral dose is half as potent as injected dose.
• Rotate injection sites.
• Has cumulative effect; marked sedation can occur after repeated doses.
• Monitor circulatory and respiratory status and bowel function.
• Warn ambulatory patient to avoid activities that require alertness.
• Regimented scheduling (around the clock) beneficial in severe, chronic pain. When used for severe, chronic pain, tolerance may develop with long-term use, requiring a higher dose to achieve the same degree of analgesia. This is *not* a sign of addiction.
• Give methadone maintenance doses as oral liquid. Completely dissolve tablets in 120 ml of orange juice or powdered citrus drink.
• Constipation often severe with maintenance. Make sure stool softener or other laxative is ordered.
• Patient treated for narcotic abstinence syndrome will usually require an additional analgesic if pain control is necessary.
• If used with general anesthetics, tranquilizers, sedatives, hypnotics, alcohol, tricyclic antidepressants or MAO inhibitors, respiratory depression, hypotension, profound sedation, or coma may occur. Use together with extreme caution. Monitor patient's response.
• Liquid form available for patients who are unable to swallow tablets.

morphine sulfate
Controlled Substance Schedule II
Duramorph PF, Epimorph, MS Contin, RMS, Roxanol, Roxanol SR
Pregnancy Category: B (D for prolonged use or use of high doses at term)

MECHANISM OF ACTION
Binds with opiate receptors at many sites in the central nervous system (brain, brain stem, and spinal cord), altering both perception of and emotional response to pain through an unknown mechanism.

INDICATIONS & DOSAGE
Severe pain—
Adults: 4 to 15 mg S.C. or I.M., or 30 to 60 mg P.O. or by rectum q 4 hours, p.r.n. or around the clock. May be injected slow I.V. (over 4 to 5 minutes) diluted in 4 to 5 ml water for injection. May also administer controlled-release tablets q 8 to 12 hours. As an epidural injection, 5 mg via an epidural catheter every 24 hours.
Children: 0.1 to 0.2 mg/kg dose S.C. Maximum 15 mg.
In some situations, morphine may be administered by continuous I.V. infusion or by intraspinal and intrathecal injection.

ADVERSE REACTIONS
CNS: *sedation, somnolence, clouded sensorium, euphoria,* convulsions with large doses, *nightmares* (with long-acting forms).
CV: *hypotension,* bradycardia.
GI: *nausea, vomiting, constipation,*

ileus.
GU: *urinary retention.*
Other: *respiratory depression, physical dependence, pruritus and skin flushing* (with epidural administration).

INTERACTIONS
Alcohol, CNS depressants: additional effects. Use together cautiously.

NURSING CONSIDERATIONS
• Use with extreme caution in patients with head injury, increased intracranial pressure, seizures, asthma, COPD, alcoholism, prostatic hypertrophy, severe hepatic or renal disease, acute abdominal conditions, hypothyroidism, Addison's disease, increased cerebrospinal fluid pressure, urethral stricture, cardiac arrhythmias, reduced blood volume, toxic psychosis, and in elderly or debilitated patients.
• Warn ambulatory patient to avoid activities that require alertness.
• Monitor circulatory and respiratory status and bowel function. Don't give if respirations are below 12/minute.
• Drug of choice in relieving pain of myocardial infarction. May cause transient decrease in blood pressure.
• Keep narcotic antagonist (naloxone) and resuscitative equipment available.
• Constipation often severe with maintenance. Make sure stool softener or other laxative is ordered.
• Respiratory depression, hypotension, profound sedation, or coma may occur if used with general anesthetics, tranquilizers, sedatives, hypnotics, alcohol, tricyclic antidepressants, or MAO inhibitors. Reduce morphine dose. Use together with extreme caution. Monitor patient's response.
• Regimented scheduling (around the clock) beneficial in severe, chronic pain.
• When used postoperatively, encourage turning, coughing, and deep

breathing to avoid atelectasis.
• Oral solutions of various concentrations are available, as well as a new intensified oral solution (20 mg/ml). Be sure to note the strength you are administering.
• Sublingual administration may be ordered. Measure out oral solution with tuberculin syringe. Administer dose a few drops at a time to allow maximal sublingual absorption and to minimize swallowing.
• Rectal suppository available in 5-, 10-, and 20-mg dosages. Refrigeration is not necessary. Note that in some patients, rectal and oral absorption may not be equivalent.
• Preservative-free preparations now available for epidural and intrathecal administration. The popularity of the epidural route is constantly increasing.
• When given epidurally, monitor closely for respiratory depression up to 24 hours after the injection. Check respiratory rate and depth every 30 to 60 minutes for 24 hours.
• May worsen or mask gallbladder pain.

nalbuphine hydrochloride
Nubain♦
Pregnancy Category: B (D for prolonged use or use of high doses at term)

MECHANISM OF ACTION
Binds with opiate receptors at many sites in the central nervous system (brain, brain stem, and spinal cord), altering both perception of and emotional response to pain through an unknown mechanism.

INDICATIONS & DOSAGE
Moderate to severe pain—
Adults: 10 to 20 mg S.C., I.M., or I.V. q 3 to 6 hours, p.r.n. or around the clock. Maximum daily dose 160 mg.

Italicized side effects are common or life-threatening.
*Liquid form contains alcohol.   **May contain tartrazine.

ADVERSE REACTIONS
CNS: *sedation,* nervousness, depression, restlessness, crying, euphoria, hostility, unusual dreams, confusion, hallucinations, delusions.
GI: cramps, dyspepsia, bitter taste, *nausea, vomiting,* constipation.
GU: urinary urgency.
Skin: itching, burning, urticaria.
Other: *respiratory depression.*

INTERACTIONS
Alcohol, CNS depressants: additive effects. Use together cautiously.
Narcotic analgesics: avoid concomitant use. Possible decreased analgesic effect.

NURSING CONSIDERATIONS
• Contraindicated in emotional instability, drug abuse, head injury, increased intracranial pressure. Use cautiously in patients with hepatic and renal disease. These patients may overreact to customary doses.
• Causes respiratory depression, which at 10 mg is equal to the respiratory depression produced by 10 mg of morphine.
• Psychological and physiologic dependence may occur.
• Respiratory depression can be reversed with naloxone.
• Also acts as a narcotic antagonist; may precipitate abstinence syndrome in narcotic-dependent patients.
• Warn patient to avoid activities that require alertness until CNS response to drug is determined.

oxycodone hydrochloride
Controlled Substance Schedule II
Oxycodone Oral Solution,
Supeudol♦♦
Combinations:
The following contain acetaminophen: Percocet♦, Percocet-Demi♦, Tylox
The following contain aspirin: Codoxy, Percodan♦, Percodan-Demi♦
Pregnancy Category: B (D for prolonged use or use of high doses at term)

MECHANISM OF ACTION
Binds with opiate receptors at many sites in the central nervous system (brain, brain stem, and spinal cord), altering both perception of and emotional response to pain through an unknown mechanism.

INDICATIONS & DOSAGE
Moderate to severe pain—
Adults: available in combination with other drugs, such as aspirin (Codoxy, Percodan, Percodan-Demi), or acetaminophen (Percocet, Tylox). One to 2 tablets P.O. q 6 hours, p.r.n. or around the clock. Or 5 mg (5 ml) of Oxycodone oral solution or tablets P.O. q 6 hours.
Adults: (Supeudol) 1 to 3 suppositories rectally daily, p.r.n. or around the clock.
Children: (Percodan-Demi) ¼ to ½ tablet P.O. q 6 hours, p.r.n. or around the clock.

ADVERSE REACTIONS
CNS: *sedation, somnolence, clouded sensorium, euphoria,* convulsions with large doses.
CV: *hypotension,* bradycardia.
GI: *nausea, vomiting, constipation,* ileus.
GU: *urinary retention.*
Other: *respiratory depression,* physical dependence.

INTERACTIONS

Anticoagulants: oxycodone hydrochloride products containing aspirin may increase anticoagulant effect. Monitor clotting times. Use together cautiously.

Alcohol, CNS depressants: additive effects. Use together cautiously.

NURSING CONSIDERATIONS

• Use with extreme caution in patients with head injury, increased intracranial pressure, increased cerebrospinal fluid pressure, seizures, asthma, COPD, alcoholism, prostatic hypertrophy, severe hepatic or renal disease, acute abdominal conditions, urethral stricture, hypothyroidism, Addison's disease, cardiac arrhythmias, reduced blood volume, toxic psychosis, and in elderly or debilitated patients.

• Don't give to children, except for Percodan-Demi and Percocet-Demi.

• Warn ambulatory patient to avoid activities that require alertness.

• Monitor circulatory and respiratory status and bowel function. Do not give if respirations are below 12/minute.

• For full analgesic effect, give before patient has intense pain.

• Give after meals or with milk.

• If used with general anesthetics, other narcotic analgesics, tranquilizers, sedatives, hypnotics, alcohol, tricyclic antidepressants, or MAO inhibitors, CNS depression is increased. Reduce oxycodone dose. Use together with extreme caution. Monitor patient's response.

• Single-agent oxycodone solution or tablets are especially good for patients who shouldn't take aspirin or acetaminophen.

• Has high abuse potential.

oxymorphone hydrochloride

Controlled Substance Schedule II
Numorphan♦
Pregnancy Category: B (D for prolonged use or use of high doses at term)

MECHANISM OF ACTION

Binds with opiate receptors at many sites in the central nervous system (brain, brain stem, and spinal cord), altering both perception of and emotional response to pain through an unknown mechanism.

INDICATIONS & DOSAGE

Moderate to severe pain—
Adults: 1 to 1.5 mg I.M. or S.C. q 4 to 6 hours, p.r.n. or around the clock, or 0.5 mg I.V. q 4 to 6 hours, p.r.n. or around the clock, or 2.5 to 5 mg rectally q 4 to 6 hours, p.r.n. or around the clock.

ADVERSE REACTIONS

CNS: *sedation, somnolence, clouded sensorium, euphoria,* convulsions with large doses.
CV: *hypotension,* bradycardia.
GI: *nausea, vomiting, constipation,* ileus.
GU: *urinary retention.*
Other: *respiratory depression,* physical dependence.

INTERACTIONS

Alcohol, CNS depressants: additive effects. Use together cautiously.

NURSING CONSIDERATIONS

• Use with extreme caution in patients with head injury, increased intracranial pressure, seizures, asthma, COPD, alcoholism, increased cerebrospinal fluid pressure, acute abdominal conditions, prostatic hypertrophy, severe hepatic or renal disease, urethral stricture, CNS depression, respiratory depression, hypothy-

---

Italicized side effects are common or life-threatening.
*Liquid form contains alcohol.   **May contain tartrazine.

roidism, Addison's disease, cardiac arrhythmias, reduced blood volume, toxic psychosis, and in elderly or debilitated patients.
• Warn ambulatory patient to avoid activities that require alertness.
• Monitor cardiovascular and respiratory status. Don't give if respirations are below 12/minute.
• Well absorbed rectally. Alternative to narcotics with more limited dosage forms.
• Keep narcotic antagonist (naloxone) and resuscitative equipment available.
• If used with general anesthetics, tranquilizers, sedatives, hypnotics, alcohol, tricyclic antidepressants, or MAO inhibitors, CNS depression is increased. Reduce oxymorphone dose. Use together with extreme caution. Monitor patient's response.
• For better analgesic effect, give before patient has intense pain.
• When used postoperatively, encourage turning, coughing, and deep breathing to avoid atelectasis.
• Not intended for mild to moderate pain. May worsen gallbladder pain.

pentazocine hydrochloride

pentazocine lactate
Controlled Substance Schedule IV
Talwin♦, Talwin-Nx
Pregnancy Category: B (D for prolonged use or use of high doses at term)

MECHANISM OF ACTION
Binds with opiate receptors at many sites in the central nervous system (brain, brain stem, and spinal cord), altering both perception of and emotional response to pain through an unknown mechanism.

INDICATIONS & DOSAGE
Moderate to severe pain—
Adults: 50 to 100 mg P.O. q 3 to 4

hours, p.r.n. or around the clock. Maximum 600 mg daily or 30 mg I.M., I.V., or S.C. q 3 to 4 hours, p.r.n. or around the clock. Maximum 360 mg daily. Doses above 30 mg I.V. or 60 mg I.M. or S.C. not recommended.

ADVERSE REACTIONS
CNS: *sedation,* visual disturbances, *hallucinations,* drowsiness, dizziness, light-headedness, confusion, euphoria, headache, *psychotomimetic effects.*
GI: nausea, vomiting, dry mouth.
GU: urinary retention.
Local: induration, nodules, sloughing, and sclerosis of injection site.
Other: *respiratory depression,* physical and psychological dependence.

INTERACTIONS
Alcohol, CNS depressants: additive effects. Use together cautiously.
Narcotic analgesics: avoid concomitant use. Possible decreased analgesic effect.

NURSING CONSIDERATIONS
• Contraindicated in emotional instability, drug abuse, head injury, increased intracranial pressure. Use cautiously in hepatic or renal disease.
• Tablets not well absorbed.
• Possesses narcotic antagonist properties. May precipitate abstinence syndrome in narcotic-dependent patients.
• Psychological and physiologic dependence may occur.
• Respiratory depression can be reversed with naloxone.
• Do not mix in same syringe with soluble barbiturates.
• Warn ambulatory patient to avoid activities that require alertness.
• Talwin-Nx, the available oral pentazocine, contains the narcotic antagonist naloxone. This prevents illicit intravenous use.

propoxyphene hydrochloride

Controlled Substance Schedule IV
Darvon♦, Dolene, Doraphen,
Myospaz, Pargesic 65, Pro-Pox 65,
Proxagesic, Ropoxy, Scrip-Dyne,
SK-65, S-Pain-65, 642♦♦

propoxyphene napsylate

Controlled Substance Schedule IV
Darvocet-N, Darvon-N♦
Pregnancy Category: C (D for
prolonged use)

MECHANISM OF ACTION

Binds with opiate receptors at many
sites in the central nervous system
(brain, brain stem, and spinal cord),
altering both perception of and emotional response to pain through an unknown mechanism.

INDICATIONS & DOSAGE

Mild to moderate pain—
Adults: 65 mg (hydrochloride) P.O. q
4 hours, p.r.n.
Mild to moderate pain—
Adults: 100 mg (napsylate) P.O. q 4
hours, p.r.n.

ADVERSE REACTIONS

CNS: *dizziness,* headache, sedation,
euphoria, paradoxical excitement, insomnia.
GI: nausea, vomiting, constipation.
Other: psychological and physical dependence.

INTERACTIONS

Alcohol, CNS depressants: additive
effects. Use together cautiously.

NURSING CONSIDERATIONS

• Not to be prescribed for maintenance purposes in narcotic addiction.
• Warn ambulatory patient to avoid
activities that require alertness until
CNS response to drug has been established.
• Warn patient not to exceed recom-

mended dosage.
• Do not use caffeine or amphetamines to treat overdose: may cause
fatal convulsions. Use narcotic antagonist instead.
• May cause false decreases in urinary steroid excretion tests.
• 65 mg propoxyphene HCl equals
100 mg propoxyphene napsylate.
• Can be considered a mild narcotic
analgesic, but pain relief is equivalent
to aspirin.
• Advise patients to limit their alcohol intake when taking this drug.

sufentanil citrate

Controlled Substance Schedule II
Sufenta
Pregnancy Category:
C (D for prolonged use or use of
high doses at term)

MECHANISM OF ACTION

Binds with opiate receptors at many
sites in the central nervous system
(brain, brain stem, and spinal cord),
altering both perception of and emotional response to pain through an unknown mechanism.

INDICATIONS & DOSAGE

Adjunct to general anesthetic—
Adults: 1 to 8 mcg/kg I.V. administered with nitrous oxide/oxygen.
As a primary anesthetic—
Adults: 8 to 30 mcg/kg I.V. administered with 100% oxygen and a muscle
relaxant.

ADVERSE REACTIONS

CNS: chills.
CV: *hypotension,* hypertension, bra-
dycardia, tachycardia.
GI: nausea, vomiting.
Skin: itching.
Other: *chest wall rigidity,* intraopera-
tive muscle movement, *respiratory
depression.*

INTERACTIONS
Alcohol, CNS depressants: additive effects. Use together cautiously.

NURSING CONSIDERATIONS
• Use cautiously in patients with pulmonary disease or decreased respiratory reserve.
• Should only be administered by persons specifically trained in the use of intravenous anesthetics.
• When used at doses of greater than 8 mcg/kg, postoperative mechanical ventilation and observation are essential because of extended postoperative respiratory depression.
• Keep narcotic antagonist (naloxone) and resuscitative equipment available when giving drug.
• Dose should be reduced in elderly and debilitated patients.
• Monitor vital signs routinely.
• Compared to fentanyl, sufentanil has a more rapid onset and shorter duration of action.
• High doses can produce muscle rigidity. This effect can be reversed by administration of neuromuscular blocking agents.

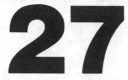

Narcotic antagonists

naloxone hydrochloride
naltrexone hydrochloride

COMBINATION PRODUCTS
None.

---

naloxone hydrochloride
Narcan♦
Pregnancy Category: B

MECHANISM OF ACTION
Displaces previously administered
narcotic analgesics from their receptors (competitive antagonism). Has
no pharmacologic activity of its own.

INDICATIONS & DOSAGE
*Known or suspected narcotic-induced
respiratory depression, including that
due to pentazocine and propoxyphene—*
Adults: 0.4 to 2 mg I.V., S.C., or
I.M. May repeat q 2 to 3 minutes,
p.r.n. If no response is observed after
10 mg has been administered, the diagnosis of narcotic-induced toxicity
should be questioned.
Postoperative narcotic depression—
Adults: 0.1 to 0.2 mg I.V. q 2 to 3
minutes, p.r.n. Adult concentration is
0.4 mg/ml.
Children: 0.01 mg/kg dose I.M.,
I.V., or S.C. May repeat q 2 to 3 minutes.
Note: If initial dose 0.01 mg/kg does
not result in clinical improvement, up
to 10 times this dose (0.1 mg/kg) may
be needed to be effective.
Neonates (asphyxia neonatorum):
0.01 mg/kg I.V. into umbilical vein.

May repeat q 2 to 3 minutes for 3
doses. Neonatal concentration (for
children also) is 0.02 mg/ml.

ADVERSE REACTIONS
With higher-than-recommended doses:
nausea, vomiting.
In narcotic-dependent patients: withdrawal symptoms.

INTERACTIONS
None significant.

NURSING CONSIDERATIONS
• Use cautiously in patients with cardiac irritability and narcotic addiction.
• Safest drug to use when cause of respiratory depression is uncertain.
• Monitor respiratory depth and rate.
Be prepared to provide oxygen, ventilation, and other resuscitative measures.
• Respiratory rate increases within 1
to 2 minutes. Effect lasts 1 to 4 hours.
• Duration of narcotic may exceed
that of the naloxone. Patient may relapse into respiratory depression.
• May be administered by continuous
I.V. infusion, which is often necessary
to control the adverse effects of epidurally administered morphine.
• Can see "overshoot" effect—respiratory rate exceeds the rate before respiratory depression.
• Although generally believed to be
ineffective in respiratory depression
caused by nonnarcotics, recent reports indicate that it may reverse
coma induced by alcohol intoxication.
• Does *not* reverse respiratory de-

Italicized side effects are common or life-threatening.
*Liquid form contains alcohol.   **May contain tartrazine.

pression secondary to diazepam.
• May dilute adult concentration (0.4 mg) by mixing 0.5 ml with 9.5 ml sterile water or saline solution for injection to make neonatal concentration (0.02 mg/ml).
• Now available in 1-ml prefilled disposable syringes, 1-ml ampules, and 10-ml vials.
• Naloxone has been successfully used investigationally to treat the senile dementia of Alzheimer's disease. Also has been shown to improve circulation in refractory shock. Used by some researchers to relieve certain cases of chronic constipation.

naltrexone hydrochloride
Trexan
Pregnancy Category: C

MECHANISM OF ACTION
Reversibly blocks the subjective effects of intravenously administered opioids by occupying opiate receptors in the brain.

INDICATIONS & DOSAGE
As an adjunct for maintenance of an opioid free state in detoxified individuals—
Adults: initially, 25 mg P.O. If no withdrawal signs occur within 1 hour, administer an additional 25 mg. Once patient has been started on 50 mg q 24 hours, flexible maintenance schedule may be used. From 50 to 150 mg may be given daily, depending on the schedule prescribed.

ADVERSE REACTIONS
CNS: *insomnia, anxiety,* nervousness, headache, depression.
GI: *nausea, vomiting,* anorexia, *abdominal pain.*
Hepatic: hepatotoxicity.
Other: *muscle and joint pain.*

INTERACTIONS
None significant.

NURSING CONSIDERATIONS
• Contraindicated in patients receiving opioid analgesics, opioid-dependent patients, patients in acute opioid withdrawal, and in anyone with positive urine screen for opioids or acute hepatitis or liver failure.
• Treatment shouldn't begin until patient receives Narcan challenge. If signs of opioid withdrawal persist after Narcan challenge, don't administer naltrexone.
• Use cautiously in patients with mild liver disease or history of recent liver disease.
• Patients must be completely free of opioids before taking naltrexone, or they may experience severe withdrawal symptoms. Those who have been addicted to short-acting opioids (such as heroin and meperidine) must wait at least 7 days after the last opioid dose before starting naltrexone. Those who have been addicted to longer-acting opioids (such as methadone) should wait at least 10 days.
• In an emergency that requires opioid analgesia, a patient receiving naltrexone can be given an opioid analgesic. However, the dose must be higher than usual to surmount naltrexone's effect. Monitor for respiratory depression from the opioid, which may be longer and deeper.
• Naltrexone should be used only as part of a comprehensive rehabilitation program.
• A suggested flexible maintenance dosage regimen: 100 mg on Monday and Wednesday; 150 mg on Friday. This schedule would be preferred for those who are deemed to be poor medication compliers.
• Advise the patient to carry a medical identification card. Warn him to tell medical personnel that he is taking naltrexone, if he needs medical treatment.
• Give patient the names of nonopioid drugs that he can continue to take for pain, diarrhea, or cough.

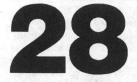

Sedative-Hypnotics

amobarbital
amobarbital sodium
butabarbital
butabarbital sodium
chloral hydrate
ethchlorvynol
flurazepam hydrochloride
glutethimide
methotrimeprazine
  hydrochloride
methyprylon
midazolam hydrochloride
paraldehyde
  (See Chapter 29, ANTICONVULSANTS.)
pentobarbital
pentobarbital sodium
phenobarbital sodium
  (See Chapter 29, ANTICONVULSANTS.)
quazepam
secobarbital
secobarbital sodium
temazepam
triazolam

COMBINATION PRODUCTS
Barbiturates
TRI-BARBS CAPSULE: phenobarbital
32 mg, butabarbital sodium 32 mg,
and secobarbital sodium 32 mg.
TUINAL 50 MG PULVULES: amobarbital sodium 25 mg and secobarbital sodium 25 mg.
TUINAL 100 MG PULVULES♦: amobarbital sodium 50 mg and secobarbital
sodium 50 mg.
TUINAL 200 MG PULVULES♦: amobarbital sodium 100 mg and secobarbital
sodium 100 mg.

amobarbital
Amytal♦

amobarbital sodium
Controlled Substance Schedule II
Amytal Sodium♦
Pregnancy Category: B (according
to manufacturer)

MECHANISM OF ACTION
Probably interferes with transmission
of impulses from the thalamus to the
cortex of the brain. A barbiturate.

INDICATIONS & DOSAGE
Sedation—
Adults: usually 30 to 50 mg P.O.
b.i.d. or t.i.d. but may range from 15
to 120 mg b.i.d. to q.i.d.
Children: 3 to 6 mg/kg daily P.O. di-
vided into 4 equal doses.
Insomnia—
Adults: 65 to 200 mg P.O. or deep
I.M. at bedtime; I.M. injection not to
exceed 5 ml in any one site. Maxi-
mum dose 500 mg.
Children: 3 to 5 mg/kg deep I.M. at
bedtime; I.M. injection not to exceed
5 ml in any one site.
Preanesthetic sedation—
Adults and children: 200 mg P.O. or
I.M. 1 to 2 hours before surgery.
*Manic reactions, as an adjunct in psy-
chotherapy, anticonvulsant—*
Adults and children over 6 years: 65
to 500 mg slow I.V.; rate not to exceed
100 mg/minute. Maximum dose 1 g.
Children under 6 years: 3 to 5 mg/
kg slow I.V. or I.M.

ADVERSE REACTIONS

CNS: *drowsiness, lethargy, hangover,* paradoxical excitement in elderly patients.
GI: nausea, vomiting.
Skin: rash, urticaria.
Local: pain, irritation, sterile abscess at injection site.
Other: *Stevens-Johnson syndrome,* angioedema, exacerbation of porphyria.

INTERACTIONS

Alcohol or other CNS depressants, including other narcotic analgesics: excessive CNS and respiratory depression. Use together cautiously.
MAO inhibitors: inhibit metabolism of barbiturates; may cause prolonged CNS depression. Reduce barbiturate dosage.
Rifampin: may decrease barbiturate levels. Monitor for decreased effect.

NURSING CONSIDERATIONS

• Contraindicated in patients with uncontrolled severe pain, respiratory disease with dyspnea or obstruction, hypersensitivity to barbiturates, previous addiction to sedatives, porphyria. Use with caution in hepatic or renal impairment.
• Elderly patients are more sensitive to the drug's effects.
• Use injection solution within 30 minutes after opening container to minimize deterioration. Don't use cloudy or precipitated solution. Don't shake solution; mix with sterile water only.
• Reserve I.V. injection for emergency treatment. Give under close supervision. Be prepared to give artificial respiration. Administer slowly I.V.; not to exceed 100 mg/minute.
• Administer I.M. injection deeply. Superficial injection may cause pain, sterile abscess, and sloughing.
• Because barbiturates potentiate narcotics, reduce dose when giving during labor. Excessive dose may cause respiratory depression in neonate.
• Remove cigarettes of patient receiving hypnotic dose.
• Supervise walking; raise bed rails, especially for elderly patients.
• Long-term high dosage may cause drug dependence and severe withdrawal symptoms. Withdraw barbiturates gradually.
• Prevent hoarding or self-overdosing by patients who are depressed, suicidal, or drug-dependent, or who have a history of drug abuse.
• Watch for signs of barbiturate toxicity: coma, pupillary constriction, cyanosis, clammy skin, hypotension. Overdose can be fatal.
• Monitor prothrombin times carefully when patient on amobarbital starts or ends anticoagulant therapy. Anticoagulant dose may need to be adjusted.
• Morning "hangover" common after hypnotic dose. Hypnotic doses suppress REM sleep. When drug is discontinued, patient may experience increased dreaming.
• Used in psychiatric settings as an "Amytal interview" to elicit information that patient can't or won't offer when fully conscious.

---

butabarbital
Butisol, Day-Barb♦♦, Medarsed, Neo-Barb♦♦

butabarbital sodium
Controlled Substance Schedule III
Butisol Sodium♦* **
Pregnancy Category: D

MECHANISM OF ACTION
Probably interferes with transmission of impulses from the thalamus to the cortex of the brain. A barbiturate.

INDICATIONS & DOSAGE
Sedation—
Adults: 15 to 30 mg P.O. t.i.d. or q.i.d.

Children: 6 mg/kg P.O. divided t.i.d. Dosage range 7.5 to 30 mg P.O. t.i.d.
Preoperatively—
Adults: 50 to 100 mg P.O. 60 to 90 minutes before surgery.
Insomnia—
Adults: 50 to 100 mg P.O. at bedtime.

ADVERSE REACTIONS

CNS: *drowsiness, lethargy, hangover,* paradoxical excitement in elderly patients.
GI: nausea, vomiting.
Skin: rash, urticaria.
Other: *Stevens-Johnson syndrome,* angioedema, exacerbation of porphyria.

INTERACTIONS

Alcohol or other CNS depressants, including narcotic analgesics: excessive CNS and respiratory depression. Use together cautiously.
MAO inhibitors: inhibit the metabolism of barbiturates; may cause prolonged CNS depression. Reduce barbiturate dosage.
Rifampin: may decrease barbiturate levels. Monitor for decreased effect.

NURSING CONSIDERATIONS

• Contraindicated in patients with uncontrolled severe pain, respiratory disease with dyspnea or obstruction, hypersensitivity to barbiturates, previous addiction to sedatives, porphyria. Use with caution in hepatic or renal impairment.
• Elderly patients are more sensitive to the drug's effects.
• Remove cigarettes of patient receiving hypnotic dose.
• Supervise walking; raise bed rails, especially for elderly patients.
• Long-term high dosage may cause drug dependence and severe withdrawal symptoms. Withdraw barbiturates gradually.
• Prevent hoarding or self-overdosing by patients who are depressed, suicidal, or drug-dependent, or who have

a history of drug abuse.
• Butisol sodium elixir is sugar-free.
• Monitor prothrombin times carefully when patient on butabarbital starts or ends anticoagulant therapy. Anticoagulant dose may need to be adjusted.
• Watch for signs of barbiturate toxicity: coma, pupillary constriction, cyanosis, clammy skin, hypotension. Overdose can be fatal.
• Prolonged administration is not recommended: drug not shown to be effective after 14 days. A drug-free interval of at least 1 week is advised.
• Morning "hangover" common after hypnotic dose.
• Hypnotic doses suppress REM sleep. When drug is discontinued, patient may experience increased dreaming.

---

chloral hydrate
Controlled Substance Schedule IV
Cohidrate, Noctec♦,
Novochlorhydrate♦♦, SK-Chloral Hydrate
Pregnancy Category: C

MECHANISM OF ACTION
Unknown.

INDICATIONS & DOSAGE
Sedation—
Adults: 250 mg P.O. or rectally t.i.d. after meals.
Children: 8 mg/kg P.O. t.i.d. Maximum 500 mg t.i.d.
Insomnia—
Adults: 500 mg to 1 g P.O. or rectally 15 to 30 minutes before bedtime.
Children: 50 mg/kg single dose. Maximum dose 1 g.
Premedication for EEG—
Children: 25 mg/kg single dose. Maximum dose 1 g.

ADVERSE REACTIONS
Blood: eosinophilia.
CNS: *hangover, drowsiness,* night-

Italicized side effects are common or life-threatening.
*Liquid form contains alcohol.   **May contain tartrazine.

mares, dizziness, ataxia, paradoxical
excitement.
GI: *nausea,* vomiting, diarrhea, flatulence.
Skin: hypersensitivity reactions.

INTERACTIONS
*Alcohol or other CNS depressants, in-
cluding narcotic analgesics:* excessive
CNS depression or vasodilation reaction. Use together cautiously.
Furosemide I.V.: sweating, flushes,
variable blood pressure, uneasiness.
Use together cautiously. Use a different hypnotic drug.

NURSING CONSIDERATIONS
• Contraindicated in patients with
marked hepatic or renal impairment,
hypersensitivity to chloral hydrate or
triclofos. Oral administration contraindicated in gastric disorders. Use
with caution in severe cardiac disease,
mental depression, suicidal tendencies.
• Dilute or administer with liquid to
minimize unpleasant taste and stomach irritation. Administer after meals.
• Prevent hoarding by patients who
are depressed, suicidal, or drug-dependent, or who have a history of
drug abuse.
• Remove cigarettes of patient receiving hypnotic dose.
• Supervise walking; raise bed rails,
especially for elderly patients.
• Large dosage may raise BUN level.
• May interfere with fluorometric
tests for urine catecholamines and
Reddy, Jenkins, Thorn test for urine
17-hydroxycorticosteroids. Do not
administer drug for 48 hours before
fluorometric test.
• Aqueous solutions incompatible
with alkaline substances.
• Store in dark container. Store suppositories in refrigerator.
• If patient is given anticoagulant,
monitor for increased prothrombin
times during the first several days of
therapy. Anticoagulant dose may need

to be adjusted.

ethchlorvynol
Controlled Substance Schedule IV
Placidyl♦**
Pregnancy Category: C

MECHANISM OF ACTION
Unknown.

INDICATIONS & DOSAGE
Sedation—
Adults: 100 to 200 mg P.O. b.i.d. or
t.i.d.
Insomnia—
Adults: 500 mg to 1 g P.O. at bed-
time. May repeat 100 to 200 mg if
awakened in early a.m.

ADVERSE REACTIONS
Blood: thrombocytopenia.
CNS: facial numbness, drowsiness,
fatigue, nightmares, dizziness, resid-
ual sedation, muscular weakness, syn-
cope, ataxia.
CV: hypotension.
EENT: unpleasant aftertaste, blurred
vision.
GI: distress, nausea, vomiting.
Skin: rashes, urticaria.

INTERACTIONS
*Alcohol or other CNS depressants, in-
cluding narcotic analgesics; MAO inhibitors:* excessive CNS depression.
Use together cautiously.

NURSING CONSIDERATIONS
• Contraindicated in patients with uncontrolled pain and porphyria. Use
cautiously in hepatic or renal impairment; in elderly or debilitated patients; in mental depression with suicidal tendencies; if patient has previously overreacted to barbiturates or
alcohol.
• Give with milk or food to minimize
transient dizziness or ataxia caused by
rapid absorption.
• May cause dependence and severe

withdrawal symptoms. Withdraw
gradually.
• Prevent hoarding or self-overdosing
by patients who are depressed, suicidal, or drug-dependent, or who have
a history of drug abuse. Overdosage
very difficult to treat and has a high
mortality.
• Watch for signs of toxicity, such as
poor muscle coordination, confusion,
hypothermia, speech or vision disturbances, tremors, or weakness.
• 750-mg strength contains tartrazine
dye. May cause allergic reactions in
susceptible patients.
• Remove cigarettes of patient receiving hypnotic dose.
• Supervise walking; raise bed rails,
especially for elderly patients.
• Slight darkening of liquid from exposure to air and light doesn't affect
safety or potency, but store in tight,
light-resistant container to avoid possible deterioration.
• Monitor prothrombin times carefully when patient on ethchlorvynol
starts or ends anticoagulant therapy.
Anticoagulant dose may need to be
adjusted.
• Drug is effective for short-term use
only; treatment period should not exceed 1 week.

---

flurazepam hydrochloride
Controlled Substance Schedule IV
Dalmane♦, Somnol♦♦
Pregnancy Category: NR

MECHANISM OF ACTION
Acts on the limbic system, thalamus,
and hypothalamus of the central nervous system to produce hypnotic effects. A benzodiazepine.

INDICATIONS & DOSAGE
Insomnia—
Adults: 15 to 30 mg P.O. at bedtime.
May repeat dose once.
Adults over 65: 15 mg P.O. at bed-
time.

ADVERSE REACTIONS
Blood: leukopenia, granulocytopenia.
CNS: *daytime sedation, dizziness,
drowsiness, disturbed coordination,*
lethargy, confusion, *headache.*

INTERACTIONS
Cimetidine: increased sedation. Monitor carefully.
*Alcohol or other CNS depressants, in-
cluding narcotic analgesics:* excessive
CNS depression. Use together cautiously.

NURSING CONSIDERATIONS
• Use cautiously in patients with impaired hepatic or renal function, mental depression, suicidal tendencies, or
history of drug abuse.
• Elderly patients are more sensitive
to the CNS effects.
• Prevent hoarding or self-overdosing
by patients who are depressed, suicidal, or drug-dependent, or who have
a history of drug abuse.
• Remove cigarettes of patient receiving drug.
• Supervise walking; raise bed rails,
especially for elderly patients.
• Dependence is possible with long-
term use.
• More effective on second, third,
and fourth nights of use because active metabolite accumulates. Encourage patient to continue drug if it
doesn't work the first night.

---

glutethimide
Controlled Substance Schedule III
Doriden♦, Rolathimide
Pregnancy Category: C

MECHANISM OF ACTION
Unknown.

INDICATIONS & DOSAGE
Insomnia—
Adults: 250 to 500 mg P.O. at bedtime. May be repeated, but not less
than 4 hours before intended awaken-

Italicized side effects are common or life-threatening.
*Liquid form contains alcohol.   **May contain tartrazine.

ing. Total daily dose should not exceed 1 g.

ADVERSE REACTIONS
CNS: *residual sedation, dizziness, ataxia,* paradoxical excitation, headache, vertigo.
EENT: dry mouth, blurred vision.
GI: irritation, nausea.
GU: bladder atony.
Skin: rash, urticaria.

INTERACTIONS
Alcohol or other CNS depressants, including narcotic analgesics: excessive CNS depression. Use together cautiously.

NURSING CONSIDERATIONS
• Contraindicated in uncontrolled pain, severe renal impairment, porphyria. Use cautiously in patients with mental depression, suicidal tendencies, history of drug abuse, prostatic hypertrophy, stenosing peptic ulcer, pyloroduodenal or bladder-neck obstruction, narrow-angle glaucoma, cardiac arrhythmias.
• Drug is effective for short-term use only.
• Remove cigarettes of patient receiving drug.
• Supervise walking; raise bed rails, especially for elderly patients.
• Prevent hoarding or self-overdosing by patients who are depressed, suicidal, or drug-dependent, or who have a history of drug abuse.
• Abrupt withdrawal may produce nausea, vomiting, nervousness, tremors, chills, fever, nightmares, insomnia, tachycardia, delirium, numbness of extremities, hallucinations, dysphagia, convulsions. Withdraw gradually.
• Monitor prothrombin times carefully when patient on glutethimide starts or ends anticoagulant therapy. Anticoagulant dose may need to be adjusted.
• Suppresses REM sleep, as do barbiturates. Patient may experience increased dreaming after drug is discontinued.

methotrimeprazine hydrochloride
Levoprome, Nozinan♦♦
Pregnancy Category: C

MECHANISM OF ACTION
Acts on the limbic system, thalamus, and hypothalamus of the central nervous system to produce hypnotic effects. A phenothiazine.

INDICATIONS & DOSAGE
Postoperative analgesia—
Adults and children over 12 years: initially, 2.5 to 7.5 mg I.M. q 4 to 6 hours, then adjust dose.
Preanesthetic medication—
Adults and children over 12 years: 2 to 20 mg I.M. 45 minutes to 3 hours before surgery.
Sedation, analgesia—
Adults and children over 12 years: 10 to 20 mg deep I.M. q 4 to 6 hours as required.
Elderly: 5 to 10 mg I.M. q 4 to 6 hours.

ADVERSE REACTIONS
Blood: agranulocytosis and other dyscrasias after long-term high dosage.
CNS: *orthostatic hypotension, fainting, weakness, dizziness,* drowsiness, excessive sedation, amnesia, disorientation, euphoria, headache, slurred speech.
CV: *drop in blood pressure,* palpitations.
EENT: dry mouth, nasal congestion.
GI: nausea, vomiting, abdominal discomfort.
GU: difficulty urinating.
Local: *pain, inflammation, swelling at injection site.*

INTERACTIONS
All antihypertensive agents: increased

orthostatic hypotension. Don't use together.

NURSING CONSIDERATIONS
• Contraindicated in patients receiving concurrent antihypertensive drug therapy, including MAO inhibitors; also, in patients with history of convulsive disorders; hypersensitivity to phenothiazines; severe cardiac, hepatic, or renal disease; previous overdose of CNS depressant; coma. Use with extreme caution in elderly or debilitated patient with cardiac disease or in any patient who may suffer serious consequences from a sudden drop in blood pressure.
• Use low initial dose in susceptible patient; increase gradually while frequently checking pulse rate, blood pressure, and circulation.
• Expect drop in blood pressure 10 to 20 minutes after I.M. injection.
• Keep patient in bed or closely supervised for 6 to 12 hours after each of the first several injections because orthostatic hypotension may occur. If hypotension is severe, combat with phenylephrine, methoxamine, or levarterenol. Don't use epinephrine.
• Don't use for longer than 30 days except in terminal illness or when narcotics are contraindicated.
• In prolonged use, monitor liver function and blood studies periodically.
• Inject I.M. into large muscle masses. Rotate sites. Do not administer subcutaneously, as local irritation results. I.V. injection not recommended.
• May be mixed in same syringe with reduced dose of atropine and scopolamine. Do not mix with other drugs. Protect solution from light.

methyprylon
Controlled Substance Schedule III
Noludar♦
Pregnancy Category: B

MECHANISM OF ACTION
Raises threshold of arousal centers in the brain stem.

INDICATIONS & DOSAGE
Insomnia—
Adults: 200 to 400 mg P.O. 15 minutes before bedtime.
Children over 3 months: 50 mg P.O. at bedtime, increased to 200 mg, if necessary. Maximum 400 mg daily.

ADVERSE REACTIONS
CNS: *morning drowsiness, dizziness,* headache, paradoxical excitation.
GI: nausea, vomiting, diarrhea, esophagitis.
Skin: rash.

INTERACTIONS
Alcohol or other CNS depressants, including narcotic analgesics: excessive CNS and respiratory depression. Use together cautiously.

NURSING CONSIDERATIONS
• Contraindicated in intermittent porphyria. Use cautiously in patients with renal or hepatic impairment.
• Periodic blood counts are advisable during repeated or long-term use.
• Long-term high dosage may cause drug dependence and severe life-threatening withdrawal symptoms. Withdrawal should be gradual and closely monitored.
• Prevent hoarding or self-overdosing by patients who are depressed, suicidal, or drug-dependent, or who have a history of drug abuse.
• Remove cigarettes of patient receiving drug.
• Supervise walking; raise bed rails, especially for elderly patients.
• Value of this drug as a sedative has

not been established.
• Overdosage symptoms include somnolence, confusion, constricted pupils, respiratory depression, hypotension, coma. Hemodialysis is useful in severe intoxication.
• Suppresses REM sleep, as do barbiturates. Patient may experience increased dreaming after drug is discontinued.

midazolam hydrochloride
Controlled Substance Schedule IV
Versed
Pregnancy Category: D

MECHANISM OF ACTION
Depresses the CNS at the limbic and subcortical levels of the brain.

INDICATIONS & DOSAGE
Preoperative sedation (to induce sleepiness or drowsiness and relieve apprehension)—
Adults: 0.07 mg to 0.08 mg/kg I.M. approximately 1 hour before surgery. May be administered with atropine or scopolamine and reduced doses of narcotics.
Conscious sedation before short diagnostic or endoscopic procedures—
Adults: 0.1 to 0.15 mg/kg by slow I.V. injection immediately before the procedure. May give up to 0.2 mg/kg when concomitant narcotics are omitted.
Induction of general anesthesia—
Adults: 0.3 to 0.35 mg/kg I.V. over 20 to 30 seconds. Additional increments of 25% of the initial dose may be needed to complete induction. Up to 0.6 mg/kg total dose may be given.

ADVERSE REACTIONS
CNS: headache, oversedation.
CV: variations in blood pressure and pulse rate.
GI: nausea, vomiting, hiccups.
Local: pain and tenderness at injection site.

Other: *decreased respiratory rate, apnea.*

INTERACTIONS
CNS depressants: may increase the risk of apnea. Prepare to adjust drug dosage.

NURSING CONSIDERATIONS
• Contraindicated in patients with acute narrow-angle glaucoma. Don't give to patients in shock, coma, or acute alcohol intoxication.
• Before administering midazolam intravenously, have oxygen and resuscitative equipment available in case of severe respiratory depression.
• Monitor blood pressure during procedure, especially in patients who have also been premedicated with narcotics.
• Midazolam has a beneficial amnestic effect, which diminishes patient's recall of perioperative events. This drug offers advantages over diazepam, hydrozyzine, and barbiturates, which are also prescribed for similar indications.
• When injecting I.M., give deep into a large muscle mass.
• May be mixed in the same syringe with morphine sulfate, meperidine, atropine sulfate, or scopolamine.
• When administering intravenously, take care to avoid extravasation.

pentobarbital
Controlled Substance Schedule II
Nebralin

pentobarbital sodium
Maso-Pent, Nembutal Sodium♦*, Nova-Rectal♦♦, Penital, Pentogen♦♦
Pregnancy Category: D

MECHANISM OF ACTION
Probably interferes with transmission of impulses from the thalamus to the cortex of the brain. A barbiturate.

INDICATIONS & DOSAGE

Sedation—
Adults: 20 to 40 mg P.O. b.i.d.,
t.i.d., or q.i.d.
Children: 6 mg/kg daily P.O. in divided doses.
Insomnia—
Adults: 100 to 200 mg P.O. at bedtime or 150 to 200 mg deep I.M.; 100 mg initially, I.V., then additional doses up to 500 mg; 120 to 200 mg rectally.
Children: 3 to 5 mg/kg I.M. Maximum dose: 100 mg. Rectal dosages: 2 months to 1 year, 30 mg; 1 to 4 years, 30 to 60 mg; 5 to 12 years, 60 mg; 12 to 14 years, 60 to 120 mg.
Preanesthetic medication—
Adults: 150 to 200 mg I.M. or P.O. in 2 divided doses.

ADVERSE REACTIONS

CNS: *drowsiness, lethargy, hangover,* paradoxical excitement in elderly patients.
GI: nausea, vomiting.
Skin: rash, urticaria.
Other: *Stevens-Johnson syndrome,* angioedema, exacerbation of porphyria.

INTERACTIONS

Alcohol or other CNS depressants, including narcotic analgesics: excessive CNS and respiratory depression. Use together cautiously.
MAO inhibitors: inhibit metabolism of barbiturates; may cause prolonged CNS depression. Reduce barbiturate dosage.
Rifampin: may decrease barbiturate levels. Monitor for decreased effect.

NURSING CONSIDERATIONS

• Contraindicated in patients with uncontrolled severe pain, respiratory disease with dyspnea or obstruction, hypersensitivity to barbiturates, previous addiction to sedatives, or porphyria. Use with caution in hepatic or renal impairment.

• Elderly patients are more sensitive to the drug's effects.
• Use injection solution within 30 minutes after opening container to minimize deterioration. Don't use cloudy solution.
• Parenteral solution alkaline. Avoid extravasation; may cause tissue necrosis.
• I.V. injection should be reserved for emergency treatment and should be given under close supervision. Be prepared to give artificial respiration.
• Administer I.M. injection deeply. Superficial injection may cause pain, sterile abscess, and slough.
• Do not mix with other medication.
• Remove cigarettes of patient receiving hypnotic dose.
• Supervise walking; raise bed rails, especially for elderly patients.
• Long-term high dosage may cause drug dependence and severe withdrawal symptoms. Withdraw barbiturates gradually.
• Prevent hoarding or self-overdosing by patients who are depressed, suicidal, or drug-dependent, or who have a history of drug abuse.
• No analgesic effect. May cause restlessness or delirium in presence of pain.
• Monitor prothrombin times carefully when patient on pentobarbital starts or ends anticoagulant therapy. Anticoagulant dose may need to be adjusted.
• Watch for signs of barbiturate toxicity: coma, pupillary constriction, cyanosis, clammy skin, hypotension. Overdose can be fatal.
• To ensure accurate dosage, don't divide rectal suppositories.
• Nembutal sodium contains tartrazine dye; may cause allergic reactions in susceptible persons.
• Morning "hangover" common after hypnotic dose.
• Hypnotic doses suppress REM sleep. When drug is discontinued, patient may experience increased

---

Italicized side effects are common or life-threatening.
*Liquid form contains alcohol.   **May contain tartrazine.

dreaming.

quazepam
Dormalin
Pregnancy Category: NR

MECHANISM OF ACTION
Acts on the limbic system, thalamus, and hypothalamus of the central nervous system to produce hypnotic effects. A benzodiazepine.

INDICATIONS & DOSAGE
Insomnia—
Adults: 15 to 30 mg P.O. at bedtime.

ADVERSE REACTIONS
CNS: *somnolence, fatigue, dizziness,* headache, *disturbed coordination.*

INTERACTIONS
Cimetidine: increased sedation. Monitor carefully.
Alcohol or other CNS depressants, including narcotic analgesics: excessive CNS depression. Use together cautiously.

NURSING CONSIDERATIONS
• Use cautiously in patients with impaired hepatic or renal function, mental depression, suicidal tendencies, or history of drug abuse. Use carefully at low end of dosage range for elderly or debilitated patients.
• Prevent hoarding or self-overdosing by patients who are depressed, suicidal, or drug-dependent, or who have a history of drug abuse.
• Remove cigarettes of hospitalized patient receiving drug.
• Supervise walking; raise bed rails, especially for elderly patients.
• Dependence is possible with long-term use.
• More effective on second, third, and fourth nights of use because, as with flurazepam, active metabolite accumulates. Encourage patient to continue drug if it doesn't work the

first night.
• Similar to flurazepam. Some patients may tolerate or respond to one or the other better.

secobarbital
Seconal*

secobarbital sodium
Controlled Substance Schedule II
Secogen Sodium♦♦, Seconal
Sodium♦, Seral♦♦
Pregnancy Category: D

MECHANISM OF ACTION
Probably interferes with transmission of impulses from the thalamus to the cortex of the brain. A barbiturate.

INDICATIONS & DOSAGE
Sedation, preoperatively—
Adults: 200 to 300 mg P.O. 1 to 2 hours before surgery.
Children: 50 to 100 mg P.O. or 4 to 5 mg/kg rectally 1 to 2 hours before surgery.
Insomnia—
Adults: 100 to 200 mg P.O. or I.M.
Children: 3 to 5 mg/kg I.M., not to exceed 100 mg, with no more than 5 ml injected in any one site. 4 to 5 mg/kg rectally.
Acute tetanus convulsion—
Adults and children: 5.5 mg/kg I.M. or slow I.V., repeated q 3 to 4 hours, if needed; I.V. injection rate not to exceed 50 mg per 15 seconds.
Acute psychotic agitation—
Adults: 50 mg/minute I.V. up to 250 mg I.V. initially, additional doses given cautiously after 5 minutes if desired response is not obtained. Not to exceed 500 mg total.
Status epilepticus—
Adults and children: 250 to 350 mg I.M. or I.V.

ADVERSE REACTIONS
CNS: *drowsiness, lethargy, hangover,* paradoxical excitement in elderly pa-

tients.
GI: nausea, vomiting.
Skin: rash, urticaria.
Other: *Stevens-Johnson syndrome,* angioedema, exacerbation of porphyria.

INTERACTIONS
Alcohol or other CNS depressants, including narcotic analgesics: excessive CNS and respiratory depression. Use together cautiously.
MAO inhibitors: inhibit metabolism of barbiturates; may cause prolonged CNS depression. Reduce barbiturate dosage.
Rifampin: may decrease barbiturate levels. Monitor for decreased effect.

NURSING CONSIDERATIONS
• Contraindicated in uncontrolled severe pain, respiratory disease with dyspnea or obstruction, hypersensitivity to barbiturates, previous addiction to sedatives, porphyria. Use with caution in patients with hepatic or renal impairment; also, in pregnant women with toxemia or history of bleeding.
• Elderly patients are more sensitive to the drug's effects.
• Use injection solution within 30 minutes after opening container to minimize deterioration. Don't use cloudy solution.
• I.V. injection should be reserved for emergency treatment and should be given under close supervision. Be prepared to give artificial respiration.
• Give I.M. injection deeply. Superficial injection may cause pain, sterile abscess, and slough.
• Because barbiturates potentiate narcotics, reduce dose when giving during labor. Excessive dose may cause respiratory depression in neonate.
• Remove cigarettes of patient receiving hypnotic dose.
• Supervise walking; raise bed rails, especially for elderly patients.
• Long-term high dosage may cause drug dependence and severe withdrawal symptoms. Withdraw barbiturates gradually.
• Prevent hoarding or self-overdosing by patients who are depressed, suicidal, or drug-dependent, or who have a history of drug abuse.
• If patient has renal insufficiency, use sterile drug reconstituted with sterile water for injection. Avoid commercial solution containing polyethylene glycol; it may irritate kidneys.
• Secobarbital in polyethylene glycol must be refrigerated.
• Secobarbital sodium injection not compatible with lactated Ringer's solution.
• Sterile secobarbital sodium compatible with Ringer's injection and normal saline solution. Don't mix with acidic solutions.
• To reconstitute, rotate ampul. Do not shake.
• Monitor prothrombin times carefully when patient on secobarbital starts or ends anticoagulant therapy. Anticoagulant dose may need to be adjusted.
• Watch for signs of barbiturate toxicity: coma, pupillary construction, cyanosis, clammy skin, hypotension. Overdose can be fatal.
• Morning "hangover" common after hypnotic dose.
• Hypnotic doses suppress REM sleep. When drug is discontinued, patient may experience increased dreaming.

temazepam
Controlled Substance Schedule IV
Restoril♦
Pregnancy Category: X

MECHANISM OF ACTION
Acts on the limbic system, thalamus, and hypothalamus of the central nervous system to produce hypnotic effects. A benzodiazepine.

Italicized side effects are common or life-threatening.
*Liquid form contains alcohol.   **May contain tartrazine.

INDICATIONS & DOSAGE
Insomnia—
Adults: 15 to 30 mg P.O. at bedtime.
Adults over 65: 15 mg P.O. at bedtime.

ADVERSE REACTIONS
CNS: *drowsiness, dizziness, lethargy,* disturbed coordination, daytime sedation, confusion.
GI: anorexia, diarrhea.

INTERACTIONS
None significant.

NURSING CONSIDERATIONS
• Use cautiously in patients with impaired hepatic or renal function; in patients with mental depression or suicidal tendencies; and in patients with history of drug abuse. Use caution and low end of dosage range for elderly or debilitated patients.
• Elderly patients are more sensitive to the CNS effects.
• Prevent hoarding or self-overdosing by patients who are depressed, suicidal, or drug-dependent, or who have a history of drug abuse. Warn about increased alcohol effects and against hazardous activity requiring alertness or skill.
• Remove cigarettes of patient receiving drug.
• Supervise walking; raise bed rails, especially for elderly patients.
• May have less residual sedative effects ("hangover") the next day than flurazepam and diazepam. Relatively short acting.
• May take as long as 2 to 2½ hours for onset of action.

triazolam
Controlled Substance Schedule IV
Halcion♦
Pregnancy Category: X

MECHANISM OF ACTION
Acts on the limbic system, thalamus, and hypothalamus of the central nervous system to produce hypnotic effects. A benzodiazepine.

INDICATIONS & DOSAGE
Insomnia—
Adults: 0.125 to 0.5 mg P.O. at bedtime.
Adults over 65: 0.125 mg P.O. at bedtime. May give up to 0.25 mg.

ADVERSE REACTIONS
CNS: *drowsiness, dizziness, headache,* rebound insomnia, amnesia, light-headedness, lack of coordination, mental confusion.
GI: nausea, vomiting.

INTERACTIONS
Alcohol or other CNS depressants, including narcotic analgesics: excessive CNS depression. Use together cautiously.
Cimetidine: may cause prolonged triazolam blood levels. Monitor for increased sedation.

NURSING CONSIDERATIONS
• Use cautiously in patients with impaired hepatic or renal function, mental depression, suicidal tendencies, or history of drug abuse.
• Elderly patients are more sensitive to the CNS effects.
• Prevent hoarding or self-overdosing by patients who are depressed, suicidal, or drug-dependent, or who have a history of drug abuse.
• Remove cigarettes of patient receiving drug.
• Supervise walking; raise bed rails, especially for elderly patients.
• Dependence is possible with long-term use.
• Triazolam is a benzodiazepine compound with similarities to flurazepam. However, it is very short-acting and therefore has less tendency to cause morning drowsiness.
• Faster-acting than temazepam, another benzodiazepine derivative.

• Warn patient not to take more than the prescribed amount since overdosage can occur at a total daily dose of 2 mg (or four times the highest recommended amount).

• Tell patient that rebound insomnia may develop for one or two nights after stopping therapy.

Italicized side effects are common or life-threatening.
*Liquid form contains alcohol.   **May contain tartrazine.

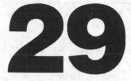

Anticonvulsants

acetazolamide sodium
(See Chapter 62, DIURETICS.)
carbamazepine
clonazepam
diazepam
(See Chapter 31, ANTIANXIETY AGENTS.)
ethosuximide
ethotoin
magnesium sulfate
mephenytoin
mephobarbital
methsuximide
paraldehyde
paramethadione
phenacemide
phenobarbital
phenobarbital sodium
phensuximide
phenytoin sodium
phenytoin sodium (extended)
phenytoin sodium (prompt)
primidone
valproate sodium
valproate sodium–valproic acid
(divalproex sodium)
valproic acid

COMBINATION PRODUCTS
DILANTIN WITH PHENOBARBITAL♦:
phenytoin sodium 100 mg and phenobarbital 16 mg.
DILANTIN WITH PHENOBARBITAL♦:
phenytoin sodium 100 mg and phenobarbital 32 mg.

carbamazepine
Mazepine♦♦, Tegretol♦
Pregnancy Category: C

MECHANISM OF ACTION
Stabilizes neuronal membranes and limits seizure activity by either increasing efflux or decreasing influx of sodium ions across cell membranes in the motor cortex during generation of nerve impulses.

INDICATIONS & DOSAGE
Generalized tonic-clonic (grand mal), complex-partial (psychomotor), mixed seizure patterns—
Adults and children over 12 years: 200 mg P.O. b.i.d. on day 1. May increase by 200 mg P.O. per day, in divided doses at 6- to 8-hour intervals. Adjust to minimum effective level when control achieved.
Children under 12 years: 10 to 20 mg/kg P.O. daily in 2 to 4 divided doses.
Trigeminal neuralgia—
Adults: 100 mg P.O. b.i.d. with meals on day 1. Increase by 100 mg q 12 hours until pain relieved. Don't exceed 1.2 g daily. Maintenance dose 200 to 400 mg P.O. b.i.d.

ADVERSE REACTIONS
Blood: *aplastic anemia, agranulocytosis,* eosinophilia, leukocytosis, *thrombocytopenia.*
CNS: dizziness, *vertigo, drowsiness,* fatigue, *ataxia,* worsening of seizures.
CV: congestive heart failure, hyper-

tension, hypotension, aggravation of coronary artery disease.
EENT: conjunctivitis, dry mouth and pharynx, blurred vision, diplopia, nystagmus.
GI: *nausea,* vomiting, abdominal pain, diarrhea, anorexia, *stomatitis,* glossitis, *dry mouth.*
GU: urinary frequency or retention, impotence, albuminuria, glycosuria, elevated BUN.
Hepatic: abnormal liver function tests, hepatitis.
Metabolic: water intoxication.
Skin: *rash,* urticaria, erythema multiforme, *Stevens-Johnson syndrome.*
Other: diaphoresis, fever, chills, pulmonary hypersensitivity.

INTERACTIONS

Troleandomycin, erythromycin, isoniazid: may increase carbamazepine blood levels. Use cautiously.
Propoxyphene: may raise carbamazepine levels. Use another analgesic.
Nicotinic acid: may decrease carbamazepine levels. Monitor for lack of therapeutic effect.

NURSING CONSIDERATIONS

● Contraindicated in patients with bone-marrow depression, hypersensitivity to carbamazepine or tricyclic antidepressants. Use cautiously in cardiac, renal, or hepatic damage, or increased intraocular pressure.
● Warn patient to avoid activities that require alertness and good psychomotor coordination until CNS response to drug has been determined.
● May cause mild-to-moderate dizziness and drowsiness when first taken. Effect usually disappears within 3 to 4 days. Should be taken three times a day, when possible, to provide consistent blood levels.
● Observe for signs of anorexia or subtle appetite changes, which may indicate excessive blood levels.
● Never stop the drug suddenly when treating seizures or status epilepticus.

Notify doctor immediately if side effects occur.
● Obtain CBC, platelet and reticulocyte counts, and serum iron levels weekly for first 3 months, then monthly. If bone-marrow depression develops, stop drug. Obtain urinalysis, BUN, and liver function tests every 3 months. Periodic eye examinations are recommended.
● Tell patient to notify doctor immediately if fever, sore throat, mouth ulcers, or easy bruising occurs.
● Therapeutic anticonvulsant blood level is 3 to 9 mcg/ml.
● Monitor blood levels and effects closely. Ask patient when last dose of medication was taken to approximately evaluate blood levels.
● When used for trigeminal neuralgia, an attempt should be made every 3 months to decrease dose or stop drug.
● Chewable tablets are available for children.
● Generally reserved for seizures unresponsive to other anticonvulsants.
● Adverse reactions may be minimized by increasing dosage gradually.
● An alternative to lithium in treatment of some affective disorders.
● Patient may take with food to minimize GI distress.

---

clonazepam
Controlled Substance Schedule IV
Klonopin, Rivotril◆
Pregnancy Category: C

MECHANISM OF ACTION
Appears to act on the limbic system, thalamus, and hypothalamus to produce anticonvulsant effects. A benzodiazepine.

INDICATIONS & DOSAGE
Absence (petit mal) and atypical absence seizures; akinetic and myoclonic seizures—
Adults: initial dose should not exceed

1.5 mg P.O. per day, divided into 3 doses. May be increased by 0.5 to 1 mg q 3 days until seizures controlled. Maximum recommended daily dose is 20 mg.
Children up to 10 years or 30 kg: 0.01 to 0.03 mg/kg P.O. daily (not to exceed 0.05 mg/kg daily), divided q 8 hours. Increase dosage by 0.25 to 0.5 mg q third day to a maximum maintenance dose of 0.1 to 0.2 mg/kg daily.

ADVERSE REACTIONS
Blood: leukopenia, thrombocytopenia, eosinophilia.
CNS: *drowsiness, ataxia, behavioral disturbances (especially in children),* slurred speech, tremor, confusion.
EENT: *increased salivation,* diplopia, nystagmus, abnormal eye movements.
GI: constipation, gastritis, change in appetite, nausea, abnormal thirst, sore gums.
GU: dysuria, enuresis, nocturia, urinary retention.
Skin: rash.
Other: respiratory depression.

INTERACTIONS
None significant.

NURSING CONSIDERATIONS
• Contraindicated in hepatic disease; chlordiazepoxide, diazepam, or other benzodiazepine sensitivity; acute narrow-angle glaucoma. Use with caution in chronic respiratory disease, impaired renal function, open-angle glaucoma.
• Elderly patients are more sensitive to the CNS effects.
• Warn patient to avoid activities that require alertness and good psychomotor coordination until CNS response to drug has been determined.
• Never withdraw drug suddenly. Call doctor at once if side effects develop.
• Obtain periodic CBC and liver function tests.
• Monitor patient for oversedation.

• Withdrawal symptoms similar to those of barbiturates.

ethosuximide
Zarontin♦
Pregnancy Category: C

MECHANISM OF ACTION
Increases seizure threshold. Reduces the paroxysmal spike-and-wave pattern of absence seizures by depressing nerve transmission in the motor cortex. Succinimide derivative.

INDICATIONS & DOSAGE
Absence (petit mal) seizure—
Adults and children over 6 years: initially, 250 mg P.O. b.i.d. May increase by 250 mg q 4 to 7 days up to 1.5 g daily.
Children 3 to 6 years: 250 mg P.O. daily or 125 mg P.O. b.i.d. May increase by 250 mg q 4 to 7 days up to 1.5 g daily.

ADVERSE REACTIONS
Blood: leukopenia, eosinophilia, *agranulocytosis,* pancytopenia, *aplastic anemia.*
CNS: *drowsiness,* headache, *fatigue, dizziness,* ataxia, irritability, hiccups, *euphoria, lethargy.*
EENT: myopia.
GI: *nausea, vomiting,* diarrhea, gum hypertrophy, weight loss, cramps, tongue swelling, *anorexia, epigastric and abdominal pain.*
GU: vaginal bleeding.
Skin: urticaria, pruritic and erythematous rashes, hirsutism.

INTERACTIONS
None significant.

NURSING CONSIDERATIONS
• Contraindicated in hypersensitivity to succinimide derivatives. Use cautiously in hepatic or renal disease.
• Never withdraw drug suddenly. Abrupt withdrawal may precipitate

absence seizures. Call doctor immediately if adverse effects develop.
- Warn patient to avoid activities that require alertness and good psychomotor coordination until CNS response to drug has been determined.
- Obtain CBC every 3 months.
- Therapeutic blood levels 40 to 80 mcg/ml.
- May increase frequency of grand mal seizures when used alone in patients who have mixed types of seizures.
- May cause positive direct Coombs' test.
- Currently the drug of choice for treating absence seizures.
- Patient may take with food to minimize GI distress.

ethotoin
Peganone
Pregnancy Category: D

MECHANISM OF ACTION
Stabilizes neuronal membranes and limits seizure activity by either increasing efflux or decreasing influx of sodium ions across cell membranes in the motor cortex during generation of nerve impulses. Hydantoin derivative.

INDICATIONS & DOSAGE
Generalized tonic-clonic (grand mal) or complex-partial (psychomotor) seizures—
Adults: initially, 250 mg P.O. q.i.d. after meals. May increase slowly over several days to 3 g daily divided q.i.d.
Children: initially, 250 mg P.O. b.i.d. May increase up to 250 mg P.O. q.i.d.

ADVERSE REACTIONS
Blood: thrombocytopenia, leukopenia, *agranulocytosis,* pancytopenia, megaloblastic anemia.
CNS: fatigue, insomnia, dizziness, headache, numbness.
CV: chest pain.

EENT: diplopia, nystagmus.
GI: *nausea, vomiting, diarrhea,* gingival hyperplasia (rare).
Skin: rash.
Other: fever, lymphadenopathy.

INTERACTIONS
Alcohol, folic acid: monitor for decreased ethotoin activity.
Oral anticoagulants, antihistamines, chloramphenicol, cimetidine, diazepam, diazoxide, disulfiram, isoniazid, phenylbutazone, salicylates, sulfamethizole, valproate: monitor for increased ethotoin activity and toxicity.

NURSING CONSIDERATIONS
- Contraindicated in patients with hydantoin hypersensitivity and in hepatic or hematologic disorders. Use cautiously in patients receiving other hydantoin derivatives.
- Never withdraw drug suddenly. Call doctor at once if side effects develop.
- Warn patient to avoid activities that require alertness and good psychomotor coordination until CNS response to drug has been determined.
- Obtain CBC and urinalysis when therapy starts and monthly thereafter.
- Give after meals. Schedule doses as evenly as possible over 24 hours.
- Stop at once if lymphadenopathy or lupus-like syndrome develops.
- Heavy use of alcohol may diminish benefits of drug.
- Hydantoin derivative of choice in young adults who are prone to gingival hyperplasia caused by phenytoin. Otherwise, infrequently used in the treatment of epilepsy.
- Ethotoin generally produces milder adverse effects than phenytoin; however, the large doses required to maintain its therapeutic effect frequently cause GI distress.

Italicized side effects are common or life-threatening.
*Liquid form contains alcohol.   **May contain tartrazine.

magnesium sulfate
Pregnancy Category: B

MECHANISM OF ACTION
May decrease acetylcholine released by nerve impulse, but its anticonvulsant mechanism is unknown.

INDICATIONS & DOSAGE
Hypomagnesemic seizures—
Adults: 1 to 2 g (as 10% solution) I.V. over 15 minutes, then 1 g I.M. q 4 to 6 hours, based on patient's response and magnesium blood levels.
Seizures secondary to hypomagnesemia in acute nephritis—
Children: 0.2 ml/kg of 50% solution I.M. q 4 to 6 hours, p.r.n. or 100 mg/kg of 10% solution I.V. very slowly. Titrate dosage according to magnesium blood levels and seizure response.
Prevention or control of seizures in preeclampsia or eclampsia—
Women: initially, 4 g I.V. in 250 ml dextrose 5% in water and 4 g deep I.M. each buttock; then 4 g deep I.M. into alternate buttock q 4 hours, p.r.n. Alternatively, 4 g I.V. loading dose followed by 1 to 4 g hourly as an I.V. infusion.

ADVERSE REACTIONS
CNS: *sweating,* drowsiness, *depressed reflexes,* flaccid paralysis, hypothermia.
CV: *hypotension, flushing, circulatory collapse,* depressed cardiac function, *heart block.*
Other: *respiratory paralysis,* hypocalcemia.

INTERACTIONS
Neuromuscular blocking agents: may cause increased neuromuscular blockade. Use cautiously.

NURSING CONSIDERATIONS
• Use cautiously in patients with impaired renal function, myocardial damage, heart block, and in women in labor.
• Magnesium sulfate can decrease the frequency and force of uterine contractions.
• Keep I.V. calcium gluconate available to reverse magnesium intoxication; however, use cautiously in patient undergoing digitalization due to danger of arrhythmias.
• Monitor vital signs every 15 minutes when giving drug I.V.
• Watch for respiratory depression and signs of heart block. Respirations should be approximately 16 per minute before each dose given.
• Monitor intake and output. Urinary output should be 100 ml or more in 4-hour period before each dose.
• Check magnesium blood levels after repeated doses. Disappearance of knee-jerk and patellar reflexes is a sign of pending magnesium toxicity.
• Maximum infusion rate is 150 mg/minute. Rapid drip will induce uncomfortable feeling of heat.
• Especially when given I.V. to toxemic mothers within 24 hours before delivery, observe newborn for signs of magnesium toxicity, including neuromuscular or respiratory depression.
• Signs of hypermagnesemia begin to appear at blood levels of 4 mEq/liter.
• Has been used as a tocolytic agent (suppresses uterine contractions) to inhibit premature labor.

mephenytoin
Mesantoin♦
Pregnancy Category: C

MECHANISM OF ACTION
Stabilizes neuronal membranes and limits seizure activity by either increasing efflux or decreasing influx of sodium ions across cell membranes in the motor cortex during generation of nerve impulses. Hydantoin derivative.

INDICATIONS & DOSAGE
Generalized tonic-clonic (grand mal) or complex-partial (psychomotor) seizures—
Adults: 50 to 100 mg P.O. daily. May increase by 50 to 100 mg at weekly intervals up to 200 mg P.O. t.i.d.
Children: initial dose 50 to 100 mg P.O. daily or 100 to 450 mg/m² P.O. daily in 3 divided doses. May increase slowly by 50 to 100 mg at weekly intervals up to 200 mg P.O. t.i.d., divided q 8 hours. Dosage must be adjusted individually.

ADVERSE REACTIONS
Blood: *leukopenia,* neutropenia, *agranulocytosis,* thrombocytopenia, pancytopenia, eosinophilia.
CNS: ataxia, *drowsiness,* fatigue, irritability, choreiform movements, depression, tremor, sleeplessness, dizziness (usually transient).
EENT: photophobia, conjunctivitis, diplopia, nystagmus.
GI: gingival hyperplasia, nausea and vomiting (with prolonged use).
Skin: *rashes, exfoliative dermatitis.*
Other: hypertrichosis, edema, dysarthria, lymphadenopathy, polyarthropathy, pulmonary fibrosis.

INTERACTIONS
Alcohol, folic acid: monitor for decreased mephenytoin activity.
Oral anticoagulants, antihistamines, chloramphenicol, cimetidine, diazepam, diazoxide, disulfiram, isoniazid, phenylbutazone, salicylates, sulfamethizole, valproate: monitor for increased mephenytoin activity and toxicity.

NURSING CONSIDERATIONS
• Contraindicated in hydantoin hypersensitivity. Use cautiously in patients receiving other hydantoin derivatives.
• Tell patient to notify doctor if fever, sore throat, bleeding, or rash occurs.
• Check CBC and platelet count initially and every 2 weeks thereafter, up to 2 weeks after full dose is attained; then monthly for first year and every 3 months thereafter. Stop drug if neutrophil count becomes less than 1,600/mm³.
• Never withdraw drug suddenly. Call doctor if side effects develop.
• Warn patient to avoid activities that require alertness and good psychomotor coordination until CNS response to drug has been determined.
• Therapeutic blood level of mephenytoin and its active metabolite 25 to 40 mcg/ml.
• Heavy use of alcohol may diminish benefit of drug.
• Potentially life-threatening blood dyscrasias limit this drug's usefulness.

mephobarbital
Controlled Substance Schedule IV
Mebaral♦, Mentabal, Mephoral
Pregnancy Category: D

MECHANISM OF ACTION
Depresses monosynaptic and polysynaptic transmission in the CNS and increases the threshold for seizure activity in the motor cortex. Barbiturate.

INDICATIONS & DOSAGE
Generalized tonic-clonic (grand mal) or absence (petit mal) seizures—
Adults: 400 to 600 mg P.O. daily or in divided doses.
Children: 6 to 12 mg/kg P.O. daily, divided q 6 to 8 hours (smaller doses are given initially and increased over 4 to 5 days as needed).

ADVERSE REACTIONS
Blood: megaloblastic anemia, agranulocytosis, thrombocytopenia.
CNS: dizziness, headache, hangover, confusion, paradoxical excitation, exacerbation of existing pain, drowsiness.
CV: hypotension.

Italicized side effects are common or life-threatening.
*Liquid form contains alcohol.   **May contain tartrazine.

GI: nausea, vomiting, epigastric pain.
Skin: urticaria, morbilliform rash, blisters, purpura, erythema multiforme.
Other: allergic reactions (facial edema).

INTERACTIONS

Alcohol and other CNS depressants, including narcotic analgesics: excessive CNS depression. Use cautiously.
MAO inhibitors: potentiated barbiturate effect. Monitor patient for increased CNS and respiratory depression.
Rifampin: may decrease barbiturate levels. Monitor for decreased effect.

NURSING CONSIDERATIONS

• Contraindicated in barbiturate hypersensitivity, porphyria, and respiratory disease with dyspnea or obstruction. Use cautiously in hepatic, renal, cardiac, or respiratory function impairment, and in myasthenia gravis and myxedema.
• Never withdraw drug suddenly. Call doctor at once if side effects develop.
• Warn patient to avoid activities that require alertness and good psychomotor coordination until CNS response to drug has been determined.
• Store in light-resistant container.
• In adults, give total or largest dose at night if seizures occur then.
• Three quarters of drug metabolized to phenobarbital; therapeutic blood levels as phenobarbital are 15 to 40 mcg/ml.
• Monitor prothrombin times carefully when patient on mephobarbital starts or ends anticoagulant therapy. Anticoagulant dose may need to be adjusted.
• Suppresses REM sleep, as do other barbiturates.

methsuximide

Celontin♦
Pregnancy Category: C

MECHANISM OF ACTION

Increases seizure threshold. Reduces the paroxysmal spike-and-wave pattern of absence seizures by depressing nerve transmission in the motor cortex. Succinimide derivative.

INDICATIONS & DOSAGE

Refractory absence (petit mal) seizures—
Adults and children: initially, 300 mg P.O. daily. May increase by 300 mg weekly. Maximum daily dosage of 1.2 g in divided doses.

ADVERSE REACTIONS

Blood: eosinophilia, leukopenia, monocytosis, pancytopenia.
CNS: *drowsiness, ataxia, dizziness,* irritability, nervousness, headache, insomnia, confusion, depression, aggressiveness.
EENT: blurred vision, photophobia, periorbital edema.
GI: *nausea, vomiting, anorexia,* diarrhea, weight loss, abdominal or epigastric pain.
Skin: urticaria, pruritic and erythematous rashes.

INTERACTIONS

None significant.

NURSING CONSIDERATIONS

• Contraindicated in hypersensitivity to succinimide derivatives. Use cautiously in hepatic or renal dysfunction.
• Never change or withdraw drug suddenly. Abrupt withdrawal may precipitate petit mal seizures. Call doctor immediately if side effects develop.
• Warn patient to avoid activities that require alertness and good psychomotor coordination until CNS response to drug has been determined.

- Obtain CBC every 3 months; urinalysis and liver function tests every 6 months.
- May color urine pink or brown.
- Not as popular an anticonvulsant as ethosuximide.

paraldehyde
Controlled Substance Schedule IV
Paral
Pregnancy Category: C

MECHANISM OF ACTION
Unknown.

INDICATIONS & DOSAGE
Refractory generalized tonic-clonic (grand mal) seizures, status epilepticus—
Adults: 5 to 10 ml I.M. (divide 10 ml dose into 2 injections); 0.2 to 0.4 ml/kg in 0.9% saline injection I.V.
Children: 0.15 ml/kg dose deep I.M. q 4 to 6 hours, p.r.n.; or 0.3 ml/kg rectally in olive oil q 4 to 6 hours; or 1 ml per year of age not to exceed 5 ml, repeated in 1 hour, p.r.n.; or dilute 5 ml in 95 ml 0.9% saline injection for I.V. infusion and titrate dose beginning at 5 ml/hour.
Sedation—
Adults: 4 to 10 ml P.O. or rectally; or 5 ml deep I.M. in upper outer quadrant of buttock. 3 to 5 ml I.V. (in emergency only).
Children: 0.15 ml/kg P.O., rectally, or deep I.M.
Insomnia—
Adults: 10 to 30 ml P.O. or rectally; 10 ml I.M. or I.V.
Children: 0.3 ml/kg P.O., rectally, or deep I.M.
Alcohol withdrawal syndrome—
Adults: 5 to 10 ml P.O. or rectally; or 5 ml deep I.M. q 4 to 6 hours for the first 24 hours, not to exceed a total of 60 ml P.O. or 30 ml I.M.; then q 6 hours on following days, not to exceed 40 ml P.O. or 20 ml I.M. per 24 hours.

Tetanus—
Adults: 4 to 5 ml I.V. (well diluted) or 12 ml (diluted 1:10) via gastric tube q 4 hours, p.r.n.; 5 to 10 ml I.M., p.r.n. to control seizures.

ADVERSE REACTIONS
CV: *I.V. administration may cause pulmonary edema or hemorrhage,* dilatation of right side of heart, *circulatory collapse.*
GI: irritation, *foul breath odor.*
GU: nephrosis with prolonged use.
Skin: *erythematous rash.*
Local: *pain,* sterile abscesses, sloughing of skin, fat necrosis, muscular irritation, nerve damage (if injection is near nerve trunk) at I.M. injection site.
Other: respiratory depression.

INTERACTIONS
Alcohol: increased CNS depression. Use with caution.
Disulfiram: increased paraldehyde and acetaldehyde blood levels; possible toxic disulfiram reaction. Use together cautiously.

NURSING CONSIDERATIONS
- Contraindicated in gastroenteritis with ulceration. Use cautiously in impaired hepatic function or in asthma or other pulmonary disease.
- Use fresh supply. Don't expose to air. Don't use if liquid is brown or has a vinegary odor, or if container has been open longer than 24 hours.
- Watch closely for respiratory depression, especially in repeated doses.
- Drug reacts with plastic. Use glass syringe and bottle for parenteral dose. Prepare fresh I.V. solution every 4 hours. I.V. administration very hazardous.
- Give I.M. dose deeply, away from nerve trunks; massage injection site.
- Dilute paraldehyde in olive oil or cottonseed oil 1:2 for rectal administration. Give as retention enema. May also use 200 ml normal saline solution

---

Italicized side effects are common or life-threatening.
*Liquid form contains alcohol.   **May contain tartrazine.

to prepare enema.
• Keep patient's room well ventilated to remove exhaled paraldehyde.
• Long-term high dosage may cause drug dependence and severe withdrawal symptoms.
• Oral or rectal administration of decomposed paraldehyde may cause severe corrosion of stomach or rectum.
• Dilute oral dose with iced juice or milk to mask taste and odor and to reduce GI distress.

paramethadione
Paradione♦* **
Pregnancy Category: D

MECHANISM OF ACTION
Raises the threshold for cortical seizure but does not modify seizure pattern. Decreases projection of focal activity and reduces both repetitive spinal-cord transmission and spike-and-wave patterns of absence (petit mal) seizures.

INDICATIONS & DOSAGE
Refractory absence (petit mal) seizures—
Adults: initially, 300 mg P.O. t.i.d. May increase by 300 mg weekly, up to 600 mg q.i.d., if needed.
Children over 6 years: 0.9 g P.O. daily in divided doses t.i.d. or q.i.d.
Children 2 to 6 years: 0.6 g P.O. daily in divided doses t.i.d. or q.i.d.
Children under 2 years: 0.3 g P.O. daily in divided doses b.i.d.

ADVERSE REACTIONS
Blood: neutropenia, leukopenia, eosinophilia, thrombocytopenia, pancytopenia, *agranulocytosis, hypoplastic and aplastic anemia.*
CNS: *drowsiness,* fatigue, vertigo, headache, paresthesias, irritability.
CV: hypertension, hypotension.
EENT: hemeralopia, photophobia, diplopia, epistaxis, retinal hemorrhage.
GI: nausea, vomiting, abdominal pain, weight loss, bleeding gums.
GU: albuminuria, vaginal bleeding.
Hepatic: abnormal liver function tests.
Skin: acneiform or morbilliform rash, *exfoliative dermatitis,* erythema multiforme, petechiae, alopecia.
Other: lymphadenopathy, lupus erythematosus.

INTERACTIONS
None significant.

NURSING CONSIDERATIONS
• Contraindicated in renal and hepatic dysfunction, severe blood dyscrasias. Use cautiously in retinal or optic nerve diseases.
• Never withdraw drug suddenly. Call doctor at once if side effects develop.
• Stop drug if scotomata or signs of hepatitis, systemic lupus erythematosus, lymphadenopathy, skin rash, nephrosis, hair loss, or grand mal seizures appear.
• Tell patient to report sore throat, fever, malaise, bruises, petechiae, or epistaxis to doctor immediately. Advise patient to wear dark glasses if photophobia occurs. Warn him not to drive car or operate machinery until CNS response to drug has been determined.
• Obtain liver function studies and urinalysis before therapy; then monthly.
• Dilute oral solution with water before giving because it contains 65% alcohol.
• Monitor CBC. Discontinue drug if neutrophil count falls below 2,500/mm^3.

phenacemide
Phenurone
Pregnancy Category: D

MECHANISM OF ACTION
Stabilizes neuronal membranes and

limits seizure activity by either increasing efflux or decreasing influx of sodium ions across cell membranes in the motor cortex during generation of nerve impulses. Hydantoin derivative.

INDICATIONS & DOSAGE
Refractory, complex-partial (psychomotor), generalized tonic-clonic (grand mal), absence (petit mal), and atypical absence seizures—
Adults: 500 mg P.O. t.i.d. May increase by 500 mg weekly up to 5 g daily, p.r.n.
Children 5 to 10 years: 250 mg P.O. t.i.d. May increase by 250 mg weekly, up to 1.5 g daily, p.r.n.

ADVERSE REACTIONS
Blood: *aplastic anemia, agranulocytosis,* leukopenia.
CNS: drowsiness, dizziness, insomnia, headaches, paresthesias, *depression, suicidal tendencies,* aggressiveness.
GI: anorexia, weight loss.
GU: nephritis with marked albuminuria.
Hepatic: hepatitis, jaundice.
Skin: rashes.

INTERACTIONS
None significant.

NURSING CONSIDERATIONS
• Contraindicated in patients with preexisting personality disturbances or in patients achieving satisfactory seizure control with other anticonvulsants. Use with caution in patients with hepatic dysfunction or history of allergy, and when a hydantoin derivative is used concomitantly.
• Obtain liver function tests, CBCs, and urinalyses before and at monthly intervals during therapy.
• Tell patient to report sore throat or fever to doctor immediately.
• Warn patient to avoid activities that require alertness or good psychomotor coordination until CNS response

to drug has been determined.
• Never withdraw drug suddenly. Call doctor at once if side effects develop.
• Tell patient's family to watch for personality or psychological changes and report them to doctor at once.
• Extremely toxic. Use drug only when other anticonvulsants are ineffective.
• When phenacemide replaces another anticonvulsant, phenacemide dosage should be increased slowly while the dosage of the drug being discontinued should be decreased slowly. This will maintain adequate seizure control.
• Notify doctor if patient develops jaundice or other signs of hepatitis, abnormal urinary findings, or WBC below 4,000/mm^3.

phenobarbital
Bar, Barbita, Eskabarb, Floramine, Gardenal♦♦, Henomint, Orprine, PB, PBR, Solfoton, Solu-Barb, Stental

phenobarbital sodium
Controlled Substance Schedule IV
Luminal Sodium♦
Pregnancy Category: D

MECHANISM OF ACTION
Depresses monosynaptic and polysynaptic transmission in the CNS and increases the threshold for seizure activity in the motor cortex. As a sedative, probably interferes with transmission of impulses from the thalamus to the cortex of the brain. A barbiturate.

INDICATIONS & DOSAGE
All forms of epilepsy, febrile seizures in children—
Adults: 100 to 200 mg P.O. daily, divided t.i.d. or given as single dose at bedtime.
Children: 4 to 6 mg/kg P.O. daily, usually divided q 12 hours. It can,

---

Italicized side effects are common or life-threatening.
*Liquid form contains alcohol.   **May contain tartrazine.

ANTICONVULSANTS **265**

however, be administered once daily.
Status epilepticus—
Adults: 10 mg/kg as I.V. infusion no
faster than 50 mg/minute. May give
up to 20 mg/kg total. Administer in
acute care or emergency area only.
Children: 5 to 10 mg/kg I.V. May re-
peat q 10 to 15 minutes up to total of
20 mg/kg. I.V. injection rate should
not exceed 50 mg/minute.
Sedation—
Adults: 30 to 120 mg P.O. daily in 2
or 3 divided doses.
Children: 6 mg/kg P.O. divided t.i.d.
Insomnia—
Adults: 100 to 320 mg P.O. or I.M.
Children: 3 to 6 mg/kg.
Preoperative sedation—
Adults: 100 to 200 mg I.M. 60 to 90
minutes before surgery.
Children: 16 to 100 mg I.M. 60 to 90
minutes before surgery.
Hyperbilirubinemia—
Neonates: 7 mg/kg daily P.O. from
first to fifth day of life; or 5 mg/kg
daily I.M. on first day, repeated P.O.
on second to seventh days.
Chronic cholestasis—
Adults: 90 to 180 mg P.O. daily in 2
or 3 divided doses.
Children under 12 years: 3 to 12
mg/kg daily P.O. in 2 or 3 divided
doses.

ADVERSE REACTIONS
CNS: *drowsiness, lethargy, hangover,*
paradoxical excitement in elderly pa-
tients.
GI: nausea, vomiting.
Skin: rash, Stevens-Johnson syn-
drome, urticaria.
Local: pain, swelling, thrombophle-
bitis, necrosis, nerve injury.
Other: angioedema.

INTERACTIONS
Alcohol and other CNS depressants,
including narcotic analgesics: excessive CNS depression. Use cautiously.
MAO inhibitors: potentiated barbiturate effect. Monitor for increased

CNS and respiratory depression.
Rifampin: may decrease barbiturate
levels. Monitor for decreased effect.
Primidone: monitor for excessive phenobarbital blood levels.
Valproic acid: increased phenobarbital levels. Monitor for toxicity.
Diazepam: increased effects of both
drugs. Use together cautiously.

NURSING CONSIDERATIONS
• Contraindicated in patients with
barbiturate hypersensitivity, porphyria, hepatic dysfunction, respiratory disease with dyspnea or obstruction, nephritis, and in lactating
women. Use cautiously in patients
with hyperthyroidism, diabetes mellitus, anemia, and in elderly or debilitated patients.
• Elderly patients are more sensitive
to the drug's effects.
• I.V. injection should be reserved for
emergency treatment and should be
given slowly under close supervision.
Monitor respirations closely.
• When administering I.V., do not
give more than 60 mg/minute.
• Give I.M. injection deeply. Superficial injection may cause pain, sterile
abscess, and tissue sloughing.
• Do not use injectable solution if it
contains a precipitate.
• Do not mix parenteral form with
acidic solutions: precipitation may result.
• Watch for barbiturate toxicity signs,
such as coma, asthmatic breathing,
cyanosis, clammy skin, hypotension.
Overdose can be fatal.
• Warn patient to avoid activities that
require alertness and good psychomotor coordination until CNS response
to drug is determined.
• Don't stop drug abruptly. Call doctor immediately if side effects develop.
• Full therapeutic effects not seen for
2 to 3 weeks, except when loading
dose is used.
• Therapeutic blood levels are 15 to

40 mg/ml.
• Monitor prothrombin times carefully when patient on phenobarbital starts or ends anticoagulant therapy. Anticoagulant dose may need to be adjusted.
• Phenobarbital is available in different milligram strengths and sizes: make sure patient is aware.
• Suppresses REM sleep, as do other barbiturates.

• Obtain CBCs every 3 months; urinalyses and liver function tests every 6 months.
• May color urine pink or red to reddish brown.
• Therapeutic blood level 40 to 80 mcg/ml.
• May increase incidence of generalized tonic-clonic seizures if used alone to treat patients with mixed seizure types.

phensuximide
Milontin♦
Pregnancy Category: D

MECHANISM OF ACTION
Increases seizure threshold. Reduces the paroxysmal spike-and-wave pattern of absence seizures by depressing nerve transmission in the motor cortex. Succinimide derivative.

INDICATIONS & DOSAGE
Absence (petit mal) seizures—
Adults and children: 500 mg to 1 g P.O. b.i.d. to t.i.d.

ADVERSE REACTIONS
Blood: transient leukopenia, pancytopenia, *agranulocytosis.*
CNS: muscular weakness, *drowsiness,* dizziness, ataxia, headache.
GI: nausea, vomiting, anorexia.
GU: urinary frequency, renal damage, hematuria.
Skin: pruritus, eruptions, erythema.

INTERACTIONS
None significant.

NURSING CONSIDERATIONS
• Contraindicated in hypersensitivity to succinimide derivatives. Use cautiously in patients with hepatic or renal disease.
• Never withdraw drug suddenly. Abrupt withdrawal may precipitate petit mal seizures. Call doctor immediately if side effects develop.

phenytoin sodium
Dilantin♦

phenytoin sodium (extended)
Dilantin Capsules♦

phenytoin sodium (prompt)
Di-Phen, Diphenylan
Pregnancy Category: D

MECHANISM OF ACTION
Stabilizes neuronal membranes and limits seizure activity by either increasing efflux or decreasing influx of sodium ions across cell membranes in the motor cortex during generation of nerve impulses. Produces antiarrhythmic effect by normalizing sodium influx to Purkinje's fibers when used to treat digitalis-induced arrhythmias. Hydantoin derivative.

INDICATIONS & DOSAGE
Generalized tonic-clonic (grand mal) seizures, status epilepticus, nonepileptic seizures (post-head trauma, Reye's syndrome)—
Adults: loading dose 900 mg to 1.5 g I.V. at 50 mg/minute or P.O. divided t.i.d., then start maintenance dose of 300 mg P.O. daily (extended only) or divided t.i.d. (extended or prompt).
Children: loading dose 15 mg/kg I.V. at 50 mg/minute or P.O. divided q 8 to 12 hours, then start maintenance dose of 5 to 7 mg/kg P.O. or I.V. daily, divided q 12 hours.

Italicized side effects are common or life-threatening.
*Liquid form contains alcohol.   **May contain tartrazine.

If patient has not received phenytoin previously or has no detectable blood level, use loading dose—
Adults: 900 mg to 1.5 g I.V. divided into t.i.d. at 50 mg/minute. Do not exceed 500 mg each dose.
Children: 15 mg/kg I.V. at 50 mg/minute.
If patient has been receiving phenytoin but has missed one or more doses and has subtherapeutic levels—
Adults: 100 to 300 mg I.V. at 50 mg/minute.
Children: 5 to 7 mg/kg I.V. at 50 mg/minute. May repeat lower dose in 30 minutes if needed.
Neuritic pain (migraine, trigeminal neuralgia, Bell's palsy)—
Adults: 200 to 400 mg P.O. daily.
Ventricular arrhythmias unresponsive to lidocaine or procainamide; supraventricular and ventricular arrhythmias induced by cardiac glycosides—
Adults: loading dose 1 g P.O. divided over first 24 hours, followed by 500 mg daily for 2 days, then maintenance dose 300 mg P.O. daily; 250 mg I.V. over 5 minutes until arrhythmias subside, adverse effects develop, or 1 g has been given. Infusion rate should never exceed 50 mg/minute (slow I.V. push).
Alternate method: 100 mg I.V. q 15 minutes until adverse effects develop, arrhythmias are controlled, or 1 g has been given. May also administer entire loading dose of 1 g I.V. slowly at 25 mg/minute. Can be diluted in normal saline solution. I.M. dose not recommended because of pain and erratic absorption.
Children: 3 to 8 mg/kg P.O. or slow I.V. daily or 250 mg/m² daily given as single dose or divided in 2 doses.

ADVERSE REACTIONS
Blood: thrombocytopenia, leukopenia, *agranulocytosis,* pancytopenia, macrocytosis, megaloblastic anemia.
CNS: *ataxia, slurred speech, confusion,* dizziness, insomnia, nervous-

ness, twitching, headache.
CV: hypotension, *ventricular fibrillation.*
EENT: *nystagmus, diplopia,* blurred vision.
GI: *nausea, vomiting, gingival hyperplasia (especially children).*
Hepatic: *toxic hepatitis.*
Skin: scarlatiniform or morbilliform rash; bullous, *exfoliative,* or purpuric *dermatitis;* Stevens-Johnson syndrome; lupus erythematosus; *hirsutism; toxic epidermal necrolysis;* photosensitivity.
Local: pain, necrosis, and inflammation at injection site, purple glove syndrome.
Other: periarteritis nodosa, lymphadenopathy, hyperglycemia, osteomalacia, hypertrichosis.

INTERACTIONS
Alcohol, dexamethasone, folic acid: monitor for decreased phenytoin activity.
Oral anticoagulants, antihistamines, amiodarone, chloramphenicol, cimetidine, diazepam, diazoxide, disulfiram, influenza vaccine, isoniazid, phenylbutazone, salicylates, sulfamethizole, valproate: monitor for increased phenytoin activity and toxicity.
Oral tube feedings with Osmolite or Isocal: may interfere with absorption of oral phenytoin. Separate feedings as far as possible from drug administration.

NURSING CONSIDERATIONS
• Contraindicated in phenacemide or hydantoin hypersensitivity, bradycardia, SA and AV block, Stokes-Adams syndrome. Use cautiously in patients with hepatic or renal dysfunction, hypotension, myocardial insufficiency, respiratory depression, and in elderly or debilitated patients, or patients receiving other hydantoin derivatives.
• Elderly patients tend to metabolize phenytoin slowly. Therefore, they

may require lower dosages.

• Phenytoin requirements usually increase during pregnancy. Monitor serum levels closely.

• Don't withdraw drug suddenly. Call doctor at once if side effects develop.

• Warn patient to avoid activities that require alertness and good psychomotor coordination until CNS response to drug is determined.

• Don't mix drug with dextrose 5% in water because it will precipitate. Clear I.V. tubing first with normal saline solution. Never use cloudy solution. May mix with normal saline solution if necessary and give as an infusion. Administer infusion over 30 to 60 minutes, when possible. Infusion must begin within 1 hour after preparation and should run through an in-line filter. Discard 4 hours after preparation. Preferably, administer slowly (50 mg/minute) as an I.V. bolus.

• Do not give I.M. unless dosage adjustments are made. Drug may precipitate at injection site, cause pain, and give erratic blood levels.

• Obtain CBC and serum calcium every 6 months. Doctor may order folic acid and vitamin B_{12} if megaloblastic anemia is evident.

• Drug may color urine pink or red to reddish brown.

• Tell patient to carry identification stating that he's taking phenytoin.

• Stress importance of good oral hygiene and regular dental examinations. Gingivectomy may be necessary periodically.

• Drug should be stopped if rash appears. If rash is scarlet or measles-like, drug may be resumed after rash clears. If rash reappears, therapy should be stopped. If rash is exfoliative, purpuric, or bullous, don't resume drug.

• Use only clear solution for injection. Slight yellow color acceptable. Don't refrigerate.

• Avoid administering I.V. push phenytoin injections into veins in the back of the hand. Inject into larger veins to avoid discoloration known as "purple glove" syndrome.

• Divided doses given with or after meals may decrease GI side effects.

• Available as suspension. Shake well before each dose. Use solid form (chewable tablets or capsules) if possible.

• Therapeutic blood level is 10 to 20 mcg/ml.

• Heavy use of alcohol may diminish benefits of drug.

• Phenytoin levels may be decreased in mononucleosis. Monitor for increased seizure activity.

• Dilantin brand and Bolar generic capsules are the only oral form that can be given on a once-daily basis. Toxic levels may result if any other brand is given once daily. Dilantin brand tablets and oral suspension should not be taken once daily.

• Advise patient not to change brands or dosage forms once stabilized on therapy.

• Suspension available as 30 mg/5 ml or 125 mg/5 ml. Read label carefully.

• The drug was formerly known as diphenylhydantoin.

• Also used to treat neuralgia and migraine headache.

---

primidone
Mysoline♦, Sertan♦♦
Pregnancy Category: D

MECHANISM OF ACTION
Unknown, but some activity may be due to phenobarbital, which is an active metabolite.

INDICATIONS & DOSAGE
Generalized tonic-clonic (grand mal) seizures, complex-partial (psychomotor) seizures—
Adults and children over 8 years: 250 mg P.O. daily. Increase by 250 mg weekly, up to maximum 2 g daily, divided q.i.d.

Italicized side effects are common or life-threatening.
*Liquid form contains alcohol.   **May contain tartrazine.

Children under 8 years: 125 mg
P.O. daily. Increase by 125 mg
weekly, up to maximum 1 g daily, divided q.i.d.

ADVERSE REACTIONS
Blood: leukopenia, eosinophilia.
CNS: *drowsiness, ataxia,* emotional
disturbances, vertigo, hyperirritabil-
ity, fatigue.
EENT: *diplopia,* nystagmus, edema
of the eyelids.
GI: anorexia, *nausea, vomiting.*
GU: impotence, polyuria.
Skin: morbilliform rash, alopecia.
Other: edema, thirst.

INTERACTIONS
Phenytoin: stimulated conversion of
primidone to phenobarbital. Observe
for increased phenobarbital effect.
Carbamezepine: increased primidone
levels. Observe for toxicity.

NURSING CONSIDERATIONS
• Contraindicated in phenobarbital
hypersensitivity, porphyria.
• Don't withdraw drug suddenly. Call
doctor at once if side effects develop.
• Warn patient to avoid activities that
require alertness and good psychomotor coordination until CNS response
to drug has been determined.
• Therapeutic blood levels of primidone 5 to 12 mcg/ml. Therapeutic
blood levels of phenobarbital 15 to 40
mcg/ml.
• CBC and routine blood chemistry
should be done every 6 months.
• Partially converted to phenobarbital; use cautiously with phenobarbital.
• Shake liquid suspension well.

valproate sodium
Depakene Syrup♦

valproate sodium–valproic acid (divalproex sodium)
Depakote♦

valproic acid
Depakene♦
Pregnancy Category: D

MECHANISM OF ACTION
Increases brain levels of gamma-ami-
nobutyric acid, which transmits in-
hibitory nerve impulses in the CNS.

INDICATIONS & DOSAGE
*Simple and complex absence seizures
(including petit mal), mixed seizure
types (including absence seizures), investigationally in major motor (grand
mal, tonic-clonic) seizures—*
Adults and children: initially, 15
mg/kg P.O. daily divided b.i.d. or
t.i.d.; then may increase by 5 to 10
mg/kg daily at weekly intervals up to
maximum of 60 mg/kg daily, divided
b.i.d. or t.i.d.

ADVERSE REACTIONS
Because drug usually used in combination with other anticonvulsants,
side effects reported may not be
caused by valproic acid alone.
Blood: *inhibited platelet aggregation,
thrombocytopenia, increased bleeding
time.*
CNS: *sedation,* emotional upset, depression, psychosis, aggression, hyperactivity, behavioral deterioration,
muscle weakness, tremors.
EENT: stomatitis.
GI: *nausea, vomiting,* indigestion,
diarrhea, abdominal cramps, constipation, increased appetite and weight
gain, *anorexia,* pancreatitis. (*Note:*
Lower incidence of GI effects with divalproex.)
Hepatic: *enzyme elevations, toxic
hepatitis.*

Unmarked trade names available in the United States only.
♦Also available in Canada.   ♦♦Available in Canada only.

Metabolic: *elevated serum ammonia levels.*
Other: alopecia.

INTERACTIONS
Antacids, aspirin: May cause valproic acid toxicity. Use together cautiously and monitor blood levels.

NURSING CONSIDERATIONS
- Contraindicated in hepatic dysfunction.
- Don't withdraw suddenly. Call doctor at once if side effects develop.
- Obtain liver function studies, platelet counts, and prothrombin time before starting drug and every month thereafter. This is especially important during the first 6 months of therapy.
- Serious or fatal hepatotoxicity may be preceded by nonspecific symptoms, such as malaise, fever, and lethargy.
- Warn patient to avoid activities that require alertness and good psychomotor coordination until CNS response to drug is determined.
- May give drug with food or milk to reduce GI side effects. Advise against chewing capsules; causes irritation of mouth and throat.
- Tremors may indicate the need for dosage reduction.
- May produce false-positive test results for ketones in urine.
- Available as tasty red syrup. Keep out of reach of children.
- Syrup is more rapidly absorbed. Peak effect within 15 minutes.
- Syrup shouldn't be mixed with carbonated beverages; may be irritating to mouth and throat.
- Don't administer syrup to patients who need sodium restriction. Check with doctor.
- Divalproex, a combination of valproic acid and valproate sodium, is available as an enteric-coated tablet. Divalproex minimizes GI intolerance.
- Valproic acid has been used investigationally to prevent recurrent febrile seizures in children.

Italicized side effects are common or life-threatening.
*Liquid form contains alcohol.   **May contain tartrazine.

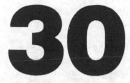

Antidepressants

Monoamine oxidase inhibitors
isocarboxazid
phenelzine sulfate
tranylcypromine sulfate

Tricyclic antidepressants
amitriptyline hydrochloride
amoxapine
desipramine hydrochloride
doxepin hydrochloride
imipramine hydrochloride
imipramine pamoate
maprotiline hydrochloride
nortriptyline hydrochloride
protriptyline hydrochloride
trimipramine maleate

Miscellaneous
trazodone hydrochloride

COMBINATION PRODUCTS
ETRAFON 2-10♦: perphenazine 2 mg and amitripyline HCl 10 mg.
ETRAFON: perphenazine 2 mg and amitriptyline HCl 25 mg.
ETRAFON-A: perphenazine 4 mg and amitriptyline 10 mg.
ETRAFON-FORTE: perphenazine 4 mg and amitriptyline 25 mg.
LIMBITROL 10-25: chlordiazepoxide 10 mg and amitriptyline (as HCl) 25 mg.
LIMBITROL 5-12.5: chlordiazepoxide 5 mg and amitriptyline (as HCl) 12.5 mg.
TRIAVIL 2-10, TRIAVIL 4-10, TRIAVIL 2-25, TRIAVIL 4-25 are products identical to the Etrafon products listed above. Triavil is also available as TRIAVIL 4-50 (perphenazine 4 mg and amitriptyline HCl 50 mg).

amitriptyline hydrochloride
Amitril, Elavil♦, Emitrip, Endep, Enovil, Levate♦♦, Meravil♦♦, Novotriptyn♦♦, Rolavil
Pregnancy Category: D

MECHANISM OF ACTION
Increases the amount of norepinephrine or serotonin, or both, in the central nervous system by blocking their reuptake by the presynaptic neurons. This action allows these neurotransmitters to accumulate.

INDICATIONS & DOSAGE
Treatment of depression—
Adults: 50 to 100 mg P.O. h.s., increasing to 200 mg daily; maximum 300 mg daily if needed; or 20 to 30 mg I.M. q.i.d. Alternatively, the entire dosage can be given at bedtime.
Elderly and adolescents: 30 mg P.O. daily in divided doses. May be increased to 150 mg.

ADVERSE REACTIONS
CNS: *drowsiness, dizziness,* excitation, tremors, weakness, confusion, headache, nervousness.
CV: *orthostatic hypotension, tachycardia, EKG changes,* hypertension.
EENT: *blurred vision,* tinnitus, mydriasis.
GI: *dry mouth, constipation,* nausea, vomiting, anorexia, paralytic ileus.
GU: *urinary retention.*
Skin: rash, urticaria.
Other: *sweating,* allergy.
After abrupt withdrawal of long-term therapy: nausea, headache,

malaise. (Does not indicate addiction.)

INTERACTIONS
MAO inhibitors: may cause severe excitation, hyperpyrexia, convulsions, usually with high dose. Use together cautiously.
Epinephrine, norepinephrine: increase hypertensive effect. Use with caution.
Barbiturates: decrease TCA blood levels. Monitor for decreased antidepressant effect.
Methylphenidate: increases TCA blood levels. Monitor for enhanced antidepressant effect.

NURSING CONSIDERATIONS
• Contraindicated during acute recovery phase of myocardial infarction, in patients with history of seizure disorders, and in patients with prostatic hypertrophy. Use with caution in patients who are suicide risks; in patients with urinary retention, narrow-angle glaucoma, increased intraocular pressure, cardiovascular disease, impaired hepatic function, or hyperthyroidism; and in patients receiving thyroid medications, electroshock therapy, or elective surgery.
• Reduce dose in elderly or debilitated persons and adolescents.
• Do not withdraw abruptly.
• If psychotic signs increase, dose should be reduced. Chart mood changes. Watch for suicidal tendencies. Allow minimum supply of tablets to lessen suicide risk.
• Check for urinary retention and constipation. Increase fluids to lessen constipation. Suggest stool softener, if needed.
• Warn patient to avoid activities that require alertness and good psychomotor coordination until CNS response to drug is determined. Drowsiness and dizziness usually subside after first few weeks.
• Has strong anticholinergic effects;

one of the most sedating tricyclic antidepressants. Avoid combining with alcohol or other depressants.
• Expect time lag of up to 10 to 14 days before noticeable effect. Full effect usually appears in 30 days.
• Dry mouth may be relieved with sugarless hard candy or gum.
• Advise the patient not to take any other drugs (prescription or over-the-counter) without first consulting the doctor.
• Whenever possible, patient should take full dose at bedtime.
• Has been used successfully to treat intractable hiccups and chronic pain associated with post-herpetic neuralgia.

amoxapine
Asendin♦
Pregnancy Category: C

MECHANISM OF ACTION
Increases the amount of norepinephrine or serotonin, or both, in the central nervous system by blocking their reuptake by the presynaptic neurons. This action allows these neurotransmitters to accumulate.

INDICATIONS & DOSAGE
Treatment of depression—
Adults: initial dose 50 mg P.O. t.i.d. May increase to 100 mg t.i.d. on third day of treatment. Increases above 300 mg daily should be made only if 300 mg daily has been ineffective during a trial period of at least 2 weeks. When effective dosage is established, entire dosage (not exceeding 300 mg) may be given at bedtime. Maximum 600 mg in hospitalized patients.

ADVERSE REACTIONS
CNS: *drowsiness, dizziness,* excitation, tremors, weakness, confusion, headache, nervousness, *tardive dyskinesia* (especially in elderly women).
CV: *orthostatic hypotension, tachy-*

Italicized side effects are common or life-threatening.
*Liquid form contains alcohol.   **May contain tartrazine.

ANTIDEPRESSANTS 273

cardia, EKG changes, hypertension.
EENT: *blurred vision,* tinnitus, mydriasis.
GI: *dry mouth, constipation,* nausea, vomiting, anorexia, paralytic ileus.
GU: *urinary retention, acute renal failure.*
Skin: rash, urticaria.
Other: *sweating,* weight gain and craving for sweets, allergy.
After abrupt withdrawal of long-term therapy: nausea, headache, malaise. (Does not indicate addiction.)

INTERACTIONS
MAO inhibitors: may cause severe excitation, hyperpyrexia, convulsions, usually with high dose. Use together cautiously.
Epinephrine, norepinephrine: increase hypertensive effect. Use with caution.
Barbiturates: decrease TCA blood levels. Monitor for decreased antidepressant effect.
Methylphenidate: increases TCA blood levels. Monitor for enhanced antidepressant effect.
Cimetidine: may increase amoxapine serum levels. Monitor for increased adverse effects.

NURSING CONSIDERATIONS
• Contraindicated in acute recovery phase of myocardial infarction, in patients with history of seizure disorders, and in patients with prostatic hypertrophy. Use with caution in patients who are suicide risks; in patients with urinary retention, narrow-angle glaucoma, increased intraocular pressure, cardiovascular disease, impaired hepatic function, or hyperthyroidism; and in patients receiving thyroid medications, electroshock therapy, or elective surgery.
• Monitor for signs and symptoms of tardive dyskinesia, especially in elderly women.
• Reduce dose in elderly or debili-

tated persons and adolescents.
• Do not withdraw abruptly.
• If psychotic signs increase, reduce dose. Chart mood changes. Watch for suicidal tendencies. Allow minimum supply of tablets to lessen suicide risk.
• Check for urinary retention and constipation. Increase fluids to lessen constipation. Suggest stool softener, if needed.
• Warn patient to avoid activities that require alertness and good psychomotor coordination until CNS response to drug is determined. Drowsiness and dizziness usually subside after first few weeks.
• Dry mouth may be relieved with sugarless hard candy or gum.
• Whenever possible, patient should take full dose at bedtime.

desipramine hydrochloride
Norpramin♦**, Pertofrane♦
Pregnancy Category: C

MECHANISM OF ACTION
Increases the amount of norepinephrine or serotonin, or both, in the central nervous system by blocking their reuptake by the presynaptic neurons. This action allows these neurotransmitters to accumulate.

INDICATIONS & DOSAGE
Treatment of depression—
Adults: 75 to 150 mg P.O. daily in divided doses, increasing to maximum 300 mg daily. Alternatively, the entire dosage can be given at bedtime.
Elderly and adolescents: 25 to 50 mg P.O. daily, increasing gradually to maximum 100 mg daily.

ADVERSE REACTIONS
CNS: *drowsiness, dizziness,* excitation, tremors, weakness, confusion, headache, nervousness.
CV: *orthostatic hypotension, tachycardia, EKG changes,* hypertension.
EENT: *blurred vision,* tinnitus, my-

driasis.
GI: *dry mouth, constipation,* nausea, vomiting, anorexia, *paralytic ileus.*
GU: *urinary retention.*
Skin: rash, urticaria.
Other: *sweating,* allergy.
After abrupt withdrawal of long-term therapy: nausea, headache, malaise. (Does not indicate addiction.)

INTERACTIONS
MAO inhibitors: may cause severe excitation, hyperpyrexia, convulsions, usually with high dose. Use together cautiously.
Epinephrine, norepinephrine: increase hypertensive effect. Use with caution.
Barbiturates: decrease TCA blood levels. Monitor for decreased antidepressant effect.
Methylphenidate: increases TCA blood levels. Monitor for enhanced antidepressant effect.
Cimetidine: may increase desipramine serum levels. Monitor for increased adverse effects.

NURSING CONSIDERATIONS
• Contraindicated during acute recovery phase of myocardial infarction, in patients with history of seizure disorders, and in patients with prostatic hypertrophy. Use with caution in patients with cardiovascular disease, urinary retention, narrow-angle glaucoma, thyroid disease, blood dyscrasias, or impaired hepatic function; in patients who are suicide risks; and in those receiving electroshock therapy, thyroid medication, or elective surgery.
• Reduce dose in elderly or debilitated persons, and adolescents.
• Do not withdraw abruptly.
• Orthostatic hypotension not as severe with this drug compared to that with other tricyclic antidepressants.
• If psychotic signs increase, dose should be decreased. Chart mood

changes. Watch for suicidal tendencies. To lessen suicide risk, allow minimum supply of tablets.
• Check for urinary retention and constipation. Increase fluids to lessen constipation. Suggest stool softener, if needed.
• Warn patient to avoid activities that require alertness and good psychomotor coordination until response to drug is determined. Drowsiness and dizziness usually subside after a few weeks.
• Dry mouth may be relieved with sugarless hard candy or gum.
• Drug has anticholinergic effect, is a metabolite of imipramine, and produces less sedation than amitriptyline or doxepin. Alcohol may antagonize effects of desipramine.
• Because it produces less tachycardia and other anticholinergic effects compared with other tricyclics, desipramine is often prescribed for cardiac patients.
• Expect time lag of 10 to 14 days before noticeable effects. Full effect usually appears in 30 days.
• Advise patient not to take any other drugs (prescription or over-the-counter) without first consulting the doctor.
• Whenever possible, patient should take full dose at bedtime.

---

doxepin hydrochloride
Adapin******, Sinequan◆
Pregnancy Category: C

MECHANISM OF ACTION
Increases the amount of norepinephrine or serotonin, or both, in the central nervous system by blocking their reuptake by the presynaptic neurons. This action allows these neurotransmitters to accumulate.

INDICATIONS & DOSAGE
Treatment of depression—
Adults: initially, 50 to 75 mg P.O.

daily in divided doses, to maximum 300 mg daily. Alternatively, entire dosage may be given at bedtime.

ADVERSE REACTIONS
CNS: *drowsiness, dizziness,* excitation, tremors, weakness, confusion, headache, nervousness.
CV: *orthostatic hypotension, tachycardia, EKG changes,* hypertension.
EENT: *blurred vision,* tinnitus, glossitis, mydriasis.
GI: *dry mouth, constipation,* nausea, vomiting, anorexia, paralytic ileus.
GU: *urinary retention.*
Skin: rash, urticaria.
Other: *sweating,* allergy.
After abrupt withdrawal of long-term therapy: nausea, headache, malaise. (Does not indicate addiction.)

INTERACTIONS
MAO inhibitors: may cause severe excitation, hyperpyrexia, convulsions, usually with high dose. Use together cautiously.
Barbiturates: decrease TCA blood levels. Monitor for decreased antidepressant effect.
Methylphenidate: increases TCA blood levels. Monitor for enhanced antidepressant effect.
Cimetidine: may increase doxepin serum levels. Monitor for increased adverse effects.

NURSING CONSIDERATIONS
• Contraindicated in patients with urinary retention, narrow-angle glaucoma, or prostatic hypertrophy. Use with caution in suicide risks.
• Reduce dose in elderly or debilitated persons, adolescents, and those receiving other medications (especially anticholinergics).
• Dilute oral concentrate with 120 ml water, milk, or juice (orange, grapefruit, tomato, prune, or pineapple). Incompatible with carbonated beverages.

• If psychotic symptoms increase, dose should be decreased. Chart mood changes. Watch for suicidal tendencies.
• Check for urinary retention and constipation. Increase fluids to lessen constipation. Suggest stool softener, if needed.
• Warn patient to avoid activities that require alertness and good psychomotor coordination until CNS response to drug is determined. Drowsiness and dizziness usually subside after a few days.
• Expect time lag of 10 to 14 days before effect is noticeable. Full effect usually appears within 30 days.
• Dry mouth may be relieved with sugarless hard candy or gum.
• Has strong anticholinergic effects; one of the most sedating tricyclic antidepressants. Avoid combining with alcohol or other depressants.
• Advise patient not to take any other drugs (over-the-counter or prescription) without first consulting the doctor.
• Liquid formulation available.
• Whenever possible, patient should take full dose at bedtime.
• Especially well tolerated by geriatric patients.

imipramine hydrochloride
Impril♦♦, Janimine**, Novopramine♦♦, Presamine, Ropramine, SK-Pramine, Tipramine, Tofranil♦**

imipramine pamoate
Tofranil-PM**
Pregnancy Category: D

MECHANISM OF ACTION
Increases the amount of norepinephrine or serotonin, or both, in the central nervous system by blocking their reuptake by the presynaptic neurons. This action allows these neurotransmitters to accumulate.

INDICATIONS & DOSAGE

Treatment of depression—
Adults: 75 to 100 mg P.O. or I.M. daily in divided doses, with 25- to 50-mg increments up to 200 mg. Maximum 300 mg daily. Alternatively, the entire dosage may be given at bedtime. (I.M. route rarely used.)
Childhood enuresis—
25 to 75 mg P.O. daily.

ADVERSE REACTIONS

CNS: *drowsiness, dizziness,* excitation, tremors, weakness, confusion, headache, nervousness.
CV: *orthostatic hypotension, tachycardia, EKG changes,* hypertension.
EENT: *blurred vision,* tinnitus, mydriasis.
GI: *dry mouth, constipation,* nausea, vomiting, anorexia, paralytic ileus.
GU: *urinary retention.*
Skin: rash, urticaria.
Other: *sweating,* allergy.
After abrupt withdrawal of long-term therapy: nausea, headache, malaise. (Does not indicate addiction.)

INTERACTIONS

MAO inhibitors: may cause severe excitation, hyperpyrexia, convulsions, usually with high dose. Use together cautiously.
Epinephrine, norepinephrine: increase hypertensive effect. Use with caution.
Barbiturates: decrease TCA blood levels. Monitor for decreased antidepressant effect.
Methylphenidate: increases TCA blood levels. Monitor for enhanced antidepressant effect.
Cimetidine: may increase imipramine serum levels. Monitor for increased adverse effects.

NURSING CONSIDERATIONS

• Contraindicated during acute recovery phase of myocardial infarction, in patients with prostatic hypertrophy, and in patients with history of seizure disorders. Use with extreme caution in patients with cardiovascular disease, urinary retention, narrow-angle glaucoma or increased intraocular pressure, thyroid disease, blood dyscrasias, or impaired hepatic function; in patients who are suicide risks; and in those receiving electroshock therapy, thyroid medication, or elective surgery.
• Reduce dose in elderly or debilitated persons, adolescents, and patients with aggravated psychotic symptoms.
• Do not withdraw abruptly.
• If psychotic signs increase, dose should be reduced. Chart mood changes. Watch for suicidal tendencies. To lessen suicide risk, allow minimum tablet supply.
• Check for urinary retention and constipation. Increase fluids to lessen constipation. Suggest stool softener, if needed.
• Warn patient to avoid activities that require alertness and good psychomotor coordination until CNS response to drug is determined. Drowsiness and dizziness usually subside after a few weeks.
• Expect time lag of 10 to 14 days before noticeable effect. Full effect usually appears in 30 days.
• Dry mouth may be relieved with sugarless hard candy or gum.
• Avoid combining with alcohol or other depressants.
• Advise patient not to take any other drugs (prescription or over-the-counter) without first consulting the doctor.
• Whenever possible, patient should take full dose at bedtime.

Italicized side effects are common or life-threatening.
*Liquid form contains alcohol.   **May contain tartrazine.

isocarboxazid
Marplan♦
Pregnancy Category: C

MECHANISM OF ACTION
Promotes accumulation of neurotransmitters by inhibiting monoamine oxidase.

INDICATIONS & DOSAGE
Treatment of depression—
Adults: 30 mg P.O. daily in divided doses. Reduce to 10 to 20 mg daily when condition improves. Not recommended for children under 16 years.

ADVERSE REACTIONS
CNS: *dizziness,* vertigo, weakness, headache, overactivity, hyperreflexia, tremors, muscle twitching, mania, *insomnia,* confusion, memory impairment, fatigue.
CV: *orthostatic hypotension,* arrhythmias, paradoxical hypertension.
EENT: blurred vision.
GI: dry mouth, *anorexia,* nausea, diarrhea, constipation.
GU: altered libido.
Skin: rash.
Other: peripheral edema, sweating, weight changes.

INTERACTIONS
Amphetamines, ephedrine, levodopa, meperidine, metaraminol, methotrimeprazine, methylphenidate, phenylephrine, phenylpropanolamine: pressor effects of these drugs are enhanced by isocarboxazid. Use together very cautiously.
Alcohol, barbiturates, and other sedatives; narcotics; dextromethorphan; tricyclic antidepressants: unpredictable interaction. Use with caution and in reduced dosage.

NURSING CONSIDERATIONS
• Contraindicated in elderly or debilitated patients, and in patients with severe hepatic or renal impairment; congestive heart failure; pheochromocytoma; hypertensive, cardiovascular, or cerebrovascular disease; severe or frequent headaches. Also contraindicated with foods containing tryptophan or tyramine. Also during therapy with other MAO inhibitor (including pargyline HCl, phenelzine sulfate, tranylcypromine sulfate) or within 10 days of such therapy; within 10 days of elective surgery requiring general anesthetic, cocaine, or local anesthetic containing sympathomimetic vasoconstrictors. Use cautiously with other psychotropic drugs or with spinal anesthetic; in hyperactive, agitated, or schizophrenic patients; in suicide risks; and in patients with diabetes or epilepsy.
• Drug is an MAO inhibitor and is generally less effective than tricyclic antidepressants. Avoid combining with alcohol or other depressant.
• Recommended only when TCA or electroshock therapy is ineffective or contraindicated.
• If patient develops symptoms of overdosage (palpitations or frequent headaches, or severe orthostatic hypotension), hold dose and notify doctor.
• Watch for suicidal tendencies.
• Dose is usually reduced to maintenance level as soon as possible.
• Do not withdraw drug abruptly.
• Weigh patient biweekly; check for edema and urinary retention.
• Warn patient to avoid foods high in tyramine or tryptophan (aged cheese, Chianti wine, beer, avocados, chicken livers, chocolate, bananas, soy sauce, meat tenderizers, salami, bologna); large amounts of caffeine; and self-medication with over-the-counter cold, hay fever, or diet preparations.
• Incidence of orthostatic hypotension is high. Supervise walking. Tell patient to get out of bed slowly, sitting up first for 1 minute.
• Have phentolamine (Regitine) available to counteract severe hyper-

tension.

• Continue precautions 10 days after stopping drug; long-lasting effects.

• Expect time lag of 1 to 4 weeks before noticeable effect.

• Obtain baseline blood pressure readings, CBC, and liver function tests before beginning therapy, and continue to monitor throughout treatment.

---

maprotiline hydrochloride
Ludiomil♦
Pregnancy Category: B

MECHANISM OF ACTION
Increases the amount of norepinephrine or serotonin, or both, in the central nervous system by blocking their reuptake by the presynaptic neurons. This action allows these neurotransmitters to accumulate.

INDICATIONS & DOSAGE
Treatment of depression—
Adults: initial dose of 75 mg daily for patients with mild to moderate depression. The dosage may be increased as required to a dose of 150 mg daily. Maximum dose is 225 mg in patients who are not hospitalized. More severely depressed, hospitalized patients may receive up to 300 mg daily.

ADVERSE REACTIONS
CNS: *drowsiness, dizziness,* excitation, *seizures,* tremors, weakness, confusion, headache, nervousness.
CV: *orthostatic hypotension, tachycardia, EKG changes,* hypertension.
EENT: *blurred vision,* tinnitus, mydriasis.
GI: *dry mouth, constipation,* nausea, vomiting, anorexia, paralytic ileus.
GU: *urinary retention.*
Skin: rash, urticaria.
Other: *sweating,* allergy.
After abrupt withdrawal of long-term therapy: nausea, headache, malaise. (Does not indicate addiction.)

INTERACTIONS
MAO inhibitors: may cause severe excitation, hyperpyrexia, convulsions, usually with high dose. Use together cautiously.
Epinephrine, norepinephrine: increase hypertensive effect. Use with caution.
Barbiturates: decrease maprotiline blood levels. Monitor for decreased antidepressant effect.
Methylphenidate: increases maprotiline blood levels. Monitor for enhanced antidepressant effect.
Cimetidine: may increase maprotiline serum levels. Monitor for increased adverse effects.

NURSING CONSIDERATIONS
• Contraindicated during acute recovery phase of myocardial infarction, in patients with prostatic hypertrophy, and in patients with history of seizure disorders. Use with caution in cardiovascular disease, urinary retention, narrow-angle glaucoma, thyroid disease or medication, blood dyscrasias, and impaired hepatic funct on; in patients who are suicide risks; and in those receiving electroshock therapy or elective surgery.

• Reduce dose in elderly or debilitated persons, and adolescents.

• Do not withdraw abruptly.

• If psychotic signs increase, reduce dose. Chart mood changes. Watch for suicidal tendencies. To lessen suicide risk, allow minimum supply of tablets.

• Check for urinary retention and constipation. Increase fluids to lessen constipation. Suggest stool softener, if needed.

• Warn patient to avoid activities that require alertness and good psychomotor coordination until CNS response to drug is determined. Drowsiness and dizziness usually subside after a

---

Italicized side effects are common or life-threatening.
*Liquid form contains alcohol.   **May contain tartrazine.

few weeks.
- Dry mouth may be relieved with sugarless hard candy or gum.
- Whenever possible, patient should take full dose at bedtime.
- The first "tetracyclic" antidepressant.

---

nortriptyline hydrochloride
Aventyl♦*, Pamelor
Pregnancy Category: D

MECHANISM OF ACTION
Increases the amount of norepinephrine or serotonin, or both, in the central nervous system by blocking their reuptake by the presynaptic neurons. This action allows these neurotransmitters to accumulate.

INDICATIONS & DOSAGE
Treatment of depression—
Adults: 25 mg P.O. t.i.d. or q.i.d., gradually increasing to maximum 150 mg daily. Alternatively, entire dose may be given at bedtime.

ADVERSE REACTIONS
CNS: *drowsiness, dizziness,* excitation, seizures, tremors, weakness, confusion, headache, nervousness.
CV: *tachycardia, EKG changes,* hypertension.
EENT: *blurred vision,* tinnitus, mydriasis.
GI: *dry mouth, constipation,* nausea, vomiting, anorexia, paralytic ileus.
GU: *urinary retention.*
Skin: rash, urticaria.
Other: *sweating,* allergy.
After abrupt withdrawal of long-term therapy: nausea, headache, malaise. (Does not indicate addiction.)

INTERACTIONS
MAO inhibitors: may cause severe excitation, hyperpyrexia, convulsions, usually with high dose. Use together cautiously.
Epinephrine, norepinephrine: increase hypertensive effect. Use with caution.
Barbiturates: decrease TCA blood levels. Monitor for decreased antidepressant effect.
Methylphenidate: increases TCA blood levels. Monitor for enhanced antidepressant effect.
Cimetidine: may increase nortriptyline serum levels. Monitor for increased adverse effects.

NURSING CONSIDERATIONS
- Contraindicated during acute recovery phase of myocardial infarction, in patients with prostatic hypertrophy, and in patients with history of seizure disorders. Use with caution in patients with cardiovascular disease, urinary retention, glaucoma, thyroid disease, impaired hepatic function, or blood dyscrasias; in patients who are suicide risks; or in those receiving electroshock therapy, thyroid medication, or elective surgery.
- Reduce dose in elderly or debilitated persons, and adolescents.
- Do not withdraw abruptly.
- If psychotic signs increase, dose should be reduced. Chart mood changes. Watch for suicidal tendencies. To lessen suicide risk, allow minimum tablet supply.
- Check for urinary retention and constipation. Increase fluids to lessen constipation. Suggest stool softener, if needed.
- Warn patient to avoid activities that require alertness and good psychomotor coordination until CNS response to drug is determined. Drowsiness and dizziness usually subside after a few weeks.
- Expect time lag of 10 to 14 days before noticeable effects. Full effect usually appears in 30 days.
- Dry mouth may be relieved with sugarless hard candy or gum.
- Drug is tricyclic antidepressant, similar in anticholinergic effects to

---

Unmarked trade names available in the United States only.
♦ Also available in Canada.   ♦ ♦ Available in Canada only.

other cyclics. Avoid combining with alcohol or other depressants.
• Advise patient not to use other drugs (prescription or over-the-counter) without first consulting the doctor.
• Liquid formulation available.
• Whenever possible, patient should take full dose at bedtime.

---

phenelzine sulfate
Nardil♦
Pregnancy Category: C

MECHANISM OF ACTION
Promotes accumulation of neurotransmitters by inhibiting monoamine oxidase.

INDICATIONS & DOSAGE
Treatment of depression—
Adults: 45 mg P.O. daily in divided doses, increasing rapidly to 60 mg daily. Then dose can usually be reduced to 15 mg daily. Maximum 90 mg daily.

ADVERSE REACTIONS
CNS: *dizziness,* vertigo, headache, overactivity, hyperreflexia, tremors, muscle twitching, mania, jitters, *insomnia,* confusion, memory impairment, drowsiness, weakness, fatigue.
CV: paradoxical hypertension, *orthostatic hypotension,* arrhythmias.
GI: dry mouth, *anorexia,* nausea, constipation.
Other: peripheral edema, sweating, weight changes.

INTERACTIONS
Amphetamines, ephedrine, levodopa, meperidine, metaraminol, methotrimeprazine, methylphenidate, phenylephrine, phenylpropanolamine: enhance pressor effects. Use together cautiously.
Alcohol, barbiturates, and other sedatives; narcotics; dextromethorphan; tricyclic antidepressants: unpredict-

able interaction. Use with caution and in reduced dosage.

NURSING CONSIDERATIONS
• Contraindicated in elderly or debilitated patients, and in patients with hepatic impairment, congestive heart failure, pheochromocytoma, hypertension, cardiovascular or cerebrovascular disease, or severe or frequent headaches. Also contraindicated with foods containing tryptophan (broad beans) or tyramine; during therapy with other MAO inhibitors (including pargyline HCl, isocarboxazid, tranylcypromine sulfate) or within 10 days of such therapy; within 10 days of elective surgery requiring general anesthetic, cocaine, or local anesthetic containing sympathomimetic vasoconstrictors; and in hyperactive, agitated, or schizophrenic patients. Use cautiously with antihypertensive drugs containing thiazide diuretics or with spinal anesthetic; and in patients with suicide risk or diabetes.
• Drug is an MAO inhibitor and is generally less effective than tricyclic antidepressants. Avoid combining with alcohol or other depressant.
• Use only when TCA or electroshock therapy is ineffective or contraindicated.
• If patient develops symptoms of overdose (severe hypotension, palpitations, or frequent headaches), hold dose and notify doctor.
• Watch for suicidal tendencies.
• Dose is usually reduced to maintenance level as soon as possible.
• Store drug in tight container, away from heat and light.
• Have phentolamine (Regitine) available to counteract severe hypertension.
• Warn patient to avoid foods high in tyramine or tryptophan (aged cheese, Chianti wine, beer, avocados, chicken livers, chocolate, bananas, soy sauce, meat tenderizers, salami, bologna) and self-medication with over-the-

---

counter cold, hay fever, or diet preparations.
• Incidence of orthostatic hypotension is high. Supervise walking. Tell patient to get out of bed slowly, sitting up first for 1 minute.
• Continue precautions 10 days after stopping drug; long-lasting effects.
• Expect time lag of 1 to 4 weeks before noticeable effect.
• Obtain baseline blood pressure readings, CBC, and liver function tests before beginning therapy, and continue to monitor throughout treatment.

protriptyline hydrochloride
Triptil♦♦, Vivactil
Pregnancy Category: C

MECHANISM OF ACTION
Increases the amount of norepinephrine or serotonin, or both, in the central nervous system by blocking their reuptake by the presynaptic neurons. This action allows these neurotransmitters to accumulate.

INDICATIONS & DOSAGE
Treatment of depression—
Adults: 15 to 40 mg P.O. daily in divided doses, increasing gradually to maximum 60 mg daily.

ADVERSE REACTIONS
CNS: excitation, seizures, tremors, weakness, confusion, headache, nervousness.
CV: *orthostatic hypotension, tachycardia, EKG changes,* hypertension.
EENT: *blurred vision,* tinnitus, mydriasis.
GI: *dry mouth, constipation,* nausea, vomiting, anorexia, paralytic ileus.
GU: *urinary retention.*
Skin: rash, urticaria.
Other: *sweating,* allergy.
After abrupt withdrawal of long-term therapy: nausea, headache, malaise. (Does not indicate addiction.)

INTERACTIONS
MAO inhibitors: may cause severe excitation, hyperpyrexia, convulsions, and death, usually with high dose. Use together cautiously.
Epinephrine, norepinephrine: increase hypertensive effect. Use with caution.
Barbiturates: decrease TCA blood levels. Monitor for decreased antidepressant effect.
Methylphenidate: increases TCA blood levels. Monitor for enhanced antidepressant effect.
Cimetidine: may increase protriptyline serum levels. Monitor for increased adverse effects.

NURSING CONSIDERATIONS
• Contraindicated during acute recovery phase of myocardial infarction, in patients with prostatic hypertrophy, and in patients with history of seizure disorders. Use with caution in elderly patients and in those with cardiovascular disease, urinary retention, increased intraocular tension, thyroid disease, or blood dyscrasias; in suicide risks; and in those receiving electroshock therapy, thyroid medication, or elective surgery.
• Reduce dose in elderly or debilitated persons, and adolescents.
• Do not withdraw abruptly.
• Watch for increased psychotic signs, anxiety, agitation, or cardiovascular reactions; dose should be reduced if they occur. Chart mood changes. Watch for suicidal tendencies. To lessen suicide risk, allow minimum supply of tablets.
• Check for urinary retention and constipation. Increase fluids to lessen constipation. Suggest stool softener, if needed.
• Warn patient to avoid activities that require alertness and good psychomotor coordination until CNS response to drug is determined. Drowsiness

and dizziness usually subside after a few weeks.
- Dry mouth may be relieved with sugarless hard candy or gum.
- Expect time lag of 7 to 14 days before effect is noticeable.
- Drug is possibly the most rapid-acting but least sedating tricyclic antidepressant. May even have an amphetamine-like effect. Avoid combining with alcohol or other depressants.
- Do not give entire dose at bedtime as patient may develop insomnia.
- Advise patient not to use other drugs (prescription or over-the-counter) without first consulting the doctor.
- Used investigationally to treat obstructive sleep apnea.

---

tranylcypromine sulfate
Parnate♦
Pregnancy Category: C

MECHANISM OF ACTION
Promotes accumulation of neurotransmitters by inhibiting monoamine oxidase.

INDICATIONS & DOSAGE
Treatment of depression—
Adults: 10 mg P.O. b.i.d. Increase to maximum 30 mg daily, if necessary, after 2 weeks. Not recommended for children under 16 years.

ADVERSE REACTIONS
CNS: *dizziness,* vertigo, headache, overactivity, hyperreflexia, tremors, muscle twitching, mania, jitters, confusion, memory impairment, fatigue.
CV: *orthostatic hypotension,* arrhythmias, paradoxical hypertension.
EENT: blurred vision.
GI: dry mouth, *anorexia,* nausea, diarrhea, constipation, abdominal pain.
GU: changed libido, impotence.
Skin: rash.
Other: peripheral edema, sweating, weight changes, chills.

INTERACTIONS
Amphetamines, ephedrine, levodopa, meperidine, metaraminol, methotrimeprazine, methylphenidate, phenylephrine, phenylpropanolamine: pressor effects of these drugs are enhanced by tranylcypromine. Use together cautiously.
Alcohol, barbiturates, and other sedatives; narcotics; dextromethorphan; tricyclic antidepressants: use with caution and in reduced dosage.

NURSING CONSIDERATIONS
- Contraindicated in patients with severe hepatic or renal impairment; congestive heart failure; pheochromocytoma, hypertension, or cardiovascular or cerebrovascular disease; severe or frequent headaches; in patients taking antihypertensive drugs or diuretics; in elderly or debilitated patients; in patients for whom close supervision is not possible; and in hyperactive, agitated, or schizophrenic patients. Also contraindicated with foods containing tryptophan or tyramine. Also contraindicated during therapy with other MAO inhibitors (including pargyline HCl, phenelzine sulfate, isocarboxazid) or within 7 days of such therapy; within 7 days of elective surgery requiring general anesthetic, cocaine, or local anesthetic containing sympathomimetic vasoconstrictors. Use cautiously with anti-Parkinson drugs, spinal anesthetic; in renal disease, diabetes, epilepsy, hyperthyroidism; and in suicide risks.
- MAO inhibitor most often reported to cause hypertensive crisis in presence of high-tyramine ingestion. Generally less effective than a tricyclic antidepressant. Avoid combining with alcohol or other depressants.
- Use only when TCA or electroshock therapy is ineffective or contraindicated.
- If patient develops symptoms of

Italicized side effects are common or life-threatening.
*Liquid form contains alcohol.   **May contain tartrazine.

overdose (palpitations, severe ortho-static hypotension), hold dose and no-tify doctor.
• Watch for suicidal tendencies.
• Dose is usually reduced to mainte-nance level as soon as possible.
• Do not withdraw drug abruptly.
• Have phentolamine (Regitine) available to counteract severe hyper-tension.
• Warn patient to avoid foods high in tyramine or tryptophan (aged cheese, Chianti wine, beer, avocados, chicken livers, chocolate, bananas, soy sauce, meat tenderizers, salami, bologna) and self-medication with over-the-counter cold, hay fever, or reducing preparations.
• Tell patient to get out of bed slowly, sitting up for 1 minute.
• Continue precautions for 7 days af-ter stopping drug; effects last that long.
• Expect time lag of 1 to 3 weeks be-fore effect is noticeable.
• More rapid onset of action than iso-carboxazid or phenelzine sulfate.
• Obtain baseline blood pressure readings, CBC, and liver function tests before beginning therapy, and continue to monitor throughout treat-ment.

trazodone hydrochloride
Desyrel♦
Pregnancy Category: C

MECHANISM OF ACTION
Inhibits serotonin uptake in the brain.

INDICATIONS & DOSAGE
Treatment of depression—
Adults: Initial dosage is 150 mg daily in divided doses, which can be in-creased by 50 mg per day q 3 to 4 days. Average dose ranges from 150 mg to 400 mg daily. Maximum dose 600 mg.

ADVERSE REACTIONS
CNS: *drowsiness, dizziness,* nervous-ness, fatigue, confusion, tremors, weakness.
CV: orthostatic hypotension, tachy-cardia.
EENT: blurred vision, tinnitus.
GI: dry mouth, constipation, nausea, vomiting, anorexia.
GU: urinary retention, priapism pos-sibly leading to impotence.
Skin: rash, urticaria.
Other: sweating.

INTERACTIONS
Antihypertensives: added hypotensive effect of trazodone. Dose of antihy-pertensive drug may have to be de-creased.
MAO inhibitors: No clinical experi-ence. Use together very cautiously.

NURSING CONSIDERATIONS
• Should not be used during initial re-covery phase of myocardial infarc-tion. Avoid concurrent administration with electroshock therapy.
• Use cautiously in patients with pre-existing cardiac disease.
• Priapism may be more common than first suspected in males taking trazodone. Be sure to note if patient complains of prolonged and painful erections.
• Watch for suicidal tendencies and chart mood changes. Allow minimum amount of tablets to lessen suicide risk.
• Warn patient to avoid activities that require alertness and good psychomo-tor coordination until CNS response to drug is determined. Drowsiness and dizziness usually subside after the first few weeks.
• Administer after meals or a light snack for optimal absorption and to decrease incidence of dizziness.
• Not chemically related to tricyclic antidepressants or MAO inhibitors.
• Anticholinergic and adverse cardiac effects are minimal.

• Expect similar lag time as with tricyclic antidepressants. Expect lag time of up to 10 to 14 days before noticeable effect. Full effect appears in 30 days.
• Avoid combining with alcohol or other depressants.

trimipramine maleate
Surmontil♦
Pregnancy Category: C

MECHANISM OF ACTION
Increases the amount of norepinephrine or serotonin, or both, in the central nervous system by blocking their reuptake by the presynaptic neurons. This action allows these neurotransmitters to accumulate.

INDICATIONS & DOSAGE
Treatment of depression—
Adults: 75 mg daily in divided doses, increased to 200 mg per day. Dosages over 300 mg per day not recommended.
Enuresis—
Children over 6 years: initial dose 25 mg P.O. 1 hour before bedtime; if no response, increase dose to 50 mg in children under 12 years, and to 75 mg in children over 12 years.

ADVERSE REACTIONS
CNS: *drowsiness, dizziness,* excitation, seizures, tremors, weakness, confusion, headache, nervousness.
CV: *orthostatic hypotension, tachycardia, EKG changes,* hypertension.
EENT: *blurred vision,* tinnitus, mydriasis.
GI: *dry mouth, constipation,* nausea, vomiting, anorexia, paralytic ileus.
GU: *urinary retention.*
Skin: rash, urticaria.
Other: *sweating,* allergy.
After abrupt withdrawal of long-term therapy: nausea, headache, malaise. (Does not indicate addiction.)

INTERACTIONS
MAO inhibitors: may cause severe excitation, hyperpyrexia, convulsions, usually with high dose. Use together cautiously.
Epinephrine, norepinephrine: increase hypertensive effect. Use with caution.
Barbiturates: decrease TCA blood levels. Monitor for decreased antidepressant effect.
Methylphenidate: increases TCA blood levels. Monitor for enhanced antidepressant effects.
Cimetidine: may increase trimipramine serum levels. Monitor for increased adverse effects.

NURSING CONSIDERATIONS
• Contraindicated during acute recovery phase of myocardial infarction, in patients with prostatic hypertrophy, and in patients with history of seizure disorders. Use with extreme caution in patients with cardiovascular disease, urinary retention, narrow-angle glaucoma or increased intraocular pressure, thyroid disease, blood dyscrasias, or impaired hepatic function. Also contraindicated in patients who are suicide risks and in those receiving electroshock therapy, thyroid medicaton, or elective surgery.
• Reduce dose in elderly or debilitated persons, and adolescents.
• Do not withdraw abruptly.
• Watch for increased psychotic signs; dose should be reduced if they occur. Chart mood changes. Watch for suicidal tendencies. Allow only minimum supply of tablets to lessen suicide risk.
• Check for urinary retention and constipation. Increase fluids to lessen constipation. Suggest stool softener, if necessary.
• Warn patient to avoid activities that require alertness and good psychomotor coordination until CNS response to drug has been determined. Drowsiness and dizziness usually subside af-

---

Italicized side effects are common or life-threatening.
*Liquid form contains alcohol.   **May contain tartrazine.

ter a few weeks.

• Don't combine with alcohol or other depressants.

• Expect time lag of 10 to 14 days before noticeable effect. Full effect usually appears in 30 days.

• Dry mouth may be relieved with sugarless hard candy or gum.

• Effectiveness in enuresis may decrease over time. Similar in anticholinergic effects to other tricyclic antidepressants.

• Advise patient not to use other drugs (prescription or over-the-counter) without first consulting the doctor.

• Whenever possible, patient should take full dose at bedtime.

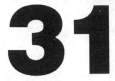

Antianxiety agents

alprazolam
buspirone hydrochloride
chlordiazepoxide hydrochloride
clorazepate dipotassium
diazepam
halazepam
hydroxyzine hydrochloride
hydroxyzine pamoate
lorazepam
meprobamate
oxazepam
prazepam

COMBINATION PRODUCTS
DEPROL**: meprobamate 400 mg and
benactyzine HCl 1 mg.
EQUAGESIC: meprobamate 200 mg
and aspirin 325 mg.
LIBRAX CAPSULES: chlordiazepoxide
hydrochloride 5 mg and clidinium
bromide 2.5 mg.
LIMBITROL 5-12.5: chlordiazepoxide
5 mg and amitriptyline (as HCl) 12.5
mg.
LIMBITROL 10-25: chlordiazepoxide
10 mg and amitriptyline (as HCl) 25
mg.
MENRIUM 5-2: chlordiazepoxide 5 mg
and esterified estrogens 0.2 mg.
MENRIUM 5-4: chlordiazepoxide 5 mg
and esterified estrogens 0.4 mg.
MENRIUM 10-4: chlordiazepoxide
10 mg and esterified estrogens 0.4
mg.
MILPREM-200: meprobamate 200 mg
and conjugated estrogens 0.45 mg.
MILPREM-400: meprobamate 400 mg
and conjugated estrogens 0.45 mg.
PMB 200: meprobamate 200 mg and
conjugated estrogens 0.45 mg.
PMB 400: meprobamate 400 mg and
conjugated estrogens 0.45 mg.

alprazolam
Controlled Substance Schedule IV
Xanax♦
Pregnancy Category: D

MECHANISM OF ACTION
Depresses the CNS at the limbic and
subcortical levels of the brain.

INDICATIONS & DOSAGE
Anxiety and tension—
Adults: Usual starting dose is 0.25 to
0.5 mg t.i.d. Maximum total daily
dosage is 4 mg in divided doses. In elderly or debilitated patients, usual
starting dose is 0.25 mg b.i.d. or
t.i.d.

ADVERSE REACTIONS
CNS: *drowsiness, light-headedness,*
headache, confusion, hostility.
CV: transient hypotension.
EENT: dry mouth.
GI: nausea, vomiting, discomfort.

INTERACTIONS
Cimetidine: increased sedation. Monitor carefully.

NURSING CONSIDERATIONS
• Contraindicated in acute narrow-
angle glaucoma, psychoses, and anxiety-free psychiatric disorders.
• Reduce dosage in elderly or debilitated patients.
• Do not withdraw drug abruptly.
Abuse or addiction is possible. Withdrawal symptoms may occur.

Italicized side effects are common or life-threatening.
*Liquid form contains alcohol.   **May contain tartrazine.

- Warn patient not to combine drug with alcohol or other depressants, and also to avoid activities that require alertness and psychomotor coordination until response to drug is determined.
- Caution patient against giving medication to others.
- Drug should not be prescribed for everyday stress.
- Drug is not for long-term use (more than 4 months).
- Warn patient not to continue drug without doctor's approval.
- Alprazolam is the first of a new type of benzodiazepine, known as a triazolo-benzodiazepine. It's more rapidly metabolized and excreted than most of the other drugs in the benzodiazepine class and has a lower incidence of lethargy than other drugs of this class.
- May also be effective for treatment of depression.

buspirone hydrochloride
Buspar
Pregnancy Category: B

MECHANISM OF ACTION
Unknown. However, the drug may inhibit neuronal firing and reduce 5-HT turnover in cortical, amygdaloid, and septohippocampal tissue.

INDICATIONS & DOSAGE
Management of anxiety disorders; short-term relief of anxiety—
Adults: initially, 5 mg P.O. t.i.d. Dosage may be increased at 3-day intervals. Usual maintenance dosage is 20 to 30 mg daily in divided doses.

ADVERSE REACTIONS
CNS: *dizziness, drowsiness,* nervousness, insomnia, headache.
GI: nausea, dry mouth, diarrhea.
Other: fatigue.

INTERACTIONS
None reported.

NURSING CONSIDERATIONS
- Although buspirone is less sedating than other anxiolytics and does not produce any serious functional impairment, CNS effects in an individual patient may be unpredictable. Therefore, warn patients to avoid hazardous activities that require alertness and neuromuscular coordination until their CNS response to this drug has been determined.
- Unlike the benzodiazepines, buspirone is not an effective anticonvulsant or skeletal muscle relaxant. Its use is limited to the treatment of anxiety.
- Advise patient to take the drug with food.
- Before initiating buspirone therapy in patients already being treated with benzodiazepines, warn them against stopping the benzodiazepine abruptly. Abrupt discontinuation may cause a benzodiazepine withdrawal reaction.
- Signs of improvement with buspirone are usually evident within 7 to 10 days; optimal results are achieved after 3 to 4 weeks of therapy.
- This drug has shown no potential for abuse and has not been classified as a controlled substance.

chlordiazepoxide hydrochloride
Controlled Substance Schedule IV
A-poxide, C-Tran♦♦, J-Liberty, Libritabs, Librium♦, Medilium♦♦, Novopoxide♦♦, Relaxil♦♦, SK-Lygen, Solium♦♦
Pregnancy Category: D

MECHANISM OF ACTION
Depresses the CNS at the limbic and subcortical levels of the brain.

INDICATIONS & DOSAGE
Mild to moderate anxiety and tension—

Adults: 5 to 10 mg t.i.d. or q.i.d.
Children over 6 years: 5 mg P.O.
b.i.d. to q.i.d. Maximum 10 mg P.O.
b.i.d. to t.i.d.
Severe anxiety and tension—
Adults: 20 to 25 mg t.i.d. or q.i.d.
Withdrawal symptoms of acute alcoholism—
Adults: 50 to 100 mg P.O., I.M., or
I.V. Maximum 300 mg daily.
Preoperative apprehension and anxiety—
Adults: 5 to 10 mg P.O. t.i.d. or
q.i.d. on day preceding surgery; or 50
to 100 mg I.M. 1 hour before surgery.
Note: parenteral form not recommended in children under 12 years.

ADVERSE REACTIONS
CNS: *drowsiness, lethargy, hangover,*
fainting.
CV: transient hypotension.
GI: nausea, vomiting, abdominal discomfort.
Local: *pain at injection site.*

INTERACTIONS
Cimetidine: increased sedation. Monitor carefully.

NURSING CONSIDERATIONS
• Use with caution in patients with
mental depression, blood dyscrasias,
hepatic or renal disease, or in those
undergoing anticoagulant therapy.
• Dosage should be reduced in elderly or debilitated patients.
• Possibility of abuse and addiction.
Do not withdraw drug abruptly; withdrawal symptoms may occur.
• Warn patient to avoid activities that
require alertness and good psychomotor coordination until CNS response
to drug is determined.
• Warn patient not to combine drug
with alcohol or other depressants.
• Although package recommends
I.M. use only, this drug may be given
I.V.
• Injectable form (as hydrochloride)
comes as two ampuls—diluent and

powdered drug. Read directions carefully. For I.M., add 2 ml of diluent to
powder and agitate gently until clear.
Use immediately. I.M. form may be
erratically absorbed.
• For I.V., use 5 ml of saline injection
or sterile water for injection as diluent; do not give packaged diluent I.V.
Give slowly over 1 minute.
• Keep powder away from light; mix
just before use; discard remainder.
• Do not mix injectable form with
any other parenteral drug.
• Caution patient against giving medication to others.
• Drug should not be prescribed regularly for everyday stress.

clorazepate dipotassium
Controlled Substance Schedule IV
Tranxene♦
Pregnancy Category: C

MECHANISM OF ACTION
Depresses the CNS at the limbic and
subcortical levels of the brain. As an
anticonvulsant, suppresses the spread
of seizure activity produced by epileptogenic foci in the cortex, thalamus, and limbic structures.

INDICATIONS & DOSAGE
Acute alcohol withdrawal—
Adults: Day 1—30 mg P.O. initially,
followed by 30 to 60 mg P.O. in divided doses; Day 2—45 to 90 mg P.O.
in divided doses; Day 3—22.5 to 45
mg P.O. in divided doses; Day 4—15
to 30 mg P.O. in divided doses; gradually reduce daily dose to 7.5 to 15
mg.
Anxiety—
Adults: 15 to 60 mg P.O. daily.
As an adjunct in epilepsy—
Adults and children over 12 years:
Maximum recommended initial dosage is 7.5 mg P.O. t.i.d. Dosage increases should be no greater than 7.5
mg/week. Maximum daily dosage
should not exceed 90 mg daily.

Italicized side effects are common or life-threatening.
*Liquid form contains alcohol.   **May contain tartrazine.

Children between 9 and 12 years:
Maximum recommended initial dosage is 7.5 mg P.O. b.i.d. Dosage increases should be no greater than 7.5 mg/week. Maximum daily dosage should not exceed 60 mg/day.

ADVERSE REACTIONS
CNS: *drowsiness, lethargy, hangover,* fainting.
CV: transient hypotension.
GI: nausea, vomiting, abdominal discomfort.

INTERACTIONS
Cimetidine: increased sedation. Monitor carefully.

NURSING CONSIDERATIONS
• Contraindicated in patients with acute narrow-angle glaucoma, depressive neuroses, psychotic reactions, and in children under 18 years. Use with caution when hepatic or renal damage is present.
• Dosage should be reduced in elderly or debilitated patients.
• Possibility of abuse and addiction exists. Do not withdraw drug abruptly; withdrawal symptoms may occur.
• Warn patient to avoid activities requiring alertness and good psychomotor coordination until CNS response to drug is determined.
• Warn patient not to combine drug with alcohol or other depressants.
• Suggest sugarless chewing gum or hard candy to relieve dry mouth.
• Caution patient against giving medication to others.
• Drug should not be prescribed regularly for everyday stress.

diazepam
Controlled Substance Schedule IV
D-Tran♦♦, E-Pam♦♦, Meval♦♦,
Novodipam♦♦, Stress-Pam♦♦,
Valium♦, Valrelease, Vivol♦♦
Pregnancy Category: D

MECHANISM OF ACTION
Depresses the CNS at the limbic and subcortical levels of the brain. As an anticonvulsant, suppresses the spread of seizure activity produced by epileptogenic foci in the cortex, thalamus, and limbic structures.

INDICATIONS & DOSAGE
Tension, anxiety, adjunct in convulsive disorders or skeletal muscle spasm—
Adults: 2 to 10 mg P.O. t.i.d. or q.i.d. Or, 15 to 30 mg of extended-release capsule once daily.
Children over 6 months: 1 to 2.5 mg P.O. t.i.d. or q.i.d.
Tension, anxiety, muscle spasm, endoscopic procedures, seizures—
Adults: 5 to 10 mg I.V. initially, up to 30 mg in 1 hour or possibly more for cardioversion or status epilepticus, depending on response.
Children 5 years and older: 1 mg I.V. or I.M. slowly q 2 to 5 minutes to maximum 10 mg. Repeat q 2 to 4 hours.
Children 30 days to 5 years: 0.2 to 0.5 mg I.V. or I.M. slowly q 2 to 5 minutes to maximum 5 mg. Repeat q 2 to 4 hours.
Tetanic muscle spasms—
Children over 5 years: 5 to 10 mg I.M. or I.V. q 3 to 4 hours, p.r.n.
Infants over 30 days: 1 to 2 mg I.M. or I.V. q 3 to 4 hours, p.r.n.
Status epilepticus—
Adults: 5 to 20 mg slow I.V. push 2 to 5 mg/minute; may repeat q 5 to 10 minutes up to maximum total dose of 60 mg. Use 2 to 5 mg in elderly or debilitated patients. May repeat therapy in 20 to 30 minutes with caution if

seizures recur.
Children: 0.1 to 0.3 mg/kg slow I.V. push (1 mg/minute over 3 minutes). May repeat q 15 minutes for 2 doses. Maximum single dose: children under 5 years— 5 mg; children over 5 years—10 mg.
Adjunctive use in convulsive disorders—
Adults and children: 2 to 10 mg P.O. b.i.d. to q.i.d. Or 15 to 30 mg of extended-release capsule once daily.

ADVERSE REACTIONS

CNS: *drowsiness, lethargy, hangover, ataxia,* fainting, slurred speech, tremor.
CV: transient hypotension, bradycardia, *cardiovascular collapse.*
EENT: diplopia, blurred vision, nystagmus.
GI: nausea, vomiting, abdominal discomfort.
Skin: rash, urticaria.
Local: desquamation, *pain, phlebitis at injection site.*
Other: respiratory depression.

INTERACTIONS

Cimetidine: increased sedation. Monitor carefully.
Phenobarbital: increased effects of both drugs. Use together cautiously.

NURSING CONSIDERATIONS

• Contraindicated in shock, coma, acute alcohol intoxication, acute narrow-angle glaucoma, psychoses, myasthenia gravis; in oral form for children under 6 months. Use with caution in patients with blood dyscrasias, hepatic or renal damage, depression, open-angle glaucoma; in elderly and debilitated patients; and in those with limited pulmonary reserve.
• Dosage should be reduced in elderly or debilitated patients.
• Possibility of abuse and addiction exists. Do not withdraw drug abruptly; withdrawal symptoms may occur.

• Warn patient to avoid activities that require alertness and good psychomotor coordination until CNS response to drug is determined.
• Warn patient not to combine drug with alcohol or other depressants.
• Do not dilute with solutions or mix with other drugs: incompatible.
• Avoid extravasation. Do not inject into small veins.
• Watch daily for phlebitis at injection site.
• Give I.V. slowly, at rate not exceeding 5 mg per minute. When injecting I.V., best to administer directly into the vein. If this is not possible, inject slowly through the infusion tubing as close as possible to the vein insertion site.
• Monitor respirations every 5 to 15 minutes and before each I.V.-repeated dose. Have emergency resuscitative equipment and oxygen at bedside. Note that naloxone does not reverse the respiratory depression produced by diazepam.
• I.V. route is more reliable; I.M. administration is not recommended because absorption is variable and injection is painful (because the solution is highly alkaline).
• Drug of choice (I.V. form) for status epilepticus.
• Seizures may recur within 20 to 30 minutes of initial control, because of redistribution of the drug.
• Continuous infusions of 1 to 10 mg hourly have been used to prevent seizure recurrence.
• Do not store diazepam in plastic syringes.
• Caution patient against giving medication to others.
• Drug should not be prescribed regularly for everyday stress.

Italicized side effects are common or life-threatening.
*Liquid form contains alcohol.   **May contain tartrazine.

halazepam
Controlled Substance Schedule IV
Paxipam
Pregnancy Category: D

MECHANISM OF ACTION
Depresses the CNS at the limbic and subcortical levels of the brain.

INDICATIONS & DOSAGE
Relief of anxiety and tension—
Adults: Usual dose is 20 to 40 mg P.O. t.i.d. or q.i.d.
Optimal daily dosage is generally 80 to 160 mg. Daily doses up to 600 mg have been given. In elderly or debilitated patients, initial dosage is 20 mg once or twice daily.

ADVERSE REACTIONS
CNS: *drowsiness, lethargy, hangover,* fainting.
CV: transient hypotension.
EENT: dry mouth.
GI: nausea and vomiting, discomfort.

INTERACTIONS
Cimetidine: possible increased sedation. Monitor carefully.

NURSING CONSIDERATIONS
• Contraindicated in acute narrow-angle glaucoma, psychoses, and anxiety-free psychiatric disorders. Use with caution in hepatorenal impairment.
• Reduce dosage in elderly or debilitated patients.
• Do not withdraw drug abruptly.
• Abuse and addiction are possible. Withdrawal symptoms may occur.
• Warn patient not to combine drug with alcohol or other depressants, and also to avoid activities that require alertness and psychomotor coordination until response to drug is determined.
• Caution patient against giving medication to others.
• Drug should not be prescribed for everyday stress.
• Halazepam is not for long-term use (more than 4 months).

hydroxyzine hydrochloride
Atarax♦*, Durrax, Hyzine-50, Orgatrax, Quiess, Vistaril (parenteral)

hydroxyzine pamoate
Vistaril (oral)
Pregnancy Category: C

MECHANISM OF ACTION
Depresses the CNS at the limbic and subcortical levels of the brain.

INDICATIONS & DOSAGE
Anxiety and tension—
Adults: 25 to 100 mg P.O. t.i.d. or q.i.d.
Anxiety, tension, hyperkinesia—
Children over 6 years: 50 to 100 mg P.O. daily in divided doses.
Children under 6 years: 50 mg P.O. daily in divided doses.
Preoperative and postoperative adjunctive therapy—
Adults: 25 to 100 mg I.M. q 4 to 6 hours.
Children: 1.1 mg/kg I.M. q 4 to 6 hours.

ADVERSE REACTIONS
CNS: *drowsiness,* involuntary motor activity.
GI: *dry mouth.*
Local: marked discomfort at site of I.M. injection.

INTERACTIONS
None significant.

NURSING CONSIDERATIONS
• Contraindicated in patients in shock or comatose states.
• Dosage should be reduced in elderly or debilitated patients.
• Warn patient to avoid activities that require alertness and good psychomo-

tor coordination until CNS response to drug is determined.
• Warn patient not to combine drug with alcohol or other depressants.
• Observe for excessive sedation due to potentiation with other CNS drugs.
• Used as an antiemetic and antianxiety drug.
• Used in psychogenically induced allergic conditions, such as chronic urticaria and pruritus.
• Parenteral form (hydroxyzine HCl) for I.M. use only, never I.V. "Z-track" injection is preferred.
• Aspirate injection carefully to prevent inadvertent intravascular injection. Inject deep into a large muscle.
• Suggest sugarless hard candy or gum to relieve dry mouth.

lorazepam
Controlled Substance Schedule IV
Ativan♦
Pregnancy Category: D

MECHANISM OF ACTION
Depresses the CNS at the limbic and subcortical levels of the brain.

INDICATIONS & DOSAGE
Anxiety, tension, agitation, irritability, especially in anxiety neuroses or organic (especially GI or CV) disorders—
Adults: 2 to 6 mg P.O. daily in divided doses. Maximum 10 mg daily.
Insomnia—
Adults: 2 to 4 mg P.O. h.s.
Premedication before operative procedure—
Adults: 2 to 4 mg I.M. or I.V.

ADVERSE REACTIONS
CNS: *drowsiness, lethargy, hangover,* fainting.
CV: transient hypotension.
GI: abdominal discomfort.

INTERACTIONS
None significant.

NURSING CONSIDERATIONS
• Contraindicated in acute narrow-angle glaucoma, psychoses, mental depression. Use with caution in organic brain syndrome, myasthenia gravis, renal or hepatic impairment.
• Dosage should be reduced in elderly or debilitated patients.
• Possibility of abuse and addiction exists. Do not withdraw drug abruptly: withdrawal symptoms may occur.
• When administering I.M., inject deep into muscle mass. Don't dilute.
• When administering I.V., dilute with an equal volume of sterile water for injection, sodium chloride injection, or dextrose 5% injection.
• Warn patient to avoid activities that require alertness or good psychomotor coordination until CNS response to drug is determined.
• Warn patient not to combine drug with alcohol or other depressants.
• Caution patient against giving medication to others.
• Drug should not be prescribed regularly for everyday stress.
• Fewer cumulative effects than other benzodiazepines, due to short half-life.
• Store parenteral form in refrigerator to prolong shelf life.

meprobamate
Controlled Substance Schedule IV
Arcoban, Equanil♦**, Kalmm, Maso-Bamate, Meditran♦, Mep-E, Meprocon, Meprotabs, Meribam, Miltown♦, Neo-Tran♦♦, Novomepro♦♦, Pax-400, Saronil, Sedabamate, Tranmep
Pregnancy Category: D

MECHANISM OF ACTION
Depresses the CNS at the limbic and subcortical levels of the brain.

INDICATIONS & DOSAGE
Anxiety and tension—

Italicized side effects are common or life-threatening.
*Liquid form contains alcohol.   **May contain tartrazine.

Adults: 1.2 to 1.6 g P.O. in 3 or 4 equally divided doses. Maximum 2.4 g daily.
Children 6 to 12 years: 100 to 200 mg P.O. b.i.d. or t.i.d. Not recommended for children under 6 years.

ADVERSE REACTIONS
Blood: *thrombocytopenia, leukopenia,* eosinophilia.
CNS: *drowsiness,* ataxia, dizziness, slurred speech, headache, vertigo.
CV: palpitation, tachycardia, hypotension.
GI: anorexia, nausea, vomiting, diarrhea, stomatitis.
Skin: pruritus, urticaria, erythematous maculopapular rash.

INTERACTIONS
None significant.

NURSING CONSIDERATIONS
• Contraindicated in patients with hypersensitivity to meprobamate, carisoprodol, mebutamate, tybamate, carbromal; and in those with renal insufficiency or porphyria. Use with caution in patients with impaired hepatic or renal function and in patients with suicidal tendencies.
• Dosage should be reduced in elderly or debilitated patients.
• Possibility of abuse and addiction exists. Withdraw drug gradually (over 2 weeks) or withdrawal symptoms may occur, including severe grand mal seizures.
• Warn patient to avoid activities that require alertness or good psychomotor coordination until CNS response to drug is determined.
• Warn patient not to combine drug with alcohol or other depressants.
• Give I.M. deep into muscle.
• Give P.O. with meals to reduce gastric distress.
• Therapeutic blood levels 0.5 to 2 mg/100 ml; levels above 20 mg/100 ml may cause coma and death.
• Periodic evaluation of CBC and liver function tests are indicated in patients receiving high doses.

---

oxazepam
Controlled Substance Schedule IV
Serax♦**
Pregnancy Category: C

MECHANISM OF ACTION
Depresses the CNS at the limbic and subcortical levels of the brain.

INDICATIONS & DOSAGE
Alcohol withdrawal—
Adults: 15 to 30 mg P.O. t.i.d. or q.i.d.
Severe anxiety—
Adults: 15 to 30 mg P.O. t.i.d. or q.i.d.
Tension, mild to moderate anxiety—
Adults: 10 to 15 mg P.O. t.i.d. or q.i.d.

ADVERSE REACTIONS
CNS: *drowsiness, lethargy, hangover,* fainting.
CV: transient hypotension.
GI: nausea, vomiting, abdominal discomfort.

INTERACTIONS
None significant.

NURSING CONSIDERATIONS
• Contraindicated in psychoses. Use cautiously in patients with history of convulsive disorders, drug allergies, blood dyscrasias, renal disease, depression.
• Dose should be reduced in elderly or debilitated patients.
• Possibility of abuse and addiction exists. Don't stop drug abruptly; withdrawal symptoms may occur.
• Warn patient to avoid activities that require alertness or good psychomotor coordination until CNS response to drug is determined.
• Warn patient not to combine drug with alcohol or other depressants.

- Fewer cumulative effects than many other benzodiazepines due to short half-life.
- Caution patient against giving medication to others.
- Not for everyday stress.

with alcohol or other depressants.
- Caution patient against giving medication to others.
- Not for everyday stress.

prazepam
Controlled Substance Schedule IV
Centrax
Pregnancy Category: C

MECHANISM OF ACTION
Depresses the CNS at the limbic and subcortical levels of the brain.

INDICATIONS & DOSAGE
Anxiety—
Adults: 30 mg P.O. in divided doses. Range 20 to 60 mg daily. May be administered as single daily dose at bedtime. Start with 20 mg.

ADVERSE REACTIONS
CNS: *drowsiness, lethargy, hangover,* fainting.
CV: transient hypotension.
GI: nausea, vomiting, abdominal discomfort.

INTERACTIONS
Cimetidine: increased sedation. Monitor carefully.

NURSING CONSIDERATIONS
- Contraindicated in patients with acute narrow-angle glaucoma, psychoses, and psychiatric disorders not showing anxiety. Use with caution in renal or hepatic impairment.
- Dosage should be reduced in elderly or debilitated patients.
- Possibility of abuse and addiction exists. Don't stop drug abruptly: withdrawal symptoms may occur.
- Warn patient to avoid activities that require alertness and good psychomotor coordination until CNS response to drug is determined.
- Warn patient not to combine drug

Italicized side effects are common or life-threatening.
*Liquid form contains alcohol.   **May contain tartrazine.

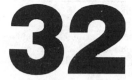

Antipsychotics

acetophenazine maleate
chlorpromazine hydrochloride
chlorprothixene
fluphenazine decanoate
fluphenazine enanthate
fluphenazine hydrochloride
haloperidol
haloperidol decanoate
loxapine succinate
mesoridazine besylate
molindone hydrochloride
perphenazine
pimozide
promazine hydrochloride
thioridazine hydrochloride
thiothixene
thiothixene hydrochloride
trifluoperazine hydrochloride
triflupromazine hydrochloride

COMBINATION PRODUCTS

ETRAFON 2-10: perphenazine 2 mg
and amitriptyline HCl 10 mg.
ETRAFON-A: perphenazine 2 mg and
amitriptyline HCl 25 mg.
ETRAFON-FORTE: perphenazine 4 mg
and amitriptyline HCl 25 mg.
TRIAVIL 2-10, TRIAVIL 4-10, TRIAVIL
2-25 are identical to Etrafon products
above; TRIAVIL 4-50: perphenazine 4
mg and amitriptyline HCl 50 mg.

acetophenazine maleate
Tindal
Pregnancy Category: C

MECHANISM OF ACTION
Blocks postsynaptic dopamine receptors in the brain. Piperazine phenothiazine.

INDICATIONS & DOSAGE
Psychotic disorders—
Adults: initially, 20 mg P.O. t.i.d. or
q.i.d. Daily dosage ranges from 40 to
80 mg in outpatients, or 80 to 120 mg
in hospitalized patients, but in severe
psychotic states up to 600 mg daily
has been safely administered. Smallest effective dose should be used at all
times.

ADVERSE REACTIONS
Blood: *transient leukopenia, agranulocytosis.*
CNS: *extrapyramidal reactions (high
incidence), tardive dyskinesia,* sedation (low incidence), pseudoparkinsonism, EEG changes, dizziness.
CV: *orthostatic hypotension,* tachycardia, EKG changes.
EENT: *ocular changes, blurred vision.*
GI: *dry mouth, constipation.*
GU: *urinary retention,* dark urine,
menstrual irregularities, gynecomastia, inhibited ejaculation.
Hepatic: *cholestatic jaundice, abnormal liver function tests.*
Metabolic: hyperprolactinemia.
Skin: *mild photosensitivity,* dermal
allergic reactions.
Other: weight gain, increased appetite.
**After abrupt withdrawal of long-
term therapy:** gastritis, nausea, vomiting, dizziness, tremors, feeling of
warmth or cold, sweating, tachycardia, headache, insomnia.

INTERACTIONS
Antacids: inhibit absorption of oral

phenothiazines. Separate antacid and phenothiazine doses by at least 2 hours.
Barbiturates: may decrease phenothiazine effect. Observe patient.

NURSING CONSIDERATIONS
• Contraindicated in CNS depression, bone-marrow depression, subcortical damage, and coma; also with use of spinal or epidural anesthetic, or adrenergic blocking agents. Use cautiously with other CNS depressants, anticholinergics; in elderly or debilitated patients; and in patients with hepatic disease, arteriosclerosis or cardiovascular disease (may cause sudden drop in blood pressure), exposure to extreme heat or cold (including antipyretic therapy), respiratory disorders, hypocalcemia, convulsive disorders (may lower seizure threshold), severe reactions to insulin or electroshock therapy, suspected brain tumor or intestinal obstruction, glaucoma, or prostatic hypertrophy.
• Tardive dyskinesia may occur after prolonged use. It may not appear until months or years later and may disappear spontaneously or persist for life.
• Hold dose and notify doctor if patient develops symptoms of blood dyscrasias (fever, sore throat, infection, cellulitis, weakness), persistent (longer than a few hours) extrapyramidal reactions, or any such reaction during pregnancy.
• Dose of 20 mg is therapeutic equivalent of 100 mg chlorpromazine.
• Monitor therapy by weekly bilirubin tests during first month; periodic blood tests (CBC, liver function); and ophthalmic tests (long-term use).
• Check intake/output for urinary retention or constipation.
• Tell patient to use sunscreening agents and protective clothing to avoid photosensitivity reactions.
• Warn against activities requiring alertness or good psychomotor coordination until CNS response to drug is determined.
• Obtain baseline measures of blood pressure before starting therapy and monitor routinely. Watch for orthostatic hypotension. Advise patient to get up slowly.
• Dry mouth may be relieved with sugarless gum, sour hard candy, or rinsing with mouthwash.
• Avoid combining with alcohol or other depressants.
• Do not withdraw drug abruptly unless required by severe side effects.
• Patient on maintenance may take medication at bedtime to facilitate sleep and decrease sedation during daytime.

chlorpromazine hydrochloride
Chlor-Promanyl♦♦, Chlorzine, Klorazine, Largactil♦♦, Ormazine, Promachlor, Promapar, Promaz, Sonazine, Terpium, Thoradex, Thorazine
Pregnancy Category: C

MECHANISM OF ACTION
Blocks postsynaptic dopamine receptors in the brain. As an antiemetic, inhibits the medullary chemoreceptor trigger zone. Aliphatic phenothiazine.

INDICATIONS & DOSAGE
Intractable hiccups—
Adults: 25 to 50 mg P.O. or I.M. t.i.d. or q.i.d.
Mild alcohol withdrawal, acute intermittent porphyria, and tetanus—
Adults: 25 to 50 mg I.M. t.i.d. or q.i.d.
Psychosis—
Adults: 500 mg P.O. daily in divided doses, increasing gradually to 2 g; or 25 to 50 mg I.M. q 1 to 4 hours, p.r.n.
Children: 0.25 mg/kg P.O. q 4 to 6 hours; or 0.25 mg/kg I.M. q 6 to 8 hours; or 0.5 mg/kg rectally q 6 to 8 hours. Maximum dose is 40 mg in children under 5 years, and 75 mg in

---

Italicized side effects are common or life-threatening.
*Liquid form contains alcohol.   **May contain tartrazine.

children 5 to 12 years.
Nausea and vomiting—
Adults: 10 to 225 mg P.O. or I.M. q 4 to 6 hours, p.r.n.; or 50 to 100 mg rectally q 6 to 8 hours, p.r.n.
Children: 0.25 mg/kg P.O. q 4 to 6 hours; or 0.25 mg/kg I.M. q 6 to 8 hours; or 0.5 mg/kg rectally q 6 to 8 hours.

ADVERSE REACTIONS
Blood: *transient leukopenia, agranulocytosis.*
CNS: *extrapyramidal reactions (moderate incidence), sedation (high incidence), tardive dyskinesia,* pseudoparkinsonism, EEG changes, dizziness.
CV: *orthostatic hypotension,* tachycardia, EKG changes.
EENT: *ocular changes, blurred vision.*
GI: *dry mouth, constipation.*
GU: *urinary retention,* dark urine, menstrual irregularities, gynecomastia, inhibited ejaculation.
Hepatic: *cholestatic jaundice, abnormal liver function tests.*
Metabolic: hyperprolactinemia.
Skin: *mild photosensitivity,* dermal allergic reactions.
Local: pain on I.M. injection, sterile abscess.
Other: weight gain, increased appetite.
After abrupt withdrawal of long-term therapy: gastritis, nausea, vomiting, dizziness, tremors, feeling of warmth or cold, sweating, tachycardia, headache, insomnia.

INTERACTIONS
Antacids: inhibit absorption of oral phenothiazines. Separate antacid and phenothiazine doses by at least 2 hours.
Anticholinergics (including antidepressant and antiparkinson agents): increased anticholinergic activity, aggravated parkinson-like symptoms. Use with caution.

Barbiturates: may decrease phenothiazine effect. Observe patient.
Lithium: possible decreased response to chlorpromazine. Observe patient.

NURSING CONSIDERATIONS
• Contraindicated in CNS depression, bone-marrow depression, subcortical damage, Reye's syndrome, and coma; also contraindicated with use of spinal or epidural anesthetic, or adrenergic blocking agents. Use cautiously with other CNS depressants, anticholinergics; in elderly or debilitated patients; in patients with hepatic disease, arteriosclerosis or cardiovascular disease (may cause sudden drop in blood pressure), exposure to extreme heat or cold (including antipyretic therapy), respiratory disorders, hypocalcemia, convulsive disorders (may lower seizure threshold), severe reactions to insulin or electroshock therapy, suspected brain tumor or intestinal obstruction, glaucoma, or prostatic hypertrophy; and in acutely ill or dehydrated children.
• Tardive dyskinesia may occur after prolonged use. It may not appear until months or years later and may disappear spontaneously or persist for life.
• Hold dose and notify doctor if patient develops jaundice, symptoms of blood dyscrasias (fever, sore throat, infection, cellulitis, weakness), persistent (longer than a few hours) extrapyramidal reactions, or any such reaction in pregnancy or in children.
• Monitor therapy by weekly bilirubin tests during first month; periodic blood tests (CBC, liver function); and ophthalmic tests (long-term use).
• Check intake/output for urinary retention or constipation.
• Tell patient to use sunscreening agents and protective clothing to avoid photosensitivity reactions. Chlorpromazine causes higher incidence of photosensitivity than any other drug in its class.
• Warn against activities that require

alertness or good psychomotor coordination until CNS response to drug is determined. Drowsiness and dizziness usually subside after first few weeks.
• Obtain baseline measures of blood pressure before starting therapy and monitor regularly. Watch for orthostatic hypotension, especially with parenteral administration. Monitor blood pressure before and after I.M. administration. Keep patient supine for 1 hour afterward. Advise patient to get up slowly.
• Avoid combining with alcohol or other depressants.
• Also available as a rectal suppository.
• Give deep I.M. only in upper outer quadrant of buttocks. Massage slowly afterward to prevent sterile abscess. Injection stings.
• Liquid (oral) and parenteral forms of drug can cause contact dermatitis. If susceptible, wear gloves when preparing solutions of this drug, and prevent any contact with skin and clothing.
• Protect liquid concentrate from light. Dilute with fruit juice, milk, or semisolid food just before administration.
• Slight yellowing of injection or concentrate is common; does not affect potency. Discard markedly discolored solutions.
• Do not withdraw drug abruptly unless required by severe side effects.
• Dry mouth may be relieved by sugarless gum, sour hard candy, or rinsing with mouthwash.

---

chlorprothixene
Taractan**, Tarasan♦♦
Pregnancy Category: C

MECHANISM OF ACTION
Blocks postsynaptic dopamine receptors in the brain. A thioxanthene.

INDICATIONS & DOSAGE
Psychotic disorders—
Adults: initially, 10 mg P.O. t.i.d. or q.i.d. Increase gradually to maximum 600 mg daily.
Children over 6 years: 10 to 25 mg P.O. t.i.d. or q.i.d.
Agitation of severe neurosis, depression, schizophrenia—
Adults: 25 to 50 mg P.O. or I.M. t.i.d. or q.i.d. Increase as needed up to maximum 600 mg.

ADVERSE REACTIONS
Blood: *transient leukopenia, agranulocytosis.*
CNS: extrapyramidal reactions (low incidence), tardive dyskinesia, sedation, pseudoparkinsonism, EEG changes, dizziness.
CV: *orthostatic hypotension,* tachycardia, EKG changes.
EENT: *ocular changes, blurred vision.*
GI: *dry mouth, constipation.*
GU: *urinary retention,* dark urine, menstrual irregularities, gynecomastia, inhibited ejaculation.
Hepatic: *cholestatic jaundice, abnormal liver function tests.*
Metabolic: hyperprolactinemia.
Skin: *mild photosensitivity,* dermal allergic reactions.
Local: pain on I.M. injection, sterile abscess.
Other: weight gain, increased appetite.
After abrupt withdrawal of long-term therapy: gastritis, nausea, vomiting, dizziness, tremors, feeling of warmth or cold, sweating, tachycardia, headache, insomnia.

INTERACTIONS
None significant.

NURSING CONSIDERATIONS
• Contraindicated in coma, CNS depression, bone-marrow depression, circulatory collapse, congestive failure, cardiac decompensation, coro-

---

nary artery or cerebral vascular disorders, subcortical damage; with use of spinal or epidural anesthetic, or adrenergic blocking agents. Use cautiously with other CNS depressants, anticholinergics; in elderly or debilitated patients; in patients with hepatic or renal disease, arteriosclerosis or cardiovascular disease (may cause sudden drop in blood pressure), exposure to extreme heat or cold (including antipyretic therapy), respiratory disorders, hypocalcemia, convulsive disorders (may lower seizure threshold), severe reactions to insulin or electroshock therapy, suspected brain tumor or intestinal obstruction, glaucoma, or prostatic hypertrophy; and in acutely ill or dehydrated children.

• Tardive dyskinesia may occur after prolonged use. It may not appear until months or years later and may disappear spontaneously or persist for life.

• Hold dose and notify doctor if patient develops symptoms of blood dyscrasias (fever, sore throat, infection, cellulitis, weakness), jaundice, persistent (longer than a few hours) extrapyramidal reactions, or any such reactions in children.

• Monitor therapy by weekly bilirubin tests during first month; periodic blood tests (CBC, liver function) before and during therapy; and ophthalmic tests (long-term therapy).

• Check intake/output for urinary retention or constipation.

• Tell patient to use sunscreening agents and protective clothing to avoid photosensitivity reactions.

• Warn against activities that require alertness or good psychomotor coordination until CNS response to drug is determined. Drowsiness and dizziness usually subside after first few weeks.

• Obtain baseline measures of blood pressure before starting therapy and monitor regularly. Watch for orthostatic hypotension, especially with parenteral administration, since adrenergic blockage is high. Keep pa-

tient in a supine position for 1 hour afterward. Advise patient to change positions slowly.

• Avoid combining with alcohol or other depressants.

• Give deep I.M. only in upper outer quadrant of buttocks or midlateral thigh. Massage slowly afterward to prevent sterile abscess. Injection stings.

• Dilute liquid concentrate with fruit juice, milk, or semisolid food just before administration.

• Protect medication from light. Slight yellowing of injection or concentrate is common; does not affect potency. Discard markedly discolored solutions.

• Do not withdraw drug abruptly unless required by severe side effects.

• Prevent contact dermatitis by keeping drug off patient's skin and clothes. Wear gloves when preparing liquid forms of the drug.

• Dry mouth may be relieved by sugarless gum, sour hard candy, or rinsing with mouthwash.

• Dose of 100 mg is the therapeutic equivalent of 100 mg chlorpromazine.

fluphenazine decanoate
Modecate Decanoate♦♦, Prolixin Decanoate

fluphenazine enanthate
Moditen Enanthate♦♦, Prolixin Enanthate

fluphenazine hydrochloride
Moditen Hydrochloride♦♦, Permitil Hydrochloride♦* **, Prolixin Hydrochloride* **
Pregnancy Category: C

MECHANISM OF ACTION
Blocks postsynaptic dopamine receptors in the brain. Piperazine phenothiazine.

INDICATIONS & DOSAGE

Psychotic disorders—
Adults: initially, 0.5 to 10 mg fluphenazine HCl P.O. daily in divided doses q 6 to 8 hours; may increase cautiously to 20 mg. Higher doses (50 to 100 mg) have been given. Maintenance: 1 to 5 mg P.O. daily. I.M. doses are ⅓ to ½ oral doses. Lower doses for geriatric patients (1 to 2.5 mg daily).
Children: 0.25 to 3.5 mg fluphenazine HCl P.O. daily in divided doses q 4 to 6 hours; or ⅓ to ½ of oral dose I.M.; maximum 10 mg daily.
Adults and children over 12 years: 12.5 to 25 mg of long-acting esters (fluphenazine decanoate and enanthate) I.M. or S.C. q 1 to 6 weeks. Maintenance: 25 to 100 mg, p.r.n.

ADVERSE REACTIONS

Blood: *transient leukopenia, agranulocytosis.*
CNS: *extrapyramidal reactions (high incidence), tardive dyskinesia,* sedation (low incidence), pseudoparkinsonism, EEG changes, dizziness.
CV: orthostatic hypotension, tachycardia, EKG changes.
EENT: *ocular changes, blurred vision.*
GI: *dry mouth, constipation.*
GU: *urinary retention,* dark urine, menstrual irregularities, gynecomastia, inhibited ejaculation.
Hepatic: *cholestatic jaundice, abnormal liver function tests.*
Metabolic: hyperprolactinemia.
Skin: *mild photosensitivity,* dermal allergic reactions.
Other: weight gain, increased appetite.
After abrupt withdrawal of long-term therapy: gastritis, nausea, vomiting, dizziness, tremors, feeling of warmth or cold, sweating, tachycardia, headache, insomnia.

INTERACTIONS

Antacids: inhibit absorption of oral phenothiazines. Separate antacid and phenothiazine doses by at least 2 hours.
Barbiturates: may decrease phenothiazine effect. Observe patient.

NURSING CONSIDERATIONS

• Contraindicated in coma, CNS depression, bone-marrow depression or other blood dyscrasia, subcortical damage, hepatic damage, renal insufficiency; and with use of spinal or epidural anesthetic, or adrenergic blocking agents. Use cautiously with other CNS depressants, anticholinergics; in elderly or debilitated patients; in acutely ill or dehydrated children; and in patients with hepatic disease, pheochromocytoma, arteriosclerotic, cerebrovascular, or cardiovascular disease (may cause sudden drop in blood pressure), peptic ulcer, exposure to extreme heat or cold (including antipyretic therapy), respiratory disorders, hypocalcemia, convulsive disorders (may lower seizure threshold), severe reactions to insulin or electroshock therapy, suspected brain tumor or intestinal obstruction, glaucoma, or prostatic hypertrophy.
• Tardive dyskinesia may occur after prolonged use. It may not appear until months or years later and may disappear spontaneously or persist for life.
• Hold dose and notify doctor if patient develops symptoms of blood dyscrasias (fever, sore throat, infection, cellulitis, weakness), persistent (longer than a few hours) extrapyramidal reactions, or any such reactions in pregnancy or in children.
• Monitor therapy by weekly bilirubin tests during first month; periodic blood tests (CBC, liver function); periodic renal function and ophthalmic tests (long-term use).
• Check intake/output for urinary retention or constipation.
• Tell patient to use sunscreening agents and protective clothing to avoid photosensitivity reactions.

• Warn against activities that require alertness and good psychomotor coordination until CNS response to drug is determined. Drowsiness and dizziness usually subside after first few weeks.
• Avoid combining with alcohol or other depressants.
• Decanoate and enanthate may be given subcutaneously.
• For long-acting forms (decanoate and enanthate), which are oil preparations, use a dry needle of at least 21 gauge. Allow 24 to 96 hours for onset of action. Important: Note and report adverse side effects in patients taking the long-acting drug forms.
• Liquid (oral) and parenteral forms can cause contact dermatitis. If susceptible, wear gloves when preparing solutions of this drug, and prevent any contact with skin and clothing.
• Dilute liquid concentrate with water, fruit juice, milk, or semisolid food just before administration.
• Protect medication from light. Slight yellowing of injection or concentrate is common; does not affect potency. Discard markedly discolored solutions.
• Dry mouth may be relieved by sugarless gum, sour hard candy, or rinsing with mouthwash.
• Do not withdraw drug abruptly unless required by severe side effects.
• Dose of 2 mg is therapeutic equivalent of 100 mg chlorpromazine.
• Note that Permitil Concentrate is 10 times more concentrated than Prolixin Elixir (5 mg/ml vs. 0.5 mg/ml).

haloperidol
Haldol♦**

haloperidol decanoate
Haldol Decanoate
Pregnancy Category: C

MECHANISM OF ACTION
Blocks postsynaptic dopamine receptors in the brain. A butyrophenone.

INDICATIONS & DOSAGE
Psychotic disorders—
Adults: dosage varies for each patient. Initial range is 0.5 to 5 mg P.O. b.i.d. or t.i.d.; or 2 to 5 mg I.M. q 4 to 8 hours, increasing rapidly if necessary for prompt control. Maximum 100 mg P.O. daily. Doses over 100 mg have been used for patients with severely resistant conditions.
Chronic psychotic patients who require prolonged therapy—
Adults: 50 to 100 mg I.M. haloperidol decanoate every 4 weeks.
Control of tics, vocal utterances in Gilles de la Tourette's syndrome—
Adults: 0.5 to 5 mg P.O. b.i.d. or t.i.d., increasing p.r.n.

ADVERSE REACTIONS
Blood: transient leukopenia and leukocytosis.
CNS: *high incidence of severe extrapyramidal reactions, tardive dyskinesia,* low incidence of sedation.
CV: low incidence of cardiovascular effects with therapeutic dosages.
EENT: blurred vision, dry mouth.
GU: urinary retention, menstrual irregularities, gynecomastia.
Skin: rash.

INTERACTIONS
Lithium: lethargy and confusion with high doses. Observe patient.
Methyldopa: possible symptoms of dementia. Observe patient.

NURSING CONSIDERATIONS
• Contraindicated in parkinsonism, coma, or CNS depression. Use with caution in elderly and debilitated patients; in severe cardiovascular disorders, allergies, glaucoma, urinary retention; and in conjunction with anticonvulsant, anticoagulant, antiparkinson, or lithium medications.
• Tardive dyskinesia may occur after prolonged use. It may not appear until months or years later and may disappear spontaneously or persist for life.

• Elderly patients usually require lower initial doses and a more gradual dosage titration.
• Warn patient against activities that require alertness and good psychomotor coordination until CNS response to drug is determined. Drowsiness and dizziness usually subside after a few weeks.
• Avoid combining with alcohol or other depressants.
• Protect medication from light. Slight yellowing of injection or concentrate is common; does not affect potency. Discard markedly discolored solutions.
• Do not withdraw drug abruptly unless required by severe side effects.
• Dry mouth may be relieved by sugarless gum, sour hard candy, and rinsing with mouthwash.
• Dose of 2 mg is therapeutic equivalent of 100 mg chlorpromazine.
• Especially useful for agitation associated with senile dementia.
• When changing from tablets to decanoate injection, patient should receive 10 to 15 times the oral dose once a month (maximum 100 mg).
• Don't administer the decanoate form I.V.

loxapine succinate
Loxapac♦♦, Loxitane, Loxitane-C
Pregnancy Category: C

MECHANISM OF ACTION
Blocks postsynaptic dopamine receptors in the brain. A dibenzoxazepine.

INDICATIONS & DOSAGE
Psychotic disorders—
Adults: 10 mg P.O. or I.M. b.i.d. to q.i.d., rapidly increasing to 60 to 100 mg P.O. daily for most patients; dose varies from patient to patient.

ADVERSE REACTIONS
Blood: *transient leukopenia.*
CNS: *extrapyramidal reactions (mod-*
erate incidence), sedation (moderate incidence), tardive dyskinesia, pseudoparkinsonism, EEG changes, dizziness.
CV: *orthostatic hypotension,* tachycardia, EKG changes.
EENT: *blurred vision.*
GI: *dry mouth, constipation.*
GU: *urinary retention,* dark urine, menstrual irregularities, gynecomastia.
Skin: *mild photosensitivity,* dermal allergic reactions.
Other: weight gain, increased appetite.

INTERACTIONS
None significant.

NURSING CONSIDERATIONS
• Contraindicated in coma, severe CNS depression, drug-induced depressed states. Use with caution in epilepsy, cardiovascular disorders, glaucoma, urinary retention, suspected intestinal obstruction or brain tumor, renal damage.
• Tardive dyskinesia may occur after prolonged use. It may not appear until months or years later and may disappear spontaneously or persist for life.
• Warn against activities that require alertness and good psychomotor coordination until CNS response to drug is determined. Drowsiness and dizziness usually subside after first few weeks.
• Avoid combining with alcohol or other depressants.
• Obtain baseline measures of blood pressure before starting therapy and monitor regularly. Advise patient to get up slowly to avoid orthostatic hypotension.
• Dilute liquid concentrate with orange or grapefruit juice just before giving.
• Dry mouth may be relieved by sugarless gum, sour hard candy, or rinsing with mouthwash.
• Periodic ophthalmic tests recommended.

Italicized side effects are common or life-threatening.
*Liquid form contains alcohol.   **May contain tartrazine.

- Tricyclic dibenzoxazepine; the only dibenzoxazepine derivative.
- Dose of 10 mg is therapeutic equivalent of 100 mg chlorpromazine.

mesoridazine besylate
Serentil♦* **
Pregnancy Category: C

MECHANISM OF ACTION
Blocks postsynaptic dopamine receptors in the brain. Piperidine phenothiazine.

INDICATIONS & DOSAGE
Alcoholism—
Adults and children over 12 years: 25 mg P.O. b.i.d. up to maximum 200 mg daily.
Behavioral problems associated with chronic brain syndrome—
Adults and children over 12 years: 25 mg P.O. t.i.d. up to maximum of 300 mg daily.
Psychoneurotic manifestations (anxiety)—
Adults and children over 12 years: 10 mg P.O. t.i.d. up to maximum 150 mg daily.
Schizophrenia—
Adults and children over 12 years: initially, 50 mg P.O. t.i.d. or 25 mg I.M. repeated in 30 to 60 minutes, p.r.n.

ADVERSE REACTIONS
Blood: *transient leukopenia, agranulocytosis.*
CNS: extrapyramidal reactions (low incidence), *tardive dyskinesia, sedation (high incidence),* EEG changes, dizziness.
CV: *orthostatic hypotension,* tachycardia, EKG changes.
EENT: *ocular changes, blurred vision,* pigmentary retinopathy.
GI: *dry mouth, constipation.*
GU: *urinary retention,* dark urine, menstrual irregularities, gynecomastia, inhibited ejaculation.

Hepatic: *cholestatic jaundice, abnormal liver function tests.*
Metabolic: hyperprolactinemia.
Skin: *mild photosensitivity,* dermal allergic reactions.
Local: pain at I.M. injection site, sterile abscess.
Other: weight gain, increased appetite.
After abrupt withdrawal of long-term therapy: gastritis, nausea, vomiting, dizziness, tremors, feeling of warmth or cold, sweating, tachycardia, headache, insomnia.

INTERACTIONS
Antacids: inhibit absorption of oral phenothiazines. Separate antacid and phenothiazine doses by at least 2 hours.
Barbiturates: may decrease phenothiazine effect. Observe patient.

NURSING CONSIDERATIONS
- Contraindicated in coma, CNS depression, bone-marrow depression, subcortical damage, and with use of spinal or epidural anesthetic or adrenergic blocking agents. Use cautiously with other CNS depressants, anticholinergics; in elderly or debilitated patients; in acutely ill or dehydrated children; and in patients with hepatic disease, arteriosclerosis or cardiovascular disease (may cause sudden drop in blood pressure), exposure to extreme heat or cold (including antipyretic therapy), respiratory disorders, hypocalcemia, convulsive disorders, severe reactions to insulin or electroshock therapy, suspected brain tumor or intestinal obstruction, glaucoma, or prostatic hypertrophy.
- Tardive dyskinesia may occur after prolonged use. It may not appear until months or years later and may disappear spontaneously or persist for life.
- Hold dose and notify doctor if patient develops jaundice, symptoms of blood dyscrasias (fever, sore throat, infection, cellulitis, weakness), per-

sistent (longer than a few hours) extrapyramidal reactions, or any such reactions in pregnancy or in children over 12 years.
• Monitor therapy by weekly bilirubin tests during first month; periodic blood tests (CBC, liver function); and ophthalmic tests (long-term use).
• Check intake/output for urinary retention or constipation.
• Tell patient to use sunscreening agents and protective clothing to avoid photosensitivity reactions.
• Warn against activities that require alertness and good psychomotor coordination until CNS response to drug is determined. Drowsiness and dizziness usually subside after a few weeks.
• Avoid combining with alcohol or other depressants.
• Obtain baseline measures of blood pressure before starting therapy and monitor regularly. Watch for orthostatic hypotension, especially with parenteral administration. Advise patient to change positions slowly.
• Give deep I.M. only in upper outer quadrant of buttocks. Massage slowly afterward to prevent sterile abscess. Injection may sting.
• Protect medication from light. Slight yellowing of injection or concentrate is common; does not affect potency. Discard markedly discolored solutions.
• Liquid (oral) and parenteral forms may cause contact dermatitis. If susceptible, wear gloves when preparing solutions of this drug, and prevent contact with skin and clothing.
• Dry mouth may be relieved with sugarless gum, sour hard candy, or rinsing with mouthwash.
• Do not withdraw drug abruptly unless required by severe side effects.
• Dose of 50 mg is therapeutic equivalent of 100 mg chlorpromazine.

molindone hydrochloride
Moban
Pregnancy Category: C

MECHANISM OF ACTION
Blocks postsynaptic dopamine receptors in the brain. A dihydroindolone.

INDICATIONS & DOSAGE
Psychotic disorders—
Adults: 50 to 75 mg P.O. daily, increasing to maximum 225 mg daily. Doses up to 400 mg may be required.

ADVERSE REACTIONS
Blood: *transient leukopenia.*
CNS: *extrapyramidal reactions (moderate incidence), tardive dyskinesia, sedation (moderate incidence),* pseudoparkinsonism, EEG changes, dizziness.
CV: orthostatic hypotension, tachycardia, EKG changes.
EENT: *blurred vision.*
GI: *dry mouth, constipation.*
GU: *urinary retention,* dark urine, menstrual irregularities, gynecomastia, inhibited ejaculation.
Hepatic: *cholestatic jaundice, abnormal liver function tests.*
Metabolic: hyperprolactinemia.
Skin: *mild photosensitivity,* dermal allergic reactions.

INTERACTIONS
None significant.

NURSING CONSIDERATIONS
• Contraindicated in coma or severe CNS depression. Use with caution when increased physical activity would be harmful, as this agent increases activity; in seizures (may lower seizure threshold), suicide risk, suspected brain tumor, or intestinal obstruction.
• Tardive dyskinesia may occur after prolonged use. It may not appear until months or years later and may disappear spontaneously or persist for life.

Italicized side effects are common or life-threatening.
*Liquid form contains alcohol.   **May contain tartrazine.

- Warn against activities that require alertness or good psychomotor coordination until CNS response to drug is determined. Drowsiness and dizziness usually subside after first few weeks.
- Avoid combining with alcohol or other depressants.
- Dry mouth may be relieved with sugarless gum, sour hard candy, or rinsing with mouthwash.
- Drug is the only dihydroindolone derivative.
- Dose of 20 mg is therapeutic equivalent of 100 mg chlorpromazine.
- No injection available.
- Liquid oral concentrate is available.
- Lidone capsules contain tartrazine dye. May cause allergy in susceptible patients.
- May be administered in a single daily dose.

perphenazine
Phenazine♦♦, Trilafon♦
Pregnancy Category: C

MECHANISM OF ACTION
Blocks postsynaptic dopamine receptors in the brain. As an antiemetic, inhibits the medullary chemoreceptor trigger zone.

INDICATIONS & DOSAGE
Hospitalized psychiatric patients—
Adults: initially, 8 to 16 mg P.O. b.i.d., t.i.d., or q.i.d., increasing to 64 mg daily.
Children over 12 years: 6 to 12 mg P.O. daily in divided doses.
Mental disturbances, acute alcoholism, nausea, vomiting, hiccups—
Adults and children over 12 years: 5 to 10 mg I.M., p.r.n. Maximum 15 mg daily in ambulatory patients, 30 mg daily in hospitalized patients.

ADVERSE REACTIONS
Blood: *transient leukopenia, agranulocytosis.*
CNS: *extrapyramidal reactions (high incidence), tardive dyskinesia,* sedation (low incidence), pseudoparkinsonism, EEG changes, dizziness.
CV: *orthostatic hypotension,* tachycardia, EKG changes.
EENT: *ocular changes, blurred vision.*
GI: *dry mouth, constipation.*
GU: *urinary retention,* dark urine, menstrual irregularities, gynecomastia, inhibited ejaculation.
Hepatic: *cholestatic jaundice, abnormal liver function tests.*
Metabolic: hyperprolactinemia.
Skin: *mild photosensitivity,* dermal allergic reactions.
Local: pain at I.M. injection site, sterile abscess.
Other: weight gain, increased appetite.
After abrupt withdrawal of long-term therapy: gastritis, nausea, vomiting, dizziness, tremors, feeling of warmth or cold, sweating, tachycardia, headache, insomnia.

INTERACTIONS
Antacids: inhibit absorption of oral phenothiazines. Separate antacid and phenothiazine doses by at least 2 hours.
Barbiturates: may decrease phenothiazine effect. Observe patient.

NURSING CONSIDERATIONS
- Contraindicated in coma, CNS depression, bone-marrow depression, subcortical damage, use of spinal or epidural anesthetic or adrenergic blocking agents. Use cautiously with other CNS depressants, anticholinergics; in elderly or debilitated patients; in acutely ill or dehydrated children; and in patients with hepatic disease, arteriosclerosis or cardiovascular disease (may cause sudden drop in blood pressure), exposure to extreme heat or cold (including antipyretic therapy), respiratory disorders, hypocalcemia, convulsive disorders (may lower seizure threshold), severe reactions to

insulin or electroshock therapy, suspected brain tumor or intestinal obstruction, glaucoma, prostatic hypertrophy.
• Tardive dyskinesia may occur after prolonged use. It may not appear until months or years later and may disappear spontaneously or persist for life.
• Hold dose and notify doctor if patient develops jaundice, symptoms of blood dyscrasias (fever, sore throat, infection, cellulitis, weakness), persistent (longer than a few hours) extrapyramidal reactions, or any such reactions in pregnancy or in children.
• Monitor therapy by weekly bilirubin tests during first month; periodic blood tests (CBC, liver function); and ophthalmic tests (long-term use).
• Check intake/output for urinary retention or constipation.
• Tell patient to use sunscreening agents and protective clothing to avoid photosensitivity reactions.
• Warn against activities that require alertness or good psychomotor coordination until CNS response to drug is determined. Drowsiness and dizziness usually subside after a few weeks.
• Avoid combining with alcohol or other depressants.
• Obtain baseline measures of blood pressure before starting therapy and monitor regularly. Watch for orthostatic hypotension, especially with parenteral administration. Keep patient supine for 1 hour afterward. Advise patient to change positions slowly.
• Give deep I.M. only in upper outer quadrant of buttocks. Massage slowly afterward to prevent sterile abscess. Injection may sting.
• Do not withdraw drug abruptly unless required by severe side effects.
• Protect drug from light. Slight yellowing of injection or concentrate is common; does not affect potency. Discard markedly discolored solutions.
• Prevent contact dermatitis by keeping drug off patient's skin and clothes. Wear gloves when preparing liquid forms of the drug.
• Dilute liquid concentrate with fruit juice, milk, carbonated beverage, or semisolid food just before giving. Exceptions: Oral concentrate causes turbidity or precipitation in colas, black coffee, grape or apple juice, or tea. Do not mix with these liquids.
• Dry mouth may be relieved with sugarless gum, sour hard candy, or rinsing with mouthwash.
• Dose of 8 mg is therapeutic equivalent of 100 mg chlorpromazine.

pimozide
Orap
Pregnancy Category: C

MECHANISM OF ACTION
Blocks dopaminergic receptors.

INDICATIONS & DOSAGE
Suppression of severe motor and phonic tics in patients with Tourette's disorder—
Adults and children over 12 years: initially, 1 to 2 mg daily in divided doses. Then, increase dose every other day. Maintenance dose ranges from 7 to 16 mg daily.

ADVERSE REACTIONS
CNS: *Parkinson-like symptoms,* other extrapyramidal symptoms (dystonia, akathisia, hyperreflexia, opisthotonus, oculogyric crisis), *tardive dyskinesia, sedation.*
CV: *EKG changes (prolonged Q-T interval),* hypotension.
EENT: visual disturbances.
GI: *dry mouth,* constipation.
GU: impotence.
Other: *neuroleptic malignant syndrome (hyperpyrexia),* muscle tightness.

INTERACTIONS
None significant.

Italicized side effects are common or life-threatening.
*Liquid form contains alcohol.   **May contain tartrazine.

NURSING CONSIDERATIONS
- Contraindicated in patients with congenital long Q-T syndrome or history of cardiac arrhythmias, in patients with severe toxic CNS depression, or in those in comatose states.
- Tardive dyskinesia may occur after prolonged use. It may not appear until months or years later and may disappear spontaneously or persist for life.
- Pimozide is not recommended for treatment of simple tics except those associated with Tourette's disorder. Don't use in drug-induced motor and phonic tics.
- Avoid concurrent administration of other drugs that prolong the Q-T interval, such as antiarrhythmic agents.
- Perform an EKG before treatment begins and periodically thereafter. Monitor for prolonged Q-T interval.
- Monitor patients who are also taking anticonvulsants for increased seizure activity. Pimozide may lower the seizure threshold.
- Because pimozide may cause serious adverse effects, the patient and his family should be thoroughly informed before deciding whether he should take the drug. Pimozide is indicated only in patients who have failed to respond satisfactorily to standard treatment.
- Warn patient not to stop taking drug abruptly and not to exceed prescribed dose.
- Offer him sugarless hard candy, gum, and liquids, as needed, to relieve dry mouth.

promazine hydrochloride
Promanyl♦♦, Sparine♦**
Pregnancy Category: C

MECHANISM OF ACTION
Blocks postsynaptic dopamine receptors in the brain. Aliphatic phenothiazine.

INDICATIONS & DOSAGE
Psychosis—
Adults: 25 to 200 mg P.O. or I.M. q 4 to 6 hours, up to 1 g daily. I.V. dose in concentrations no greater than 25 mg/ml for acutely agitated patients. Initial dose 50 to 150 mg; repeat within 5 to 10 minutes if necessary.
Children over 12 years: 10 to 25 mg P.O. or I.M. q 4 to 6 hours.

ADVERSE REACTIONS
Blood: *transient leukopenia, agranulocytosis.*
CNS: *extrapyramidal reactions (moderate incidence), tardive dyskinesia, sedation (high incidence),* pseudoparkinsonism, EEG changes, dizziness.
CV: *orthostatic hypotension,* tachycardia, EKG changes.
EENT: *ocular changes, blurred vision.*
GI: *dry mouth, constipation.*
GU: *urinary retention,* dark urine, menstrual irregularities, gynecomastia, inhibited ejaculation.
Hepatic: *cholestatic jaundice, abnormal liver function tests.*
Metabolic: hyperprolactinemia.
Skin: *mild photosensitivity,* dermal allergic reactions.
Local: pain at I.M. injection site, sterile abscess.
Other: weight gain, increased appetite.
After abrupt withdrawal of long-term therapy: gastritis, nausea, vomiting, dizziness, tremors, feeling of warmth or cold, sweating, tachycardia, headache, insomnia.

INTERACTIONS
Antacids: inhibit absorption of oral phenothiazines. Separate antacid and phenothiazine doses by at least 2 hours.
Anticholinergics (including antidepressant and antiparkinson agents): increased anticholinergic activity, aggravated parkinson-like symptoms. Use with caution.

Barbiturates: may decrease phenothiazine effect. Observe patient.

NURSING CONSIDERATIONS

• Contraindicated in coma, CNS depression, bone-marrow depression, subcortical damage, and with use of spinal or epidural anesthetic or adrenergic blocking agents. Use cautiously with other CNS depressants, anticholinergics; in elderly or debilitated patients; in patients with hepatic disease, arteriosclerosis or cardiovascular disease (may cause sudden drop in blood pressure), exposure to extreme heat or cold (including antipyretic therapy), respiratory disorders, hypocalcemia, convulsive disorders (may lower seizure threshold), severe reactions to insulin or electroshock therapy, suspected brain tumor or intestinal obstruction, glaucoma, prostatic hypertrophy; and in acutely ill or dehydrated children.

• Tardive dyskinesia may occur after prolonged use. It may not appear until months or years later and may disappear spontaneously or persist for life.

• Hold dose and notify doctor if patient develops jaundice, symptoms of blood dyscrasias (fever, sore throat, infection, cellulitis, weakness), persistent (longer than a few hours) extrapyramidal reactions, or such reactions during pregnancy or in children.

• Monitor therapy by weekly bilirubin tests during first month; periodic blood tests (CBC, liver function); and ophthalmic tests (long-term use).

• Check intake/output for urinary retention or constipation.

• Tell patient to use sunscreening agents and protective clothing to avoid photosensitivity reactions.

• Warn against activities that require alertness or good psychomotor coordination until CNS response to drug is determined. Drowsiness and dizziness usually subside after a few weeks.

• Avoid combining with alcohol or other depressants.

• Monitor blood pressure with patient lying and standing before starting therapy, and routinely throughout course of treatment.

• Watch for orthostatic hypotension, especially with parenteral administration. Keep patient supine for 1 hour afterward. Advise patient to change positions slowly.

• Give deep I.M. only in upper outer quadrant of buttocks. Massage slowly afterward to prevent sterile abscess. Injection may sting.

• Protect drug from light. Slight yellowing of injection or concentrate is common; does not affect potency. Discard markedly discolored solutions.

• Prevent contact dermatitis by keeping drug off patient's skin and clothes. Wear gloves when preparing liquid forms of the drug.

• Dilute liquid concentrate with fruit juice, milk, semisolid food, or chocolate-flavored drinks just before giving. For best taste, use at least 10 ml diluent per 25 mg drug.

• Do not withdraw drug abruptly unless required by severe side effects.

• Dry mouth may be relieved with sugarless gum, sour hard candy, or rinsing with mouthwash.

---

thioridazine hydrochloride
Mellaril♦*, Novoridazine♦♦, SE
Thioridazine
Pregnancy Category: C

MECHANISM OF ACTION
Blocks postsynaptic dopamine receptors in the brain. Piperidine phenothiazine.

INDICATIONS & DOSAGE
Psychosis—
Adults: initially, 50 to 100 mg P.O. t.i.d., with gradual increments up to 800 mg daily in divided doses, if needed. Dosage varies.
Adults over 65: initial dose, 25 mg

Italicized side effects are common or life-threatening.
*Liquid form contains alcohol.   **May contain tartrazine.

t.i.d.

Depressive neurosis, alcohol withdrawal, dementia in geriatric patients, behavioral problems in children—
Adults: initially, 25 mg P.O. t.i.d. Maintenance dose is 20 to 200 mg daily.
Children over 2 years: 0.5 to 3 mg/kg daily in divided doses.

ADVERSE REACTIONS
Blood: *transient leukopenia, agranulocytosis.*
CNS: extrapyramidal reactions (low incidence), *tardive dyskinesia, sedation (high incidence)*, EEG changes, dizziness.
CV: *orthostatic hypotension*, tachycardia, EKG changes.
EENT: *ocular changes, blurred vision*, pigmentary retinopathy.
GI: *dry mouth, constipation.*
GU: *urinary retention*, dark urine, menstrual irregularities, gynecomastia, inhibited ejaculation.
Hepatic: *cholestatic jaundice.*
Metabolic: hyperprolactinemia.
Skin: *mild photosensitivity*, dermal allergic reactions.
Other: weight gain, increased appetite.
After abrupt withdrawal of long-term therapy: gastritis, nausea, vomiting, dizziness, tremors, feeling of warmth or cold, sweating, tachycardia, headache, insomnia.

INTERACTIONS
Antacids: inhibit absorption of oral phenothiazines. Separate antacid and phenothiazine doses by at least 2 hours.
Barbiturates: may decrease phenothiazine effect. Observe patient.

NURSING CONSIDERATIONS
• Contraindicated in coma, CNS depression, bone-marrow depression, hypertensive or hypotensive cardiac disease, subcortical damage, and with use of spinal or epidural anesthetic or adrenergic blocking agents. Use cautiously with other CNS depressants, anticholinergics; in elderly or debilitated patients; in patients with hepatic disease, arteriosclerosis or cardiovascular disease (may cause sudden drop in blood pressure), exposure to extreme heat or cold (including antipyretic therapy), respiratory disorders, hypocalcemia, convulsive disorders, severe reactions to insulin or electroshock therapy, suspected brain tumor or intestinal obstruction, glaucoma, or prostatic hypertrophy; and in acutely ill or dehydrated children.
• Tardive dyskinesia may occur after prolonged use. It may not appear until months or years later and may disappear spontaneously or persist for life.
• Hold dose and notify doctor if patient develops jaundice, symptoms of blood dyscrasias (fever, sore throat, infection, cellulitis, weakness), persistent (longer than a few hours) extrapyramidal reactions, or such reactions during pregnancy or in children.
• Monitor therapy by weekly bilirubin tests during first month; periodic blood tests (CBC, liver function); and ophthalmic tests (long-term therapy).
• Check intake/output for urinary retention or constipation.
• Watch for blurred vision, dry mouth; high incidence of anticholinergic effects.
• Tell patient to use sunscreening agents and protective clothing to avoid photosensitivity reactions.
• Monitor blood pressure.
• Warn against activities that require alertness or good psychomotor coordination until response to drug is determined. Drowsiness and dizziness usually subside after a few weeks.
• Avoid combining with alcohol or other depressants.
• Watch for orthostatic hypotension, especially with parenteral administration. Advise patient to change positions slowly.

- Prevent contact dermatitis by keeping drug off patient's skin and clothes. Wear gloves when preparing liquid forms of the drug.
- Caution: There are four different liquid formulations available (two concentrates and two suspensions).
- Not available in injectable form. Mesoridazine is prescribed when parenteral use of a thioridazine-like drug is desirable.
- Dilute liquid concentrate with water or fruit juice just before giving.
- Do not withdraw abruptly unless required by severe side effects.
- Dry mouth may be relieved with sugarless gum, sour hard candy, or rinsing with mouthwash.
- A piperidine phenothiazine.
- Dose of 100 mg is the therapeutic equivalent of 100 mg chlorpromazine.
- Dose above 800 mg may be associated with ocular toxicity (pigmentary retinopathy).

thiothixene

thiothixene hydrochloride
Navane♦*
Pregnancy Category: C

MECHANISM OF ACTION
Blocks postsynaptic dopamine receptors in the brain. A thioxanthene.

INDICATIONS & DOSAGE
Acute agitation—
Adults: 4 mg I.M. b.i.d. to q.i.d. Maximum 30 mg daily I.M. Change to P.O. as soon as possible.
Mild to moderate psychosis—
Adults: initially, 2 mg P.O. t.i.d. May increase gradually to 15 mg daily.
Severe psychosis—
Adults: initially, 5 mg P.O. b.i.d. May increase gradually to 15 to 30 mg daily. Maximum recommended daily dose 60 mg. Not recommended in children under 12 years.

ADVERSE REACTIONS
Blood: *transient leukopenia, agranulocytosis.*
CNS: *extrapyramidal reactions (high incidence), tardive dyskinesia,* sedation (low incidence), pseudoparkinsonism, EEG changes, dizziness.
CV: *orthostatic hypotension,* tachycardia, EKG changes.
EENT: *ocular changes, blurred vision.*
GI: *dry mouth, constipation.*
GU: *urinary retention,* dark urine, menstrual irregularities, gynecomastia, inhibited ejaculation.
Hepatic: *cholestatic jaundice.*
Metabolic: hyperprolactinemia.
Skin: *mild photosensitivity,* dermal allergic reactions.
Local: pain at I.M. injection site, sterile abscess.
Other: weight gain, increased appetite.
After abrupt withdrawal of long-term therapy: gastritis, nausea, vomiting, dizziness, tremors, feeling of warmth or cold, sweating, tachycardia, headache, insomnia.

INTERACTIONS
None significant.

NURSING CONSIDERATIONS
- Contraindicated in convulsive seizures, circulatory collapse, coma, CNS depression, blood dyscrasias, bone-marrow depression, alcohol withdrawal, akathisia or restlessness, subcortical damage, and with use of spinal or epidural anesthetic or adrenergic blocking agents. Use cautiously with other CNS depressants, anticholinergics; in elderly or debilitated patients; and in patients with hepatic disease, arteriosclerosis or cardiovascular disease (may cause sudden drop in blood pressure), exposure to extreme heat or cold (including antipyretic therapy) or undue sunlight, respiratory disorders, hypocalcemia, severe reactions to insulin or electro-

Italicized side effects are common or life-threatening.
*Liquid form contains alcohol.   **May contain tartrazine.

shock therapy, suspected brain tumor or intestinal obstruction, glaucoma, or prostatic hypertrophy.

• Tardive dyskinesia may occur after prolonged use. It may not appear until months or years later and may disappear spontaneously or persist for life.

• Hold dose and notify doctor if patient develops jaundice, symptoms of blood dyscrasias (fever, sore throat, infection, cellulitis, weakness), persistent (longer than a few hours) extrapyramidal reactions, or any such reactions during pregnancy.

• Monitor therapy by weekly bilirubin tests during first month; periodic blood tests (CBC, liver function); and ophthalmic tests (long-term therapy).

• Check intake/output for urinary retention or constipation.

• Tell patient to use sunscreening agents and protective clothing to avoid photosensitivity reactions.

• Warn against activities that require alertness or good psychomotor coordination until CNS response to drug is determined. Drowsiness and dizziness usually subside after a few weeks.

• Avoid combining with alcohol or other depressants.

• Watch for orthostatic hypotension, especially with parenteral administration. Keep patient in a supine position for 1 hour afterward. Advise patient to change positions slowly.

• Give I.M. only in upper outer quadrant of buttocks or midlateral thigh. Massage slowly afterward to prevent sterile abscess. Injection may sting.

• I.M. form must be stored in refrigerator.

• Slight yellowing of injection or concentrate is common; does not affect potency. Discard markedly discolored solutions.

• Prevent contact dermatitis by keeping drug off patient's skin and clothes. Wear gloves when preparing liquid forms of the drug.

• Dilute liquid concentrate with fruit juice, milk, or semisolid food just before giving.

• Do not withdraw abruptly unless required by severe side effects.

• Dry mouth may be relieved with sugarless gum, sour hard candy, or rinsing with mouthwash.

• Drug is a thioxanthene derivative but produces responses similar to phenothiazines and butyrophenones.

• Dose of 4 mg is therapeutic equivalent of 100 mg chlorpromazine.

trifluoperazine hydrochloride
Novoflurazine♦♦, Solazine♦♦, Stelazine♦, Terfluzine♦♦, Triflurin♦♦
Pregnancy Category: C

MECHANISM OF ACTION
Blocks postsynaptic dopamine receptors in the brain. Piperazine phenothiazine.

INDICATIONS & DOSAGE
Anxiety states—
Adults: 1 to 2 mg P.O. b.i.d.
Schizophrenia and other psychotic disorders—
Adults:
outpatients—1 to 2 mg P.O. b.i.d., up to 4 mg daily; *hospitalized*—2 to 5 mg P.O. b.i.d.; may gradually increase to 40 mg daily. 1 to 2 mg I.M. q 4 to 6 hours, p.r.n.
Children 6 to 12 years (hospitalized or under close supervision): 1 mg P.O. daily or b.i.d.; may increase gradually to 15 mg daily.

ADVERSE REACTIONS
Blood: *transient leukopenia, agranulocytosis.*
CNS: *extrapyramidal reactions (high incidence), tardive dyskinesia,* sedation (low incidence), pseudoparkinsonism, EEG changes, dizziness.
CV: *orthostatic hypotension,* tachycardia, EKG changes.
EENT: *ocular changes, blurred vision.*

GI: *dry mouth, constipation.*
GU: *urinary retention,* dark urine, menstrual irregularities, gynecomastia, inhibited ejaculation.
Hepatic: *cholestatic jaundice.*
Metabolic: hyperprolactinemia.
Skin: *mild photosensitivity,* dermal allergic reactions.
Local: pain at I.M. injection site, sterile abscess.
Other: weight gain, increased appetite.
After abrupt withdrawal of long-term therapy: gastritis, nausea, vomiting, dizziness, tremors, feeling of warmth or cold, sweating, tachycardia, headache, insomnia.

INTERACTIONS

Antacids: inhibit absorption of oral phenothiazines. Separate antacid and phenothiazine doses by at least 2 hours.
Barbiturates: may decrease phenothiazine effect. Observe patient.

NURSING CONSIDERATIONS

• Contraindicated in coma, CNS depression, bone-marrow depression, subcortical damage, and with use of spinal or epidural anesthetic or adrenergic blocking agents. Use cautiously with other CNS depressants, anticholinergics; in elderly or debilitated patients; in patients with hepatic disease, arteriosclerosis or cardiovascular disease (may cause drop in blood pressure), exposure to extreme heat or cold (including antipyretic therapy), respiratory disorders, hypocalcemia, convulsive disorders, severe reactions to insulin or electroshock therapy, suspected brain tumor or intestinal obstruction, glaucoma, or prostatic hypertrophy; and in acutely ill or dehydrated children.
• Tardive dyskinesia may occur after prolonged use. It may not appear until months or years later and may disappear spontaneously or persist for life.
• Hold dose and notify doctor if patient develops jaundice, symptoms of blood dyscrasias (fever, sore throat, infection, cellulitis, weakness), persistent (longer than a few hours) extrapyramidal reactions, or any such reactions during pregnancy or in children.
• Monitor therapy by weekly bilirubin tests during first month; periodic blood tests (CBC, liver function); and ophthalmic tests (long-term therapy).
• Check intake/output for urinary retention or constipation.
• Tell patient to use sunscreening agents and protective clothing to avoid photosensitivity reactions.
• Warn against activities that require alertness or good psychomotor coordination until CNS response to drug is determined. Drowsiness and dizziness usually subside after a few weeks.
• Avoid combining with alcohol or other depressants.
• Watch for orthostatic hypotension, especially with parenteral administration. Keep patient supine for 1 hour afterward. Advise patient to change positions slowly.
• Give deep I.M. only in upper outer quadrant of buttocks. Massage slowly afterward to prevent sterile abscess. Injection may sting.
• Protect drug from light. Slight yellowing of injection or concentrate is common; does not affect potency. Discard markedly discolored solutions.
• Prevent contact dermatitis by keeping drug off patient's skin and clothes. Wear gloves when preparing liquid forms of the drug.
• Dilute liquid concentrate with 60 ml tomato or fruit juice, carbonated beverages, coffee, tea, milk, water, or semisolid food just before giving.
• Do not withdraw abruptly unless required by severe side effects.
• Dry mouth may be relieved with sugarless gum, sour hard candy, or rinsing with mouthwash.
• Drug is a prototype piperazine phe-

Italicized side effects are common or life-threatening.
*Liquid form contains alcohol.   **May contain tartrazine.

nothiazine.
• Dose of 5 mg is therapeutic equivalent of 100 mg chlorpromazine.

triflupromazine hydrochloride
Vesprin**
Pregnancy Category: C

MECHANISM OF ACTION
Blocks postsynaptic dopamine receptors in the brain. Aliphatic phenothiazine.

INDICATIONS & DOSAGE
Acute, severe agitation—
Adults: 60 to 150 mg I.M. in 2 or 3 divided doses.
Children over 2½ years: 0.2 to 0.25 mg/kg in divided doses. Maximum dose 10 mg daily.
Nausea and vomiting—
Adults: 20 to 30 mg P.O. daily; or 1 to 3 mg I.V. daily; or 5 to 15 mg I.M. daily up to maximum 60 mg daily.
Children: 0.2 mg/kg P.O. or I.M. up to maximum 10 mg daily.
Psychotic disorders (mild to moderate symptoms)—
Adults: 10 to 25 mg P.O. b.i.d.
Children over 2½ years: 10 mg P.O. t.i.d.
Elderly, debilitated patients: 10 mg b.i.d. or t.i.d.; increase gradually to desired effect.
Severe symptoms—
Adults: 50 mg P.O. b.i.d. or t.i.d.
Children over 2½ years: 2 mg/kg P.O. in 3 divided doses; may increase gradually to 150 mg daily.

ADVERSE REACTIONS
Blood: *transient leukopenia, agranulocytosis.*
CNS: *extrapyramidal reactions (moderate incidence), tardive dyskinesia, sedation (high incidence),* pseudoparkinsonism, EEG changes, dizziness.
CV: *orthostatic hypotension,* tachycardia, EKG changes.

EENT: *ocular changes, blurred vision.*
GI: *dry mouth, constipation.*
GU: *urinary retention,* dark urine, menstrual irregularities, gynecomastia, inhibited ejaculation.
Hepatic: *cholestatic jaundice.*
Metabolic: hyperprolactinemia.
Skin: *mild photosensitivity,* dermal allergic reactions.
Local: pain at I.M. injection site, sterile abscess.
Other: weight gain, increased appetite.
After abrupt withdrawal of long-term therapy: gastritis, nausea, vomiting, dizziness, tremors, feeling of warmth or cold, sweating, tachycardia, headache, insomnia.

INTERACTIONS
Antacids: inhibit absorption of oral phenothiazines. Separate antacid and phenothiazine doses by at least 2 hours.
Anticholinergics (including antidepressant and antiparkinson agents): increased anticholinergic activity, aggravated parkinson-like symptoms. Use with caution.
Barbiturates: may decrease phenothiazine effect. Observe patient.

NURSING CONSIDERATIONS
• Contraindicated in coma, CNS depression, blood dyscrasias, bone-marrow depression, subcortical brain damage, and with use of spinal or epidural anesthetic or adrenergic blocking agents. Use cautiously with other CNS depressants, anticholinergics; in elderly or debilitated patients; in patients with hepatic disease, arteriosclerosis or cardiovascular disease (may cause sudden drop in blood pressure), exposure to extreme heat or cold (including antipyretic therapy), respiratory disorders, pheochromocytoma, hypocalcemia, convulsive disorders, severe reactions to insulin or electroshock therapy, suspected brain

tumor or intestinal obstruction, glaucoma, prostatic hypertrophy; and in acutely ill or dehydrated children.

• Tardive dyskinesia may occur after prolonged use. It may not appear until months or years later and may disappear spontaneously or persist for life.

• Hold dose and notify doctor if patient develops jaundice, symptoms of blood dyscrasias (fever, sore throat, infection, cellulitis, weakness), persistent (longer than a few hours) extrapyramidal reactions, or any such reactions during pregnancy or in children.

• Monitor therapy by weekly bilirubin tests during first month; periodic blood tests (CBC, liver function); and ophthalmic tests in long-term therapy.

• Check intake/output for urinary retention or constipation.

• Tell patient to use sunscreening agents and protective clothing to avoid photosensitivity reactions.

• Warn against activities that require alertness or good psychomotor coordination until response to drug is determined. Drowsiness and dizziness usually subside after a few weeks.

• Avoid combining with alcohol or other depressants.

• Watch for orthostatic hypotension, especially with parenteral administration. Keep patient supine for 1 hour afterward. Advise patient to change positions slowly.

• Give I.M. only in upper outer quadrant of buttocks. Massage slowly afterward to prevent sterile abscess. Injection may sting.

• Protect drug from light. Slight yellowing of injection or concentrate is common; does not affect potency. Discard markedly discolored solutions.

• Keep liquid suspension tightly closed.

• Prevent contact dermatitis by keeping drug off patient's skin and clothes. Wear gloves when preparing liquid forms of the drug.

• Do not withdraw abruptly unless required by severe side effects.

• Dry mouth may be relieved with sugarless gum, sour hard candy, or rinsing with mouthwash.

• Dose of 25 mg is therapeutic equivalent of 100 mg chlorpromazine.

Italicized side effects are common or life-threatening.
*Liquid form contains alcohol.   **May contain tartrazine.

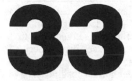

Miscellaneous psychotherapeutics

lithium carbonate
lithium citrate

COMBINATION PRODUCTS
None.

lithium carbonate
Carbolith♦♦, Duralith♦♦, Eskalith, Eskalith CR, Lithane♦**, Lithizine♦♦, Lithobid, Lithonate, Lithotabs

lithium citrate
Cibalith-S
Pregnancy Category: D

MECHANISM OF ACTION
Alters chemical transmitters in the central nervous system, possibly by interfering with ionic pump mechanisms in brain cells. Its exact mechanism of action in mania, however, is unknown.

INDICATIONS & DOSAGE
Prevention or control of mania—
Adults: 300 to 600 mg P.O. up to four times daily, increasing on the basis of blood levels to achieve optimal dosage. Recommended therapeutic lithium blood levels: 1 to 1.5 mEq/liter for acute mania; 0.6 to 1.2 mEq/liter for maintenance therapy; and 2 mEq/liter as maximum.
Adults: 5 ml lithium citrate (liquid) contains 8 mEq lithium equal to 300 mg lithium carbonate.

ADVERSE REACTIONS
Blood: *leukocytosis of 14,000 to 18,000 (reversible).*
CNS: tremors, drowsiness, headache, confusion, restlessness, dizziness, psychomotor retardation, stupor, lethargy, coma, blackouts, epileptiform seizures, EEG changes, worsened organic brain syndrome, impaired speech, ataxia, muscle weakness, incoordination, hyperexcitability.
CV: *reversible EKG changes,* arrhythmia, hypotension, peripheral circulatory collapse, allergic vasculitis, ankle and wrist edema.
EENT: tinnitus, impaired vision.
GI: nausea, vomiting, anorexia, diarrhea, dry mouth, *thirst,* metallic taste.
GU: *polyuria,* glycosuria, incontinence, renal toxicity with long-term use.
Metabolic: transient hyperglycemia, goiter, hypothyroidism (lowered T_3, T_4, and PBI, but elevated ^{131}I uptake), hyponatremia.
Skin: pruritus, rash, diminished or lost sensation, drying and thinning of hair.

INTERACTIONS
Diuretics: increased reabsorption of lithium by kidneys, with possible toxic effect. Use with extreme caution, and monitor lithium and electrolyte levels (especially sodium).
Haloperidol and thioridazine: encephalopathic syndrome (lethargy, tremors, extrapyramidal symptoms). Watch for syndrome, and stop drug if it occurs.
Aminophylline, sodium bicarbonate, and sodium chloride: ingestion of

---

these salts increases lithium excretion. Avoid salt loads and monitor lithium levels.
Carbamazepine, probenecid, indomethacin, methyldopa and piroxicam: increased effect of lithium. Monitor for lithium toxicity.

NURSING CONSIDERATIONS

• Contraindicated if therapy cannot be closely monitored. Use with caution with haloperidol, other antipsychotics, neuromuscular blocking agents, and diuretics; in elderly or debilitated persons; and in thyroid disease, epilepsy, renal or cardiovascular disease, brain damage, severe debilitation or dehydration, and sodium depletion.
• Monitor baseline EKG, thyroid, and renal studies, and electrolyte levels. Monitor lithium blood levels 8 to 12 hours after first dose, usually before morning dose, two or three times weekly first month, then weekly to monthly on maintenance.
• Determination of lithium blood concentration is crucial to the safe use of the drug. Shouldn't be used in patients who can't have regular lithium blood level checks.
• Explain to patient that lithium has a narrow therapeutic margin of safety. A blood level that is even slightly too high can be dangerous.
• When blood levels of lithium are below 1.5 mEq/liter, side effects generally remain mild.
• Check fluid intake and output, especially when surgery is scheduled.
• Warn patient and family to watch for signs of toxicity (diarrhea, vomiting, drowsiness, muscular weakness, ataxia) and to expect transient nausea, polyuria, thirst, and discomfort during first few days. Patient should withhold one dose and call doctor if toxic symptoms appear, but not stop drug abruptly.
• Expect lag of 1 to 3 weeks before drug's beneficial effects are noticed.

• Weigh patient daily; check for signs of edema or sudden weight gain.
• Adjust fluid and salt ingestion to compensate if excessive loss occurs through protracted sweating or diarrhea. Under normal conditions, patients should have fluid intake of 2,500 to 3,000 ml daily and a balanced diet with adequate salt intake.
• Have outpatient follow-up of thyroid and renal functions every 6 to 12 months. Palpate thyroid to check for enlargement.
• Patient should carry identification/instruction card (available from pharmacy) with toxicity and emergency information.
• Warn ambulatory patient to avoid activities that require alertness and good psychomotor coordination until CNS response to drug is determined.
• Administer with plenty of water, and after meals to minimize GI upset.
• Check urine for specific gravity and report level below 1.005, which may indicate diabetes insipidus syndrome.
• May alter glucose tolerance in diabetics. Monitor blood glucose closely.
• Tell patient not to switch brands of lithium or to take other drugs (prescription or over-the-counter) without doctor's guidance.
• Investigationally used to increase white cells in patients undergoing cancer chemotherapy.
• Also used investigationally for treatment of cluster headaches, aggression, organic brain syndrome, and tardive dyskinesia. Has been used to treat syndrome of inappropriate ADH.

Italicized side effects are common or life-threatening.
*Liquid form contains alcohol.   **May contain tartrazine.

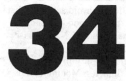

Cerebral stimulants

amphetamine sulfate
benzphetamine hydrochloride
caffeine
dextroamphetamine sulfate
diethylpropion hydrochloride
fenfluramine hydrochloride
mazindol
methamphetamine hydrochloride
methylphenidate hydrochloride
pemoline
phenmetrazine hydrochloride
phentermine hydrochloride

COMBINATION PRODUCTS
BIPHETAMINE 12½: dextroamphetamine 6.25 mg and amphetamine
6.25 mg.
BIPHETAMINE 20: dextroamphetamine
10 mg and amphetamine 10 mg.

amphetamine sulfate
Controlled Substance Schedule II
Pregnancy Category: C

MECHANISM OF ACTION
Main site of activity appears to be the
cerebral cortex and the reticular activating system. Promotes nerve impulse transmission by releasing stored
norepinephrine from nerve terminals
in the brain. In children with hyperkinesia, amphetamines have a paradoxical calming effect.

INDICATIONS & DOSAGE
Attention deficit disorder with hyper-
activity (ADDH)—
Children 6 years and older: 5 mg
P.O. daily, with 5-mg increments
weekly, p.r.n.

Children 3 to 5 years: 2.5 mg P.O.
daily, with 2.5-mg increments
weekly, p.r.n.
Narcolepsy—
Adults: 5 to 60 mg P.O. daily in divided doses.
Children over 12 years: 10 mg P.O.
daily, with 10-mg increments weekly,
p.r.n.
Children 6 to 12 years: 5 mg P.O.
daily, with 5-mg increments weekly,
p.r.n.
Short-term adjunct in exogenous obe-
sity—
Adults: single 10- or 15-mg long-acting capsule daily, or 2 if needed, up to
30 mg daily; or 5 to 30 mg daily in divided doses 30 to 60 minutes before
meals. Not recommended for children
under age 12.

ADVERSE REACTIONS
CNS: *restlessness,* tremor, *hyperactiv-*
ity, talkativeness, insomnia, irritability, dizziness, headache, chills, overstimulation, dysphoria.
CV: *tachycardia, palpitations,* hypertension, hypotension.
GI: nausea, vomiting, cramps, dry
mouth, diarrhea, constipation, metallic taste, anorexia, weight loss.
Other: urticaria, impotence, changes
in libido.

INTERACTIONS
MAO inhibitors: severe hypertension;
possible hypertensive crisis. Don't
use together.
Antacids, sodium bicarbonate, acet-
azolamide: increased renal reabsorption. Monitor for enhanced effect.

Ammonium chloride, ascorbic acid: observe for decreased amphetamine effect.

Phenothiazines, haloperidol: observe for decreased amphetamine effect.

NURSING CONSIDERATIONS
• Contraindicated in symptomatic cardiovascular diseases, hyperthyroidism, nephritis, angina pectoris, moderate to severe hypertension, parkinsonism due to arteriosclerosis, certain types of glaucoma, advanced arteriosclerosis, agitated states, or patients with history of drug abuse. Use with caution in patients with diabetes mellitus and in elderly, debilitated, or hyperexcitable patients.
• Use cautiously in children with Gilles de la Tourette's disorder.
• Psychic dependence or habituation may occur, especially in patients with history of drug addiction. Avoid prolonged administration. When used long-term, lower dosage gradually to prevent acute rebound depression.
• Not recommended for first-line treatment of obesity. Use as an anorexigenic agent is prohibited in some states.
• When used for obesity, make sure patient is also on a weight-reduction program. Give drug 30 to 60 minutes before meals. Monitor dietary intake. Do calorie counts, if necessary.
• Fatigue may result as drug effects wear off. Patient will need more rest.
• Tell patient to avoid drinks containing caffeine, which increase the effects of amphetamines and related amines.
• Check vital signs regularly for signs of excessive stimulation.
• Urinary acidification enhances renal excretion; urinary alkalinization enhances renal reabsorption and recycling.
• When tolerance to anorexigenic effect develops, dosage should not be increased, but drug discontinued.
• Discourage use to combat fatigue.

• Warn patient to avoid activities that require alertness or good psychomotor coordination until CNS response to drug is determined.
• May alter daily insulin needs in patients with diabetes. Monitor blood and urine sugars.
• Use as analeptic is usually discouraged, since CNS stimulation superimposed on CNS depression can lead to neuronal instability and seizures.
• May reverse beneficial effect of antihypertensives. Monitor blood pressure.
• Give at least 6 hours before bedtime to avoid sleep interference.

benzphetamine hydrochloride
Controlled Substance Schedule III
Didrex**
Pregnancy Category: X

MECHANISM OF ACTION
Main site of activity appears to be the cerebral cortex and the reticular activating system. Promotes nerve impulse transmission by releasing stored norepinephrine from nerve terminals in the brain.

INDICATIONS & DOSAGE
Short-term adjunct in exogenous obesity—
Adults: 25 to 50 mg P.O. daily, b.i.d., or t.i.d.

ADVERSE REACTIONS
CNS: *restlessness,* tremor, *hyperactivity, talkativeness, insomnia,* irritability, dizziness, headache, chills, overstimulation, dysphoria.
CV: *tachycardia, palpitations,* hypertension, hypotension.
GI: nausea, vomiting, cramps, dry mouth, diarrhea, constipation, metallic taste, anorexia, weight loss.
Skin: urticaria.
Other: impotence, changes in libido.

Italicized side effects are common or life-threatening.
*Liquid form contains alcohol.   **May contain tartrazine.

INTERACTIONS
MAO inhibitors: severe hypertension; possible hypertensive crisis. Don't use together.
Antacids, sodium bicarbonate, acetazolamide: increased renal reabsorption. Monitor for enhanced effects.
Ammonium chloride, ascorbic acid: observe for decreased benzphetamine effects.
Phenothiazines, haloperidol: observe for decreased benzphetamine effects.

NURSING CONSIDERATIONS
• Contraindicated in symptomatic cardiovascular diseases, hyperthyroidism, nephritis, angina pectoris, moderate to severe hypertension, parkinsonism due to arteriosclerosis, certain types of glaucoma, advanced arteriosclerosis, agitated states, or patients with history of drug abuse. Use with caution in patients with diabetes mellitus and in elderly, debilitated, or hyperexcitable patients.
• Psychic dependence or habituation may occur, especially in patients with history of drug addiction. Avoid prolonged administration. When used long-term, lower dosage gradually to prevent acute rebound depression.
• Use in conjunction with weight-reduction program. Monitor dietary intake. Do calorie counts, if necessary. Give 30 to 60 minutes before meals.
• Fatigue may result as drug effects wear off. Patient will need more rest.
• Tell patient to avoid caffeine-containing drinks, which increase the effects of amphetamines and related amines.
• Check vital signs regularly for signs of excessive stimulation.
• Urinary acidification enhances renal excretion; urinary alkalinization enhances renal reabsorption and recycling.
• When tolerance to anorexigenic effect develops, dosage should not be increased, but drug discontinued.

• Warn patient to avoid activities that require alertness or good psychomotor coordination until CNS response to drug is determined.
• May alter daily insulin needs in patients with diabetes. Monitor blood and urine sugars.
• Give at least 6 hours before bedtime to avoid sleep interference.

caffeine
No Doz, Tirend, Vivarin♦
Pregnancy Category: B

MECHANISM OF ACTION
Inhibits phosphodiesterase, the enzyme that degrades cyclic AMP.

INDICATIONS & DOSAGE
Central nervous system stimulant—
Adults: 100 to 200 mg anhydrous caffeine P.O.

ADVERSE REACTIONS
CNS: *stimulation, insomnia,* restlessness, nervousness, mild delirium, headache, excitement, agitation, muscle tremors, twitches.
CV: *tachycardia.*
GI: nausea, vomiting.
GU: *diuresis.*
Skin: hyperesthesia.

INTERACTIONS
None significant.

NURSING CONSIDERATIONS
• Contraindicated in patients with gastric or duodenal ulcer.
• Caffeine-containing beverages should be restricted in patients who experience arrhythmic symptoms.
• Tolerance or psychological dependence may develop.
• Be alert for signs of overdose: GI pain, mild delirium, insomnia, diuresis, dehydration, and fever. Treat with short-acting barbiturates, gastric emesis, or lavage.
• Single dose should not exceed 1 g.

• Caffeine content in cola beverages, 17 to 55 mg/180 ml; tea, 40 to 100 mg/180 ml; instant coffee, 60 to 180 mg/180 ml; brewed coffee, 100 to 150 mg/180 ml; decaffeinated coffee, 1 to 6 mg/180 ml.

• Caffeine does not reverse alcohol intoxication or depressant effects of alcohol. Overvigorous therapy with caffeine may aggravate depression in an already depressed patient.

• Sudden discontinuation of caffeine may cause headache and irritability.

• Caffeine is included in many OTC analgesic preparations. There's conflicting evidence regarding whether it increases pain relief.

---

dextroamphetamine sulfate
Controlled Substance Schedule II
Dexampex**, Dexedrine•* **,
Ferndex, Robese, Spancap #1
Pregnancy Category: C

MECHANISM OF ACTION
Main site of activity appears to be the cerebral cortex and the reticular activating system. Promotes nerve impulse transmission by releasing stored norepinephrine from nerve terminals in the brain. In children with hyperkinesia, amphetamines have a paradoxical calming effect.

INDICATIONS & DOSAGE
Narcolepsy—
Adults: 5 to 60 mg P.O. daily in divided doses.
Children over 12 years: 10 mg P.O. daily, with 10-mg increments weekly, p.r.n.
Children 6 to 12 years: 5 mg P.O. daily, with 5-mg increments weekly, p.r.n.
Short-term adjunct in exogenous obesity—
Adults: single 10- to 15-mg long-acting capsule, up to 30 mg daily; or in divided doses, 5 to 10 mg ½ hour before meals.

Attention deficit disorders with hyperactivity (ADDH)—
Children 6 years and older: 5 mg once daily or b.i.d., with 5-mg increments weekly, p.r.n.
Children 3 to 5 years: 2.5 mg P.O. daily, with 2.5-mg increments weekly, p.r.n.

ADVERSE REACTIONS
CNS: *restlessness*, tremor, *hyperactivity, talkativeness, insomnia*, irritability, dizziness, headache, chills, overstimulation, dysphoria.
CV: *tachycardia, palpitations*, hypertension, hypotension.
GI: nausea, vomiting, cramps, dry mouth, diarrhea, constipation, metallic taste, anorexia, weight loss.
Skin: urticaria.
Other: impotence, changes in libido.

INTERACTIONS
MAO inhibitors: severe hypertension; possible hypertensive crisis. Don't use together.
Antacids, sodium bicarbonate, acetazolamide: increased renal reabsorption. Monitor for enhanced amphetamine effects.
Ammonium chloride, ascorbic acid: observe for decreased amphetamine effects.
Phenothiazines, haloperidol: observe for decreased amphetamine effects.

NURSING CONSIDERATIONS
• Contraindicated in patients with hyperthyroidism, nephritis, severe hypertension, angina pectoris or other severe cardiovascular disease, some types of glaucoma, or history of drug abuse. Use with caution in patients with diabetes mellitus and in elderly, debilitated, or hyperexcitable patients.
• Use cautiously in children with Gilles de la Tourette's disorder.
• Psychic dependence or habituation may occur, especially in patients with history of drug addiction. Avoid pro-

---

Italicized side effects are common or life-threatening.
*Liquid form contains alcohol.   **May contain tartrazine.

longed administration. When used long-term, lower dosage gradually to prevent acute rebound depression.

• Not recommended for first-line treatment of obesity. Use as an anorexigenic agent is prohibited in some states.

• When used for obesity, be sure patient is also on a weight-reduction program. Give 30 to 60 minutes before meals. Avoid giving within 6 hours of bedtime.

• Fatigue may result as drug effects wear off. Patient will need more rest.

• Tell patient to avoid drinks containing caffeine, which increase the effects of amphetamines and related amines.

• Check vital signs regularly. Observe for signs of excessive stimulation.

• Urinary acidification enhances renal excretion; urinary alkalinization enhances renal reabsorption and recycling.

• When tolerance to anorexigenic effect develops, dosage should not be increased, but drug discontinued.

• Discourage use to combat fatigue.

• Warn patient to avoid activities that require alertness or good psychomotor coordination until CNS response to drug is determined.

• May alter daily insulin needs in patients with diabetes. Monitor blood and urine sugars.

• Use as analeptic is usually discouraged, since CNS stimulation superimposed on CNS depression can lead to neuronal instability and seizures.

• Give at least 6 hours before bedtime to avoid sleep interference.

diethylpropion hydrochloride

Controlled Substance Schedule IV
Nobesine♦♦, Nu-Dispoz,
Regibon♦♦, Ro-Diet, Tenuate♦,
Tepanil
Pregnancy Category: B

MECHANISM OF ACTION
Main site of activity appears to be the cerebral cortex and the reticular activating system. Promotes nerve impulse transmission by releasing stored norepinephrine from nerve terminals in the brain.

INDICATIONS & DOSAGE
Short-term adjunct in exogenous obesity—
Adults: 25 mg P.O. before meals, t.i.d.; or 75 mg controlled-release tablet P.O. in midmorning.

ADVERSE REACTIONS
CNS: headache, *nervousness,* dizziness.
CV: *tachycardia, palpitations,* rise in blood pressure.
EENT: blurred vision.
GI: nausea, abdominal cramps, dry mouth, diarrhea, constipation.
Skin: urticaria.
Other: impotence, libido changes, menstrual upset.

INTERACTIONS
MAO inhibitors: hypertension; possible hypertensive crisis. Don't use together.

NURSING CONSIDERATIONS
• Contraindicated in patients with hyperthyroidism, hypertension, angina pectoris, severe cardiovascular disease, glaucoma, or history of drug abuse. Use with caution in epilepsy, diabetes mellitus, or hyperexcitability states. May alter insulin requirements. Monitor blood and urine sugars.
• When tolerance to anorexigenic ef-

fect develops, dosage should not be increased, but drug discontinued.
• Habituation or psychic dependence may occur.
• Be sure patient is also on a weight-reduction program.
• Can be used to stop nighttime eating. Rarely causes insomnia.
• Fatigue may result as drug effects wear off. Patient will need more rest.
• Tell patient to avoid drinks containing caffeine, which increase the effects of amphetamines and related amines.
• Check vital signs regularly. Observe for signs of excessive stimulation.
• Urinary acidification enhances renal excretion; urinary alkalinization enhances renal reabsorption and recycling.
• Use as analeptic is usually discouraged, since CNS stimulation superimposed on CNS depression can lead to neuronal instability and seizures.
• Give at least 6 hours before bedtime to avoid sleep interference.

---

fenfluramine hydrochloride
Controlled Substance Schedule IV
Ponderal♦♦, Pondimin♦
Pregnancy Category: C

MECHANISM OF ACTION
Stimulates ventromedial nucleus of the hypothalamus. May also affect serotonin metabolism.

INDICATIONS & DOSAGE
Short-term adjunct in exogenous obesity—
Adults: initially, 20 mg P.O. t.i.d. before meals. Maximum 40 mg t.i.d. Adjust dosage according to patient's response.

ADVERSE REACTIONS
CNS: *drowsiness,* dizziness, incoordination, headache, euphoria or depression, anxiety, *insomnia,* weakness or fatigue, agitation.
CV: *palpitations,* hypotension, hypertension, chest pain.
EENT: eye irritation, blurred vision.
GI: *diarrhea, dry mouth,* nausea, vomiting, abdominal pain, constipation.
GU: dysuria, increased urinary frequency, impotence, increased libido.
Skin: rashes, urticaria, burning sensation.
Other: sweating, chills, fever.

INTERACTIONS
MAO inhibitors: severe hypertension; possible hypertensive crisis. Don't use together.

NURSING CONSIDERATIONS
• Contraindicated in patients with glaucoma, hypersensitivity to sympathomimetic amines, symptomatic cardiovascular disease, alcoholism, or history of drug abuse. Use with caution in patients with hypertension, history of mental depression, diabetes mellitus.
• Because of possible hypoglycemia, patients with diabetes may have altered insulin or sulfonylurea requirements. Monitor blood and urine sugars.
• Differs pharmacologically from amphetamines in that it produces CNS depression more often than stimulation.
• Check vital signs regularly. Observe patient for signs of excessive sedation, depression, or excessive stimulation. Closely monitor blood pressure.
• Be sure patient is on a weight-reduction program.
• Tolerance or dependence may occur. Avoid prolonged administration.
• Tell patient to avoid drinks containing caffeine, which increase the effects of amphetamines and related amines.
• Fenfluramine should not be discontinued abruptly; may precipitate an

---

Italicized side effects are common or life-threatening.
*Liquid form contains alcohol.   **May contain tartrazine.

acute depressive reaction.
• Has been proven effective for treating autistic children.

mazindol
Controlled Substance Schedule IV
Mazanor, Sanorex♦
Pregnancy Category: C

MECHANISM OF ACTION
Inhibits neuronal uptake of norepinephrine and dopamine.

INDICATIONS & DOSAGE
Short-term adjunct in exogenous obesity—
Adults: 1 mg t.i.d. 1 hour before meals, or 2 mg daily 1 hour before lunch. Use lowest effective dose.

ADVERSE REACTIONS
CNS: *nervousness,* restlessness, dizziness, *insomnia,* dysphoria, headache, depression, drowsiness, weakness, tremors.
CV: *palpitations, tachycardia.*
GI: dry mouth, nausea, constipation, diarrhea, unpleasant taste.
GU: difficulty initiating micturition, impotence, libido changes.
Skin: rash, clamminess, pallor.
Other: shivering, excessive sweating.

INTERACTIONS
MAO inhibitors: severe hypertension; possible hypertensive crisis. Don't use together.

NURSING CONSIDERATIONS
• Contraindicated in patients with glaucoma, cardiovascular disease including arrhythmias, agitated states, and history of drug abuse. Use with caution in diabetes mellitus, hypertension, hyperexcitability states.
• Warn patient to avoid activities that require alertness or good psychomotor coordination until CNS response to drug has been determined.
• Fatigue may result as drug effects

wear off. Patient will need more rest.
• Tell patient to avoid caffeine-containing drinks, which increase the effects of amphetamines and related amines.
• Check vital signs regularly. Observe for signs of excessive stimulation.
• Tolerance or dependence may develop. Avoid prolonged use.
• Be sure patient is also on a weight-reduction program.
• May alter insulin needs in patients with diabetes. Monitor blood and urine sugars.
• Give at least 6 hours before bedtime to avoid sleep interference.

methamphetamine hydrochloride
Controlled Substance Schedule II
Desoxyn, Methampex
Pregnancy Category: C

MECHANISM OF ACTION
Main site of activity appears to be the cerebral cortex and the reticular activating system. Promotes nerve impulse transmission by releasing stored norepinephrine from nerve terminals in the brain. In children with hyperkinesia, amphetamines have a paradoxical calming effect.

INDICATIONS & DOSAGE
Attention deficit disorder with hyperactivity (ADDH)—
Children 6 years and older: 2.5 to 5 mg P.O. once daily or b.i.d., with 5-mg increments weekly, p.r.n. Usual effective dosage is 20 to 25 mg daily.
Short-term adjunct in exogenous obesity—
Adults: 2.5 to 5 mg P.O. once to t.i.d. 30 minutes before meals; or 1 long-acting 5- to 15-mg tablet daily before breakfast.

ADVERSE REACTIONS
CNS: *nervousness, insomnia,* irrita-

bility, *talkativeness,* dizziness, headache, hyperexcitability, tremors.
CV: hypertension or hypotension, *tachycardia, palpitations,* cardiac arrhythmias.
EENT: blurred vision, mydriasis.
GI: nausea, vomiting, abdominal cramps, diarrhea or constipation, dry mouth, anorexia, metallic taste.
Skin: urticaria.
Other: impotence, libido changes.

INTERACTIONS

MAO inhibitors: severe hypertension; possible hypertensive crisis. Don't use together.
Antacids, sodium bicarbonate, acetazolamide: increased renal reabsorption. Monitor for enhanced effects.
Ammonium chloride, ascorbic acid: observe for decreased amphetamine effects.
Phenothiazines, haloperidol: observe for decreased amphetamine effects.

NURSING CONSIDERATIONS

• Contraindicated in patients with hypertension, hyperthyroidism, nephritis, angina pectoris or other severe cardiovascular disease, glaucoma, parkinsonism due to arteriosclerosis, agitated states, or history of drug abuse. Use with caution in patients with diabetes mellitus; and in patients who are elderly, debilitated, asthenic, psychopathic, or who have a history of suicidal or homicidal tendencies.
• Use cautiously in children with Gilles de la Tourette's disorder.
• Warn that potential for abuse is high. Discourage use to combat fatigue.
• May alter insulin needs in patients with diabetes. Monitor blood and urine sugars.
• Not recommended for first-line treatment of obesity. Use as an anorexigenic agent is prohibited in some states.
• When used for obesity, be sure patient is on a weight-reduction pro-

gram.
• Tell patient to avoid caffeinic drinks, which increase the effects of amphetamines and related amines.
• Check vital signs regularly. Observe for signs of excessive stimulation.
• Urinary acidification enhances renal excretion; urinary alkalinization enhances renal reabsorption and recycling.
• When tolerance to anorexigenic effect develops, dosage should not be increased, but drug discontinued.
• Warn patient to avoid activities that require alertness or good psychomotor coordination until CNS response to drug is determined.
• Give at least 6 hours before bedtime to avoid sleep interference.

methylphenidate hydrochloride

Controlled Substance Schedule II
Methidate♦♦, Ritalin♦, Ritalin SR
Pregnancy Category: C

MECHANISM OF ACTION

Main site of activity appears to be the cerebral cortex and the reticular activating system. Promotes nerve impulse transmission by releasing stored norepinephrine from nerve terminals in the brain. In children with hyperkinesia, amphetamines have a paradoxical calming effect.

INDICATIONS & DOSAGE

Attention deficit disorder with hyperactivity (ADDH)—
Children 6 years and older: initial dose 5 to 10 mg P.O. daily before breakfast and lunch, with 5- to 10-mg increments weekly as needed, up to 60 mg daily.
Narcolepsy—
Adults: 10 mg P.O. b.i.d. or t.i.d. ½ hour before meals. Dosage varies with patient needs. Dosage range is 5 to 50 mg daily.

Italicized side effects are common or life-threatening.
*Liquid form contains alcohol.   **May contain tartrazine.

ADVERSE REACTIONS
CNS: *nervousness, insomnia,* dizziness, headache, akathisia, dyskinesia, *Tourette's disorder.*
CV: *palpitations,* angina, *tachycardia,* changes in blood pressure and pulse rate.
EENT: difficulty with accommodation and blurring of vision.
GI: nausea, dry throat, abdominal pain, anorexia, weight loss.
Skin: rash, urticaria, *exfoliative dermatitis,* erythema multiforme.
Other: growth suppression.

INTERACTIONS
MAO inhibitors: severe hypertension; possible hypertensive crisis. Don't use together.

NURSING CONSIDERATIONS
• Contraindicated in patients with symptomatic cardiac disease; hyperthyroidism; moderate to severe hypertension; angina pectoris; advanced arteriosclerosis; severe depression of either endogenous or exogenous form; glaucoma; parkinsonism; history of drug abuse or dependency; history of marked anxiety, tension, or agitation. Use with caution in elderly, debilitated, or hyperexcitable patients and those with history of cardiovascular disease, diabetes, or seizures.
• May precipitate Tourette's disorder in children. Monitor especially at start of therapy.
• Closely monitor blood pressure. Observe for signs of excessive stimulation.
• Discourage use to combat fatigue.
• Observe for interactions, as treatment of other disease states may be affected. May alter daily insulin needs in patients with diabetes. Monitor blood and urine sugars. May decrease seizure threshold in patients with seizure disorders.
• Drug of choice for ADDH. Usually stopped postpuberty.
• Periodic CBC, differential, and platelet counts advised with long-term use.
• Tolerance, psychic dependence, or habituation may develop, especially in patients with history of drug addiction. High abuse potential. Avoid prolonged administration. When used long-term, lower dosage gradually to prevent acute rebound depression.
• Fatigue may result as drug effects wear off. Patient will need more rest.
• Tell patient to avoid drinks containing caffeine, which increase the effects of amphetamines and related amines.
• Warn patient to avoid activities that require alertness or good psychomotor coordination until CNS response to drug is determined.
• Monitor height and weight in children on prolonged therapy because drug has been associated with growth suppression.
• Now available in a sustained-release form (duration, 6 to 8 hours). Warn patient against chewing these tablets.
• Give at least 6 hours before bedtime to prevent insomnia. Administer after meals to reduce appetite suppressive effects.

pemoline
Controlled Substance Schedule IV
Cylert
Pregnancy Category: B

MECHANISM OF ACTION
Main site of activity appears to be the cerebral cortex and the reticular activating system. Promotes nerve impulse transmission by releasing stored norepinephrine from nerve terminals in the brain.

INDICATIONS & DOSAGE
Attention deficit disorder with hyperactivity (ADDH)—
Children 6 years and older: initially, 37.5 mg P.O. given in the morning. Daily dose can be raised by 18.75 mg

weekly. Effective dosage range 56.25 to 75 mg daily; maximum is 112.5 mg daily.

ADVERSE REACTIONS
CNS: *insomnia,* malaise, irritability, fatigue, mild depression, dizziness, headache, drowsiness, hallucinations, nervousness (large doses), seizures, *Tourette's disorder,* psychosis.
CV: tachycardia (large doses).
GI: anorexia, abdominal pain, nausea, diarrhea.
Hepatic: liver enzyme elevations.
Skin: rash.

INTERACTIONS
None significant.

NURSING CONSIDERATIONS
• Use with caution in patients with impaired renal function. Drug may accumulate.
• May precipitate Tourette's disorder in children. Monitor especially at start of therapy.
• Closely monitor patients on long-term therapy for possible hepatic function abnormalities and for growth suppression.
• Structurally dissimilar to amphetamines or methylphenidate. However, may produce similar adverse reactions. Also, has a greater potential for drug abuse and dependence than previously thought.
• Therapeutic effects may not be evident for up to 3 to 4 weeks.
• Give at least 6 hours before bedtime to avoid sleep interference.

---

phenmetrazine hydrochloride
Controlled Substance Schedule II
Preludin**
Pregnancy Category: C

MECHANISM OF ACTION
Main site of activity appears to be the cerebral cortex and the reticular activating system. Promotes nerve impulse transmission by releasing stored norepinephrine from nerve terminals in the brain.

INDICATIONS & DOSAGE
Short-term adjunct in exogenous obesity—
Adults: 25 mg P.O. b.i.d. or t.i.d. 1 hour before meals, up to 75 mg daily; or single 50- to 75-mg extended-release tablet daily in midmorning.

ADVERSE REACTIONS
CNS: *nervousness,* dizziness, *insomnia,* headache.
CV: *tachycardia, palpitations,* increased blood pressure.
EENT: blurred vision.
GI: dry mouth, nausea, abdominal cramps, constipation.
Skin: urticaria.
Other: libido changes, impotence.

INTERACTIONS
MAO inhibitors: severe hypertension; possible hypertensive crisis. Don't use together.
Antacids, sodium bicarbonate, acetazolamide: increased renal reabsorption. Monitor for enhanced effects.
Ammonium chloride, ascorbic acid: observe for decreased phenmetrazine effects.
Phenothiazines, haloperidol: observe for decreased effect.

NURSING CONSIDERATIONS
• Contraindicated in patients with hyperthyroidism, hypertension, angina pectoris or other cardiovascular disease, glaucoma, or history of drug addiction. Use with caution in hyperexcitability states.
• Tolerance or dependence may develop. High abuse potential. Not advised for prolonged use.
• Be sure patient is also following weight-reduction program.
• Fatigue may result as drug effects wear off. Patient will need more rest.

• Tell patient to avoid drinks containing caffeine, which increase the effects of amphetamines and related amines.
• Check vital signs regularly. Observe for signs of excessive stimulation.
• Urinary acidification enhances renal excretion; urinary alkalinization enhances renal reabsorption and recycling.

phentermine hydrochloride
Controlled Substance Schedule IV
Anoxine, Fastin♦, Ionamin♦,
Parmine, Phentrol, Rolaphent,
Wilpowr
Pregnancy Category: C

MECHANISM OF ACTION
Main site of activity appears to be the cerebral cortex and the reticular activating system. Promotes nerve impulse transmission by releasing stored norepinephrine from nerve terminals in the brain.

INDICATIONS & DOSAGE
Short-term adjunct in exogenous obesity—
Adults: 8 mg P.O. t.i.d. ½ hour before meals; or 15 to 30 mg daily before breakfast (resin complex).

ADVERSE REACTIONS
CNS: *nervousness,* dizziness, *insomnia.*
CV: *palpitations, tachycardia,* increased blood pressure.
GI: dry mouth, unpleasant taste, nausea, constipation, diarrhea.
Skin: urticaria.
Other: libido changes, impotence.

INTERACTIONS
MAO inhibitors: severe hypertension; possible hypertensive crisis. Don't use together.
Antacids, sodium bicarbonate, acetazolamide: increased renal reabsorp-

tion. Monitor for enhanced effects.
Ammonium chloride, ascorbic acid: observe for decreased phentermine effects.
Phenothiazines, haloperidol: observe for decreased effects.

NURSING CONSIDERATIONS
• Contraindicated in hyperthyroidism, hypertension, angina pectoris or other severe cardiovascular disease, glaucoma. Use with caution in hyperexcitability states or patients with history of drug addiction.
• Tolerance or dependence may develop. Avoid prolonged administration.
• Use with weight-reduction program. Give 30 minutes before meals.
• Fatigue may result as drug effects wear off. Patient will need more rest.
• Tell patient to avoid caffeine drinks, which increase the effects of amphetamines and related amines.
• Check vital signs regularly. Observe for signs of excessive stimulation.
• Urinary acidification enhances renal excretion; urinary alkalinization enhances renal reabsorption and recycling.
• Give at least 6 hours before bedtime to avoid sleep interference.

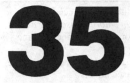

Respiratory stimulants

ammonia, aromatic spirits
doxapram hydrochloride

COMBINATION PRODUCTS
None.

---

ammonia, aromatic spirits
Pregnancy Category: C

MECHANISM OF ACTION
Irritates the sensory receptors in the nasal membranes, producing reflex stimulation of the respiratory centers.

INDICATIONS & DOSAGE
Fainting—
Adults and children: inhale as needed.

ADVERSE REACTIONS
None reported.

INTERACTIONS
None significant.

NURSING CONSIDERATIONS
• Stimulates mucous membranes of upper respiratory tract.

---

doxapram hydrochloride
Dopram♦
Pregnancy Category: C

MECHANISM OF ACTION
Acts either directly on the central respiratory centers in the medulla or indirectly on the chemoreceptors.

INDICATIONS & DOSAGE
Postanesthesia respiratory stimulation, drug-induced central nervous system depression, and chronic pulmonary disease associated with acute hypercapnia—
Adults: 0.5 to 1 mg/kg of body weight (up to 2 mg/kg in CNS depression), I.V. injection or infusion. Maximum 4 mg/kg, up to 3 g in 1 day. Infusion rate 1 to 3 mg/minute (initial: 5 mg/minute for postanesthesia).
Chronic obstructive pulmonary disease—
Adults: infusion, 1 to 2 mg/minute. Maximum 3 mg/minute for a maximum duration of 2 hours.

ADVERSE REACTIONS
CNS: *seizures, headache,* dizziness, apprehension, disorientation, pupillary dilation, bilateral Babinski's signs, flushing, sweating, paresthesias.
CV: *chest pain and tightness, variations in heart rate, hypertension,* lowered T waves.
GI: nausea, vomiting, diarrhea.
GU: urinary retention, or stimulation of the bladder with incontinence.
Other: sneezing, coughing, laryngospasm, bronchospasm, hiccups, rebound hypoventilation, pruritus.

INTERACTIONS
MAO inhibitors: potentiate adverse cardiovascular effects. Use together cautiously.

NURSING CONSIDERATIONS
• Contraindicated in convulsive dis-

Italicized side effects are common or life-threatening.
*Liquid form contains alcohol.   **May contain tartrazine.

orders; head injury; cardiovascular disorders; frank uncompensated heart failure; severe hypertension; cerebrovascular accidents; respiratory failure or incompetence secondary to neuromuscular disorders, muscle paresis, flail chest, obstructed airway, pulmonary embolism, pneumothorax, restrictive respiratory disease, acute bronchial asthma, extreme dyspnea; hypoxia not associated with hypercapnia. Use with caution in bronchial asthma, severe tachycardia or cardiac arrhythmias, cerebral edema or increased cerebrospinal fluid pressure, hyperthyroidism, pheochromocytoma, or metabolic disorders.

• Doxapram's use as an analeptic is strongly discouraged by most doctors.

• Establish adequate airway before administering drug. Prevent patient from aspirating vomitus by placing him on his side.

• Monitor blood pressure, heart rate, deep tendon reflexes, and arterial blood gases before giving drug and every 30 minutes afterward.

• Be alert for signs of overdosage: hypertension, tachycardia, arrhythmias, skeletal muscle hyperactivity, dyspnea. Discontinue if patient shows signs of increased arterial carbon dioxide or oxygen tension, or if mechanical ventilation is started. May give I.V. injection of anticonvulsant.

• Use only in surgical or emergency room situations.

• Do not combine with alkaline solutions such as thiopental sodium; doxapram is acidic.

Cholinergics (parasympathomimetics)

ambenonium chloride
bethanechol chloride
edrophonium chloride
neostigmine bromide
neostigmine methylsulfate
physostigmine salicylate
pyridostigmine bromide

COMBINATION PRODUCTS
None.

ambenonium chloride
Mytelase♦
Pregnancy Category: C

MECHANISM OF ACTION
Inhibits the destruction of acetylcholine released from the parasympathetic and somatic efferent nerves. Acetylcholine accumulates, promoting increased stimulation of the receptor.

INDICATIONS & DOSAGE
Symptomatic treatment of myasthenia gravis in patients who cannot take neostigmine bromide and pyridostigmine bromide—
Adults: dose must be individualized for each patient, but usually ranges from 5 to 25 mg P.O. 3 to 4 times a day. Starting dose usually 5 mg P.O. 3 to 4 times a day. Increase gradually and adjust at 1- to 2-day intervals to avoid drug accumulation and overdosage. May range from 5 mg to as much as 75 mg per dose.

ADVERSE REACTIONS
CNS: headache, dizziness, muscle weakness, convulsions, mental confusion, jitters, sweating.
CV: bradycardia, hypotension.
EENT: miosis, blurred vision.
GI: *nausea, vomiting, diarrhea, abdominal cramps,* increased salivation.
GU: urinary frequency, incontinence.
Other: bronchospasm, *muscle cramps,* bronchoconstriction, increased bronchial secretions, *respiratory paralysis.*

INTERACTIONS
Procainamide, quinidine: may reverse cholinergic effect on muscle. Observe for lack of drug effect.

NURSING CONSIDERATIONS
• Contraindicated in patients with mechanical obstruction of intestine or urinary tract, bradycardia, hypotension.
• Use with extreme caution in patients with bronchial asthma.
• Use cautiously in patients with epilepsy, recent coronary occlusion, vagotonia, hyperthyroidism, cardiac arrhythmias, peptic ulcer.
• Avoid large dose in patients with decreased gastrointestinal motility or megacolon.
• Discontinue all other cholinergics before administering this drug.
• Watch patient very closely for side effects, particularly if total dose is greater than 200 mg daily. Side effects may indicate drug toxicity. Notify doctor immediately if they develop.
• Monitor and document vital signs frequently, being especially careful to

---

Italicized side effects are common or life-threatening.
*Liquid form contains alcohol.   **May contain tartrazine.

check respirations. Always have atropine injection readily available and be prepared to give atropine 0.5 mg subcutaneously or slow I.V. push as ordered, and provide respiratory support as needed.
• Administer each dose exactly as ordered, on time. Amount and frequency of dosage should vary with patient's activity level. The doctor will probably order larger doses to be given when patient is fatigued, for example, in the afternoon and at mealtime.
• If muscle weakness is severe, doctor must determine if this is caused by drug toxicity or exacerbation of myasthenia gravis. A test dose of edrophonium I.V. will aggravate drug-induced weakness but will temporarily relieve weakness that results from the disease.
• Weakness occurring 30 to 60 minutes after taking dose is a warning sign of drug toxicity. Notify doctor immediately.
• Observe and record the patient's variations in muscle strength. Show him how to do it himself.
• When given for myasthenia gravis, explain to patient that this drug will relieve symptoms of ptosis, double vision, difficulty in chewing and swallowing, and trunk and limb weakness. Stress the importance of taking this drug exactly as ordered. Explain to patient and his family that he may have to take this drug for the rest of his life. Teach them about the disease and the drug's effect on symptoms.
• Monitor intake and output.
• Patient may develop resistance to drug.
• Seek approval when indicated for hospitalized patient to have bedside supply of tablets to take himself. Patients with long-standing disease often insist on this.
• Give with milk or food to produce fewer muscarinic side effects.
• Advise patient to wear identifica-

tion tag indicating he has myasthenia gravis.

---

bethanechol chloride
Duvoid♦, Myotonachol,
Urecholine♦
Pregnancy Category: C

MECHANISM OF ACTION
Binds to cholinergic (muscarinic) receptors, mimicking the action of acetylcholine.

INDICATIONS & DOSAGE
Acute postoperative and postpartum nonobstructive (functional) urinary retention, neurogenic atony of urinary bladder with retention, abdominal distention, megacolon—
Adults: 10 to 30 mg P.O. t.i.d. or q.i.d. Or, 2.5 to 10 mg S.C. Never give I.M. or I.V. When used for urinary retention, some patients may require 50 to 100 mg P.O. per dose. Use such doses with extreme caution.
Test dose: 2.5 mg S.C. repeated at 15- to 30-minute intervals to total of 4 doses to determine the minimal effective dose; then use minimal effective dose q 6 to 8 hours. All doses must be adjusted individually.

ADVERSE REACTIONS
Dose-related:
CNS: headache, malaise.
CV: bradycardia, hypotension, *cardiac arrest,* reflex tachycardia.
EENT: lacrimation, miosis.
GI: *abdominal cramps, diarrhea,* salivation, nausea, vomiting, belching, borborygmus.
GU: urinary urgency.
Skin: flushing, sweating.
Other: bronchoconstriction, increased bronchial secretions.

INTERACTIONS
Procainamide, quinidine: may reverse cholinergic effects on muscle. Observe for lack of drug effect.

NURSING CONSIDERATIONS

• Contraindicated in patients with uncertain strength or integrity of bladder wall; when increased muscular activity of GI or urinary tract is harmful; in mechanical obstructions of GI or urinary tract; in hyperthyroidism, peptic ulcer, latent or active bronchial asthma, cardiac or coronary artery disease, vagotonia, epilepsy, Parkinson's disease, bradycardia, chronic obstructive pulmonary disease, hypotension. Use cautiously in hypertension, vasomotor instability, peritonitis, or other acute inflammatory conditions of GI tract.

• *Never* give I.M. or I.V.; could cause circulatory collapse, hypotension, severe abdominal cramping, bloody diarrhea, shock, or cardiac arrest.

• Should stop all other cholinergics before giving this drug.

• Watch closely for side effects that may indicate drug toxicity, especially with subcutaneous administration.

• Monitor vital signs frequently, being especially careful to check respirations. Always have atropine injection readily available and be prepared to give atropine 0.5 mg subcutaneously or slow I.V. push as ordered, and provide respiratory support if needed.

• If used to treat urinary retention, make sure bedpan is readily available. Monitor intake and output.

• When used to prevent abdominal distention and GI distress, the doctor may also order a rectal tube inserted to help passage of gas.

• Poor and variable oral absorption requires larger oral doses. Oral and subcutaneous doses are *not* interchangeable.

• Drug usually effective 5 to 15 minutes after injection and 30 to 90 minutes after oral use.

• Give on empty stomach; if taken after meals, may cause nausea and vomiting.

edrophonium chloride
Tensilon♦
Pregnancy Category: C

MECHANISM OF ACTION
Inhibits the destruction of acetylcholine released from the parasympathetic and somatic efferent nerves. Acetylcholine accumulates, promoting increased stimulation of the receptor.

INDICATIONS & DOSAGE
As a curare antagonist (to reverse neuromuscular blocking action)—
Adults: 10 mg I.V. given over 30 to 45 seconds. Dose may be repeated as necessary to 40 mg maximum dose. Larger doses may potentiate rather than antagonize effect of curare.
Diagnostic aid in myasthenia gravis (the Tensilon test)—
Adults: 1 to 2 mg I.V. within 15 to 30 seconds, then 8 mg if no response (increase in muscular strength).
Children over 34 kg: 2 mg I.V. If no response within 45 seconds, give 1 mg q 45 seconds to maximum of 10 mg.
Children up to 34 kg: 1 mg I.V. If no response within 45 seconds, give 1 mg q 45 seconds to maximum of 5 mg.
Infants: 0.5 mg I.V.
To differentiate myasthenic crisis from cholinergic crisis—
Adults: 1 mg I.V. If no response in 1 minute, repeat dose once. Increased muscular strength confirms myasthenic crisis; no increase or exaggerated weakness confirms cholinergic crisis.
Paroxysmal supraventricular tachycardia—
Adults: 10 mg I.V. given over 1 minute or less.

ADVERSE REACTIONS
CNS: weakness, respiratory paralysis, sweating.

CV: hypotension, bradycardia.
EENT: miosis.
GI: nausea, vomiting, *diarrhea, abdominal cramps,* excessive salivation.
Other: increased bronchial secretions, bronchospasm, muscle cramps, muscle fasciculation.

INTERACTIONS
Procainamide, quinidine: may reverse cholinergic effects on muscle. Observe for lack of drug effect.

NURSING CONSIDERATIONS
• Contraindicated in mechanical obstruction of intestine or urinary tract, bradycardia, hypotension. Use cautiously in hyperthyroidism, cardiac disease, peptic ulcer, bronchial asthma.
• Should stop all other cholinergics before giving this drug.
• Watch closely for side effects; may indicate toxicity.
• Monitor vital signs frequently, being especially careful to check respirations. Always have atropine injection readily available and be prepared to give atropine 0.5 mg subcutaneously or slow I.V. push as ordered, and provide respiratory support as needed.
• When giving drug to differentiate myasthenic crisis from cholinergic crisis, observe patient's muscle strength closely.
• Edrophonium not effective against muscle relaxation induced by decamethonium bromide and succinylcholine chloride.
• This cholinergic has the most rapid onset but shortest duration; therefore, not used for treatment of myasthenia gravis.
• For easier parenteral administration, use a tuberculin syringe with an I.V. needle.
• I.M. route may be used in children due to difficulty with I.V. route: for children under 34 kg, inject 2 mg I.M.; children over 34 kg, 5 mg I.M.

Expect same reactions as with I.V. test, but these appear after 2- to 10-minute delay.

neostigmine bromide
Prostigmin Bromide♦

neostigmine methylsulfate
Prostigmin♦
Pregnancy Category: C

MECHANISM OF ACTION
Inhibits the destruction of acetylcholine released from the parasympathetic and somatic efferent nerves. Acetylcholine accumulates, promoting increased stimulation of the receptor.

INDICATIONS & DOSAGE
Antidote for tubocurarine—
Adults: 0.5 to 2 mg I.V. slowly. Repeat p.r.n. Give 0.6 to 1.2 mg atropine sulfate I.V. before antidote dose.
Postoperative abdominal distention and bladder atony—
Adults: 0.5 to 1 mg I.M. or S.C. q 4 to 6 hours.
Postoperative ileus—
Adults: 0.25 to 1 mg I.M. or S.C. q 4 to 6 hours.
Treatment of myasthenia gravis—
Adults: 15 to 30 mg t.i.d. (range 15 to 375 mg daily); or 0.5 to 2 mg I.M. or I.V. q 1 to 3 hours. Dose must be individualized, depending on response and tolerance of side effects. Therapy may be required day and night.
Children: 7.5 to 15 mg P.O. t.i.d. to q.i.d.
Note: 1:1,000 solution of injectable solution contains 1 mg/1 ml; 1:2,000 solution contains 0.5 mg/ml.

ADVERSE REACTIONS
CNS: dizziness, muscle weakness, mental confusion, jitters, sweating, respiratory depression.
CV: bradycardia, hypotension.

EENT: miosis.
GI: *nausea, vomiting, diarrhea, abdominal cramps,* excessive salivation.
Skin: rash (bromide).
Other: bronchospasm, *muscle cramps,* bronchoconstriction.

INTERACTIONS
Procainamide, quinidine: may reverse cholinergic effect on muscle. Observe for lack of drug effect.

NURSING CONSIDERATIONS
• Contraindicated in hypersensitivity to cholinergics or to bromide, mechanical obstruction of the intestine or urinary tract, bradycardia, hypotension. Use with extreme caution in bronchial asthma. Use cautiously in epilepsy, recent coronary occlusion, peritonitis, vagotonia, hyperthyroidism, cardiac arrhythmias, or peptic ulcer.
• Should stop all other cholinergics before giving this drug.
• Monitor vital signs frequently, being especially careful to check respirations. Have atropine injection readily available and be prepared to give as ordered, and provide respiratory support as needed.
• Difficult to judge optimum dose. Help doctor by documenting patient's response after each dose. Observe closely for improvement in strength, vision, and ptosis 45 to 60 minutes after each dose. Show patient how to observe and record variations in muscle strength.
• When using for myasthenia gravis, explain that this drug will relieve ptosis, double vision, difficulty in chewing and swallowing, trunk and limb weakness. Stress importance of taking drug exactly as ordered. Explain that drug may have to be taken for life.
• In myasthenia gravis, schedule the largest dose before periods of fatigue. For example, if patient has dysphagia, schedule dose 30 minutes before each meal.

• When used to prevent abdominal distention and GI distress, the doctor may order a rectal tube inserted to help passage of gas.
• Patients sometimes develop a resistance to neostigmine.
• If muscle weakness is severe, doctor determines if it is caused by drug-induced toxicity or exacerbation of myasthenia gravis. Test dose of edrophonium I.V. will aggravate drug-induced weakness but will temporarily relieve weakness caused by disease.
• Hospitalized patient with long-standing myasthenia may request bedside supply of tablets. This will enable patient to take each dose precisely as ordered. Seek approval for self-medication program according to hospital policy, but continue to oversee medication regimen.
• GI side effects may be reduced by taking drug with milk or food.
• Advise patient to wear an identification tag indicating that he has myasthenia gravis.
• I.M. neostigmine may be used instead of edrophonium to diagnose myasthenia gravis. May be preferable to edrophonium when limb weakness is the only symptom.

physostigmine salicylate
Antilirium♦
Pregnancy Category: C

MECHANISM OF ACTION
Inhibits the destruction of acetylcholine released from the parasympathetic and somatic efferent nerves. Acetylcholine accumulates, promoting increased stimulation of the receptor.

INDICATIONS & DOSAGE
Tricyclic antidepressant and anticholinergic poisoning—
Adults: 0.5 to 3 mg P.O., I.M., or I.V. (1 mg/minute I.V.) repeated as necessary if life-threatening signs recur

---

Italicized side effects are common or life-threatening.
*Liquid form contains alcohol.   **May contain tartrazine.

(coma, convulsions, arrhythmias).

ADVERSE REACTIONS
CNS: hallucinations, muscular twitching, muscle weakness, ataxia, *restlessness, excitability, sweating.*
CV: irregular pulse, palpitations.
EENT: miosis.
GI: nausea, vomiting, epigastric pain, *diarrhea, excessive salivation.*
Other: bronchospasm, bronchial constriction, dyspnea.

INTERACTIONS
Procainamide, quinidine: may reverse cholinergic effects on muscle. Observe for lack of drug effect.

NURSING CONSIDERATIONS
• Use cautiously in preexisting conditions: mechanical obstruction of intestine or urogenital tract, bronchial asthma, gangrene, diabetes, cardiovascular disease, vagotonia, bradycardia, hypotension, epilepsy, Parkinson's disease, hyperthyroidism, peptic ulcer.
• Watch closely for side effects, particularly CNS disturbances. Use side rails if patient becomes restless or hallucinates. Side effects may indicate drug toxicity.
• Monitor vital signs frequently, being especially careful to check respirations. Position patient to make breathing easier. Always have atropine injection readily available and be prepared to give atropine 0.5 mg subcutaneously or slow I.V. push as ordered, and provide respiratory support as needed. Best administered in presence of doctor.
• Use only clear solution. Darkening may indicate loss of potency.
• Give I.V. at controlled rate; use slow, direct injection at no more than 1 mg/minute.
• Only cholinergic that crosses blood-brain barrier; therefore the only one useful for treating CNS effects of anticholinergic or tricyclic antidepressant

toxicity.
• Effectiveness often immediate and dramatic but may be transient and may require repeat dose.

---

pyridostigmine bromide
Mestinon♦*, Regonol♦
Pregnancy Category: C

MECHANISM OF ACTION
Inhibits the destruction of acetylcholine released from the parasympathetic and somatic efferent nerves. Acetylcholine accumulates, promoting increased stimulation of the receptor.

INDICATIONS & DOSAGE
Curariform antagonist postoperatively—
Adults: 10 to 30 mg I.V. preceded by atropine sulfate 0.6 to 1.2 mg I.V.
Myasthenia gravis—
Adults: 60 to 180 mg P.O. b.i.d. or q.i.d. Usual dose 600 mg daily but higher doses may be needed (up to 1,500 mg daily). Give ⅟₃₀ of oral dose I.M. or I.V. Dose must be adjusted for each patient, depending on response and tolerance of side effects.

ADVERSE REACTIONS
CNS: headache (with high doses), weakness, sweating, convulsions.
CV: bradycardia, hypotension.
EENT: miosis.
GI: abdominal cramps, nausea, vomiting, diarrhea, excessive salivation.
Skin: rash.
Local: thrombophlebitis.
Other: bronchospasm, bronchoconstriction, increased bronchial secretions, muscle cramps.

INTERACTIONS
Procainamide, quinidine: may reverse cholinergic effects on muscle. Observe for lack of drug effect.

NURSING CONSIDERATIONS

• Contraindicated in mechanical obstruction of intestine or urinary tract, bradycardia, hypotension. Use with extreme caution in bronchial asthma. Use cautiously in epilepsy, recent coronary occlusion, vagotonia, hyperthyroidism, cardiac arrhythmias, peptic ulcer. Avoid large doses in decreased gastrointestinal motility.

• Difficult to judge optimum dosage. Help doctor by recording patient's response after each dose.

• Should stop all other cholinergics before giving this drug.

• Monitor vital signs frequently, being especially careful to check respirations. Position patient to make breathing easier. Have atropine injection readily available and be prepared to give as ordered, and provide respiratory support as needed.

• If muscle weakness is severe, doctor determines if it is caused by drug-induced toxicity or exacerbation of myasthenia gravis. Test dose of edrophonium I.V. will aggravate drug-induced weakness but will temporarily relieve weakness caused by disease.

• When using for myasthenia gravis, stress importance of taking drug exactly as ordered, on time, in evenly spaced doses. If doctor has ordered extended-release tablets, explain how these work. Patient must take them at the same time each day, at least 6 hours apart. Explain that he may have to take this drug for life.

• Has longest duration of the cholinergics used for myasthenia gravis.

• Used by the oral route in the treatment of senility associated with Alzheimer's disease.

• Don't crush the Timespan tablets.

• Available as a syrup for patients who have difficulty swallowing. Syrup is very sweet; give over ice chips if patient can't tolerate flavor.

• Store tablets in a tightly capped bottle, away from moisture.

Italicized side effects are common or life-threatening.
*Liquid form contains alcohol.   **May contain tartrazine.

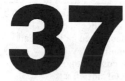

Cholinergic blockers (parasympatholytics)

atropine sulfate
(See Chapter 19, ANTIARRHYTHMICS.)
benztropine mesylate
biperiden hydrochloride
biperiden lactate
glycopyrrolate
ipratropium bromide
procyclidine hydrochloride
scopolamine hydrobromide
trihexyphenidyl hydrochloride

COMBINATION PRODUCTS
Cholinergic blocking agents are available in tablets and capsules, combined with varying amounts of sedatives.

benztropine mesylate
Cogentin♦
Pregnancy Category: C

MECHANISM OF ACTION
Blocks central cholinergic receptors, helping to balance cholinergic activity in the basal ganglia.

INDICATIONS & DOSAGE
Acute dystonic reaction—
Adults: 2 mg I.V. or I.M. followed by 1 to 2 mg P.O. b.i.d. to prevent recurrence.
Parkinsonism—
Adults: 0.5 to 6 mg P.O. daily. Initial dose 0.5 mg to 1 mg. Increase 0.5 mg every 5 to 6 days. Adjust dosage to meet individual requirements.

ADVERSE REACTIONS
CNS: disorientation, restlessness, irritability, incoherence, hallucinations, headache, sedation, depression, muscular weakness.
CV: palpitations, tachycardia, paradoxical bradycardia.
EENT: dilated pupils, blurred vision, photophobia, difficulty swallowing.
GI: *constipation, mouth dryness,* nausea, vomiting, epigastric distress.
GU: urinary hesitancy or retention.
Some side effects may be due to pending atropine-like toxicity and are dose related.

INTERACTIONS
Amantadine: anticholinergic side effects, such as confusion and hallucinations. Reduce dosage before administering amantadine.

NURSING CONSIDERATIONS
● Contraindicated in narrow-angle glaucoma. Use cautiously in patients with prostatic hypertrophy, tendency to tachycardia, and in elderly or debilitated patients; produces atropine-like side effects.
● Monitor vital signs carefully. Watch closely for side effects, especially in elderly or debilitated patients. Call doctor promptly.
● Never discontinue this drug abruptly. Dosage must be reduced gradually.
● Warn patient to avoid activities that require alertness until CNS response to drug is determined. If patient is to receive single daily dose, give at bedtime.
● Explain that drug may take 2 to 3 days to exert full effect.
● Monitor intake/output; urinary hesitancy and retention may develop.

- Watch for intermittent constipation, distention, abdominal pain; may be onset of paralytic ileus.
- Relieve dry mouth with cool drinks, ice chips, sugarless gum, or hard candy.
- To help prevent gastric irritation, administer after meals.

biperiden hydrochloride
Akineton♦

biperiden lactate
Akineton Lactate
Pregnancy Category: C

MECHANISM OF ACTION
Blocks central cholinergic receptors, helping to balance cholinergic activity in the basal ganglia.

INDICATIONS & DOSAGE
Extrapyramidal disorders—
Adults: 2 to 6 mg P.O. daily, b.i.d., or t.i.d., depending on severity. Usual dose is 2 mg daily, or 2 mg I.M. or I.V. q ½ hour, not to exceed 4 doses or 8 mg total daily.
Parkinsonism—
Adults: 2 mg P.O. t.i.d. to q.i.d.

ADVERSE REACTIONS
CNS: disorientation, euphoria, restlessness, irritability, incoherence, dizziness, increased tremor.
CV: transient postural hypotension.
EENT: blurred vision.
GI: *constipation, mouth dryness,* nausea, vomiting, epigastric distress.
GU: urinary hesitancy or retention. Side effects are dose-related and may resemble atropine toxicity.

INTERACTIONS
None significant.

NURSING CONSIDERATIONS
- Use with caution in prostatism, cardiac arrhythmias, narrow-angle glaucoma.

- Monitor vital signs carefully. Watch closely for side effects, especially in elderly or debilitated patients. Call doctor promptly.
- Give oral doses with or after meals to decrease GI side effects.
- When giving parenterally, keep patient in a supine position. Parenteral administration may cause transient postural hypotension and coordination disturbances.
- I.V. injections should be made very slowly.
- Because of possible dizziness, help patient when he gets out of bed.
- Tolerance may develop, requiring increased dosage.
- In severe parkinsonism, tremors may increase as spasticity is relieved.
- Warn patient to avoid activities that require alertness until CNS response to drug is determined.
- Monitor intake/output; urinary hesitancy and retention may develop.
- Relieve dry mouth with cool drinks, ice chips, sugarless gum, or hard candy.

glycopyrrolate
Robinul♦, Robinul Forte♦
Pregnancy Category: B

MECHANISM OF ACTION
Inhibits cholinergic (muscarinic) actions of acetylcholine on autonomic effectors innervated by postganglionic cholinergic nerves.

INDICATIONS & DOSAGE
To reverse neuromuscular blockade—
Adults: 0.2 mg I.V. for each 1 mg neostigmine or equivalent dose of pyridostigmine. May be given intravenously without dilution or may be added to dextrose injection and given by infusion.
Preoperatively to diminish secretions and block cardiac vagal reflexes—
Adults: 0.002 mg/lb of body weight I.M. 30 to 60 minutes before anesthe-

Italicized side effects are common or life-threatening.
*Liquid form contains alcohol.   **May contain tartrazine.

sia.

Adjunctive therapy in peptic ulcers and other gastrointestinal disorders—
Adults: 1 to 2 mg P.O. t.i.d. or 0.1 mg I.M. t.i.d. or q.i.d. Dosage should be individualized.

ADVERSE REACTIONS
CNS: disorientation, irritability, incoherence, weakness, nervousness, drowsiness, dizziness, headache.
CV: palpitations, tachycardia, paradoxical bradycardia.
EENT: *dilated pupils, blurred vision,* photophobia, increased intraocular pressure, difficulty swallowing.
GI: *constipation, mouth dryness,* nausea, vomiting, epigastric distress.
GU: *urinary hesitancy or retention.*
Skin: urticaria, decreased sweating or anhidrosis, other dermal manifestations.
Local: burning at injection site.
Other: bronchial plugging, fever.

INTERACTIONS
None significant.

NURSING CONSIDERATIONS
• Contraindicated in narrow-angle glaucoma, obstructive uropathy, obstructive disease of the GI tract, myasthenia gravis, paralytic ileus, intestinal atony, unstable cardiovascular status in acute hemorrhage, toxic megacolon. Use with caution in patients with autonomic neuropathy, hyperthyroidism, coronary artery disease, cardiac arrhythmias, congestive heart failure, hypertension; hiatal hernia associated with reflux esophagitis, hepatic or renal disease, ulcerative colitis; and in patients over 40 years because of increased incidence of glaucoma. Use with caution in hot or humid environments. Drug-induced heatstroke possible.
• Check all dosages carefully. Even slight overdose could lead to toxicity.
• Don't mix with I.V. solution containing sodium chloride or bicarbon-

ate.
• Monitor vital signs carefully. Watch closely for side effects, especially in elderly or debilitated patients. Call doctor promptly.
• Monitor intake/output. Causes urinary retention or hesitancy.
• Warn patient to avoid activities that require alertness until CNS response to drug is determined.
• Administer 30 minutes to 1 hour before meals.
• Administer smaller doses to elderly patients.

ipratropium bromide
Atrovent
Pregnancy Category: B

MECHANISM OF ACTION
Inhibits vagally mediated reflexes by antagonizing acetylcholine. An anticholinergic.

INDICATIONS & DOSAGE
Maintenance treatment of bronchospasm associated with chronic obstructive pulmonary disease—
Adults: 2 inhalations (26 mcg) q.i.d. Additional inhalations may be needed. However, total inhalations should not exceed 12 in 24 hrs.

ADVERSE REACTIONS
CNS: nervousness, dizziness, headache.
CV: palpitations.
GI: nausea, GI distress, dry mouth.
Other: cough.

INTERACTIONS
None significant.

NURSING CONSIDERATIONS
• Use cautiously in patients with narrow-angle glaucoma, prostatic hypertrophy, or bladder-neck obstruction.
• Warn patient that this is not effective in the treatment of acute episodes

of bronchospasm where rapid response is required.

• Teach patient to use the inhaler correctly, as follows: Enclose mouthpiece with lips and hold the base of the canister vertically. Exhale deeply, then inhale slowly through the mouth and, at the same time, firmly press once on the up-ended canister base. Hold your breath for a few seconds, then remove mouthpiece from the mouth and exhale slowly. Wait 15 seconds, then repeat inhalation.

• Tell patient to avoid accidentally spraying into eyes. Temporary blurring of vision may result.

• Ipratropium is the first anticholinergic bronchodilator available as an aerosol. Works by a different mechanism from either the adrenergics or theophylline compounds.

procyclidine hydrochloride
Kemadrin♦, Procyclid♦♦
Pregnancy Category: C

MECHANISM OF ACTION
Blocks central cholinergic receptors, helping to balance cholinergic activity in the basal ganglia.

INDICATIONS & DOSAGE
Parkinsonism, muscle rigidity—
Adults: initially, 2 to 2.5 mg P.O. t.i.d., after meals. Increase as needed to maximum 60 mg daily.

Also used to relieve extrapyramidal dysfunction that accompanies treatment with phenothiazines and rauwolfia derivatives. Also controls excessive salivation from neuroleptic medications.

ADVERSE REACTIONS
CNS: light-headedness, giddiness.
EENT: blurred vision, mydriasis.
GI: *constipation, mouth dryness,* nausea, vomiting, epigastric distress.
Skin: rash.

INTERACTIONS
None significant.

NURSING CONSIDERATIONS
• Contraindicated in narrow-angle glaucoma. Use cautiously in tachycardia, hypotension, urinary retention, or prostatic hypertrophy.

• Watch closely for mental confusion, disorientation, agitation, hallucinations, and psychotic symptoms, especially in the elderly. Call doctor promptly if these occur.

• In severe parkinsonism, tremors may increase as spasticity is relieved.

• Give after meals to minimize GI distress.

• Warn patient to avoid activities that require alertness until CNS response to drug is determined.

• Relieve dry mouth with cool drinks, ice chips, sugarless gum, or hard candy.

scopolamine hydrobromide
Pregnancy Category: C

MECHANISM OF ACTION
Inhibits muscarinic actions of acetylcholine on autonomic effectors innervated by postganglionic cholinergic nerves.

INDICATIONS & DOSAGE
Postencephalitic parkinsonism and other spastic states—
Adults: 0.5 to 1 mg P.O. t.i.d. to q.i.d.; 0.3 to 0.6 mg S.C., I.M., or I.V. (with suitable dilution) t.i.d. to q.i.d.
Children: 0.006 mg/kg P.O. or S.C. t.i.d. to q.i.d.; or 0.2 mg/m^2.
Preoperatively to reduce secretions—
Adults: 0.4 to 0.6 mg S.C.

ADVERSE REACTIONS
CNS: disorientation, restlessness, irritability, incoherence, headache.
CV: palpitations, tachycardia, paradoxical bradycardia.

Italicized side effects are common or life-threatening.
*Liquid form contains alcohol.   **May contain tartrazine.

EENT: dilated pupils, blurred vision, photophobia, increased intraocular pressure, difficulty swallowing.
GI: *constipation, mouth dryness, nausea, vomiting, epigastric distress.*
GU: urinary hesitancy or retention.
Skin: flushing, dryness.
Other: bronchial plugging, fever, depressed respirations.

Side effects may be due to pending atropine-like toxicity and are dose related. Individual tolerance varies greatly.

INTERACTIONS
None significant.

NURSING CONSIDERATIONS
• Contraindicated in narrow-angle glaucoma, obstructive uropathy, obstructive disease of the GI tract, asthma, chronic pulmonary disease, myasthenia gravis, paralytic ileus, intestinal atony, unstable cardiovascular status in acute hemorrhage, or toxic megacolon. Use with caution in patients with autonomic neuropathy, hyperthyroidism, coronary artery disease, cardiac arrhythmias, congestive heart failure, hypertension, hiatal hernia associated with reflux esophagitis, hepatic or renal disease, ulcerative colitis; in patients over 40 years because of the increased incidence of glaucoma; and in children under 6 years. Use with caution in hot or humid environments. Drug-induced heatstroke possible.
• Some patients become temporarily excited or disoriented. Symptoms disappear when sedative effect is complete. Use bed rails as precaution.
• In therapeutic doses, scopolamine may produce amnesia, drowsiness, and euphoria. These effects are desirable when used as an adjunct to anesthesia. May need to reorient patient.
• Warn patient to avoid activities requiring alertness until CNS response to drug is determined.
• Monitor intake/output; urinary hes-

itancy or retention may develop.
• Tolerance may develop when given over a long period of time.
• Many of the side effects (such as dry mouth, constipation) are an extension of the drug's pharmacologic activity and may be expected.
• To determine m² for dosage calculation in children, use a nomogram.

trihexyphenidyl hydrochloride
Aparkane♦♦, Artane♦*, Hexaphen, Novohexidyl♦♦, T.H.P., Trihexane, Trihexidyl
Pregnancy Category: C

MECHANISM OF ACTION
Blocks central cholinergic receptors, helping to balance cholinergic activity in the basal ganglia.

INDICATIONS & DOSAGE
Drug-induced parkinsonism—
Adults: 1 mg P.O. 1st day, 2 mg 2nd day, then increase 2 mg every 3 to 5 days until total of 6 to 10 mg is given daily. Usually given t.i.d. with meals and, if needed, q.i.d. (last dose should be before bedtime). Postencephalitic parkinsonism may require 12 to 15 mg total daily dose.

ADVERSE REACTIONS
CNS: nervousness, dizziness, headache, restlessness, agitation, hallucinations, euphoria, delusion, amnesia.
CV: tachycardia.
EENT: blurred vision, mydriasis, increased intraocular pressure.
GI: constipation, *dry mouth, nausea.*
GU: urinary hesitancy or retention.
Side effects are dose related.

INTERACTIONS
Amantadine: anticholinergic side effects, such as confusion and hallucinations. Reduce dosage before administering amantadine.

NURSING CONSIDERATIONS
• Use cautiously in patients with narrow-angle glaucoma; cardiac, hepatic, or renal disorders; hypertension; obstructive disease of the gastrointestinal and the genitourinary tracts; possible prostatic hypertrophy; patients over 60 years; and those with arteriosclerosis or history of drug hypersensitivities.
• Warn patient to avoid activities that require alertness until CNS response to drug is determined.
• Causes nausea if given before meals.
• Relieve dry mouth with cool drinks, ice chips, sugarless gum, or hard candy.
• Patient may develop a tolerance to this drug.
• Monitor intake/output; urinary hesitancy or retention may develop.
• Gonioscopic evaluation and close monitoring of intraocular pressures advised, especially in patients over 40 years.

Adrenergics (sympathomimetics)

albuterol
bitolterol mesylate
dobutamine hydrochloride
dopamine hydrochloride
ephedrine sulfate
epinephrine
epinephrine bitartrate
epinephrine hydrochloride
isoetharine hydrochloride 1%
isoetharine mesylate
isoproterenol hydrochloride
isoproterenol sulfate
metaproterenol sulfate
metaraminol bitartrate
norepinephrine injection
  (formerly levarterenol
  bitartrate)
phenylephrine hydrochloride
pseudoephedrine hydrochloride
pseudoephedrine sulfate
terbutaline sulfate

COMBINATION PRODUCTS
Only a few of the many combinations are included here as examples of this group.
Inhalants
DUO-MEDIHALER: isoproterenol hydrochloride 0.16 mg and phenylephrine bitartrate 0.24 mg per dose.
Oral bronchodilators
BRONCHOBID DURACAPS: theophylline 260 mg and ephedrine HCl 35 mg.
MARAX♦*: theophylline 130 mg, ephedrine sulfate 25 mg, and hydroxyzine HCl 10 mg.
QUADRINAL♦: theophylline calcium salicylate 65 mg, ephedrine hydrochloride 24 mg, potassium iodide 320 mg, and phenobarbital 24 mg.

QUIBRON PLUS*: theophylline 150 mg, ephedrine hydrochloride 25 mg, guaifenesin 100 mg, and butabarbital 20 mg.
TEDRAL SA♦: theophylline 180 mg, ephedrine hydrochloride 48 mg, and phenobarbital 25 mg.
(OTC) TEDRAL: theophylline 130 mg, ephedrine hydrochloride 24 mg, and phenobarbital 8 mg.
(OTC) THALFED: theophylline 120 mg, ephedrine hydrochloride 25 mg, and phenobarbital 8 mg.
Decongestants
(OTC) ACTIFED: pseudoephedrine hydrochloride 60 mg and triprolidine hydrochloride 2.5 mg.
CONGESPRIN: phenylephrine hydrochloride 1.25 mg and aspirin 81 mg.
DRISTAN: phenylephrine hydrochloride 5 mg, chlorpheniramine maleate 2 mg, aspirin 325 mg, and caffeine 16.2 mg.
HISTASPAN-PLUS: phenylephrine hydrochloride 20 mg and chlorpheniramine maleate 8 mg.
NALDECON: phenylpropanolamine hydrochloride 40 mg, phenylephrine hydrochloride 10 mg, chlorpheniramine maleate 5 mg, and phenyltoloxamine citrate 15 mg.
(OTC) ORNEX: phenylpropanolamine hydrochloride 18 mg and acetaminophen 325 mg.
PHENERGAN-D: pseudoephedrine hydrochloride 60 mg and promethazine hydrochloride 6.25 mg.
(OTC) TRIAMINIC: phenylpropanolamine hydrochloride 50 mg, pyrilamine maleate 25 mg, and pheniramine maleate 25 mg.

albuterol
Proventil, Proventil Syrup, Ventolin♦
Pregnancy Category: C

MECHANISM OF ACTION
Relaxes bronchial smooth muscle by
acting on beta$_2$-adrenergic receptors.

INDICATIONS & DOSAGE
*Prevention and treatment of broncho-
spasm in patients with reversible obstructive airway disease—*
Adults and children over 13 years: 1
to 2 inhalations q 4 to 6 hours. More
frequent administration or a greater
number of inhalations is not recommended.
Oral tablets—2 to 4 mg t.i.d. or q.i.d.
Maximum 8 mg q.i.d.
Children 6 to 13 years: 2 mg (1 teaspoonful) t.i.d. or q.i.d.
Children 2 to 5 years: 0.1 mg/kg
t.i.d., not to exceed 2 mg (1 teaspoonful) t.i.d.
Adults over 65: 2 mg t.i.d. or q.i.d.
To prevent exercise-induced asthma—
Adults: 2 inhalations 15 minutes before exercise.

ADVERSE REACTIONS
CNS: *tremor, nervousness,* dizziness,
insomnia, headache.
CV: tachycardia, palpitations, hyper-
tension.
EENT: drying and irritation of nose
and throat (with inhaled form).
GI: heartburn, nausea, vomiting.
Other: muscle cramps.

INTERACTIONS
Propranolol and other beta blockers:
blocked bronchodilating effect of albuterol. Monitor patient carefully.

NURSING CONSIDERATIONS
• Use cautiously in patients with cardiovascular disorders, including coronary insufficiency and hypertension;
in patients with hyperthyroidism or
diabetes mellitus; and in patients who
arc unusually responsive to adrenergics.
• Warn patient about the possibility
of paradoxical bronchospasm. If this
occurs, the drug should be discontinued immediately.
• Patients may use tablets and aerosol
concomitantly. Monitor closely for
toxicity.
• Albuterol reportedly produces less
cardiac stimulation than other sympathomimetics, especially isoproterenol.
• Elderly patients usually require a
lower dose.
• Teach patient how to administer
metered dose correctly. Have him
shake container; exhale through nose;
administer aerosol while inhaling
deeply on mouthpiece of inhaler; hold
breath for a few seconds, then exhale
slowly. Tell him to allow 2 minutes
between inhalations.
• Pleasant-tasting syrup may be taken
by children as young as age 2. Contains no alcohol or sugar.
• Store drug in light-resistant container.

bitolterol mesylate
Tornalate
Pregnancy Category: C

MECHANISM OF ACTION
Relaxes bronchial smooth muscle by
acting on beta$_2$-adrenergic receptors.

INDICATIONS & DOSAGE
*To prevent and treat bronchial asthma
and bronchospasm—*
Adults and children over 12 years:
to treat bronchospasm, two inhalations at an interval of at least 1 to 3
minutes followed by a third inhalation, if needed. To prevent bronchospasm, the usual dose is two inhalations q 8 hours. In either case, dose
should never exceed three inhalations
q 6 hours or two inhalations q 4 hours.

Italicized side effects are common or life-threatening.
*Liquid form contains alcohol.   **May contain tartrazine.

ADVERSE REACTIONS

CNS: *tremors,* nervousness, headache, dizziness, light-headedness.
CV: palpitations, chest discomfort, tachycardia.
EENT: throat irritation.
Other: coughing, dyspnea, *hypersensitivity.*

INTERACTIONS

None significant.

NURSING CONSIDERATIONS

• Use cautiously in patients with ischemic heart disease or hypertension, hyperthyroidism, diabetes mellitus, cardiac arrhythmias, and convulsive disorders.
• Monitor blood pressure regularly.
• Advise patients not to exceed recommended dosages. Too frequent use may cause tachycardia.
• Remind patients that beneficial effects last for up to 8 hours, longer than most other similar bronchodilators.
• Has rapid onset of action (about 3 to 4 minutes). Peak effect occurs in 30 to 60 minutes.
• Show patient how to use inhaler correctly.

dobutamine hydrochloride

Dobutrex♦
Pregnancy Category: C

MECHANISM OF ACTION

Directly stimulates beta₁ receptors of the heart to increase myocardial contractility and stroke volume, resulting in increased cardiac output.

INDICATIONS & DOSAGE

Refractory heart failure and as adjunct in cardiac surgery—
Adults: 2.5 to 10 mcg/kg/minute as an I.V. infusion. Rarely, infusion rates up to 40 mcg/kg/minute may be needed.

ADVERSE REACTIONS

CNS: headache.
CV: *increased heart rate, hypertension, premature ventricular beats,* angina, nonspecific chest pain.
GI: nausea, vomiting.
Other: shortness of breath.

INTERACTIONS

Beta blockers: may make dobutamine ineffective. Do not use together.

NURSING CONSIDERATIONS

• Contraindicated in idiopathic hypertrophic subaortic stenosis.
• A unique agent. Increases contractility of failing heart without inducing marked tachycardia, except at high doses.
• Hypovolemia should be corrected with plasma volume expanders before initiating therapy with dobutamine.
• Dobutamine is chemical modification of isoproterenol.
• Often used with nitroprusside for additive effects.
• EKG, blood pressure, pulmonary wedge pressure, and cardiac output should be monitored continuously. Also monitor urinary output.
• Incompatible with alkaline solutions. Do not mix with sodium bicarbonate injection.
• Infusions of up to 72 hours produce no more adverse effects than shorter infusions.
• Oxidation of drug may slightly discolor admixtures containing dobutamine. This does not indicate a significant loss of potency.
• Intravenous solutions remain stable for 24 hours.

dopamine hydrochloride

Dopastat, Intropin♦, Revimine♦♦
Pregnancy Category: C

MECHANISM OF ACTION

Stimulates dopaminergic, beta-adrenergic, and alpha-adrenergic receptors of the sympathetic nervous system.

INDICATIONS & DOSAGE

To treat shock and correct hemodynamic imbalances; to improve perfusion to vital organs, increase cardiac output; to correct hypotension—
Adults: 2 to 5 mcg/kg/minute I.V. infusion, up to 50 mcg/kg/minute. Titrate the dosage to the desired hemodynamic and/or renal response.

ADVERSE REACTIONS

CNS: headache.
CV: ectopic beats, tachycardia, anginal pain, palpitations, *hypotension*. Less frequently, bradycardia, widening of QRS complex, conduction disturbances, vasoconstriction.
GI: nausea, vomiting.
Local: necrosis and tissue sloughing with extravasation.
Other: piloerection, dyspnea.

INTERACTIONS

Ergot alkaloids: extreme elevations in blood pressure. Don't use together.
Phenytoin: may lower blood pressure of dopamine-stabilized patients. Monitor carefully.
MAO inhibitors: may cause hypertensive crisis. Avoid if possible.

NURSING CONSIDERATIONS

• Contraindicated in uncorrected tachyarrhythmias, pheochromocytoma, ventricular fibrillation. Use cautiously in patients with occlusive vascular disease, cold injuries, diabetic endarteritis, arterial embolism; also, in pregnant patients and those taking MAO inhibitors.
• Not a substitute for blood or fluid volume deficit. If volume deficit exists, it should be replaced before vasopressors are administered.
• Use large vein, as in antecubital fossa, to minimize risk of extravasation. Watch site carefully for signs of extravasation. If it occurs, stop infusion immediately and call doctor. He may want to counteract effect by infiltrating the area with 5 to 10 mg phentolamine and 10 to 15 ml normal saline solution.
• Check blood pressure, pulse rate, urinary output, and extremity color and temperature often during infusion. Titrate infusion rate according to findings, using doctor's guidelines. Use a microdrip or infusion pump to regulate flow rate.
• Observe patient closely for side effects. If adverse effects develop, dosage may need to be adjusted or discontinued.
• If a disproportionate rise in the diastolic pressure (a marked decrease in pulse pressure) is observed in patients receiving dopamine, decrease infusion rate and observe carefully for further evidence of predominant vasoconstrictor activity, unless such an effect is desired.
• Most patients satisfactorily maintained on less than 20 mcg/kg/minute.
• If doses exceed 50 mcg/kg/minute, check urinary output often. If urine flow decreases without hypotension, consider reducing dose.
• If drug is stopped, watch closely for sudden drop in blood pressure.
• Don't mix with alkaline solutions. Use dextrose 5% in water, normal saline solution, or combination of dextrose 5% in water and saline solution. Mix just before use.
• Dopamine solutions deteriorate after 24 hours. Discard at that time or earlier if solution is discolored.
• Do not mix other drugs in bottle containing dopamine.
• Do not give alkaline drugs (sodium bicarbonate, phenytoin sodium) through I.V. line containing dopamine.
• Acidosis decreases effectiveness of dopamine.

Italicized side effects are common or life-threatening.
*Liquid form contains alcohol.   **May contain tartrazine.

ephedrine sulfate
Pregnancy Category: C

MECHANISM OF ACTION
Both a direct-acting and indirect-acting sympathomimetic that stimulates alpha- and beta-adrenergic receptors.

INDICATIONS & DOSAGE
To correct hypotensive states; to support ventricular rate in Adams-Stokes syndrome—
Adults: 25 to 50 mg I.M. or S.C., or 10 to 25 mg I.V. p.r.n. to maximum 150 mg/24 hours.
Children: 3 mg/kg S.C. or I.V. daily, divided into 4 to 6 doses.
Bronchodilator or nasal decongestant—
Adults: 12.5 to 50 mg P.O. b.i.d., t.i.d., or q.i.d. Maximum 400 mg daily in 6 to 8 divided doses.
Children: 2 to 3 mg/kg P.O. daily in 4 to 6 divided doses.

ADVERSE REACTIONS
CNS: *insomnia, nervousness,* dizziness, headache, muscle weakness, sweating, euphoria, confusion, delirium.
CV: *palpitations,* tachycardia, hypertension.
EENT: dryness of nose and throat.
GI: nausea, vomiting, anorexia.
GU: urinary retention, painful urination due to visceral sphincter spasm.

INTERACTIONS
MAO inhibitors and tricyclic antidepressants: when given with sympathomimetics, may cause severe hypertension (hypertensive crisis). Don't use together.
Methyldopa: may inhibit effect of ephedrine. Give together cautiously.

NURSING CONSIDERATIONS
• Contraindicated in patients with porphyria, severe coronary artery disease, cardiac arrhythmias, narrow-angle glaucoma, psychoneurosis, and in patients on MAO-inhibitor therapy. Use with caution in elderly patients and those with hypertension, hyperthyroidism, nervous or excitable states, cardiovascular disease, or prostatic hypertrophy.
• Not a substitute for blood or fluid volume deficit. Volume deficit should be replaced before vasopressors are administered.
• Give I.V. injection slowly.
• Hypoxia, hypercapnia, and acidosis, which may reduce effectiveness or increase the incidence of adverse effects, must be identified and corrected before or during ephedrine administration.
• Effectiveness decreases after 2 to 3 weeks. Then increased dosage may be needed. Tolerance develops, but drug is not known to cause addiction.
• To prevent insomnia, avoid giving within 2 hours before bedtime.
• Warn patient not to take over-the-counter drugs that contain ephedrine without informing doctor.

epinephrine
Inhalants:
Bronkaid Mist♦, Primatene Mist

epinephrine bitartrate
Inhalants:
AsthmaHaler, Medihaler-Epi♦

epinephrine hydrochloride
Adrenalin♦, Sus-Phrine♦
Pregnancy Category: C

MECHANISM OF ACTION
Stimulates alpha- and beta-adrenergic receptors within the sympathetic nervous system.

INDICATIONS & DOSAGE
Bronchospasm, hypersensitivity reactions, and anaphylaxis—
Adults: 0.1 to 0.5 ml of 1:1,000 S.C. or I.M. Repeat q 10 to 15 minutes,

p.r.n. Or 0.1 to 0.25 ml 1:1,000 I.V.
Children: 0.01 ml (10 mcg) of
1:1,000/kg S.C. Repeat q 20 minutes
to 4 hours, p.r.n.; 0.005 ml/kg of
1:200 (Sus-Phrine). Repeat q 8 to 12
hours, p.r.n.
Hemostatic—
Adults: 1:50,000 to 1:1,000, applied
topically.
Acute asthmatic attacks (inhalation)—
Adults and children: 1 or 2 inhalations of 1:100 or 2.25% racemic, every 1 to 5 minutes until relief is obtained; 0.2 mg/dose usual content.
To prolong local anesthetic effect—
Adults and children: 0.2 to 0.4 ml of
1:1,000 intraspinal; 1:500,000 to
1:50,000 local mixed with local anesthetic.
*To restore cardiac rhythm in cardiac
arrest—*
Adults: 0.5 to 1 mg I.V. or into endotracheal tube. May be given intracardiac if no I.V. route or intratracheal
route available. Following initial I.V.
administration, may be infused I.V. at
a rate of 1 to 4 mcg/minute.
Children: 10 mcg/kg I.V. or 5 to 10
mcg (0.05 to 0.1 ml of 1:10,000)/kg
intracardiac.
Note: 1 mg = 1 ml of 1:1,000 or 10
ml of 1:10,000.

ADVERSE REACTIONS
CNS: *nervousness,* tremor, euphoria,
anxiety, coldness of extremities, vertigo, *headache,* sweating, cerebral
hemorrhage, disorientation, agitation.
In patients with Parkinson's disease,
the drug increases rigidity and tremor.
CV: *palpitations;* widened pulse pressure; hypertension; *tachycardia; ventricular fibrillation; CVA;* anginal
pain; EKG changes, including a decrease in the T-wave amplitude.
Metabolic: *hyperglycemia,* glycosuria.
Other: pulmonary edema, dyspnea,
pallor.

INTERACTIONS
Tricyclic antidepressants: when given
with sympathomimetics, may cause
severe hypertension (hypertensive
crisis). Don't give together.
Propranolol: vasoconstriction and reflex bradycardia. Monitor patient
carefully.

NURSING CONSIDERATIONS
• Contraindicated in narrow-angle
glaucoma, shock (other than anaphylactic shock), organic brain damage,
cardiac dilatation, and coronary insufficiency. Also during general anesthesia with halogenated hydrocarbons
or cyclopropane and in labor (may delay second stage). Use with extreme
caution in patients with long-standing
bronchial asthma and emphysema
who have developed degenerative
heart disease. Use with caution in elderly patients, and those with hyperthyroidism, angina, hypertension,
psychoneurosis, diabetes.
• Don't mix with alkaline solutions.
Use dextrose 5% in water, normal saline solution, or a combination of dextrose 5% in water and saline solution.
Mix just before use.
• Epinephrine is rapidly destroyed by
oxidizing agents, such as iodine, chro-
mates, nitrates, nitrites, oxygen, and
salts of easily reducible metals such
as iron.
• Epinephrine solutions deteriorate
after 24 hours. Discard after that time
or before if solution is discolored or
contains precipitate. Keep solution in
light-resistant container, and don't remove before use.
• Massage site after injection to
counteract possible vasoconstriction.
Repeated local injection can cause necrosis at site due to vasoconstriction.
• Avoid intramuscular administration
of oil injection into buttocks. Gas
gangrene may occur because epinephrine reduces oxygen tension of the tissues, encouraging the growth of con-
taminating organisms.

Italicized side effects are common or life-threatening.
*Liquid form contains alcohol.   **May contain tartrazine.

- This drug may widen patient's pulse pressure.
- In the event of a sharp blood pressure rise, rapid-acting vasodilators, such as the nitrites or alpha-adrenergic blocking agents, can be given to counteract the marked pressor effect of large doses of epinephrine.
- Observe patient closely for side effects. If adverse effects develop, dosage may need to be adjusted or discontinued.
- If patient has acute hypersensitivity reactions, it may be necessary to instruct him to self-inject epinephrine at home.
- Drug of choice in emergency treatment of acute anaphylactic reactions, including anaphylactic shock.

isoetharine hydrochloride 1%
Beta-Z Solution, Bronkosol

isoetharine mesylate
Bronkometer
Pregnancy Category: C

MECHANISM OF ACTION
Relaxes bronchial smooth muscle by acting on beta$_2$-adrenergic receptors.

INDICATIONS & DOSAGE
Bronchial asthma and reversible bronchospasm that may occur with bronchitis and emphysema—
Adults (hydrochloride): administered by hand nebulizer, oxygen aerosolization, or IPPB.

Method	Dose	Dilution
Hand	3 to 7 inhalations	undiluted
Oxygen aerosolization	0.5 ml	1:3 with saline
IPPB	0.5 ml	1:3 with saline

Adults (mesylate): 1 to 2 inhalations. Occasionally, more may be required.

ADVERSE REACTIONS
CNS: *tremor, headache,* dizziness, excitement.
CV: *palpitations,* increased heart rate.
GI: nausea, vomiting.

INTERACTIONS
Propranolol and other beta blockers: blocked bronchodilating effect of isoetharine. Monitor patient carefully if used together.

NURSING CONSIDERATIONS
- Use cautiously in patients with hyperthyroidism, hypertension, coronary disease, or those with sensitivity to sympathomimetics.
- Excessive use can lead to decreased effectiveness.
- Monitor for severe paradoxical bronchoconstriction after excessive use. Discontinue immediately if bronchoconstriction occurs.
- Although isoetharine has minimal effects on the heart, use cautiously in patients receiving general anesthetics that sensitize the myocardium to sympathomimetic drugs.
- Instruct patient in the use of aerosol and mouthpiece.
- Due to oxidation of drug when diluted with water, pink sputum mimicking hemoptysis may occur after inhaling isoetharine solution. Tell patient not to be concerned.

isoproterenol hydrochloride
Isuprel♦*, Proternol (tabs)
Inhalants: Norisodrine, Vapo-Iso

isoproterenol sulfate
Iso-Autohaler, Luf-Iso Inhalation, Medihaler-Iso♦, Norisodrine
Pregnancy Category: C

MECHANISM OF ACTION
Relaxes bronchial smooth muscle by acting on beta$_2$-adrenergic receptors. As a cardiac stimulant, acts on beta$_1$-

adrenergic receptors in the heart.

INDICATIONS & DOSAGE

Bronchial asthma and reversible bronchospasm (hydrochloride)—
Adults: 10 to 20 mg S.L. q 6 to 8 hours.
Children: 5 to 10 mg S.L. q 6 to 8 hours. Not recommended for children under 6 years.
Bronchospasm (sulfate)—
Adults and children: acute dyspneic episodes: 1 inhalation initially. May repeat if needed after 2 to 5 minutes. Maintenance: 1 to 2 inhalations q.i.d. to 6 times daily. May repeat once more 10 minutes after second dose. Not more than 3 doses should be administered for each attack.
Heart block and ventricular arrhythmias (hydrochloride)—
Adults: initially, 0.02 to 0.06 mg I.V. Subsequent doses 0.01 to 0.2 mg I.V. or 5 mcg/minute I.V.; or 0.2 mg I.M. initially, then 0.02 to 1 mg, p.r.n.
Children: may give ½ of initial adult dose.
Shock (hydrochloride)—
Adults and children: 0.5 to 5 mcg/minute by continuous I.V. infusion. Usual concentration: 1 mg (5 ml) in 500 ml dextrose 5% in water. Adjust rate according to heart rate, central venous pressure, blood pressure, and urine flow.

ADVERSE REACTIONS

CNS: *headache,* mild tremor, weakness, dizziness, nervousness, insomnia.
CV: *palpitations, tachycardia, anginal pain; blood pressure may be elevated and then fall.*
GI: nausea, vomiting.
Metabolic: hyperglycemia.
Other: sweating, flushing of face, bronchial edema and inflammation.

INTERACTIONS

Propranolol and other beta blockers: blocked bronchodilating effect of iso-

proterenol. Monitor patient carefully if used together.

NURSING CONSIDERATIONS

• Contraindicated in tachycardia caused by digitalis intoxication and in patients with preexisting arrhythmias, especially tachycardia, because chronotropic effect on the heart may aggravate such disorders. Contraindicated in recent myocardial infarction. Use cautiously in coronary insufficiency, diabetes, hyperthyroidism.
• Not a substitute for blood or fluid volume deficit. If deficit exists, it should be replaced before vasopressors are administered.
• If heart rate exceeds 110 beats/minute, it may be advisable to decrease infusion rate or temporarily stop infusion. Doses sufficient to increase the heart rate to more than 130 beats/minute may induce ventricular arrhythmias.
• If precordial distress or anginal pain occurs, stop drug immediately.
• When administering I.V. isoproterenol for shock, closely monitor blood pressure, CVP, EKG, arterial blood gas measurements, and urinary output. Carefully adjust infusion rate according to these measurements.
• Oral and sublingual tablets are poorly and erratically absorbed.
• Teach patient how to take sublingual tablet properly. Tell him to hold tablet under tongue until it dissolves and is absorbed and not to swallow saliva until that time. Prolonged use of sublingual tablets can cause tooth decay. Instruct patient to rinse mouth with water between doses. Will also help prevent dryness of oropharynx.
• If possible, don't give at bedtime because it interrupts sleep patterns.
• This drug may cause slight rise in systolic blood pressure and slight to marked drop in diastolic blood pressure.
• Use a microdrip or infusion pump to regulate infusion flow rate.

Italicized side effects are common or life-threatening.
*Liquid form contains alcohol.   **May contain tartrazine.

- Observe patient closely for side effects. Dosage may need to be adjusted or discontinued.
- Teach patient to perform oral inhalation correctly. Give the following instructions for using a metered-dose nebulizer:
    —Clear nasal passages and throat.
    —Breathe out, expelling as much air from lungs as possible.
    —Place mouthpiece well into mouth as dose from nebulizer is released, and inhale deeply.
    —Hold breath for several seconds, remove mouthpiece, and exhale slowly.
- Instructions for metered powder nebulizer are the same, except that deep inhalation is not necessary.
- Patient may develop a tolerance to this drug. Warn against overuse.
- Warn patient using oral inhalant that drug may turn sputum and saliva pink.
- May aggravate ventilation perfusion abnormalities; even while ease of breathing is improved, arterial oxygen tension may fall paradoxically.
- Discard inhalation solution if it is discolored or contains precipitate.

metaproterenol sulfate
Alupent♦, Metaprel
Pregnancy Category: C

MECHANISM OF ACTION
Relaxes bronchial smooth muscle by acting on beta$_2$-adrenergic receptors.

INDICATIONS & DOSAGE
Acute episodes of bronchial asthma—
Adults and children: 2 to 3 inhalations. Should not repeat inhalations more often than q 3 to 4 hours. Should not exceed 12 inhalations daily.
Bronchial asthma and reversible bronchospasm—
Adults: 20 mg P.O. q 6 to 8 hours.
Children over 9 years or over 27 kg: 20 mg P.O. q 6 to 8 hours. (0.4 mg to

0.9 mg/kg/dose t.i.d.)
Children 6 to 9 years or less than 27 kg: 10 mg P.O. q 6 to 8 hours. (0.4 mg to 0.9 mg/kg/dose t.i.d.)
Not recommended for children under 6 years.

ADVERSE REACTIONS
CNS: nervousness, weakness, drowsiness, tremor.
CV: tachycardia, hypertension, palpitations; *with excessive use, cardiac arrest.*
GI: vomiting, nausea, bad taste in mouth.
Other: paradoxical bronchiolar constriction with excessive use.

INTERACTIONS
Propranolol and other beta blockers: blocked bronchodilating effect of metaproterenol. Monitor patient carefully if used together.

NURSING CONSIDERATIONS
- Contraindicated in tachycardia, and in arrhythmias associated with tachycardia. Use with caution in hypertension, coronary artery disease, hyperthyroidism, diabetes.
- Safe use of inhalant in children under 12 years not established.
- Teach patient how to administer metered dose correctly. Instructions: shake container; exhale through nose; administer aerosol while inhaling deeply on mouthpiece of inhaler; hold breath for a few seconds, then exhale slowly. Allow 2 minutes between inhalations. Store drug in light-resistant container.
- Metaproterenol inhalations should precede steroid inhalations (when prescribed) by 10 to 15 minutes to maximize therapy.
- Warn patient about the possibility of paradoxical bronchospasm. If this occurs, the drug should be discontinued immediately.
- Patients may use tablets and aerosol concomitantly. Monitor closely for

toxicity.
• Metaproterenol reportedly produces less cardiac stimulation than other sympathomimetics, especially isoproterenol.
• Inhalant solution can be administered by IPPB diluted in saline solution or via a hand nebulizer at full strength.
• Tell patient to notify doctor if no response is derived from dosage. Warn against changing dose without calling doctor.

metaraminol bitartrate
Aramine
Pregnancy Category: D

MECHANISM OF ACTION
Predominantly stimulates alpha-adrenergic receptors within the sympathetic nervous system.

INDICATIONS & DOSAGE
Prevention of hypotension—
Adults: 2 to 10 mg I.M. or S.C.
Severe shock—
Adults: 0.5 to 5 mg direct I.V. followed by I.V. infusion.
Treatment of hypotension due to shock—
Adults: 15 to 100 mg in 500 ml normal saline solution or dextrose 5% in water I.V. infusion. Adjust rate to maintain blood pressure.
All indications—
Children: 0.01 mg/kg as single I.V. injection; 1 mg/25 ml dextrose 5% in water as I.V. infusion. Adjust rate to maintain blood pressure in normal range. 0.1 mg/kg I.M. as single dose, p.r.n. Allow at least 10 minutes to elapse before increasing dose because maximum effect is not immediately apparent.

ADVERSE REACTIONS
CNS: apprehension, restlessness, dizziness, headache, tremor, weakness; with excessive use, convulsions.

CV: hypertension; hypotension; precordial pain; palpitations; arrhythmias, including sinus or ventricular tachycardia; bradycardia; premature supraventricular beats; atrioventricular dissociation.
GI: nausea, vomiting.
GU: decreased urinary output.
Metabolic: hyperglycemia.
Skin: flushing, pallor, sweating.
Local: irritation upon extravasation.
Other: *metabolic acidosis in hypovolemia, increased body temperature, respiratory distress.*

INTERACTIONS
MAO inhibitors: may cause severe hypertension (hypertensive crisis). Don't use together.

NURSING CONSIDERATIONS
• Contraindicated in peripheral or mesenteric thrombosis, pulmonary edema, hypercarbia, and acidosis; also during anesthesia with cyclopropane and halogenated hydrocarbon anesthetics. Use cautiously in patients with hypertension, thyroid disease, diabetes, cirrhosis, or malaria, and those receiving digitalis.
• Not a substitute for blood or fluid volume deficit. Fluid deficit should be replaced before vasopressors are administered.
• Keep solution in light-resistant container, away from heat.
• Use large veins, as in antecubital fossa, to minimize risk of extravasation. Watch infusion site carefully for signs of extravasation. If it occurs, stop infusion immediately and call doctor.
• During infusion, check blood pressure every 5 minutes until stabilized; then every 15 minutes. Check pulse rates, urinary output, and color and temperature of extremities. Titrate infusion rate according to findings, using doctor's guidelines.
• Use a microdrip or infusion pump to regulate infusion flow rate.

Italicized side effects are common or life-threatening.
*Liquid form contains alcohol.   **May contain tartrazine.

- Observe patient closely for side effects. If adverse effects develop, dosage may need to be adjusted or discontinued.
- For I.V. therapy, use two-bottle setup so I.V. can continue if this drug is stopped.
- Blood pressure should be raised to slightly less than the patient's normal level. Be careful to avoid excessive blood pressure response. Rapidly induced hypertensive response can cause acute pulmonary edema, arrhythmias, and cardiac arrest.
- Because of prolonged action, a cumulative effect is possible. With an excessive vasopressor response, elevated blood pressure may persist after the drug is stopped.
- Urinary output may decrease initially, then increase as blood pressure reaches normal level. Report persistent decreased urinary output.
- When discontinuing therapy with this drug, slow infusion rate gradually. Continue monitoring vital signs, watching for possible severe drop in blood pressure. Keep equipment nearby to start drug again, if necessary. Pressor therapy should not be reinstated until the systolic blood pressure falls below 70 to 80 mm Hg.
- Keep emergency drugs on hand to reverse effects of metaraminol: atropine for reflex bradycardia; phentolamine to decrease vasopressor effects; propranolol for arrhythmias.
- Closely monitor patients with diabetes. Adjustment in insulin dose may be needed.
- Metaraminol should not be mixed with other drugs.

norepinephrine injection (formerly levarterenol bitartrate)
Levophed♦
Pregnancy Category: D

MECHANISM OF ACTION
Stimulates alpha- and beta-adrenergic receptors within the sympathetic nervous system.

INDICATIONS & DOSAGE
To restore blood pressure in acute hypotensive states—
Adults: initially, 8 to 12 mcg/minute I.V. infusion, then adjust to maintain normal blood pressure. Average maintenance dose 2 to 4 mcg/minute.

ADVERSE REACTIONS
CNS: *headache,* anxiety, weakness, dizziness, tremor, restlessness, insomnia.
CV: bradycardia, severe hypertension, marked increase in peripheral resistance, decreased cardiac output, arrhythmias, *ventricular tachycardia, fibrillation,* bigeminal rhythm, atrioventricular dissociation, precordial pain.
GU: *decreased urinary output.*
Metabolic: *metabolic acidosis,* hyperglycemia, increased glycogenolysis.
Local: irritation with extravasation.
Other: fever, respiratory difficulty.

INTERACTIONS
Tricyclic antidepressants: when given with sympathomimetics, may cause severe hypertension (hypertensive crisis). Don't give together.

NURSING CONSIDERATIONS
- Contraindicated in mesenteric or peripheral vascular thrombosis, pregnancy, profound hypoxia, hypercarbia, hypotension from blood volume deficits, or during cyclopropane and halothane anesthesia. Use cautiously

in hypertension, hyperthyroidism, severe cardiac disease. Use with extreme caution in patients receiving MAO inhibitors or tricyclic antidepressants.

• Not a substitute for blood or fluid volume deficit. If deficit exists, it should be replaced before vasopressors are administered.

• Norepinephrine solutions deteriorate after 24 hours.

• Use large vein, as in antecubital fossa, to minimize risk of extravasation. Check site frequently for signs of extravasation. If it occurs, stop infusion immediately and call doctor. He may counteract effect by infiltrating area with 5 to 10 mg phentolamine and 10 to 15 ml normal saline solution. Also check for blanching along course of infused vein; may progress to superficial slough.

• During infusion, check blood pressure every 2 minutes until stabilized; then every 5 minutes. Also check pulse rates, urinary output, and color and temperature of extremities. Titrate infusion rate according to findings, using doctor's guidelines. In previously hypertensive patients, blood pressure should be raised no more than 40 mm Hg below preexisting systolic pressure.

• Never leave patient unattended during infusion.

• Use a microdrip or infusion pump to regulate infusion flow rate.

• For I.V. therapy, use two-bottle setup with Y-port so I.V. can continue if norepinephrine is stopped.

• Report decreased urinary output to doctor immediately.

• If prolonged I.V. therapy is necessary, change injection site frequently.

• When stopping drug, slow infusion rate gradually. Monitor vital signs, even after drug is stopped. Watch for severe drop in blood pressure.

• Keep emergency drugs on hand to reverse effects of norepinephrine: atropine for reflex bradycardia; propranolol for arrhythmias; phentolamine for increased vasopressor effects.

• Administer in dextrose and saline solution; saline solution alone is not recommended.

phenylephrine hydrochloride
Neo-Synephrine♦
Pregnancy Category: C

MECHANISM OF ACTION
Predominantly stimulates alpha-adrenergic receptors in the sympathetic nervous system.

INDICATIONS & DOSAGE
Hypotensive emergencies during spinal anesthesia—
Adults: initially, 0.2 mg I.V., then subsequent doses of 0.1 to 0.2 mg.
Maintenance of blood pressure during spinal or inhalation anesthesia—
Adults: 2 to 3 mg S.C. or I.M. 3 or 4 minutes before anesthesia.
Children: 0.04 mg to 0.088 mg/kg S.C. or I.M.
Mild to moderate hypotension—
Adults: 2 to 5 mg S.C. or I.M.; 0.1 to 0.5 mg I.V. Not to be repeated more often than 10 to 15 minutes.
Paroxysmal supraventricular tachycardia—
Adults: initially, 0.5 mg rapid I.V.; subsequent doses should not exceed the preceding dose by more than 0.1 to 0.2 mg and should not exceed 1 mg.
Prolongation of spinal anesthesia—
Adults: 2 to 5 mg added to anesthetic solution.
Severe hypotension and shock (including drug-induced)—
Adults: 10 mg in 500 ml dextrose 5% in water. Start 100 to 180 drops per minute I.V. infusion, then 40 to 60 drops per minute. Adjust to patient response.
Vasoconstrictor for regional anesthe-

sia—
Adults: 1 mg phenylephrine added to 20 ml local anesthetic.

ADVERSE REACTIONS
CNS: *trembling, sweating, pallor,* sense of fullness in head, *tingling in extremities,* sleeplessness, dizziness, *paresthesia in extremities from injection,* light-headedness, weakness.
CV: palpitations, tachycardia, extrasystoles, short paroxysms of ventricular tachycardia, hypertension, anginal pain.
EENT: blurred vision.
Skin: gooseflesh, feeling of coolness.
Local: tissue sloughing with extravasation.
Other: tachyphylaxis may occur with continued use.

INTERACTIONS
MAO inhibitors: may cause severe hypertension (hypertensive crisis). Don't use together.
Tricyclic antidepressants: increased pressor response. Observe patient.

NURSING CONSIDERATIONS
• Contraindicated in narrow-angle glaucoma; with MAO inhibitors, tricyclic antidepressants; hypotension; ventricular tachycardia; severe coronary disease or cardiovascular disease (including myocardial infarction). Use with extreme caution in heart disease, hyperthyroidism, diabetes, severe atherosclerosis, bradycardia, partial heart block, myocardial disease, and the elderly.
• Longer acting than ephedrine and epinephrine.
• Causes little or no CNS stimulation.
• Monitor blood pressure frequently. Avoid excessive rise in blood pressure. Maintain blood pressure at slightly below the patient's normal level. In previously normotensive patients, maintain systolic blood pressure at 80 to 100 mm Hg; in previously hypertensive patients, maintain

systolic blood pressure at 30 to 40 mm Hg below their usual level.
• May reverse severe increase in blood pressure with phentolamine.
• With I.V. infusions, avoid abrupt withdrawal. Monitor blood pressure throughout. Reverse therapy if blood pressure falls too rapidly.

---

pseudoephedrine hydrochloride
Besan, Cenafed, Eltor♦♦, First Sign, Gyrocaps, Robidrine♦♦, Ro-Fedrin, Sudabid, Sudafed♦, Sudafed SA

pseudoephedrine sulfate
Afrinol Repetabs
Pregnancy Category: C

MECHANISM OF ACTION
Stimulates alpha-adrenergic receptors in the respiratory tract, producing vasoconstriction.

INDICATIONS & DOSAGE
Nasal and eustachian tube decongestant—
Adults: 60 mg P.O. q 4 hours. Maximum dose 240 mg daily.
Children 6 to 12 years: 30 mg P.O. q 4 hours. Maximum 120 mg daily.
Children 2 to 6 years: 15 mg P.O. q 4 hours. Maximum 60 mg/day.
Extended-relief tablets and capsules:
Adults and children over 12 years: 60 to 120 mg P.O. q 12 hours. This form contraindicated for children under 12 years.
Relief of nasal congestion—
Adults: 120 mg every 12 hours.

ADVERSE REACTIONS
CNS: *anxiety,* transient stimulation, tremors, dizziness, headache, insomnia, *nervousness.*
CV: arrhythmias, *palpitations,* tachycardia.
GI: anorexia, nausea, vomiting, dry mouth.

GU: difficulty in urinating.
Skin: pallor.

INTERACTIONS
MAO inhibitors: may cause severe hypertension (hypertensive crisis). Don't use together.

NURSING CONSIDERATIONS
• Contraindicated in patients with severe hypertension or severe coronary artery disease; in those receiving MAO inhibitors; and in breast-feeding mothers. Use cautiously in hypertension, cardiac disease, diabetes, glaucoma, hyperthyroidism, or prostatic hypertrophy.
• Elderly patients are more sensitive to the drug's effects.
• Tell patient to stop drug if he becomes unusually restless and to notify doctor promptly.
• Warn against using over-the-counter products containing other sympathomimetic amines.
• Tell patient not to take drug within 2 hours of bedtime because it can cause insomnia.
• Tell patient he can relieve dry mouth with sugarless gum or sour hard candy.

---

terbutaline sulfate
Brethaire, Brethine, Bricanyl◆
Pregnancy Category: B

MECHANISM OF ACTION
Relaxes bronchial smooth muscle by acting on beta$_2$-adrenergic receptors. Also relaxes uterine muscle.

INDICATIONS & DOSAGE
Relief of bronchospasm in patients with reversible obstructive airway disease—
Adults and children over 11 years: 2 inhalations separted by a 60-second interval, repeated every 4 to 6 hours. May also administer 2.5 to 5 mg P.O. q 8 hours or 0.25 mg S.C.

Treatment of premature labor—
0.01 mg/minute by I.V. infusion. Increase by 0.005 mg q 10 minutes up to 0.025 mg/minute or until contractions cease. Or, give 0.25 mg S. C. hourly until contractions cease. Maintenance dose: 5 mg P.O. q 4 hours for 48 hours, then 5 mg q 6 hours.

ADVERSE REACTIONS
CNS: *nervousness, tremors, headache,* drowsiness, sweating.
CV: palpitations, increased heart rate.
EENT: drying and irritation of nose and throat (with inhaled form).
GI: vomiting, nausea.

INTERACTIONS
MAO inhibitors: when given with sympathomimetics, may cause severe hypertension (hypertensive crisis). Don't use together.
Propranolol and other beta blockers: blocked bronchodilating effects of terbutaline.

NURSING CONSIDERATIONS
• Use cautiously in patients with diabetes, hypertension, hyperthyroidism, severe cardiac disease, or cardiac arrhythmias.
• Protect injection from light. Do not use if discolored.
• Make sure patient and his family understand why drug is necessary.
• Give subcutaneous injections in lateral deltoid area.
• Tolerance may develop with prolonged use.
• Warn patient about the possibility of paradoxical bronchospasm. If this occurs, the drug should be discontinued immediately.
• Patients may use tablets and aerosol concomitantly. Monitor closely for toxicity.
• Teach patient how to administer metered dose correctly. Have him shake container; exhale through nose;

---

administer aerosol while inhaling
deeply on mouthpiece of inhaler; hold
breath for a few seconds, then exhale
slowly.
• Although not approved by the FDA
for treatment of preterm labor, it is
considered very effective and is used
in many hospitals.

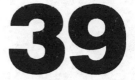

Adrenergic blockers (sympatholytics)

dihydroergotamine mesylate
ergotamine tartrate
methysergide maleate
phenoxybenzamine
   hydrochloride
   (See Chapter 21, ANTIHYPERTENSIVES.)
propranolol hydrochloride
   (See Chapter 20, ANTIANGINALS.)

COMBINATION PRODUCTS
CAFERGOT: ergotamine tartrate 1 mg
and caffeine 100 mg.
CAFERGOT SUPPOSITORIES: ergotamine tartrate 2 mg and caffeine 100
mg.
ERGOCAFF: ergotamine tartrate 1 mg
and caffeine 100 mg.
MIGRAL: ergotamine tartrate 1 mg,
caffeine 50 mg, and cyclizine HCl 25
mg.
WIGRAINE♦: ergotamine tartrate 1
mg, caffeine 100 mg, levorotatory
belladonna alkaloids 0.1 mg, and
phenacetin 130 mg.
WIGRAINE SUPPOSITORIES: ergotamine tartrate 2 mg, caffeine 100 mg,
and tartaric acid 21.5 mg.

---

dihydroergotamine mesylate
D.H.E. 45
Pregnancy Category: X

MECHANISM OF ACTION
Inhibits the effects of epinephrine,
norepinephrine, and other sympathomimetic amines. Also has antiserotonin effects.

INDICATIONS & DOSAGE
Vascular or migraine headache—
Adults: 1 mg I.M. or I.V. May repeat
q 1 to 2 hours, p.r.n., up to total of 3
mg. Maximum weekly dose is 6 mg.

ADVERSE REACTIONS
CV: numbness and tingling in fingers
and toes, *transient tachycardia or bradycardia*, precordial distress and
pain, increased arterial pressure.
GI: nausea, vomiting.
Skin: itching.
Other: weakness in legs, muscle
pains in extremities, localized edema.

INTERACTIONS
Propranolol and other beta blockers:
blocked natural pathway for vasodilation in patients receiving ergot alkaloids and thus could result in excessive vasoconstriction. Watch closely if
drugs are used together.

NURSING CONSIDERATIONS
• Contraindicated in pregnancy and
in patients with peripheral and occlusive vascular disease, coronary artery
disease, hypertension, hepatic or
renal dysfunction, sepsis.
• Avoid prolonged administration;
don't exceed recommended dosage.
• Tell patient to report any feeling of
coldness in extremities or tingling of
fingers and toes due to vasoconstriction. Severe vasoconstriction may result in tissue damage.
• Most effective when used at first
sign of migraine or soon after onset.
Provide a quiet, low-light environment to help patient relax.

Italicized side effects are common or life-threatening.
*Liquid form contains alcohol.   **May contain tartrazine.

- Help patient evaluate underlying causes of stress.
- Protect ampules from heat and light. Discard if solution is discolored.
- Best results are obtained by adjusting the dose in order to determine the most effective, minimal dose.
- Ergotamine rebound, or an increase in frequency and duration of headache, may occur when the drug is stopped.
- For short-term use only.

ergotamine tartrate
Ergomar♦, Ergostat, Medihaler-Ergotamine♦, Wigrettes
Pregnancy Category: X

MECHANISM OF ACTION
Inhibits the effects of epinephrine, norepinephrine, and other sympathomimetic amines. Also has antiserotonin effects.

INDICATIONS & DOSAGE
Vascular or migraine headache—
Adults: initially, 2 mg P.O. S.L., then 1 to 2 mg P.O. q hour or S.L. q ½ hour, to maximum 6 mg daily and 10 mg weekly. Maximum dose 0.5 mg/24 hours and 1 mg/week; or 1 inhalation initially; if not relieved in 5 minutes, use another inhalation. May repeat inhalations at least 5 minutes apart up to maximum of 6 per 24 hours. As a suppository, 2 mg initially; if not relieved, give another 2 mg in 1 hour. Maximum, 4 mg per attack or 10 mg per week.

ADVERSE REACTIONS
CV: numbness and tingling in fingers and toes, transient tachycardia or bradycardia, precordial distress and pain, increased arterial pressure, angina pectoris.
GI: nausea, vomiting, diarrhea, abdominal cramps.
Skin: itching.

Other: weakness in legs, muscle pains in extremities, localized edema.

INTERACTIONS
Propranolol and other beta blockers: blocked natural pathway for vasodilation in patients receiving ergot alkaloids and thus could result in excessive vasoconstriction. Watch closely if drugs are used together.

NURSING CONSIDERATIONS
- Contraindicated in pregnancy and in patients with peripheral and occlusive vascular diseases, coronary artery disease, hypertension, hepatic or renal dysfunction, sepsis.
- Avoid prolonged administration; don't exceed recommended dosage.
- Most effective when used during prodromal stage of headache or as soon as possible after onset.
- Provide a quiet, low-light environment to help patient relax.
- Help patient evaluate underlying causes of physical or emotional stress, which may precipitate attacks.
- Prolonged exposure to cold weather should be avoided whenever possible. Cold may increase many of the side effects.
- Instruct patient on long-term therapy to check for and report feeling of coldness in extremities or tingling of fingers and toes due to vasoconstriction. Severe vasoconstriction may result in tissue damage.
- Store drug in light-resistant container.
- Sublingual tablet is preferred during early stage of attack because of its rapid absorption.
- Warn patient not to increase dosage without first consulting the doctor.
- Obtain an accurate dietary history from patient to determine if a relationship exists between certain foods and onset of headache.
- Ergotamine rebound, or an increase in frequency and duration of headache, may occur if the drug is

stopped.
• Instruct patient how to use the inhaler correctly.

methysergide maleate
Sansert♦**
Pregnancy Category: C

MECHANISM OF ACTION
Specifically blocks serotonin (a neurotransmitter).

INDICATIONS & DOSAGE
Prevention of frequent, severe, uncontrollable, or disabling migraine or vascular headache—
Adults: 4 to 8 mg P.O. daily with meals.

ADVERSE REACTIONS
Blood: neutropenia, eosinophilia.
CNS: insomnia, drowsiness, *euphoria, vertigo,* ataxia, *light-headedness,* hyperesthesia, weakness, *hallucinations or feelings of dissociation.*
CV: *fibrotic thickening of cardiac valves and aorta, inferior vena cava, and common iliac branches (retroperitoneal fibrosis);* vasoconstriction, causing chest pain, abdominal pain, vascular insufficiency of lower limbs; cold, numb, painful extremities with or without paresthesias and diminished or absent pulses; postural hypotension; tachycardia; peripheral edema; murmurs; bruits.
EENT: nasal stuffiness.
GI: nausea, vomiting, diarrhea, constipation, epigastric pain.
Skin: hair loss, dermatitis, sweating, flushing, rash.
Other: *retroperitoneal fibrosis,* causing general malaise, fatigue, weight gain, backache, low-grade fever, urinary obstruction; *pulmonary fibrosis,* causing dyspnea, tightness and pain in chest, pleural friction rubs and effusion, arthralgia, myalgia.

INTERACTIONS
None significant.

NURSING CONSIDERATIONS
• Contraindicated in patients with severe hypertension, arteriosclerosis, peripheral vascular insufficiency, renal or hepatic disease, severe coronary artery diseases, thromboembolic disorders, phlebitis or cellulitis of lower limbs, fibrotic processes, valvular heart disease; and in debilitated patients. Use cautiously in patients with peptic ulcers or suspected coronary artery disease. EKG and cardiac status evaluation advisable before giving to patients over 40 years.
• GI effects may be prevented by gradual introduction of medication and by administering with meals.
• Obtain laboratory studies of cardiac and renal function, blood count, and sedimentation rate before and during therapy.
• Stop drug every 6 months; then restart after at least 3 or 4 weeks.
• Tell patient not to stop drug abruptly; may cause rebound headaches. Stop gradually over 2 to 3 weeks.
• Patient should keep daily weight record and report unusually rapid weight gain. Teach him to check for peripheral edema. Explain and suggest low-salt diet if necessary.
• Give drug for 3 weeks before evaluating effectiveness.
• Tell patient to report to doctor promptly if he experiences cold, numb, or painful hands and feet; leg cramps when walking; pelvic, chest, or flank pain.
• Not for treatment of migraine or vascular headache in progress, or for treatment of tension (muscle contraction) headaches.
• Indicated only for patients who are unresponsive to other drugs and who can be kept under close medical supervision.

Italicized side effects are common or life-threatening.
*Liquid form contains alcohol.   **May contain tartrazine.

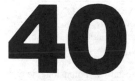

Skeletal muscle relaxants

baclofen
carisoprodol
chlorphenesin carbamate
chlorzoxazone
cyclobenzaprine
dantrolene sodium
methocarbamol
orphenadrine citrate

COMBINATION PRODUCTS
BLANEX: chlorzoxazone 250 mg and acetaminophen 300 mg.
CHLOROFON-F: chlorzoxazone 250 mg and acetaminophen 300 mg.
CHLORZONE FORTE: chlorzoxazone 250 mg and acetaminophen 300 mg.
FLEXAPHEN: chlorzoxazone 250 mg and acetaminophen 300 mg.
LOBAC: chlorzoxazone 250 mg and acetaminophen 300 mg.
MUS-LAX: chlorzoxazone 250 mg and acetaminophen 300 mg.
NORGESIC: orphenadrine citrate 25 mg, aspirin 385 mg, and caffeine 30 mg.
NORGESIC FORTE: orphenadrine citrate 50 mg, aspirin 770 mg, and caffeine 60 mg.
PARACET FORTE: chlorzoxazone 250 mg and acetaminophen 300 mg.
PARAFON FORTE♦*: chlorzoxazone 250 mg and acetaminophen 300 mg.
POLYFLEX: chlorzoxazone 250 mg and acetaminophen 300 mg.
ROBAXISAL♦: methocarbamol 400 mg and aspirin 325 mg.
SOMA COMPOUND♦: carisoprodol 200 mg and aspirin 325 mg.
SOMA COMPOUND WITH CODEINE: carisoprodol 200 mg, aspirin 325 mg, caffeine 32 mg, and codeine phosphate 16 mg.
ZOXAPHEN: chlorzoxazone 250 mg and acetaminophen 300 mg.

baclofen
Lioresal♦, Lioresal DS
Pregnancy Category: C

MECHANISM OF ACTION
Reduces transmission of impulses from the spinal cord to skeletal muscle.

INDICATIONS & DOSAGE
Spasticity in multiple sclerosis, spinal cord injury—
Adults: initially, 5 mg t.i.d. for 3 days, 10 mg t.i.d. for 3 days, 15 mg t.i.d. for 3 days, 20 mg t.i.d. for 3 days. Increase according to response up to maximum of 80 mg daily.

ADVERSE REACTIONS
CNS: *drowsiness, dizziness,* headache, *weakness, fatigue,* confusion, insomnia.
CV: hypotension.
EENT: nasal congestion.
GI: *nausea,* constipation.
GU: urinary frequency.
Hepatic: increased SGOT, alkaline phosphatase.
Metabolic: hyperglycemia.
Skin: rash, pruritus.
Other: ankle edema, excessive perspiration, weight gain.

INTERACTIONS
Alcohol, CNS depressants: increased

CNS depression.

NURSING CONSIDERATIONS
• Use cautiously in patients with impaired renal function, stroke (minimal benefit, poor tolerance), epilepsy, and when spasticity is used to maintain motor function.
• Give with meals or milk to prevent gastric distress.
• Amount of relief determines if dosage (and drowsiness) can be reduced.
• Tell patient to avoid activities that require alertness until CNS response to drug is determined. Drowsiness is usually transient.
• Watch for increased incidence of seizures in epileptics.
• Watch for sensitivity reactions such as fever, skin eruptions, respiratory distress.
• Advise patient to follow doctor's orders regarding rest, physical therapy.
• Do not withdraw abruptly unless required by severe side effects; may precipitate hallucinations or rebound spasticity.
• Overdosage treatment is supportive only; do not induce emesis or use a respiratory stimulant in obtunded patients.
• Used investigationally for treatment of unstable bladder.

carisoprodol
Rela, Soma♦
Pregnancy Category: C

MECHANISM OF ACTION
Reduces transmission of impulses from the spinal cord to skeletal muscle.

INDICATIONS & DOSAGE
As an adjunct in acute, painful musculoskeletal conditions—
Adults and children over 12 years:
350 mg P.O. t.i.d. and at bedtime. Not recommended for children under 12 years.

ADVERSE REACTIONS
CNS: *drowsiness, dizziness,* vertigo, ataxia, tremor, agitation, irritability, headache, depressive reactions, insomnia.
CV: orthostatic hypotension, tachycardia, facial flushing.
GI: nausea, vomiting, hiccups, increased bowel activity, epigastric distress.
Skin: rash, *erythema multiforme,* pruritus.
Other: asthmatic episodes, fever, angioneurotic edema, *anaphylaxis.*

INTERACTIONS
Alcohol, CNS depressants: increased CNS depression.

NURSING CONSIDERATIONS
• Contraindicated in hypersensitivity to related compounds (including meprobamate, tybamate); or intermittent porphyria. Use with caution in impaired hepatic or renal function.
• Watch for idiosyncratic reactions after first to fourth dose (weakness, ataxia, visual and speech difficulties, fever, skin eruptions, mental changes) or severe reactions, including bronchospasm, hypotension, anaphylactic shock. Hold dose and notify doctor immediately of any unusual reactions.
• Record amount of relief to determine whether dosage can be reduced.
• Warn patient to avoid activities that require alertness until CNS response to drug is determined. Drowsiness is transient.
• Avoid combining with alcohol or other depressants.
• Advise patient to follow doctor's orders regarding rest, physical therapy.
• Do not stop drug abruptly; mild withdrawal effects such as insomnia, headache, nausea, abdominal cramps may result.

Italicized side effects are common or life-threatening.
*Liquid form contains alcohol. **May contain tartrazine.

chlorphenesin carbamate
Maolate**
Pregnancy Category: C

MECHANISM OF ACTION
Reduces transmission of impulses from the spinal cord to skeletal muscle.

INDICATIONS & DOSAGE
As an adjunct in short-term, acute, painful musculoskeletal conditions—
Adults: initial dose 800 mg P.O. t.i.d. Maintenance 400 mg P.O. q.i.d. for maximum of 8 weeks.

ADVERSE REACTIONS
Blood: blood dyscrasia.
CNS: *drowsiness, dizziness,* confusion, headache, weakness. Dose-related side effects include paradoxical stimulation, agitation, insomnia, nervousness, headache.
GI: *nausea, epigastric distress.*
Other: *anaphylaxis.*

INTERACTIONS
Alcohol and CNS depressants: increased CNS depression.

NURSING CONSIDERATIONS
• Use cautiously in hepatic disease or impaired renal function.
• Use cautiously in patients hypersensitive to aspirin.
• Safe use for periods over 8 weeks not established.
• Take with meals or milk to prevent gastric distress.
• Amount of relief determines if dosage (and drowsiness) can be reduced.
• Watch for sensitivity reactions such as fever, skin eruptions, and respiratory distress. Hold dose and notify doctor of unusual reactions.
• Monitor blood studies.
• Watch for unusual bleeding and infections that may indicate blood dyscrasia.

chlorzoxazone
Paraflex**
Pregnancy Category: C

MECHANISM OF ACTION
Reduces transmission of impulses from the spinal cord to skeletal muscle.

INDICATIONS & DOSAGE
As an adjunct in acute, painful musculoskeletal conditions—
Adults: 250 to 750 mg t.i.d. or q.i.d.
Children: 20 mg/kg daily divided t.i.d. or q.i.d.

ADVERSE REACTIONS
CNS: *drowsiness, dizziness, lightheadedness,* malaise, headache, overstimulation.
GI: anorexia, nausea, vomiting, heartburn, abdominal distress, constipation, diarrhea.
GU: urine discoloration (orange or purple-red).
Hepatic: hepatic dysfunction.
Skin: urticaria, redness, itching, petechiae, bruising.

INTERACTIONS
Alcohol and CNS depressants: increased CNS depression.

NURSING CONSIDERATIONS
• Contraindicated in impaired hepatic function. Use cautiously in patients with a history of drug allergies.
• Record amount of relief to determine whether dosage can be reduced.
• Watch for signs of hepatic dysfunction. Hold dose and notify doctor.
• Warn patient to avoid activities that require alertness until CNS response to drug is determined. Drowsiness is transient.
• Avoid combining with alcohol or other depressants.
• Tell patient that the drug may discolor urine orange or purple-red.
• Advise patient to follow doctor's or-

ders regarding rest, physical therapy.
• Give with meals or milk to prevent gastric distress.

cyclobenzaprine
Flexeril♦
Pregnancy Category: B

MECHANISM OF ACTION
Reduces transmission of impulses from the spinal cord to skeletal muscle.

INDICATIONS & DOSAGE
Short-term treatment of muscle spasm—
Adults: 10 mg P.O. t.i.d. for 7 days. Maximum 60 mg daily for 2 to 3 weeks.

ADVERSE REACTIONS
CNS: *drowsiness,* euphoria, weakness, headache, insomnia, nightmares, paresthesias, dizziness.
CV: tachycardia.
EENT: blurred vision.
GI: abdominal pain, dyspepsia, peculiar taste, constipation, dry mouth.
GU: urinary retention.
Skin: rash, urticaria, pruritus.
Other: in high doses, watch for side effects like those of other tricyclic drugs (amitriptyline, imipramine).

INTERACTIONS
None significant.

NURSING CONSIDERATIONS
• Contraindicated in patients who have received MAO inhibitors within 14 days; during acute recovery phase of myocardial infarction; in heart block, arrhythmias, conduction disturbances, or congestive heart failure. Use cautiously in patients with urinary retention, narrow-angle glaucoma, increased intraocular pressure, cardiovascular disease, impaired hepatic function, seizures; and in elderly or debilitated patients.

• Withdrawal symptoms (nausea, headache, malaise) may occur if drug is stopped abruptly after long-term use.
• Watch for symptoms of overdose, including possible cardiotoxicity. Notify doctor immediately and have physostigmine available.
• Check intake and output. Be alert for urinary retention. If constipation is a problem, increase fluid intake and get an order for a stool softener.
• Warn patient to avoid activities that require alertness until CNS response to drug is determined. Drowsiness and dizziness usually subside after 2 weeks.
• Avoid combining alcohol or other depressants with cyclobenzaprine.
• Tell patient that dry mouth may be relieved with sugarless candy or gum.

dantrolene sodium
Dantrium♦, Dantrium I.V.♦
Pregnancy Category: C

MECHANISM OF ACTION
Acts directly on skeletal muscle to interfere with intracellular calcium movement.

INDICATIONS & DOSAGE
Spasticity and sequelae secondary to severe chronic disorders (multiple sclerosis, cerebral palsy, spinal cord injury, stroke)—
Adults: 25 mg P.O. daily. Increase gradually in increments of 25 mg at 4- to 7-day intervals, up to 100 mg b.i.d. to q.i.d., to maximum of 400 mg daily.
Children: 1 mg/kg daily P.O. b.i.d. to q.i.d. Increase gradually as needed by 1 mg/kg daily to maximum of 100 mg q.i.d.
Management of malignant hyperthermia—
Adults and children: 1 mg/kg I.V. initially; may repeat dose up to cumulative dose of 10 mg/kg.

Italicized side effects are common or life-threatening.
*Liquid form contains alcohol.   **May contain tartrazine.

Prevention or attenuation of malignant hyperthermia in susceptible patients who require surgery—
Adults: 4 to 8 mg/kg/day P.O. given in 3 to 4 divided doses for 1 to 2 days before procedure. Administer final dose 3 to 4 hours before procedure.
Prevention of recurrence of malignant hyperthermia—
Adults: 4 to 8 mg/kg/day given in 4 divided doses for up to 3 days following hyperthermic crisis.

ADVERSE REACTIONS

CNS: *muscle weakness, drowsiness,* dizziness, light-headedness, malaise, headache, confusion, nervousness, insomnia.
CV: tachycardia, blood pressure changes.
EENT: excessive tearing, visual disturbances.
GI: anorexia, constipation, cramping, dysphagia, *severe diarrhea.*
GU: urinary frequency, incontinence, nocturia, dysuria, crystalluria, difficulty achieving erection.
Hepatic: *hepatitis.*
Skin: eczematoid eruption, pruritus, urticaria, photosensitivity.
Other: abnormal hair growth, drooling, sweating, pleural effusion, myalgia, chills, fever.

INTERACTIONS

Alcohol, CNS depressants: increased CNS depression. Monitor for decreased alertness.
Verapamil (I.V.): may result in cardiovascular collapse. Stop drug before administering I.V. dantrolene.

NURSING CONSIDERATIONS

The following are considerations for the P.O. form only:
• Contraindicated when spasticity is used to maintain motor function; in spasms in rheumatic disorders; and in lactation. Use with caution in patients with severely impaired cardiac or pulmonary function or preexisting he-

patic disease; in females; and in patients over 35 years.
• Safety and efficacy in long-term use not established; value may be determined by therapeutic trial. Do not give more than 45 days if no benefits obtained.
• Give with meals or milk to prevent gastric distress.
• Prepare oral suspension for single dose by dissolving capsule contents in juice or other suitable liquid. For multiple dose, use acid vehicle, such as citric acid in USP Syrup; refrigerate. Use in several days.
• Record amount of relief to determine whether dosage can be reduced.
• Liver function tests should be performed at the beginning of therapy.
• Watch for hepatitis (fever, jaundice), severe diarrhea or weakness, or sensitivity reactions (fever, skin eruptions). Hold dose and notify doctor.
• Warn patient to avoid driving and other hazardous activities until CNS response to drug is determined. Side effects should subside after 4 days.
• Tell patient to avoid combining with alcohol or other depressants; to avoid photosensitivity reactions by using sunscreening agents and protective clothing; to report abdominal discomfort or GI problems immediately; and to follow doctor's orders regarding rest, physical therapy.
The following are considerations for the I.V. form only:
• Administer as soon as malignant hyperthermia reaction is recognized.
• Reconstitute each vial by adding 60 ml of sterile water for injection and shaking vial until clear. Don't use a diluent that contains a bacteriostatic agent.
• Protect contents from light and use within 6 hours.
• Be careful to avoid extravasation.

methocarbamol
Delaxin, Forbaxin, Robamol, Robaxin♦, Romethocarb, SK-Methocarbamol, Spenaxin
Pregnancy Category: C

MECHANISM OF ACTION
Reduces transmission of impulses from the spinal cord to skeletal muscle.

INDICATIONS & DOSAGE
As an adjunct in acute, painful musculoskeletal conditions—
Adults: 1.5 g P.O. for 2 to 3 days, then 1 g P.O. q.i.d., or not more than 500 mg (5 ml) I.M. into each gluteal region. May repeat q 8 hours. Or 1 to 3 g daily (10 to 30 ml) I.V. directly into vein at 3 ml/minute, or 10 ml may be added to no more than 250 ml of dextrose 5% in water or normal saline solution. Maximum dose 3 g daily.
Supportive therapy in tetanus management—
Adults: 1 to 2 g into tubing of running I.V. or 1 to 3 g in infusion bottle q 6 hours.
Children: 15 mg/kg I.V. q 6 hours.

ADVERSE REACTIONS
Blood: hemolysis, increased hemoglobin (I.V. only).
CNS: drowsiness, dizziness, lightheadedness, headache, vertigo, mild muscular incoordination (I.M. or I.V. only), convulsions (I.V. only).
CV: hypotension, bradycardia (I.M. or I.V. only).
GI: *nausea, anorexia, GI upset*.
GU: red blood cells in urine (I.V. only), discoloration of urine.
Skin: urticaria, pruritus, rash.
Local: thrombophlebitis, extravasation (I.V. only).
Other: fever, metallic taste, flushing, *anaphylactic reactions* (I.M. or I.V. only).

INTERACTIONS
Alcohol and CNS depressants: increased CNS depression.

NURSING CONSIDERATIONS
• Contraindicated in patients with impaired renal function (injectable form), myasthenia gravis, epilepsy (injectable form); in children under 12 years (except in tetanus); and in patients receiving anticholinesterase agents.
• I.V. irritates veins, may cause phlebitis, aggravates seizures, may cause fainting if injected rapidly.
• Give I.V. slowly. Maximum rate 300 mg (3 ml)/minute. Give I.M. deeply, only in upper outer quadrant of buttocks, with maximum of 5 ml in each buttock, and inject slowly. Do not give subcutaneously.
• In tetanus management, use methocarbamol with tetanus antitoxin, penicillin, tracheotomy, and aggressive supportive care. Long course of I.V. methocarbamol required.
• Watch for sensitivity reactions such as fever, skin eruptions.
• Warn patient to avoid activities that require alertness until CNS response to drug is determined. Drowsiness subsides.
• Avoid combining with alcohol or other depressants.
• Advise patient to follow doctor's orders regarding rest, physical therapy.
• Tell patient urine may turn green, black, or brown.
• Give with meals or milk to prevent gastric distress.
• Watch for orthostatic hypotension, especially with parenteral administration. Keep patient supine for 15 minutes afterward, and supervise ambulation. Advise patient to get up slowly.
• Have epinephrine, antihistamines, corticosteroids available.
• Prepare liquid by crushing tablets into water or saline solution. Give through nasogastric tube.
• Obtain WBC count periodically

Italicized side effects are common or life-threatening.
*Liquid form contains alcohol.   **May contain tartrazine.

during prolonged therapy.

orphenadrine citrate
Banflex, Flexon, Myolin, Norflex♦,
Ro-Orphena, X-Otag
Pregnancy Category: C

MECHANISM OF ACTION
Reduces transmission of impulses
from the spinal cord to skeletal muscle.

INDICATIONS & DOSAGE
*Adjunctive treatment in painful, acute
musculoskeletal conditions—*
Adults: 100 mg P.O. b.i.d., or 60 mg
I.V. or I.M. q 12 hours, p.r.n.
For maintenance, switch to oral ther-
apy beginning 12 hours after last par-
enteral dose.

ADVERSE REACTIONS
CNS: disorientation, restlessness, irritability, weakness, *drowsiness,*
headache.
CV: palpitations, tachycardia.
EENT: dilated pupils, blurred vision,
difficulty swallowing.
GI: constipation, *dry mouth,* nausea,
vomiting, paralytic ileus, epigastric
distress.
GU: urinary hesitancy or retention.

INTERACTIONS
Alcohol and CNS depressants: increased CNS depression.

NURSING CONSIDERATIONS
• Contraindicated in patients with
narrow-angle glaucoma; prostatic hypertrophy; pyloric, duodenal, or bladder-neck obstruction; myasthenia
gravis; tachycardia; severe hepatic or
renal disease; ulcerative colitis. Use
cautiously in elderly or debilitated patients with cardiac disease, arrhythmias; and in those exposed to high
temperatures.
• Check all dosages carefully. Even a
slight overdose can lead to toxicity.

Early signs are excessive dry mouth,
dilated pupils, blurred vision, skin
flushing, fever.
• Monitor vital signs carefully.
• With I.V. administration, inject the
drug over a period of approximately 5
minutes while patient is lying down.
Wait 5 to 10 minutes and then help patient to sit up.
• When given I.V., may cause paradoxical initial bradycardia. Usually
disappears in 2 minutes.
• Monitor intake and output. Orphenadrine is an anticholinergic. It causes
urinary retention and hesitancy; have
patient void before taking the drug.
• Relieve dry mouth with cool drinks,
sugarless gum, or hard candy.

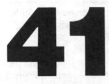

Neuromuscular blockers

atracurium besylate
gallamine triethiodide
metocurine iodide
pancuronium bromide
succinylcholine chloride
tubocurarine chloride
vecuronium bromide

COMBINATION PRODUCTS
None.

atracurium besylate
Tracrium
Pregnancy Category: C

MECHANISM OF ACTION
Prevents acetylcholine from binding to the receptors on the muscle end plate, thus blocking depolarization. Nondepolarizing agent.

INDICATIONS & DOSAGE
Adjunct to general anesthesia, to facilitate endotracheal intubation and to provide skeletal muscle relaxation during surgery or mechanical ventilation—
Dose depends on anesthetic used, individual needs, and response. Doses are representative and must be adjusted.
Adults and children over 2 years: 0.4 to 0.5 mg/kg by I.V. bolus. Maintenance dose of 0.08 to 0.10 mg/kg within 20 to 45 minutes of initial dose should be administered during prolonged surgical procedures. Maintenance doses may be administered q 12 to 25 minutes in patients receiving balanced anesthesia.

Children 1 month to 2 years: initial dose, 0.3 to 0.4 mg/kg. Frequent maintenance doses may be needed.

ADVERSE REACTIONS
CV: bradycardia.
Skin: skin flush, erythema, pruritus, urticaria.
Other: *prolonged dose-related apnea.*

INTERACTIONS
Aminoglycoside antibiotics (including amikacin, gentamicin, kanamycin, neomycin, streptomycin); polymyxin antibiotics (polymyxin B sulfate, colistin); clindamycin; quinidine; local anesthetics: potentiated neuromuscular blockade, leading to increased skeletal muscle relaxation and possible respiratory paralysis. Use cautiously during surgical and postoperative periods.
Lithium, narcotic analgesics: potentiated neuromuscular blockade, leading to increased skeletal muscle relaxation and possible respiratory paralysis. Use with extreme caution and reduce dose of atracurium.

NURSING CONSIDERATIONS
• Use cautiously in patients with cardiovascular disease, severe electrolyte disorders, and neuromuscular diseases.
• Prior administration of succinylcholine does not prolong duration of action, but it quickens onset and may deepen neuromuscular blockade.
• Atracurium facilitates intubation within 2 to 2½ minutes. The duration of effect is 20 to 35 minutes.

Italicized side effects are common or life-threatening.
*Liquid form contains alcohol.   **May contain tartrazine.

• Once spontaneous recovery starts, atracurium-induced neuromuscular blockade may be reversed with an anticholinesterase agent, together with an anticholinergic drug.
• Don't administer by I.M. injection.
• Atracurium has a longer duration of action than succinylcholine and a shorter duration of action than d-tubocurarine or pancuronium.

gallamine triethiodide
Flaxedil♦
Pregnancy Category: C

MECHANISM OF ACTION
Prevents acetylcholine from binding to the receptors on the muscle end plate, thus blocking depolarization. Nondepolarizing agent.

INDICATIONS & DOSAGE
Adjunct to anesthesia to induce skeletal muscle relaxation; facilitate intubation, reduction of fractures and dislocations; lessen muscle contractions in pharmacologically or electrically induced convulsions; assist with mechanical ventilation—
Dose depends on anesthetic used, individual needs, and response. Doses are representative and must be adjusted.
Adults and children over 1 month: initially, l mg/kg I.V. to maximum of 100 mg, regardless of patient's weight; then 0.5 mg to 1 mg/kg q 30 to 40 minutes.
Children under 1 month but over 5 kg (11 lbs): initially, 0.25 to 0.75 mg/kg I.V., then may give additional doses of 0.1 to 0.5 mg/kg q 30 to 40 minutes.

ADVERSE REACTIONS
CV: tachycardia.
Other: *respiratory paralysis, dose-related prolonged apnea,* residual muscle weakness, increased oropharyngeal secretions, allergic or idiosyncratic hypersensitivity reactions.

INTERACTIONS
Aminoglycoside antibiotics (amikacin, gentamicin, kanamycin, neomycin, streptomycin); polymyxin antibiotics (polymyxin B sulfate, colistin); clindamycin; quinidine; local anesthetics: potentiated neuromuscular blockade, leading to increased skeletal muscle relaxation and possible respiratory paralysis. Use cautiously during surgical and postoperative periods.
Narcotic analgesics: potentiated neuromuscular blockade, leading to increased skeletal muscle relaxation and possible respiratory paralysis. Use with extreme caution, and reduce dose of gallamine.

NURSING CONSIDERATIONS
• Contraindicated in patients with hypersensitivity to iodides, impaired renal function, myasthenia gravis; patients in shock; and patients in whom tachycardia may be hazardous. Use cautiously in elderly or debilitated patients; those with hepatic or pulmonary impairment, respiratory depression, myasthenic syndrome of lung cancer, dehydration, thyroid disorders, collagen diseases, porphyria, and electrolyte disturbances; and in patients undergoing cesarean section.
• Monitor baseline electrolyte determinations (electrolyte imbalance can potentiate neuromuscular effects).
• Take vital signs every 15 minutes, especially for developing tachycardia. Notify doctor immediately of significant changes.
• Measure intake/output (renal dysfunction prolongs duration of action, since drug is unchanged before excretion).
• Keep airway clear. Have emergency respiratory support (endotracheal equipment, ventilator, oxygen, atropine, neostigmine) on hand.
• Determine whether patient has iodide allergy.

• Protect drug from light or excessive heat; use only fresh solutions.
• Do not mix solution with meperidine HCl or barbiturate solutions.
• Give I.V. slowly (over 30 to 90 seconds).
• Do not give without direct supervision of doctor.
• May be preferred in patients who have bradycardia.
• Neostigmine or edrophonium (Tensilon) may be used to reverse the effects.

---

metocurine iodide
Metubine♦
Pregnancy Category: C

MECHANISM OF ACTION
Prevents acetylcholine from binding to the receptors on the muscle end plate, thus blocking depolarization. Nondepolarizing agent.

INDICATIONS & DOSAGE
Adjunct to anesthesia to induce skeletal muscle relaxation; facilitate intubation, reduction of fractures and dislocations—
Dose depends on anesthetic used, individual needs, and response. Doses are representative and must be adjusted. Administer as sustained injection over 30 to 60 seconds.
Adults: given cyclopropane: 2 to 4 mg I.V. (2.68 mg average).
Given ether: 1.5 to 3 mg I.V. (2.1 mg average).
Given nitrous oxide: 4 to 7 mg I.V. (4.79 mg average). Supplemental injections of 0.5 to 1 mg in 25 to 90 minutes, repeated p.r.n.
Lessen muscle contractions in pharmacologically or electrically induced convulsions—
Adults: 1.75 to 5.5 mg I.V.

ADVERSE REACTIONS
CV: hypotension secondary to histamine release, ganglionic blockade in rapid dose or overdose.
Other: *dose-related prolonged apnea,* residual muscle weakness, increased oropharyngeal secretions, allergic or idiosyncratic hypersensitivity reactions, *bronchospasm.*

INTERACTIONS
Aminoglycoside antibiotics (including amikacin, gentamicin, kanamycin, neomycin, streptomycin); polymyxin antibiotics (polymyxin B sulfate, colistin); clindamycin; quinidine; local anesthetics: potentiated neuromuscular blockade, leading to increased skeletal muscle relaxation and possible respiratory paralysis. Use cautiously during surgical and postoperative periods.
Narcotic analgesics: potentiated neuromuscular blockade, leading to increased skeletal muscle relaxation and possible respiratory paralysis. Use with extreme caution, and reduce dose of metocurine iodide.

NURSING CONSIDERATIONS
• Contraindicated in patients with hypersensitivity to iodides; and in whom histamine release is a hazard (asthmatic or atopic patients). Use cautiously in elderly or debilitated patients; and in renal, hepatic, or pulmonary impairment, respiratory depression, myasthenia gravis, myasthenic syndrome of lung cancer, dehydration, thyroid disorders, collagen diseases, porphyria, electrolyte disturbances, hyperthermia, and (in large doses) cesarean section.
• Neostigmine and edrophonium may be used to reverse effects of metocurine.
• Dose of 1 mg is the therapeutic equivalent of 3 mg *d*-tubocurarine chloride.
• Monitor baseline electrolyte determinations (electrolyte imbalance, especially potassium, calcium, and magnesium, can potentiate neuromuscular effects) and vital signs, espe-

---

Italicized side effects are common or life-threatening.
*Liquid form contains alcohol.   **May contain tartrazine.

cially respiration.
• Measure intake and output (renal dysfunction prolongs duration of action, since drug is mainly unchanged before excretion).
• Keep airway clear. Have emergency respiratory support (endotracheal equipment, ventilator, oxygen, atropine, edrophonium, epinephrine, and neostigmine) on hand.
• Determine whether patient has iodide allergy.
• Store solution away from heat, sunlight; do not mix with barbiturates, methohexital, or thiopental (precipitate will form). Use fresh solutions only.
• Do not give without direct supervision of doctor.

---

pancuronium bromide
Pavulon♦
Pregnancy Category: C

MECHANISM OF ACTION
Prevents acetylcholine from binding to the receptors on the muscle end plate, thus blocking depolarization. Nondepolarizing agent.

INDICATIONS & DOSAGE
Adjunct to anesthesia to induce skeletal muscle relaxation; facilitate intubation; lessen muscle contractions in pharmacologically or electrically induced convulsions; assist with mechanical ventilation—
Dose depends on anesthetic used, individual needs, and response. Doses are representative and must be adjusted.
Adults: initially, 0.04 to 0.1 mg/kg I.V.; then 0.01 mg/kg q 30 to 60 minutes.
Children over 10 years: initially, 0.04 to 0.1 mg/kg I.V., then ⅕ initial dose q 30 to 60 minutes.

ADVERSE REACTIONS
CV: tachycardia, increased blood pressure.
Local: burning sensation.
Skin: transient rashes.
Other: excessive sweating and salivation, *prolonged dose-related apnea,* residual muscle weakness, allergic or idiosyncratic hypersensitivity reactions.

INTERACTIONS
Aminoglycoside antibiotics (including amikacin, gentamicin, kanamycin, neomycin, streptomycin); polymyxin antibiotics (polymyxin B sulfate, colistin); clindamycin; quinidine; local anesthetics: potentiated neuromuscular blockade, leading to increased skeletal muscle relaxation and possible respiratory paralysis. Use cautiously during surgical and postoperative periods.
Lithium, narcotic analgesics: potentiated neuromuscular blockade, leading to increased skeletal muscle relaxation and possible respiratory paralysis. Use with extreme caution, and reduce dose of pancuronium.

NURSING CONSIDERATIONS
• Contraindicated in hypersensitivity to bromides; preexisting tachycardia; and in patients for whom even a minor increase in heart rate is undesirable. Use cautiously in elderly or debilitated patients; renal, hepatic, or pulmonary impairment; respiratory depression; myasthenia gravis; myasthenic syndrome of lung cancer; dehydration; thyroid disorders; collagen diseases; porphyria; electrolyte disturbances; hyperthermia; toxemic states; and (in large doses) cesarean section.
• Causes no histamine release or hypotension.
• Dose of 1 mg is the approximate therapeutic equivalent of 5 mg *d*-tubocurarine chloride.
• Monitor baseline electrolyte determinations (electrolyte imbalance can potentiate neuromuscular effects) and

vital signs (watch respiration and heart rate closely).
• Measure intake and output (renal dysfunction may prolong duration of action, since 25% of the drug is unchanged before excretion).
• Have emergency respiratory support (endotracheal equipment, ventilator, oxygen, atropine, neostigmine) on hand.
• Allow succinylcholine effects to subside before giving pancuronium.
• Store in refrigerator. Do not store in plastic containers or syringes, although plastic syringes may be used for administration.
• Do not mix with barbiturate solutions; use only fresh solutions.
• Do not give without direct supervision of doctor.
• Neostigmine or edrophonium (Tensilon) may be used to reverse the effects.

succinylcholine chloride
Anectine♦, Anectine Flo-Pack Powder
Pregnancy Category: C

MECHANISM OF ACTION
Prolongs depolarization of the muscle end plate. Depolarizing agent.

INDICATIONS & DOSAGE
Adjunct to anesthesia to induce skeletal muscle relaxation; facilitate intubation and assist with mechanical ventilation or orthopedic manipulations (drug of choice); lessen muscle contractions in pharmacologically or electrically induced convulsions—
Dose depends on anesthetic used, individual needs, and response. Doses are representative and must be adjusted.
Adults: 25 to 75 mg I.V., then 2.5 mg/minute, p.r.n., or 2.5 mg/kg I.M. up to maximum 150 mg I.M. in deltoid muscle.
Children: 1 to 2 mg/kg I.M. or I.V.

Maximum I.M. dose 150 mg. (Children may be less sensitive to succinylcholine than adults.)

ADVERSE REACTIONS
CV: bradycardia, tachycardia, hypertension, hypotension, arrhythmias.
EENT: increased intraocular pressure.
Other: *prolonged respiratory depression, apnea, malignant hyperthermia,* muscle fasciculation, *postoperative muscle pain,* myoglobinemia, excessive salivation, allergic or idiosyncratic hypersensitivity reactions.

INTERACTIONS
Aminoglycoside antibiotics (including amikacin, gentamicin, kanamycin, neomycin, streptomycin); polymyxin antibiotics (polymyxin B sulfate, colistin); echothiophate; local anesthetics: potentiated neuromuscular blockade, leading to increased skeletal muscle relaxation and possible respiratory paralysis. Use cautiously during surgical and postoperative periods.
Narcotic analgesics, methotrimeprazine: potentiated neuromuscular blockade, leading to increased skeletal muscle relaxation and possible respiratory paralysis. Use with extreme caution.
MAO inhibitors, lithium, cyclophosphamide: prolonged apnea. Use with caution.
Magnesium sulfate (parenterally): potentiated neuromuscular blockade, increased skeletal muscle relaxation, and possible respiratory paralysis. Use with caution, preferably with reduced doses.
Cardiac glycosides: possible cardiac arrhythmias. Use together cautiously.

NURSING CONSIDERATIONS
• Contraindicated in abnormally low plasma pseudocholinesterase levels. Use with caution in patients with personal or family history of malignant hypertension or hyperthermia; elderly

or debilitated patients; hepatic, renal, or pulmonary impairment; and in respiratory depression, severe burns or trauma, electrolyte imbalances, quinidine or digitalis therapy, hyperkalemia, paraplegia, spinal neuraxis injury, degenerative or dystrophic neuromuscular disease, myasthenia gravis, myasthenic syndrome of lung cancer, dehydration, thyroid disorders, collagen diseases, porphyria, fractures, muscle spasms, glaucoma, eye surgery or penetrating eye wounds, pheochromocytoma, and (in large doses) cesarean section.

• Drug of choice for short procedures (less than 3 minutes) and for orthopedic manipulations; use caution in fractures or dislocations.

• Duration of action prolonged to 20 minutes by continuous I.V. infusion or single-dose administration, along with hexafluorenium bromide.

• Repeated or continuous infusions of succinylcholine alone not advised; may cause reduced response or prolonged apnea.

• Monitor baseline electrolyte determinations and vital signs (check respiration every 5 to 10 minutes during infusion).

• Keep airway clear. Have emergency respiratory support (endotracheal equipment, ventilator, oxygen, atropine, neostigmine) on hand.

• Reassure patient that postoperative stiffness is normal and will soon subside.

• Store injectable form in refrigerator. Store powder form at room temperature, tightly closed. Use immediately after reconstitution. Do not mix with alkaline solutions (thiopental, sodium bicarbonate, barbiturates).

• Give test dose (10 mg I.M. or I.V.) after patient has been anesthetized. Normal response (no respiratory depression or transient depression lasting less than 5 minutes) indicates drug may be given. Do not give if patient develops respiratory paralysis suffi-

cient to permit endotracheal intubation. (Recovery within 30 to 60 minutes.)

• Do not give without direct supervision of doctor.

• Give deep I.M., preferably high into the deltoid muscle.

tubocurarine chloride
Tubarine♦♦
Pregnancy Category: C

MECHANISM OF ACTION
Prevents acetylcholine from binding to the receptors on the muscle end plate, thus blocking depolarization. Nondepolarizing agent.

INDICATIONS & DOSAGE
Adjunct to anesthesia to induce skeletal muscle relaxation; facilitate intubation, orthopedic manipulations—
Dose depends on anesthetic used, individual needs, and response. Doses listed are representative and must be adjusted.
Adults: 1 unit/kg or 0.15 mg/kg I.V. slowly over 60 to 90 seconds. Average, initially, 40 to 60 units I.V. May give 20 to 30 units in 3 to 5 minutes. For longer procedures, give 20 units, p.r.n.
Children: 1 unit/kg or 0.15 mg/kg.
Assist with mechanical ventilation—
Adults and children: initially, 0.0165 mg/kg I.V. (average 1 mg or 7 units), then adjust subsequent doses to patient's response.
Lessen muscle contractions in pharmacologically or electrically induced convulsions—
Adults and children: 1 unit/kg or 0.15 mg/kg slowly over 60 to 90 seconds. Initial dose 20 units (3 mg) less than calculated dose.

ADVERSE REACTIONS
CV: hypotension, circulatory depression.
Other: profound and prolonged mus-

cle relaxation, *respiratory depression to the point of apnea,* hypersensitivity, idiosyncrasy, residual muscle weakness, *bronchospasm.*

INTERACTIONS
Aminoglycoside antibiotics (including amikacin, gentamicin, kanamycin, neomycin, streptomycin); polymyxin antibiotics (polymyxin B sulfate, colistin); local anesthetics: potentiated neuromuscular blockade, leading to increased skeletal muscle relaxation and possible respiratory paralysis. Use cautiously during surgical and postoperative periods.
Quinidine: prolonged neuromuscular blockade. Use together with caution. Monitor closely.
Thiazide diuretics, furosemide, ethacrynic acid, amphotericin B, propranolol, methotrimeprazine, narcotic analgesics: potentiated neuromuscular blockade, leading to increased respiratory paralysis. Use with extreme caution during surgical and postoperative periods.

NURSING CONSIDERATIONS
• Contraindicated in patients for whom histamine release is a hazard (asthmatics). Use cautiously in elderly or debilitated patients; in hepatic or pulmonary impairment, respiratory depression, myasthenia gravis, myasthenic syndrome of lung cancer, dehydration, thyroid disorders, collagen diseases, porphyria, electrolyte disturbances, fractures, muscle spasms, and (in large doses) cesarean section.
• Small margin of safety between therapeutic dose and dose causing respiratory paralysis.
• Allow succinylcholine effects to subside before giving tubocurarine.
• Monitor baseline electrolyte determinations (electrolyte imbalance can potentiate neuromuscular effects).
• Watch respirations closely for early symptoms of paralysis—inability to

keep eyelids open and eyes focused, or difficulty in swallowing and speaking. Notify doctor immediately.
• Check vital signs every 15 minutes. Notify doctor at once of changes.
• Measure intake and output (renal dysfunction prolongs duration of action, since much of drug is unchanged before excretion).
• Keep airway clear. Have emergency respiratory support (endotracheal equipment, ventilator, oxygen, atropine, edrophonium, epinephrine, and neostigmine) on hand.
• Decrease dose if inhalation anesthetics are used.
• Do not mix with barbiturates. Use only fresh solutions and discard if discolored.
• Give I.V. slowly (60 to 90 seconds); give deep I.M. in deltoid muscle.
• Do not give without direct supervision of doctor.
• Neostigmine or edrophonium (Tensilon) may be used to reverse the effects.

---

vecuronium bromide
Norcuron
Pregnancy Category: C

MECHANISM OF ACTION
Prevents acetylcholine from binding to the receptors on the muscle end plate, thus blocking depolarization. Nondepolarizing agent.

INDICATIONS & DOSAGE
Adjunct to general anesthesia, to facilitate endotracheal intubation and to provide skeletal muscle relaxation during surgery or mechanical ventilation—
Dose depends on anesthetic used, individual needs, and response. Doses are representative and must be adjusted.
Adults and children over 9 years: Initially, 0.08 to 0.10 mg/kg I.V. bolus. Maintenance doses of 0.010 to

0.015 mg/kg within 25 to 40 minutes of initial dose should be administered during prolonged surgical procedures. Maintenance doses may be given q 12 to 15 minutes in patients receiving balanced anesthesia.

Children under 10 years may require a slightly higher initial dose and may also require supplementation slightly more often than adults.

ADVERSE REACTIONS
Other: *prolonged dose-related apnea.*

INTERACTIONS
Aminoglycoside antibiotics (including amikacin, gentamicin, kanamycin, neomycin, streptomycin); polymyxin antibiotics (polymyxin B sulfate, colistin); clindamycin; quinidine; local anesthetics: potentiated neuromuscular blockade, leading to increased skeletal muscle relaxation and possible respiratory paralysis. Use cautiously during surgical and postoperative periods.
Narcotic analgesics: potentiated neuromuscular blockade, leading to increased skeletal muscle relaxation and possible respiratory paralysis. Use with extreme caution, and reduce dose of vecuronium.

NURSING CONSIDERATIONS
• Contraindicated in hypersensitivity to bromides. Use cautiously in patients with altered circulation time due to cardiovascular disease, old age, and edematous states; in hepatic disease; in severe obesity; and in neuromuscular disease.
• Unlike other nondepolarizing neuromuscular blockers, vecuronium has no effect on cardiovascular system. Also, the drug causes no histamine release and therefore no histamine-related hypersensitivity reactions such as bronchospasm, hypotension, or tachycardia.
• The drug is well tolerated in patients with renal failure.

• Prior administration of succinylcholine may enhance the neuromuscular blocking effect and duration of action.
• Vecuronium provides conditions for intubation within 2½ to 3 minutes. The duration of effect is 25 to 40 minutes.
• Once spontaneous recovery starts, vecuronium-induced neuromuscular blockade may be reversed with an anticholinesterase agent, together with an anticholinergic drug.
• Have emergency respiratory support (endotracheal equipment, ventilator, oxygen, atropine, neostigmine) on hand.
• Store reconstituted solution in refrigerator. Discard after 24 hours.

42

Antihistamines

azatadine maleate
brompheniramine maleate
carbinoxamine maleate
chlorpheniramine maleate
clemastine fumarate
cyproheptadine hydrochloride
dexchlorpheniramine maleate
diphenhydramine hydrochloride
methdilazine hydrochloride
promethazine hydrochloride
terfenadine
trimeprazine tartrate
tripelennamine hydrochloride
triprolidine hydrochloride

COMBINATION PRODUCTS

ALLEREST TABLETS: phenylpropanolamine hydrochloride 18.7 mg and chlorpheniramine maleate 2 mg.

ALLERGESIC: phenylpropanolamine 18.7 mg and chlorpheniramine maleate 2 mg.

CHLOR-TRIMETON DECONGESTANT: chlorpheniramine maleate 4 mg and pseudoephedrine sulfate 60 mg.

CHLOR-TRIMETON DECONGESTANT REPETABS: chlorpheniramine maleate 8 mg and pseudoephedrine sulfate 120 mg.

CODIMAL DH*: hydrocodone bitartrate 1.66 mg, phenylephrine hydrochloride 5 mg, pyrilamine maleate 8.33 mg, potassium guaiacolsulfonate 83.3 mg, sodium citrate 216 mg, and citric acid 50 mg.

CONDRIN-LA: phenylpropanolamine HCl 75 mg and chlorpheniramine maleate 12 mg.

CONTAC: phenylpropanolamine 75 mg and chlorpheniramine maleate 8 mg.

CORICIDIN TABLETS: chlorpheniramine maleate 2 mg and aspirin 325 mg.

COTROL-D: pseudoephedrine HCl 60 mg and chlorpheniramine maleate 4 mg.

DECONADE: phenylpropanolamine HCl 75 mg and chlorpheniramine maleate 12 mg.

DECONAMINE: pseudoephedrine HCl 60 mg and chlorpheniramine maleate 4 mg.

DIMETAPP EXTENTABS: brompheniramine maleate 12 mg, and phenylpropanolamine hydrochloride 75 mg.

DISOPHROL CHRONOTAB: dexbrompheniramine maleate 6 mg and pseudoephedrine sulfate 120 mg.

DRIXORAL♦: dexbrompheniramine maleate 6 mg and pseudoephedrine sulfate 120 mg.

DRIZE: phenylpropanolamine HCl 75 mg and chlorpheniramine maleate 12 mg.

FEDAHIST: pseudoephedrine HCl 60 mg and chlorpheniramine maleate 4 mg.

HISTABID DURACAPS: phenylpropanolamine 75 mg and chlorpheniramine maleate 8 mg.

HISTASPAN-D: chlorpheniramine maleate 8 mg, phenylephrine hydrochloride 20 mg, and methscopolamine nitrate 2.5 mg.

NALDECON: phenylephrine hydrochloride 10 mg, phenylpropanolamine hydrochloride 40 mg, phenyltoloxamine citrate 15 mg, and chlorpheniramine maleate 5 mg.

NEOTEP: chlorpheniramine maleate 9 mg and phenylephrine hydrochloride 21 mg.

Italicized side effects are common or life-threatening.
*Liquid form contains alcohol.   **May contain tartrazine.

NOLAMINE: chlorpheniramine maleate 4 mg, phenindamine tartrate 24 mg, and phenylpropanolamine hydrochloride 50 mg.

NOVAFED A: pseudoephedrine hydrochloride 120 mg and chlorpheniramine maleate 8 mg.

NOVAHISTINE COLD TABLETS: phenylpropanolamine 18.7 mg and chlorpheniramine maleate 2 mg.

NOVAHISTINE ELIXIR*: phenylpropanolamine hydrochloride 18.7 mg, chlorpheniramine maleate 2 mg, and alcohol 5%/5 ml.

ORAHIST: phenylpropanolamine HCl 75 mg and chlorpheniramine 12 mg.

ORNADE: phenylpropanolamine hydrochloride 75 mg and chlorpheniramine maleate 12 mg.

RHINEX D-LAY: acetaminophen 300 mg, salicylamide 300 mg, phenylpropanolamine hydrochloride 60 mg, and chlorpheniramine maleate 4 mg.

RONDEC: carbinoxamine maleate 4 mg and pseudoephedrine hydrochloride 60 mg.

SUDAFED PLUS: pseudoephedrine HCl 60 mg and chlorpheniramine maleate 4 mg.

TRIAMINIC-12: phenylpropanolamine HCl 75 mg and chlorpheniramine maleate 12 mg.

TRIAMINIC TABLETS: phenylpropanolamine hydrochloride 50 mg, pheniramine maleate 25 mg, and pyrilamine maleate 25 mg.

azatadine maleate
Optimine♦
Pregnancy Category: B

MECHANISM OF ACTION
Competes with histamine for H_1-receptor sites on effector cells. Prevents but does not reverse histamine-mediated responses.

INDICATIONS & DOSAGE
Rhinitis, allergy symptoms, chronic urticaria—

Adults: 1 to 2 mg P.O. b.i.d. Maximum 4 mg daily.
Not intended for children under 12 years.

ADVERSE REACTIONS
Blood: thrombocytopenia.
CNS: (especially in the elderly) *drowsiness, dizziness,* vertigo, disturbed coordination.
CV: hypotension, palpitations.
GI: anorexia, nausea, vomiting, *dry mouth and throat.*
GU: urinary retention.
Skin: urticaria, rash.
Other: thick bronchial secretions.

INTERACTIONS
CNS depressants: increased sedation. Use together cautiously.

NURSING CONSIDERATIONS
• Contraindicated in acute asthmatic attack. Use cautiously in elderly patients and in patients with increased intraocular pressure, hyperthyroidism, cardiovascular or renal disease, hypertension, bronchial asthma, urinary retention, prostatic hypertrophy, bladder-neck obstruction, and stenosing peptic ulcers.
• Warn patient against drinking alcoholic beverages during therapy and against activities that require alertness until CNS response to drug is determined.
• Reduce GI distress by giving with food or milk.
• Coffee or tea may reduce drowsiness. Sugarless gum, sour hard candy, or ice chips may relieve dry mouth.
• If tolerance develops, another antihistamine may be substituted.
• Warn patient to stop taking drug 4 days before allergy skin tests to preserve accuracy of tests.
• Monitor blood counts during long-term therapy; watch for signs of blood dyscrasias.

brompheniramine maleate
Brombay, Dimetane*♦, Dimetane-Ten, Rolabromophen, Spentane, Veltane
Pregnancy Category: C

MECHANISM OF ACTION
Competes with histamine for H_1-receptor sites on effector cells. Prevents but does not reverse histamine-mediated responses.

INDICATIONS & DOSAGE
Rhinitis, allergy symptoms—
Adults: 4 to 8 mg P.O. t.i.d. or q.i.d.; or (timed-release) 8 to 12 mg P.O. b.i.d. or t.i.d.; or 5 to 20 mg q 6 to 12 hours I.M., I.V., or S.C. Maximum 40 mg daily.
Children over 6 years: 2 to 4 mg t.i.d. or q.i.d.; or (timed-release) 8 to 12 mg q 12 hours; or 0.5 mg/kg daily I.M., I.V., or S.C. divided t.i.d. or q.i.d.
Children under 6 years: 0.5 mg/kg daily P.O., I.M., I.V., or S.C. divided t.i.d. or q.i.d.

ADVERSE REACTIONS
Blood: thrombocytopenia, *agranulocytosis.*
CNS: (especially in the elderly) dizziness, tremors, irritability, insomnia, *drowsiness, stimulation.*
CV: hypotension, palpitations.
GI: anorexia, nausea, vomiting, *dry mouth and throat.*
GU: urinary retention.
Skin: urticaria, rash.
After parenteral administration: local reaction, sweating, syncope.

INTERACTIONS
CNS depressants: increased sedation. Use together cautiously.

NURSING CONSIDERATIONS
• Contraindicated in acute asthmatic attack. Use cautiously in elderly patients, and in patients with increased intraocular pressure, hyperthyroidism, cardiovascular or renal disease, hypertension, bronchial asthma, urinary retention, prostatic hypertrophy, bladder-neck obstruction, and stenosing peptic ulcers.
• Warn patient against drinking alcoholic beverages during therapy and against activities that require alertness.
• Reduce GI distress by giving with food or milk.
• Causes less drowsiness than some other antihistamines.
• Coffee or tea may reduce drowsiness. Sugarless gum, sour hard candy, or ice chips may relieve dry mouth.
• If tolerance develops, another antihistamine may be substituted.
• Warn patient to stop taking drug 4 days before allergy skin tests to preserve accuracy of tests.
• Injectable form containing 10 mg/ml can be given diluted or undiluted very slowly I.V. The 100 mg/ml injection should not be given I.V.
• Monitor blood count during long-term therapy; observe for signs of blood dyscrasias.

carbinoxamine maleate
Clistin*
Pregnancy Category: C

MECHANISM OF ACTION
Competes with histamine for H_1-receptor sites on effector cells. Prevents but does not reverse histamine-mediated responses.

INDICATIONS & DOSAGE
Rhinitis, allergy symptoms—
Adults: 4 to 8 mg P.O. t.i.d. or q.i.d., or (timed-release) 8 to 12 mg q 8 to 12 hours.
Children over 6 years: 4 to 6 mg P.O. t.i.d. or q.i.d.
Children 3 to 6 years: 2 to 4 mg P.O. t.i.d. or q.i.d.
Children 1 to 3 years: 2 mg P.O.

Italicized side effects are common or life-threatening.
*Liquid form contains alcohol.   **May contain tartrazine.

t.i.d. or q.i.d.

ADVERSE REACTIONS
CNS: (especially in the elderly) *drowsiness, dizziness, stimulation.*
GI: anorexia, nausea, vomiting, *dry mouth.*
GU: urinary retention.

INTERACTIONS
CNS depressants: increased sedation. Use together cautiously.

NURSING CONSIDERATIONS
• Contraindicated in acute asthmatic attack. Use cautiously in elderly patients, and in patients with increased intraocular pressure, hyperthyroidism, cardiovascular or renal disease, hypertension, bronchial asthma, urinary retention, prostatic hypertrophy, bladder-neck obstruction, and stenosing peptic ulcers.
• Warn patient against drinking alcoholic beverages during therapy and against driving or other activities that require alertness until CNS response to drug is determined.
• Reduce GI distress by giving with food or milk.
• Coffee or tea may reduce drowsiness. Sugarless gum, sour hard candy, or ice chips may relieve dry mouth.
• If tolerance develops, another antihistamine may be substituted.
• Warn patient to stop taking drug 4 days before allergy skin tests to preserve accuracy of tests.

---

chlorpheniramine maleate
AL-R, Chlormene, Chlortab, Chlor-Trimeton*, Chlor-Tripolon♦♦,
Histaspan, Novopheniram♦♦,
Pyranistan, Teldrin
Pregnancy Category: B

MECHANISM OF ACTION
Competes with histamine for H_1-receptor sites on effector cells. Prevents but does not reverse histamine-me-diated responses.

INDICATIONS & DOSAGE
Rhinitis, allergy symptoms—
Adults: 2 to 4 mg P.O. t.i.d. or q.i.d.; or (timed-release) 8 to 12 mg P.O. b.i.d. or t.i.d.; or 5 to 40 mg I.M., I.V., or S.C. daily. Give I.V. injection over 1 minute.
Not recommended for children under 12 years, except under medical supervision.

ADVERSE REACTIONS
CNS: *stimulation,* sedation, *drowsiness* (especially in the elderly), excitability (in children).
CV: hypotension, palpitations.
GI: epigastric distress, *dry mouth.*
GU: urinary retention.
Skin: rash, urticaria.
Other: thick bronchial secretions.
After parenteral administration: local stinging, burning sensation, pallor, weak pulse, transient hypotension.

INTERACTIONS
CNS depressants: increased sedation. Use together cautiously.

NURSING CONSIDERATIONS
• Contraindicated in acute asthmatic attack. Use cautiously in elderly patients, and in patients with increased intraocular pressure, hyperthyroidism, cardiovascular or renal disease, hypertension, bronchial asthma, urinary retention, prostatic hypertrophy, bladder-neck obstruction.
• Warn patient against drinking alcoholic beverages and using other CNS depressants during therapy and against driving or other activities that require alertness until CNS response to drug is determined.
• Coffee or tea may reduce drowsiness. Sugarless gum, sour hard candy, or ice chips may relieve dry mouth.
• If tolerance develops, another antihistamine may be substituted.
• Warn patient to stop taking drug 4

days before allergy skin tests to preserve accuracy of tests.
• Only injectable forms *without* preservatives can be given I.V. Give *slowly*.
• If symptoms occur during or after parenteral dose, stop drug. Notify doctor.

clemastine fumarate
Tavist♦, Tavist-1
Pregnancy Category: C

MECHANISM OF ACTION
Competes with histamine for H_1-receptor sites on effector cells. Prevents but does not reverse histamine-mediated responses.

INDICATIONS & DOSAGE
Rhinitis, allergy symptoms—
Adults: 1.34 to 2.68 mg P.O. b.i.d. or t.i.d. Maximum recommended daily dosage is 8.04 mg.
Allergic skin manifestation of urticaria and angioedema—
Adults: 2.68 mg up to t.i.d. maximum.

ADVERSE REACTIONS
Blood: hemolytic anemia, thrombocytopenia, *agranulocytosis.*
CNS: (especially in the elderly) *sedation, drowsiness.*
CV: hypotension, palpitations, tachycardia.
GI: epigastric distress, anorexia, nausea, vomiting, constipation, *dry mouth.*
GU: urinary retention.
Skin: rash, urticaria.
Other: thick bronchial secretions.

INTERACTIONS
CNS depressants: increased sedation. Use together cautiously.

NURSING CONSIDERATIONS
• Contraindicated in acute asthmatic attack. Use cautiously in elderly pa-

tients, and in patients with increased intraocular pressure, hyperthyroidism, cardiovascular or renal disease, hypertension, bronchial asthma, urinary retention, prostatic hypertrophy, bladder-neck obstruction, and stenosing peptic ulcers.
• Warn patient against drinking alcoholic beverages during therapy and against driving or other activities that require alertness until CNS response to drug is determined.
• Coffee or tea may reduce drowsiness. Sugarless gum, sour hard candy, or ice chips may relieve dry mouth.
• If tolerance develops, another antihistamine may be substituted.
• Warn patient to stop taking drug 4 days before allergy skin tests to preserve accuracy of tests.
• Monitor blood counts during long-term therapy; observe for signs of blood dyscrasias.

cyproheptadine hydrochloride
Periactin♦, Vimicon♦♦
Pregnancy Category: B

MECHANISM OF ACTION
Competes with histamine for H_1-receptor sites on effector cells. Prevents but does not reverse histamine-mediated responses.

INDICATIONS & DOSAGE
Allergy symptoms, pruritus—
Adults: 4 mg P.O. t.i.d. or q.i.d. Maximum 0.5 mg/kg daily.
Children 7 to 14 years: 4 mg P.O. b.i.d. or t.i.d. Maximum 16 mg daily.
Children 2 to 6 years: 2 mg P.O. b.i.d. or t.i.d. Maximum 12 mg daily.

ADVERSE REACTIONS
CNS: (especially in the elderly) *drowsiness,* dizziness, headache, fatigue.
GI: nausea, vomiting, *dry mouth.*
GU: urinary retention.

Skin: rash.
Other: weight gain.

INTERACTIONS
CNS depressants: increased sedation. Use together cautiously.

NURSING CONSIDERATIONS
• Contraindicated in acute asthmatic attack. Use cautiously in elderly patients, and in patients with increased intraocular pressure, hyperthyroidism, cardiovascular or renal disease, hypertension, bronchial asthma, urinary retention, prostatic hypertrophy, bladder-neck obstruction, and stenosing peptic ulcers.
• Warn patient against drinking alcoholic beverages during therapy and against driving or other activities that require alertness until CNS response to drug is determined.
• Reduce GI distress by giving with food or milk.
• Coffee or tea may reduce drowsiness. Sugarless gum, sour hard candy, or ice chips may relieve dry mouth.
• If tolerance develops, another antihistamine may be substituted.
• Warn patient to stop taking drug 4 days before allergy skin tests to preserve accuracy of tests.
• Used experimentally to stimulate appetite and increase weight gain in children.

---

dexchlorpheniramine maleate
Polaramine♦
Pregnancy Category: B

MECHANISM OF ACTION
Competes with histamine for H_1-receptor sites on effector cells. Prevents but does not reverse histamine-mediated responses.

INDICATIONS & DOSAGE
Rhinitis, allergy symptoms, contact dermatitis, pruritus—

Adults: 1 to 2 mg P.O. t.i.d. or q.i.d.; or (timed-release) 4 to 6 mg b.i.d. or t.i.d.
Children under 12 years: 0.15 mg/kg P.O. daily divided into 4 doses. Do not use timed-release tablets for children younger than 6 years.

ADVERSE REACTIONS
CNS: (especially in the elderly) *drowsiness,* dizziness, *stimulation.*
GI: nausea, *dry mouth.*
GU: polyuria, dysuria, urinary retention.

INTERACTIONS
CNS depressants: increased sedation. Use together cautiously.

NURSING CONSIDERATIONS
• Contraindicated in acute asthmatic attack. Use cautiously in elderly patients, and in patients with increased intraocular pressure, hyperthyroidism, cardiovascular or renal disease, hypertension, bronchial asthma, urinary retention, prostatic hypertrophy, bladder-neck obstruction, and stenosing peptic ulcers.
• Warn patient against drinking alcoholic beverages during therapy and against driving or other activities that require alertness until CNS response to drug is determined.
• Causes less drowsiness than some other antihistamines.
• Coffee or tea may reduce drowsiness. Sugarless gum, sour hard candy, or ice chips may relieve dry mouth.
• If tolerance develops, another antihistamine may be substituted.
• Warn patient to stop taking drug 4 days before allergy skin tests to preserve accuracy of tests.

diphenhydramine hydrochloride
Allerdryl♦, Baramine, Bax*,
Benachlor, Benadryl♦*, Benahist,
Ben-Allergin, Bentrac, Bonyl,
Compoz♦, Diphenacen, Nordryl,
Nytol with DPH♦, Rodryl, Rohydra,
Sominex Formula 2♦, Span-Lanin,
Valdrene, Wehdryl
Pregnancy Category: C

MECHANISM OF ACTION
Competes with histamine for H_1-receptor sites on effector cells. Prevents but does not reverse histamine-mediated responses, particularly histamine's effects on the smooth muscle of the bronchial tubes, gastrointestinal tract, uterus, and blood vessels. Structurally related to local anesthetics, diphenhydramine provides local anesthesia by preventing initiation and transmission of nerve impulses. Also suppresses the cough reflex by a direct effect in the medulla of the brain.

INDICATIONS & DOSAGE
Rhinitis, allergy symptoms, nighttime sedation, motion sickness, antiparkinsonism—
Adults: 25 to 50 mg P.O. t.i.d. or q.i.d.; or 10 to 50 mg deep I.M. or I.V. Maximum 400 mg daily.
Children under 12 years: 5 mg/kg daily P.O., deep I.M., or I.V. divided q.i.d. Maximum 300 mg daily.
Sedation—
Adults: 25 to 50 mg P.O., deep I.M., p.r.n.
As a nighttime sleep aid—
Adults: 50 mg P.O. h.s.
Nonproductive cough—
Adults: 25 mg P.O. q 4 hours (not to exceed 100 mg daily).
Children 6 to 12 years: 12.5 mg P.O. q 4 hours (not to exceed 50 mg daily).
Children 2 to 6 years: 6.25 mg P.O. q 4 hours (not to exceed 25 mg daily).

ADVERSE REACTIONS
CNS: (especially in the elderly) *drowsiness,* confusion, insomnia, headache, vertigo.
CV: palpitations.
EENT: photosensitivity, diplopia, nasal stuffiness.
GI: *nausea,* vomiting, diarrhea, *dry mouth,* constipation.
GU: dysuria, urinary retention.
Skin: urticaria.

INTERACTIONS
CNS depressants: increased sedation. Use together cautiously.

NURSING CONSIDERATIONS
• Contraindicated in acute asthmatic attack. Use cautiously in narrow-angle glaucoma, prostatic hypertrophy, pyloroduodenal and bladder-neck obstruction, and stenosing peptic ulcers; in newborns; and in asthmatic, hypertensive, or cardiac patients.
• Alternate injection sites to prevent irritation. Administer deep I.M. into large muscle.
• Warn patient against drinking alcoholic beverages during therapy and against driving or other hazardous activities until CNS response to drug is determined.
• Reduce GI distress by giving with food or milk.
• Coffee or tea may reduce drowsiness. Sugarless gum, sour hard candy, or ice chips may relieve dry mouth.
• If tolerance develops, another antihistamine may be substituted.
• Warn patient to stop taking drug 4 days before allergy skin tests to preserve accuracy of tests.
• Used with epinephrine in anaphylaxis.
• One of most sedating antihistamines; often used as a hypnotic.

Italicized side effects are common or life-threatening.
*Liquid form contains alcohol.   **May contain tartrazine.

methdilazine hydrochloride
Dilosyn♦♦, Tacaryl
Pregnancy Category: C

MECHANISM OF ACTION
Competes with histamine for H$_1$-receptor sites on effector cells. Prevents but does not reverse histamine-mediated responses.

INDICATIONS & DOSAGE
Pruritus—
Adults: 8 mg P.O. b.i.d. to q.i.d. or (chewable tablets) 7.2 mg P.O. b.i.d. to q.i.d.
Children over 3 years: 4 mg P.O. b.i.d. to q.i.d. or (chewable tablets) 3.6 mg P.O. b.i.d. to q.i.d.

ADVERSE REACTIONS
CNS: (especially in the elderly) *drowsiness,* dizziness, headache.
GI: nausea, *dry mouth and throat.*
GU: urinary retention.
Hepatic: cholestatic jaundice.
Skin: rash.

INTERACTIONS
Phenothiazines: increased effects. Don't use together.
CNS depressants: increased sedation. Use together cautiously.

NURSING CONSIDERATIONS
• Contraindicated in acute asthmatic attack. Use cautiously in elderly or debilitated patients; acutely ill or dehydrated children; and in patients with pulmonary, hepatic, or cardiovascular disease, asthma, hypertension, prostatic hypertrophy, bladder-neck obstruction, CNS depression, and stenosing peptic ulcers.
• Warn patient against drinking alcoholic beverages during therapy and against driving or other activities that require alertness until CNS response to drug is determined.
• Reduce GI distress by giving with food or milk.

• Coffee or tea may reduce drowsiness. Sugarless gum, sour hard candy, or ice chips may relieve dry mouth.
• If tolerance develops, another antihistamine may be substituted.
• Available as chewable tablet for children. Instruct child to chew completely and swallow promptly; may cause local anesthetic effect in mouth, which increases the risk of choking.
• Warn patient to stop taking drug 4 days before allergy skin tests to preserve accuracy of tests.

promethazine hydrochloride
K-Phen, Methazine, Pentazine, Phencen-50, Phenergan♦*, Promethamead, Promethazine, Prorex, Provigan, Remsed, Rolamethazine*, Sigazine
Pregnancy Category: C

MECHANISM OF ACTION
Competes with histamine for H$_1$-receptor sites on effector cells. Prevents but does not reverse histamine-mediated responses.

INDICATIONS & DOSAGE
Motion sickness—
Adults: 25 mg P.O. b.i.d.
Children: 12.5 to 25 mg P.O., I.M., or rectally b.i.d.
Nausea—
Adults: 12.5 to 25 mg P.O., I.M., or rectally q 4 to 6 hours, p.r.n.
Children: 0.25 to 0.5 mg/kg I.M. or rectally q 4 to 6 hours, p.r.n.
Rhinitis, allergy symptoms—
Adults: 12.5 mg P.O. q.i.d.; or 25 mg P.O. at bedtime.
Children: 6.25 to 12.5 mg P.O. t.i.d. or 25 mg P.O. or rectally at bedtime.
Sedation—
Adults: 25 to 50 mg P.O. or I.M. at bedtime or p.r.n.
Children: 12.5 to 25 mg P.O., I.M., or rectally at bedtime.

Unmarked trade names available in the United States only.
♦ Also available in Canada.   ♦♦ Available in Canada only.

Routine preoperative or postoperative sedation or as an adjunct to analgesics—
Adults: 25 to 50 mg I.M., I.V., or P.O.
Children: 12.5 to 25 mg I.M., I.V., or P.O.

ADVERSE REACTIONS
Blood: leukopenia, *agranulocytosis.*
CNS: (especially in the elderly) *sedation,* confusion, restlessness, tremors, *drowsiness.*
CV: hypotension.
EENT: transient myopia, nasal congestion.
GI: anorexia, nausea, vomiting, constipation, *dry mouth.*
GU: urinary retention.
Other: *photosensitivity.*

INTERACTIONS
Phenothiazines: increased effects. Don't give together.
CNS depressants: increased sedation. Use together cautiously.

NURSING CONSIDERATIONS
• Contraindicated in patients with increased intraocular pressure, intestinal obstruction, prostatic hypertrophy, bladder-neck obstruction, epilepsy, bone-marrow depression, coma, CNS depression, stenosing peptic ulcers, and in newborns and acutely ill or dehydrated children. Use cautiously in pulmonary, hepatic, or cardiovascular disease; asthma; hypertension; bone-marrow depression; and in elderly or debilitated patients.
• Warn patient against drinking alcoholic beverages during therapy and against driving or other activities that require alertness until CNS response to drug is determined.
• Reduce GI distress by giving with food or milk.
• Coffee or tea may reduce drowsiness. Sugarless gum, sour hard candy, or ice chips may relieve dry mouth.
• Warn patient to stop taking drug 4

days before allergy skin tests to preserve accuracy of tests.
• Pronounced sedative effect limits use in many ambulatory patients.
• May cause false-positive immunologic urine pregnancy test (Gravindex). Also may interfere with blood grouping in ABO system.
• When treating motion sickness, tell patient to take first dose 30 to 60 minutes before travel. On succeeding days of travel, he should take dose upon arising and with evening meal.
• Inject deep I.M. into large muscle mass. Don't administer S.C. Rotate injection sites.
• May be administered I.V., but don't give in a concentration greater than 25 mg/ml, nor at a rate exceeding 25 mg/minute. Shield I.V. infusion from direct light.
• May be safely mixed with meperidine (Demerol) in the same syringe.
• Warn patient about possible photosensitivity and precautions to avoid it.

terfenadine
Seldane
Pregnancy Category: C

MECHANISM OF ACTION
Competes with histamine for H_1-receptor sites on effector cells. Prevents but does not reverse histamine-mediated responses.

INDICATIONS & DOSAGE
Rhinitis, allergy symptoms—
Adults and children 12 years or older: 60 mg P.O. b.i.d.
Children 6 to 12 years: 30 to 60 mg P.O. b.i.d.
Children 3 to 5 years: 15 mg P.O. b.i.d.

ADVERSE REACTIONS
CNS: fatigue, dizziness, headache.
GI: abdominal distress, nausea.
EENT: dry throat and mouth, nasal stuffiness.

Italicized side effects are common or life-threatening.
*Liquid form contains alcohol.   **May contain tartrazine.

INTERACTIONS
None significant.

NURSING CONSIDERATIONS
• May cause a mild anticholinergic drying effect in patients with lower airway disease, such as asthma. Keep patients well hydrated.
• Instruct patients not to exceed prescribed dose.
• Relief of symptoms begins within 1 hour.
• Terfenadine is a new, distinctly different antihistamine. Significant lack of adverse reactions also makes it unique.
• Does not cause drowsiness and sedation associated with other antihistamines because drug does not cross blood-brain barrier; its anticholinergic and antiserotonin effects are mild.

---

trimeprazine tartrate
Panectyl♦♦, Temaril♦
Pregnancy Category: C

MECHANISM OF ACTION
Competes with histamine for H_1-receptor sites on effector cells. Prevents but does not reverse histamine-mediated responses.

INDICATIONS & DOSAGE
Pruritus—
Adults: 2.5 mg P.O. q.i.d.; or (timed-release) 5 mg P.O. b.i.d.
Children 3 to 12 years: 2.5 mg P.O. h.s. or t.i.d., p.r.n.
Children 6 months to 3 years: 1.25 mg P.O. h.s. or t.i.d., p.r.n.

ADVERSE REACTIONS
Blood: *agranulocytosis,* leukopenia.
CNS: *(especially in the elderly) drowsiness,* dizziness, confusion, headache, restlessness, tremors, irritability, insomnia; (in children) paradoxical excitation.
CV: hypotension, palpitations, tachycardia.

GI: anorexia, nausea, vomiting, *dry mouth and throat.*
GU: urinary frequency or retention.
Skin: urticaria, rash, *photosensitivity.*

INTERACTIONS
Phenothiazines: increased effects. Don't use together.
CNS depressants: increased sedation. Use together cautiously.

NURSING CONSIDERATIONS
• Contraindicated in acute asthmatic attack. Use cautiously in pulmonary, hepatic, or cardiovascular disease; asthma; hypertension; narrow-angle glaucoma; intestinal obstruction; prostatic hypertrophy; bladder-neck obstruction; epilepsy; bone-marrow depression; coma; CNS depression; stenosing peptic ulcers; in elderly or debilitated patients, and acutely ill or dehydrated children.
• Warn patient against drinking alcoholic beverages during therapy and against driving or other activities that require alertness until CNS response to drug is determined.
• Reduce GI distress by giving with food or milk.
• Coffee or tea may reduce drowsiness. Sugarless gum, sour hard candy, or ice chips may relieve dry mouth.
• Warn patient to stop taking drug 4 days before allergy skin tests to preserve accuracy of tests.
• Monitor blood counts during long-term therapy.
• Warn patient about risk of photosensitivity. Recommend use of a sunscreen. If photosensitivity occurs, tell patient to stop taking the drug and call the doctor.

tripelennamine hydrochloride
PBZ-SR, Pyribenzamine♦, Ro-Hist
Pregnancy Category: B

MECHANISM OF ACTION
Competes with histamine for H_1-receptor sites on effector cells. Prevents but does not reverse histamine-mediated responses.

INDICATIONS & DOSAGE
Rhinitis, allergy symptoms—
Adults: 25 to 50 mg P.O. q 4 to 6 hours; or (timed-release) 100 mg b.i.d. or t.i.d. Maximum 600 mg daily.
Children over 5 years: 50 mg P.O. q 8 to 12 hours (timed-release).
Children under 5 years: 5 mg/kg daily P.O. in 4 to 6 divided doses. Maximum 300 mg daily.

ADVERSE REACTIONS
CNS: (especially in the elderly) *drowsiness,* dizziness, confusion, restlessness, tremors, irritability, insomnia.
CV: palpitations.
GI: anorexia, diarrhea or constipation, *nausea, vomiting, dry mouth.*
GU: urinary frequency or retention.
Skin: urticaria, rash.
Other: thick bronchial secretions.

INTERACTIONS
CNS depressants: increased sedation. Use together cautiously.

NURSING CONSIDERATIONS
• Contraindicated in acute asthmatic attack. Use cautiously in elderly patients, and in patients with increased intraocular pressure, hyperthyroidism, cardiovascular or renal disease, hypertension, or bronchial asthma, urinary retention, prostatic hypertrophy, bladder-neck obstruction, and stenosing peptic ulcers.
• Warn patient against drinking alcoholic beverages during therapy and against driving or other activities that require alertness until CNS response to drug is determined.
• Reduce GI distress by giving with food or milk.
• Coffee or tea may reduce drowsiness. Sugarless gum, sour hard candy, or ice chips may relieve dry mouth.
• If tolerance develops, another antihistamine may be substituted.
• Warn patient to stop taking drug 4 days before allergy skin tests to preserve accuracy of tests.

triprolidine hydrochloride
Actidil♦, Bayidyl
Pregnancy Category: C

MECHANISM OF ACTION
Competes with histamine for H_1-receptor sites on effector cells. Prevents but does not reverse histamine-mediated responses.

INDICATIONS & DOSAGE
Colds and allergy symptoms—
Adults: 2.5 mg P.O. t.i.d. or q.i.d.
Children over 6 years: 1.25 mg t.i.d. or q.i.d.
Children 4 to 6 years: 0.9 mg t.i.d. or q.i.d.
Children 2 to 4 years: 0.6 mg t.i.d. or q.i.d.
Children 4 months to 2 years: 0.3 mg t.i.d. or q.i.d.

ADVERSE REACTIONS
CNS: (especially in the elderly) *drowsiness,* dizziness, confusion, restlessness, insomnia, *stimulation.*
GI: anorexia, diarrhea or constipation, nausea, vomiting, *dry mouth.*
GU: urinary frequency or retention.
Skin: urticaria, rash.

INTERACTIONS
CNS depressants: increased sedation.

Italicized side effects are common or life-threatening.
*Liquid form contains alcohol.   **May contain tartrazine.

NURSING CONSIDERATIONS
• Contraindicated in acute asthma. Use cautiously in elderly patients, and in patients with increased intraocular pressure, hyperthyroidism, cardiovascular or renal disease, hypertension, diabetes mellitus, bronchial asthma, urinary retention, prostatic hypertrophy, bladder-neck obstruction, and stenosing peptic ulcers.
• Warn patient against drinking alcoholic beverages during therapy and against driving or other activities that require alertness until CNS response to drug is determined.
• Reduce GI distress by giving with food or milk.
• Coffee or tea may reduce drowsiness. Sugarless gum, sour hard candy, or ice chips may relieve dry mouth.
• Warn patient to stop taking drug 4 days before allergy skin tests to preserve accuracy of tests.

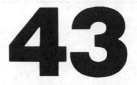

Expectorants and antitussives

Expectorants
acetylcysteine
ammonium chloride
(See Chapter 103, ACIDIFIERS AND
ALKALINIZERS.)
**guaifenesin (formerly glyceryl
guaiacolate)**
iodinated glycerol
potassium iodide (SSKI)
terpin hydrate

Antitussives
benzonatate
codeine phosphate
(See Chapter 26, NARCOTIC AND OPIOID
ANALGESICS.)
codeine sulphate
(See Chapter 26, NARCOTIC AND OPIOID
ANALGESICS.)
**dextromethorphan
hydrobromide**
diphenhydramine hydrochloride
(See Chapter 42, ANTIHISTAMINES.)
hydromorphone hydrochloride
(See Chapter 26, NARCOTIC AND OPIOID
ANALGESICS.)

COMBINATION PRODUCTS
Preparations are available in the following combinations:
• expectorants with decongestants or
antihistamines, or both
• antitussives with decongestants or
antihistamines, or both
• expectorants and antitussives
• expectorants and antitussives with
decongestants or antihistamines, or
both.

acetylcysteine
Airbron♦♦, Mucomyst♦
Pregnancy Category: B

MECHANISM OF ACTION
Increases production of respiratory
tract fluids to help liquefy and reduce
the viscosity of thick, tenacious secretions. Also restores liver stores of
glutathione in the treatment of acetaminophen toxicity.

INDICATIONS & DOSAGE
*Pneumonia, bronchitis, tuberculosis,
cystic fibrosis, emphysema, atelectasis
(adjunct), complications of thoracic
surgery and CV surgery—*
Adults and children: 1 to 2 ml 10%
to 20% solution by direct instillation
into trachea as often as every hour; or
3 to 5 ml 20% solution, or 6 to 10 ml
10% solution, by mouthpiece t.i.d. or
q.i.d.
Acetaminophen toxicity—
140 mg/kg initially P.O., followed by
70 mg/kg q 4 hours for 17 doses (a total of 1,330 mg/kg).

ADVERSE REACTIONS
EENT: *rhinorrhea, hemoptysis.*
GI: *stomatitis, nausea.*
Other: *bronchospasm (especially in
asthmatics).*

INTERACTIONS
Activated charcoal: don't use together
in treating acetaminophen toxicity.
Limits acetylcysteine's effectiveness.

Italicized side effects are common or life-threatening.
*Liquid form contains alcohol.   **May contain tartrazine.

NURSING CONSIDERATIONS

• Use cautiously in patients with asthma or severe respiratory insufficiency; in elderly or debilitated patients.
• Classified as a mucolytic.
• Use plastic, glass, stainless steel, or another nonreactive metal when administering by nebulization. Hand bulb nebulizers not recommended because output is too small and particle size too large.
• After opening, store in refrigerator; use within 96 hours.
• Incompatible with oxytetracycline, tetracycline, erythromycin lactobionate, amphotericin B, ampicillin, iodized oil, chymotrypsin, trypsin, and hydrogen peroxide. Administer separately.
• Monitor cough type and frequency. For maximum effect, instruct patient to clear his airway by coughing before aerosol administration.
• Large doses are used P.O. to treat acetaminophen overdose. Dilute with cola, fruit juice, or water.

benzonatate
Tessalon♦
Pregnancy Category: C

MECHANISM OF ACTION
Suppresses the cough reflex by direct action on the cough center in the medulla (brain). Also has local anesthetic action.

INDICATIONS & DOSAGE
Nonproductive cough—
Adults and children over 10 years: 100 mg P.O. t.i.d.; up to 600 mg daily.
Children under 10 years: 8 mg/kg P.O. in 3 to 6 divided doses.

ADVERSE REACTIONS
CNS: dizziness, drowsiness, headache.
EENT: nasal congestion, sensation of burning in eyes.
GI: nausea, constipation.
Skin: rash.
Other: chills.

INTERACTIONS
None significant.

NURSING CONSIDERATIONS
• Patient should not chew capsules or leave in mouth to dissolve; local anesthesia will result. If capsules dissolve in mouth, CNS stimulation may cause restlessness, tremors, and possibly convulsions.
• A cough suppressant; don't use when cough is valuable as diagnostic sign or is beneficial (as after thoracic surgery).
• Monitor cough type and frequency.
• Use with percussion and chest vibration.
• Maintain fluid intake to help liquefy sputum.

dextromethorphan hydrobromide
Balminil DM♦♦, Broncho-Grippol-DM♦♦, Delsym♦, Pertussin 8-hour, St. Joseph's Cough Syrup for Children, Silence Is Golden. More commonly available in combination products such as Benylin-DM, Coryban-D Cough Syrup*, Dimacol*, 2G-DM, Naldetuss, Novahistine DMX, Ornacol, Phenergan Expectorant with Dextromethorphan*, Robitussin DM*, Rondec-DM*, Triaminicol, Trind-DM*, Tussi-Organidin-DM*
Pregnancy Category: C

MECHANISM OF ACTION
Suppresses the cough reflex by direct action on the cough center in the medulla (brain).

INDICATIONS & DOSAGE
Nonproductive cough—
Adults: 10 to 20 mg q 4 hours, or 30

mg q 6 to 8 hours. Or the controlled-release liquid twice daily (60 mg b.i.d.). Maximum 120 mg daily.
Children 6 to 12 years: 5 to 10 mg q 4 hours, or 15 mg q 6 to 8 hours. Or the controlled-release liquid twice daily (30 mg b.i.d.). Maximum 60 mg daily.
Children 2 to 6 years: 2.5 to 5 mg q 4 hours, or 7.5 mg q 6 to 8 hours. Maximum 30 mg daily.

ADVERSE REACTIONS
CNS: drowsiness, dizziness.
GI: nausea.

INTERACTIONS
MAO inhibitors: hypotension, coma, hyperpyrexia, and death have occurred. Do not use together.

NURSING CONSIDERATIONS
• Contraindicated in patients currently taking or within 2 weeks of stopping MAO inhibitors.
• Produces no analgesia or addiction and little or no CNS depression.
• An antitussive; don't use when cough is valuable diagnostic sign or beneficial (as after thoracic surgery).
• Use with percussion and chest vibration.
• Monitor cough type and frequency.
• Available in most over-the-counter cough medicines.
• 15 to 30 mg dextromethorphan is equivalent to 8 to 15 mg codeine as an antitussive.

guaifenesin (formerly glyceryl guaiacolate)
Anti-Tuss, Balminil♦♦, Bowtussin, Breonesin, Colrex*, Cosin-GG, Dilyn, 2/G, G-100, GG-CEN, Glycotuss, Gly-O-Tussin, Glytuss, G-Tussin, Guaiatussin*, Hytuss, Malotuss, Nortussin, Proco, Recsei-Tuss, Resyl♦♦, Robitussin♦*, Tursen, Wal-Tussin DM
Pregnancy Category: C

MECHANISM OF ACTION
Increases production of respiratory tract fluids to help liquefy and reduce the viscosity of thick, tenacious secretions.

INDICATIONS & DOSAGE
As expectorant—
Adults: 100 to 200 mg P.O. q 2 to 4 hours. Maximum 800 mg daily.
Children: 12 mg/kg P.O. daily in 6 divided doses.

ADVERSE REACTIONS
CNS: drowsiness.
GI: vomiting and nausea occur with large doses.

INTERACTIONS
None significant.

NURSING CONSIDERATIONS
• May interfere with certain laboratory tests for 5-hydroxyindoleacetic acid and vanillylmandelic acid.
• Watch for bleeding gums, hematuria, and bruising if given to patients on heparin. Should such symptoms appear, guaifenesin should be discontinued.
• Liquefies thick, tenacious sputum; maintain fluid intake. Advise patient to take with a glass of water whenever possible.
• Monitor cough type and frequency.
• Encourage deep-breathing exer-

Italicized side effects are common or life-threatening.
*Liquid form contains alcohol.   **May contain tartrazine.

cises.
- Although a popular expectorant, its efficacy has not been established.

iodinated glycerol
Organidin♦*
Pregnancy Category: X

MECHANISM OF ACTION
Increases production of respiratory tract fluids to help liquefy and reduce the viscosity of thick, tenacious secretions.

INDICATIONS & DOSAGE
Bronchial asthma, bronchitis, emphysema (adjunct)—
Adults: 60 mg P.O. q.i.d. (tablets), or 20 drops (solution) P.O. q.i.d. with fluids, or 5 ml (elixir) P.O. q.i.d.
Children: up to ½ adult dose based on child's weight.

ADVERSE REACTIONS
After long-term use:
GI: *nausea,* gastrointestinal distress.
Skin: *eruptions.*
Other: acute parotitis, thyroid enlargement, hypothyroidism.

INTERACTIONS
None significant.

NURSING CONSIDERATIONS
- Contraindicated in hypothyroidism, iodine sensitivity, and during pregnancy and lactation.
- Skin rash or other hypersensitivity reaction may require stopping drug.
- May liquefy thick, tenacious sputum; maintain fluid intake.
- Monitor cough type and frequency.
- Encourage deep-breathing exercises.

potassium iodide (SSKI)
Pregnancy Category: D

MECHANISM OF ACTION
Increases production of respiratory tract fluids to help liquefy and reduce the viscosity of thick secretions.

INDICATIONS & DOSAGE
As expectorant, chronic bronchitis, chronic pulmonary emphysema, bronchial asthma—
Adults: 0.3 to 0.6 ml P.O. q 4 to 6 hours.
Children: 0.25 to 0.5 ml of saturated solution (1 g/ml) b.i.d. to q.i.d.
Nuclear radiation protection—
Adults and children: 0.13 ml P.O. of SSKI immediately before or after initial exposure will block 90% of radioactive iodine. Same dose given 3 to 4 hours after exposure will provide 50% block. Should be administered for up to 10 days under medical supervision.
Infants under 1 year: ½ adult dose.

ADVERSE REACTIONS
GI: *nausea,* vomiting, *epigastric pain,* metallic taste.
Metabolic: goiter, hyperthyroid adenoma, hypothyroidism (with excessive use), collagen disease-like syndrome.
Skin: rash.
Other: drug fever.
Prolonged use: chronic iodine poisoning, soreness of mouth, coryza, sneezing, swelling of eyelids.

INTERACTIONS
Lithium carbonate: may cause hypothyroidism. Don't use together.

NURSING CONSIDERATIONS
- Contraindicated in iodine hypersensitivity, tuberculosis, hyperkalemia, acute bronchitis, hyperthyroidism.
- Maintain fluid intake.
- Has strong, salty, metallic taste. Dilute with milk, fruit juice, or broth to

reduce GI distress and disguise taste.
• Sudden withdrawal may precipitate thyroid storm.
• If skin rash appears, discontinue use. Contact doctor.

terpin hydrate
Pregnancy Category: C

MECHANISM OF ACTION
Increases production of respiratory tract fluids to help liquefy and reduce the viscosity of thick secretions.

INDICATIONS & DOSAGE
Excessive bronchial secretions—
Adults: 5 to 10 ml P.O. of elixir q 4 to 6 hours.

ADVERSE REACTIONS
GI: nausea, vomiting.

INTERACTIONS
None significant.

NURSING CONSIDERATIONS
• Contraindicated in peptic ulcer or severe diabetes mellitus.
• Don't give in large doses; *high alcoholic content of elixir* (86 proof).
• Monitor cough type and frequency.

Italicized side effects are common or life-threatening.
*Liquid form contains alcohol.   **May contain tartrazine.

44

Antacids, adsorbents, and antiflatulents

activated charcoal
aluminum carbonate
aluminum hydroxide
aluminum phosphate
calcium carbonate
dihydroxyaluminum sodium carbonate
magaldrate (aluminum-magnesium complex)
magnesia magma (MOM) (magnesium hydroxide)
(See Chapter 47, LAXATIVES.)
magnesium trisilicate
simethicone
sodium bicarbonate
(See Chapter 103, ACIDIFIERS AND ALKALINIZERS.)

COMBINATION PRODUCTS

ALKA-SELTZER WITHOUT ASPIRIN: sodium bicarbonate 958 mg, citric acid 832 mg, and potassium bicarbonate 312 mg.
ALUDROX SUSPENSION: aluminum hydroxide 307 mg, magnesium hydroxide 103 mg.
ALUDROX TABLETS: aluminum hydroxide 233 mg, magnesium hydroxide 83 mg.
CAMALOX♦: aluminum hydroxide 225 mg, magnesium hydroxide 200 mg, and calcium carbonate 250 mg.
DELCID SUSPENSION: aluminum hydroxide 600 mg, magnesium hydroxide 665 mg.
DI-GEL: aluminum hydroxide and magnesium carbonate 282 mg, magnesium hydroxide 87 mg, simethicone 20 mg.
GAVISCON♦: aluminum hydroxide 31.7 mg, magnesium carbonate 137 mg.
GELUSIL♦: aluminum hydroxide 200 mg, magnesium hydroxide 200 mg, simethicone 25 mg.
GELUSIL-II: aluminum hydroxide 400 mg, magnesium hydroxide 400 mg, simethicone 30 mg.
GELUSIL-M: aluminum hydroxide 300 mg, magnesium hydroxide 200 mg, simethicone 25 mg.
KOLANTYL WAFERS♦: aluminum hydroxide 180 mg and magnesium hydroxide 170 mg.
MAALOX NO. 1: aluminum hydroxide 200 mg and magnesium hydroxide 200 mg.
MAALOX NO. 2: aluminum hydroxide 400 mg and magnesium hydroxide 400 mg.
MAALOX PLUS♦: aluminum hydroxide 200 mg, magnesium hydroxide 200 mg, simethicone 25 mg.
MAALOX THERAPEUTIC CONCENTRATE: aluminum hydroxide 600 mg, magnesium hydroxide 300 mg.
MAGNATRIL: aluminum hydroxide 260 mg, magnesium hydroxide 130 mg, and magnesium trisilicate 455 mg.
MYLANTA♦: aluminum hydroxide 200 mg, magnesium hydroxide 200 mg, simethicone 20 mg.
MYLANTA-II♦: aluminum hydroxide 400 mg, magnesium hydroxide 400 mg, simethicone 30 mg.
RIOPAN PLUS CHEW TABLETS: magaldrate 540 mg, simethicone 20 mg.
RIOPAN PLUS SUSPENSION; magaldrate 540 mg, simethicone 20 mg.
SILAIN-GEL: aluminum hydroxide 282 mg, magnesium hydroxide 285

Unmarked trade names available in the United States only.
♦Also available in Canada. ♦♦Available in Canada only.

mg, simethicone 25 mg.
SIMECO SUSPENSION: aluminum hydroxide 365 mg, magnesium hydroxide 300 mg, simethicone 30 mg.
TITRALAC LIQUID: calcium carbonate 1,000 mg, glycine 300 mg.
TITRALAC TABLETS: calcium carbonate 420 mg, glycine 180 mg.
UNIVOL♦♦: aluminum hydroxide and magnesium carbonate co-dried gel 300 mg and magnesium hydroxide 100 mg.
WINGEL: aluminum hydroxide 180 mg, magnesium hydroxide 160 mg.

activated charcoal
Arm-a-char, Charcoaide, Charcocaps, Charcodote, Charcotabs, Digestalin
Pregnancy Category: C

MECHANISM OF ACTION
Adheres to many drugs and chemicals, inhibiting their absorption from the GI tract. An adsorbent.

INDICATIONS & DOSAGE
Flatulence or dyspepsia—
Adults: 600 mg to 5 g P.O. t.i.d. or q.i.d.
Poisoning—
Adults and children: 5 to 10 times estimated weight of drug or chemical ingested. Minimum dose 30 g in 250 ml water to make a slurry.
Give orally, preferably within 30 minutes of poisoning. Larger doses are necessary if food is in the stomach. For treatment of poisoning or overdosage with acetaminophen, amphetamines, aspirin, antimony, atropine, arsenic, barbiturates, camphor, cocaine, cardiac glycosides, glutethimide, ipecac, malathion, morphine, poisonous mushrooms, opium, oxalic acid, parathion, phenol, phenothiazines, potassium permanganate, propoxyphene, quinine, strychnine, sulfonamides, or cyclic antidepressants.

ADVERSE REACTIONS
GI: black stools, nausea.

INTERACTIONS
Ipecac: Ipecac rendered ineffective. Don't administer together.

NURSING CONSIDERATIONS
• Don't use in semiconscious or unconscious persons.
• Because activated charcoal absorbs and inactivates syrup of ipecac, give after emesis is complete.
• Don't give in ice cream, milk, or sherbert. Reduces absorptive capacity.
• Powder form most effective. Mix with tap water to form consistency of thick syrup. May add small amount of fruit juice or flavoring to make more palatable.
• May need to repeat dose if patient vomits shortly after administration.
• Space doses at least 1 hour apart from other drugs if activated charcoal is being used for any indication other than poisoning.
• Warn patient that feces will be black.

aluminum carbonate
Basaljel
Pregnancy Category: C

MECHANISM OF ACTION
Reduces total acid load in the GI tract and elevates gastric pH to reduce pepsin activity. Also strengthens the gastric mucosal barrier and increases esophageal sphincter tone. An antacid.

INDICATIONS & DOSAGE
As antacid—
Adults: suspension: 5 to 10 ml, p.r.n. Extra-strength suspension: 2.5 to 5 ml, p.r.n. Tablets: 1 to 2, p.r.n. Capsules: 1 to 2, p.r.n.
To prevent formation of urinary phosphate stones (with low-phosphate

diet)—
Adults: suspension: 15 to 30 ml suspension in water or juice 1 hour after meals and h.s.; 5 to 15 ml extrastrength in water or juice 1 hour after meals and h.s.; 2 to 6 tablets or capsules 1 hour after meals and h.s.

ADVERSE REACTIONS
GI: anorexia, *constipation,* intestinal obstruction.
Metabolic: hypophosphatemia.

INTERACTIONS
Tetracyclines: Decreased antibiotic effect. Separate administration times.

NURSING CONSIDERATIONS
• Use cautiously in elderly patients, especially those with decreased GI motility (those receiving antidiarrheals, antispasmodics, or anticholinergics), dehydration, fluid restriction, chronic renal disease, and suspected intestinal obstruction.
• Record amount and consistency of stools. Manage constipation with laxatives or stool softeners; alternate with magnesium-containing antacids (if patient does not have renal disease).
• Shake suspension well; give with small amount of water or fruit juice to assure passage to stomach. When administering through nasogastric tube, be sure tube is placed correctly and is patent; follow antacid with water to clear tube.
• Watch long-term–high-dose use in patient on restricted sodium intake.
• Warn patient not to take aluminum carbonate indiscriminately and not to switch antacids without doctor's advice.
• Because it contains aluminum, it is used in patients with renal failure to help control hyperphosphatemia. Binds phosphate in GI tract.
• Monitor serum phosphate levels.
• Watch for symptoms of hypophosphatemia with prolonged use (an-

orexia, malaise, muscle weakness); can also lead to resorption of calcium and bone demineralization.
• May cause enteric-coated drugs to be released prematurely in stomach. Separate doses by 1 hour.
• Basaljel liquid contains no sugar.

aluminum hydroxide
ALternaGEL, Alu-Cap, Alugel♦♦, Aluminett, Amphojel♦, Basaljel♦♦, Dialume
Pregnancy Category: C

MECHANISM OF ACTION
Reduces total acid load in the GI tract and elevates gastric pH to reduce pepsin activity. Also strengthens the gastric mucosal barrier and increases esophageal sphincter tone. An antacid.

INDICATIONS & DOSAGE
Antacid—
Adults: 600 mg P.O. (5 to 10 ml of most products) 1 hour after meals and h.s.; 300- or 600-mg tablet, chewed before swallowing, taken with milk or water 5 to 6 times daily after meals and h.s.
Hyperphosphatemia in renal failure—
Adults: 500 mg to 2 g b.i.d. to q.i.d.

ADVERSE REACTIONS
GI: anorexia, *constipation,* intestinal obstruction.
Metabolic: hypophosphatemia.

INTERACTIONS
Tetracyclines: Decreased antibiotic effect. Separate administration times.

NURSING CONSIDERATIONS
• Use cautiously in elderly patients, especially those with decreased GI motility (those receiving antidiarrheals, antispasmodics, or anticholinergics), dehydration, fluid restriction, chronic renal disease, and suspected intestinal obstruction.

• Record amount and consistency of stools. Manage constipation with laxatives or stool softeners; alternate with magnesium-containing antacids (if patient does not have renal disease).

• Shake suspension well; give with small amount of milk or water to assure passage to stomach. When administering through nasogastric tube, be sure tube is placed correctly and is patent. After instilling antacid, flush tube with water.

• Watch long-term–high-dose use in patient on restricted sodium intake.

• Warn patient not to take aluminum hydroxide indiscriminately or switch antacids without doctor's advice.

• Because it contains aluminum, it is used in patients with renal failure to help control hyperphosphatemia. Binds phosphate in the GI tract.

• Monitor serum phosphate levels.

• Watch for symptoms of hypophosphatemia with prolonged use (anorexia, malaise, muscle weakness); can also lead to resorption of calcium and bone demineralization.

• May cause enteric-coated drugs to be released prematurely in stomach. Separate doses by 1 hour.

aluminum phosphate
Phosphaljel♦
Pregnancy Category: C

MECHANISM OF ACTION
Reduces total acid load in the GI tract and elevates gastric pH to reduce pepsin activity. Also strengthens the gastric mucosal barrier and increases esophageal sphincter tone. An antacid.

INDICATIONS & DOSAGE
Antacid—
Adults: 15 to 30 ml undiluted q 2 hours between meals and h.s.

ADVERSE REACTIONS
GI: *constipation,* intestinal obstruction.

INTERACTIONS
Tetracyclines: Decreased antibiotic effect. Separate administration times.

NURSING CONSIDERATIONS
• Use cautiously in elderly patients, especially those with decreased GI motility (those receiving antidiarrheals, antispasmodics, or anticholinergics), dehydration, fluid restriction, chronic renal disease, and suspected intestinal obstruction.

• Record amount and consistency of stools. Manage constipation with laxatives or stool softeners; alternate with magnesium-containing antacids (if patient does not have renal disease).

• Shake well; give alone or with small amount of milk or water. When administering through nasogastric tube, be sure tube is placed correctly and is patent; after instilling, flush tube with water to facilitate passage to stomach and maintain tube patency.

• Watch long-term–high-dose use in patient on restricted sodium intake.

• Warn patient not to take aluminum phosphate indiscriminately and not to switch antacids without doctor's advice.

• This drug is a very weak antacid.

• Can reverse hypophosphatemia induced by aluminum hydroxide.

• May cause enteric-coated drugs to be released prematurely in stomach. Separate doses by 1 hour.

• Phosphaljel contains no sugar.

Italicized side effects are common or life-threatening.
*Liquid form contains alcohol.   **May contain tartrazine.

calcium carbonate
Alka-2, Amitone, Calcilac,
Calglycine, Dicarbosil, Equilet,
Gustalac, Mallamint, P.H. Tablets,
Titracid, Titralac, Tums
Pregnancy Category: C

MECHANISM OF ACTION
Reduces total acid load in the GI tract
and elevates gastric pH to reduce pepsin activity. Also strengthens the gastric mucosal barrier and increases
esophageal sphincter tone. An antacid.

INDICATIONS & DOSAGE
Antacid—
Adults: 1-g tablet, 4 to 6 times daily,
chewed well and taken with water; or
1 g of suspension (5 ml of most products), 1 hour after meals and h.s.

ADVERSE REACTIONS
GI: *constipation,* gastric distention,
flatulence, acid-rebound, *nausea.*
Metabolic: *hypercalcemia, hypophosphatemia;* if taken with milk—milk-
alkali syndrome.

INTERACTIONS
Tetracyclines: Decreased antibiotic
effect. Separate administration times.

NURSING CONSIDERATIONS
• Contraindicated in severe renal disease. Use cautiously in elderly patients, especially those with decreased
GI motility (those receiving antidiarrheals, antispasmodics, anticholinergics), dehydration, fluid restriction,
chronic renal disease, and suspected
intestinal obstruction.
• Do not administer with milk or
other foods high in vitamin D. Can
cause milk-alkali syndrome (headache, confusion, distaste for food,
nausea, vomiting, hypercalcemia, hypercalciuria, calcinosis, hypophosphatemia).
• Record amount and consistency of
stools. Manage constipation with laxatives or stool softeners.
• Watch for symptoms of hypercalcemia (nausea, vomiting, headache,
mental confusion, anorexia).
• Monitor serum calcium levels, especially in mild renal impairment.
• Warn patient not to take calcium
carbonate indiscriminately and not to
switch antacids without doctor's advice.
• Has been known to cause rebound
hyperacidity.
• Emphasize that it is *not* candy.
• May cause enteric-coated tablets to
be released prematurely in stomach.
Separate doses by 1 hour.

dihydroxyaluminum sodium carbonate
Rolaids♦
Pregnancy Category: C

MECHANISM OF ACTION
Reduces total acid load in the GI tract
and elevates gastric pH to reduce pepsin activity. Also strengthens the gastric mucosal barrier and increases
esophageal sphincter tone. An antacid.

INDICATIONS & DOSAGE
Antacid—
Adults: chew 1 to 2 tablets (334 to
668 mg), p.r.n.

ADVERSE REACTIONS
GI: anorexia, *constipation,* intestinal
obstruction.

INTERACTIONS
Tetracyclines: Decreased antibiotic
effect. Separate administration times.

NURSING CONSIDERATIONS
• Use cautiously in elderly patients,
especially those with decreased GI
motility (those receiving antidiarrheals, antispasmodics, or anticholinergics), dehydration, fluid restric-

tion, chronic renal disease, and suspected intestinal obstruction.
• Has high sodium content and may increase sodium and water retention.
• Record amount and consistency of stools. Manage constipation with laxatives or stool softeners; alternate with magnesium-containing antacids (if patient does not have renal disease).
• Watch long-term–high-dose use in patient on restricted sodium intake.
• Warn patient not to take dihydroxyaluminum sodium carbonate indiscriminately.
• Emphasize that it is *not* candy.
• May cause enteric-coated drugs to be released prematurely in stomach. Separate doses by 1 hour.

---

magaldrate (aluminum-magnesium complex)
Riopan♦, Riopan Plus
Pregnancy Category: C

MECHANISM OF ACTION
Reduces total acid load in the GI tract and elevates gastric pH to reduce pepsin activity. Also strengthens the gastric mucosal barrier and increases esophageal sphincter tone. An antacid.

INDICATIONS & DOSAGE
Antacid—
Adults: suspension: 400 to 800 mg (5 to 10 ml) between meals and h.s. with water. Tablet: 400 to 800 mg (1 to 2 tablets) P.O. with water between meals and h.s. Chewable tablet: 400 to 800 mg (1 to 2 tablets) chewed before swallowing, between meals and h.s.

ADVERSE REACTIONS
GI: mild constipation or diarrhea.

INTERACTIONS
Tetracyclines: Decreased antibiotic effect. Separate administration times.

NURSING CONSIDERATIONS
• Contraindicated in severe renal disease. Use cautiously in elderly patients, especially those with decreased GI motility (those receiving antidiarrheals, antispasmodics, or anticholinergics), dehydration, fluid restriction, and mild renal impairment.
• Record amount and consistency of stools.
• Shake suspension well; give with a little water to assure passage to stomach. When giving through nasogastric tube, be sure tube is placed properly and is patent. After instilling, flush tube with water to assure passage to stomach and maintain tube patency.
• Monitor serum magnesium in patients with mild renal impairment. Symptomatic hypermagnesemia usually occurs only in severe renal failure.
• Not usually used in patients with renal failure (although it contains aluminum) to help control hypophosphatemia, since it contains magnesium, which may accumulate in renal failure.
• Good for patient on restricted sodium intake; very low sodium content.
• Warn patient not to take magaldrate indiscriminately and not to switch antacids without doctor's advice.
• May cause enteric-coated drugs to be released prematurely in stomach. Separate doses by 1 hour.
• Riopan, Riopan Plus liquid, and Riopan Swallow Tablet contain no sugar. Chewable tablets contain sugar.

---

magnesium trisilicate
Trisomin
Pregnancy Category: C

MECHANISM OF ACTION
Reduces total acid load in the GI tract and elevates gastric pH to reduce pepsin activity. Also strengthens the gastric mucosal barrier and increases

---

Italicized side effects are common or life-threatening.
*Liquid form contains alcohol.   **May contain tartrazine.

esophageal sphincter tone. An antacid.

INDICATIONS & DOSAGE
Antacid—
Adults: 1- to 4-g tablet t.i.d. chewed well and taken with ½ glass of water.

ADVERSE REACTIONS
GI: *diarrhea,* gastric distention, flatulence, nausea, abdominal pain.
GU: possible formation of silica renal calculi with prolonged use.
Metabolic: hypermagnesemia.

INTERACTIONS
Tetracyclines: Decreased antibiotic effect. Separate administration times.

NURSING CONSIDERATIONS
• Contraindicated in severe renal disease. Use cautiously in elderly patients, and in patients with mild renal impairment.
• With prolonged use and some degree of renal impairment, watch for symptoms of hypermagnesemia (hypotension, nausea, vomiting, depressed reflexes, respiratory depression, coma). Monitor serum magnesium levels.
• If diarrhea occurs on antacid doses, suggest alternate preparation.
• Warn patient not to take magnesium trisilicate indiscriminately.
• Tell patient to chew tablet before swallowing.
• May cause enteric-coated drugs to be released prematurely in stomach. Separate doses by 1 hour.

---

simethicone
Mylicon, Ovol♦♦, Silain
Pregnancy Category: C

MECHANISM OF ACTION
By its defoaming action, disperses or prevents formation of mucus-surrounded gas pockets in the GI tract.

INDICATIONS & DOSAGE
Flatulence, functional gastric bloating—
Adults and children over 12 years: 40 to 100 mg after each meal and h.s.

ADVERSE REACTIONS
GI: expulsion of excessive liberated gas as belching, rectal flatus.

INTERACTIONS
None significant.

NURSING CONSIDERATIONS
• Warn patient not to take simethicone indiscriminately.
• Tell patient to chew tablet before swallowing.

Unmarked trade names available in the United States only.
♦Also available in Canada.   ♦♦Available in Canada only.

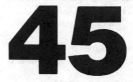

Digestants

bentiromide
bile salts
chenodiol
dehydrocholic acid
glutamic acid hydrochloride
monooctanoin
pancreatin
pancrelipase

COMBINATION PRODUCTS
ACCELERASE-PB CAPSULES: lipase
4,000 units, amylase 15,000 units,
protease 15,000 units, cellulase 2 mg,
mixed conjugated bile salts 65 mg,
calcium carbonate 20 mg, l-alkaloids
of belladonna 0.2 mg, and phenobarbital 16 mg.
BILRON♦: bile salts and iron.
CHOLAN-HMB TABLETS: dehydrocholic acid 250 mg, homatropine
methylbromide 2.5 mg, and phenobarbital 8 mg.
COTAZYM-B TABLETS: lipase 4,000
units, amylase 15,000 units, protease
15,000 units, cellulase 2 mg, and
mixed conjugated bile salts 65 mg.
DONNAZYME TABLETS: pancreatin
300 mg, pepsin 150 mg, bile salts
150 mg, hyoscyamine sulfate 0.0518
mg, atropine sulfate 0.0097 mg,
hyoscine hydrobromide 0.0033 mg,
and phenobarbital 8.1 mg.
ENTOZYME TABLETS♦: pancreatin
300 mg, pepsin 250 mg, and bile salts
150 mg.

bentiromide
Chymex
Pregnancy Category: B

MECHANISM OF ACTION
Biochemically broken down by pancreatic enzymes.

INDICATIONS & DOSAGE
*As a screening test for pancreatic exo-
crine insufficiency—*
Adults and children over 12 years:
Following overnight fast and morning
void, administer a single 500-mg dose
P.O. and follow with an 8-oz glass of
water.
Children under 12 years: Dose is 14
mg/kg followed with an 8-oz glass of
water.
Give patient another glass of water 2
hours after dose. An additional 2
glasses of water are recommended
during post-dosing hours 2 to 6.

ADVERSE REACTIONS
CNS: *headache*.
GI: *diarrhea*, flatulence, nausea,
vomiting.
Other: weakness.

INTERACTIONS
None significant.

NURSING CONSIDERATIONS
• Effective use requires close attention to technical details of drug administration and urine collection,
handling and assay of arylamine levels.
• Encourage your patient to drink wa-

---

ter during post-dosing period to promote diuresis.
• Collect urine during 0 to 6 hours post-dosing. Measure volume of the collection and retain a 10-ml sample for analysis.
• If subsequent retesting is necessary, wait at least 7 days.
• When testing diabetic patients, insulin dose may have to be adjusted during the fasting procedure.

bile salts
Bilron♦, Ox-Bile Extract Enseals
Pregnancy Category: C

MECHANISM OF ACTION
Stimulate bile flow from the liver, promoting normal digestion and absorption of fats, fat-soluble vitamins, and cholesterol.

INDICATIONS & DOSAGE
Uncomplicated constipation—
Adults and children: 300 to 500 mg (enteric-coated tablets) b.i.d. or t.i.d. after meals; or 150 to 450 mg capsules with or after meals.

ADVERSE REACTIONS
GI: loose stools and mild cramping (with large doses).

INTERACTIONS
None significant.

NURSING CONSIDERATIONS
• Contraindicated in marked hepatic dysfunction and complete biliary obstruction, except in malnutrition with steatorrhea and vitamin K deficiency with hypoprothrombinemia.
• Use Ox-Bile Extract cautiously in obstructive jaundice.
• Don't use Ox-Bile Extract if other preparations are available, since it doesn't provide an adequate amount of conjugated bile salts.
• Has not been shown to effectively treat bile salt deficiency.

chenodiol
Chenix
Pregnancy Category: X

MECHANISM OF ACTION
Suppresses hepatic synthesis of both cholesterol and cholic acid. These actions contribute to biliary cholesterol desaturation and gradual dissolution of gallstones.

INDICATIONS & DOSAGE
Dissolution of radiolucent cholesterol stones (gallstones) when systemic disease or age precludes surgery—
Adults: 250 mg b.i.d. for the first 2 weeks, followed, as tolerated, by weekly increases of 250 mg/day, up to 13 to 16 mg/kg/day for up to 24 months.

ADVERSE REACTIONS
GI: *diarrhea,* cramps, heartburn, constipation, nausea, vomiting, anorexia, epigastric distress.
Hepatic: *hepatic enzyme elevations, possible liver toxicity.*

INTERACTIONS
Cholestyramine, colestinol, estrogens, oral contraceptives, clofibrate: decreased chenodiol effect. Monitor patient carefully.

NURSING CONSIDERATIONS
• Contraindicated in patients with known hepatocyte dysfunction; a gallbladder confirmed as nonvisualizing after two consecutive single doses of dye; radiopaque or radiolucent bile pigment stones; or gallstone complications or compelling reasons for gallbladder surgery, including unremitting acute cholecystitis, cholangitis, biliary obstruction, gallstone pancreatitis, or biliary GI fistula.
• Chenodiol treatment should be reserved for carefully selected patients.
• The drug is particularly effective in the dissolution of small, floatable

gallstones.
- Monitor serum transaminase levels monthly for the first 3 months and thereafter every 3 months for duration of therapy.
- The final dosage shouldn't be less than 10 mg/kg/day; lower dosages are usually ineffective.
- Diarrhea occurs in 30% to 40% of all patients. Doctor may reduce dosage until diarrhea subsides. Antidiarrheals may also be prescribed. In some patients, however, persistent diarrhea will require discontinuation of chenodiol therapy.
- Monitor oral cholecystogram or ultrasonogram every 6 to 9 months to observe for gallstone dissolution.

dehydrocholic acid
Cholan-DH, Decholin,
Dycholium♦♦, Hepahydrin
Pregnancy Category: C

MECHANISM OF ACTION
Stimulates bile flow from the liver, promoting normal digestion and absorption of fats, fat-soluble vitamins, and cholesterol.

INDICATIONS & DOSAGE
Constipation, biliary tract conditions—
Adults: 250 to 500 mg P.O. b.i.d. or t.i.d. after meals for 4 to 6 weeks.

ADVERSE REACTIONS
GI: diarrhea with weakness (in large doses).

INTERACTIONS
None significant.

NURSING CONSIDERATIONS
- Contraindicated in complete mechanical biliary obstruction.
- Do not use when patient is nauseated or vomiting, or has abdominal pain.
- Simultaneous administration of bile

salts may be needed in biliary fistula.
- Used to prevent bacterial accumulation after biliary tract surgery.
- Probably much less effective than natural bile salts in lowering surface tension and promoting absorption.
- Don't use dehydrocholic acid to accelerate healing in jaundiced patients.
- Frequent use may result in dependence on laxatives.

glutamic acid hydrochloride
Acidulin♦
Pregnancy Category: C

MECHANISM OF ACTION
Replaces gastric acid.

INDICATIONS & DOSAGE
Hypoacidity—
Adults: 1 to 3 capsules P.O. t.i.d. before meals.

ADVERSE REACTIONS
Metabolic: systemic acidosis in massive overdose.

INTERACTIONS
None significant.

NURSING CONSIDERATIONS
- Contraindicated in gastric hyperacidity or peptic ulcer.
- Use instead of hydrochloric acid so tooth enamel won't be damaged; however, glutamic acid HCl is not as effective in decreasing gastric pH.
- Gastric acidifier.

monooctanoin
Moctanin
Pregnancy Category: C

MECHANISM OF ACTION
Dissolves gallstones by rendering them more soluble.

INDICATIONS & DOSAGE
To solubilize cholesterol gallstones that

---

are retained in the biliary tract after cholecystectomy—
Adults: Administered as a continuous perfusion through a catheter inserted directly into the common bile duct via a T tube. Perfusion rate should not exceed 3 to 5 ml/hour at a pressure of 10 cm water. Duration of perfusion is 7 to 21 days.

ADVERSE REACTIONS
GI: *gastrointestinal pain and discomfort, nausea, vomiting,* diarrhea, anorexia, indigestion.
Other: metabolic acidosis.

INTERACTIONS
None reported.

NURSING CONSIDERATIONS
• Contraindicated in patients with clinical jaundice, significant biliary tract infection, or a history of recent duodenal ulcer or jejunitis.
• Because impaired liver function may lead to metabolic acidosis during administration of this drug, routine liver function tests should be done before perfusion therapy begins.
• Monooctanoin should only be started by individuals experienced in perfusion therapy.
• Not to be administered parenterally. For biliary tract perfusion only.
• Perfusion pressure *must* be kept below 15 cm H₂O. Keeping the perfusion pressure at 10 cm H₂O will help minimize gastrointestinal and biliary tract irritation.
• Use a peristaltic infusion pump to regulate the perfusion. Outpatients may use a battery-operated portable pump.
• Warm the solution to 60 to 80°F. before perfusion. Temperature of the solution should not fall below 65°F. during administration.
• Gastrointestinal symptoms may be reduced by slowing the perfusion rate or discontinuing the perfusion during meals.

pancreatin
Fortezyme♦♦
Pregnancy Category: C

MECHANISM OF ACTION
Replaces endogenous exocrine pancreatic enzymes and aids digestion of starches, fats, and proteins.

INDICATIONS & DOSAGE
Exocrine pancreatic secretion insufficiency, digestive aid in cystic fibrosis—
Adults and children: 325 mg to 1 g P.O. with meals.

ADVERSE REACTIONS
GI: nausea, diarrhea with high doses.
Other: hyperuricosuria (with high doses).

INTERACTIONS
Antacids: may negate pancreatin's beneficial effect. Don't use together.

NURSING CONSIDERATIONS
• Use cautiously in patients who are hypersensitive to pork. Bovine preparations are available for these patients, but are less effective.
• Balance fat, protein, and starch intake properly to avoid indigestion. Dosage varies according to degree of maldigestion and malabsorption, amount of fat in diet, and enzyme activity of individual preparations.
• Adequate replacement decreases number of bowel movements and improves stool consistency.
• Use only after confirmed diagnosis of exocrine pancreatic insufficiency. Not effective in GI disorders unrelated to pancreatic enzyme deficiency.
• For infants, mix powder with applesauce and give with meals. Avoid inhalation of powder. Older children may swallow capsules with food.
• Enteric coating on some products may reduce availability of enzyme in

upper portion of jejunum.
• Store in tight containers at room temperature.
• Note that Viokase is now a brand of pancrelipase, not pancreatin, due to a formulation change.

pancrelipase
Cotazym♦, Cotazyme-S, Ilozyme, Ku-Zyme HP, Pancrease♦, Viokase
Pregnancy Category: C

MECHANISM OF ACTION
Replaces endogenous exocrine pancreatic enzymes and aids digestion of starches, fats, and proteins.

INDICATIONS & DOSAGE
Dose must be titrated to patient's response. Exocrine pancreatic secretion insufficiency, cystic fibrosis in adults and children, steatorrhea and other disorders of fat metabolism secondary to insufficient pancreatic enzymes—
Adults and children: dosage range 1 to 3 capsules or tablets P.O. before or with meals and 1 capsule or tablet with snack; or 1 to 2 powder packets before meals or snacks.

ADVERSE REACTIONS
GI: *nausea,* diarrhea with high doses.

INTERACTIONS
Antacids: may negate pancrelipase's beneficial effect. Don't use together.

NURSING CONSIDERATIONS
• Contraindicated in patients with severe pork hypersensitivity.
• Use only after confirmed diagnosis of exocrine pancreatic insufficiency. Not effective in GI disorders unrelated to enzyme deficiency.
• Lipase activity greater than with other pancreatic enzymes.
• For infants, mix powder from capsules with applesauce and give at mealtime. Avoid inhalation of powder. Older children may swallow capsules with food.
• Dosage varies with degree of maldigestion and malabsorption, amount of fat in diet, and enzyme activity of individual preparations.
• Adequate replacement decreases number of bowel movements and improves stool consistency.
• Enteric coating on some products may reduce availability of enzyme in upper portion of jejunum.
• Crushing or chewing of capsule interferes with the enteric coating.

Italicized side effects are common or life-threatening.
*Liquid form contains alcohol.   **May contain tartrazine.

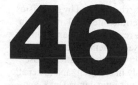

Antidiarrheals

bismuth subgallate
bismuth subsalicylate
calcium polycarbophil
(See Chapter 47, LAXATIVES.)
diphenoxylate hydrochloride
(with atropine sulfate)
kaolin and pectin mixtures
lactobacillus
loperamide
opium tincture
opium tincture, camphorated

COMBINATION PRODUCTS

DONNAGEL-PG*: powdered opium 24 mg, kaolin 6 g, pectin 142.8 mg, hyoscyamine sulfate 0.1037 mg, atropine sulfate 0.0194 mg, hyoscine hydrobromide 0.0065 mg, and alcohol 5% in 30-ml suspension.
DONNAGEL SUSPENSION♦*: kaolin 6 g, pectin 142.8 mg, hyoscyamine sulfate 0.1037 mg, atropine sulfate 0.0194 mg, hyoscine hydrobromide 0.0065 mg, and alcohol 3.8% in 30-ml suspension.
PAREPECTOLIN*: opium 15 mg (equivalent to paregoric 3.7 ml), kaolin 5.85 g, pectin 162 mg, and alcohol 0.69% in 30-ml suspension.

---

bismuth subgallate
Devrom♦

bismuth subsalicylate
Pepto-Bismol
Pregnancy Category: NR

MECHANISM OF ACTION

Has a mild water-binding capacity; also may adsorb toxins and provide protective coating for mucosa.

INDICATIONS & DOSAGE

Mild, nonspecific diarrhea—
Adults: 1 to 2 tablets chewed or swallowed whole t.i.d. (subgallate).
Adults: 30 ml or 2 tablets q ½ to 1 hour up to a maximum of 8 doses and for no longer than 2 days (subsalicylate).
Children 10 to 14 years: 20 ml.
Children 6 to 10 years: 10 ml.
Children 3 to 6 years: 5 ml.
Prevention and treatment of traveler's diarrhea (turista)—
Adults: Prophylactically, 60 ml (Pepto-Bismol) q.i.d. during the first 2 weeks of travel. During acute illness, 30 to 60 ml q 30 minutes for a total of 8 doses. Alternatively, 2 tablets P.O. q.i.d. for up to 3 weeks.

ADVERSE REACTIONS

GI: temporary darkening of tongue and stools.
Other: salicylism (high doses).

INTERACTIONS
None significant.

NURSING CONSIDERATIONS

• Warn patient that bismuth subsalicylate contains a large amount of salicylate. Should be used cautiously in patients already taking aspirin.
• Instruct patient to chew tablets well.
• Both the liquid and tablet forms of Pepto-Bismol are effective against traveler's diarrhea. Tablets may be more convenient to carry.

Unmarked trade names available in the United States only.
♦ Also available in Canada. ♦ ♦ Available in Canada only.

diphenoxylate hydrochloride (with atropine sulfate)

Controlled Substance Schedule V
Lofene, Lomotil♦*, Lotrol, SK-Diphenoxylate
Pregnancy Category: C

MECHANISM OF ACTION
Increases smooth-muscle tone in the GI tract, inhibits motility and propulsion, and diminishes secretions.

INDICATIONS & DOSAGE
Acute, nonspecific diarrhea—
Adults: initially, 5 mg P.O. q.i.d., then adjust dose.
Children 2 to 12 years: 0.3 to 0.4 mg/kg P.O. daily in divided doses, using liquid form only. For maintenance, initial dose may be reduced by as much as 75%.
Don't use in children under 2 years.

ADVERSE REACTIONS
CNS: *sedation, dizziness,* headache, drowsiness, lethargy, restlessness, depression, euphoria.
CV: tachycardia.
EENT: mydriasis.
GI: *dry mouth,* nausea, vomiting, abdominal discomfort or distention, *paralytic ileus,* anorexia, fluid retention in bowel (may mask depletion of extracellular fluid and electrolytes, especially in young children treated for acute gastroenteritis).
GU: urinary retention.
Skin: pruritus, giant urticaria, rash.
Other: possibly physical dependence in long-term use, angioedema, respiratory depression.

INTERACTIONS
None significant.

NURSING CONSIDERATIONS
• Contraindicated in acute diarrhea resulting from poison until toxic material is eliminated from GI tract; in acute diarrhea caused by organisms that penetrate intestinal mucosa; in diarrhea resulting from antibiotic-induced pseudomembranous enterocolitis; and in jaundiced patients. Use cautiously in children, and in hepatic disease, narcotic dependence, and pregnancy. Use cautiously in acute ulcerative colitis. Stop therapy immediately if abdominal distention or other signs of toxic megacolon develop.
• Risk of physical dependence increases with high dosage and long-term use. Atropine sulfate is included to discourage abuse.
• Don't use for more than 2 days when treating acute diarrhea.
• Warn patient not to exceed recommended dosage.
• Dehydration, especially in young children, may increase risk of delayed toxicity. Correct fluid and electrolyte disturbances before starting drug.
• Dose of 2.5 mg as effective as 5 ml camphorated tincture of opium.
• Not indicated in treatment of antibiotic-induced diarrhea.
• Not likely to be effective if there is no response within 48 hours.

kaolin and pectin mixtures

Kaoparin, Kaopectate♦, Pectokay
Pregnancy Category: C

MECHANISM OF ACTION
Decrease the stool's fluid content, although *total* water loss seems to remain the same.

INDICATIONS & DOSAGE
Mild, nonspecific diarrhea—
Adults: 60 to 120 ml after each bowel movement.
Children over 12 years: 60 ml after each bowel movement.
Children 6 to 12 years: 30 to 60 ml after each bowel movement.
Children 3 to 6 years: 15 to 30 ml after each bowel movement.

Italicized side effects are common or life-threatening.
*Liquid form contains alcohol.   **May contain tartrazine.

ADVERSE REACTIONS
GI: drug absorbs nutrients, drugs, and enzymes; fecal impaction or ulceration in infants, elderly, debilitated patients after chronic use; constipation.

INTERACTIONS
None significant.

NURSING CONSIDERATIONS
• Contraindicated in suspected obstructive bowel lesions.
• Don't use for more than 2 days.
• Don't use in place of specific therapy for underlying cause.
• May reduce absorption of other P.O. drugs, requiring dosage adjustments.
• GI absorbent.

lactobacillus
Bacid♦, Dofus, Lactinex♦
Pregnancy Category: NR

MECHANISM OF ACTION
Suppresses the growth of pathogenic microorganisms to help reestablish normal intestinal flora.

INDICATIONS & DOSAGE
Diarrhea, especially that caused by antibiotics—
Adults: 2 capsules (Bacid) P.O. b.i.d., t.i.d., or q.i.d., preferably with milk; or 4 tablets or 1 packet (Lactinex) P.O. t.i.d. or q.i.d., preferably with food, milk, or juice; or 1 capsule (Dofus) P.O. daily before meals.

ADVERSE REACTIONS
GI: (with Bacid and Dofus) increased intestinal flatus at beginning of therapy; subsides with continued therapy.

INTERACTIONS
None significant.

NURSING CONSIDERATIONS
• Bacid and Dofus contraindicated in fever.
• Don't use Bacid for more than 2 days.
• Store in refrigerator.
• Diet containing large amounts of carbohydrate (up to 400 g), such as lactose, lactulose, and dextrin, may be more effective than lactobacillus in reestablishing normal flora after antibiotic therapy.
• Controversial form of diarrhea treatment.
• May be used prophylactically in patients with history of antibiotic-induced diarrhea.

loperamide
Imodium♦
Pregnancy Category: B

MECHANISM OF ACTION
Inhibits peristaltic activity, prolonging transit of intestinal contents.

INDICATIONS & DOSAGE
Acute, nonspecific diarrhea—
Adults: initially, 4 mg P.O., then 2 mg after each unformed stool. Maximum 16 mg daily.
Children 2 to 5 years: 5 ml t.i.d. on first day.
Children 5 to 8 years: 10 ml b.i.d. on first day.
Children 8 to 12 years: 10 ml t.i.d. on first day. (Subsequent doses of 5 ml per 10 kg of body weight may be administered after each unformed stool.)
Chronic diarrhea—
Adults: initially, 4 mg P.O., then 2 mg after each unformed stool until diarrhea subsides. Adjust dose to individual response.

ADVERSE REACTIONS
CNS: drowsiness, fatigue, dizziness.
GI: dry mouth; abdominal pain, distention, or discomfort; *constipation;*

Unmarked trade names available in the United States only.
♦Also available in Canada.   ♦♦Available in Canada only.

nausea; vomiting.
Skin: rash.

INTERACTIONS
None significant.

NURSING CONSIDERATIONS
• Contraindicated in acute diarrhea resulting from poison until toxic material is removed from GI tract, when constipation must be avoided, and in acute diarrhea caused by organisms that penetrate intestinal mucosa. Use cautiously in patients with severe prostatic hypertrophy, hepatic disease, and history of narcotic dependence.
• Stop drug immediately if abdominal distention or other symptoms develop in patients with acute colitis.
• In acute diarrhea, stop drug if no improvement within 48 hours; in chronic diarrhea, stop drug if no improvement after giving 16 mg daily for at least 10 days.
• Warn patient not to exceed recommended dosage.
• Produces antidiarrheal action similar to diphenoxylate HCl but without as many CNS side effects.

---

opium tincture

opium tincture, camphorated
Controlled Substance Schedule III
Paregoric♦
Pregnancy Category: B (D for prolonged use or high doses at term)

MECHANISM OF ACTION
Increases smooth-muscle tone in the GI tract, inhibits motility and propulsion, and diminishes secretions.

INDICATIONS & DOSAGE
Acute, nonspecific diarrhea—
Adults: 0.6 ml opium tincture (range 0.3 to 1 ml) P.O. q.i.d. Maximum

dose 6 ml daily; or 5 to 10 ml camphorated opium tincture daily b.i.d., t.i.d., or q.i.d. until diarrhea subsides.
Children: 0.25 to 0.5 ml/kg camphorated opium tincture daily, b.i.d., t.i.d., or q.i.d. until diarrhea subsides.

ADVERSE REACTIONS
GI: nausea, vomiting.
Other: physical dependence after long-term use.

INTERACTIONS
None significant.

NURSING CONSIDERATIONS
• Contraindicated in acute diarrhea resulting from poisons until toxic material is removed from GI tract, and in diarrhea caused by organisms that penetrate intestinal mucosa. Use cautiously in asthma, prostatic hypertrophy, hepatic disease, narcotic dependence.
• Risk of physical dependence increases with long-term use.
• Don't use for more than 2 days.
• An effective and prompt-acting antidiarrheal; but unique because dose can be adjusted precisely to patient's needs.
• Opium content of opium tincture 25 times greater than camphorated tincture of opium. Camphorated opium tincture is more dilute, and teaspoonful doses easier to measure than dropper quantities of opium tincture.
• Milky fluid forms when camphorated opium tincture is added to water.
• Camphorated opium tincture 0.06 to 0.5 ml daily has been used to treat infants with mild narcotic physical dependence.
• Store in tightly capped, light-resistant container.
• Mix with sufficient water to ensure passage to stomach.
• Narcotic antagonist naloxone can reverse the respiratory depression resulting from overdose.

Italicized side effects are common or life-threatening.
*Liquid form contains alcohol.   **May contain tartrazine.

47

Laxatives

bisacodyl
calcium polycarbophil
cascara sagrada
cascara sagrada aromatic fluidextract
cascara sagrada fluidextract
castor oil
docusate calcium (formerly dioctyl calcium sulfosuccinate)
docusate potassium (formerly dioctyl potassium sulfosuccinate)
docusate sodium (formerly dioctyl sodium sulfosuccinate)
glycerin
lactulose
magnesium salts
methylcellulose
mineral oil
phenolphthalein
psyllium
senna
sodium biphosphate
sodium phosphate

COMBINATION PRODUCTS

AGORAL: mineral oil 28% and white phenolphthalein 1.3% in emulsion, with tragacanth, agar, egg albumin, acacia, and glycerin.
CORRECTOL: yellow phenolphthalein 64.8 mg and docusate sodium 100 mg.
DIALOSE: docusate sodium 100 mg and sodium carboxymethylcellulose 400 mg.
DIALOSE-PLUS: docusate sodium 100 mg and casanthranol 30 mg.
DORBANTYL: docusate sodium 50 mg and danthron 25 mg.
DORBANTYL FORTE: docusate sodium 100 mg and danthron 50 mg.
DOXIDAN♦: docusate calcium 60 mg and danthron 50 mg.
D-S-S PLUS: docusate sodium 100 mg and casanthranol 30 mg.
HALEY'S M-O: mineral oil (25%) and magnesium hydroxide.
HYDROCIL, FORTIFIED: blond psyllium coating 50% and casanthranol (with dextrose) 30 mg/6 g.
KONDREMUL WITH CASCARA♦: heavy mineral oil 55%, cascara sagrada extract 660 mg/15 ml, and Irish moss as emulsifier.
KONDREMUL WITH PHENOLPHTHALEIN♦: heavy mineral oil 55%, white phenolphthalein 150 mg/15 ml, and Irish moss as emulsifier.
PERI-COLACE♦ (capsules): docusate sodium 100 mg and casanthranol 30 mg.
PERI-COLACE (syrup): docusate sodium 60 mg and casanthranol 30 mg/15 ml.
PETROGALAR WITH PHENOLPHTHALEIN: mineral oil 65% and phenolphthalein 0.3%.
SENOKOT-S♦: docusate sodium 50 mg and standardized senna concentrate 187 mg.

bisacodyl

Biscolax♦**, Dulcolax♦, Fleet Bisacodyl
Pregnancy Category: C

MECHANISM OF ACTION

Increases peristalsis by direct effect

Unmarked trade names available in the United States only.
♦Also available in Canada. ♦♦Available in Canada only.

on the smooth muscle of the intestine. Thought either to irritate the musculature or to stimulate the colonic intramural plexus. Also promotes fluid accumulation in the colon and small intestine. A stimulant laxative.

INDICATIONS & DOSAGE
Chronic constipation; preparation for delivery, surgery, or rectal or bowel examination—
Adults: 10 to 15 mg P.O. in evening or before breakfast. Up to 30 mg may be used for thorough evacuation needed for examinations or surgery.
Children over 3 years: 5 to 10 mg P.O.
Rectal:
Adults and children over 2 years: 10 mg.
Children under 2 years: 5 mg.
Enema:
Adults: 1.25 oz.
Children under 6 years: approximately ½ contents of micro enema.

ADVERSE REACTIONS
CNS: muscle weakness in excessive use.
GI: *nausea, vomiting, abdominal cramps,* diarrhea in high doses, *burning sensation in rectum with suppositories.*
Metabolic: alkalosis, hypokalemia, tetany, protein-losing enteropathy in excessive use, fluid and electrolyte imbalance.
Other: laxative dependence in long-term or excessive use.

INTERACTIONS
None significant.

NURSING CONSIDERATIONS
• Contraindicated in patients with abdominal pain, nausea, vomiting, or other symptoms of appendicitis or acute surgical abdomen, or in rectal fissures or ulcerated hemorrhoids.
• Tell patient to swallow enteric-coated tablet whole to avoid GI irrita-

tion. Don't give within one hour of milk or antacid intake. Begins to act 6 to 12 hours after oral administration.
• Soft, formed stool usually produced 15 to 60 minutes after rectal administration. Time administration of drug so as not to interfere with scheduled activities or sleep.
• Tablets and suppositories may be used together to cleanse colon before and after surgery and before barium enema.
• Use for short-term treatment. Stimulant laxative, class of laxative most abused. Discourage excessive use.
• Before giving for constipation, determine if patient has adequate fluid intake, exercise, and diet. Tell him that dietary sources of bulk include bran and other cereals, fresh fruit, and vegetables.
• Store tablets and suppositories at temperature below 86° F. (30° C.).
• Tell patient to report adverse effects to the doctor.

calcium polycarbophil
Mitrolan♦
Pregnancy Category: C

MECHANISM OF ACTION
Absorbs water and expands to increase bulk and moisture content of the stool. The increased bulk encourages peristalsis and bowel movement. A bulk-forming laxative. As an antidiarrheal, absorbs free fecal water, thereby producing formed stools.

INDICATIONS & DOSAGE
Constipation (tablets must be chewed before swallowing)—
Adults: 1 g P.O. q.i.d. as required. Maximum 6 g in 24-hour period.
Children 6 to 12 years: 500 mg P.O. t.i.d. as required. Maximum 3 g in 24-hour period.
Children 3 to 6 years: 500 mg P.O. b.i.d. as required. Maximum 1.5 g in 24-hour period.

Italicized side effects are common or life-threatening.
*Liquid form contains alcohol.   **May contain tartrazine.

Diarrhea associated with irritable bowel syndrome, as well as acute nonspecific diarrhea (tablets must be chewed before swallowing)—
Adults: 1 g P.O. q.i.d. as required. Maximum 6 g in 24-hour period.
Children 6 to 12 years: 500 mg P.O. t.i.d. as required. Maximum 3 g in 24-hour period.
Children 3 to 6 years: 500 mg P.O. b.i.d. as required. Maximum 1.5 g in 24-hour period.

ADVERSE REACTIONS
GI: abdominal fullness and increased flatus, intestinal obstruction.
Other: laxative dependence in long-term or excessive use.

INTERACTIONS
None significant.

NURSING CONSIDERATIONS
• Contraindicated in patients with signs of GI obstruction.
• Rectal bleeding or failure to respond to therapy may indicate need for surgery.
• Before giving for constipation, determine if patient has adequate fluid intake, sufficient exercise, and proper diet. Tell him that dietary sources of bulk include bran and other cereals, fresh fruit, and vegetables.
• Advise patient to chew the tablets thoroughly and drink a full glass of water with each dose. However, when used as an antidiarrheal, tell patient *not* to drink a glass of water.
• For episodes of severe diarrhea, the dose may be repeated every half hour, but maximum daily dosage should not be exceeded.

cascara sagrada
cascara sagrada aromatic fluidextract
cascara sagrada fluidextract
Pregnancy Category: C

MECHANISM OF ACTION
Increases peristalsis by direct effect on the smooth muscle of the intestine. Thought either to irritate the musculature or to stimulate the colonic intramural plexus. Also promotes fluid accumulation in the colon and small intestine. A stimulant laxative.

INDICATIONS & DOSAGE
Acute constipation; preparation for bowel or rectal examination—
Adults: 325 mg cascara sagrada tablets P.O. h.s.; or 1 ml fluidextract daily; or 5 ml aromatic fluidextract daily.
Children 2 to 12 years: ½ adult dose.
Children under 2 years: ¼ adult dose.

ADVERSE REACTIONS
GI: *nausea;* vomiting; diarrhea; loss of normal bowel function with excessive use; *abdominal cramps,* especially in severe constipation; malabsorption of nutrients; "cathartic colon" (syndrome resembling ulcerative colitis radiologically and pathologically) after chronic misuse; discoloration of rectal mucosa after long-term use.
Metabolic: hypokalemia, protein enteropathy, electrolyte imbalance in excessive use.
Other: laxative dependence in long-term or excessive use.

INTERACTIONS
None significant.

NURSING CONSIDERATIONS

• Contraindicated in abdominal pain, nausea, vomiting, or other symptoms of appendicitis or acute surgical abdomen; in acute surgical delirium, fecal impaction, intestinal obstruction or perforation. Use cautiously when rectal bleeding is present.
• Aromatic cascara fluidextract is less active and less bitter than nonaromatic fluidextract.
• Liquid preparations more reliable than solid dosage forms.
• Before giving for constipation, determine if patient has adequate fluid intake, exercise, and diet. Tell him that dietary sources of bulk include bran and other cereals, fresh fruit, and vegetables.
• May turn alkaline urine red-pink and acidic urine yellow-brown.
• Monitor serum electrolytes during prolonged use.
• Onset of action is 6 to 12 hours.

castor oil
Alphamul, Neoloid♦, Purge
Pregnancy Category: X

MECHANISM OF ACTION
Increases peristalsis by direct effect on the smooth muscle of the intestine. Thought either to irritate the musculature or to stimulate the colonic intramural plexus. Also promotes fluid accumulation in the colon and small intestine. A stimulant laxative.

INDICATIONS & DOSAGE
Preparation for rectal or bowel examination, or surgery; acute constipation (rarely)—
Adults: 15 to 60 ml P.O. as liquid or 1.25 to 3.7 mg P.O. as tablet.
Children over 2 years: 5 to 15 ml P.O.
Children under 2 years: 1.25 to 7.5 ml P.O.
Infants: up to 4 ml P.O. Increased dose produces no greater effect.

ADVERSE REACTIONS
GI: *nausea;* vomiting; diarrhea; loss of normal bowel function with excessive use; *abdominal cramps,* especially in severe constipation; malabsorption of nutrients; "cathartic colon" (syndrome resembling ulcerative colitis radiologically and pathologically) in chronic misuse. May cause constipation after catharsis.
GU: pelvic congestion in menstruating women.
Metabolic: hypokalemia, protein enteropathy, other electrolyte imbalance in excessive use.
Other: laxative dependence in long-term or excessive use.

INTERACTIONS
None significant.

NURSING CONSIDERATIONS
• Contraindicated in ulcerative bowel lesions; during menstruation; in abdominal pain, nausea, vomiting, or other symptoms of appendicitis or acute surgical abdomen; in anal or rectal fissures; fecal impaction; intestinal obstruction or perforation; and in pregnancy. Use cautiously in rectal bleeding.
• Failure to respond may indicate acute condition requiring surgery.
• Give with juice or carbonated beverage to mask oily taste. Patient should stir mixture and drink it promptly. Ice held in mouth before taking drug will help prevent tasting it.
• Shake emulsion well. Store below 40° F. (4.4° C.). Don't freeze.
• Give on empty stomach for best results.
• Produces complete evacuation after 3 hours. Tell patient that after castor oil has emptied bowel he will not have bowel movement for 1 to 2 days.
• Time drug administration so that it doesn't interfere with scheduled activities or sleep.
• Monitor serum electrolytes during

Italicized side effects are common or life-threatening.
*Liquid form contains alcohol.   **May contain tartrazine.

prolonged use.
- Generally used before diagnostic testing or therapy requiring thorough evacuation of GI tract.
- Use for short-term treatment. Not recommended for routine use; useful for acute constipation not responsive to milder laxatives.
- Before giving for constipation, determine if patient has adequate fluid intake, exercise, and diet. Tell him that dietary sources of bulk include bran and other cereals, fresh fruit, and vegetables.
- Increased intestinal motility lessens absorption of concomitantly administered P.O. drugs. Reschedule dose.
- Castor oil affects the small intestine. Regular use may cause excessive loss of water and salt.
- Castor oil emulsion is better tolerated but is more expensive.

docusate calcium (formerly dioctyl calcium sulfosuccinate)
Surfak♦

docusate potassium (formerly dioctyl potassium sulfosuccinate)
Kasof

docusate sodium (formerly dioctyl sodium sulfosuccinate)
Colace♦*, Doxinate, D.S.S., Laxinate, Regutol
Pregnancy Category: C

MECHANISM OF ACTION
Reduces surface tension of interfacing liquid contents of the bowel. This detergent activity promotes incorporation of additional liquid into the stool, forming a softer mass. A stool softener.

INDICATIONS & DOSAGE
Stool softener—

Adults and older children: 50 to 300 mg (docusate sodium) P.O. daily or 240 mg (docusate calcium and docusate potassium) P.O. daily until bowel movements are normal.
Children 6 to 12 years: 40 to 120 mg (docusate sodium) P.O. daily.
Children 3 to 6 years: 20 to 60 mg (docusate sodium) P.O. daily.
Children under 3 years: 10 to 40 mg (docusate sodium) P.O. daily.
Higher doses are for initial therapy. Adjust dose to individual response. Usual dose in children and adults with minimal needs: 50 to 150 mg (docusate calcium) P.O. daily.

ADVERSE REACTIONS
EENT: throat irritation.
GI: bitter taste, mild abdominal cramping, diarrhea.
Other: laxative dependence in long-term or excessive use.

INTERACTIONS
None significant.

NURSING CONSIDERATIONS
- Should only be used occasionally. Don't use for more than 1 week without doctor's knowledge.
- Give liquid in milk, fruit juice, or infant formula to mask bitter taste.
- Not for use in treating existing constipation, but prevents constipation from developing.
- Laxative of choice in patients who should not strain during defecation, such as those recovering from myocardial infarction or rectal surgery; in disease of rectum and anus that makes passage of firm stool difficult; or postpartum constipation.
- Acts within 24 to 48 hours to produce firm, semisolid stool.
- Instruct patient that dietary sources of bulk include bran and other cereals, fresh fruit, and vegetables.
- Doesn't stimulate intestinal peristaltic movements.
- Discontinue if severe cramping oc-

curs.
- Store at 59° to 86° F. (15° to 30° C.). Protect liquid from light.
- Many doctors feel that the minimum effective dose is 300 mg daily. A lower dose may not produce satisfactory results.

glycerin
Pregnancy Category: C

MECHANISM OF ACTION
Draws water from the tissues into the feces and thus stimulates evacuation. Hyperosmolar laxative.

INDICATIONS & DOSAGE
Constipation—
Adults and children over 6 years: 3 g as a suppository; or 5 to 15 ml as an enema.
Children under 6 years: 1 to 1.5 g as a suppository; or 2 to 5 ml as an enema.

ADVERSE REACTIONS
GI: *cramping pain,* rectal discomfort, hyperemia of rectal mucosa.

INTERACTIONS
None significant.

NURSING CONSIDERATIONS
- A hyperosmolar laxative used mainly to reestablish proper toilet habits in laxative-dependent patients.
- Usually acts within 1 hour.

lactulose
Cephulac♦, Chronulac♦
Pregnancy Category: C

MECHANISM OF ACTION
Produces an osmotic effect in the colon. Resultant distention promotes peristalsis. Also decreases blood ammonia, probably as a result of bacterial degradation, which decreases the pH of colon contents.

INDICATIONS & DOSAGE
Treatment of constipation—
Adults: 15 to 30 ml P.O. daily.
To prevent and treat portal-systemic encephalopathy, including hepatic precoma and coma in patients with severe hepatic disease—
Adults: initially, 20 to 30 g P.O. (30 to 45 ml) t.i.d. or q.i.d., until two or three soft stools are produced daily. Usual dose is 60 to 100 g daily in divided doses. Can also be given by retention enema in at least 100 ml of fluid.

ADVERSE REACTIONS
GI: abdominal cramps, belching, diarrhea, gaseous distention, flatulence.
Metabolic: hypernatremia.

INTERACTIONS
None significant.

NURSING CONSIDERATIONS
- Contraindicated in patients who need low-galactose diet. Use cautiously in diabetes mellitus.
- Reduce dosage if diarrhea occurs. Replace fluid loss.
- Monitor serum sodium for possible hypernatremia, especially when giving in higher doses to treat hepatic encephalopathy.
- Minimize drug's sweet taste by diluting with water or fruit juice or giving with food.
- Store at room temperature, preferably below 86° F. (30° C.). Don't freeze.

magnesium salts
Concentrated Milk of Magnesia, Magnesium Citrate, Magnesium Sulfate, Milk of Magnesia
Pregnancy Category: B

MECHANISM OF ACTION
Produces an osmotic effect in the small intestine by drawing water into

the intestinal lumen. A saline laxative.

INDICATIONS & DOSAGE
Constipation, to evacuate bowel before surgery—
Adults and children over 6 years: 15 g magnesium sulfate P.O. in glass of water; or 10 to 20 ml concentrated milk of magnesia P.O.; or 15 to 60 ml milk of magnesia P.O.; or 5 to 10 oz magnesium citrate at bedtime.
Laxative—
Adults: 30 to 60 ml, usually h.s., Milk of Magnesia P.O.
Children 6 to 12 years: 15 to 30 ml P.O. Milk of Magnesia.
Children 2 to 6 years: 5 to 15 ml P.O. Milk of Magnesia.

ADVERSE REACTIONS
GI: *abdominal cramping, nausea.*
Metabolic: fluid and electrolyte disturbances if used daily.
Other: laxative dependence in long-term or excessive use.

INTERACTIONS
None significant.

NURSING CONSIDERATIONS
• Contraindicated in abdominal pain, nausea, vomiting, or other symptoms of appendicitis or acute surgical abdomen; in myocardial damage, heart block, imminent delivery, fecal impaction, rectal fissures, intestinal obstruction or perforation, renal disease. Use cautiously in rectal bleeding.
• Shake suspension well; give with large amount of water when used as laxative. When administering through nasogastric tube, be sure tube is placed properly and is patent. After instilling, flush tube with water to assure passage to stomach and maintain tube patency.
• For short-term therapy; don't use longer than 1 week.
• When used as laxative, don't give oral drugs 1 to 2 hours before or after.

• Saline laxative; produces watery stool in 3 to 6 hours. Time drug administration so that it doesn't interfere with scheduled activities or sleep.
• Magnesium sulfate is more potent than other saline laxatives.
• Before giving for constipation, determine if patient has adequate fluid intake, exercise, and diet. Tell him that dietary sources of bulk include bran and other cereals, fresh fruit, and vegetables.
• Magnesium may accumulate in renal insufficiency.
• Chilling before use may make magnesium citrate more palatable.
• Monitor serum electrolytes during prolonged use.
• Frequent or prolonged use as a laxative may cause dependence.

methylcellulose
Cologel
Pregnancy Category: C

MECHANISM OF ACTION
Absorbs water and expands to increase bulk and moisture content of the stool. The increased bulk encourages peristalsis and bowel movement. A bulk-forming laxative.

INDICATIONS & DOSAGE
Chronic constipation—
Adults: 5 to 20 ml liquid P.O. t.i.d. with a glass of water; or 15 ml syrup P.O. morning and evening.
Children: 5 to 10 ml P.O. daily or b.i.d.

ADVERSE REACTIONS
GI: *nausea,* vomiting, diarrhea (all after excessive use); esophageal, gastric, small intestinal, or colonic strictures when drug is chewed or taken in dry form; *abdominal cramps,* especially in severe constipation.
Other: laxative dependence in long-term or excessive use.

INTERACTIONS
None significant.

NURSING CONSIDERATIONS
• Contraindicated in abdominal pain, nausea, vomiting, or other symptoms of appendicitis or acute surgical abdomen; and in intestinal obstruction or ulceration, disabling adhesion, or difficulty swallowing.
• Laxative effect usually takes 12 to 24 hours, but may be delayed 3 days.
• Tell patient to take drug with at least 8 oz (240 ml) of pleasant-tasting liquid to mask grittiness.
• Especially useful in postpartum constipation, debilitated patients, chronic laxative abuse, irritable bowel syndrome, diverticular disease, colostomies, and to empty colon before barium enema examinations.
• Before giving for constipation, determine if patient has adequate fluid intake, exercise, and diet. Tell him that dietary sources of bulk include bran and other cereals, fresh fruit, and vegetables.
• Not absorbed systemically; nontoxic.

---

mineral oil
Agoral Plain♦, Fleet Mineral Oil Enema, Kondremul Plain♦, Neo-Cultol, Petrogalar Plain
Pregnancy Category: C

MECHANISM OF ACTION
Increases water retention in the stool by creating a barrier between colon wall and feces that prevents colonic reabsorption of fecal water. A lubricant laxative.

INDICATIONS & DOSAGE
Constipation; preparation for bowel studies or surgery—
Adults: 15 to 30 ml P.O. h.s.; or 4 oz enema.
Children: 5 to 15 ml P.O. h.s.; or 1 to 2 oz enema.

ADVERSE REACTIONS
GI: *nausea;* vomiting; diarrhea in excessive use; *abdominal cramps,* especially in severe constipation; decreased absorption of nutrients and fat-soluble vitamins, resulting in deficiency; and slowed healing after hemorrhoidectomy.
Other: laxative dependence in long-term or excessive use and pruritus.

INTERACTIONS
Docusate salts: may increase mineral oil absorption and cause lipoid pneumonia. Don't administer together.

NURSING CONSIDERATIONS
• Contraindicated in abdominal pain, nausea, vomiting, or other symptoms of appendicitis or acute surgical abdomen; in fecal impaction, intestinal obstruction or perforation. Use cautiously in young children; in elderly or debilitated patients due to susceptibility to lipid pneumonitis through aspiration, absorption, and transport from intestinal mucosa; in rectal bleeding. Enema contraindicated in children under 2 years.
• Don't give drug with meals or immediately after, as it delays passage of food from stomach. More active on an empty stomach.
• To be taken only at bedtime. Warn patient not to take for more than 1 week.
• A lubricant laxative.
• Give with fruit juices or carbonated drinks to disguise taste.
• Use when patient needs to ease the strain of evacuation.
• Warn patient of possible rectal leakage so he can avoid soiling clothing.
• Before giving for constipation, determine if patient has adequate fluid intake, exercise, and diet. Tell him that dietary sources of bulk include bran and other cereals, fresh fruit, and vegetables.
• Onset of action 6 to 8 hours.

---

phenolphthalein
Alophen**, Espotabs, Evac-U-Gen,
Evac-U-Lax, Ex-Lax, Feen-A-Mint,
Phenolax
Pregnancy Category: NR

MECHANISM OF ACTION
Increases peristalsis by direct effect
on the smooth muscle of the intestine.
Thought either to irritate the musculature or to stimulate the colonic intramural plexus. Also promotes fluid
accumulation in the colon and small
intestine. A stimulant laxative.

INDICATIONS & DOSAGE
Constipation—
Adults: 60 to 200 mg P.O., preferably
h.s.

ADVERSE REACTIONS
GI: diarrhea; *colic in large doses;* fac-
titious nausea; vomiting; loss of normal bowel function in excessive use;
abdominal cramps, especially in severe constipation; malabsorption of
nutrients; "cathartic colon" (syndrome resembling ulcerative colitis
radiologically and pathologically) in
chronic misuse; reddish discoloration
in alkaline feces or urine.
Skin: dermatitis, pruritus, rash, pigmentation.
Other: laxative dependence in long-
term or excessive use, *hypersensitivity.*

INTERACTIONS
None significant.

NURSING CONSIDERATIONS
• Contraindicated in abdominal pain,
nausea, vomiting, or other symptoms
of appendicitis or acute surgical abdomen; in fecal impaction, intestinal obstruction or perforation. Use cautiously in rectal bleeding.
• Laxative effect may last up to 3 to 4
days.
• Produces semisolid stool within 6

to 8 hours. Time drug administration
so that it doesn't interfere with scheduled activities or sleep.
• Warn patient with rash to avoid sun
and discontinue use. Don't use any
other product containing phenolphthalein.
• Before giving for constipation, determine if patient has adequate fluid
intake, exercise, and diet. Tell him
that dietary sources of bulk include
bran and other cereals, fresh fruit,
and vegetables.
• May discolor alkaline urine red-
pink and acidic urine yellow-brown.
• Drug is available in many dosage
forms. Most popular over-the-counter
laxative.
• Children may mistake for candy.
Keep out of reach.

psyllium
Effersyllium Instant Mix, Hydrocil
Instant Powder, Konsyl, L.A.
Formula, Metamucil♦, Metamucil
Instant Mix♦, Metamucil Sugar
Free, Modane Bulk, Mucilose, Plain
Hydrocil, Siblin♦, Syllact
Pregnancy Category: C

MECHANISM OF ACTION
Absorbs water and expands to increase bulk and moisture content of
the stool. The increased bulk encourages peristalsis and bowel movement.
A bulk-forming laxative.

INDICATIONS & DOSAGE
Constipation; bowel management—
Adults: 1 to 2 rounded teaspoonfuls
P.O. in full glass of liquid daily, b.i.d.
or t.i.d., followed by second glass of
liquid; or 1 packet P.O. dissolved in
water daily, b.i.d. or t.i.d.
Children over 6 years: 1 level teaspoonful P.O. in ½ glass of liquid h.s.

ADVERSE REACTIONS
GI: nausea, vomiting, diarrhea, all
after excessive use; esophageal, gas-

Unmarked trade names available in the United States only.
♦Also available in Canada.   ♦♦Available in Canada only.

tric, small intestinal, or colonic strictures when drug taken in dry form; abdominal cramps, especially in severe constipation.

INTERACTIONS
None significant.

NURSING CONSIDERATIONS
• Contraindicated in abdominal pain, nausea, vomiting, or other symptoms of appendicitis; and in intestinal obstruction or ulceration, disabling adhesion, or difficulty swallowing.
• Metamucil Instant Mix (effervescent form) contains a significant amount of sodium and should not be used for patients on sodium-restricted diets.
• In diabetic patients, use brand of psyllium that does not contain sugar. Check label.
• Mix with at least 8 oz (240 ml) of cold, pleasant-tasting liquid such as orange juice to mask grittiness, and stir only a few seconds. Patient should drink it immediately or mixture will congeal. Follow with additional glass of liquid.
• Before giving for constipation, determine if patient has adequate fluid intake, exercise, and diet. Tell him that dietary sources of bulk include bran and other cereals, fresh fruit, and vegetables.
• May reduce appetite if taken before meals.
• Laxative effect usually seen in 12 to 24 hours, but may be delayed 3 days.
• Highly refined, purified vegetable mucilloid; from seeds of plantago plant.
• Not absorbed systemically; nontoxic. Especially useful in postpartum constipation, debilitated patients, chronic laxative abuse, irritable bowel syndrome, diverticular disease, and in combination with other laxatives to empty colon before barium enema examinations.

senna
Black Draught, Senokot♦, X-Prep*
Pregnancy Category: C

MECHANISM OF ACTION
Increases peristalsis by direct effect on the smooth muscle of the intestine. Thought either to irritate the musculature or to stimulate the colonic intramural plexus. Also promotes fluid accumulation in the colon and small intestine. A stimulant laxative.

INDICATIONS & DOSAGE
Acute constipation, preparation for bowel or rectal examination—
Adults: Dosage range for Senokot: 1 to 8 tablets P.O.; ½ to 4 teaspoonfuls of granules added to liquid; 1 to 2 suppositories h.s.; 1 to 4 teaspoonfuls syrup h.s. Black Draught: 2 tablets or ¼ to ½ level teaspoonfuls of granules mixed with water.
Children over 27 kg: ½ adult dose of tablets, granules, or syrup (except Black Draught tablets and granules not recommended for children).
Children 1 month to 1 year: 1.25 to 2.5 ml Senokot syrup P.O. h.s.
X-Prep used solely as single dose for preradiographic bowel evacuation. Give ¾ oz powder dissolved in juice or 2.5 oz liquid between 2 p.m. and 4 p.m. on day before X-ray procedure. May be given in divided doses for elderly or debilitated patients.

ADVERSE REACTIONS
GI: *nausea;* vomiting; diarrhea; loss of normal bowel function in excessive use; *abdominal cramps,* especially in severe constipation; malabsorption of nutrients; "cathartic colon" (syndrome resembling ulcerative colitis radiologically) in chronic misuse: senna may cause constipation after catharsis; yellow, yellow-green cast feces; diarrhea in nursing infants of mothers on senna; darkened pigmentation of rectal mucosa in long-term

use, which is usually reversible within 4 to 12 months after stopping drug.
GU: red-pink discoloration in alkaline urine; yellow-brown color to acidic urine.
Metabolic: hypokalemia, protein enteropathy, electrolyte imbalance with excessive use.
Other: laxative dependence in long-term or excessive use.

INTERACTIONS
None significant.

NURSING CONSIDERATIONS
• Contraindicated in ulcerative bowel lesions; in nausea, vomiting, abdominal pain, or other symptoms of appendicitis or acute surgical abdomen; and in fecal impaction, intestinal obstruction, or perforation.
• Use for short-term treatment.
• More potent than cascara sagrada. Acts in 6 to 10 hours. X-Prep gives thorough, strong bowel action beginning in 6 hours.
• Avoid exposing to excessive heat or light.
• Before giving for constipation, determine if patient has adequate fluid intake, exercise, and diet. Tell him that dietary sources of bulk include bran and other cereals, fresh fruit, and vegetables.
• After X-Prep liquid is taken, diet should be confined to clear liquids.
• Senna is one of the most effective laxatives for counteracting constipation caused by narcotic analgesics.

---

sodium biphosphate
Fleet Enema♦, Phospho-Soda**

sodium phosphate
Pregnancy Category: C

MECHANISM OF ACTION
Produces an osmotic effect in the small intestine by drawing water into the intestinal lumen. A saline laxative.

INDICATIONS & DOSAGE
Constipation—
Adults: 5 to 20 ml liquid P.O. with water; or 4 g powder P.O. dissolved in warm water; or 20 to 46 ml solution mixed with 4 oz cold water; or 2 to 4.5 oz enema.

ADVERSE REACTIONS
GI: *abdominal cramping.*
Metabolic: fluid and electrolyte disturbances (hypernatremia, hyperphosphatemia) if used daily.
Other: laxative dependence in long-term or excessive use.

INTERACTIONS
None significant.

NURSING CONSIDERATIONS
• Contraindicated in abdominal pain, nausea, vomiting, or other symptoms of appendicitis or acute surgical abdomen; in intestinal obstruction or perforation; edema; congestive heart failure; megacolon; impaired renal function; and in patients on salt-restricted diets.
• Use with caution for patients with large hemorrhoids or anal excoriations.
• Available in oral and rectal forms.
• Before giving for constipation, determine if patient has adequate fluid intake, exercise, and diet. Tell him that dietary sources of bulk include bran and other cereals, fresh fruit, and vegetables.
• Saline laxative; up to 10% of sodium content may be absorbed.
• Enema form elicits response in 5 to 10 minutes.
• Used in preparation for barium enema, sigmoidoscopy, and for treatment of fecal impaction.
• Also prescribed in the treatment of hypercalcemia or as a phosphate replacement.

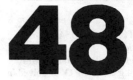

Emetics and antiemetics

apomorphine hydrochloride
benzquinamide hydrochloride
buclizine hydrochloride
chlorpromazine hydrochloride
   (See Chapter 32, ANTIPSYCHOTICS.)
cyclizine hydrochloride
cyclizine lactate
dimenhydrinate
dronabinol (THC)
ipecac syrup
meclizine hydrochloride
metoclopramide hydrochloride
nabilone
prochlorperazine edisylate
prochlorperazine maleate
scopolamine
trimethobenzamide
   hydrochloride

COMBINATION PRODUCTS
None.

apomorphine hydrochloride
Controlled Substance Schedule II
Pregnancy Category: C

MECHANISM OF ACTION
Acts directly on the chemoreceptor trigger zone in the medulla oblongata to induce vomiting.

INDICATIONS & DOSAGE
To induce vomiting in poisoning—
Adults: 2 to 10 mg S.C. or I.M. preceded by 200 to 300 ml water or, preferably, evaporated milk. Don't repeat.
Children over 1 year: 0.07 mg/kg S.C. or I.M. preceded by up to 2 glasses of water or, preferably, evapo-

rated milk.
Children under 1 year: 0.07 mg/kg S.C. preceded by ½ to 1 glass of water or, preferably, evaporated milk.

ADVERSE REACTIONS
CNS: *depression, euphoria,* restlessness, tremors.
CV: *acute circulatory failure in elderly or debilitated patients,* tachycardia.
Other: *depressed respiratory center in large or repeated doses.*

INTERACTIONS
None significant.

NURSING CONSIDERATIONS
• Contraindicated in patients with hypersensitivity to narcotics; impending shock; corrosive poisoning; narcosis resulting from opiates, barbiturates, alcohol, or other CNS depressants; and in patients too inebriated to stand unaided. Use cautiously in children and in patients who are debilitated, have cardiac decompensation, or are predisposed to nausea and vomiting.
• Don't give after ingestion of petroleum distillates (for example, kerosene, gasoline) or volatile oils; retching and vomiting may cause aspiration and lead to bronchospasm, pulmonary edema, or aspiration pneumonitis. Vegetable oil will delay absorption of these substances.
• Emetic action is increased if dose is followed immediately by water or evaporated milk. Evaporated milk is preferred because studies show that water may increase absorption of

---

Italicized side effects are common or life-threatening.
*Liquid form contains alcohol.   **May contain tartrazine.

toxic substances.
• Don't give after ingestion of caustic substances, such as lye; additional injury to the esophagus and mediastinum can occur.
• Keep narcotic antagonists, such as naloxone, available to help stop vomiting and to alleviate drowsiness.
• If delay in giving emetic is expected, give activated charcoal P.O. immediately. When absorbable poison is ingested, give activated charcoal P.O. immediately after apomorphine hydrochloride.
• Vomiting occurs in 5 to 10 minutes in adults. If vomiting doesn't occur within 15 minutes, gastric lavage should begin. Apomorphine HCl is emetic of choice when rapid removal of poisons is necessary, and when identification of enteric-coated tablets or other ingested toxic material in vomitus is important. Stomach contents are usually expelled completely; vomitus may also contain material from upper portion of intestinal tract.
• Don't administer if solution for injection is discolored green, or if precipitate is present.

benzquinamide hydrochloride
Emete-Con
Pregnancy Category: C

MECHANISM OF ACTION
Acts on the chemoreceptor trigger zone to inhibit nausea and vomiting.

INDICATIONS & DOSAGE
Nausea and vomiting associated with anesthesia and surgery—
Adults: 50 mg I.M. (0.5 mg/kg to 1 mg/kg). May repeat in 1 hour, and thereafter q 3 to 4 hours, p.r.n.; or 25 mg (0.2 mg/kg to 0.4 mg/kg) I.V. as single dose, administered slowly.

ADVERSE REACTIONS
CNS: *drowsiness,* fatigue, insomnia, restlessness, headache, excitation, tremors, twitching, dizziness.
CV: sudden rise in blood pressure and transient arrhythmias (premature atrial and ventricular contractions, atrial fibrillation) after I.V. administration; hypertension; hypotension.
EENT: dry mouth, salivation, blurred vision.
GI: anorexia, nausea.
Skin: urticaria, rash.
Other: muscle weakness, flushing, hiccups, sweating, chills, fever. May mask signs of overdose of toxic agents or underlying conditions (intestinal obstruction, brain tumor).

INTERACTIONS
None significant.

NURSING CONSIDERATIONS
• I.V. use contraindicated in cardiovascular disease. Don't give I.V. within 15 minutes of preanesthetic or cardiovascular drugs.
• Give I.M. injections in large muscle mass. Use deltoid area only if well developed. Be sure to aspirate syringe for I.M. injection to avoid inadvertent intravenous injection.
• Reconstituted solution stable for 14 days at room temperature. Store dry powder and reconstituted solution in light-resistant container.
• Precipitation occurs if reconstituted with 0.9% sodium chloride injection.
• Monitor blood pressure frequently.
• Excellent alternative if prochlorperazine (Compazine) is contraindicated.

buclizine hydrochloride
Bucladin-S**, Softran
Pregnancy Category: C

MECHANISM OF ACTION
May affect neural pathways originating in the labyrinth to inhibit nausea and vomiting, but the exact mechanism of action is unknown.

INDICATIONS & DOSAGE

Motion sickness (prevention)—
Adults: 50 mg P.O. at least ½ hour
before beginning travel. If needed,
may repeat another 50 mg P.O. after 4
to 6 hours.
Vertigo—
Adults: 50 mg P.O., up to 150 mg
P.O. daily in severe cases. Maintenance dose is 50 mg b.i.d.

ADVERSE REACTIONS

CNS: *drowsiness,* headache, dizziness, jitters.
EENT: blurred vision, dry mouth.
GU: urinary retention.
Other: may mask symptoms of ototoxicity, intestinal obstruction, or
brain tumor.

INTERACTIONS

None significant.

NURSING CONSIDERATIONS

• Use cautiously in patients with
glaucoma, GU or GI obstruction, and
in elderly males with possible prostatic hypertrophy.
• Warn patient against driving and
other activities that require alertness
until CNS response to drug is established.
• Tablets may be placed in mouth and
allowed to dissolve without water.
May also be chewed or swallowed
whole.
• Classified as an antihistamine.

---

cyclizine hydrochloride

cyclizine lactate

Marezine, Marzine♦♦
Pregnancy Category: B

MECHANISM OF ACTION

May affect neural pathways originating in the labyrinth to inhibit nausea
and vomiting, but the exact mechanism of action is unknown.

INDICATIONS & DOSAGE

*Motion sickness (prevention and treat-
ment)—*
Adults: 50 mg P.O. (hydrochloride)
½ hour before travel, then q 4 to 6
hours, p.r.n., to maximum of 200 mg
daily; or 50 mg I.M. (lactate) q 4 to 6
hours, p.r.n.
Postoperative vomiting (prevention)—
Adults: 50 mg I.M. (lactate) preoperatively or 20 to 30 minutes before expected termination of surgery; then
postoperatively 50 mg I.M. (lactate) q
4 to 6 hours, p.r.n.
*Motion sickness and postoperative
vomiting—*
Children 6 to 12 years: 3 mg/kg (lactate) I.M. divided t.i.d., or 25 mg
(hydrochloride) P.O. q 4 to 6 hours
p.r.n. to a maximum of 75 mg daily.

ADVERSE REACTIONS

CNS: *drowsiness,* dizziness, auditory
and visual hallucinations.
CV: hypotension.
EENT: blurred vision, dry mouth.
GI: constipation.
GU: urinary retention.
Other: may mask symptoms of oto-
toxicity, brain tumor, or intestinal ob-
struction.

INTERACTIONS

None significant.

NURSING CONSIDERATIONS

• Use cautiously in patients with
glaucoma, in patients with GU or GI
obstruction, and in elderly males with
possible prostatic hypertrophy.
• Warn patient against driving and
other activities that require alertness
until CNS response to drug is determined.
• Classified as an antihistamine.
• Store in cool place. When stored at
room temperature, injection may turn
slightly yellow, but this color change
does not indicate loss of potency.

Italicized side effects are common or life-threatening.
*Liquid form contains alcohol.   **May contain tartrazine.

dimenhydrinate
Dimentabs, Dipendrate, Dramaject, Dramamine♦*, Dramamine Junior, Dymenate, Gravol♦♦, Hydrate, Marmine, Nauseal♦♦, Nauseatol♦♦, Novodimenate♦♦, Ram, Reidamine, Signate, Travamine♦♦, Trav-Arex, Traveltabs♦, Wehamine
Pregnancy Category: B

MECHANISM OF ACTION
May affect neural pathways originating in the labyrinth to inhibit nausea and vomiting, but the exact mechanism of action is unknown.

INDICATIONS & DOSAGE
Nausea, vomiting, dizziness of motion sickness (treatment and prevention)—
Adults: 50 mg P.O. q 4 hours, or 100 mg q 4 hours if drowsiness is not objectionable; or 100 mg rectally daily or b.i.d. if oral route is not practical; or 50 mg I.M., p.r.n.; or 50 mg I.V. diluted in 10 ml NaCl solution, injected over 2 minutes.
Children: 5 mg/kg P.O. or I.M., divided q.i.d. Maximum 300 mg daily. Don't use in children less than 2 years old.

ADVERSE REACTIONS
CNS: *drowsiness*, headache, incoordination, dizziness.
CV: palpitations, hypotension.
EENT: blurred vision, tinnitus, dry mouth and respiratory passages.
Other: may mask symptoms of ototoxicity, brain tumor, or intestinal obstruction.

INTERACTIONS
None significant.

NURSING CONSIDERATIONS
• Use cautiously in seizures, narrow-angle glaucoma, enlargement of prostate gland.
• Undiluted solution is irritating to veins; may cause sclerosis.

• Classified as an antihistamine.
• Warn patient against driving and other activities that require alertness until CNS response to drug is determined.
• May mask ototoxicity of aminoglycoside antibiotics.
• Avoid mixing parenteral preparation with other drugs; incompatible with many solutions.

dronabinol (THC)
Controlled Substance Schedule II
Marinol
Pregnancy Category: B

MECHANISM OF ACTION
Unknown.

INDICATIONS & DOSAGE
Treatment of nausea and vomiting associated with cancer chemotherapy—
Adults: 5 mg/m^2 P.O. 1 to 3 hours before administration of chemotherapy. Then give same dose q 2 to 4 hours after chemotherapy is administered for a total of 4 to 6 doses per day. Dose may be increased in increments of 2.5 mg/m^2 to a maximum of 15 mg/m^2 per dose.

ADVERSE REACTIONS
CNS: *drowsiness, euphoria, dizziness, anxiety, muddled thinking, perceptual difficulties, impaired coordination,* irritability, depression, weakness, headache, hallucinations, ataxia, paresthesias, visual distortions, confusion.
CV: tachycardia, orthostatic hypotension.
GI: dry mouth, diarrhea.
Other: muscular pains.

INTERACTIONS
CNS depressants: may increase CNS adverse reactions. Avoid concomitant use.

NURSING CONSIDERATIONS

• Contraindicated for nausea and vomiting from any cause other than cancer chemotherapy; contraindicated in patients hypersensitive to sesame oil.

• Use cautiously in elderly patients and those with hypertension, heart disease, or psychiatric illness.

• Warn patients not to drive a car or engage in any activity that requires sound judgment and unimpaired coordination while taking this drug.

• This drug is to be prescribed only for patients who have not responded satisfactorily to other antiemetics.

• Effects of this drug may persist for days after treatment ends. Duration of persistent effect varies greatly among patients. Therefore, patients should be supervised for untoward responses until it's certain that they're no longer experiencing the drug's effects. There's considerable patient variation regarding the persistance of dronabinol's effect.

• Dronabinol is the principal active substance present in *Cannabis sativa* (marijuana). Therefore, this can produce both physical and psychological dependence and has high potential for abuse.

• CNS effects are intensified at higher drug dosages.

• To prevent panic and anxiety, tell patients this drug may induce unusual changes in mood or other adverse behavioral effects.

• Impress upon family members that patient should be under supervision by a responsible person during and immediately after the treatment.

---

ipecac syrup
Pregnancy Category: C

MECHANISM OF ACTION
Induces vomiting by acting locally on the gastric mucosa and centrally on the chemoreceptor trigger zone.

INDICATIONS & DOSAGE
To induce vomiting in poisoning—
Adults: 15 ml P.O., followed by 200 to 300 ml of water.
Children 1 year or older: 15 ml P.O., followed by about 200 ml of water or milk.
Children under 1 year: 5 to 10 ml P.O., followed by 100 to 200 ml of water or milk. May repeat dose once after 20 minutes, if necessary.

ADVERSE REACTIONS
CNS: depression.
CV: *cardiac arrhythmias, bradycardia, hypotension, atrial fibrillation, or fatal myocarditis* if drug is absorbed (e.g., if patient doesn't vomit within 30 minutes) or after ingestion of excessive dose.
GI: *diarrhea.*

INTERACTIONS
Activated charcoal: neutralized emetic effect. Don't give together but may give activated charcoal after vomiting has occurred.

NURSING CONSIDERATIONS
• Contraindicated in semicomatose or unconscious patients, or those with severe inebriation, convulsions, shock, loss of gag reflex.

• Don't give after ingestion of petroleum distillates (for example, kerosene, gasoline) or volatile oils; retching and vomiting may cause aspiration and lead to bronchospasm, pulmonary edema, or aspiration pneumonitis. Vegetable oil will delay absorption of these substances.

• Don't give after ingestion of caustic substances, such as lye; additional injury to the esophagus and mediastinum can occur.

• Clearly indicate ipecac *syrup,* not single word "ipecac," to avoid confusion with fluidextract. Fluidextract is 14 times more concentrated and, if inadvertently used instead of syrup, may cause death.

• Induces vomiting within 30 minutes in more than 90% of patients; average time usually less than 20 minutes.
• Stomach is usually emptied completely; vomitus may contain some intestinal material as well.
• In antiemetic toxicity, ipecac syrup is usually effective if less than 1 hour has passed since ingestion of antiemetic.
• Recommend that 1 oz of syrup be readily available in the home when child becomes 1 year old for immediate use in case of emergency.
• No systemic toxicity with doses of 30 ml or less.
• If two doses do not induce vomiting, gastric lavage is necessary.
• Now commonly abused by bulimics who practice "binge-purge." Suspect young adult females and watch your unit supply.

meclizine hydrochloride
Antivert♦, Bonamine♦♦, Bonine, Rhu-Vert-M, Whevert
Pregnancy Category: B

MECHANISM OF ACTION
May affect neural pathways originating in the labyrinth to inhibit nausea and vomiting, but the exact mechanism of action is unknown.

INDICATIONS & DOSAGE
Dizziness—
Adults: 25 to 100 mg P.O. daily in divided doses. Dose varies with patient response.
Motion sickness—
Adults: 25 to 50 mg P.O. 1 hour before travel, repeated daily for duration of journey.

ADVERSE REACTIONS
CNS: *drowsiness,* fatigue.
EENT: dry mouth, blurred vision.
Other: may mask symptoms of ototoxicity, brain tumor, or intestinal obstruction.

INTERACTIONS
CNS depressants: increased drowsiness.

NURSING CONSIDERATIONS
• Use cautiously in patients with glaucoma, GU or GI obstruction, and in elderly males with possible prostatic hypertrophy.
• Warn patient against driving and other activities that require alertness until CNS response to drug is determined.
• Antihistamine with a slower onset and longer duration of action than other antihistamine antiemetics.

metoclopramide hydrochloride
Maxeran♦♦, Reglan♦
Pregnancy Category: B

MECHANISM OF ACTION
Stimulates motility of the upper GI tract by increasing lower esophageal sphincter tone. Also blocks dopamine receptors at the chemoreceptor trigger zone.

INDICATIONS & DOSAGE
Preventing or reducing nausea and vomiting induced by cisplatin and other chemotherapy—
Adults: 2 mg/kg I.V. q 2 hours for 5 doses, beginning 30 minutes prior to cisplatin administration.
To facilitate small-bowel intubation and to aid in radiologic examinations—
Adults: 10 mg (2 ml) I.V. as a single dose over 1 to 2 minutes.
Children 6 to 14 years: 2.5 to 5 mg (0.5 to 1 ml).
Children under 6 years: 0.1 mg/kg.
Delayed gastric emptying secondary to diabetic gastroparesis—
Adults: 10 mg P.O. 30 minutes before meals and at bedtime for 2 to 8 weeks, depending on response.
Treatment of gastroesophageal re-

flux—
Adults: 10 to 15 mg P.O. q.i.d.,
p.r.n. Take 30 minutes before meals.

ADVERSE REACTIONS
CNS: *restlessness, anxiety, drowsiness,* fatigue, *lassitude,* insomnia, headache, dizziness, *extrapyramidal symptoms, tardive dyskinesia, dystonic reactions,* sedation.
CV: transient hypertension.
Endocrine: prolactin secretion, loss of libido.
GI: nausea, bowel disturbances.
Skin: rash.
Other: fever.

INTERACTIONS
Anticholinergics, narcotic analgesics: antagonize effects of metoclopramide. Use together cautiously.

NURSING CONSIDERATIONS
• Contraindicated whenever stimulation of GI motility might be dangerous (hemorrhage, obstruction, perforation), and in pheochromocytoma and epilepsy.
• Diphenhydramine 25 mg I.V. may be prescribed to counteract the extrapyramidal side effects associated with high metoclopramide doses.
• Elderly patients are more likely to experience extrapyramidal symptoms and tardive dyskinesia.
• Should not be taken for longer than 12 weeks.
• Monitor blood pressure frequently in patients receiving I.V. dosage.
• Intravenous infusions should be given slowly over at least 15 minutes. Protection from light is unnecessary if the infusion mixture is administered within 24 hours.
• Warn patient to avoid activities requiring alertness for 2 hours after taking each dose.
• Now available in syrup form. Contains 5 mg/5 ml.
• Oral form is being used investigationally to treat nausea and vomiting.

nabilone
Controlled Substance Schedule II
Cesamet
Pregnancy Category: NR

MECHANISM OF ACTION
Unknown.

INDICATIONS & DOSAGE
Treatment of nausea and vomiting associated with cancer chemotherapy—
Adults: 1 to 2 mg P.O. b.i.d. On the day of chemotherapy, the first dose should be given 1 to 3 hours before chemotherapy is administered. Maximum daily dose is 6 mg divided t.i.d.

ADVERSE REACTIONS
CNS: *drowsiness, vertigo, euphoria, anxiety, decreased ability to concentrate, disorientation, depression,* ataxia, headache, visual disturbances, paresthesias, hallucinations.
CV: orthostatic hypotension, tachycardia.
GI: *dry mouth,* increased appetite.

INTERACTIONS
CNS depressants: may increase CNS adverse reactions. Avoid concomitant use.

NURSING CONSIDERATIONS
• Contraindicated for nausea and vomiting from any cause other than cancer chemotherapy.
• Use cautiously in elderly patients and those with hypertension, heart disease, or psychiatric illness.
• Warn patients not to drive a car or engage in any activity that requires sound judgment and unimpaired coordination while taking this drug.
• This drug is to be prescribed only for patients who have not responded satisfactorily to other antiemetics.
• Effects of nabilone may persist for a variable and unpredictable period of time after its administration. Adverse psychological reactions can persist for

Italicized side effects are common or life-threatening.
*Liquid form contains alcohol.   **May contain tartrazine.

48 to 72 hours after treatment ends.
- Nabilone is a synthetic cannabinoid. It is chemically similar to tetrahydrocannabinol, the active substance in marijuana.
- CNS effects are intensified at higher dosages.
- To prevent panic and anxiety, tell patients this drug may induce unusual changes in mood or other adverse behavioral effects.
- Impress upon family members that patient should be under supervision by a responsible person during and immediately after the treatment.

---

prochlorperazine edisylate

prochlorperazine maleate
Compazine**, Stemetil♦♦
Pregnancy Category: C

MECHANISM OF ACTION
Acts on the chemoreceptor trigger zone to inhibit nausea and vomiting, and in larger doses, partially depresses the vomiting center as well.

INDICATIONS & DOSAGE
Preoperative nausea control—
Adults: 5 to 10 mg I.M. 1 to 2 hours before induction of anesthetic, repeat once in 30 minutes, if necessary; or 5 to 10 mg I.V. 15 to 30 minutes before induction of anesthetic (repeat once if necessary); or 20 mg/liter dextrose 5% and sodium chloride 0.9% solution by I.V. infusion, added to infusion 15 to 30 minutes before induction. Maximum parenteral dose 40 mg daily.
Severe nausea, vomiting—
Adults: 5 to 10 mg P.O. t.i.d. or q.i.d.; or 15 mg sustained-release form P.O. on arising; or 10 mg sustained-release form P.O. q 12 hours; or 25 mg rectally b.i.d. or 5 to 10 mg I.M. injected deeply into upper outer quadrant of gluteal region. Repeat q 3 to 4 hours, p.r.n. Maximum I.M. dose

40 mg daily.
Children 18 to 39 kg: 2.5 mg P.O. or rectally t.i.d.; or 5 mg P.O. or rectally b.i.d. Maximum 15 mg daily; or 0.132 mg/kg deep I.M. injection. (Control usually obtained with 1 dose.)
Children 14 to 17 kg: 2.5 mg P.O. or rectally b.i.d. or t.i.d. Maximum 10 mg daily; or 0.132 mg/kg deep I.M. injection. (Control usually obtained with 1 dose.)
Children 9 to 13 kg: 2.5 mg P.O. or rectally daily or b.i.d. Maximum 7.5 mg daily; or 0.132 mg/kg deep I.M. injection. (Control usually obtained with 1 dose.)

ADVERSE REACTIONS
Blood: *transient leukopenia, agranulocytosis.*
CNS: *extrapyramidal reactions (high incidence),* sedation (low incidence), pseudoparkinsonism, EEG changes, dizziness.
CV: *orthostatic hypotension,* tachycardia, EKG changes.
EENT: *ocular changes, blurred vision.*
GI: *dry mouth, constipation.*
GU: *urinary retention,* dark urine, menstrual irregularities, gynecomastia, inhibited ejaculation.
Hepatic: *cholestatic jaundice.*
Metabolic: hyperprolactinemia.
Skin: *mild photosensitivity,* dermal allergic reactions, *exfoliative dermatitis.*
Other: weight gain, increased appetite.

INTERACTIONS
Anticholinergics, including antidepressant and antiparkinson agents: increased anticholinergic activity, aggravated parkinson-like symptoms. Use together cautiously.
Antacids: inhibited absorption of oral phenothiazines. Separate antacid and phenothiazine dosage by at least 2 hours.

Barbiturates: may decrease phenothiazine effect. Monitor patient for decreased antiemetic effect.

NURSING CONSIDERATIONS

• Contraindicated in phenothiazine hypersensitivity, coma, depression, CNS depression, bone-marrow depression, subcortical damage; during pediatric surgery, use of spinal or epidural anesthetic or adrenergic blocking agents, alcohol usage. Use with caution in combination with other CNS depressants; in hepatic disease, arteriosclerosis or cardiovascular disease (may cause sudden drop in blood pressure), exposure to extreme heat or cold (including antipyretic therapy), respiratory disorders, hypocalcemia, vomiting in children, convulsive disorders or severe reactions to insulin or electroshock therapy, suspected brain tumor or intestinal obstruction, glaucoma, or prostatic hypertrophy; in acutely ill or dehydrated children; and in elderly or debilitated patients.

• Elderly patients should usually receive dosages in the lower range.

• Store in light-resistant container. Slight yellowing does not affect potency; discard very discolored solutions.

• Since drug has a very long duration of action, timed-release capsules have no significant advantage over ordinary oral dosage forms.

• Use only when vomiting can't be controlled by other measures, or when only a few doses are required. If more than 4 doses needed in 24-hour period, notify doctor.

• Not effective in motion sickness.

• To prevent contact dermatitis, avoid getting concentrate or injection solution on hands or clothing.

• Dilute oral solution with tomato or fruit juice, milk, coffee, carbonated beverage, tea, water, soup, or pudding.

• Monitor CBC and liver function studies during prolonged therapy.

Warn patients to wear protective clothing when exposed to sunlight.

• Watch for orthostatic hypotension, especially when giving I.V.

• Do not give subcutaneously or mix in syringe with another drug. Give deep I.M.

---

scopolamine
Transderm-Scop♦
Pregnancy Category: C

MECHANISM OF ACTION
May affect neural pathways originating in the labyrinth to inhibit nausea and vomiting, but the exact mechanism of action is unknown.

INDICATIONS & DOSAGE
Prevention of nausea and vomiting associated with motion sickness—
Adults: One Transderm-Scop system (a circular flat unit) programmed to deliver 0.5 mg scopolamine over 3 days (72 hours), applied to the skin behind the ear several hours before the antiemetic is required.
Not recommended for children.

ADVERSE REACTIONS
CNS: *drowsiness,* restlessness, disorientation, confusion.
EENT: *dry mouth,* transient impairment of eye accommodation.

INTERACTIONS
None significant.

NURSING CONSIDERATIONS
• Use cautiously in patients with glaucoma, pyloric obstruction, or urinary bladder-neck obstruction.

• Wash and dry hands thoroughly before applying the system on dry skin behind the ear. After removing the system, discard it, then wash both the hands and application site thoroughly.

• If the system becomes displaced, remove and replace it with another system on a fresh skin site in the post-

---

Italicized side effects are common or life-threatening.
*Liquid form contains alcohol.   **May contain tartrazine.

auricular area.
• Caution patient to wash hands after applying transdermal patch particularly before touching eye. May cause pupil to dilate.
• A patient brochure is available with this product; tell patient to request it from the pharmacist.
• Warn patient against driving and other activities that require alertness until response to drug is determined.
• Sugarless hard candy may be helpful in minimizing dry mouth.
• Transderm-Scop is effective if applied 2 to 3 hours before experiencing motion, but more effective if used 12 hours before. Therefore, advise patient to apply system the night before a planned trip.
• Transdermal method of administration releases a controlled therapeutic amount of scopolamine.

---

trimethobenzamide hydrochloride
Ticon, Tigan♦, Tiject-20
Pregnancy Category: C

MECHANISM OF ACTION
Acts on the chemoreceptor trigger zone to inhibit nausea and vomiting.

INDICATIONS & DOSAGE
Nausea and vomiting (treatment)—
Adults: 250 mg P.O. t.i.d. or q.i.d.; or 200 mg I.M. or rectally t.i.d. or q.i.d.
Postoperative nausea and vomiting (prevention)—
Adults: 200 mg I.M. or rectally (single dose) before or during surgery; may repeat 3 hours after termination of anesthesia, p.r.n.
Children 13 to 40 kg: 100 to 200 mg P.O. or rectally t.i.d. or q.i.d.
Children under 13 kg: 100 mg rectally t.i.d. or q.i.d. Limited to prolonged vomiting of known etiology.

ADVERSE REACTIONS
CNS: *drowsiness,* dizziness (in large doses).
CV: hypotension.
GI: diarrhea, exaggeration of preexisting nausea (in large doses).
Hepatic: *liver toxicity.*
Local: pain, stinging, burning, redness, swelling at I.M. injection site.
Skin: skin hypersensitivity reactions.
Other: antiemetic effect may mask signs of overdosage of toxic agents, or intestinal obstruction, brain tumor, or other conditions.

INTERACTIONS
None significant.

NURSING CONSIDERATIONS
• Contraindicated in children with viral illness (a possible cause of vomiting in children); may contribute to the development of Reye's syndrome, a potentially fatal acute childhood encephalopathy, characterized by fatty degeneration of the liver.
• Suppositories contraindicated in hypersensitivity to benzocaine hydrochloride or similar local anesthetic.
• Stop drug if allergic skin reaction occurs.
• Give I.M. dose by deep injection into upper outer quadrant of gluteal region to reduce pain and local irritation.
• Warn patient of the possibility of drowsiness and dizziness, and caution him against driving or other activities requiring alertness until CNS response to drug is determined.
• Store suppositories in refrigerator.
• Has little or no value in preventing motion sickness; limited value as antiemetic.

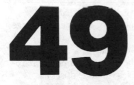

Gastrointestinal anticholinergics

Belladonna alkaloids
atropine sulfate
(See Chapter 19, ANTIARRHYTHMICS.)
belladonna leaf
hyoscyamine sulfate
levorotatory alkaloids of
belladonna

Quaternary anticholinergics
anisotropine methylbromide
clidinium bromide
glycopyrrolate
(See Chapter 37, CHOLINERGIC
BLOCKERS.)
hexocyclium methylsulfate
isopropamide iodide
mepenzolate bromide
methantheline bromide
methscopolamine bromide
oxyphenonium bromide
propantheline bromide

Tertiary synthetics
(antispasmodics)
dicyclomine hydrochloride
oxyphencyclimine hydrochloride

COMBINATION PRODUCTS
BARBIDONNA ELIXIR*: atropine sulfate 0.034 mg/5 ml, phenobarbital 21.6 mg/5 ml, hyoscyamine hydrobromide or sulfate 0.174 mg/5 ml, hyoscine hydrobromide 0.01 mg/5 ml, and alcohol 15%.
BARBIDONNA TABLETS: atropine sulfate 0.025 mg, hyoscine hydrobromide 0.0074 mg, hyoscyamine hydrobromide or sulfate 0.1286 mg, and phenobarbital 16 mg.
BARBIDONNA #2 TABLETS: atropine sulfate 0.025 mg, hyoscine hydrobromide 0.0074 mg, hyoscyamine hydrobromide or sulfate 0.1286 mg, and phenobarbital 32 mg.
BELLADENAL TABLETS♦: L-alkaloids of belladonna 0.25 mg and phenobarbital 50 mg.
BENTYL WITH PHENOBARBITAL SYRUP*: dicyclomine hydrochloride 10 mg/5 ml, phenobarbital 15 mg/5 ml, and alcohol 19%.
BENTYL 10 MG WITH PHENOBARBITAL CAPSULES: dicyclomine hydrochloride 10 mg and phenobarbital 15 mg.
BENTYL 20 MG WITH PHENOBARBITAL TABLETS: dicyclomine hydrochloride 20 mg and phenobarbital 15 mg.
BUTIBEL ELIXIR*: belladonna extract 15 mg/5 ml, butabarbital sodium 15 mg/5 ml, and alcohol 7%.
BUTIBEL TABLETS: belladonna extract 15 mg and butabarbital sodium 15 mg.
CHARDONNA-2: belladonna extract 15 mg and phenobarbital 15 mg.
COMBID SPANSULES♦: isopropamide iodide 5 mg and prochlorperazine maleate 10 mg.
DARICON PB TABLETS: oxyphencyclimine hydrochloride 5 mg and phenobarbital 15 mg.
DONNATAL ELIXIR♦*: atropine sulfate 0.0194 mg/5 ml, hyoscine hydrobromide 0.0065 mg/5 ml, alcohol 23%, hyoscyamine hydrobromide or sulfate 0.1037 mg/5 ml and phenobarbital 16 mg/5 ml.
DONNATAL EXTENTABS♦: atropine sulfate 0.0582 mg, hyoscine hydrobromide 0.0195 mg, hyoscyamine sulfate 0.3111 mg, and phenobarbital 48.6 mg.

DONNATAL TABLETS AND CAP-
SULES♦: atropine sulfate 0.0194 mg,
hyoscine hydrobromide 0.0065 mg,
hyoscyamine hydrobromide or sulfate
0.1037 mg, and phenobarbital 16 mg.
DONNATAL #2 TABLETS: atropine sulfate 0.0194 mg, hyoscine hydrobromide 0.0065 mg, hyoscyamine hydrobromide or sulfate 0.1037 mg, and
phenobarbital 32.4 mg.
ENARAX 5 TABLETS: oxyphencyclimine hydrochloride 5 mg and hydroxyzine hydrochloride 25 mg.
ENARAX 10 TABLETS: oxyphencyclimine hydrochloride 10 mg and hydroxyzine hydrochloride 25 mg.
HYBEPHEN ELIXIR*: atropine sulfate
0.0233 mg/5 ml, hyoscine hydrobromide 0.0094 mg/5 ml, hyoscyamine
hydrobromide or sulfate 0.1277 mg/5
ml, phenobarbital 15 mg/5 ml, and alcohol 16.5%.
KINESED TABLETS: atropine sulfate
0.02 mg, hyoscine hydrobromide
0.007 mg, hyoscyamine hydrobromide or sulfate 0.1 mg, and phenobarbital 16 mg.
LIBRAX CAPSULES: clidinium bromide
2.5 mg and chlordiazepoxide hydrochloride 5 mg.
PATHIBAMATE 200 TABLETS: tridihex-
ethyl chloride 25 mg and meprobamate 200 mg.
PATHIBAMATE 400 TABLETS: tridihex-
ethyl chloride 25 mg and meprobamate 400 mg.
PRO-BANTHINE WITH PHENOBARBITAL
TABLETS♦: propantheline bromide
15 mg and phenobarbital 15 mg.
ROBINUL PH FORTE TABLETS♦: glycopyrrolate 2 mg and phenobarbital
16.2 mg.
ROBINUL PH TABLETS♦: glycopyrrolate 1 mg and phenobarbital 16.2 mg.
VISTRAX 10 TABLETS: oxyphencyclimine hydrochloride 10 mg and hydroxyzine hydrochloride 25 mg.

anisotropine methylbromide
Valpin 50♦
Pregnancy Category: C

MECHANISM OF ACTION
Competitively blocks acetylcholine,
which decreases GI motility and inhibits gastric acid secretion.

INDICATIONS & DOSAGE
Adjunctive treatment of peptic ulcer—
Adults: 50 mg P.O. t.i.d. To be effective should be titrated to individual
patient needs.

ADVERSE REACTIONS
CNS: headache, insomnia, drowsiness, dizziness, *confusion or excitement in elderly patients,* nervousness,
weakness.
CV: *palpitations,* tachycardia.
EENT: *blurred vision,* mydriasis, increased ocular tension, cycloplegia,
photophobia.
GI: *dry mouth,* dysphagia, heartburn,
loss of taste, nausea, vomiting, *paralytic ileus, constipation.*
GU: *urinary hesitancy and retention,*
impotence.
Skin: urticaria, decreased sweating
and possible anhidrosis, other dermal
manifestations.
Other: fever, allergic reactions.
Overdosage may cause curare-like
symptoms.

INTERACTIONS
None significant.

NURSING CONSIDERATIONS
• Contraindicated in narrow-angle
glaucoma, obstructive uropathy, obstructive disease of the GI tract, severe ulcerative colitis, myasthenia
gravis, hypersensitivity to anticholinergics, paralytic ileus, intestinal
atony, unstable cardiovascular status
in acute hemorrhage, and toxic megacolon. Use cautiously in autonomic

neuropathy, hyperthyroidism, coronary artery disease, cardiac arrhythmias, congestive heart failure, hypertension, hiatal hernia associated with reflux esophagitis, hepatic or renal disease, ulcerative colitis, or in patients over 40 years because of increased incidence of glaucoma.

• Use with caution in hot or humid environments. Drug-induced heatstroke can develop.

• Give 30 minutes to 1 hour before meals.

• Administer smaller doses to the elderly.

• Monitor patient's vital signs and urinary output carefully.

• Instruct patient to avoid driving and other hazardous activities if he is drowsy, dizzy, or has blurred vision; to drink plenty of fluids to help prevent constipation; to report any skin rash or local eruption.

• Gum or sugarless hard candy may relieve mouth dryness.

---

belladonna leaf
(used to prepare extract and tincture)
Belladonna Tincture USP
Pregnancy Category: C

MECHANISM OF ACTION
Competitively blocks acetylcholine, which decreases GI motility and inhibits gastric acid secretion.

INDICATIONS & DOSAGE
Adjunctive therapy for peptic ulcer, irritable bowel syndrome, functional gastrointestinal disorders, and neurogenic bowel disturbances—
Adults: 10.8 to 21.6 mg P.O. t.i.d. or q.i.d. of the extract; 0.3 to 1 ml t.i.d. or q.i.d. of tincture.

ADVERSE REACTIONS
CNS: headache, insomnia, drowsiness, dizziness, *confusion or excitement in elderly patients,* nervousness,

weakness.
CV: *palpitations,* tachycardia.
EENT: *blurred vision,* mydriasis, increased ocular tension, cycloplegia, photophobia.
GI: *dry mouth,* dysphagia, heartburn, loss of taste, *constipation,* nausea, vomiting.
GU: *urinary hesitancy and retention,* impotence.
Skin: urticaria, decreased sweating or anhidrosis, other dermal manifestations.
Other: fever, allergic reactions. Overdosage may cause curare-like symptoms.

INTERACTIONS
None significant.

NURSING CONSIDERATIONS
• Contraindicated in narrow-angle glaucoma, obstructive uropathy, obstructive disease of GI tract, severe ulcerative colitis, myasthenia gravis, hypersensitivity to anticholinergics, paralytic ileus, intestinal atony, unstable cardiovascular status in acute hemorrhage, and toxic megacolon. Use cautiously in autonomic neuropathy, hyperthyroidism, coronary artery disease, cardiac arrhythmias, congestive heart failure, hypertension, hiatal hernia associated with reflux esophagitis, hepatic or renal disease, ulcerative colitis, or in patients over 40 years because of increased incidence of glaucoma.

• Give 30 minutes to 1 hour before meals and at bedtime. Bedtime dose can be larger and should be given at least 2 hours after last meal of day.

• Administer smaller doses to the elderly.

• Use with caution in hot or humid environments. Drug-induced heatstroke can develop.

• Monitor patient's vital signs and urinary output carefully.

• Instruct patient to avoid driving and other hazardous activities if he is

---

Italicized side effects are common or life-threatening.
*Liquid form contains alcohol.   **May contain tartrazine.

drowsy, dizzy, or has blurred vision; to drink plenty of fluids to help prevent constipation; to report skin rash.
• Gum or sugarless hard candy may relieve mouth dryness.

clidinium bromide
Quarzan
Pregnancy Category: C

MECHANISM OF ACTION
Competitively blocks acetylcholine, which decreases GI motility and inhibits gastric acid secretion.

INDICATIONS & DOSAGE
Adjunctive therapy for peptic ulcers— Dosage should be individualized according to severity of symptoms and occurrence of side effects.
Adults: 2.5 to 5 mg P.O. t.i.d. or q.i.d. before meals and at bedtime.
Geriatric or debilitated patients: 2.5 mg P.O. t.i.d. before meals.

ADVERSE REACTIONS
CNS: headache, insomnia, drowsiness, dizziness, *confusion or excitement in elderly patients,* nervousness, weakness.
CV: *palpitations,* tachycardia.
EENT: *blurred vision,* mydriasis, increased ocular tension, cycloplegia, photophobia.
GI: *dry mouth,* dysphagia, heartburn, loss of taste, nausea, vomiting, *paralytic ileus, constipation.*
GU: *urinary hesitancy and retention,* impotence.
Skin: urticaria, decreased sweating or anhidrosis, other dermal manifestations.
Other: fever, allergic reactions. Overdosage may cause curare-like symptoms.

INTERACTIONS
None significant.

NURSING CONSIDERATIONS
• Contraindicated in narrow-angle glaucoma, obstructive uropathy, obstructive disease of GI tract, severe ulcerative colitis, myasthenia gravis, hypersensitivity to anticholinergics, paralytic ileus, intestinal atony, unstable cardiovascular status in acute hemorrhage, and toxic megacolon. Use cautiously in autonomic neuropathy, hyperthyroidism, coronary artery disease, cardiac arrhythmias, congestive heart failure, hypertension, hiatal hernia associated with reflux esophagitis, hepatic or renal disease, ulcerative colitis, or in patients over 40 years, because of increased incidence of glaucoma.
• Give 30 minutes to 1 hour before meals and at bedtime. Bedtime dose can be larger and should be given at least 2 hours after last meal of day.
• Use with caution in hot or humid environments. Drug-induced heatstroke may develop.
• Monitor patient's vital signs and urinary output carefully.
• Instruct patient to avoid driving and other hazardous activities if he is drowsy, dizzy, or has blurred vision; to drink plenty of fluids to help prevent constipation; and to report any skin rash or local eruption.
• Gum or sugarless hard candy may relieve mouth dryness.
• Dysphagia may cause aspiration.
• There is no conclusive evidence that clidinium aids in healing, decreases recurrence of, or prevents complications of peptic ulcers.

dicyclomine hydrochloride
Antispas, Bentyl, Bentylol♦♦,
Dibent, Dicen, Formulex♦♦,
Neoquess, Nospaz, Or-Tyl,
Rocyclo, Rotyl HCl, Stannitol,
Viscerol♦♦
Pregnancy Category: B

MECHANISM OF ACTION
Exerts a nonspecific, direct spasmolytic action on smooth muscle. Also possesses local anesthetic properties that may be partly responsible for the spasmolysis.

INDICATIONS & DOSAGE
Adjunctive therapy for peptic ulcers and other functional gastrointestinal disorders—
Adults: 10 to 20 mg P.O. t.i.d. or q.i.d.; 20 mg I.M. q 4 to 6 hours.
Children: 10 mg P.O. t.i.d. or q.i.d.
Infant colic—
Infants: 5 mg P.O. t.i.d. or q.i.d.
Always adjust dosage according to patient's needs and response.

ADVERSE REACTIONS
CNS: *headache,* insomnia, drowsiness, *dizziness.*
CV: *palpitations,* tachycardia.
GI: nausea, *constipation,* vomiting, *paralytic ileus.*
GU: urinary hesitancy and retention, impotence.
Skin: urticaria, decreased sweating or anhidrosis, other dermal manifestations.
Other: fever, allergic reactions. Overdosage may cause curare-like symptoms.

INTERACTIONS
None significant.

NURSING CONSIDERATIONS
• Contraindicated in obstructive uropathy, obstructive disease of GI tract, severe ulcerative colitis, myasthenia gravis, hypersensitivity to anticholinergics, paralytic ileus, intestinal atony, unstable cardiovascular status in acute hemorrhage, and toxic megacolon. Use cautiously in autonomic neuropathy, narrow-angle glaucoma, hyperthyroidism, coronary artery disease, cardiac arrhythmias, congestive heart failure, hypertension, hiatal hernia associated with reflux esophagitis, hepatic or renal disease, ulcerative colitis.
• Use with caution in hot or humid environments. Drug-induced heatstroke can develop.
• Give 30 minutes to 1 hour before meals and at bedtime. Bedtime dose can be larger and should be given at least 2 hours after last meal of day.
• Monitor patient's vital signs and urinary output carefully.
• Instruct patient to avoid driving and other hazardous activities if he is drowsy, dizzy, or has blurred vision; to drink plenty of fluids to help prevent constipation; and to report any skin rash.
• Gum or sugarless hard candy may relieve mouth dryness.
• A synthetic tertiary derivative that may have fewer atropine-like side effects.
• Not for I.V. use.

hexocyclium methylsulfate
Tral**
Pregnancy Category: C

MECHANISM OF ACTION
Competitively blocks acetylcholine, which decreases GI motility and inhibits gastric acid secretion.

INDICATIONS & DOSAGE
Adjunctive therapy in peptic ulcer and other gastrointestinal disorders—
Adults: 25 mg q.i.d. before meals and h.s.; 50 mg (timed release) daily, in the morning or b.i.d.

Italicized side effects are common or life-threatening.
*Liquid form contains alcohol.   **May contain tartrazine.

ADVERSE REACTIONS

CNS: headache, insomnia, drowsiness, dizziness, *confusion or excitement in elderly patients*, nervousness, weakness.
CV: *palpitations,* tachycardia.
EENT: *blurred vision,* mydriasis, increased ocular tension, cycloplegia, photophobia.
GI: *dry mouth,* dysphagia, heartburn, loss of taste, nausea, *constipation,* vomiting, *paralytic ileus.*
GU: *urinary hesitancy and retention,* impotence.
Skin: urticaria, decreased sweating or anhidrosis, other dermal manifestations.
Other: fever, allergic reactions. Overdosage may cause curare-like symptoms.

INTERACTIONS
None significant.

NURSING CONSIDERATIONS
• Contraindicated in narrow-angle glaucoma, obstructive uropathy, obstructive disease of GI tract, severe ulcerative colitis, myasthenia gravis, hypersensitivity to anticholinergics, paralytic ileus, intestinal atony, unstable cardiovascular status in acute hemorrhage, and toxic megacolon. Use cautiously in autonomic neuropathy, hyperthyroidism, coronary artery disease, cardiac arrhythmias, congestive heart failure, hypertension, hiatal hernia associated with reflux esophagitis, hepatic or renal disease, ulcerative colitis, or in patients over 40 years because of increased incidence of glaucoma.
• Use with caution in hot or humid environments. Drug-induced heatstroke can develop.
• Give 30 minutes to 1 hour before meals and at bedtime. Bedtime dose can be larger and should be given at least 2 hours after last meal of day.
• Monitor patient's vital signs and urinary output carefully.

• Instruct patient to avoid driving and other hazardous activities if he is drowsy, dizzy, or has blurred vision; to drink plenty of fluids to help prevent constipation; and to report any skin rash.
• Gum or sugarless hard candy may relieve mouth dryness.
• Tablets contain tartrazine dye. May cause allergy in susceptible patients.

hyoscyamine sulfate
Anaspaz, Levsin, Levsinex, Levsinex Time Caps
Pregnancy Category: C

MECHANISM OF ACTION
Competitively blocks acetylcholine, which decreases GI motility and inhibits gastric acid secretion.

INDICATIONS & DOSAGE
Treatment of gastrointestinal tract disorders due to spasm; adjunctive therapy for peptic ulcers—
Adults: 0.125 to 0.25 mg P.O. or S.L. t.i.d. or q.i.d. before meals and at bedtime; sustained-release form 0.375 mg P.O. q 12 hours; or 0.25 to 0.5 mg (1 or 2 ml) I.M., I.V., or S.C. q 6 hours. (Substitute oral medication when symptoms are controlled.)
Children 2 to 10 years: ½ adult dose P.O.
Children under 2 years: ¼ adult dose P.O.

ADVERSE REACTIONS
CNS: headache, insomnia, drowsiness, dizziness, *confusion or excitement in elderly patients,* nervousness, weakness.
CV: *palpitations,* tachycardia.
EENT: *blurred vision,* mydriasis, increased ocular tension, cycloplegia, photophobia.
GI: *dry mouth,* dysphagia, *constipation,* heartburn, loss of taste, nausea, vomiting, *paralytic ileus.*
GU: *urinary hesitancy and retention,*

impotence.
Skin: urticaria, decreased sweating or anhidrosis, other dermal manifestations.
Other: fever, allergic reactions. Overdosage may cause curare-like symptoms.

INTERACTIONS
None significant.

NURSING CONSIDERATIONS
• Contraindicated in narrow-angle glaucoma, obstructive uropathy, obstructive disease of GI tract, severe ulcerative colitis, myasthenia gravis, hypersensitivity to anticholinergics, paralytic ileus, intestinal atony, unstable cardiovascular status in acute hemorrhage, and toxic megacolon. Use cautiously in autonomic neuropathy, hyperthyroidism, coronary artery disease, cardiac arrhythmias, congestive heart failure, hypertension, hiatal hernia associated with reflux esophagitis, hepatic or renal disease, ulcerative colitis, or in patients over 40 years, because of the increased incidence of glaucoma.
• Use with caution in hot or humid environments. Drug-induced heatstroke can develop.
• Give 30 minutes to 1 hour before meals and at bedtime. Bedtime dose can be larger and should be given at least 2 hours after the last meal of the day.
• Monitor patient's vital signs and urinary output carefully.
• Instruct patient to avoid driving and other hazardous activities if he is drowsy, dizzy, or has blurred vision; to drink plenty of fluids to help prevent constipation; and to report any skin rash.
• Gum or sugarless hard candy may relieve mouth dryness.

isopropamide iodide
Darbid♦
Pregnancy Category: C

MECHANISM OF ACTION
Competitively blocks acetylcholine, which decreases GI motility and inhibits gastric acid secretion.

INDICATIONS & DOSAGE
Adjunctive therapy for peptic ulcer, irritable bowel syndrome—
Adults and children over 12 years: 5 mg P.O. q 12 hours. Some patients may require 10 mg or more b.i.d. Dose should be individualized to patient's need.

ADVERSE REACTIONS
CNS: headache, insomnia, drowsiness, dizziness, *confusion or excitement in elderly patients,* nervousness, weakness.
CV: *palpitations,* tachycardia.
EENT: *blurred vision,* mydriasis, increased ocular tension, cycloplegia, photophobia.
GI: *dry mouth,* dysphagia, heartburn, loss of taste, nausea, vomiting, *constipation, paralytic ileus.*
GU: *urinary hesitancy and retention,* impotence.
Skin: urticaria, decreased sweating or anhidrosis, other dermal manifestations, iodine skin rash.
Other: fever, allergic reactions. Overdosage may cause curare-like symptoms.

INTERACTIONS
None significant.

NURSING CONSIDERATIONS
• Contraindicated in hypersensitivity to iodine, narrow-angle glaucoma, obstructive uropathy, obstructive disease of GI tract, severe ulcerative colitis, myasthenia gravis, hypersensitivity to anticholinergics, paralytic ileus, intestinal atony, unstable car-

diovascular status in acute hemorrhage, and toxic megacolon. Use cautiously in autonomic neuropathy, hyperthyroidism, coronary artery disease, cardiac arrhythmias, congestive
heart failure, hypertension, hiatal
hernia associated with reflux esophagitis, hepatic or renal disease, ulcerative colitis, or in patients over 40
years because of increased incidence
of glaucoma.
• Use with caution in hot or humid
environments. Drug-induced heat-
_____ before
can be larger and should be given at
least 2 hours after the last meal of the
day.
• Monitor patient's vital signs and
urinary output carefully.
• Instruct patient to avoid driving and
other hazardous activities if he is
drowsy, dizzy, or has blurred vision;
to drink plenty of fluids to help prevent constipation; and to report any
skin rash.
• Gum or sugarless hard candy may
relieve mouth dryness.
• Single dose produces 10- to 12-hour
antisecretory effect and gastrointestinal antispasmodic effect.
• Discontinue 1 week before thyroid
function tests.

levorotatory alkaloids of belladonna
(as maleate salts)
Bellafoline
Pregnancy Category: C

MECHANISM OF ACTION
Competitively blocks acetylcholine,
which decreases GI motility and inhibits gastric acid secretion.

INDICATIONS & DOSAGE
*Adjunctive therapy for peptic ulcer, ir-
ritable bowel syndrome, and functional gastrointestinal disorders—*

Adults: 0.25 to 0.5 mg P.O. t.i.d.; or
0.125 to 0.5 mg S.C. daily or b.i.d.
Children over 6 years: 0.125 to 0.25
mg P.O. t.i.d.

ADVERSE REACTIONS
CNS: headache, insomnia, drowsiness, dizziness, *confusion or excitement in elderly patients,* nervousness,
weakness.
CV: *palpitations,* tachycardia.
EENT: *blurred vision,* mydriasis, increased ocular tension, cycloplegia,
photophobia.
GI: *dry mouth,* dysphagia, heartburn,
loss of taste, *constipation, paralytic
ileus.*
GU: *urinary hesitancy and retention,*
impotence.
Skin: urticaria, decreased sweating or
anhidrosis, other dermal manifestations.
Other: fever, allergic reactions.
Overdosage may cause curare-like
symptoms.

INTERACTIONS
None significant.

NURSING CONSIDERATIONS
• Contraindicated in narrow-angle
glaucoma, obstructive uropathy, obstructive disease of GI tract, severe
ulcerative colitis, myasthenia gravis,
hypersensitivity to anticholinergics,
paralytic ileus, intestinal atony, unstable cardiovascular status in acute
hemorrhage, and toxic megacolon.
Use cautiously in autonomic neuropathy, hyperthyroidism, coronary artery
disease, cardiac arrhythmias, congestive heart failure, hypertension, hiatal
hernia associated with reflux esophagitis, hepatic or renal disease, ulcerative colitis, or in patients over 40
years, because of increased incidence
of glaucoma.
• Use with caution in hot or humid
environments. Drug-induced heatstroke can develop.
• Administer 30 minutes to 1 hour

before meals.
• Monitor patient's vital signs and urinary output carefully.
• Instruct patient to avoid driving and other hazardous activities if he is drowsy, dizzy, or has blurred vision; to drink plenty of fluids to help prevent constipation; to report any skin rash.
• Gum or sugarless hard candy may relieve mouth dryness.

mepenzolate bromide
Cantil**
Pregnancy Category: C

MECHANISM OF ACTION
Competitively blocks acetylcholine, which decreases GI motility and inhibits gastric acid secretion.

INDICATIONS & DOSAGE
Adjunctive therapy in treating peptic ulcer, irritable bowel syndrome, and neurologic bowel disturbances—
Adults: 25 to 50 mg P.O. q.i.d. with meals and at bedtime. Adjust dosage to individual patient's needs.

ADVERSE REACTIONS
CNS: headache, insomnia, drowsiness, dizziness, *confusion or excitement in elderly patients*, nervousness, weakness.
CV: *palpitations*, tachycardia.
EENT: *blurred vision*, mydriasis, increased ocular tension, cycloplegia, photophobia.
GI: *dry mouth*, dysphagia, heartburn, loss of taste, nausea, *constipation*, vomiting, *paralytic ileus*.
GU: *urinary hesitancy and retention*, impotence.
Skin: urticaria, decreased sweating or anhidrosis, other dermal manifestations.
Other: fever, allergic reactions. Overdosage may cause curare-like symptoms.

INTERACTIONS
None significant.

NURSING CONSIDERATIONS
• Contraindicated in narrow-angle glaucoma, obstructive uropathy, obstructive disease of GI tract, severe ulcerative colitis, myasthenia gravis, hypersensitivity to anticholinergics, paralytic ileus, intestinal atony, unstable cardiovascular status in acute hemorrhage, and toxic megacolon. Use cautiously in autonomic neuropathy, hyperthyroidism, coronary artery disease, cardiac arrhythmias, tive heart failure or renal disease, ulcerative colitis, or in patients over 40 years, because of increased incidence of glaucoma.
• Use with caution in hot or humid environments. Drug-induced heatstroke can develop.
• Give with meals and at bedtime.
• Monitor patient's vital signs and urinary output carefully.
• Instruct patient to avoid driving and other hazardous activities if he is drowsy, dizzy, or has blurred vision; to drink plenty of fluids to help prevent constipation; and to report any skin rash.
• Gum or sugarless hard candy may relieve mouth dryness.

methantheline bromide
Banthine
Pregnancy Category: C

MECHANISM OF ACTION
Competitively blocks acetylcholine, which decreases GI motility and inhibits gastric acid secretion.

INDICATIONS & DOSAGE
Adjunctive therapy in peptic ulcer, pylorospasm, spastic colon, biliary dyskinesia, pancreatitis, and certain forms of gastritis—

Italicized side effects are common or life-threatening.
*Liquid form contains alcohol. **May contain tartrazine.

diovascular status in acute hemorrhage, and toxic megacolon. Use cautiously in autonomic neuropathy, hyperthyroidism, coronary artery disease, cardiac arrhythmias, congestive heart failure, hypertension, hiatal hernia associated with reflux esophagitis, hepatic or renal disease, ulcerative colitis, or in patients over 40 years because of increased incidence of glaucoma.

• Use with caution in hot or humid environments. Drug-induced heatstroke can develop.

• Give 30 minutes to 1 hour before meals and at bedtime. Bedtime dose can be larger and should be given at least 2 hours after the last meal of the day.

• Monitor patient's vital signs and urinary output carefully.

• Instruct patient to avoid driving and other hazardous activities if he is drowsy, dizzy, or has blurred vision; to drink plenty of fluids to help prevent constipation; and to report any skin rash.

• Gum or sugarless hard candy may relieve mouth dryness.

• Single dose produces 10- to 12-hour antisecretory effect and gastrointestinal antispasmodic effect.

• Discontinue 1 week before thyroid function tests.

---

levorotatory alkaloids of belladonna
(as maleate salts)
Bellafoline
Pregnancy Category: C

MECHANISM OF ACTION
Competitively blocks acetylcholine, which decreases GI motility and inhibits gastric acid secretion.

INDICATIONS & DOSAGE
Adjunctive therapy for peptic ulcer, irritable bowel syndrome, and functional gastrointestinal disorders—

Adults: 0.25 to 0.5 mg P.O. t.i.d.; or 0.125 to 0.5 mg S.C. daily or b.i.d.
Children over 6 years: 0.125 to 0.25 mg P.O. t.i.d.

ADVERSE REACTIONS
CNS: headache, insomnia, drowsiness, dizziness, *confusion or excitement in elderly patients,* nervousness, weakness.
CV: *palpitations,* tachycardia.
EENT: *blurred vision,* mydriasis, increased ocular tension, cycloplegia, photophobia.
GI: *dry mouth,* dysphagia, heartburn, loss of taste, *constipation, paralytic ileus.*
GU: *urinary hesitancy and retention,* impotence.
Skin: urticaria, decreased sweating or anhidrosis, other dermal manifestations.
Other: fever, allergic reactions. Overdosage may cause curare-like symptoms.

INTERACTIONS
None significant.

NURSING CONSIDERATIONS
• Contraindicated in narrow-angle glaucoma, obstructive uropathy, obstructive disease of GI tract, severe ulcerative colitis, myasthenia gravis, hypersensitivity to anticholinergics, paralytic ileus, intestinal atony, unstable cardiovascular status in acute hemorrhage, and toxic megacolon. Use cautiously in autonomic neuropathy, hyperthyroidism, coronary artery disease, cardiac arrhythmias, congestive heart failure, hypertension, hiatal hernia associated with reflux esophagitis, hepatic or renal disease, ulcerative colitis, or in patients over 40 years, because of increased incidence of glaucoma.

• Use with caution in hot or humid environments. Drug-induced heatstroke can develop.

• Administer 30 minutes to 1 hour

---

before meals.
• Monitor patient's vital signs and urinary output carefully.
• Instruct patient to avoid driving and other hazardous activities if he is drowsy, dizzy, or has blurred vision; to drink plenty of fluids to help prevent constipation; to report any skin rash.
• Gum or sugarless hard candy may relieve mouth dryness.

mepenzolate bromide
Cantil**
Pregnancy Category: C

MECHANISM OF ACTION
Competitively blocks acetylcholine, which decreases GI motility and inhibits gastric acid secretion.

INDICATIONS & DOSAGE
Adjunctive therapy in treating peptic ulcer, irritable bowel syndrome, and neurologic bowel disturbances—
Adults: 25 to 50 mg P.O. q.i.d. with meals and at bedtime. Adjust dosage to individual patient's needs.

ADVERSE REACTIONS
CNS: headache, insomnia, drowsiness, dizziness, *confusion or excitement in elderly patients,* nervousness, weakness.
CV: *palpitations,* tachycardia.
EENT: *blurred vision,* mydriasis, increased ocular tension, cycloplegia, photophobia.
GI: *dry mouth,* dysphagia, heartburn, loss of taste, nausea, *constipation,* vomiting, *paralytic ileus.*
GU: *urinary hesitancy and retention,* impotence.
Skin: urticaria, decreased sweating or anhidrosis, other dermal manifestations.
Other: fever, allergic reactions. Overdosage may cause curare-like symptoms.

INTERACTIONS
None significant.

NURSING CONSIDERATIONS
• Contraindicated in narrow-angle glaucoma, obstructive uropathy, obstructive disease of GI tract, severe ulcerative colitis, myasthenia gravis, hypersensitivity to anticholinergics, paralytic ileus, intestinal atony, unstable cardiovascular status in acute hemorrhage, and toxic megacolon. Use cautiously in autonomic neuropathy, hyperthyroidism, coronary artery disease, cardiac arrhythmias, congestive heart failure, hypertension, hiatal hernia associated with reflux esophagitis, hepatic or renal disease, ulcerative colitis, or in patients over 40 years, because of increased incidence of glaucoma.
• Use with caution in hot or humid environments. Drug-induced heatstroke can develop.
• Give with meals and at bedtime.
• Monitor patient's vital signs and urinary output carefully.
• Instruct patient to avoid driving and other hazardous activities if he is drowsy, dizzy, or has blurred vision; to drink plenty of fluids to help prevent constipation; and to report any skin rash.
• Gum or sugarless hard candy may relieve mouth dryness.

methantheline bromide
Banthine
Pregnancy Category: C

MECHANISM OF ACTION
Competitively blocks acetylcholine, which decreases GI motility and inhibits gastric acid secretion.

INDICATIONS & DOSAGE
Adjunctive therapy in peptic ulcer, pylorospasm, spastic colon, biliary dyskinesia, pancreatitis, and certain forms of gastritis—

Italicized side effects are common or life-threatening.
*Liquid form contains alcohol.   **May contain tartrazine.

Adults: 50 to 100 mg P.O. q 6 hours.
Children over 1 year: 12.5 to 50 mg
q.i.d.
Children under 1 year: 12.5 to 25
mg q.i.d.
Neonates: 12.5 mg b.i.d., then t.i.d.

ADVERSE REACTIONS
CNS: headache, insomnia, drowsiness, dizziness, *confusion or excitement in elderly patients,* nervousness,
weakness.
CV: *palpitations,* tachycardia.
EENT: *blurred vision,* mydriasis, increased ocular tension, cycloplegia,
photophobia.
GI: *dry mouth,* dysphagia, *constipation,* heartburn, loss of taste, nausea,
vomiting, *paralytic ileus.*
GU: *urinary hesitancy and retention,*
impotence.
Skin: urticaria, decreased sweating or
anhidrosis, other dermal manifestations.
Other: fever, allergic reactions.
Overdosage may cause curare-like
symptoms.

INTERACTIONS
None significant.

NURSING CONSIDERATIONS
• Contraindicated in narrow-angle
glaucoma, obstructive uropathy, obstructive disease of GI tract, severe
ulcerative colitis, myasthenia gravis,
hypersensitivity to anticholinergics,
paralytic ileus, intestinal atony, unstable cardiovascular status in acute
hemorrhage, and toxic megacolon.
Use cautiously in autonomic neuropathy, hyperthyroidism, coronary artery
disease, cardiac arrhythmias, congestive heart failure, hypertension, hiatal
hernia associated with reflux esophagitis, hepatic or renal disease, ulcerative colitis, or in patients over 40
years, because of the increased incidence of glaucoma.
• Use with caution in hot or humid
environments. Drug-induced heat-

stroke can develop.
• Give 30 minutes to 1 hour before
meals and at bedtime. Bedtime dose
can be larger and should be given at
least 2 hours after the last meal of the
day.
• If patient is also taking antihistamines, he may experience increased
dryness of mouth.
• Monitor patient's vital signs and
urinary output carefully.
• Instruct patient to avoid driving and
other hazardous activities if he is
drowsy, dizzy, or has blurred vision;
to drink plenty of fluids to help prevent constipation; and to report any
skin rash.
• Gum or sugarless hard candy may
relieve mouth dryness.
• Therapeutic effects appear in 30 to
45 minutes; persist for 4 to 6 hours after oral administration.

methscopolamine bromide
Pamine, Scoline
Pregnancy Category: C

MECHANISM OF ACTION
Competitively blocks acetylcholine,
which decreases GI motility and inhibits gastric acid secretion.

INDICATIONS & DOSAGE
Adjunctive therapy in peptic ulcer—
Adults: 2.5 to 5 mg P.O. ½ hour be-
fore meals and h.s.

ADVERSE REACTIONS
CNS: headache, insomnia, dizziness,
*confusion or excitement in elderly pa-
tients,* nervousness, weakness.
CV: *palpitations,* tachycardia.
EENT: *blurred vision,* mydriasis, increased ocular tension, cycloplegia,
photophobia.
GI: *dry mouth,* dysphagia, *constipation,* heartburn, loss of taste, nausea,
vomiting, *paralytic ileus.*
GU: *urinary hesitancy and retention,*
impotence.

Skin: urticaria, decreased sweating or anhidrosis, other dermal manifestations.
Other: fever, allergic reactions. Overdosage may cause curare-like symptoms.

INTERACTIONS
None significant.

NURSING CONSIDERATIONS
• Contraindicated in narrow-angle glaucoma, obstructive uropathy, obstructive disease of GI tract, severe ulcerative colitis, myasthenia gravis, hypersensitivity to anticholinergics, paralytic ileus, intestinal atony, unstable cardiovascular status in acute hemorrhage, and toxic megacolon. Use cautiously in autonomic neuropathy, hyperthyroidism, coronary artery disease, cardiac arrhythmias, congestive heart failure, hypertension, hiatal hernia associated with reflux esophagitis, hepatic or renal disease, ulcerative colitis, or in patients over 40 years, because of increased incidence of glaucoma.
• Use with caution in hot or humid environments. Drug-induced heatstroke can develop.
• Give 30 minutes to 1 hour before meals and at bedtime. Bedtime dose can be larger and should be given at least 2 hours after the last meal of the day.
• Monitor patient's vital signs and urinary output carefully.
• Instruct patient to avoid driving and other hazardous activities if he is drowsy, dizzy, or has blurred vision; to drink plenty of fluids to help prevent constipation; and to report any skin rash.
• Gum or sugarless hard candy may relieve mouth dryness.

oxyphencyclimine hydrochloride
Daricon♦
Pregnancy Category: C

MECHANISM OF ACTION
Exerts a nonspecific, direct spasmolytic action on smooth muscle. Also possesses local anesthetic properties that may be partly responsible for the spasmolysis.

INDICATIONS & DOSAGE
Adjunctive treatment of peptic ulcer—
Adults: 10 mg P.O. b.i.d. in the morning and h.s., or 5 mg b.i.d. or t.i.d.

ADVERSE REACTIONS
CNS: *headache,* insomnia, drowsiness, *dizziness.*
CV: *palpitations,* tachycardia.
EENT: *blurred vision,* mydriasis, increased ocular tension, cycloplegia, photophobia.
GI: *constipation,* nausea, vomiting, *paralytic ileus.*
GU: urinary hesitancy and retention, impotence.
Skin: urticaria, decreased sweating or anhidrosis, other dermal manifestations.
Other: fever, allergic reactions. Overdosage may cause curare-like symptoms.

INTERACTIONS
None significant.

NURSING CONSIDERATIONS
• Contraindicated in narrow-angle glaucoma, obstructive uropathy, obstructive disease of GI tract, severe ulcerative colitis, myasthenia gravis, hypersensitivity to anticholinergics, paralytic ileus, intestinal atony, unstable cardiovascular status in acute hemorrhage, and toxic megacolon. Use cautiously in autonomic neuropathy, hyperthyroidism, coronary artery

disease, cardiac arrhythmias, congestive heart failure, hypertension, hiatal hernia associated with reflux esophagitis, hepatic or renal disease, ulcerative colitis, or in patients over 40 years, because of increased incidence of glaucoma.
• Use with caution in hot or humid environments. Drug-induced heatstroke can develop.
• Give 30 minutes to 1 hour before breakfast and at bedtime.
• Monitor patient's vital signs and urinary output carefully.
• Instruct patient to avoid driving and other hazardous activities if he is drowsy, dizzy, or has blurred vision; to drink plenty of fluids to help prevent constipation; and to report any skin rash.
• Gum or sugarless hard candy may relieve mouth dryness.
• Synthetic tertiary derivative that may have fewer atropine-like side effects.

oxyphenonium bromide
Antrenyl
Pregnancy Category: C

MECHANISM OF ACTION
Competitively blocks acetylcholine, which decreases GI motility and inhibits gastric acid secretion.

INDICATIONS & DOSAGE
Adjunctive treatment of peptic ulcer—
Adults: 10 mg P.O. q.i.d. for several days, then reduced according to patient response.

ADVERSE REACTIONS
CNS: headache, insomnia, drowsiness, dizziness, *confusion or excitement in elderly patients,* nervousness, weakness.
CV: *palpitations,* tachycardia.
EENT: *blurred vision,* mydriasis, increased ocular tension, cycloplegia, photophobia.

GI: *dry mouth,* dysphagia, *constipation,* heartburn, loss of taste, nausea, vomiting, *paralytic ileus.*
GU: *urinary hesitancy and retention,* impotence.
Skin: urticaria, decreased sweating or anhidrosis, other dermal manifestations.
Other: fever, allergic reactions. Overdosage may cause curare-like symptoms.

INTERACTIONS
None significant.

NURSING CONSIDERATIONS
• Contraindicated in narrow-angle glaucoma, obstructive uropathy, obstructive disease of GI tract, severe ulcerative colitis, myasthenia gravis, hypersensitivity to anticholinergics, paralytic ileus, intestinal atony, unstable cardiovascular status in acute hemorrhage, and toxic megacolon. Use cautiously in autonomic neuropathy, hyperthyroidism, coronary artery disease, cardiac arrhythmias, congestive heart failure, hypertension, hiatal hernia associated with reflux esophagitis, hepatic or renal disease, ulcerative colitis, or in patients over 40 years, because of increased incidence of glaucoma.
• Use with caution in hot or humid environments. Drug-induced heatstroke can develop.
• Give 30 minutes to 1 hour before meals and at bedtime. Bedtime dose can be larger and should be given at least 2 hours after the last meal of the day.
• Monitor patient's vital signs and urinary output.
• Instruct patient to avoid driving and other hazardous activities if he is drowsy, dizzy, or has blurred vision; to drink plenty of fluids to help prevent constipation; and to report any skin rash.
• Gum or sugarless hard candy may relieve mouth dryness.

propantheline bromide
Banlin♦♦, Norpanth, Pro-Banthine♦,
Propanthel♦♦, Robantaline, SK-
Propantheline Bromide
Pregnancy Category: C

MECHANISM OF ACTION
Competitively blocks acetylcholine,
which decreases GI motility and inhibits gastric acid secretion.

INDICATIONS & DOSAGE
*Adjunctive treatment of peptic ulcer,
irritable bowel syndrome, and other
gastrointestinal disorders; to reduce
duodenal motility during diagnostic
radiologic procedures—*
Adults: 15 mg P.O. t.i.d. before
meals, and 30 mg at bedtime up to 60
mg q.i.d. For elderly patients, 7.5 mg
P.O. t.i.d. before meals.

ADVERSE REACTIONS
CNS: headache, insomnia, drowsiness, dizziness, *confusion or excitement in elderly patients,* nervousness,
weakness.
CV: *palpitations,* tachycardia.
EENT: *blurred vision,* mydriasis, increased ocular tension, cycloplegia,
photophobia.
GI: *dry mouth,* dysphagia, constipation, heartburn, loss of taste, nausea,
vomiting, paralytic ileus.
GU: *urinary hesitancy and retention,*
impotence.
Skin: urticaria, decreased sweating or
anhidrosis, other dermal manifestations.
Other: fever, allergic reactions.
Overdosage may cause curare-like
symptoms.

INTERACTIONS
None significant.

NURSING CONSIDERATIONS
• Contraindicated in narrow-angle
glaucoma, obstructive uropathy, obstructive disease of GI tract, severe

ulcerative colitis, myasthenia gravis,
hypersensitivity to anticholinergics,
paralytic ileus, intestinal atony, unstable cardiovascular status in acute
hemorrhage, and toxic megacolon.
Use cautiously in autonomic neuropathy, hyperthyroidism, coronary artery
disease, cardiac arrhythmias, congestive heart failure, hypertension, hiatal
hernia associated with reflux esophagitis, hepatic or renal disease, ulcerative colitis, or in patients over 40
years, because of the increased incidence of glaucoma.
• Use with caution in hot or humid
environments. Drug-induced heatstroke can develop.
• Give 30 minutes to 1 hour before
meals and at bedtime. Bedtime dose
can be larger and should be given at
least 2 hours after the last meal of the
day.
• Monitor patient's vital signs and
urinary output carefully.
• Instruct patient to avoid driving and
other hazardous activities if he is
drowsy, dizzy, or has blurred vision;
to drink plenty of fluids to help prevent constipation; and to report any
skin rash.
• Gum or sugarless hard candy may
relieve mouth dryness.

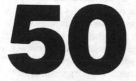

H₂ receptor antagonists and sucralfate

cimetidine
famotidine
ranitidine
sucralfate

COMBINATION PRODUCTS
None.

cimetidine
Tagamet♦
Pregnancy Category: B

MECHANISM OF ACTION
Competitively inhibits the action of histamine (H_2) at receptor sites of the parietal cells, decreasing gastric acid secretion.

INDICATIONS & DOSAGE
Duodenal ulcer (short-term treatment)—
Adults and children over 16 years: 300 mg P.O. q.i.d. with meals and h.s. for maximum therapy of 8 weeks. Alternatively, may give 400 mg P.O. b.i.d. or 800 mg once daily at bedtime. When healing occurs, stop treatment or give bedtime dose only to control nocturnal hypersecretion. Parenteral: 300 mg diluted to 20 ml with 0.9% normal saline solution or other compatible I.V. solution by I.V. push over 1 to 2 minutes q 6 hours. Or 300 mg diluted in 100 ml dextrose 5% solution or other compatible I.V. solution by I.V. infusion over 15 to 20 minutes q 6 hours. Or 300 mg I.M. q 6 hours (no dilution necessary). To increase dose, give 300 mg doses more frequently to maximum daily dose of 2,400 mg.
Duodenal ulcer prophylaxis—
Adults and children over 16 years: 400 mg P.O. h.s.
Active benign gastric ulcer—
Adults: 300 mg q.i.d. with meals and at bedtime for up to 8 weeks.
Pathologic hypersecretory conditions (such as Zollinger-Ellison syndrome, systemic mastocytosis, and multiple endocrine adenomas)—
Adults and children over 16 years: 300 mg P.O. q.i.d. with meals and h.s.; adjust to individual needs. Maximum daily dose 2,400 mg.
Parenteral: 300 mg diluted to 20 ml with 0.9% normal saline solution or other compatible I.V. solutions by I.V. push over 1 to 2 minutes q 6 hours. Or 300 mg diluted in 100 ml dextrose 5% solution or other compatible I.V. solution by I.V. infusion over 15 to 20 minutes q 6 hours. To increase dose, give 300 mg doses more frequently to maximum daily dose of 2,400 mg.

ADVERSE REACTIONS
Blood: *agranulocytosis, neutropenia, thrombocytopenia, aplastic anemia.*
CNS: *mental confusion, dizziness,* headaches, depression.
CV: bradycardia.
GI: *mild and transient diarrhea,* perforation of chronic peptic ulcers after abrupt cessation of drug, phytobezoars in the elderly.
GU: interstitial nephritis, *transient elevations in BUN and serum creatinine,* reduced sperm count, impotence.
Hepatic: jaundice.

Skin: acne-like rash, urticaria, *exfoliative dermatitis*.
Other: hypersensitivity, muscle pain, mild gynecomastia after use longer than 1 month, hypospermia.

INTERACTIONS
Antacids: interfere with absorption of cimetidine. Separate cimetidine and antacids by at least 1 hour if possible.

NURSING CONSIDERATIONS
• I.M. route of administration may be painful.
• I.V. solutions compatible for dilution with cimetidine: 0.9% sodium chloride solution, dextrose 5% and 10% (and combinations of these) solutions, lactated Ringer's solution, and 5% sodium bicarbonate injection. Do not dilute with sterile water for injection.
• Hemodialysis reduces blood levels of cimetidine. Schedule cimetidine dose at end of hemodialysis treatment.
• Up to 10 g overdosage has been reported without untoward effects.
• Effectiveness in treatment of gastric ulcers not as great as in duodenal ulcer. Cimetidine may prove useful but is still unapproved in pancreatic insufficiency, short-bowel syndrome, psoriasis, prevention and treatment of GI bleeding, relief of symptoms and acid sensitivity in reflux esophagitis, and prevention of gastric inactivation of oral enzyme preparations by gastric acid and pepsin.
• Taking tablets with meals will ensure a more consistent therapeutic effect.
• Remind patient that if he's taking cimetidine once daily, he should take it at bedtime for best results.
• Large parenteral doses should be avoided in asthmatics.
• Blue dye in Tagamet tablets may produce a false-positive Hemoccult test for blood in gastric juice. This can be avoided by administering the tablet at least 15 minutes before obtaining gastric juice by aspiration.
• Elderly patients more susceptible to cimetidine-induced mental confusion. Dose should be decreased in elderly and in patients with hepatic or renal insufficiency.
• I.V. cimetidine often used in critically ill patients prophylactically to prevent GI bleeding.
• Don't infuse I.V. too rapidly. May cause bradycardia.
• Urge your patient to avoid smoking cigarettes. Smoking causes cimetidine to work less effectively.
• Cimetidine is being used investigationally to treat chronic hives.
• When administering cimetidine I.V. in 100 ml of diluent solution, do not infuse so rapidly that circulatory overload is produced. Some authorities recommend that the drug be infused over at least 30 minutes, to minimize the risk of adverse cardiac effects.
• Available in liquid form (300 mg/5 ml).
• Tablets available in four strengths: 200 mg, 300 mg, 400 mg and 800 mg. All tablets are pale blue-green. Identify tablet when obtaining a drug history.
• Has many investigational uses. Used before the introduction of anesthesia for prophylaxis of aspiration pneumonitis; also used to treat hyperparathyroidism and herpes zoster.

famotidine
Pepcid
Pregnancy Category: B

MECHANISM OF ACTION
Competitively inhibits the action of histamine (H_2) at receptor sites of the parietal cells, decreasing gastric acid secretion.

INDICATIONS & DOSAGE
Duodenal ulcer—

Adults: For acute therapy, 40 mg P.O. once daily at bedtime. For maintenance therapy, 20 mg P.O. once daily at bedtime.
Pathologic hypersecretory conditions (such as Zollinger-Ellison syndrome)—
Adults: 20 mg P.O. q 6 hours. As much as 160 mg q 6 hours may be administered.
Hospitalized patients with intractable ulcers or hypersecretory conditions, or patients who cannot take oral medication—
Adults: 20 mg I.V. q 12 hours.

ADVERSE REACTIONS
CNS: *headache,* dizziness, hallucinations.
GI: diarrhea, constipation, nausea, flatulence.
Local: transient irritation at I.V. site.

INTERACTIONS
None significant.

NURSING CONSIDERATIONS
• Gastric malignancy must be ruled out before famotidine therapy.
• Advise patient not to take the drug for longer than 8 weeks unless doctor specifically orders it.
• Especially at the beginning of therapy when pain is severe, with doctor's knowledge, patient may take antacids concomitantly.
• Urge patient to avoid cigarette smoking as this may increase gastric acid secretion and worsen disease.
• Patient may take famotidine with a snack if he desires. Remind patient that this drug is most effective if taken at bedtime.
• Some patients may have this drug prescribed to be taken 20 mg twice daily instead of 40 mg at bedtime. This alternate dosing schedule is also effective. However, at least one dose should be taken at bedtime.
• Unlike cimetidine, which has a weak androgenic effect, famotidine has not been reported to cause gynecomastia or impotence in males. Unlike cimetidine and ranitidine, famotidine is not known to cause significant drug interactions.

ranitidine
Zantac♦
Pregnancy Category: B

MECHANISM OF ACTION
Competitively inhibits the action of histamine (H₂) at receptor sites of the parietal cells, decreasing gastric acid secretion.

INDICATIONS & DOSAGE
Duodenal and gastric ulcer (short-term treatment); pathological hypersecretory conditions, such as Zollinger-Ellison syndrome—
Adults: 150 mg P.O. b.i.d. or 300 mg once daily at bedtime. Doses up to 6 g/day may be prescribed in patients with Zollinger-Ellison syndrome. May also be administered parenterally: 50 mg I.V. or I.M. q 6 to 8 hours. When administering I.V. push, dilute to a total volume of 20 ml and inject over a period of 5 minutes. No dilution necessary when administering I.M. May also be administered by intermittent I.V. infusion. Dilute 50 mg ranitidine in 100 ml of dextrose 5% and infuse over 15 to 20 minutes.
Maintenance therapy in duodenal ulcer—
Adults: 150 mg P.O. at bedtime.
Gastroesophageal reflux disease (GERD)—
Adults: 150 mg P.O. b.i.d.

ADVERSE REACTIONS
Blood: neutropenia, thrombocytopenia.
CNS: headache, malaise, dizziness.
GI: nausea, constipation.
Hepatic: increases in liver enzymes, jaundice.
Skin: rash.

Local: burning and itching at injection site.

INTERACTIONS
Antacids: interfere with absorption of ranitidine. Separate ranitidine and antacids dosage by at least 1 hour, if possible.

NURSING CONSIDERATIONS
• Use cautiously in patients with hepatic dysfunction. Dosage should be adjusted in patients with impaired renal function.
• Does not appear to cause as many of the adverse reactions produced by cimetidine. Does not affect the action of other drugs to the extent that cimetidine does.
• Due to decreased renal clearance, the elderly are more likely to experience adverse reactions.
• Can be taken without regard to meals. Absorption not affected by food.
• Remind patient that if he's taking ranitidine once daily, he should take it at bedtime for best results.
• Urge patient to avoid smoking, which impairs effectiveness of ranitidine.
• Most patients show healing of ulcer within 4 weeks. Additional treating after this interval has not been demonstrated.

---

sucralfate
Carafate, Sulcrate♦♦
Pregnancy Category: B

MECHANISM OF ACTION
Adheres to and protects the ulcer surface by forming a barrier.

INDICATIONS & DOSAGE
Short-term (up to 8 weeks) treatment of duodenal ulcer—
Adults: 1 g P.O. q.i.d. 1 hour before meals and at bedtime.

ADVERSE REACTIONS
CNS: dizziness, sleepiness.
GI: *constipation,* nausea, gastric discomfort, diarrhea, bezoar formation.

INTERACTIONS
Antacids: May decrease binding of drug to gastroduodenal mucosa, impairing effectiveness. Don't give within 30 minutes of each other.

NURSING CONSIDERATIONS
• No known contraindications.
• Symptomatic improvement doesn't preclude possibility of gastric cancer.
• Drug is minimally absorbed. Incidence of side effects is low.
• Tell patient for best results to take sucralfate on an empty stomach (1 hour before each meal and at bedtime).
• Pain and ulcer symptoms may subside within first few weeks of therapy. However, for complete healing, be sure patient continues on prescribed regimen.
• Monitor for severe, persistent constipation.
• Studies suggest that drug is as effective as cimetidine in healing duodenal ulcers.
• Drug has been used to treat gastric ulcers, but effectiveness of this use is still under investigation.
• Drug contains aluminum, but isn't classified as an antacid.
• Don't crush tablet and place in water before administering through nasogastric tube. Sucralfate's fairly insoluble in water so a bezoar may form. Best to have pharmacist prepare a water-sorbitol suspension.

Italicized side effects are common or life-threatening.
*Liquid form contains alcohol.   **May contain tartrazine.

51

Corticosteroids

Glucocorticoids
beclomethasone dipropionate
betamethasone
**betamethasone acetate and
betamethasone sodium
phosphate**
**betamethasone disodium
phosphate**
**betamethasone sodium
phosphate**
cortisone acetate
dexamethasone
dexamethasone acetate
**dexamethasone sodium
phosphate**
flunisolide
hydrocortisone
hydrocortisone acetate
hydrocortisone retention enema
**hydrocortisone sodium
phosphate**
**hydrocortisone sodium
succinate**
methylprednisolone
methylprednisolone acetate
**methylprednisolone sodium
succinate**
paramethasone acetate
prednisolone
prednisolone acetate
prednisolone sodium phosphate
prednisolone tebutate
prednisone
triamcinolone
triamcinolone acetonide
triamcinolone diacetate
triamcinolone hexacetonide

Mineralocorticoids
desoxycorticosterone acetate
desoxycorticosterone pivalate

fludrocortisone acetate

COMBINATION PRODUCTS
DECADRON WITH XYLOCAINE: dexamethasone phosphate 4 mg and lidocaine hydrochloride 10 mg/ml.

---

beclomethasone dipropionate
Beclovent♦, Vanceril♦
Pregnancy Category: C

MECHANISM OF ACTION
Decreases inflammation, mainly by stabilizing leukocyte lysosomal membranes. Also suppresses the immune response, stimulates bone marrow, and influences protein, fat, and carbohydrate metabolism.

INDICATIONS & DOSAGE
Steroid-dependent asthma—
Adults: 2 to 4 inhalations t.i.d. or q.i.d. Maximum 20 inhalations daily.
Children 6 to 12 years: 1 to 2 inhalations t.i.d. or q.i.d. Maximum 10 inhalations daily.

ADVERSE REACTIONS
EENT: hoarseness, fungal infections of mouth and throat.
GI: dry mouth.

INTERACTIONS
None significant.

NURSING CONSIDERATIONS
• Contraindicated in status asthmaticus. Not for asthma controlled by bronchodilators or other noncortico-

---

Unmarked trade names available in the United States only.
♦Also available in Canada.   ♦♦Available in Canada only.

steroids alone, or for nonasthmatic bronchial diseases.

• Oral glucocorticoid therapy should be tapered slowly. Acute adrenal insufficiency and death have occurred in asthmatics who changed abruptly from oral corticosteroids to beclomethasone.

• During times of stress (trauma, surgery, infection) systemic corticosteroids may be needed to prevent adrenal insufficiency in previously steroid-dependent patients.

• Instruct patient to carry a card indicating his need for supplemental systemic glucocorticoids during stress.

• Patient requiring bronchodilator should use it several minutes before beclomethasone.

• Allow 1 minute to elapse before taking subsequent puffs of medication. Hold breath for a few seconds to enhance action of drug.

• Inform patient that beclomethasone doesn't provide relief for emergency asthma attack.

• Instruct patient to contact doctor if he notices a decreased response. Dose may have to be adjusted. Patient shouldn't exceed recommended dose on his own.

• Check mucous membranes frequently for signs of fungal infection.

• Oral fungal infections can be prevented by following inhalations with glass of water.

• Tell patient to keep inhaler clean and unobstructed. Wash with warm water and dry thoroughly.

betamethasone
Betnelan♦♦, Celestone♦*

betamethasone acetate and betamethasone sodium phosphate
Celestone Soluspan♦

betamethasone disodium phosphate
Betnesol♦♦

betamethasone sodium phosphate
Celestone Phosphate♦
Pregnancy Category: C

MECHANISM OF ACTION
Decreases inflammation, mainly by stabilizing leukocyte lysosomal membranes. Also suppresses the immune response, stimulates bone marrow, and influences protein, fat, and carbohydrate metabolism.

INDICATIONS & DOSAGE
Severe inflammation or immunosuppression—
Adults: 0.6 to 7.2 mg P.O. daily; or 0.5 to 9 mg (sodium phosphate) I.M., I.V., or into joint or soft tissue daily; or 1.5 to 12 mg (sodium phosphate-acetate suspension) into joint or soft tissue q 1 to 2 weeks, p.r.n.
Prevention of neonatal respiratory distress syndrome—
Adults (pregnant female): 12 mg I.M. Celestone Soluspan 36 to 48 hours before premature delivery. Repeated in 24 hours.

ADVERSE REACTIONS
Most side effects of corticosteroids are dose- or duration-dependent.
CNS: *euphoria, insomnia,* psychotic behavior, pseudotumor cerebri.
CV: *congestive heart failure,* hypertension, edema.
EENT: cataracts, glaucoma.
GI: *peptic ulcer,* gastrointestinal irri-

Italicized side effects are common or life-threatening.
*Liquid form contains alcohol.   **May contain tartrazine.

tation, increased appetite.
Metabolic: *possible hypokalemia, hyperglycemia and carbohydrate intolerance,* growth suppression in children.
Skin: delayed wound healing, acne, various skin eruptions.
Other: muscle weakness, pancreatitis, hirsutism, susceptibility to infections. Acute adrenal insufficiency may follow increased stress (infection, surgery, trauma) or abrupt withdrawal after long-term therapy.
Withdrawal symptoms: rebound inflammation, fatigue, weakness, arthralgia, fever, dizziness, lethargy, depression, fainting, orthostatic hypotension, dyspnea, anorexia, hypoglycemia. *Sudden withdrawal may be fatal.*

INTERACTIONS
Barbiturates, phenytoin, rifampin: decreased corticosteroid effect. Corticosteroid dose may need to be increased.
Indomethacin, aspirin: increased risk of GI distress and bleeding. Give together cautiously.

NURSING CONSIDERATIONS
• Contraindicated in systemic fungal infections. Use cautiously in patients with GI ulceration or renal disease, hypertension, osteoporosis, varicella, vaccinia, exanthema, diabetes mellitus, Cushing's syndrome, thromboembolic disorders, seizures, myasthenia gravis, congestive heart failure, tuberculosis, ocular herpes simplex, hypoalbuminemia, emotional instability, or psychotic tendencies.
• Don't use for alternate-day therapy.
• Adrenal suppression may last up to 1 year after drug is stopped. Gradually reduce drug dosage after long-term therapy. Tell patient not to stop drug abruptly or without doctor's consent.
• Always titrate to lowest effective dose.
• To prevent muscle atrophy, give by

deep I.M. injection.
• Monitor blood sugars, along with serum potassium, regularly.
• Teach patients about the effects and side effects of the medication. Warn patients who are on long-term therapy about cushingoid symptoms.
• Observe for signs of infection, especially after steroid withdrawal. Tell patients to report slow healing.
• Instruct patient to carry a card indicating his need for supplemental glucocorticoids during stress.
• Give once-daily doses in the morning for better results and less toxicity.
• Give with milk or food to reduce gastric irritation.
• Glucocorticoid with little mineralocorticoid effect.
• Watch for additional potassium depletion from diuretics and amphotericin B.
• Immunizations may show decreased antibody response.
• Obtain baseline weight before starting therapy, and weigh patient daily; report any sudden weight gain to doctor.
• Check for glycosuria in patients using glucose oxidase reagent sticks instead of tablets.
• Betamethasone sometimes prescribed to treat respiratory distress syndrome in premature infants.

cortisone acetate
Cortistan, Cortone♦
Pregnancy Category: D

MECHANISM OF ACTION
Decreases inflammation, mainly by stabilizing leukocyte lysosomal membranes. Also suppresses the immune response, stimulates bone marrow, and influences protein, fat, and carbohydrate metabolism.

INDICATIONS & DOSAGE
Adrenal insufficiency, allergy, inflammation—

Adults: 25 to 300 mg P.O. or I.M. daily or on alternate days. Doses highly individualized, depending on severity of disease.

ADVERSE REACTIONS
Most side effects of corticosteroids are dose- or duration-dependent.
CNS: *euphoria, insomnia,* psychotic behavior, pseudotumor cerebri.
CV: *congestive heart failure,* hypertension, edema.
EENT: cataracts, glaucoma.
GI: *peptic ulcer,* gastrointestinal irritation, increased appetite.
Metabolic: *possible hypokalemia, hyperglycemia and carbohydrate intolerance,* growth suppression in children.
Skin: delayed wound healing, acne, various skin eruptions.
Local: atrophy at I.M. injection sites.
Other: muscle weakness, pancreatitis, hirsutism, susceptibility to infections. Acute adrenal insufficiency may follow increased stress (infection, surgery, trauma) or abrupt withdrawal after long-term therapy.
Withdrawal symptoms: rebound inflammation, fatigue, weakness, arthralgia, fever, dizziness, lethargy, depression, fainting, orthostatic hypotension, dyspnea, anorexia, hypoglycemia. *Sudden withdrawal may be fatal.*

INTERACTIONS
Barbiturates, phenytoin, rifampin: decreased corticosteroid effect. Corticosteroid dose may need to be increased.
Indomethacin, aspirin: increased risk of GI distress and bleeding. Give together cautiously.

NURSING CONSIDERATIONS
• Contraindicated in systemic fungal infections. Use cautiously in patients with GI ulceration or renal disease, hypertension, osteoporosis, varicella, vaccinia, exanthema, diabetes mellitus, Cushing's syndrome, thromboembolic disorders, seizures, myasthenia gravis, congestive heart failure, tuberculosis, ocular herpes simplex, hypoalbuminemia, emotional instability, or psychotic tendencies.
• Gradually reduce drug dosage after long-term therapy. Tell patient not to discontinue drug abruptly or without doctor's consent.
• Always titrate to lowest effective dose.
• Patient may need salt-restricted diet and potassium supplement.
• I.M. route causes slow onset of action. Don't use in acute conditions where rapid effect required. May use on a b.i.d. schedule matching diurnal variation.
• Glucocorticoid with potent mineralocorticoid effect; report sudden weight gain or edema to doctor.
• Observe for signs of infection, especially after steroid withdrawal. Tell patient to report slow healing.
• Drug of choice for replacement therapy in adrenal insufficiency.
• Monitor serum electrolytes and blood sugars.
• Warn patients on long-term therapy about cushingoid symptoms.
• Give with milk or food to reduce gastric irritation.
• Instruct patient to carry a card indicating his need for supplemental glucocorticoids during stress.
• Give once-daily doses in the morning for better results and less toxicity.
• Not for I.V. use.
• Watch for additional potassium depletion from diuretics and amphotericin B.
• Immunizations may show decreased antibody response.

Italicized side effects are common or life-threatening.
*Liquid form contains alcohol.   **May contain tartrazine.

desoxycorticosterone acetate
Doca Acetate, Percorten Acetate

desoxycorticosterone pivalate
Percorten Pivalate
Pregnancy Category: C

MECHANISM OF ACTION
Increases sodium reabsorption, and potassium and hydrogen secretion at the nephron's distal convoluted tubule.

INDICATIONS & DOSAGE
Adrenal insufficiency (partial replacement), salt-losing adrenogenital syndrome—
Adults: 2 to 5 mg (acetate) I.M. daily; or 25 to 100 mg (pivalate) I.M. q 4 weeks. Or implant 1 pellet for each 0.5 mg of the daily injected maintenance dose. Pellets last for 8 to 12 months.

ADVERSE REACTIONS
CNS: headache.
CV: *sodium and water retention,* hypertension, cardiac hypertrophy, *edema*.
Metabolic: *hypokalemia*.

INTERACTIONS
None significant.

NURSING CONSIDERATIONS
• Contraindicated in hypertension, congestive heart failure, cardiac disease. Use cautiously in Addison's disease. Patients may have exaggerated side effects.
• Has no anti-inflammatory effect.
• Most potent mineralocorticoid. Has little glucocorticoid effect.
• Use with glucocorticoid for full treatment of adrenal insufficiency.
• Report significant weight gain, edema, hypertension, or cardiac symptoms to doctor.

• Establish baseline weight and blood pressure; monitor intake and output.
• Injection is sesame oil solution. Withdraw dose with 19G needle, but give with 23G needle. Inject in upper, outer quadrant of buttocks. Not for I.V. use.
• Monitor sodium and potassium levels, fluid intake. Patient may need salt-restricted diet, potassium supplement.
• Watch for additional potassium depletion from diuretics and amphotericin B.
• The repository form should be given no more frequently than once a month. Use a 20G needle and inject into upper quadrant of buttocks.

dexamethasone
Decadron♦, Dexamethasone Intensol, Dexasone♦♦, Dexone, Hexadrol♦, SK-Dexamethasone

dexamethasone acetate
Dalalone-LA, Decadron-LA, Decaject LA, Decameth-LA, Dexacen-LA, Dexasone-LA, Dexone LA

dexamethasone sodium phosphate
Decadron Phosphate♦, Decaject, Decameth, Dexacen-4, Dexasone, Dexone, Dezone, Hexadrol Phosphate♦, Savacort-D
Pregnancy Category: C

MECHANISM OF ACTION
Decreases inflammation, mainly by stabilizing leukocyte lysosomal membranes. Also suppresses the immune response, stimulates bone marrow, and influences protein, fat, and carbohydrate metabolism.

INDICATIONS & DOSAGE
Cerebral edema—
Adults: initially, 10 mg (phosphate) I.V., then 4 to 6 mg I.M. q 6 hours for

2 to 4 days, then taper over 5 to 7 days.
Children: 0.2 mg/kg P.O. daily in divided doses.
Inflammatory conditions, allergic reactions, neoplasias—
Adults: 0.25 to 4 mg P.O. b.i.d., t.i.d., or q.i.d.; or 4 to 16 mg (acetate) I.M. into joint or soft tissue q 1 to 3 weeks; or 0.8 to 1.6 mg (acetate) into lesions q 1 to 3 weeks.
Shock—
Adults: 1 to 6 mg/kg (phosphate) I.V. single dose; or 40 mg I.V. q 2 to 6 hours, p.r.n.
Dexamethasone suppression test—
0.5 mg P.O. q 6 hours for 48 hours.

ADVERSE REACTIONS
Most side effects of corticosteroids are dose- or duration-dependent.
CNS: *euphoria, insomnia,* psychotic behavior, pseudotumor cerebri.
CV: *congestive heart failure,* hypertension, edema.
EENT: cataracts, glaucoma.
GI: *peptic ulcer,* gastrointestinal irritation, increased appetite.
Metabolic: *possible hypokalemia, hyperglycemia and carbohydrate intolerance,* growth suppression in children.
Skin: delayed wound healing, acne, various skin eruptions.
Local: atrophy at I.M. injection sites.
Other: muscle weakness, pancreatitis, hirsutism, susceptibility to infections. Acute adrenal insufficiency may follow increased stress (infection, surgery, trauma) or abrupt withdrawal after long-term therapy.
Withdrawal symptoms: rebound inflammation, fatigue, weakness, arthralgia, fever, dizziness, lethargy, depression, fainting, orthostatic hypotension, dyspnea, anorexia, hypoglycemia. *Sudden withdrawal may be fatal.*

INTERACTIONS
Barbiturates, phenytoin, rifampin: decreased corticosteroid effect. Corti-

costeroid dose may need to be increased.
Indomethacin, aspirin: increased risk of GI distress and bleeding. Give together cautiously.

NURSING CONSIDERATIONS
• Contraindicated in systemic fungal infections and for alternate-day therapy. Use cautiously in patients with GI ulceration or renal disease, hypertension, osteoporosis, varicella, vaccinia, exanthema, diabetes mellitus, Cushing's syndrome, thromboembolic disorders, seizures, myasthenia gravis, metastatic cancer, congestive heart failure, tuberculosis, ocular herpes simplex, hypoalbuminemia, emotional instability or psychotic tendencies, and in children.
• Gradually reduce drug dosage after long-term therapy. Tell patient not to discontinue drug abruptly or without doctor's consent.
• Always titrate to lowest effective dose.
• Monitor patient's weight, blood pressure, serum electrolytes.
• Instruct patient to carry a card indicating his need for supplemental systemic glucocorticoids during stress, especially as dose is decreased.
• Give once-daily doses in the morning for better results and less toxicity.
• Teach patient signs of early adrenal insufficiency: fatigue, muscular weakness, joint pain, fever, anorexia, nausea, dyspnea, dizziness, fainting.
• May mask or exacerbate infections.
• Watch for depression or psychotic episodes, especially in high-dose therapy.
• Inspect patient's skin for petechiae. Warn patient about easy bruising.
• Patients with diabetes may need increased insulin; monitor blood glucose levels.
• Monitor growth in infants and children on long-term therapy.
• Give I.M. injection deep into gluteal muscle. Avoid subcutaneous in-

jection, as atrophy and sterile abscesses may occur.
• Give P.O. dose with food when possible.
• Warn patients on long-term therapy about cushingoid symptoms.
• Watch for additional potassium depletion from diuretics and amphotericin B.
• Immunizations may show decreased antibody response.
• Not used for alternate-day therapy.
• Dexamethasone most recently used in the diagnosis of depression. It is also an effective antiemetic.

fludrocortisone acetate
Florinef Acetate♦
Pregnancy Category: C

MECHANISM OF ACTION
Increases sodium reabsorption, and potassium and hydrogen secretion at the nephron's distal convoluted tubule.

INDICATIONS & DOSAGE
Adrenal insufficiency (partial replacement), salt-losing adrenogenital syndrome—
Adults: 0.1 to 0.2 mg P.O. daily.

ADVERSE REACTIONS
CV: *sodium and water retention,* hypertension, cardiac hypertrophy, edema.
Metabolic: hypokalemia.

INTERACTIONS
None significant.

NURSING CONSIDERATIONS
• Contraindicated in hypertension, congestive heart failure, cardiac disease. Use cautiously in Addison's disease.
• Monitor patient's blood pressure and serum electrolytes. Weigh patient daily; report sudden weight gain to doctor.

• Warn patient that mild peripheral edema is common.
• Unless contraindicated, give salt-restricted diet rich in potassium and protein. Potassium supplement may be needed.
• Has potent mineralocorticoid effects. Little glucocorticoid effect with usual doses.
• Used with cortisone or hydrocortisone in adrenal insufficiency.
• Watch for additional potassium depletion from diuretics and amphotericin B.
• Fludrocortisone is also prescribed to treat severe orthostatic hypotension.

flunisolide
Aerobid
Pregnancy Category: C

MECHANISM OF ACTION
Decreases inflammation, mainly by stabilizing leukocyte lysosomal membranes. Also suppresses the immune response, stimulates bone marrow, and influences protein, fat, and carbohydrate metabolism.

INDICATIONS & DOSAGE
Steroid—dependent asthma—
Adults and children over 6 years: 2 inhalations b.i.d. Don't exceed 4 inhalations b.i.d.

ADVERSE REACTIONS
EENT: hoarseness, fungal infections of mouth and throat.
GI: dry mouth.

INTERACTIONS
None significant.

NURSING CONSIDERATIONS
• Contraindicated in status asthmaticus. Not recommended for asthma controlled by bronchodilators or other noncorticosteroids alone, or for nonasthmatic bronchial diseases.

Unmarked trade names available in the United States only.
♦Also available in Canada.   ♦♦Available in Canada only.

• Oral glucocorticoid therapy should be tapered slowly.
• During times of stress (trauma, surgery, infection), systemic corticosteroids may be needed to prevent adrenal insufficiency in previously steroid-dependent patients.
• Instruct patient to carry a card indicating his need for supplemental systemic glucocorticoids during stress.
• Check mucous membranes frequently for signs of fungal infection. Prevent such infections by following inhalations with glass of water.
• Tell patient to keep inhaler clean and unobstructed. Wash with warm water and dry thoroughly after use.
• Patient requiring bronchodilator should use it several minutes before flunisolide.
• Allow 1 minute to elapse before repeating inhalations. Hold breath for a few seconds to enhance action of drug.
• Inform patient that flunisolide doesn't relieve emergency asthma attack.

hydrocortisone
Cortef♦, Hydrocortone♦

hydrocortisone acetate
Cortef Acetate, Hydrocortone Acetate♦

hydrocortisone retention enema
Cortenema, Rectoid

hydrocortisone sodium phosphate
Hydrocortone Phosphate

hydrocortisone sodium succinate
A-HydroCort, S-Cortilean♦♦, Solu-Cortef♦
Pregnancy Category: C

MECHANISM OF ACTION
Decreases inflammation, mainly by stabilizing leukocyte lysosomal membranes. Also suppresses the immune response, stimulates bone marrow, and influences protein, fat, and carbohydrate metabolism.

INDICATIONS & DOSAGE
Severe inflammation, adrenal insufficiency—
Adults: 5 to 30 mg P.O. b.i.d., t.i.d., or q.i.d. (as much as 80 mg P.O. q.i.d. may be given in acute situations); or initially, 100 to 250 mg (succinate) I.M. or I.V., then 50 to 100 mg I.M., as indicated; or 15 to 240 mg (phosphate) I.M. or I.V. q 12 hours; or 5 to 75 mg (acetate) into joints and soft tissue. Dose varies with size of joint. Often local anesthetics are injected with dose.
Shock—
Adults: 500 mg to 2 g (succinate) q 2 to 6 hours.
Children: 0.16 to 1 mg/kg (phosphate or succinate) I.M. or I.V. b.i.d. or t.i.d.
Adjunctive treatment of ulcerative co-

litis and proctitis—
Adults: 1 enema (100 mg) nightly for 21 days.

ADVERSE REACTIONS
Most side effects of corticosteroids are dose- or duration-dependent.
CNS: *euphoria, insomnia,* psychotic behavior, pseudotumor cerebri.
CV: *congestive heart failure,* hypertension, edema.
EENT: cataracts, glaucoma.
GI: *peptic ulcer,* gastrointestinal irritation, increased appetite.
Metabolic: *possible hypokalemia, hyperglycemia and carbohydrate intolerance,* growth suppression in children.
Skin: delayed wound healing, acne, various skin eruptions.
Other: muscle weakness, pancreatitis, hirsutism, susceptibility to infections. Acute adrenal insufficiency may occur with increased stress (infection, surgery, trauma) or abrupt withdrawal after long-term therapy. *Withdrawal symptoms:* rebound inflammation, fatigue, weakness, arthralgia, fever, dizziness, lethargy, depression, fainting, orthostatic hypotension, dyspnea, anorexia, hypoglycemia. *Sudden withdrawal may be fatal.*

INTERACTIONS
Barbiturates, phenytoin, rifampin: decreased corticosteroid effect. Corticosteroid dose may need to be increased.
Indomethacin, aspirin: increased risk of GI distress and bleeding. Give together cautiously.

NURSING CONSIDERATIONS
• Contraindicated in systemic fungal infections. Use cautiously in patients with GI ulceration or renal disease, hypertension, osteoporosis, varicella, vaccinia, exanthema, diabetes mellitus, Cushing's syndrome, thromboembolic disorders, seizures, myasthenia gravis, metastatic cancer, congestive heart failure, tuberculosis, ocular herpes simplex, hypoalbuminemia, emotional instability or psychotic tendencies, and in children.
• Gradually reduce drug dosage after long-term therapy. Tell patient not to discontinue drug abruptly or without doctor's consent.
• Always titrate to lowest effective dose.
• Glucocorticoid and mineralocorticoid effect.
• Monitor patient's weight, blood pressure, serum electrolytes.
• May mask or exacerbate infections.
• Stress (fever, trauma, surgery, emotional problems) may increase adrenal insufficiency. Dose may have to be increased.
• Instruct patient to carry a card identifying his need for supplemental systemic glucocorticoids during stress.
• Give once-daily doses in the morning for better results and less toxicity.
• Teach patient signs of early adrenal insufficiency: fatigue, muscular weakness, joint pain, fever, anorexia, nausea, dyspnea, dizziness, fainting.
• Watch for depression or psychotic episodes, especially in high-dose therapy.
• Inspect patient's skin for petechiae. Warn patient about easy bruising.
• Patients with diabetes may need increased insulin; monitor blood glucose levels.
• Monitor growth in infants and children on long-term therapy.
• Give I.M. injection deep into gluteal muscle. Avoid subcutaneous injection as atrophy and sterile abscesses may occur.
• Unless contraindicated, give salt-restricted diet rich in potassium and protein. Potassium supplement may be needed. Watch for additional potassium depletion from diuretics and amphotericin B.
• Give P.O. dose with food when possible.
• Warn patients on long-term therapy

about cushingoid symptoms.
- Acetate form not for I.V. use.
- Enema may produce same systemic effects as other forms of hydrocortisone. If enema therapy must exceed 21 days, discontinue gradually by reducing administration to every other night for 2 or 3 weeks.
- Immunizations may show decreased antibody response.
- Do not confuse Solu-Cortef with Solu-Medrol.
- Injectable forms not for alternate-day therapy.

methylprednisolone
Medrol♦**

methylprednisolone acetate
Depo-Medrol♦, Duralone, Medralone, Rep-Pred

methylprednisolone sodium succinate
A-Methapred, Solu-Medrol♦
Pregnancy Category: C

MECHANISM OF ACTION
Decreases inflammation, mainly by stabilizing leukocyte lysosomal membranes. Also suppresses the immune response, stimulates bone marrow, and influences protein, fat, and carbohydrate metabolism.

INDICATIONS & DOSAGE
Severe inflammation or immunosuppression—
Adults: 2 to 60 mg P.O. in four divided doses; or 40 to 80 mg (acetate) daily, I.M. or 10 to 250 mg (succinate) I.M. or I.V. q 4 hours; or 4 to 30 mg (acetate) into joints and soft tissue, p.r.n.
Children: 117 mcg to 1.66 mg/kg (succinate) I.V. in three or four divided doses.
Shock—
100 to 250 mg (succinate) I.V. at 2- to 6-hour intervals.

ADVERSE REACTIONS
Most side effects of corticosteroids are dose- or duration-dependent.
CNS: *euphoria, insomnia,* psychotic behavior, pseudotumor cerebri.
CV: *congestive heart failure,* hypertension, edema.
EENT: cataracts, glaucoma.
GI: *peptic ulcer,* gastrointestinal irritation, increased appetite.
Metabolic: *possible hypokalemia, hyperglycemia and carbohydrate intolerance,* growth suppression in children.
Skin: delayed wound healing, acne, various skin eruptions.
Other: muscle weakness, pancreatitis, hirsutism, susceptibility to infections. Acute adrenal insufficiency may occur with increased stress (infection, surgery, trauma) or abrupt withdrawal after long-term therapy. *Withdrawal symptoms:* rebound inflammation, fatigue, weakness, arthralgia, fever, dizziness, lethargy, depression, fainting, orthostatic hypotension, dyspnea, anorexia, hypoglycemia. *Sudden withdrawal may be fatal.*

INTERACTIONS
Barbiturates, phenytoin, rifampin: decreased corticosteroid effect. Corticosteroid dose may need to be increased.
Indomethacin, aspirin: increased risk of GI distress and bleeding. Give together cautiously.

NURSING CONSIDERATIONS
- Contraindicated in systemic fungal infections. Use cautiously in patients with GI ulceration or renal disease, hypertension, osteoporosis, varicella, vaccinia, exanthema, diabetes mellitus, Cushing's syndrome, thromboembolic disorders, seizures, myasthenia gravis, metastatic cancer, congestive heart failure, tuberculosis, ocular herpes simplex, hypoalbuminemia, emotional instability, or psychotic tendencies.

Italicized side effects are common or life-threatening.
*Liquid form contains alcohol.   **May contain tartrazine.

- Gradually reduce drug dosage after long-term therapy. Tell patient not to discontinue drug abruptly or without doctor's consent.
- Always titrate to lowest effective dose.
- Glucocorticoid with little mineralo-corticoid effect.
- Discard reconstituted solutions after 48 hours.
- Don't use acetate salt when immediate onset of action is needed.
- Dermal atrophy may occur with large doses of acetate salt. Use multiple small injections into lesions.
- Monitor weight, blood pressure, serum electrolytes, sleep patterns. Euphoria may initially interfere with sleep, but patient generally adjusts to the medication after 1 to 3 weeks.
- May mask or exacerbate infections.
- Instruct patient to carry a card identifying his need for supplemental systemic glucocorticoids during stress.
- Give once-daily doses in the morning for better results and less toxicity.
- Teach patient signs of early adrenal insufficiency: fatigue, muscular weakness, joint pain, fever, anorexia, nausea, dyspnea, dizziness, fainting.
- Watch for depression or psychotic episodes, especially in high-dose therapy.
- Patients with diabetes may need increased insulin; monitor blood glucose levels.
- Give I.M. injection deep into gluteal muscle. Avoid subcutaneous injection, as atrophy and sterile abscesses may occur.
- Unless contraindicated, give salt-restricted diet rich in potassium and protein. Potassium supplement may be needed. Watch for additional potassium depletion from diuretics and amphotericin B.
- Give P.O. dose with food when possible. Critically ill patients may require concomitant antacid therapy.
- Give I.V. dose slowly over 1 minute; in shock, give massive I.V. doses over at least 10 minutes to prevent cardiac arrhythmias and circulatory collapse.
- Warn patients on long-term therapy about cushingoid symptoms.
- Acetate form not for I.V. use.
- Do not confuse Solu-Medrol with Solu-Cortef.
- Immunizations may show decreased antibody response.
- May be used for alternate-day therapy.

paramethasone acetate
Haldrone
Pregnancy Category: C

MECHANISM OF ACTION
Decreases inflammation, mainly by stabilizing leukocyte lysosomal membranes. Also suppresses the immune response, stimulates bone marrow, and influences protein, fat, and carbohydrate metabolism.

INDICATIONS & DOSAGE
Inflammatory conditions—
Adults: 0.5 to 6 mg P.O. t.i.d. or q.i.d.
Children: 58 to 800 mcg/kg daily divided t.i.d. or q.i.d.

ADVERSE REACTIONS
Most side effects of corticosteroids are dose- or duration-dependent.
CNS: *euphoria, insomnia,* psychotic behavior, pseudotumor cerebri.
CV: *congestive heart failure,* hypertension, edema.
EENT: cataracts, glaucoma.
GI: *peptic ulcer,* gastrointestinal irritation, increased appetite.
Metabolic: *possible hypokalemia, hyperglycemia and carbohydrate intolerance,* growth suppression in children.
Skin: delayed wound healing, acne, various skin eruptions.
Other: muscle weakness, pancreatitis, hirsutism, susceptibility to infections. Acute adrenal insufficiency

may occur with increased stress (infection, surgery, trauma) or abrupt withdrawal after long-term therapy. *Withdrawal symptoms:* rebound inflammation, fatigue, weakness, arthralgia, fever, dizziness, lethargy, depression, fainting, orthostatic hypotension, dyspnea, anorexia, hypoglycemia. *Sudden withdrawal may be fatal.*

INTERACTIONS
Barbiturates, phenytoin, rifampin: decreased corticosteroid effect. Corticosteroid dose may need to be increased.
Indomethacin, aspirin: increased risk of GI distress and bleeding. Give together cautiously.

NURSING CONSIDERATIONS
• Contraindicated in systemic fungal infections and alternate-day therapy. Use cautiously in patients with GI ulceration or renal disease, hypertension, osteoporosis, varicella, vaccinia, exanthema, diabetes mellitus, Cushing's syndrome, thromboembolic disorders, seizures, myasthenia gravis, metastatic cancer, congestive heart failure, tuberculosis, ocular herpes simplex, hypoalbuminemia, emotional instability, or psychotic tendencies.
• Gradually reduce drug dosage after long-term therapy. Tell patient not to discontinue drug abruptly.
• Titrate to lowest effective dose.
• Has little mineralocorticoid effect.
• Monitor patient's weight, blood pressure, serum electrolytes.
• May mask or exacerbate infections.
• Instruct patient to carry a card identifying his need for supplemental systemic glucocorticoids during stress.
• Give once-daily doses in the morning for better results and less toxicity.
• Teach patient signs of early adrenal insufficiency: fatigue, muscular weakness, joint pain, fever, anorexia, nausea, dyspnea, dizziness, fainting.

• Watch for depression or psychotic episodes with high-dose therapy.
• Patients with diabetes may need increased insulin; monitor blood glucose levels.
• Monitor growth in infants and children on long-term therapy.
• Unless contraindicated, give salt-restricted diet rich in potassium and protein. Potassium supplement may be needed.
• Watch for additional hypokalemia from diuretics and amphotericin B.
• Give P.O. dose with food when possible, especially if GI irritation occurs.
• Warn patients on long-term therapy about cushingoid symptoms.
• Immunizations may show decreased antibody response.

prednisolone
Cortalone, Delta-Cortef, Predoxine

prednisolone acetate
Savacort

prednisolone sodium phosphate
Hydeltrasol, PSP-I.V.

prednisolone tebutate
Hydeltra-TBA, Metalone-TBA
Pregnancy Category: B

MECHANISM OF ACTION
Decreases inflammation, mainly by stabilizing leukocyte lysosomal membranes. Also suppresses the immune response, stimulates bone marrow, and influences protein, fat, and carbohydrate metabolism.

INDICATIONS & DOSAGE
Severe inflammation or immunosuppression—
Adults: 2.5 to 15 mg P.O. b.i.d., t.i.d., or q.i.d.; 2 to 30 mg I.M. (acetate, phosphate), or I.V. (phosphate) q 12 hours; or 2 to 30 mg (phosphate)

into joints, lesions, and soft tissue; or 4 to 40 mg (tebutate) into joints and lesions; or 0.25 to 1 ml (acetate-phosphate suspension) into joints weekly, p.r.n.

ADVERSE REACTIONS
Most side effects of corticosteroids are dose- or duration-dependent.
CNS: *euphoria, insomnia,* psychotic behavior, pseudotumor cerebri.
CV: *congestive heart failure,* hypertension, edema.
EENT: cataracts, glaucoma.
GI: *peptic ulcer,* gastrointestinal irritation, increased appetite.
Metabolic: *possible hypokalemia, hyperglycemia and carbohydrate intolerance,* growth suppression in children.
Skin: delayed wound healing, acne, various skin eruptions.
Other: muscle weakness, pancreatitis, hirsutism, susceptibility to infections. Acute adrenal insufficiency may occur with increased stress (infection, surgery, trauma) or abrupt withdrawal after long-term therapy. *Withdrawal symptoms:* rebound inflammation, fatigue, weakness, arthralgia, fever, dizziness, lethargy, depression, fainting, orthostatic hypotension, dyspnea, anorexia, hypoglycemia. *Sudden withdrawal may be fatal.*

INTERACTIONS
Barbiturates, phenytoin, rifampin: decreased corticosteroid effect. Corticosteroid dose may need to be increased.
Indomethacin, aspirin: increased risk of GI distress and bleeding. Give together cautiously.

NURSING CONSIDERATIONS
• Contraindicated in systemic fungal infections. Use cautiously in patients with GI ulceration or renal disease, hypertension, osteoporosis, varicella, vaccinia, exanthema, diabetes mellitus, Cushing's syndrome, thromboembolic disorders, seizures, myasthenia gravis, metastatic cancer, congestive heart failure, tuberculosis, ocular herpes simplex, hypoalbuminemia, emotional instability, or psychotic tendencies.
• Gradually reduce drug dosage after long-term therapy. Tell patient not to discontinue drug abruptly or without doctor's consent.
• Always titrate to lowest effective dose.
• Glucocorticoid with slight mineralocorticoid action.
• Prednisolone salts (acetate, sodium phosphate, and tebutate) are used parenterally less often than other corticosteroids that have more potent anti-inflammatory action.
• May use for alternate-day therapy.
• Monitor patient's weight, blood pressure, serum electrolytes.
• May mask or exacerbate infections. Tell patient to report slow healing.
• Instruct patient to carry a card identifying his need for supplemental systemic glucocorticoids during stress.
• Teach patient signs of early adrenal insufficiency: fatigue, muscular weakness, joint pain, fever, anorexia, nausea, dyspnea, dizziness, fainting.
• Watch for depression or psychotic episodes, especially in high-dose therapy.
• Patients with diabetes may need increased insulin; monitor blood glucose levels.
• Give I.M. injection deep into gluteal muscle. Avoid subcutaneous injection, as atrophy and sterile abscesses may occur.
• Unless contraindicated, give salt-restricted diet rich in potassium and protein. Potassium supplement may be needed.
• Give P.O. dose with food when possible, to reduce GI irritation.
• Warn patients on long-term therapy about cushingoid symptoms.
• Acetate form not for I.V. use.
• Watch for additional potassium de-

pletion from diuretics and amphotericin B.
• Immunizations may show decreased antibody response.

prednisone
Colisone♦♦, Deltasone♦, Liquid Pred, Meticorten, Orasone, Prednicen-M, SK-Prednisone, Wojtab
Pregnancy Category: B

MECHANISM OF ACTION
Decreases inflammation, mainly by stabilizing leukocyte lysosomal membranes. Also suppresses the immune response, stimulates bone marrow, and influences protein, fat, and carbohydrate metabolism.

INDICATIONS & DOSAGE
Severe inflammation or immunosuppression—
Adults: 2.5 to 15 mg P.O. b.i.d., t.i.d., or q.i.d. Maintenance dose given once daily or every other day. Dosage must be individualized.
Children: 0.14 to 2 mg/kg daily P.O. divided q.i.d.
Acute exacerbations of multiple sclerosis—
Adults: 200 mg P.O. per day for 1 week, then 80 mg every other day for 1 month.

ADVERSE REACTIONS
Most side effects of corticosteroids are dose- or duration-dependent.
CNS: *euphoria, insomnia,* psychotic behavior, pseudotumor cerebri.
CV: *congestive heart failure,* hypertension, edema.
EENT: cataracts, glaucoma.
GI: *peptic ulcer,* gastrointestinal irritation, increased appetite.
Metabolic: *possible hypokalemia, hyperglycemia and carbohydrate intolerance,* growth suppression in children.
Skin: delayed wound healing, acne, various skin eruptions.

Other: muscle weakness, pancreatitis, hirsutism, susceptibility to infections. Acute adrenal insufficiency may occur with increased stress (infection, surgery, trauma) or abrupt withdrawal after long-term therapy.
Withdrawal symptoms: rebound inflammation, fatigue, weakness, arthralgia, fever, dizziness, lethargy, depression, fainting, orthostatic hypotension, dyspnea, anorexia, hypoglycemia. *Sudden withdrawal may be fatal.*

INTERACTIONS
Barbiturates, phenytoin, rifampin: decreased corticosteroid effect. Corticosteroid dose may need to be increased.
Indomethacin, aspirin: increased risk of GI distress and bleeding. Give together cautiously.

NURSING CONSIDERATIONS
• Contraindicated in systemic fungal infections. Use cautiously in patients with GI ulceration or renal disease, hypertension, osteoporosis, varicella, vaccinia, exanthema, diabetes mellitus, Cushing's syndrome, thromboembolic disorders, seizures, myasthenia gravis, metastatic cancer, congestive heart failure, tuberculosis, ocular herpes simplex, hypoalbuminemia, emotional instability, or psychotic tendencies.
• Gradually reduce drug dosage after long-term therapy. Tell patient not to discontinue drug abruptly or without doctor's consent.
• Always titrate to lowest effective dose.
• Monitor patient's blood pressure, sleep patterns, serum potassium levels.
• Weigh patient daily; report sudden weight gain to doctor.
• May mask or exacerbate infections. Tell patient to report slow healing.
• Instruct patient to carry a card identifying his need for supplemental sys-

---

Italicized side effects are common or life-threatening.
*Liquid form contains alcohol.   **May contain tartrazine.

temic glucocorticoids during stress.
• Give once-daily doses in the morning for better results and less toxicity.
• Teach patient signs of early adrenal insufficiency: fatigue, muscular weakness, joint pain, fever, anorexia, nausea, dyspnea, dizziness, fainting.
• Watch for depression or psychotic episodes, especially in high-dose therapy.
• Patients with diabetes may need increased insulin; monitor blood glucose levels.
• Monitor growth in infants and children on long-term therapy.
• Give salt-restricted diet rich in potassium and protein. Potassium supplement may be needed.
• Unless contraindicated, give P.O. dose with food when possible, to reduce GI irritation.
• May use for alternate-day therapy.
• Watch for additional potassium depletion from diuretics and amphotericin B.
• Warn patients on long-term therapy about cushingoid symptoms.
• Immunizations may show decreased antibody response.
• Now available in oral solution form.

triamcinolone
Aristocort♦, Kenacort♦**, Spencort, Tricilone

triamcinolone acetonide
Azmacort, Kenalog♦

triamcinolone diacetate
Amcort, Aristocort Forte Parenteral, Cenocort Forte, Tracilon, Triam-Forte, Tristoject

triamcinolone hexacetonide
Aristospan♦
Pregnancy Category: C

MECHANISM OF ACTION
Decreases inflammation, mainly by stabilizing leukocyte lysosomal membranes. Also suppresses the immune response, stimulates bone marrow, and influences protein, fat, and carbohydrate metabolism.

INDICATIONS & DOSAGE
Severe inflammation or immunosuppression—
Adults: 4 to 48 mg P.O. daily divided b.i.d., t.i.d., or q.i.d., or 40 mg I.M. (diacetate or acetonide) weekly; or 5 to 48 mg (diacetate or acetonide) into lesions; or 2 to 40 mg (diacetate or acetonide) into joints and soft tissue; or up to 0.5 mg (hexacetonide) per square inch of affected skin intralesional; or 2 to 20 mg (hexacetonide) intra-articular or intrasynovial into soft tissue or into joint or lesion. Often, a local anesthetic is injected into the joint with triamcinolone.
Steroid-dependent asthma—
Adults: 2 inhalations t.i.d. to q.i.d. Maximum 16 inhalations daily.
Children 6 to 12 years: 1 to 2 inhalations t.i.d. to q.i.d. Maximum 12 inhalations daily.

ADVERSE REACTIONS
Systemic:
Most adverse reactions of corticosteroids are dose- or duration-dependent.
CNS: *euphoria, insomnia,* psychotic behavior, pseudotumor cerebri.
CV: *congestive heart failure,* hypertension, edema.
EENT: cataracts, glaucoma.
GI: *peptic ulcer,* gastrointestinal irritation, increased appetite.
Metabolic: *possible hypokalemia, hyperglycemia and carbohydrate intolerance,* growth suppression in children.
Skin: delayed wound healing, acne, various skin eruptions.
Other: muscle weakness, pancreatitis, hirsutism, susceptibility to infections. Acute adrenal insufficiency may occur with increased stress (infection, surgery, trauma) or abrupt withdrawal after long-term therapy.

Withdrawal symptoms: rebound inflammation, fatigue, weakness, arthralgia, fever, dizziness, lethargy, depression, fainting, orthostatic hypotension, dyspnea, anorexia, hypoglycemia. *Sudden withdrawal may be fatal.*
Inhalation:
EENT: hoarseness, fungal infections of mouth and throat.
GI: dry mouth.

INTERACTIONS
Systemic:
Barbiturates, phenytoin, rifampin: decreased corticosteroid effect. Corticosteroid dose may need to be increased.
Indomethacin, aspirin: increased risk of GI distress and bleeding. Give together cautiously.

NURSING CONSIDERATIONS
Systemic:
• Contraindicated in systemic fungal infections. Use cautiously in patients with GI ulceration or renal disease, hypertension, osteoporosis, varicella, vaccinia, exanthema, diabetes mellitus, Cushing's syndrome, thromboembolic disorders, seizures, myasthenia gravis, metastatic cancer, congestive heart failure, tuberculosis, ocular herpes simplex, hypoalbuminemia, emotional instability, or psychotic tendencies.
• Gradually reduce drug dosage after long-term therapy. Tell patient not to discontinue drug abruptly or without doctor's consent.
• Always titrate to lowest effective dose.
• Monitor patient's weight, blood pressure, serum electrolytes.
• May mask or exacerbate infections. Tell patient to report slow healing.
• Instruct patient to carry a card identifying his need for supplemental systemic glucocorticoids during stress.
• Give once-daily doses in the morning for better results and less toxicity.

• Teach patient signs of early adrenal insufficiency: fatigue, muscular weakness, joint pain, fever, anorexia, nausea, dyspnea, dizziness, fainting.
• Watch for depression or psychotic episodes, especially in high-dose therapy.
• Patients with diabetes may need increased insulin; monitor blood glucose levels.
• Give I.M. injection deep into gluteal muscle.
• Unless contraindicated, give salt-restricted diet rich in potassium and protein. Potassium supplement may be needed. Watch for additional potassium depletion from diuretics and amphotericin B.
• Give P.O. dose with food when possible to reduce GI irritation.
• Don't use diluents that contain preservatives. Flocculation may occur.
• Warn patients on long-term therapy about cushingoid symptoms.
• Immunizations may show decreased antibody response.
• Not for alternate-day therapy.
Inhalation:
• Contraindicated in status asthmaticus. Not for asthma controlled by bronchodilators or other noncorticosteroids alone, or for nonasthmatic bronchial diseases.
• Oral therapy should be tapered slowly.
• Instruct patient to carry a card indicating his need for supplemental systemic glucocorticoids during stress.
• Patient requiring bronchodilator should use it several minutes before triamcinolone.
• Allow 1 minute to elapse before repeat inhalations. Hold breath for a few seconds to enhance action of drug.
• Inform patient that triamcinolone doesn't provide relief for emergency asthma attack.
• Instruct patient to contact doctor if he notices a decreased response. Dose may have to be adjusted. Patient

shouldn't exceed recommended dose on his own.
• Check mucous membranes frequently for signs of fungal infection. Prevent such infections by following inhalations with glass of water.
• Tell patient to keep inhaler clean and unobstructed. Wash with warm water and dry thoroughly after use.

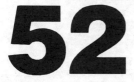

Androgens and anabolic steroids

danazol
ethylestrenol
fluoxymesterone
methyltestosterone
nandrolone decanoate
nandrolone phenpropionate
oxandrolone
oxymetholone
stanozolol
testosterone
testosterone cypionate
testosterone enanthate
testosterone propionate

COMBINATION PRODUCTS
DELADUMONE INJECTION (oil)♦: testosterone enanthate 90 mg, estradiol valerate 4 mg, and chlorobutanol 0.5%.
DEPO-TESTADIOL (oil): testosterone cypionate 50 mg, estradiol cypionate 2 mg, and chlorobutanol 0.5%.
DITATE: estradiol valerate 4 mg, and testosterone enanthate 90 mg.
DITATE-DS: estradiol valerate 8 mg, and testosterone enanthate 180 mg.
ESTRATEST H.S.: esterified estrogens 0.625 mg, and methyltestosterone 1.25 mg.
FORMATRIX: conjugated estrogens 1.25 mg, methyltestosterone 10 mg, and ascorbic acid 400 mg.
LACTOSTAT (oil)♦♦: testosterone enanthate benzilic acid hydrazone 300 mg, estradiol dienanthate 15 mg, and estradiol benzoate 6 mg.
MEDIATRIC: conjugated estrogens 0.25 mg, methyltestosterone 2.5 mg, methamphetamine HCl 1 mg, vitamin C 100 mg, thiamine 10 mg, vitamin B_{12} 2.5 mcg, ferrous sulfate 30 mg,

vitamin B_2 5 mg, vitamin B_6 3 mg, and nicotinamide 50 mg.
PREMARIN WITH METHYLTESTOSTERONE♦: conjugated estrogens 0.625 mg and methyltestosterone 5 mg.
TESTOJECT-E.P.: testosterone enanthate 200 mg, testosterone propionate 25 mg, and chlorobutanol 0.5%.

---

danazol
Cyclomen♦♦, Danocrine
Pregnancy Category: C

MECHANISM OF ACTION
Gonadotropin inhibitor that suppresses the pituitary-ovarian axis. Also acts on estrogen receptors to inhibit estrogenic effects.

INDICATIONS & DOSAGE
Endometriosis—
Women: 400 mg P.O. b.i.d. uninterrupted for 3 to 6 months; may continue for 9 months.
Fibrocystic breast disease—
Women: 100 to 400 mg P.O. daily in 2 divided doses uninterrupted for 2 to 6 months.
Prevention of hereditary angioedema—
Adults: 200 mg P.O. 2 to 3 times a day, continued until favorable response is achieved. Then dosage should be decreased by half at 1- to 3-month intervals.

ADVERSE REACTIONS
Androgenic: acne, edema, *weight gain, hirsutism,* hoarseness, clitoral enlargement, *decrease in breast size,*

Italicized side effects are common or life-threatening.
*Liquid form contains alcohol.   **May contain tartrazine.

changes in libido, male-pattern baldness, *oiliness of skin or hair*.
Blood: thrombocytopenia.
CNS: dizziness, headache, sleep disorders, fatigue, tremor, irritability, excitation, lethargy, mental depression, chills, paresthesias.
CV: elevated blood pressure.
EENT: visual disturbances.
GI: gastric irritation, nausea, vomiting, diarrhea, constipation, change in appetite.
GU: hematuria.
Hepatic: reversible jaundice.
Hypoestrogenic: flushing; sweating; vaginitis, including itching, dryness, burning, and vaginal bleeding; nervousness, emotional lability, menstrual irregularities.
Other: muscle cramps or spasms.

INTERACTIONS
None significant.

NURSING CONSIDERATIONS
• Contraindicated in patients with undiagnosed abnormal genital bleeding; impaired renal, cardiac, or hepatic function. Use cautiously in patients with epilepsy or migraine headache.
• Use with diet high in calories and protein unless contraindicated.
• Monitor closely for signs of virilization. Some androgenic effects, such as deepening of voice, may not be reversible upon discontinuation of drug.
• Advise patient who is taking danazol for fibrocystic disease to examine breasts regularly. If breast nodule enlarges during treatment, tell patient to call doctor immediately.
• Instruct patient to wear cotton underwear only.
• Washing after intercourse is recommended to decrease the risk of vaginitis.
• Has been used investigationally with impressive results in the treatment of hemophilia and Christmas disease.

ethylestrenol
Maxibolin♦*
Pregnancy Category: X

MECHANISM OF ACTION
Anabolic steroid that promotes tissue-building processes and reverses catabolism. Also stimulates erythropoiesis.

INDICATIONS & DOSAGE
Promote weight gain and combat tissue depletion, refractory anemias, catabolic effects of corticosteroid therapy, osteoporosis, prolonged immobilization, and debilitated states—
Adults: 4 to 8 mg P.O. daily, reduced to minimum levels at first evidence of clinical response.
Children: 1 to 3 mg P.O. daily; highly individualized.
A single course of therapy in both adults and children should not exceed 6 weeks; may be reinstituted after 4-week interval.

ADVERSE REACTIONS
Androgenic: in females—*acne, edema, oily skin, weight gain, hirsutism, hoarseness,* clitoral enlargement, changes in libido. In males—prepubertal: premature epiphyseal closure, acne, priapism, growth of body and facial hair, phallic enlargement; postpubertal: testicular atrophy, oligospermia, decreased ejaculatory volume, impotence, gynecomastia, epididymitis.
CV: edema.
GI: gastroenteritis, nausea, vomiting, diarrhea, constipation, change in appetite.
GU: bladder irritability.
Hepatic: reversible jaundice, hepatotoxicity.
Hypoestrogenic: in females—flushing; sweating; vaginitis with itching, drying, burning, or bleeding; menstrual irregularities.
Other: hypercalcemia.

INTERACTIONS
None significant.

NURSING CONSIDERATIONS
• Contraindicated in patients with prostatic hypertrophy with obstruction; carcinoma of male breast; hypercalcemia; prostatic cancer; cardiac, hepatic, or renal decompensation; nephrosis; and in premature infants. Use cautiously in prepubertal males; patients with diabetes or coronary disease; patients taking ACTH, corticosteroids, or anticoagulants.
• Hypercalcemia symptoms may be difficult to distinguish from symptoms of condition being treated unless anticipated and thought of as a symptom cluster. Hypercalcemia is particularly likely to occur in patients with metastatic breast cancer and may indicate bone metastases.
• Tell females to report menstrual irregularities; therapy should be discontinued pending etiologic determination.
• Watch for signs of virilization; may be irreversible despite prompt discontinuation of therapy. Doctor must decide if benefits outweigh effects.
• Closely monitor boys under 7 years for precocious development of male sexual characteristics.
• In children: therapy should be preceded by X-ray of wrist bones to establish level of bone maturation. During treatment, bone maturation may proceed more rapidly than linear growth; dosage should be intermittent and X-rays taken periodically.
• Edema is generally controllable with salt restriction and/or diuretics. Monitor weight routinely.
• Watch for symptoms of jaundice. Dose adjustment may reverse condition. If liver function tests are abnormal, discontinue therapy.
• Observe patient on concomitant anticoagulant therapy for ecchymotic areas, petechiae, or abnormal bleeding. Monitor prothrombin time.

• Watch for symptoms of hypoglycemia in patients with diabetes. Dosage of antidiabetic drug may need adjustment.
• Use with diet high in calories and protein unless contraindicated. Give small, frequent feedings.
• Take with food or meals if GI upset occurs.
• Anabolic steroids may alter many laboratory studies during therapy and for 2 to 3 weeks after therapy is stopped.
• Involve the patient, family members, and a dietitian in developing a dietary regimen suitable to the anorexic or debilitated patient.

---

fluoxymesterone
Android-F, Halotestin◆**, Oratestryl
Pregnancy Category: X

MECHANISM OF ACTION
Stimulates target tissues to develop normally in androgen-deficient males.

INDICATIONS & DOSAGE
Hypogonadism and impotence due to testicular deficiency—
Adults: 2 to 10 mg P.O. daily.
Palliation of breast cancer in women—
15 to 30 mg P.O. daily in divided doses. All dosages should be individualized and reduced to minimum when effect is noted.
Postpartum breast engorgement—
2.5 mg P.O. followed by 5 to 10 mg daily for 5 days.

ADVERSE REACTIONS
Androgenic: in females—*acne, edema, oily skin, weight gain, hirsutism, hoarseness,* clitoral enlargement, change in libido. In males—prepubertal: premature epiphyseal closure, acne, priapism, growth of body and facial hair, phallic enlargement; postpubertal: testicular atrophy, oligospermia, decreased ejaculatory volume, impotence, gynecomastia, epi-

---

Italicized side effects are common or life-threatening.
*Liquid form contains alcohol.   **May contain tartrazine.

didymitis.

CV: edema.

GI: gastroenteritis, nausea, vomiting, constipation, change in appetite, diarrhea.

GU: bladder irritability.

Hepatic: reversible jaundice.

Hypoestrogenic: in females—flushing; sweating; vaginitis with itching, drying, burning, or bleeding; menstrual irregularities; emotional lability.

Other: hypercalcemia.

INTERACTIONS

None significant.

NURSING CONSIDERATIONS

• Contraindicated in patients with prostatic hypertrophy with obstruction; carcinoma of male breast; prostatic cancer; cardiac, hepatic, or renal decompensation; nephrosis; hypercalcemia; and in premature infants. Use cautiously in prepubertal males; patients with diabetes or coronary disease; and patients taking ACTH, corticosteroids, or anticoagulants.

• Hypercalcemia symptoms may be difficult to distinguish from symptoms associated with condition being treated unless anticipated and thought of as a symptom cluster. Hypercalcemia is particularly likely to occur in patients with metastatic breast cancer and may indicate bone metastases.

• Explain to patient on drug for palliation of breast cancer that virilization usually occurs at dosage used. Give emotional support. Tell patient to report androgenic effects immediately. Stopping drug will prevent further androgenic changes but will probably not reverse those already existing.

• When used in breast cancer, subjective effects may not be seen for about 1 month; objective symptoms not for 3 months.

• Tell females to report menstrual irregularities; therapy should be dis-

continued pending etiologic determination.

• Edema is generally controllable with salt restriction and/or diuretics. Monitor weight routinely.

• Watch for symptoms of jaundice. Dose adjustment may reverse condition. If liver function tests are abnormal, therapy should be discontinued.

• Observe patient on concomitant anticoagulant therapy for ecchymotic areas, petechiae, or abnormal bleeding. Monitor prothrombin time.

• Watch for symptoms of hypoglycemia in patients with diabetes. Dosage of antidiabetic drug may need adjustment.

• Use with diet high in calories and protein unless contraindicated. Give small, frequent feedings.

• Take with food or meals if GI upset occurs.

methyltestosterone

Android-5, Android-10,
Metandren♦**, Oreton-Methyl,
Testred, Virilon
Pregnancy Category: X

MECHANISM OF ACTION

Stimulates target tissues to develop normally in androgen-deficient males.

INDICATIONS & DOSAGE

Adults:

Breast engorgement of nonnursing mothers—80 mg P.O. daily, or 40 mg buccal daily for 3 to 5 days.

Breast cancer in women 1 to 5 years postmenopausal—200 mg P.O. daily; or 100 mg buccal daily.

Eunuchoidism and eunuchism, male climacteric symptoms—10 to 40 mg P.O. daily; or 5 to 20 mg buccal daily.

Postpubertal cryptorchidism—30 mg P.O. daily; or 15 mg buccal daily.

ADVERSE REACTIONS

Androgenic: in females—*acne, edema, oily skin, weight gain, hirsut-*

---

ism, hoarseness, clitoral enlargement, changes in libido. In males—prepubertal: premature epiphyseal closure, acne, priapism, growth of body and facial hair, phallic enlargement; postpubertal: testicular atrophy, oligospermia, decreased ejaculatory volume, impotence, gynecomastia, epididymitis.

CV: edema.
GI: gastroenteritis, constipation, nausea, vomiting, diarrhea, change in appetite.
GU: bladder irritability.
Hepatic: reversible jaundice.
Hypoestrogenic: in females—flushing; sweating; vaginitis with itching, drying, burning, or bleeding; menstrual irregularities.
Local: irritation of oral mucosa with buccal administration.
Other: hypercalcemia.

INTERACTIONS
None significant.

NURSING CONSIDERATIONS
• Contraindicated in women of childbearing potential (possible masculinization of female infant); in elderly, asthenic males who may react adversely to androgen overstimulation; in hypercalcemia; cardiac, hepatic, or renal decompensation; prostatic or breast cancer in males; benign prostatic hypertrophy with obstruction; conditions aggravated by fluid retention; hypertension; and in premature infants. Use cautiously in myocardial infarction or coronary artery disease.
• Treatment of breast cancer usually restricted to patients 1 to 5 years postmenopausal.
• Edema is generally controllable with salt restriction and/or diuretics.
• Periodic serum cholesterol and calcium determinations, and cardiac and liver function tests recommended. Watch closely for jaundice.
• In metastatic breast cancer, hypercalcemia may indicate progression of bone metastases. Report signs of hypercalcemia.
• Therapeutic response in breast cancer is usually apparent within 3 months. Therapy should be stopped if signs of disease progression appear.
• Enhances hypoglycemia; teach patient signs of hypoglycemia, and instruct him to report immediately if they occur.
• Watch for ecchymoses, petechiae, and abnormal bleeding in patients receiving concomitant anticoagulants.
• Promptly report signs of virilization in females.
• Use with diet high in calories and protein unless contraindicated. Give small, frequent feedings.
• Buccal tablets twice as potent as oral tablets. Tell patient to avoid eating, drinking, chewing, or smoking while buccal tablet is in place, and that tablet is not to be swallowed. Place in upper or lower buccal pouch between cheek and gum. Tablet requires 30 to 60 minutes to dissolve. Instruct patient to change tablet absorption site with each dose to minimize risk of buccal irritation.
• Erroneously thought to enhance athletic ability.

nandrolone decanoate
Androlone-D 50, Deca-Durabolin♦, Hybolin Decanoate

nandrolone phenpropionate
Anabolin, Anorolone, Durabolin♦, Hybolin Improved, Nandrobolic
Pregnancy Category: X

MECHANISM OF ACTION
Anabolic steroid that promotes tissue-building processes and reverses catabolism. Also stimulates erythropoiesis.

INDICATIONS & DOSAGE
Severe debility or disease states, refractory anemias (decanoate)—
Adults: 100 to 200 mg I.M. weekly.

Italicized side effects are common or life-threatening.
*Liquid form contains alcohol.   **May contain tartrazine.

Therapy should be intermittent.
Tissue-building (decanoate)—
Adults: 50 to 100 mg I.M. q 3 to 4
weeks.
Children 2 to 13 years: 25 to 50 mg
I.M. q 3 to 4 weeks.
*Control of metastatic breast cancer
(phenpropionate)—*
Adults: 25 to 50 mg I.M. weekly.
Children 2 to 13 years: 12.5 to 25
mg I.M. every 2 to 4 weeks.

ADVERSE REACTIONS
Androgenic: in females—*acne,
edema, oily skin, weight gain, hirsutism, hoarseness,* clitoral enlargement,
decreased or increased libido. In
males—prepubertal: premature
epiphyseal closure, acne, priapism,
growth of body and facial hair, phallic enlargement; postpubertal: testicular atrophy, oligospermia, decreased
ejaculatory volume, impotence, gynecomastia, epididymitis.
CV: edema.
GI: gastroenteritis, nausea, vomiting,
diarrhea, change in appetite.
GU: bladder irritability.
Hepatic: reversible jaundice, hepatotoxicity.
Hypoestrogenic: in females—flushing; sweating; vaginitis with itching,
drying, burning, or bleeding; menstrual irregularities with large doses.
Local: pain at injection site, induration.
Other: hypercalcemia, hypercalciuria.

INTERACTIONS
None significant.

NURSING CONSIDERATIONS
• Contraindicated in patients with
prostatic hypertrophy with obstruction; male breast and prostatic cancer;
cardiac, hepatic, or renal decompensation; nephrosis; and in premature
infants. Use cautiously in prepubertal
males; patients with diabetes or coronary disease; patients taking ACTH,

corticosteroids, or anticoagulants.
• Inject drug deep I.M., preferably
into upper outer quadrant of gluteal
muscle in adults.
• Monitor serum cholesterol in cardiac patients.
• Hypercalcemia is most likely to occur in patients with mammary carcinoma; these patients should have
quantitative urinary and serum calcium level determinations.
• Tell females to report menstrual irregularities; therapy should be discontinued pending etiologic determination.
• Watch for signs of virilization; they
may be irreversible despite prompt
discontinuation of therapy.
• Closely observe boys under 7 years
for precocious development of male
sexual characteristics.
• In children, therapy should be
preceded by X-ray of wrist bones to
establish level of bone maturation.
During treatment, bone maturation
may proceed more rapidly than linear
growth; dosage should be intermittent
and X-rays taken periodically.
• Edema is generally controllable
with salt restrictions and/or diuretics.
• Watch for symptoms of jaundice.
Dose adjustment may reverse condition. If liver function tests are abnormal, therapy should be discontinued.
• Observe patients receiving concomitant anticoagulant therapy for ecchymotic areas, petechiae, or abnormal
bleeding. Monitor prothrombin time.
• Watch for symptoms of hypoglycemia in patients with diabetes. Dosage
of antidiabetic drug may need adjustment.
• Use with diet high in calories and
protein unless contraindicated. Give
small, frequent feedings.
• Erroneously thought to enhance
athletic ability.
• Considered an adjunctive therapy.
• Anabolic steroids may alter many
laboratory studies during therapy and
for 2 to 3 weeks after therapy is

stopped.

oxandrolone
Anavar
Pregnancy Category: X

MECHANISM OF ACTION
Anabolic steroid that promotes tissue-building processes and reverses catabolism. Also stimulates erythropoiesis.

INDICATIONS & DOSAGE
To combat catabolic effects of corticosteroid therapy, osteoporosis, prolonged immobilization and debilitated states—
Adults: 2.5 mg P.O. b.i.d., t.i.d., or q.i.d.; up to 20 mg daily for 2 to 4 weeks.
Children: 0.25 mg/kg daily P.O. for 2 to 4 weeks.
Continuous therapy should not exceed 3 months.

ADVERSE REACTIONS
Androgenic: in females—*acne, edema, oily skin, weight gain, hirsutism, hoarseness,* clitoral enlargement, decreased or increased libido. In males—prepubertal: premature epiphyseal closure, acne, priapism, growth of body and facial hair, phallic enlargement; postpubertal: testicular atrophy, oligospermia, decreased ejaculatory volume, impotence, gynecomastia, epididymitis.
CV: edema.
GI: gastroenteritis, nausea, vomiting, constipation or diarrhea, change in appetite.
GU: bladder irritability.
Hepatic: reversible jaundice, hepatotoxicity.
Hypoestrogenic: in females—flushing; sweating; vaginitis with itching, drying, burning, or bleeding; menstrual irregularities.
Other: hypercalcemia.

INTERACTIONS
None significant.

NURSING CONSIDERATIONS
• Contraindicated in patients with prostatic hypertrophy with obstruction; prostatic and male breast cancer; cardiac, hepatic, or renal decompensation; nephrosis; and in premature infants. Use cautiously in prepubertal males; patients with diabetes or coronary disease; patients taking ACTH, corticosteroids, or anticoagulants.
• Hypercalcemia symptoms may be difficult to distinguish from symptoms of condition being treated unless anticipated and thought of as a cluster. Hypercalcemia most likely to occur with metastatic breast cancer and may indicate bone metastases.
• Tell females to report menstrual irregularities; therapy should be discontinued pending etiologic determination.
• Watch for signs of virilization; may be irreversible despite prompt discontinuation of therapy. Doctor must decide if benefits outweigh effects.
• Boys under 7 years should be closely observed for precocious development of male sexual characteristics.
• In children, therapy should be preceded by X-ray of wrist bones to establish level of bone maturation. During treatment, bone maturation may proceed more rapidly than linear growth; dosage should be intermittent and X-rays taken periodically.
• Edema is generally controllable with salt restriction and/or diuretics. Monitor weight routinely.
• Watch for symptoms of jaundice. Dose adjustment may reverse condition. Periodic liver function tests are recommended.
• Observe patient on concomitant anticoagulant therapy for ecchymotic areas, petechiae, or abnormal bleeding. Monitor prothrombin time.
• Watch for symptoms of hypoglyce-

Italicized side effects are common or life-threatening.
*Liquid form contains alcohol.   **May contain tartrazine.

mia in patients with diabetes. Change of dosage of antidiabetic drug may be required.
• Use with diet high in calories and protein unless contraindicated. Give small, frequent feedings.
• Take with food or meals if GI upset occurs.
• Erroneously thought to enhance athletic ability.
• Anabolic steroids may alter many laboratory studies during therapy and for 2 to 3 weeks after therapy is stopped.

oxymetholone
Adroyd, Anadrol-50, Anapolon 50♦♦
Pregnancy Category: X

MECHANISM OF ACTION
Anabolic steroid that promotes tissue-building processes and reverses catabolism. Also stimulates erythropoiesis.

INDICATIONS & DOSAGE
Aplastic anemia—
Adults and children: 1 to 5 mg/kg P.O. daily. Dose highly individualized; response not immediate. Trial of 3 to 6 months required.
Osteoporosis, catabolic conditions—
Adults: 5 to 15 mg P.O. daily, or up to 30 mg P.O. daily.
Children over 6 years: up to 10 mg P.O. daily.
Children under 6 years: 1.25 mg P.O. daily or up to q.i.d. Continuous therapy should not exceed 30 days in children; 90 days in any patient.

ADVERSE REACTIONS
Androgenic: in females—*acne, edema, oily skin, weight gain, hirsutism, hoarseness,* clitoral enlargement, decreased or increased libido, male-pattern hair loss. In males—prepubertal: premature epiphyseal closure, acne, priapism, growth of body and facial hair, phallic enlargement; post-pubertal: testicular atrophy, oligospermia, decreased ejaculatory volume, impotence, gynecomastia, epididymitis.
CV: edema.
GI: gastroenteritis, nausea, vomiting, constipation, diarrhea, change in appetite.
GU: bladder irritability.
Hepatic: reversible jaundice, hepatotoxicity.
Hypoestrogenic: in females—flushing; sweating; vaginitis with itching, drying, burning, or bleeding; menstrual irregularities.
Other: hypercalcemia.

INTERACTIONS
None significant.

NURSING CONSIDERATIONS
• Contraindicated in patients with prostatic hypertrophy with obstruction; prostatic and male breast cancer; cardiac, hepatic, or renal decompensation; nephrosis; and in premature infants. Use cautiously in prepubertal males; patients with diabetes or coronary diseases; patients taking ACTH, corticosteroids, or anticoagulants.
• Hypercalcemia symptoms may be difficult to distinguish from symptoms of condition being treated unless anticipated and thought of as a cluster. Hypercalcemia most likely to occur in metastatic breast cancer and may indicate bone metastases.
• Supportive treatment of anemias (transfusions, correction of iron, folic acid, vitamin B_{12}, or pyridoxine deficiency). Give 3 to 6 months for response.
• Effects in osteoporosis usually seen in 4 to 6 weeks.
• Tell females to report menstrual irregularities; therapy should be discontinued pending etiologic determination.
• Watch for signs of virilization; may be irreversible despite prompt stopping of therapy. Doctor must decide if

benefits outweigh effects.
• Boys under 7 years should be closely observed for precocious development of male sexual characteristics.
• In children, therapy should be preceded by X-ray of wrist bones to establish level of bone maturation. During treatment, bone maturation may proceed more rapidly than linear growth; dosage should be intermittent and X-rays taken periodically. Epiphyseal development may continue 6 months after stopping therapy.
• Edema is generally controllable with salt restriction and/or diuretics. Monitor weight routinely.
• Watch for symptoms of jaundice. Dose adjustment may reverse condition; if liver function tests are abnormal, therapy should be discontinued.
• Observe patient on concomitant anticoagulant therapy for ecchymotic areas, petechiae, or abnormal bleeding. Monitor prothrombin time.
• Watch for symptoms of hypoglycemia in patients with diabetes. Change of dosage in antidiabetic drug may be required.
• Use with diet high in calories and protein unless contraindicated. Give small, frequent feedings.
• Take with food or meals if GI upset occurs.
• Erroneously thought to enhance athletic ability.
• Anabolic steroids may alter many laboratory studies during therapy and for 2 to 3 weeks after therapy is stopped.
• Has also been used to prevent hereditary angioedema.

---

stanozolol
Winstrol♦
Pregnancy Category: X

MECHANISM OF ACTION
Anabolic steroid that promotes tissue-building processes and reverses catab-

olism. Also stimulates erythropoiesis.

INDICATIONS & DOSAGE
To increase hemoglobin in some cases of aplastic anemia—
Adults: 2 mg P.O. t.i.d.
Children 6 to 12 years: up to 2 mg P.O. t.i.d.
Children under 6 years: 1 mg P.O. b.i.d.
Therapy should be intermittent.
Prevention of hereditary angioedema—
Adults: 0.5 to 2 mg P.O. daily for 2 years.

ADVERSE REACTIONS
Androgenic: in females—*acne, edema, oily skin, weight gain, hirsutism, hoarseness,* clitoral enlargement, decreased or increased libido. In males— prepubertal: premature epiphyseal closure, acne, priapism, growth of body and facial hair, phallic enlargement; postpubertal: testicular atrophy, oligospermia, decreased ejaculatory volume, impotence, gynecomastia, epididymitis.
CV: edema.
GI: gastroenteritis, nausea, vomiting, constipation, diarrhea, change in appetite.
GU: bladder irritability.
Hepatic: reversible jaundice, hepatotoxicity.
Hypoestrogenic: in females—flushing; sweating; vaginitis with itching, drying, burning or bleeding; menstrual irregularities.
Other: hypercalcemia.

INTERACTIONS
None significant.

NURSING CONSIDERATIONS
• Contraindicated in patients with prostatic hypertrophy with obstruction; prostatic and male breast cancer; cardiac, hepatic, or renal decompensation; nephrosis; and in premature infants. Use cautiously in prepubertal

---

Italicized side effects are common or life-threatening.
*Liquid form contains alcohol.   **May contain tartrazine.

males; patients with diabetes or coronary disease; patients taking ACTH, corticosteroids, or anticoagulants.
• Hypercalcemia symptoms may be difficult to distinguish from symptoms of condition being treated unless anticipated and thought of as a cluster. Hypercalcemia most likely to occur in metastatic breast cancer and may indicate bone metastases.
• Tell females to report menstrual irregularities; therapy should be discontinued pending etiologic determination.
• Smaller dose (2 mg b.i.d.) is used in females to avoid virilization. Watch for these side effects; may be irreversible despite prompt stopping of therapy. Doctor must decide if benefits outweigh effects.
• Boys under 7 years should be closely observed for precocious development of male sexual characteristics.
• In children, therapy should be preceded by X-ray of wrist bones to establish level of bone maturation. During treatment, bone maturation may proceed more rapidly than linear growth; dosage should be intermittent and X-rays taken periodically.
• Edema is generally controllable with salt restriction and/or diuretics. Monitor weight routinely.
• Watch for symptoms of jaundice. Dose adjustment may reverse condition; check liver function tests regularly. If abnormal, therapy should be discontinued.
• Observe patient on concomitant anticoagulant therapy for ecchymotic areas, petechiae, or abnormal bleeding. Monitor prothrombin time.
• Watch for symptoms of hypoglycemia in patients with diabetes. Change of dosage of antidiabetic drug may be required.
• Use with diet high in calories and protein unless contraindicated. Give small, frequent feedings.
• Administer before or with meals to minimize GI distress.
• Monitor serum cholesterol in cardiac patients.
• Erroneously thought to enhance athletic ability.
• Anabolic steroids may alter many laboratory studies during therapy and for 2 to 3 weeks after therapy is stopped.

---

testosterone

Histerone, Malogen♦, Testoject
Pregnancy Category: X

MECHANISM OF ACTION
Stimulates target tissues to develop normally in androgen-deficient males.

INDICATIONS & DOSAGE
Eunuchoidism, eunuchism, male climacteric symptoms—
Adults: 10 to 25 mg I.M. 2 to 5 times weekly.
Breast engorgement of nonnursing mothers—
25 to 50 mg I.M. daily for 3 to 4 days, starting at delivery.
Breast cancer in women 1 to 5 years postmenopausal—
100 mg I.M. 3 times weekly as long as improvement maintained.

ADVERSE REACTIONS
Androgenic: in females—*acne, edema, oily skin, weight gain, hirsutism, hoarseness,* clitoral enlargement, decreased or increased libido. In males—prepubertal: premature epiphyseal closure, acne, priapism, growth of body and facial hair, phallic enlargement; postpubertal: testicular atrophy, oligospermia, decreased ejaculatory volume, impotence, gynecomastia, epididymitis.
CV: edema.
GI: gastroenteritis, nausea, vomiting, constipation, diarrhea, change in appetite.
GU: bladder irritability.
Hepatic: reversible jaundice.

Unmarked trade names available in the United States only.
♦Also available in Canada.   ♦♦Available in Canada only.

Hypoestrogenic: in females—flushing; sweating; vaginitis with itching, drying, burning, or bleeding; menstrual irregularities.
Local: pain at injection site, induration, irritation and sloughing with pellet implantation, edema.
Other: hypercalcemia.

INTERACTIONS
None significant.

NURSING CONSIDERATIONS
• Contraindicated in women of childbearing potential (possible masculinization of female infant); in elderly, asthenic males who may react adversely to androgen overstimulation; in hypercalcemia; cardiac, hepatic, or renal decompensation; prostatic or breast cancer in males; benign prostatic hypertrophy with obstruction; conditions aggravated by fluid retention; hypertension; and in premature infants. Use cautiously in patients with myocardial infarction or coronary artery disease, and in prepubertal males.
• Periodic liver function tests should be performed.
• In metastatic breast cancer, hypercalcemia usually indicates progression of bone metastases. Report signs of hypercalcemia.
• Therapeutic response in breast cancer is usually apparent within 3 months. Stop therapy if signs of disease progression appear.
• Enhances hypoglycemia; tell patient to report signs of hyperinsulinism.
• Instruct males to report priapism, reduced ejaculatory volume, and gynecomastia. Withdraw drug if these occur.
• Report signs of virilization in females; reevaluate treatment.
• Monitor prepubertal males by X-ray for rate of bone maturation.
• Edema is generally controllable with salt restriction and/or diuretics. Monitor weight routinely.

• Use with diet high in calories and protein unless contraindicated. Give small, frequent feedings.
• Store I.M. preparations at room temperature. If crystals appear, warming and shaking the bottle will usually disperse them.
• Inject deep into upper outer quadrant of gluteal muscle.
• Watch for ecchymotic areas, petechiae, or abnormal bleeding in patients on concomitant anticoagulant therapy. Monitor prothrombin time.
• Many laboratory studies may be altered during therapy and for 2 to 3 weeks after therapy is stopped.

---

testosterone cypionate
Andro-Cyp, Andronate, Depotest, Depo-Test, Depo-Testosterone♦, Duratest

testosterone enanthate
Android-T LA, Andro-LA, Andryl, Delatestryl♦, Everone, Malogex♦♦

testosterone propionate
Androlan, Androlin, Testex
Pregnancy Category: X

MECHANISM OF ACTION
Stimulates target tissues to develop normally in androgen-deficient males.

INDICATIONS & DOSAGE
Eunuchism, eunuchoidism, deficiency after castration and male climacteric—
Adults: 200 to 400 mg (cypionate or enanthate) I.M. q 4 weeks.
Oligospermia—
Adults: 100 to 200 mg (cypionate or enanthate) I.M. q 4 to 6 weeks for development and maintenance of testicular function.
Eunuchism and eunuchoidism, male climacteric, impotence—
Adults: 10 to 25 mg (propionate) I.M. 2 to 4 times weekly.
Metastatic breast cancer in women—

Italicized side effects are common or life-threatening.
*Liquid form contains alcohol.   **May contain tartrazine.

50 to 100 mg (propionate) I.M. 3 times weekly. 200 to 400 mg (cypionate or enanthate) I.M. every 2 to 4 weeks.
Postmenopausal or senile osteoporosis—
Adults: 200 to 400 mg (enanthate) I.M. every 4 weeks.

ADVERSE REACTIONS
Androgenic: in females—*acne, edema, oily skin, weight gain, hirsutism, hoarseness,* clitoral enlargement, changes in libido. In males—prepubertal: premature epiphyseal closure, acne, priapism, growth of body and facial hair, phallic enlargement; postpubertal: testicular atrophy, oligospermia, decreased ejaculatory volume, impotence, gynecomastia, epididymitis.
CV: edema.
GI: gastroenteritis, nausea, vomiting, constipation, diarrhea, change in appetite.
GU: bladder irritability.
Hepatic: reversible jaundice.
Local: pain at injection site, induration, postinjection furunculosis.
Other: hypercalcemia.

INTERACTIONS
None significant.

NURSING CONSIDERATIONS
• Contraindicated in women of childbearing potential (possible masculinization of female infant); in patients with hypercalcemia; cardiac, hepatic, or renal decompensation; prostatic or breast cancer in males; benign prostatic hypertrophy with obstruction; conditions aggravated by fluid retention; hypertension; elderly, asthenic males who may react adversely to androgen overstimulation; and in premature infants. Use cautiously in patients with myocardial infarction or coronary artery disease, and in prepubertal males.
• Periodic liver function tests should be performed.
• In metastatic breast cancer, hypercalcemia usually indicates progression of bone metastases. Report signs of hypercalcemia.
• Response in breast cancer is usually apparent within 3 months. Stop therapy if signs of disease progression appear.
• Enhances hypoglycemia; teach signs of hypoglycemia, and instruct the patient to report immediately if they occur.
• Instruct males to report priapism, reduced ejaculatory volume, and gynecomastia. Withdraw drug.
• Watch for signs of ecchymoses, petechiae with concomitant anticoagulant therapy. Monitor prothrombin time.
• Inject deep into upper outer quadrant of gluteal muscle. Report soreness at site; possibility of postinjection furunculosis.
• Report signs of virilization in females; reevaluate treatment.
• Monitor prepubertal males by X-ray for rate of bone maturation.
• Edema is generally controllable with salt restriction and/or diuretics. Monitor weight routinely.
• Use with diet high in calories and protein unless contraindicated. Give small, frequent feedings.
• Daily requirements best administered in divided doses.
• May alter many laboratory studies during therapy and for 2 to 3 weeks after therapy is stopped.

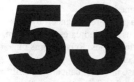

Oral contraceptives

estrogen with progestogen

COMBINATION PRODUCTS
None.

---

estrogen with progestogen
Brevicon, Demulen♦, Enovid,
Enovid-E, Loestrin 1/20, Loestrin
1.5/30♦, Lo/Ovral, Min-Ovral♦♦,
Modicon, Nordette, Norinyl 1 + 35,
Norinyl 1 + 50♦, Norinyl 1 + 80♦,
Norinyl 2 mg♦, Norlestrin♦,
Norlestrin 1/50, Norlestrin 2.5/50,
Ortho-Novum 1/50♦, Ortho-Novum
1/80♦, Ortho-Novum 2 mg♦, Ortho-
Novum 7/7/7, Ortho-Novum 10/11,
Ovcon 35**, Ovcon 50**, Ovral,
Ovulen♦, Trilevlen, Tri-Norinyl,
Triphasil
Pregnancy Category: X

MECHANISM OF ACTION
Oral contraceptives inhibit ovulation
through a negative feedback mechanism directed at the hypothalamus.
They may also prevent transport of
the ovum through the fallopian tubes.
    Estrogen suppresses secretion of
follicle-stimulating hormone, blocking follicular development and ovulation.
    Progestogen suppresses luteinizing
hormone secretion so ovulation can't
occur even if the follicle develops.
Progestogen thickens cervical mucus,
which interferes with sperm migration, and also causes endometrial
changes that prevent implantation of
the fertilized ovum.

INDICATIONS & DOSAGE
Contraception—
Women: 1 tablet P.O. daily, beginning on day 5 of menstrual cycle (first
day of menstrual flow is day 1). With
20- and 21-tablet packages, new dosing cycle begins 7 days after last tablet
taken. With 28-tablet packages, dosage is 1 tablet daily without interruption; extra tablets are placebos or contain iron. If only 1 or 2 doses are
missed, dosage may continue on
schedule. If 3 or more doses are
missed, remaining tablets in monthly
package must be discarded and another contraceptive method substituted. If next menstrual period
doesn't begin on schedule, rule out
pregnancy before starting new dosing
cycle. If menstrual period begins,
start new dosing cycle 7 days after
last tablet was taken. If all doses have
been taken on schedule and 1 menstrual period is missed, continue dosing cycle. If 2 consecutive menstrual
periods are missed, pregnancy test is
required before new dosing cycle is
started.
*Biphasic oral contraceptives (Ortho-
Novum 10/11)—*
1 color tablet daily for 10 days, then
next color tablet for 11 days.
*Triphasic oral contraceptives (Ortho-
Novum 7/7/7, Tri-Norinyl, Triphasil)—*
1 tablet daily in the sequence specified by the brand.
Hypermenorrhea—
Women: use high-dose combinations
only. Dose same as for contraception.
Endometriosis—

Women: Cyclic therapy: 1 tablet Ortho-Novum 10 mg P.O. daily for 20 days from day 5 to day 24 of menstrual cycle.

Suppressive therapy: Enovid 5 mg or 10 mg—1 tablet P.O. daily for 2 weeks starting on day 5 of menstrual cycle. Continue without interruption for 6 to 9 months, increasing dose by 5 to 10 mg q 2 weeks, up to 20 mg daily. Up to 40 mg daily may be needed if breakthrough bleeding occurs.

ADVERSE REACTIONS
CNS: *headache, dizziness,* depression, libido changes, lethargy, migraine.
CV: *thromboembolism,* hypertension, edema.
EENT: worsening of myopia or astigmatism, intolerance to contact lenses.
GI: *nausea,* vomiting, abdominal cramps, bloating, diarrhea, constipation, anorexia, changes in appetite, weight gain, *bowel ischemia,* pancreatitis.
GU: *breakthrough bleeding, granulomatous colitis,* dysmenorrhea, amenorrhea, cervical erosion or abnormal secretions, enlargement of uterine fibromas, vaginal candidiasis.
Hepatic: gallbladder disease, cholestatic jaundice, liver tumors.
Metabolic: hyperglycemia, hypercalcemia, folic acid deficiency.
Skin: rash, acne, seborrhea, oily skin, erythema multiforme, hyperpigmentation.
Other: *breast tenderness,* enlargement, secretion.
Adverse effects may be more serious, frequent, and rapid in onset with high-dose than with low-dose combinations.

INTERACTIONS
Barbiturates, anticonvulsants, rifampin: may diminish contraceptive effectiveness. Use supplemental form of contraception.

NURSING CONSIDERATIONS
• Contraindicated in thromboembolic disorders, cerebrovascular or coronary artery disease, myocardial infarction, known or suspected cancer of breasts or reproductive organs, benign or malignant liver tumors, undiagnosed abnormal vaginal bleeding, known or suspected pregnancy, lactation; and in adolescents with incomplete epiphyseal closure. Also contraindicated in women 35 years or older who smoke more than 15 cigarettes a day, and in all women over 40 years. Use cautiously in patients with systemic lupus erythematosus, hypertension, mental depression, migraine, epilepsy, asthma, diabetes mellitus, amenorrhea, scanty or irregular periods, fibrocystic breast disease, family history (mother, grandmother, sister) of breast or genital tract cancer, renal or gallbladder disease. Report development or worsening of these conditions to doctor. Prolonged therapy inadvisable in women who plan to become pregnant.
• Discontinue if patient develops granulomatous colitis while on oral contraceptives.
• Discontinue at least 1 week before surgery to decrease risk of thromboembolism. Use an alternate method of birth control.
• If one menstrual period is missed and tablets have been taken on schedule, tell patient to continue taking them. If two consecutive menstrual periods are missed, tell patient to stop drug and to have pregnancy test. Progestogens may cause birth defects if taken early in pregnancy.
• Missed doses in midcycle greatly increase likelihood of pregnancy.
• If one tablet is missed, tell patient to take it as soon as remembered, or take two tablets the next day and continue regular schedule. If patient misses 2 consecutive days, she should take two tablets daily for 2 days, and resume normal schedule. Patient

should use an additional method of birth control for 7 days after two missed doses.

• Warn patient that headache, nausea, dizziness, breast tenderness, spotting, and breakthrough bleeding are common at first. These should diminish after 3 to 6 dosing cycles (months). However, breakthrough bleeding in patients taking high-dose estrogen-progestogen combinations for menstrual disorders may necessitate dosage adjustment.

• Warn patient to immediately report abdominal pain; numbness, stiffness, or pain in legs or buttocks; pressure or pain in chest; shortness of breath; severe headache; visual disturbances, such as blind spots, blurriness, or flashing lights; undiagnosed vaginal bleeding or discharge; two consecutive missed menstrual periods; lumps in the breast; swelling of hands and feet; severe pain in the abdomen (tumor rupture in the liver).

• Advise patient to use an additional method of birth control for the first week of administration in the initial cycle. Some doctors instruct patients to also use condoms or a diaphragm with spermicide.

• Tell patient to take tablets at same time each day; nighttime dosing may reduce nausea and headaches.

• Stress importance of semiannual Pap smears and annual gynecologic examinations while taking estrogen-progestogen combinations.

• Warn the patient of possible delay in achieving pregnancy when drug is discontinued. Advise patient to check with doctor regarding how soon after hormone therapy pregnancy may be attempted.

• Teach the patient how to perform a breast self-examination.

• Advise the patient of increased risks associated with simultaneous use of cigarettes and oral contraceptives.

• Many laboratory tests are affected by oral contraceptives; some include: increase in serum bilirubin, alkaline phosphatase, SGOT, SGPT, and protein-bound iodine; decrease in glucose tolerance and urinary excretion of 17-hydroxycorticosteroids (17-OHCS).

• Estrogens and progestogens may alter glucose tolerance, thus changing requirements for antidiabetic drugs. Monitor blood glucose levels.

• Instruct patient to weigh herself at least twice a week and to report any sudden weight gain or edema to doctor.

• Warn patient to avoid exposure to ultraviolet light or prolonged exposure to sunlight.

• Many doctors recommend that women not become pregnant within 2 months after stopping drug. Advise patient to check with her doctor about how soon pregnancy may be attempted after hormonal therapy is stopped.

• Advise patient not to take same drug for longer than 18 months without consulting doctor.

• Many doctors advise women on prolonged therapy with oral contraceptives (5 years or longer) to stop drug and use other birth control methods in order to periodically reassess patient while off hormone therapy.

• The Centers for Disease Control (CDC) report that the use of oral contraceptives *may decrease* the incidence of ovarian and endometrial cancer. Also, oral contraceptives do not appear to increase a woman's risk of breast cancer. However, FDA reports that they may be linked to an increased risk of cervical cancer.

• Ovral has been prescribed as a postcoital contraceptive ("morning-after" pill). Patients are given 2 tablets at the initial visit and 2 tablets 12 hours later.

• Triphasic oral contraceptives may cause fewer side effects such as breakthrough bleeding and spotting.

Italicized side effects are common or life-threatening.
*Liquid form contains alcohol.   **May contain tartrazine.

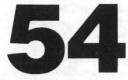

Estrogens

chlorotrianisene
dienestrol
diethylstilbestrol
diethylstilbestrol diphosphate
esterified estrogens
estradiol
estradiol cypionate
estradiol valerate
estrogenic substances,
  conjugated
estrone
ethinyl estradiol
quinestrol

COMBINATION PRODUCTS
MENRIUM 5-2♦: chlordiazepoxide 5
mg and esterified estrogens 0.2 mg.
MENRIUM 5-4♦: chlordiazepoxide 5
mg and esterified estrogens 0.4 mg.
MENRIUM 10-4♦: chlordiazepoxide
10 mg and esterified estrogens 0.4
mg.
MILPREM-200: conjugated estrogens
0.45 mg and meprobamate 200 mg.
MILPREM-400: conjugated estrogens
0.45 mg and meprobamate 400 mg.
PMB 200: conjugated estrogens 0.45
mg and meprobamate 200 mg.
PMB 400: conjugated estrogens 0.45
mg and meprobamate 400 mg.
See Chapter 52, ORAL CONTRACEP-
TIVES.

chlorotrianisene
Tace♦
Pregnancy Category: X

MECHANISM OF ACTION
Increases the synthesis of DNA,
RNA, and protein in responsive tissues. Also reduces FSH and LH release from the pituitary.

INDICATIONS & DOSAGE
Men:
Prostatic cancer—
12 to 25 mg P.O. daily.
Nonnursing mothers:
Postpartum breast engorgement—
72 mg P.O. b.i.d. for 2 days; or 50 mg
q 6 hours for 6 doses; or 12 mg q.i.d.
for 7 days. Start dosing within 8 hours
after delivery.
Women:
Menopausal symptoms—
12 to 25 mg P.O. daily for 30 days or
cyclic (3 weeks on, 1 week off).
Female hypogonadism—
12 to 25 mg P.O. for 21 days, followed by 1 dose of progesterone 100
mg I.M. or 5 days of oral progestogen
given concurrently with last 5 days of
chlorotrianisene (i.e., medroxyprogesterone 5 to 10 mg).
Atrophic vaginitis—
12 to 25 mg P.O. daily for 30 to 60
days.

ADVERSE REACTIONS
CNS: headache, dizziness, chorea,
migraine, depression, libido changes.
CV: thrombophlebitis; *thromboembolism;* hypertension; edema; *increased
risk of stroke, pulmonary embolism,
and myocardial infarction.*
EENT: worsening of myopia or astigmatism, intolerance to contact lenses.
GI: *nausea,* vomiting, abdominal
cramps, bloating, diarrhea, constipation, anorexia, increased appetite, excessive thirst, weight changes, pan-

---

creatitis.
GU: breakthrough bleeding, altered menstrual flow, dysmenorrhea, amenorrhea, cervical erosion or abnormal secretions, enlargement of uterine fibromas, vaginal candidiasis; *in males: gynecomastia, testicular atrophy, impotence.*
Hepatic: cholestatic jaundice.
Metabolic: hyperglycemia, hypercalcemia, folic acid deficiency.
Skin: melasma, urticaria, acne, seborrhea, oily skin, hirsutism or loss of hair.
Other: leg cramps, purpura, breast changes (tenderness, enlargement, secretion).

INTERACTIONS
None significant.

NURSING CONSIDERATIONS
• Contraindicated in thrombophlebitis or thromboembolic disorders; cancer of breast, reproductive organs, or genitals; undiagnosed abnormal genital bleeding. Use cautiously in patients with hypertension, asthma, mental depression, bone diseases, blood dyscrasias, gallbladder disease, migraine, seizures, diabetes mellitus, amenorrhea, heart failure, hepatic or renal dysfunction, and family history (mother, grandmother, sister) of breast or genital tract cancer. Development or worsening of these conditions may require discontinuation of the drug.
• Patient package insert that describes estrogen adverse reactions is available. However, provide verbal explanation also.
• Warn patient to report immediately: abdominal pain; pain, numbness, or stiffness in legs or buttocks; pressure or pain in chest; shortness of breath; severe headaches; visual disturbances, such as blind spots, flashing lights, blurriness; vaginal bleeding or discharge; breast lumps; swelling of hands or feet; yellow skin and sclera;

dark urine; and light-colored stools.
• Tell male patients on long-term therapy about possible gynecomastia and impotence, which will disappear when therapy is terminated.
• Not used for menstrual disorders because duration of action is very long.
• Pathologist should be advised of estrogen therapy when specimen is sent.
• Patients with diabetes should report elevated blood glucose test results so antidiabetic medication dose can be adjusted.
• Teach female patients how to perform routine breast self-examination.
• Explain to patient on cyclic therapy for postmenopausal symptoms that, although withdrawal bleeding may occur during week off drug, fertility has not been restored. Pregnancy is not possible since she has not ovulated.

---

dienestrol
Dienestrol Cream♦
Available in combination with sulfanilamide and aminacrine as AVC/Dienestrol, cream or suppositories
Pregnancy Category: X

MECHANISM OF ACTION
Increases the synthesis of DNA, RNA, and protein in responsive tissues. Also reduces FSH and LH release from the pituitary.

INDICATIONS & DOSAGE
Postmenopausal women:
Atrophic vaginitis and kraurosis vulvae—
1 to 2 applications of cream daily for 2 weeks (as directed), then half that dose for 2 more weeks; or 1 to 2 vaginal suppositories daily for 1 month, as directed.
Atrophic and senile vaginitis and kraurosis vulvae when complicated by infection—
1 application of AVC/Dienestrol

Italicized side effects are common or life-threatening.
*Liquid form contains alcohol.   **May contain tartrazine.

cream intravaginally daily or b.i.d. for 1 to 2 weeks (as directed), then every other day for 1 to 2 weeks.

ADVERSE REACTIONS
GU: vaginal discharge; with excessive use, uterine bleeding.
Local: increased discomfort, burning sensation. Systemic effects possible.
Other: breast tenderness.

INTERACTIONS
None significant.

NURSING CONSIDERATIONS
• Contraindicated in thrombophlebitis or thromboembolic disorders; cancer of breast, reproductive organs, or genitals; undiagnosed abnormal genital bleeding. Use cautiously in menstrual irregularities or endometriosis.
• Instruct patient to apply drug at bedtime to increase effectiveness.
• Prolonged therapy with estrogen-containing products is contraindicated.
• Patient package insert that describes estrogen adverse reactions is available. However, provide verbal explanation also.
• Systemic reactions possible with normal intravaginal use. Monitor closely.
• Warn patient not to exceed the prescribed dose.
• Withdrawal bleeding may occur if estrogen is suddenly stopped.
• Patient shouldn't wear tampon while receiving vaginal therapy. She may need to wear sanitary pad to protect clothing.
• Teach patient how to insert suppositories or cream. Wash vaginal area with soap and water before application.
• Instruct patient to remain recumbent for 30 minutes after administration to prevent loss of drug.
• Teach patient how to perform breast self-examination.

diethylstilbestrol
DES, Stilboestrol♦♦

diethylstilbestrol diphosphate
Honvol♦♦, Stilphostrol
Pregnancy Category: X

MECHANISM OF ACTION
Increases the synthesis of DNA, RNA, and protein in responsive tissues. Also reduces FSH and LH release from the pituitary.

INDICATIONS & DOSAGE
Women:
Hypogonadism, castration, primary ovarian failure—
0.2 to 0.5 mg P.O. daily.
Menopausal symptoms—
0.1 to 2 mg P.O. daily in cycles of 3 weeks on and 1 week off.
Postcoital contraception ("morning-after pill")—
25 mg P.O. b.i.d. for 5 days, starting within 72 hours after coitus.
Postpartum breast engorgement—
5 mg P.O. daily or t.i.d. up to total dose of 30 mg.
Men:
Prostatic cancer—
1 to 3 mg P.O. daily, initially; may be reduced to 1 mg P.O. daily, or 5 mg I.M. twice weekly initially, followed by up to 4 mg I.M. twice weekly. Or 50 to 200 mg (diphosphate) P.O. t.i.d.; or 0.25 to 1 g I.V. daily for 5 days, then once or twice weekly.
Men and postmenopausal women:
Breast cancer—
15 mg P.O. daily.

ADVERSE REACTIONS
CNS: headache, dizziness, chorea, depression, lethargy.
CV: *thrombophlebitis; thromboembolism;* hypertension; edema; *increased risk of stroke, pulmonary embolism, and myocardial infarction.*
EENT: worsening of myopia or astig-

matism, intolerance to contact lenses.
GI: *nausea,* vomiting, abdominal
cramps, bloating, diarrhea, constipation, anorexia, increased appetite, excessive thirst, weight changes, pancreatitis.
GU: breakthrough bleeding, altered
menstrual flow, dysmenorrhea, amenorrhea, cervical erosion, altered cervical secretions, enlargement of uterine fibromas, vaginal candidiasis, loss
of libido; *in males:* gynecomastia,
testicular atrophy, impotence.
Hepatic: cholestatic jaundice.
Metabolic: hyperglycemia, hypercalcemia, folic acid deficiency.
Skin: melasma, urticaria, acne, seborrhea, oily skin, hirsutism or loss of
hair.
Other: leg cramps, breast tenderness
or enlargement.

INTERACTIONS
None significant.

NURSING CONSIDERATIONS
• Contraindicated in thrombophlebitis or thromboembolic disorders; undiagnosed abnormal genital bleeding.
Use cautiously in patients with hypertension, asthma, mental depression,
bone disease, migraine, seizures,
blood dyscrasias, diabetes mellitus,
gallbladder disease, amenorrhea,
heart failure, hepatic or renal dysfunction, and family history (mother,
grandmother, sister) of breast or genital tract cancer. Development or worsening of these conditions may require
discontinuation of the drug.
• Patient package insert that describes estrogen adverse reactions is
available. However, provide verbal
explanation also.
• Only the 25-mg tablet is approved
by FDA as the "morning-after pill."
To be effective, it must be taken
within 72 hours after coitus. Nausea
and vomiting are common with this
large dose.
• Warn patient to stop taking drug

immediately if she becomes pregnant,
since it can affect the fetus adversely.
• Warn patient to report immediately:
abdominal pain; pain, numbness, or
stiffness in legs or buttocks; pressure
or pain in chest; shortness of breath;
severe headache; visual disturbances,
such as blind spots, flashing lights, or
blurriness; vaginal bleeding or discharge; breast lumps; sudden weight
gain; swelling of hands or feet; yellow
sclera or skin; dark urine or light-colored stools.
• Pathologist should be advised of estrogen therapy when specimen is sent.
• Patients with diabetes should report
elevated blood glucose test results so
antidiabetic medication dose can be
adjusted.
• High incidence of gross nonmalignant genital changes in offspring of
women taking drug during pregnancy.
Female offspring have higher than
normal risk of developing cervical
and vaginal adenocarcinoma. Male
offspring may have higher than normal risk of developing testicular tumors.
• Increased number of cardiovascular
deaths reported in men taking diethylstilbestrol tablet (5 mg daily) for prostatic cancer over long period of time.
This effect not associated with 1 mg
daily dose.
• Reassure male patients on estrogen
therapy that such side effects as gynecomastia and impotence will disappear when therapy ends.
• Teach female patients how to perform routine breast self-examination.
• Explain to patient on cyclic therapy
for postmenopausal symptoms that,
although withdrawal bleeding may occur during week off drug, fertility has
not been restored. Pregnancy is not
possible since she has not ovulated.
• Use of estrogens associated with increased risk of endometrial cancer.
Possible increased risk of breast cancer.

Italicized side effects are common or life-threatening.
*Liquid form contains alcohol.   **May contain tartrazine.

esterified estrogens
Climestrone♦♦, Estabs, Estratab,
Menest, Ms-Med, Neo-Estrone♦♦
Pregnancy Category: X

MECHANISM OF ACTION
Increases the synthesis of DNA,
RNA, and protein in responsive tissues. Also reduces FSH and LH release from the pituitary.

INDICATIONS & DOSAGE
Men:
Prostatic cancer—
1.25 to 2.5 mg P.O. t.i.d.
Men and postmenopausal women:
Breast cancer—
10 mg P.O. t.i.d. for 3 or more
months.
Women:
*Hypogonadism, castration, primary
ovarian failure—*
2.5 mg daily to t.i.d. in cycles of 3
weeks on, 1 week off.
Menopausal symptoms—
average 0.3 to 3.75 mg P.O. daily in
cycles of 3 weeks on, 1 week off.

ADVERSE REACTIONS
CNS: headache, dizziness, chorea,
depression, libido changes, lethargy.
CV: thrombophlebitis; *thromboembolism;* hypertension; edema; *increased
risk of stroke, pulmonary embolism,
and myocardial infarction.*
EENT: worsening of myopia or astigmatism, intolerance to contact lenses.
GI: *nausea,* vomiting, abdominal
cramps, bloating, diarrhea, constipation, anorexia, increased appetite,
weight changes, pancreatitis.
GU: breakthrough bleeding, altered
menstrual flow, dysmenorrhea, amenorrhea, cervical erosion, altered cervical secretions, enlargement of uterine fibromas, vaginal candidiasis; *in
males:* gynecomastia, testicular atrophy, impotence.
Hepatic: cholestatic jaundice.
Metabolic: hyperglycemia, hypercal-

cemia, folic acid deficiency.
Skin: melasma, rash, acne, hirsutism
or hair loss, seborrhea, oily skin.
Other: breast changes (tenderness,
enlargement, secretion).

INTERACTIONS
None significant.

NURSING CONSIDERATIONS
• Contraindicated in thrombophlebitis or thromboembolic disorders; undiagnosed abnormal genital bleeding.
Use cautiously in patients with history
of hypertension, mental depression,
gallbladder disease, migraine, seizures, diabetes mellitus, amenorrhea,
or family history (mother, grandmother, sister) of breast or genital
tract cancer. Development or worsening of these conditions may require
discontinuation of the drug.
• Patient package insert that describes estrogen adverse reactions is
available. However, provide verbal
explanation also.
• Warn patient to report immediately:
abdominal pain; pain, numbness, or
stiffness in legs or buttocks; pressure
or pain in chest; shortness of breath;
severe headaches; visual disturbances, such as blind spots, flashing
lights, or blurriness; vaginal bleeding
or discharge; breast lumps; swelling
of hands or feet; yellow skin or sclera;
dark urine or light-colored stools.
• Pathologist should be advised of estrogen therapy when specimen is sent.
• Patients with diabetes should report
elevated blood glucose test results so
antidiabetic medication dose can be
adjusted.
• Explain to patient on cyclic therapy
for postmenopausal symptoms that,
although she may experience withdrawal bleeding during week off drug,
fertility has not been restored. Pregnancy cannot occur since she has not
ovulated.
• Teach female patients how to perform routine breast self-examination.

Unmarked trade names available in the United States only.
♦ Also available in Canada.   ♦♦ Available in Canada only.

• Reassure male patients on estrogen therapy that such side effects as gynecomastia and impotence will disappear when therapy ends.

---

estradiol
Estrace♦**, Estrace Vaginal Cream, Estraderm

estradiol cypionate
Depo-Estradiol Cypionate, Depogen, Dura Estrin, Estro-Cyp, Estroject-L.A.

estradiol valerate
Delestrogen♦♦, Dioval, Duragen, Estradiol L.A., Estraval, Retestrin, Valergen
Pregnancy Category: X

MECHANISM OF ACTION
Increases the synthesis of DNA, RNA, and protein in responsive tissues. Also reduces FSH and LH release from the pituitary.

INDICATIONS & DOSAGE
Women:
Menopausal symptoms, hypogonadism, castration, primary ovarian failure—
1 to 2 mg P.O. daily, in cycles of 21 days on and 7 days off, or cycles of 5 days on and 2 days off; or 0.2 to 1 mg I.M. weekly.
Kraurosis vulvae—
1 to 1.5 mg I.M. once or more per week.
Atrophic vaginitis—
2 to 4 g vaginal cream daily for 1 to 2 weeks. When vaginal mucosa is restored, begin maintenance dose of 1 g one to three times weekly.
Menopausal symptoms—
1 to 5 mg (cypionate) I.M. q 3 to 4 weeks. Or 5 to 20 mg (valerate) I.M., repeated once after 2 to 3 weeks.
Postpartum breast engorgement—
10 to 25 mg (valerate) I.M. at end of first stage of labor.

Inoperable breast cancer (oral estradiol)—
10 mg t.i.d. for 3 months.
Treatment of moderate to severe symptoms of menopause, female hypogonadism, female castration, primary ovarian failure, and atrophic conditions caused by deficient endogenous estrogen production—
Place one Estraderm transdermal patch on trunk of the body twice weekly. Administer on an intermittent cyclic schedule (3 weeks of therapy followed by discontinuation for 1 week).
Men:
Inoperable prostatic cancer—
30 mg (valerate) I.M. q 1 to 2 weeks. Or, 1 to 2 mg (oral estradiol) t.i.d.

ADVERSE REACTIONS
CNS: headache, dizziness, chorea, depression, libido changes, lethargy.
CV: thrombophlebitis, *thromboembolism,* hypertension, edema.
EENT: worsening of myopia or astigmatism, intolerance to contact lenses.
GI: *nausea,* vomiting, abdominal cramps, bloating, diarrhea, constipation, anorexia, increased appetite, weight changes, pancreatitis.
GU: breakthrough bleeding, altered menstrual flow, dysmenorrhea, amenorrhea, cervical erosion, altered cervical secretions, enlargement of uterine fibromas, vaginal candidiasis; *in males:* gynecomastia, testicular atrophy, impotence.
Hepatic: cholestatic jaundice.
Metabolic: hyperglycemia, hypercalcemia, folic acid deficiency.
Skin: melasma, urticaria, acne, seborrhea, oily skin, hirsutism or hair loss.
Other: breast changes (tenderness, enlargement, secretion), leg cramps.

INTERACTIONS
None significant.

Italicized side effects are common or life-threatening.
*Liquid form contains alcohol.   **May contain tartrazine.

NURSING CONSIDERATIONS

• Contraindicated in thrombophlebitis or thromboembolic disorders; cancer of breast, reproductive organs; undiagnosed abnormal genital bleeding. Use cautiously in patients with hypertension, mental depression, bone diseases, blood dyscrasias, migraine, seizures, diabetes mellitus, amenorrhea, heart failure, hepatic or renal dysfunction, or family history (mother, grandmother, sister) of breast or genital tract cancer. Development or worsening of these conditions may require discontinuation of the drug.

• Patient package insert that describes estrogen adverse reactions is available. However, provide verbal explanation also.

• Warn patient to report immediately: abdominal pain; pain, numbness, or stiffness in legs or buttocks; pressure or pain in chest; shortness of breath; severe headaches; visual disturbances, such as blind spots, flashing lights, or blurriness; vaginal bleeding or discharge; breast lumps; swelling of hands or feet; yellow skin or sclera; dark urine or light-colored stools.

• Risk of endometrial cancer is increased in postmenopausal women who take estrogens for more than 1 year.

• Patients with diabetes should report elevated blood glucose test results so antidiabetic medication dose can be adjusted.

• Pathologist should be advised of estrogen therapy when specimen is sent.

• Estradiol available as aqueous suspension or solution in peanut oil.

• Estradiol cypionate available as solution in cottonseed oil or vegetable oil.

• Estradiol valerate available as solution in castor oil, sesame oil, and vegetable oil. Check for allergy.

• Before injection, make sure drug is well dispersed in solution by rolling vial between palms. Inject deep I.M. into large muscle.

• Reassure male patient that possible side effects of gynecomastia and impotence disappear after termination of therapy.

• In women who are currently taking oral estrogen, treatment with the Estraderm transdermal patch can begin 1 week after withdrawal of oral therapy or sooner if symptoms appear before the end of the week.

• Teach female patients how to perform routine breast self-examination.

• Explain to patient on cyclic therapy for postmenopausal symptoms that, although withdrawal bleeding may occur during week off drug, fertility has not been restored. Pregnancy cannot occur since she has not ovulated.

---

estrogenic substances, conjugated
Estrocon, Premarin♦
Pregnancy Category: X

MECHANISM OF ACTION
Increases the synthesis of DNA, RNA, and protein in responsive tissues. Also reduces FSH and LH release from the pituitary.

INDICATIONS & DOSAGE
Women:
Abnormal uterine bleeding (hormonal imbalance)—
25 mg I.V. or I.M. Repeat in 6 to 12 hours.
Breast cancer (at least 5 years after menopause)—
10 mg P.O. t.i.d. for 3 months or more.
Castration, primary ovarian failure, and osteoporosis—
1.25 mg P.O. daily in cycles of 3 weeks on, 1 week off.
Hypogonadism—
2.5 mg P.O. b.i.d. or t.i.d. for 20 consecutive days each month.
Menopausal symptoms—
0.3 to 1.25 mg P.O. daily in cycles of

3 weeks on, 1 week off.
Postpartum breast engorgement—
3.75 mg P.O. q 4 hours for 5 doses or
1.25 mg q 4 hours for 5 days.
Men:
Prostatic cancer—
1.25 to 2.5 mg P.O. t.i.d.

ADVERSE REACTIONS
CNS: headache, dizziness, chorea, depression, libido changes, lethargy.
CV: thrombophlebitis; *thromboembolism;* hypertension; edema; *increased risk of stroke, pulmonary embolism, and myocardial infarction.*
EENT: worsening of myopia or astigmatism, intolerance to contact lenses.
GI: *nausea,* vomiting, abdominal cramps, bloating, diarrhea, constipation, anorexia, increased appetite, weight changes, pancreatitis.
GU: breakthrough bleeding, altered menstrual flow, dysmenorrhea, amenorrhea, cervical erosion, altered cervical secretions, enlargement of uterine fibromas, vaginal candidiasis; *in males:* gynecomastia, testicular atrophy, impotence.
Hepatic: cholestatic jaundice.
Metabolic: hyperglycemia, hypercalcemia, folic acid deficiency.
Skin: melasma, urticaria, acne, seborrhea, oily skin, flushing (when given rapidly I.V.), hirsutism or loss of hair.
Other: breast changes (tenderness, enlargement, secretion), leg cramps.

INTERACTIONS
None significant.

NURSING CONSIDERATIONS
• Contraindicated in thrombophlebitis or thromboembolic disorders; undiagnosed abnormal genital bleeding. Use cautiously in hypertension, gallbladder disease, bone diseases, blood dyscrasias, migraine, seizures, diabetes mellitus, amenorrhea, heart failure, hepatic or renal dysfunction, or family history (mother, grandmother, sister) of breast or genital tract cancer. Development or worsening of these conditions may require discontinuation of the drug.
• Patient package insert that describes estrogen adverse reactions is available. However, provide verbal explanation also.
• Warn patient to report immediately: abdominal pain; pain, numbness, or stiffness in legs or buttocks; pressure or pain in chest; shortness of breath; severe headaches; visual disturbances, such as blind spots, flashing lights, or blurriness; vaginal bleeding or discharge; breast lumps; swelling of hands or feet; yellow skin or sclera; dark urine or light-colored stools.
• I.M. or I.V. use preferred for rapid treatment of dysfunctional uterine bleeding or reduction of surgical bleeding.
• Refrigerate before reconstituting. Agitate gently after adding diluent.
• Pathologist should be advised of estrogen therapy when specimen is sent.
• Patients with diabetes should report elevated blood glucose test results so antidiabetic medication dose can be adjusted.
• Use associated with increased risk of endometrial cancer. Possible increased risk of breast cancer.
• Teach female patients how to perform routine breast self-examination.
• Explain to patient on cyclic therapy for postmenopausal symptoms that, although withdrawal bleeding may occur during week off drug, fertility has not been restored. Pregnancy cannot occur since she has not ovulated.
• Reassure male patients that possible side effects of gynecomastia and impotence disappear after termination of therapy.

Italicized side effects are common or life-threatening.
*Liquid form contains alcohol.   **May contain tartrazine.

estrone

Bestrone, Kestrone-5, Theelin
Pregnancy Category: X

MECHANISM OF ACTION

Increases the synthesis of DNA, RNA, and protein in responsive tissues. Also reduces FSH and LH release from the pituitary.

INDICATIONS & DOSAGE

Women:
Atrophic vaginitis and menopausal symptoms—
0.1 to 0.5 mg I.M. two or three times weekly.
Female hypogonadism and primary ovarian failure—
0.1 to 1 mg I.M. weekly in single or divided doses.
Men:
Prostatic cancer—
2 to 4 mg I.M. 2 to 3 times weekly.

ADVERSE REACTIONS

CNS: headache, dizziness, chorea, depression, libido changes, lethargy.
CV: thrombophlebitis, *thromboembolism,* hypertension, edema.
EENT: worsening of myopia or astigmatism, intolerance to contact lenses.
GI: *nausea,* vomiting, abdominal cramps, bloating, diarrhea, constipation, anorexia, increased appetite, weight changes, pancreatitis.
GU: breakthrough bleeding, altered menstrual flow, dysmenorrhea, amenorrhea, cervical erosion, altered cervical secretions, enlargement of uterine fibromas, vaginal candidiasis; *in males:* gynecomastia, testicular atrophy, impotence.
Hepatic: cholestatic jaundice.
Metabolic: hyperglycemia, hypercalcemia, folic acid deficiency.
Skin: melasma, urticaria, acne, seborrhea, oily skin, hirsutism or hair loss.
Other: breast changes (tenderness, enlargement, secretion), leg cramps.

INTERACTIONS

None significant.

NURSING CONSIDERATIONS

• Contraindicated in thrombophlebitis or thromboembolic disorders; cancer of breast or reproductive organs; undiagnosed abnormal genital bleeding. Use cautiously in patients with hypertension, mental depression, migraine, seizures, diabetes mellitus, amenorrhea, hepatic or renal dysfunction, or family history (mother, grandmother, sister) of breast or genital tract cancer. Development or worsening of these conditions may require discontinuation of the drug.
• Estrone must be administered I.M.
• Patient package insert that describes estrogen adverse reactions is available. However, provide verbal explanation also.
• Warn patient to report immediately: abdominal pain; pain, numbness, or stiffness in legs or buttocks; pressure or pain in chest; shortness of breath; severe headaches; visual disturbances, such as blind spots, flashing lights, or blurriness; vaginal bleeding or discharge; breast lumps; swelling of hands or feet.
• Pathologist should be advised of estrogen therapy when specimen is sent.
• Patients with diabetes should report elevated blood glucose test results so antidiabetic medication dose can be adjusted.
• Teach female patients how to perform routine breast self-examination.
• Use of estrogens associated with increased risk of endometrial cancer. Possible increased risk of breast cancer.
• Explain to patient on cyclic therapy for postmenopausal symptoms that, although withdrawal bleeding may occur during week off drug, fertility has not been restored. Pregnancy cannot occur since she has not ovulated.
• Reassure male patients that possible side effects of gynecomastia and im-

potence disappear after termination of therapy.

ethinyl estradiol
Estinyl♦**, Feminone
Pregnancy Category: X

MECHANISM OF ACTION
Increases the synthesis of DNA, RNA, and protein in responsive tissues. Also reduces FSH and LH release from the pituitary.

INDICATIONS & DOSAGE
Women:
Breast cancer (at least 5 years after menopause)—
1 mg P.O. t.i.d.
Hypogonadism—
0.05 mg daily to t.i.d. for 2 weeks a month, followed by 2 weeks progesterone therapy; continue for 3 to 6 monthly dosing cycles, followed by 2 months off.
Menopausal symptoms—
0.02 to 0.05 mg P.O. daily for cycles of 3 weeks on, 1 week off.
Postpartum breast engorgement—
0.5 to 1 mg P.O. daily for 3 days, then taper over 7 days to 0.1 mg and discontinue.
Men:
Prostatic cancer—
0.15 to 2 mg P.O. daily.

ADVERSE REACTIONS
CNS: headache, dizziness, chorea, depression, libido changes, lethargy.
CV: thrombophlebitis, *thromboembolism,* hypertension, edema.
EENT: worsening of myopia or astigmatism, intolerance to contact lenses.
GI: *nausea,* vomiting, abdominal cramps, bloating, diarrhea, constipation, anorexia, increased appetite, weight changes.
GU: breakthrough bleeding, altered menstrual flow, dysmenorrhea, amenorrhea, cervical erosion, altered cervical secretions, enlargement of uter-

ine fibromas, vaginal candidiasis; *in males:* gynecomastia, testicular atrophy, impotence.
Hepatic: cholestatic jaundice.
Metabolic: hyperglycemia, hypercalcemia, folic acid deficiency.
Skin: melasma, urticaria, acne, seborrhea, oily skin, hirsutism or hair loss.
Other: breast changes (tenderness, enlargement, secretion), leg cramps.

INTERACTIONS
None significant.

NURSING CONSIDERATIONS
• Contraindicated in thrombophlebitis or thromboembolic disorders; undiagnosed abnormal genital bleeding. Use cautiously in patients with hypertension, mental depression, bone diseases, migraine, seizures, blood dyscrasias, diabetes mellitus, amenorrhea, heart failure, hepatic or renal dysfunction, or family history (mother, grandmother, sister) of breast or genital tract cancer. Development or worsening of these conditions may require discontinuation of the drug.
• Patient package insert that describes estrogen adverse reactions is available. However, provide verbal explanation also.
• Warn patient to report immediately: abdominal pain; pain, numbness, or stiffness in legs or buttocks; pressure or pain in chest; shortness of breath; severe headaches; visual disturbances, such as blind spots, flashing lights, or blurriness; vaginal bleeding or discharge; breast lumps; swelling of hands or feet; yellow skin or sclera; dark urine or light-colored stools.
• Pathologist should be advised of estrogen therapy when specimen is sent.
• Patients with diabetes should report elevated blood glucose test results so antidiabetic medication dose can be adjusted.
• Teach female patients how to per-

form routine breast self-examination.
• Use of estrogens associated with increased risk of endometrial cancer. Possible increased risk of breast cancer.
• Explain to patient on cyclic therapy for postmenopausal symptoms that, although withdrawal bleeding may occur during week off drug, fertility has not been restored. Pregnancy cannot occur since she has not ovulated.
• Reassure male patients that possible side effects of gynecomastia and impotence disappear after termination of therapy.

quinestrol
Estrovis
Pregnancy Category: X

MECHANISM OF ACTION
Increases the synthesis of DNA, RNA, and protein in responsive tissues. Also reduces FSH and LH release from the pituitary.

INDICATIONS & DOSAGE
Women:
Moderate to severe vasomotor symptoms associated with menopause, and for atrophic vaginitis, kraurosis vulvae, female hypogonadism, female castration, and primary ovarian failure—
100-mcg tablet once daily for 7 days, followed by 100 mcg weekly as maintenance dose beginning 2 weeks after start of treatment. Dosage may be increased to 200 mcg weekly.

ADVERSE REACTIONS
CNS: headache, dizziness, chorea, migraine, depression, libido changes.
CV: thrombophlebitis; *thromboembolism;* hypertension; edema; *increased risk of stroke, pulmonary embolism, and myocardial infarction*.
EENT: worsening of myopia or astigmatism, intolerance to contact lenses.
GI: *nausea,* vomiting, abdominal

cramps, bloating, diarrhea, constipation, anorexia, increased appetite, excessive thirst, weight changes.
GU: breakthrough bleeding, altered menstrual flow, dysmenorrhea, amenorrhea, cervical erosion or abnormal secretions, enlargement of uterine fibromas, vaginal candidiasis.
Hepatic: cholestatic jaundice.
Metabolic: hyperglycemia, hypercalcemia, folic acid deficiency.
Skin: melasma, urticaria, acne, seborrhea, oily skin, hirsutism or loss of hair.
Other: leg cramps, purpura, breast changes (tenderness, enlargement, secretion).

INTERACTIONS
None significant.

NURSING CONSIDERATIONS
• Contraindicated in thrombophlebitis or thromboembolic disorders; cancer of breast or reproductive organs; undiagnosed abnormal genital bleeding. Use cautiously in patients with hypertension, mental depression, migraine, seizures, diabetes mellitus, amenorrhea, hepatic or renal dysfunction, or family history (mother, grandmother, sister) of breast or genital tract cancer. Development or worsening of these may require discontinuation of the drug.
• Patient package insert that describes estrogen adverse reactions is available. However, provide verbal explanation also.
• Warn patient to report immediately: abdominal pain; pain, numbness, or stiffness in legs or buttocks; pressure or pain in chest; shortness of breath; severe headaches; visual disturbances, such as blind spots, flashing lights, or blurriness; vaginal bleeding or discharge; breast lumps; swelling of hands or feet; yellow skin or sclera; dark urine or light-colored stools.
• Pathologist should be advised of estrogen therapy when specimen is sent.

• Patients with diabetes should report elevated blood glucose test results so antidiabetic medication dose can be adjusted.

• Attempts to discontinue medication should be made at 3- to 6-month intervals.

• Similar in effectiveness to conjugated estrogens in treatment of postmenopausal symptoms. Biggest advantage is that quinestrol can be taken once a week.

• Use of estrogens associated with increased risk of endometrial cancer.

• Explain to patients on replacement therapy for postmenopausal symptoms that, although menstrual-like bleeding or spotting may occur, fertility has not been restored.

• Teach female patients how to perform breast self-examination.

• Reassure male patients that possible side effects of gynecomastia and impotence disappear after therapy stops.

Italicized side effects are common or life-threatening.
*Liquid form contains alcohol.   **May contain tartrazine.

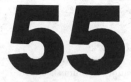

Progestogens

hydroxyprogesterone caproate
medroxyprogesterone acetate
norethindrone
norethindrone acetate
norgestrel
progesterone

COMBINATION PRODUCTS
See Chapter 53, ORAL CONTRACEP-
TIVES.

---

hydroxyprogesterone caproate
Delalutin♦, Duralutin
Pregnancy Category: X

MECHANISM OF ACTION
Suppresses ovulation, possibly by inhibiting pituitary gonadotropin secretion. Also forms a thick cervical mucus.

INDICATIONS & DOSAGE
Women:
Menstrual disorders—
125 to 375 mg I.M. q 4 weeks. Stop
after 4 cycles.
Uterine cancer—
1 to 5 g I.M. weekly.

ADVERSE REACTIONS
CNS: dizziness, migraine headache,
lethargy, depression.
CV: hypertension, thrombophlebitis,
pulmonary embolism, edema.
GI: nausea, vomiting, abdominal
cramps.
GU: breakthrough bleeding, dysmenorrhea, amenorrhea; cervical erosion
or abnormal secretions; uterine fibro-

mas; vaginal candidiasis.
Hepatic: cholestatic jaundice.
Local: irritation and pain at injection
site.
Metabolic: hyperglycemia.
Skin: melasma, rash.
Other: breast tenderness, enlarge-
ment, or secretion; decreased libido.

INTERACTIONS
Rifampin: decreased progestogen effects. Monitor for diminished therapeutic response.

NURSING CONSIDERATIONS
• Contraindicated in thromboembolic
disorders, breast cancer, undiagnosed
abnormal vaginal bleeding, severe hepatic disease, missed abortion, or
pregnancy. Use cautiously when diabetes mellitus, seizure disorder, migraine, cardiac or renal disease,
asthma, or mental illness is present.
• FDA regulations require that, before receiving first dose, patients read
package insert explaining possible
progestogen side effects. Provide verbal explanation also. Patient should
report any unusual symptoms immediately and should stop drug and call
doctor if visual disturbances or migraine occurs.
• Don't use as test for pregnancy;
drug may cause birth defects and
masculinization of female fetus.
• Warn patient that edema and weight
gain are likely.
• Give oil solutions (sesame oil and
castor oil) deep I.M. in gluteal muscle.
• Effect lasts 7 to 14 days.

- For I.M. use only.
- Teach patient how to perform a breast self-examination.
- Instruct patient that normal menstrual cycles may not resume for 2 to 3 months after drug is stopped.

medroxyprogesterone acetate
Amen, Curretab, Depo-Provera♦, Provera♦
Pregnancy Category: X

MECHANISM OF ACTION
Suppresses ovulation, possibly by inhibiting pituitary gonadotropin secretion. Also forms a thick cervical mucus.

INDICATIONS & DOSAGE
Women:
Abnormal uterine bleeding due to hormonal imbalance—
5 to 10 mg P.O. daily for 5 to 10 days beginning on the 16th day of menstrual cycle. If patient has received estrogen—10 mg P.O. daily for 10 days beginning on 16th day of cycle.
Secondary amenorrhea—
5 to 10 mg P.O. daily for 5 to 10 days.
Endometrial or renal carcinoma—
Adults: 400 to 1,000 mg/week I.M.

ADVERSE REACTIONS
CNS: dizziness, migraine headache, lethargy, depression.
CV: hypertension, thrombophlebitis, *pulmonary embolism, edema.*
GI: nausea, vomiting, abdominal cramps.
GU: breakthrough bleeding, dysmenorrhea, amenorrhea; cervical erosion or abnormal secretions; uterine fibromas, vaginal candidiasis.
Hepatic: cholestatic jaundice.
Metabolic: hyperglycemia, decreased libido.
Skin: melasma, rash.
Local: pain, induration, sterile abscesses.

Other: breast tenderness, enlargement, or secretion.

INTERACTIONS
Rifampin: decreased progestogen effects. Monitor for diminished therapeutic response.

NURSING CONSIDERATIONS
- Contraindicated in thromboembolic disorders, breast cancer, undiagnosed abnormal vaginal bleeding, pregnancy, missed abortion, hepatic dysfunction. Use cautiously when diabetes mellitus, seizure disorder, migraine, cardiac or renal disease, asthma, or mental illness is present.
- I.M. injection may be painful. Monitor sites for evidence of sterile abscess.
- FDA regulations require that, before receiving first dose, patients read package insert explaining possible progestogen side effects. Provide verbal explanation also. Patient should report any unusual symptoms immediately and should stop drug and call doctor if visual disturbances or migraine occurs.
- Don't use as test for pregnancy; drug may cause birth defects and masculinization of female fetus.
- Teach patient how to perform a breast self-examination.
- Has been used effectively to treat obstructive sleep apnea.

norethindrone
Micronor♦, Norlutin, Nor-Q.D.
Pregnancy Category: X

MECHANISM OF ACTION
Suppresses ovulation, possibly by inhibiting pituitary gonadotropin secretion. Also forms a thick cervical mucus.

INDICATIONS & DOSAGE
Women:
Amenorrhea; abnormal uterine bleed-

ing—
5 to 20 mg P.O. daily on days 5 to 25
of menstrual cycle.
Endometriosis—
10 mg P.O. daily for 14 days, then increase by 5 mg P.O. daily q 2 weeks
up to 30 mg daily.

ADVERSE REACTIONS
CNS: dizziness, migraine headache,
lethargy, depression.
CV: hypertension, thrombophlebitis,
pulmonary embolism, edema.
GI: nausea, vomiting, abdominal
cramps.
GU: breakthrough bleeding, dysmenorrhea, amenorrhea; cervical erosion
or abnormal secretions; uterine fibromas; vaginal candidiasis.
Hepatic: cholestatic jaundice.
Metabolic: hyperglycemia, decreased
libido.
Skin: melasma, rash.
Other: breast tenderness, enlargement, or secretion.

INTERACTIONS
Rifampin: decreased progestogen effects. Monitor for diminished therapeutic response.

NURSING CONSIDERATIONS
• Contraindicated in thromboembolic
disorders, breast cancer, undiagnosed
abnormal vaginal bleeding, severe hepatic disease, missed abortion, or
pregnancy. Use cautiously when diabetes mellitus, seizure disorder, migraine, cardiac or renal disease,
asthma, or mental illness is present.
• Don't use as test for pregnancy;
drug may cause birth defects and
masculinization of female fetus.
• FDA regulations require that, before receiving first dose, patients read
package insert explaining possible
progestogen side effects. Provide verbal explanation also. Patient should
report any unusual symptoms immediately and should stop drug and call
doctor if visual disturbances or mi-

graine occurs.
• Watch patient carefully for signs of
edema.
• Preliminary estrogen treatment is
usually needed in menstrual disorders.
• Teach the patient how to perform a
breast self-examination.

---

norethindrone acetate
Aygestin, Norlutate♦
Pregnancy Category: X

MECHANISM OF ACTION
Suppresses ovulation, possibly by inhibiting pituitary gonadotropin secretion. Also forms a thick cervical mucus.

INDICATIONS & DOSAGE
Women:
*Amenorrhea, abnormal uterine bleed-
ing—*
2.5 to 10 mg P.O. daily on days 5 to
25 of menstrual cycle.
Endometriosis—
5 mg P.O. daily for 14 days, then increase by 2.5 mg daily q 2 weeks up
to 15 mg daily.

ADVERSE REACTIONS
CNS: dizziness, migraine headache,
lethargy, depression.
CV: hypertension, thrombophlebitis,
pulmonary embolism, edema.
GI: nausea, vomiting, abdominal
cramps.
GU: breakthrough bleeding, dysmenorrhea, amenorrhea; cervical erosion
or abnormal secretions; uterine fibromas; vaginal candidiasis.
Hepatic: cholestatic jaundice.
Metabolic: hyperglycemia, decreased
libido.
Skin: melasma, rash.
Other: breast tenderness, enlargement, or secretion.

INTERACTIONS
Rifampin: decreased progestogen ef-

fects. Monitor for diminished therapeutic response.

NURSING CONSIDERATIONS
• Contraindicated in thromboembolic disorders, breast cancer, undiagnosed abnormal vaginal bleeding, severe hepatic disease, missed abortion, or pregnancy. Use cautiously when diabetes mellitus, seizure disorder, migraine, cardiac or renal disease, asthma, or mental illness is present.
• FDA regulations require that, before receiving first dose, patients read package insert explaining possible progestogen side effects. Provide verbal explanation also. Patient should report any unusual symptoms immediately and should stop drug and call doctor if visual disturbances or migraine occurs.
• Don't use as test for pregnancy; drug may cause birth defects and masculinization of female fetus.
• Preliminary estrogen treatment is usually needed in menstrual disorders.
• Twice as potent as norethindrone.
• Teach patient how to perform a breast self-examination.

---

norgestrel
Ovrette**
Pregnancy Category: X

MECHANISM OF ACTION
Suppresses ovulation, possibly by inhibiting pituitary gonadotropin secretion. Also forms a thick cervical mucus.

INDICATIONS & DOSAGE
Women:
Contraception—
1 tablet P.O. daily.

ADVERSE REACTIONS
CNS: cerebral thrombosis or hemorrhage, migraine headache, lethargy, depression.

CV: hypertension, thrombophlebitis, *pulmonary embolism, edema.*
GI: nausea, vomiting, abdominal cramps, gallbladder disease.
GU: *breakthrough bleeding, change in menstrual flow,* dysmenorrhea, spotting, amenorrhea; cervical erosion, vaginal candidiasis.
Hepatic: cholestatic jaundice.
Skin: melasma, rash.
Other: breast tenderness, enlargement, or secretion.

INTERACTIONS
Rifampin: decreased progestogen effects. Monitor for diminished therapeutic response.

NURSING CONSIDERATIONS
• Contraindicated in thromboembolic disorders, breast cancer, undiagnosed abnormal vaginal bleeding, severe hepatic disease, missed abortion, or pregnancy. Use cautiously when diabetes mellitus, seizure disorder, migraine, cardiac or renal disease, asthma, or mental illness is present.
• FDA regulations require that, before receiving first dose, patients read package insert explaining possible progestogen effects. Provide verbal explanation also. Patient should report any unusual symptoms immediately and should stop drug and call doctor if visual disturbances, migraine, or numbness or tingling in limbs occurs.
• Tell patient to take pill every day, even if menstruating. Pill should be taken at the same time every day.
• Progestogen-only oral contraceptive known as "minipill."
• Teach the patient how to perform a breast self-examination.
• Women using oral contraceptives should be advised of the increased risk of serious cardiovascular side effects associated with heavy cigarette smoking (15 or more cigarettes per day). These risks are quite marked in women over 35 years.

Italicized side effects are common or life-threatening.
*Liquid form contains alcohol.   **May contain tartrazine.

• Risk of pregnancy increases with each tablet missed. A patient who misses one tablet should take it as soon as she remembers; she should then take the next tablet at the regular time. A patient who misses two tablets should take one as soon as she remembers and then take the next regular dose at the usual time; she should use a nonhormonal method of contraception in addition to norgestrel until 14 tablets have been taken. A patient who misses three or more tablets should discontinue the drug and use a nonhormonal method of contraception until after her menses. If her menstrual period does not occur within 45 days, pregnancy testing is necessary.
• Instruct the patient to report immediately excessive bleeding or bleeding between menstrual cycles.

progesterone
Femotrone, Profac-O, Progelan, Progest-50, Progestaject-50, Progestasert♦
Pregnancy Category: X

MECHANISM OF ACTION
Suppresses ovulation, possibly by inhibiting pituitary gonadotropin secretion. Also forms a thick cervical mucus.

INDICATIONS & DOSAGE
Women:
Amenorrhea—
5 to 10 mg I.M. daily for 6 to 8 days.
Dysfunctional uterine bleeding—
5 to 10 mg I.M. daily for 6 doses.
Contraception (as an intrauterine device)—
Progestasert system inserted into uterine cavity. Replace after 1 year.
Management of premenstrual syndrome (PMS)—
200 to 400 mg as a suppository administered either rectally or vaginally.

ADVERSE REACTIONS
CNS: dizziness, migraine headache, lethargy, depression.
CV: hypertension, thrombophlebitis, *pulmonary embolism, edema.*
GI: nausea, vomiting, abdominal cramps.
GU: breakthrough bleeding, dysmenorrhea, amenorrhea; cervical erosion or abnormal secretions; uterine fibromas; vaginal candidiasis.
Hepatic: cholestatic jaundice.
Local: pain at injection site.
Metabolic: hyperglycemia, decreased libido.
Skin: melasma, rash.
Other: breast tenderness, enlargement, or secretion.

INTERACTIONS
Rifampin: decreased progestogen effects. Monitor for diminished therapeutic response.

NURSING CONSIDERATIONS
• Contraindicated in thromboembolic disorders, breast cancer, undiagnosed abnormal vaginal bleeding, severe hepatic disease, or missed abortion. Use cautiously when diabetes mellitus, seizure disorder, migraine, cardiac or renal disease, asthma, or mental illness is present.
• FDA regulations require that, before receiving first dose, patients read package insert explaining possible progestogen side effects. Provide verbal explanation also. Patient should report any unusual symptoms immediately and should stop drug and call doctor if visual disturbances or migraine occurs.
• Give oil solutions (peanut oil or sesame oil) deep I.M. Check sites frequently for irritation. Rotate injection sites.
• A progesterone-containing IUD (Progestasert) available that releases 65 mcg progesterone daily for 1 year.
• Instruct patient with Progestasert IUD how to check for proper IUD

placement. Also, advise patient that she may experience cramps for several days after insertion and menstrual periods may be heavier. Patient should report excessively heavy menses and bleeding between menses to the doctor.

• Tell patient with Progestasert IUD that the progesterone supply is depleted in 1 year and the device must be changed. Pregnancy risk increases after 1 year if patient relies on progesterone-depleted device for contraception.

• Patients considering IUD contraception should be advised of side effects, including uterine perforation, increased risk of infection, pelvic inflammatory disease, ectopic pregnancy, abdominal cramping, increased menstrual flow, and expulsion of the device.

• Preliminary estrogen treatment is usually needed in menstrual disorders.

• Teach the patient how to perform a breast self-examination.

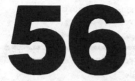

Gonadotropins

chorionic gonadotropin, human
gonadorelin hydrochloride
menotropins

COMBINATION PRODUCTS
None.

---

chorionic gonadotropin, human
Android HCG, A.P.L.♦, Chorex,
Follutein, Glukor, Gonic, Libigen,
Pregnyl, Profasi HP♦, Stemutrolin
Pregnancy Category: C

MECHANISM OF ACTION
Serves as a substitute for luteinizing
hormone (LH) to stimulate ovulation
of an HMG-prepared follicle. Also
promotes secretion of gonadal steroid
hormones by stimulating production
of androgen by the interstitial cells of
the testes (Leydig's cells).

INDICATIONS & DOSAGE
Anovulation and infertility—
Women: 10,000 units I.M. 1 day af-
ter last dose of menotropins.
Hypogonadism—
Men: 500 to 1,000 units I.M. 3 times
weekly for 3 weeks, then twice
weekly for 3 weeks; or 4,000 units
I.M. 3 times weekly for 6 to 9
months, then 2,000 units 3 times
weekly for 3 more months.
Nonobstructive cryptorchidism—
Boys 4 to 9 years: 5,000 units I.M.
every other day for 4 doses.

ADVERSE REACTIONS
CNS: headache, fatigue, irritability,
restlessness, depression.
GU: early puberty (growth of testes,
penis, pubic and axillary hair; voice
change; down on upper lip; growth of
body hair).
Local: *pain at injection site.*
Other: gynecomastia, edema.

INTERACTIONS
None significant.

NURSING CONSIDERATIONS
• Contraindicated in pituitary hypertrophy or tumor, prostatic cancer, and
early puberty (usual onset between 10
and 13 years of age). Use cautiously
in epilepsy, migraine, asthma, cardiac
or renal disease.
• When used with menotropins to induce ovulation, multiple births possible.
• Usually used only after failure of
clomiphene in anovulatory patients.
• In infertility, encourage daily intercourse from day before chorionic gonadotropin is given until ovulation occurs.
• Inspect genitalia of boys for signs of
early puberty.
• Be alert to symptoms of ectopic
pregnancy. Usually evident between
week 8 to 12 of gestation.

---

gonadorelin hydrochloride
Factrel♦
Pregnancy Category: B

MECHANISM OF ACTION
A synthetic luteinizing hormone that
releases LH.

INDICATIONS & DOSAGE
Evaluation of the functional capacity and response of gonadotropic hormones—
Adults: 100 µg S.C. or I.V. In women for whom the phase of the menstrual cycle can be established, perform the test between day 1 and day 7.

ADVERSE REACTIONS
Local: swelling, occasionally with pain and pruritus when administered S.C.; skin rash after chronic S.C. administration.
Systemic: headache, nausea, lightheadedness, abdominal discomfort.

INTERACTIONS
Levodopa, spironolactone: may elevate gonadotropin levels. Monitor results carefully.
Digoxin, oral contraceptives: may depress gonadotropin levels. Monitor results carefully.

NURSING CONSIDERATIONS
• Although no hypersensitivity reactions have been reported to date, use cautiously in patients who are allergic to other drugs. Keep epinephrine readily available.
• The gonadorelin test can be performed concomitantly with other post-treatment evaluation.
• For specific test methodology and interpretation of test results, refer to the manufacturer's full product information. Ask pharmacist for a copy.
• Reconstitute vial with 1 ml of accompanying sterile diluent. Prepare solution immediately before use. After reconstitution, store at room temperature and use within 1 day. Discard unused reconstituted solution and diluent.
• Store at room temperature.
• As a single injection, gonadorelin can evaluate the functional capacity and response of the gonadotropins of the anterior pituitary. Prolonged or repeated administration may be necessary to measure pituitary gonadotropic reserve.

menotropins
Pergonal♦
Pregnancy Category: C

MECHANISM OF ACTION
Menotropins, when administered to women who have not had primary ovarian failure, mimics follicle-stimulating hormone (FSH) in inducing follicular growth and LH in aiding follicular maturation.

INDICATIONS & DOSAGE
Anovulation—
Women: 75 international units (IU) each FSH and LH I.M. daily for 9 to 12 days, followed by 10,000 units chorionic gonadotropin I.M. 1 day after last dose of menotropins. Repeat for 1 to 3 menstrual cycles until ovulation occurs.
Infertility with ovulation—
Women: 75 IU each of FSH and LH I.M. daily for 9 to 12 days, followed by 10,000 units chorionic gonadotropin I.M. 1 day after last dose of menotropins. Repeat for 2 menstrual cycles and then increase to 150 IU each FSH and LH I.M. daily for 9 to 12 days, followed by 10,000 units chorionic gonadotropin I.M. 1 day after last dose of menotropins. Repeat for 2 menstrual cycles.
Infertility—
Men: 1 ampul I.M. 3 times weekly (given concomitantly with HCG 2,000 units twice weekly) for at least 4 months.
Menotropins are available in ampuls containing 75 IU each FSH and LH.

ADVERSE REACTIONS
Blood: hemoconcentration with fluid loss into abdomen.
GI: nausea, vomiting, diarrhea.
GU: women; *ovarian enlargement with pain and abdominal distention,*

Italicized side effects are common or life-threatening.
*Liquid form contains alcohol.   **May contain tartrazine.

multiple birth, ovarian hyperstimulation syndrome (sudden ovarian enlargement, ascites with or without pain, or pleural effusion).
GU: mcn; *gynecomastia*.
Other: fever.

INTERACTIONS
None significant.

NURSING CONSIDERATIONS
• Contraindicated in high urinary gonadotropin levels, thyroid or adrenal dysfunction, pituitary tumor, abnormal uterine bleeding, ovarian cysts or enlargement, and pregnancy.
• Tell patient that there is a possibility of multiple birth.
• In infertility, encourage daily intercourse from day before chorionic gonadotropin is given until ovulation occurs.
• Pregnancy usually occurs 4 to 6 weeks after therapy.
• Reconstitute with 1 to 2 ml sterile saline injection. Use immediately.

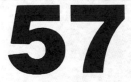

Antidiabetic agents and glucagon

acetohexamide
chlorpropamide
glipizide
glucagon
glyburide
insulins
tolazamide
tolbutamide

COMBINATION PRODUCTS
MIXTARD INJECTION: 100 mg/ml isophane purified pork insulin suspension and purified pork insulin injection.

---

acetohexamide
Dimelor◆◆, Dymelor
Pregnancy Category: D

MECHANISM OF ACTION
Stimulates insulin release from the pancreatic beta cells and reduces glucose output by the liver. An extrapancreatic effect increases peripheral sensitivity to insulin. A sulfonylurea.

INDICATIONS & DOSAGE
Adjunct to diet to lower the blood glucose in patients with non-insulin dependent diabetes mellitus (type II)—
Adults: initially, 250 mg P.O. daily before breakfast; may increase dose q 5 to 7 days (by 250 to 500 mg) as needed to maximum 1.5 g daily, divided b.i.d. to t.i.d. before meals.
To replace insulin therapy—
If insulin dose is less than 20 units daily, insulin may be stopped and oral therapy started with 250 mg P.O. daily, before breakfast, increased as

above if needed. If insulin dose is 20 to 40 units daily, start oral therapy with 250 mg P.O. daily, before breakfast, while reducing insulin dose 25% to 30% daily or every other day, depending on response to oral therapy.

ADVERSE REACTIONS
GI: nausea, heartburn, vomiting.
Metabolic: sodium loss, *hypoglycemia.*
Skin: rash, pruritus, facial flushing.
Other: hypersensitivity reactions.

INTERACTIONS
Anabolic steroids, chloramphenicol, clofibrate, guanethidine, MAO inhibitors, oral anticoagulants, phenylbutazone, salicylates, sulfonamides: increased hypoglycemic activity. Monitor blood glucose.
Beta blockers, clonidine: prolonged hypoglycemic effect and masked symptoms of hypoglycemia. Use together cautiously.
Corticosteroids, glucagon, rifampin, thiazide diuretics: decreased hypoglycemic response. Monitor blood glucose.

NURSING CONSIDERATIONS
• Contraindicated in treatment of juvenile, growth-onset, brittle, and severe diabetes; in diabetes mellitus adequately controlled by diet; and in maturity-onset diabetes complicated by ketosis, acidosis, diabetic coma, Raynaud's gangrene, renal or hepatic impairment, thyroid or other endocrine dysfunction. Use cautiously in patients with sulfonamide hypersensi-

---

Italicized side effects are common or life-threatening.
*Liquid form contains alcohol.   **May contain tartrazine.

tivity.
• Instruct patient about nature of disease; importance of following therapeutic regimen and adhering to specific diet, weight reduction, exercise, personal hygiene, and avoiding infection; how and when to perform self-blood glucose monitoring; recognition of hypoglycemia and hyperglycemia.
• Be sure patient knows that the therapy relieves symptoms but doesn't cure the disease.
• Patient transferring from another oral sulfonylurea antidiabetic drug usually needs no transition period.
• Patient transferring from insulin therapy to an oral antidiabetic requires blood glucose monitoring at least t.i.d. before meals. Patient may require hospitalization during transition.
• During periods of increased stress, such as infection, fever, surgery, or trauma, patient may require insulin therapy. Monitor patient closely for hyperglycemia in these situations.
• Advise patient to avoid moderate to large intake of alcohol; disulfiram reaction possible.
• The possibility of increased cardiovascular mortality is associated with the use of sulfonylureas.

chlorpropamide
Chloronase♦♦, Diabinese♦,
Glucamide, Novopropamide♦♦,
Stabinol♦♦
Pregnancy Category: D

MECHANISM OF ACTION
Stimulates insulin release from the pancreatic beta cells and reduces glucose output by the liver. An extrapancreatic effect increases peripheral sensitivity to insulin. Also exerts an antidiuretic effect in patients with pituitary-deficient diabetes insipidus. A sulfonylurea.

INDICATIONS & DOSAGE
Adjunct to diet to lower the blood glucose in patients with non-insulin dependent diabetes mellitus (type II)—
Adults: 250 mg P.O. daily with breakfast or in divided doses if GI disturbances occur. First dosage increase may be made after 5 to 7 days due to extended duration of action, then dose may be increased q 3 to 5 days by 50 to 125 mg, if needed, to maximum 750 mg daily. Start with dose of 100 to 125 mg in older patients.
Adults over 65: initial dose should be in the range of 100 to 125 mg daily.
To change from insulin to oral therapy—
If insulin dose less than 40 units daily, insulin may be stopped and oral therapy started as above. If insulin dose is 40 units or more daily, start oral therapy as above with insulin dose reduced 50%. Further insulin reductions should be made according to the patient's response.

ADVERSE REACTIONS
GI: nausea, heartburn, vomiting.
GU: tea-colored urine.
Metabolic: prolonged hypoglycemia, *dilutional hyponatremia.*
Skin: rash, pruritus, facial flushing.
Other: *hypersensitivity reactions.*

INTERACTIONS
Anabolic steroids, chloramphenicol, clofibrate, guanethidine, MAO inhibitors, oral anticoagulants, phenylbutazone, salicylates, sulfonamides: increased hypoglycemic activity. Monitor blood glucose.
Beta blockers, clonidine: prolonged hypoglycemic effect and masked symptoms of hypoglycemia. Use together cautiously.
Corticosteroids, glucagon, rifampin, thiazide diuretics: decreased hypoglycemic response. Monitor blood glucose.

NURSING CONSIDERATIONS
• Contraindicated in the treatment of juvenile, growth-onset, brittle, and severe diabetes.
• Contraindicated in diabetes mellitus adequately controlled by diet and in maturity-onset diabetes complicated by fever, ketosis, acidosis, diabetic coma, major surgery, severe trauma, Raynaud's gangrene, renal or hepatic impairment, thyroid or other endocrine dysfunction. Use cautiously in patients with sulfonamide hypersensitivity.
• Elderly patients may be more sensitive to this drug's adverse reactions.
• Instruct patient about nature of the disease; importance of following therapeutic regimen and adhering to specific diet, weight reduction, exercise, personal hygiene, avoiding infection; how and when to perform self-blood glucose monitoring; and recognition of and intervention for hypoglycemia and hyperglycemia.
• Make sure patient understands that therapy relieves symptoms but does not cure the disease.
• Side effects, especially hypoglycemia, may be more frequent or severe than with some other sulfonylurea drugs (acetohexamide, tolazamide, and tolbutamide) because of its long duration of effect (36 hours).
• If hypoglycemia occurs, patient should be monitored closely for a minimum of 3 to 5 days.
• Patient transferring from another oral sulfonylurea antidiabetic drug usually needs no transition period.
• Patient may require hospitalization during transition from insulin therapy to an oral antidiabetic. Monitor patient for blood glucose levels at least t.i.d., before meals; emphasize the need for a double-voided specimen.
• Drug may accumulate in patients with renal insufficiency.
• Advise patient to avoid intake of alcohol. Chlorpropamide-alcohol flush (CPAF) is characterized by facial flushing, light-headedness, headache, and occasional breathlessness. Even very small amounts of alcohol can produce this reaction.
• Watch for signs of impending renal insufficiency, such as dysuria, anuria, and hematuria, and report them to the doctor immediately.
• May potentiate antidiuretic hormone. Sometimes used to treat diabetes insipidus.
• The possibility of increased cardiovascular mortality is associated with the use of sulfonylureas.

glipizide
Glucotrol
Pregnancy Category: C

MECHANISM OF ACTION
Stimulates insulin release from the pancreatic beta cells and reduces glucose output by the liver. An extrapancreatic effect increases peripheral sensitivity to insulin. A sulfonylurea.

INDICATIONS & DOSAGE
Adjunct to diet to lower the blood glucose in patients with non-insulin-dependent diabetes mellitus (type II)—
Adults: Initially, 5 mg P.O. daily given before breakfast. Geriatric patients or those with liver disease may be started on 2.5 mg. Usual maintenance dose is 10 to 15 mg. Maximum recommended daily dose is 40 mg.
To replace insulin therapy—
If insulin dose is more than 20 units daily, patient may be started at usual dosage in addition to 50% of the insulin dose. If insulin dose is less than 20 units, insulin may be discontinued.

ADVERSE REACTIONS
CNS: dizziness.
GI: nausea, vomiting, constipation.
Hepatic: *cholestatic jaundice*.
Metabolic: *hypoglycemia*.
Skin: rash, pruritus, facial flushing.

INTERACTIONS
Anabolic steroids, chloramphenicol, clofibrate, guanethidine, MAO inhibitors, oral anticoagulants, phenylbutazone, salicylates, sulfonamides: increased hypoglycemic activity. Monitor blood glucose.

Beta blockers, clonidine: prolonged hypoglycemic effect and masked symptoms of hypoglycemia. Use together cautiously.

Corticosteroids, glucagon, rifampin, thiazide diuretics: decreased hypoglycemic response. Monitor blood glucose.

NURSING CONSIDERATIONS
• Contraindicated in patients with diabetic ketoacidosis, with or without coma. Use cautiously in patients with renal and hepatic disease and in patients with sulfonamide hypersensitivity.

• Elderly patients may be more sensitive to this drug's adverse reactions.

• Patient transferring from insulin therapy to an oral antidiabetic requires blood glucose monitoring at least t.i.d. before meals. Patient may require hospitalization during transition.

• During periods of increased stress, such as infection, fever, surgery, or trauma, patient may require insulin therapy. Monitor patient closely for hyperglycemia in these situations.

• Instruct patient about nature of disease; importance of following therapeutic regimen and adhering to specific diet, weight reduction, exercise, personal hygiene, and avoiding infection; how and when to perform self-blood glucose monitoring; recognition of hypoglycemia and hyperglycemia.

• Some patients taking glipizide may be effectively controlled on a once-a-day regimen, while others show better response with divided dosing.

• Give approximately 30 minutes before meals.

• Glipizide is a second-generation sulfonylurea oral hypoglycemic. The frequency of side effects appears to be lower than with first-generation drugs such as chlorpropamide and tolbutamide.

• Glipizide has a mild diuretic effect. May be useful in patients who have CHF or cirrhosis.

• The possibility of increased cardiovascular mortality is associated with the use of sulfonylureas.

---

glucagon
Pregnancy Category: B

MECHANISM OF ACTION
Raises blood glucose levels by promoting catalytic depolymerization of hepatic glycogen to glucose.

INDICATIONS & DOSAGE
Coma of insulin-shock therapy—
Adults: 0.5 to 1 mg S.C., I.M., or I.V. 1 hour after coma develops; may repeat within 25 minutes, if necessary. In very deep coma, also give glucose 10% to 50% I.V. for faster response. When patient responds, give additional carbohydrate immediately.

Severe insulin-induced hypoglycemia during diabetic therapy—
Adults and children: 0.5 to 1 mg S.C., I.M., or I.V.; may repeat q 20 minutes for 2 doses, if necessary. If coma persists, give glucose 10% to 50% I.V.

Diagnostic aid for radiologic examination—
Adults: 0.25 to 2 mg I.V. or I.M. prior to initiation of radiologic procedure.

ADVERSE REACTIONS
GI: nausea, vomiting.
Other: hypersensitivity.

INTERACTIONS
Phenytoin: inhibited glucagon-induced insulin release. Use cautiously.

NURSING CONSIDERATIONS
• Hypoglycemic juvenile or unstable diabetics usually do not respond to glucagon. Give dextrose I.V. instead.
• It is vital to arouse the patient from coma as quickly as possible and to give additional carbohydrates orally to prevent secondary hypoglycemic reactions.
• For I.V. drip infusion, glucagon is compatible with dextrose solution, but forms a precipitate in chloride solutions.
• Instruct the patient and family in proper glucagon administration, recognition of hypoglycemia, and urgency of calling a doctor immediately in emergencies.
• May be used as diagnostic aid in radiologic examination of the stomach, duodenum, small bowel, and colon when a hypotonic state is advantageous.
• Has a positive inotropic and chronotropic action on the heart. May be used to treat overdosage of beta-adrenergic blockers.

glyburide
Diabeta**, Micronase
Pregnancy Category: B

MECHANISM OF ACTION
Stimulates insulin release from the pancreatic beta cells and reduces glucose output by the liver. An extrapancreatic effect increases peripheral sensitivity to insulin. A sulfonylurea.

INDICATIONS & DOSAGE
Adjunct to diet to lower the blood glucose in patients with non-insulin-dependent diabetes mellitus (type II)—
Adults: Initially, 2.5 to 5 mg P.O. daily administered with breakfast. Patients who are more sensitive to hypoglycemic drugs should be started at 1.25 mg daily. Usual maintenance dose is 1.25 to 20 mg daily, given either as a single dose or in divided

doses.
To replace insulin therapy—
If insulin dose is more than 40 units daily, patient may be started on 5 mg glyburide daily in addition to 50% of the insulin dose.

ADVERSE REACTIONS
GI: nausea, epigastric fullness, heartburn.
Hepatic: *cholestatic jaundice.*
Metabolic: *hypoglycemia.*
Skin: rash, pruritus, facial flushing.

INTERACTIONS
Anabolic steroids, chloramphenicol, clofibrate, guanethidine, MAO inhibitors, oral anticoagulants, phenylbutazone, salicylates, sulfonamides: increased hypoglycemic activity. Monitor blood glucose.
Beta blockers, clonidine: prolonged hypoglycemic effect and masked symptoms of hypoglycemia. Use together cautiously.
Corticosteroids, glucagon, rifampin, thiazide diuretics: decreased hypoglycemic response. Monitor blood glucose.

NURSING CONSIDERATIONS
• Contraindicated in patients with diabetic ketoacidosis, with or without coma. Use cautiously in patients with sulfonamide hypersensitivity and in patients with severe renal impairment.
• Elderly patients may be more sensitive to this drug's adverse reactions.
• Patient transferring from insulin therapy to an oral antidiabetic requires blood glucose monitoring at least t.i.d. before meals. Patient may require hospitalization during transition.
• During periods of increased stress, such as infection, fever, surgery, or trauma, patient may require insulin therapy. Monitor patient closely for hyperglycemia in these situations.
• Instruct patient about nature of dis-

ease; importance of following therapeutic regimen and adhering to specific diet, weight reduction, exercise, personal hygiene, and avoiding infection; how and when to perform self-blood glucose monitoring; recognition of hypoglycemia and hyperglycemia.

• A maintenance dose of 5 mg glyburide provides approximately the same degree of blood glucose control as 250 to 375 mg chlorpropamide, 250 to 375 mg tolazamide, 500 to 750 mg acetohexamide, or 1,000 to 1,500 mg tolbutamide.

• Although most patients may take glyburide once a day, patients taking more than 10 mg daily may achieve better results with twice-daily dosage.

• Glyburide is a second-generation sulfonylurea oral hypoglycemic. The frequency of side effects appears to be lower than with first-generation drugs such as chlorpropamide and tolbutamide.

• Glyburide exerts a mild diuretic effect. May be useful in patients who have CHF or cirrhosis.

• The possibility of increased cardiovascular mortality is associated with the use of sulfonylureas.

insulins

regular insulin
Beef Regular Iletin II (acid neutral CZI), Humulin R♦, Iletin Regular♦♦, Novolin R, Pork Regular Iletin II♦, Regular Iletin I, Regular Pork Insulin, Velosulin♦, Velosulin Human

regular insulin concentrated
Regular (concentrated) Iletin

prompt insulin zinc suspension
Iletin Semilente♦♦, Semilente Iletin I, Semilente Insulin, Semilente Purified Pork

isophane insulin suspension (NPH)
Beef NPH Iletin II, Humulin N♦, Iletin NPH♦♦, Insulatard NPH♦, Insulatard NPH Human, NPH♦♦, NPH Iletin I, Pork NPH Iletin II♦, Protaphane NPH, Novolin N

isophane insulin suspension and regular insulin
Initard♦♦, Mixtard♦

insulin zinc suspension
Beef Lente Iletin II, Lente Iletin I, Lente Insulin♦, Pork Lente Iletin II♦, Lentard, Monotard, Novolin L, Humulin L

protamine zinc insulin suspension (PZI)
Beef Protamine Zinc Iletin II, Iletin PZI♦♦, Pork Protamine Zinc Iletin II, Protamine Zinc Iletin I

extended insulin zinc suspension
Iletin Ultralente♦♦, Ultralente♦♦, Ultralente Iletin I, Ultralente Insulin, Ultralente Purified Beef
Pregnancy Category: B

MECHANISM OF ACTION
Increases glucose transport across muscle and fat-cell membranes to reduce blood glucose levels. Promotes conversion of glucose to its storage form, glycogen; triggers amino acid uptake and conversion to protein in muscle cells and inhibits protein degradation; stimulates triglyceride formation and inhibits release of free fatty acids from adipose tissue; and stimulates lipoprotein lipase activity, which converts circulating lipoproteins to fatty acids.

INDICATIONS & DOSAGE
Diabetic ketoacidosis (use regular insulin only)—

Unmarked trade names available in the United States only.
♦ Also available in Canada.   ♦♦ Available in Canada only.

Adults: 25 to 150 units I.V. immediately, then additional doses may be given q 1 hour based on blood sugar levels until patient is out of acidosis; then give S.C. q 6 hours thereafter. Alternative dosage schedule: 50 to 100 units I.V. and 50 to 100 units S.C. stat; additional doses may be given q 2 to 6 hours based on blood sugar levels; or 0.33 units/kg I.V. bolus, followed by 7 to 10 units/hour I.V. by continuous infusion. Continue infusion until blood sugar drops to 250 mg%, then start S.C. insulin q 6 hours.

Children: 0.5 to 1 unit/kg divided into 2 doses, 1 given I.V. and the other S.C., followed by 0.5 to 1 unit/kg I.V. q 1 to 2 hours; or 0.1 unit/kg I.V. bolus, then 0.1 unit/kg hourly continuous I.V. infusion until blood sugar drops to 250 mg%, then start S.C. insulin. Preparation of infusion: add 100 units regular insulin and 1 g albumin to 100 ml 0.9% saline solution. Insulin concentration will be 1 unit/ml. (The albumin will adsorb to plastic, preventing loss of the insulin to plastic.)

Ketosis-prone and juvenile-onset diabetes mellitus, diabetes mellitus inadequately controlled by diet and oral hypoglycemics—
Adults and children: therapeutic regimen prescribed by doctor and adjusted according to patient's blood and urine glucose concentrations.

ADVERSE REACTIONS
Metabolic: *hypoglycemia, hyperglycemia (rebound, or Somogyi, effect).*
Skin: urticaria.
Local: *lipoatrophy, lipohypertrophy,* itching, swelling, redness, stinging, warmth at site of injection.
Other: *anaphylaxis.*

INTERACTIONS
Alcohol, beta blockers, clofibrate, fenfluramine, MAO inhibitors, salicylates, tetracycline: prolonged hypo-

glycemic effect. Monitor blood glucose carefully.
Corticosteroids, thiazide diuretics: diminished insulin response. Monitor for hyperglycemia.

NURSING CONSIDERATIONS
• Use only regular insulin in patients with circulatory collapse, diabetic ketoacidosis, or hyperkalemia. Do not use regular insulin concentrated, I.V. Do not use intermediate or long-acting insulins for coma or other emergency requiring rapid drug action.
• Accuracy of measurement is very important, especially with regular insulin concentrated. Aids, such as magnifying sleeve, dose magnifier, or cornwall syringe, may help improve accuracy.
• Dosage is always expressed in USP units.
• Don't interchange single-source beef or pork insulins; a dosage adjustment may be required.
• Lente, semilente, and ultralente insulins may be mixed in any proportion.
• Regular insulin may be mixed with NPH or lente insulins in any proportion.
• Regular insulin *should not* be mixed with globin insulin.
• Advise patient not to alter the order of mixing insulins or change the model or brand of syringe or needle.
• Note that switching from separate injections to a prepared mixture may alter your patient's response. Whenever NPH or lente is mixed with regular insulin in the same syringe, be sure to administer immediately to avoid binding.
• Store insulin in cool area. Refrigeration desirable but not essential, except with regular insulin concentrated.
• Don't use insulin that has changed color or becomes clumped or granular in appearance.

Italicized side effects are common or life-threatening.
*Liquid form contains alcohol.   **May contain tartrazine.

- Check expiration date on vial before using contents.
- Administration route is S.C. because absorption rate and pain are less than with I.M. injections. Ketosis-prone juvenile-onset, severely ill, and newly diagnosed diabetics with very high blood sugar levels may require hospitalization and I.V. treatment with regular fast-acting insulin. Ketosis-resistant diabetics may be treated as outpatients with intermediate-acting insulin and instructions on how to alter dosage according to self-performed blood glucose determinations. Some patients, primarily pregnant or brittle diabetics, may use reflectance meter to do fingerstick blood glucose tests at home.
- Press but do not rub site after injection. Rotate injection sites. Chart sites to avoid overuse of one area. However, unstable diabetics may achieve better control if injection site is rotated within same anatomic region.
- To mix insulin suspension, swirl vial gently or rotate between palms or between palm and thigh. Don't shake vigorously: this causes bubbling and air in syringe.
- Insulin requirements increase, sometimes drastically, in pregnant diabetics, then decline immediately postpartum.
- Be sure the patient knows that therapy relieves symptoms but doesn't cure the disease.
- Tell patient about the nature of disease, the importance of following the therapeutic regimen and specific diet, weight reduction, exercise, personal hygiene, avoiding infection, and timing of injection and eating. Emphasize that meals must not be omitted. Teach that urine tests are essential guides to dosage and success of therapy; important to recognize hypoglycemic symptoms because insulin-induced hypoglycemia is hazardous and may cause brain damage if prolonged; most side effects are self-limiting and temporary.

- Advise patient to wear medical ID always; to carry ample insulin supply and syringes on trips; to have carbohydrates (lump of sugar or candy) on hand for emergency; to take note of time zone changes for dose schedule when traveling.
- Marijuana use may increase insulin requirements.
- Cigarette smoking decreases the amount of absorption of insulin administered subcutaneously. Advise patient not to smoke within 30 minutes after insulin injection.
- Some patients may develop insulin resistance and require large insulin doses to control symptoms of diabetes. U-500 insulin is available for such patients as Purified Pork Iletin Regular Insulin, U500. Although every pharmacy may not normally stock it, it is readily available. Patient should notify pharmacist several days before refill of prescription is needed. Nurse should give hospital pharmacy sufficient notice before needing to refill in-house prescription. Never store U-500 insulin in same area with other insulin preparations because of danger of severe overdose if given accidentally to other patients. U-500 insulin must be administered with a U-100 syringe since no syringes are made for this drug.
- Human insulin may be advantageous in patients who are allergic to pork or beef forms. Otherwise, these insulins offer no advantage. Humulin is synthesized by a strain of *Escherichia coli* that has been genetically altered. Novolin brands are derived by enzymatic alteration of pork insulin.

tolazamide
Tolinase
Pregnancy Category: C

MECHANISM OF ACTION
Stimulates insulin release from the pancreatic beta cells and reduces glucose output by the liver. An extrapancreatic effect increases peripheral sensitivity to insulin. A sulfonylurea.

INDICATIONS & DOSAGE
Adjunct to diet to lower the blood glucose in patients with non-insulin dependent diabetes mellitus (type II)—
Adults: initially, 100 mg P.O. daily with breakfast if fasting blood sugar (FBS) under 200 mg%; or 250 mg if FBS is over 200 mg%. May adjust dose at weekly intervals by 100 to 250 mg. Maximum dose 500 mg b.i.d. before meals.
Adults over 65: 100 mg once daily.
To change from insulin to oral therapy—
If insulin dose under 20 units daily, insulin may be stopped and oral therapy started at 100 mg P.O. daily with breakfast. If insulin dose is 20 to 40 units daily, insulin may be stopped and oral therapy started at 250 mg P.O. daily with breakfast. If insulin dose is over 40 units daily, decrease insulin dose 50% and start oral therapy at 250 mg P.O. daily with breakfast. Increase doses as above.

ADVERSE REACTIONS
GI: nausea, vomiting.
Metabolic: hypoglycemia.
Skin: rash, urticaria, facial flushing.
Other: hypersensitivity reactions.

INTERACTIONS
Anabolic steroids, chloramphenicol, clofibrate, guanethidine, MAO inhibitors, oral anticoagulants, phenylbutazone, salicylates, sulfonamides: increased hypoglycemic activity. Monitor blood glucose.
Beta blockers, clonidine: prolonged hypoglycemic effect and masked symptoms of hypoglycemia. Use together cautiously.
Corticosteroids, glucagon, rifampin, thiazide diuretics: decreased hypoglycemic response. Monitor blood glucose.

NURSING CONSIDERATIONS
• Contraindicated in juvenile, growth-onset, and severe diabetes mellitus; diabetes mellitus adequately controlled by diet or in maturity-onset diabetes mellitus complicated by fever, ketosis, acidosis, or coma; major surgery; severe trauma; Raynaud's gangrene; renal or hepatic impairment; thyroid or other endocrine dysfunction. Use cautiously in patients with sulfonamide hypersensitivity and in elderly, debilitated, or malnourished patients.
• Elderly patients may be more sensitive to this drug's adverse reactions.
• Instruct patient about nature of disease; importance of following therapeutic regimen and specific diet, weight reduction, exercise, personal hygiene, avoiding infection; how and when to perform self-blood glucose monitoring; and recognition of hypoglycemia and hyperglycemia.
• Be sure patient knows that therapy relieves symptoms but doesn't cure disease.
• Patient transferring from another oral sulfonylurea antidiabetic drug usually needs no transition period.
• Patient transferring from insulin therapy to an oral hypoglycemic should test for blood glucose at least t.i.d. before meals. Hospitalization may be required during the transition.
• Advise patient to avoid moderate to large intake of alcohol; disulfiram reaction possible.
• The possibility of increased cardiovascular mortality is associated with the use of sulfonylureas.

Italicized side effects are common or life-threatening.
*Liquid form contains alcohol.   **May contain tartrazine.

tolbutamide

Mobenol♦♦, Novobutamide♦♦,
Orinase♦, SK-Tolbutamide,
Tolbutone♦♦
Pregnancy Category: C

MECHANISM OF ACTION

Stimulates insulin release from the
pancreatic beta cells and reduces glucose output by the liver. An extrapancreatic effect increases peripheral
sensitivity to insulin. A sulfonylurea.

INDICATIONS & DOSAGE

*Stable, maturity-onset nonketotic dia-
betes mellitus uncontrolled by diet
alone and previously untreated—*
Adults: initially, 1 to 2 g P.O. daily as
single dose or divided b.i.d. to t.i.d.
May adjust dose to maximum 3 g
daily.
*To change from insulin to oral ther-
apy—*
If insulin dose is under 20 units daily,
insulin may be stopped and oral therapy started at 1 to 2 g daily. If insulin
dose is 20 to 40 units daily, insulin
dose is reduced 30% to 50% and oral
therapy started as above. If insulin
dose is over 40 units daily, insulin
dose is decreased 20% and oral therapy started as above. Further reductions in insulin dose are based on patient's response to oral therapy.

ADVERSE REACTIONS

GI: nausea, heartburn.
Metabolic: hypoglycemia, dilutional
hyponatremia.
Skin: rash, pruritus, facial flushing.
Other: hypersensitivity reactions.

INTERACTIONS

*Anabolic steroids, chloramphenicol,
clofibrate, guanethidine, MAO inhibitors, oral anticoagulants, phenylbutazone, salicylates, sulfonamides:* increased hypoglycemic activity. Monitor blood glucose.
Beta blockers, clonidine: prolonged
hypoglycemic effect and masked
symptoms of hypoglycemia. Use together cautiously.
*Corticosteroids, glucagon, rifampin,
thiazide diuretics:* decreased hypoglycemic response. Monitor blood glucose.

NURSING CONSIDERATIONS

• Contraindicated in juvenile,
growth-onset, brittle, and severe diabetes; diabetes mellitus adequately
controlled by diet or in maturity-onset
diabetes mellitus complicated by fever, ketosis, acidosis, or coma; major
surgery; severe trauma; Raynaud's
gangrene; renal or hepatic impairment; thyroid or other endocrine dysfunction; pregnancy. Use cautiously in
patients with sulfonamide hypersensitivity.
• Elderly patients may be more sensitive to this drug's adverse reactions.
• Instruct patient about nature of disease; importance of following therapeutic regimen and specific diet,
weight reduction, exercise, personal
hygiene, and avoiding infection; how
and when to perform self-blood glucose monitoring; and recognition of
hypoglycemia and hyperglycemia.
• Be sure patient knows that therapy
relieves symptoms but doesn't cure
disease.
• Patient transferring from another
oral sulfonylurea antidiabetic drug
usually needs no transition period.
• Patient transferring from insulin
therapy to an oral hypoglycemic
should test for blood glucose at least
t.i.d. before meals. Hospitalization
may be required during the transition.
• Advise patient to avoid moderate to
large intake of alcohol: disulfiram reaction possible.
• The possibility of increased cardiovascular mortality is associated with
the use of sulfonylureas.

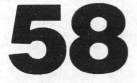

Thyroid hormones

levothyroxine sodium (T₄, or
   L-thyroxine sodium)
liothyronine sodium (T₃)
liotrix
thyroglobulin
thyroid USP (desiccated)
thyrotropin (thyroid-stimulating
   hormone, or TSH)

COMBINATION PRODUCTS
EUTHROID-½: levothyroxine sodium
30 mcg and liothyronine sodium 7.5
mcg.
EUTHROID-1: levothyroxine sodium
60 mcg and liothyronine sodium 15
mcg.
EUTHROID-2: levothyroxine sodium
120 mcg and liothyronine sodium 30
mcg.
EUTHROID-3: levothyroxine sodium
180 mcg and liothyronine sodium
45 mcg.
THYROLAR-¼: levothyroxine sodium
12.5 mcg and liothyronine sodium
3.1 mcg.
THYROLAR-½♦: levothyroxine sodium 25 mcg and liothyronine sodium
6.25 mcg.
THYROLAR-1♦: levothyroxine sodium
50 mcg and liothyronine sodium 12.5
mcg.
THYROLAR-2♦: levothyroxine sodium
100 mcg and liothyronine sodium
25 mcg.
THYROLAR-3♦: levothyroxine sodium
150 mcg and liothyronine sodium
37.5 mcg.

levothyroxine sodium
(T₄, or L-thyroxine sodium)
Eltroxin♦♦, Levoid, Levothroid,
Synthroid♦**
Pregnancy Category: A

MECHANISM OF ACTION
Stimulates the metabolism of all body
tissues by accelerating the rate of cellular oxidation.

INDICATIONS & DOSAGE
*Cretinism in children younger than 1
year*—initially, 0.025 to 0.05 mg P.O.
daily, increased by 0.05 mg P.O. q 2
to 3 weeks to total daily dose 0.1 to
0.4 mg P.O.
Myxedema coma—
Adults: 0.2 to 0.5 mg I.V. If no response in 24 hours, additional 0.1 to
0.3 mg I.V. After condition stabilized, oral maintenance.
Thyroid hormone replacement—
Adults: initially, 0.025 to 0.1 mg
P.O. daily, increased by 0.05 to 0.1
mg P.O. q 1 to 4 weeks until desired
response. Maintenance dose 0.1 to
0.4 mg daily. May be administered
I.V. or I.M. when P.O. ingestion is
precluded for long periods.
Adults over 65: 0.025 mg daily. May
be increased by 0.025 mg at 3- to 4-
week intervals depending on response.
Children: initially, maximum 0.05
mg P.O. daily, gradually increased by
0.025 to 0.05 mg P.O. q 1 to 4 weeks
until desired response.

ADVERSE REACTIONS

Side effects of thyroid hormones are extensions of their pharmacologic properties and reflect patient sensitivity to them.

Signs of overdosage:

CNS: *nervousness, insomnia, tremor.*
CV: *tachycardia, palpitations, arrhythmias, angina pectoris,* hypertension.
GI: change in appetite, nausea, diarrhea.
Other: headache, leg cramps, weight loss, sweating, heat intolerance, fever, menstrual irregularities.

INTERACTIONS

Cholestyramine and colestipol: levothyroxine absorption impaired. Separate doses by 4 to 5 hours.
I.V. phenytoin: free thyroid released. Monitor for tachycardia.

NURSING CONSIDERATIONS

• Contraindicated in myocardial infarction, thyrotoxicosis (except with antithyroid drugs), or uncorrected adrenal insufficiency (thyroid hormones increase tissue demand for adrenocortical hormone and may cause acute adrenal crisis). Use with extreme caution in angina pectoris, hypertension, or other cardiovascular disorders; renal insufficiency; or ischemic states.
• Thyroid hormone replacement requirements are about 25% lower in patients over age 60 than in young adults.
• Use carefully in myxedema; patients are unusually sensitive to thyroid hormone. Dose varies widely among patients; start at lowest and titrate in higher doses according to patient's symptoms and laboratory data until euthyroid state is reached.
• Rapid replacement in patients with arteriosclerosis may precipitate angina, coronary occlusion, or stroke. Use cautiously in such patients.
• In patients with coronary artery disease who must receive thyroid, observe carefully for possible coronary insufficiency if catecholamines must be given.
• Potentially dangerous; not indicated to relieve such vague symptoms as physical and mental sluggishness, irritability, depression, nervousness, ill-defined pains; to treat obesity in euthyroid persons; to treat metabolic insufficiency not associated with thyroid insufficiency; or to treat menstrual disorders or male infertility, unless associated with hypothyroidism.
• When changing from levothyroxine to liothyronine, stop levothyroxine and begin liothyronine. Increase in small increments after residual effects of levothyroxine have disappeared. When changing from liothyronine to levothyroxine, start levothyroxine several days before withdrawing liothyronine to avoid relapse.
• Different brands of levothyroxine may not be bioequivalent. Once the patient has been stabilized on one brand, warn him not to switch to another. Also advise him to avoid "generic" levothyroxine.
• Warn patient to tell doctor at once if chest pain (especially in elderly), palpitations, sweating, nervousness, or other signs of overdosage occur. Also notify doctor immediately if any signs of aggravated cardiovascular disease develop (chest pain, dyspnea, tachycardia).
• During first few months of therapy, children may suffer partial hair loss. Reassure patient that this is temporary.
• Tell patient to take thyroid hormones regularly, at the same time each day, to maintain constant hormone levels.
• Suggest morning dosage to prevent insomnia.
• Monitor pulse rate, blood pressure.
• Protect from moisture and light. Prepare I.V. dose immediately before injection.

• Thyroid hormones alter thyroid function test results. Monitor prothrombin time; patients taking these hormones usually require less anticoagulant. Alert patients to report unusual bleeding and bruising.
• Patients taking levothyroxine who need to have radioactive iodine uptake studies must discontinue drug 4 weeks before test.

---

liothyronine sodium (T₃)

Cytomel♦, Cytomine, Tertroxin♦♦
Pregnancy Category: A

MECHANISM OF ACTION
Stimulates the metabolism of all body tissues by accelerating the rate of cellular oxidation.

INDICATIONS & DOSAGE
Cretinism—
Children 3 years and older: 50 to 100 mcg P.O. daily.
Children under 3 years: 5 mcg P.O. daily, increased by 5 mcg q 3 to 4 days until desired response occurs.
Myxedema—
Adults: initially, 5 mcg daily, increased by 5 to 10 mcg q 1 or 2 weeks. Maintenance dose 50 to 100 mcg daily.
Nontoxic goiter—
Adults: initially, 5 mcg P.O. daily; may be increased by 12.5 to 25 mcg daily q 1 to 2 weeks. Usual maintenance dose 75 mcg daily.
Elderly: initially, 5 mcg P.O. daily, increased by 5-mcg increments at weekly intervals until desired response.
Children: initially, 5 mcg P.O. daily, increased by 5-mcg increments at weekly intervals until desired response.
Thyroid hormone replacement—
Adults: initially, 25 mcg P.O. daily, increased by 12.5 to 25 mcg q 1 to 2 weeks until satisfactory response.

Usual maintenance dose 25 to 75 mcg daily.
T₃ suppression test to differentiate hyperthyroidism from euthyroidism—
Adults: 75 to 100 mcg daily for 7 days.

ADVERSE REACTIONS
Adverse reactions of thyroid hormones are extensions of their pharmacologic properties and reflect patient sensitivity to them.
CNS: hyperirritability, *nervousness, insomnia,* twitching, *tremors,* headache.
CV: increased cardiac output, *tachycardia,* cardiac arrhythmias, *angina pectoris,* increased blood pressure, *cardiac decompensation and collapse.*
GI: diarrhea, abdominal cramps, vomiting.
Other: weight loss, heat intolerance, hyperhidrosis, menstrual irregularities; in infants and children—accelerated rate of bone maturation.

INTERACTIONS
Cholestyramine and colestipol: liothyronine absorption impaired. Separate doses by 4 to 5 hours.
I.V. phenytoin: free thyroid released. Monitor for tachycardia.

NURSING CONSIDERATIONS
• Contraindicated in myocardial infarction, thyrotoxicosis (except with antithyroid drugs), or uncorrected adrenal insufficiency (thyroid hormones increase tissue demand for adrenocortical hormone and may cause acute adrenal crisis). Use with extreme caution in angina pectoris, hypertension, or other cardiovascular disorders; renal insufficiency; or ischemic states.
• Thyroid hormone replacement requirements are about 25% lower in patients over age 60 than in young adults.
• Rapid replacement in patients with arteriosclerosis may precipitate angina, coronary occlusion, or stroke.

Italicized side effects are common or life-threatening.
*Liquid form contains alcohol.   **May contain tartrazine.

Use cautiously in such patients.
• In patients with coronary artery disease who must receive thyroid hormones, observe carefully for possible coronary insufficiency if catecholamines must be given.
• Use carefully in myxedema; patients are unusually sensitive to thyroid hormone.
• Potentially dangerous; not indicated to relieve vague symptoms, such as physical and mental sluggishness, irritability, depression, nervousness, and ill-defined aches and pains; to treat obesity in euthyroid persons; to treat metabolic insufficiency; or to treat menstrual disorders or male infertility, unless asssociated with hypothyroidism.
• When changing from levothyroxine to liothyronine, stop levothyroxine and begin liothyronine. Increase in small increments after residual effects of levothyroxine have disappeared. When changing from liothyronine to levothyroxine, start levothyroxine several days before withdrawing liothyronine to avoid relapse.
• Warn patient to tell doctor at once if chest pain (especially in elderly), palpitations, sweating, nervousness, or other signs of overdosage occur. Also notify doctor immediately if any signs of aggravated cardiovascular disease develop (chest pain, dyspnea, tachycardia).
• During first few months of therapy, children may suffer partial hair loss. Reassure patient that this is temporary.
• Tell patient to take thyroid hormones regularly, at the same time each day, to maintain constant hormone levels.
• Suggest morning dosage to prevent insomnia.
• Monitor pulse rate, blood pressure.
• Thyroid hormones alter thyroid function tests. Monitor prothrombin time; patients taking these hormones may require less anticoagulant. Alert patients to report unusual bleeding and bruising.
• Patients taking liothyronine who need to have radioactive iodine uptake studies must discontinue drug 7 to 10 days before test.

liotrix
Euthroid♦**, Thyrolar♦
Pregnancy Category: A

MECHANISM OF ACTION
Stimulates the metabolism of all body tissues by accelerating the rate of cellular oxidation.

INDICATIONS & DOSAGE
Hypothyroidism—dosages must be individualized to approximate the deficit in the patient's thyroid secretion.
Adults and children: initially, 15 to 30 mg P.O. daily, increasing by 15 to 30 mg q 1 to 2 weeks to desired response; increments in children's dose q 2 weeks.
Elderly: initially, 15 to 30 mg. Usual adult dose doubled q 6 to 8 weeks to desired response.

ADVERSE REACTIONS
Adverse reactions of thyroid hormones are extensions of their pharmacologic properties and reflect patient sensitivity to them.
CNS: hyperirritability, *nervousness, insomnia,* twitching, *tremors.*
CV: increased cardiac output, *tachycardia,* cardiac arrhythmia, *angina pectoris,* increased blood pressure, *cardiac decompensation and collapse.*
GI: diarrhea, abdominal cramps, vomiting.
Other: weight loss, menstrual irregularities, heat intolerance, hyperhidrosis; infants and children—accelerated rate of bone maturation.

INTERACTIONS
Cholestyramine and colestipol: liotrix absorption impaired. Separate doses

by 4 to 5 hours.
I.V. phenytoin: free thyroid released. Monitor for tachycardia.

NURSING CONSIDERATIONS
• Contraindicated in myocardial infarction, thyrotoxicosis (except with antithyroid drugs), or uncorrected adrenal insufficiency (thyroid hormones increase tissue demand for adrenocortical hormone and may cause acute adrenal crisis). Use with extreme caution in angina pectoris, hypertension, or other cardiovascular disorders; renal insufficiency; or ischemic states.
• Thyroid hormone replacement requirements are about 25% lower in patients over age 60 than in young adults.
• Rapid replacement in patients with arteriosclerosis may precipitate angina, coronary occlusion, or stroke. Use cautiously in such patients.
• Use carefully in myxedema; patients are unusually sensitive to thyroid hormone.
• In patients with coronary artery disease who must receive thyroid hormones, observe carefully for possible coronary insufficiency if catecholamines must be given. Also observe carefully during surgery, since cardiac arrhythmias can be precipitated.
• Potentially dangerous; not indicated to relieve vague symptoms, such as physical and mental sluggishness, irritability, depression, nervousness, ill-defined pains; to treat obesity in euthyroid persons; to treat metabolic insufficiency not associated with thyroid insufficiency; or to treat menstrual disorders for male infertility, unless associated with hypothyroidism.
• Tell patient to take thyroid hormones regularly, at the same time each day, preferably before breakfast, to maintain constant hormone levels.
• Warn patient to tell doctor at once if chest pain (especially in elderly), palpitations, sweating, nervousness, or other signs of overdosage occur. Also notify doctor immediately if any signs of aggravated cardiovascular disease develop (chest pain, dyspnea, tachycardia).
• The two commercially prepared liotrix drugs contain different amounts of each ingredient; do not change from one brand to the other without considering the differences in potency: Thyrolar-½ contains 25 mcg T_4 and 6.25 mcg T_3; Euthroid-½ contains 30 mcg T_4 and 7.5 mcg T_3.
• Monitor pulse rate, blood pressure.
• Protect from heat, light, moisture.
• Thyroid hormones alter thyroid function test results. Monitor prothrombin time; patients taking these hormones usually require less anticoagulant. Alert patients to report unusual bleeding and bruising.

thyroglobulin
Proloid♦
Pregnancy Category: A

MECHANISM OF ACTION
Stimulates the metabolism of all body tissues by accelerating the rate of cellular oxidation.

INDICATIONS & DOSAGE
Cretinism and juvenile hypothyroidism—
Children 1 year and older: dosage may approach adult dose (60 to 180 mg P.O. daily), depending on response.
Children 4 to 12 months: 60 to 80 mg P.O. daily.
Children 1 to 4 months: initially, 15 to 30 mg P.O. daily, increased at 2-week intervals. Usual maintenance dose 30 to 45 mg P.O. daily.
Hypothyroidism or myxedema—
Adults: initially, 15 to 30 mg P.O. daily, increased by 15 to 30 mg at 2-week intervals until desired response. Usual maintenance dose 60 to 180 mg P.O. daily, as a single dose.

Italicized side effects are common or life-threatening.
*Liquid form contains alcohol.   **May contain tartrazine.

Elderly: initially 7.5 to 15 mg P.O. daily; the dose is doubled at 6- to 8-week intervals until desired response is obtained.

ADVERSE REACTIONS
Side effects of thyroid hormones are extensions of their pharmacologic properties and reflect patient sensitivity to them.
CNS: hyperirritability, *nervousness, insomnia,* twitching, *tremors,* headache.
CV: increased cardiac output, *tachycardia,* cardiac arrhythmias, *angina pectoris,* increased blood pressure, *cardiac decompensation and collapse.*
GI: diarrhea, abdominal cramps, vomiting.
Other: weight loss, heat intolerance, hyperhidrosis, menstrual irregularities; in infants and children—accelerated rate of bone maturation.

INTERACTIONS
Cholestyramine and colestipol: thyroglobulin absorption impaired. Separate doses by 4 to 5 hours.
I.V. phenytoin: free thyroid released. Monitor for tachycardia.

NURSING CONSIDERATIONS
• Contraindicated in myocardial infarction, thyrotoxicosis (except with antithyroid drugs), or uncorrected adrenal insufficiency (thyroid hormones increase tissue demand for adrenocortical hormone and may cause acute adrenal crisis). Use with extreme caution in angina pectoris, hypertension, or other cardiovascular disorders; renal insufficiency; or ischemic states.
• Thyroid hormone replacement requirements are about 25% lower in patients over age 60 than in young adults.
• In patients with coronary artery disease who must receive thyroid hormones, observe carefully for possible coronary insufficiency if catecholamines must be given.

• Use carefully in myxedema; patients are unusually sensitive to thyroid hormone.
• Potentially dangerous; not indicated to relieve vague symptoms, such as physical and mental sluggishness, irritability, depression, nervousness, and ill-defined pains; to treat obesity in euthyroid persons; to treat metabolic insufficiency not associated with thyroid insufficiency; or to treat menstrual disorders or male infertility, unless associated with hypothyroidism.
• Tell patient to take thyroid hormones regularly, at the same time each day, to maintain constant hormone levels.
• Warn patient to tell doctor at once if chest pain (especially in elderly), palpitations, sweating, nervousness, or other signs of overdosage occur. Also notify doctor immediately if any signs of aggravated cardiovascular disease develop (chest pain, dyspnea, tachycardia).
• During first few months of therapy, children may suffer partial hair loss. Reassure patient that this is temporary.
• Suggest morning dosage to prevent insomnia.
• Monitor pulse rate, blood pressure.
• Thyroid hormones alter thyroid function test results. Monitor prothrombin time; patients taking these hormones usually require less anticoagulant. Alert patients to report unusual bleeding and bruising.

thyroid USP (desiccated)
S-P-T, Thyrar, Thyro-Teric
Pregnancy Category: A

MECHANISM OF ACTION
Stimulates the metabolism of all body tissues by accelerating the rate of cellular oxidation.

INDICATIONS & DOSAGE

Adult hypothyroidism—
Adults: initially, 60 mg P.O. daily, increased by 60 mg q 30 days until desired response. Usual maintenance dose 60 to 180 mg P.O. daily, as a single dose.
Elderly: 7.5 to 15 mg P.O. daily; dose is doubled at 6- to 8-week intervals.
Adult myxedema—
Adults: 16 mg P.O. daily. May double dose q 2 weeks to maximum 120 mg.
Cretinism and juvenile hypothyroidism—
Children 1 year and older: dosage may approach adult dose (60 to 180 mg) daily, depending on response.
Children 4 to 12 months: 30 to 60 mg P.O. daily.
Children 1 to 4 months: initially, 15 to 30 mg P.O. daily, increased at 2-week intervals. Usual maintenance dose 30 to 45 mg P.O. daily.

ADVERSE REACTIONS

Side effects of thyroid hormones are extensions of their pharmacologic properties and reflect patient sensitivity to them.
CNS: *hyperirritability, nervousness, insomnia,* twitching, tremors, headache.
CV: increased cardiac output, *tachycardia,* cardiac arrhythmias, *angina pectoris,* increased blood pressure, *cardiac decompensation and collapse.*
GI: diarrhea, abdominal cramps, vomiting.
Other: weight loss, heat intolerance, hyperhidrosis, menstrual irregularities; in infants and children—accelerated rate of bone maturation.

INTERACTIONS

Cholestyramine: thyroid absorption impaired. Separate doses by 4 to 5 hours.
I.V. phenytoin: free thyroid released. Monitor for tachycardia.

NURSING CONSIDERATIONS

• Contraindicated in myocardial infarction, thyrotoxicosis (except with antithyroid drugs), or uncorrected adrenal insufficiency (thyroid hormones increase tissue demand for adrenocortical hormone and may cause acute adrenal crisis). Use with extreme caution in angina pectoris, hypertension, or other cardiovascular disorders; renal insufficiency; or ischemic states.
• Thyroid hormone replacement requirements are about 25% lower in patients over age 60 than in young adults.
• Use carefully in myxedema; patients are unusually sensitive to thyroid hormone.
• In patients with coronary artery disease who must receive thyroid hormones, observe carefully for possible coronary insufficiency if catecholamines must be given.
• Potentially dangerous; not indicated to relieve vague symptoms, such as physical and mental sluggishness, irritability, depression, nervousness, ill-defined pains; to treat obesity in euthyroid persons; to treat metabolic insufficiency not associated with thyroid insufficiency; or to treat menstrual disorders or male infertility, unless associated with hypothyroidism.
• Tell patient to take thyroid hormones regularly, at the same time each day, to maintain constant hormone levels.
• Warn patient to tell doctor at once if chest pain (especially in elderly), palpitations, sweating, nervousness, or other signs of overdosage occur. Also notify doctor immediately if any signs of aggravated cardiovascular disease develop (chest pain, dyspnea, tachycardia).
• During first few months of therapy, children may suffer partial hair loss. Reassure patient that this is temporary.
• Suggest morning dosage to prevent

Italicized side effects are common or life-threatening.
*Liquid form contains alcohol.   **May contain tartrazine.

insomnia.
- Monitor pulse rate and blood pressure.
- In children, sleeping pulse rate and basal morning temperature are guides to treatment.
- Thyroid hormones alter thyroid function test results. Monitor prothrombin time; patients taking these hormones usually require less anticoagulant. Alert patients to report unusual bleeding and bruising.

thyrotropin (thyroid-stimulating hormone, or TSH)
Thytropar♦
Pregnancy Category: C

MECHANISM OF ACTION
Stimulates the uptake of radioactive iodine in patients with thyroid carcinoma. Also promotes thyroid hormone production by the anterior pituitary.

INDICATIONS & DOSAGE
Diagnosis of thyroid cancer remnant with ^{131}I after surgery—10 international units I.M. or S.C. for 3 to 7 days.
Differential diagnosis of primary and secondary hypothyroidism—10 units I.M. or S.C. for 1 to 3 days.
In PBI or ^{131}I uptake determinations for differential diagnosis of subclinical hypothyroidism or low thyroid reserve—10 units I.M. or S.C.
Therapy for thyroid carcinoma (local or metastatic) with ^{131}I—10 units I.M. or S.C. for 3 to 8 days.
To determine thyroid status of patient receiving thyroid—10 units I.M. or S.C. for 1 to 3 days.

ADVERSE REACTIONS
CNS: headache.
CV: *tachycardia,* atrial fibrillation, *angina pectoris, congestive failure,* hypotension.

GI: nausea, vomiting.
Other: thyroid hyperplasia (large doses), fever, menstrual irregularities, allergic reactions (postinjection flare, urticaria, *anaphylaxis*).

INTERACTIONS
None significant.

NURSING CONSIDERATIONS
- Contraindicated in coronary thrombosis, untreated Addison's disease. Use cautiously in angina pectoris, heart failure, hypopituitarism, adrenocortical suppression.
- May cause thyroid hyperplasia.
- Diagnostic use: to identify subclinical hypothyroidism or low thyroid reserve, to evaluate need for thyroid therapy, to distinguish between primary and secondary hypothyroidism, and to detect thyroid remnants and metastases of thyroid carcinoma.
- Therapeutic use: management of certain types of thyroid carcinoma and resulting metastases, and in conjunction with radioactive ^{131}I to enhance uptake of ^{131}I by the thyroid.
- Three-day dosage schedule may be used in long-standing pituitary myxedema or with prolonged use of thyroid medication.

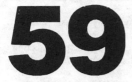

Thyroid hormone antagonists

methimazole
potassium iodide
propylthiouracil (PTU)
radioactive iodine (sodium iodide) [131]I

COMBINATION PRODUCTS
None.

---

methimazole
Tapazole♦
Pregnancy Category: D

MECHANISM OF ACTION
Inhibits oxidation of iodine in the thyroid gland, blocking iodine's ability to combine with tyrosine to form thyroxine. May also prevent the coupling of monoiodotyrosine and diiodotyrosine to form thyroxine and triiodothyronine.

INDICATIONS & DOSAGE
Hyperthyroidism—
Adults: 5 mg P.O. t.i.d. if mild; 10 to 15 mg P.O. t.i.d. if moderately severe; and 20 mg P.O. t.i.d. if severe. Continue until patient is euthyroid, then start maintenance dose of 5 mg daily to t.i.d. Maximum dose 150 mg daily.
Children: 0.4 mg/kg daily divided q 8 hours. Continue until patient is euthyroid, then start maintenance dose of 0.2 mg/kg daily divided q 8 hours.
Preparation for thyroidectomy—
Adults and children: same doses as for hyperthyroidism until patient is euthyroid; then iodine may be added for 10 days before surgery.

Thyrotoxic crisis—
Adults and children: same doses as for hyperthyroidism, with concomitant iodine therapy and propranolol.

ADVERSE REACTIONS
Blood: *agranulocytosis,* leukopenia, granulopenia, thrombocytopenia (appear to be dose-related).
CNS: headache, drowsiness, vertigo.
GI: diarrhea, nausea, vomiting (may be dose-related).
Hepatic: jaundice.
Skin: rash, urticaria, skin discoloration.
Other: arthralgia, myalgia, salivary gland enlargement, loss of taste, drug fever, lymphadenopathy.

INTERACTIONS
None significant.

NURSING CONSIDERATIONS
• Use cautiously in pregnancy. Pregnant women may require less drug as pregnancy progresses. Monitor thyroid function studies closely. Thyroid may be added to regimen. Drugs may be stopped during last few weeks of pregnancy.
• Watch for signs of hypothyroidism (mental depression; cold intolerance; hard, nonpitting edema). Dose may need to be adjusted.
• Monitor CBC periodically to detect impending leukopenia, thrombocytopenia, and agranulocytosis.
• Doses of over 30 mg/day increase the risk of granulocytosis.
• Warn patient to report immediately: fever, sore throat, or mouth sores

(possible signs of developing agranulocytosis). Agranulocytosis can develop too rapidly to be detected by periodic blood cell counts. Tell patient also to immediately report skin eruptions (sign of hypersensitivity).

• Drug should be stopped if severe rash or enlarged cervical lymph nodes develop.

• Tell patient to ask doctor about using iodized salt and eating shellfish during treatment.

• Warn patient against over-the-counter cough medicines; many contain iodine.

• Give with meals to reduce GI side effects.

• Store in light-resistant container.

potassium iodide
Potassium Iodide Solution, USP;
Strong Iodine Solution, USP
(Lugol's Solution), containing 5%
iodine and 10% potassium iodide
Pregnancy Category: D

MECHANISM OF ACTION
Inhibits thyroid hormone formation by blocking iodotyrosine and iodothyronine synthesis. It also limits iodide transport into the thyroid gland and blocks thyroid hormone release.

INDICATIONS & DOSAGE
Preparation for thyroidectomy—
Adults and children: Strong Iodine Solution, USP, 0.1 to 0.3 ml t.i.d., or Potassium Iodide Solution, USP, 5 drops in water t.i.d. after meals for 2 to 3 weeks before surgery.
Thyrotoxic crisis—
Adults and children: Strong Iodine Solution, USP, 1 ml in water P.O. t.i.d. after meals.

ADVERSE REACTIONS
EENT: acute rhinitis, inflammation of salivary glands, periorbital edema, conjunctivitis, hyperemia.
GI: burning, irritation, *nausea,* vomiting, *metallic taste.*
Skin: acneiform rash, mucous membrane ulceration.
Other: fever, frontal headache, tooth discoloration, *hypersensitivity, including symptoms resembling serum sickness.*

INTERACTIONS
Lithium carbonate: hypothyroidism may occur. Use with caution.

NURSING CONSIDERATIONS
• Contraindicated in tuberculosis, iodide hypersensitivity, hyperkalemia; after meals that contain excessive starch; in laryngeal edema, swelling of salivary glands.

• Earliest signs of delayed hypersensitivity caused by iodides are irritation and swelling of the eyelids.

• Dilute oral doses in water, milk, or fruit juice, and give after meals to prevent gastric irritation, to hydrate the patient, and to mask the very salty taste.

• Tell patient to ask the doctor about using iodized salt and eating shellfish during treatment. Iodine-rich foods may not be permitted.

• Warn the patient that sudden withdrawal may precipitate thyroid storm.

• Store in light-resistant container.

• Give iodides through straw to avoid tooth discoloration.

• Usually given with other antithyroid drugs.

propylthiouracil (PTU)
Propyl-Thyracil♦♦
Pregnancy Category: D

MECHANISM OF ACTION
Inhibits oxidation of iodine in the thyroid gland, blocking iodine's ability to combine with tyrosine to form thyroxine. May also prevent the coupling of monoiodotyrosine and diiodotyrosine to form thyroxine and triiodothyronine.

INDICATIONS & DOSAGE
Hyperthyroidism—
Adults: 100 mg P.O. t.i.d.; up to 300 mg q 8 hours have been used in severe cases. Continue until patient is euthyroid, then start maintenance dose of 100 mg daily to t.i.d.
Children over 10 years: 100 mg P.O. t.i.d. Continue until patient is euthyroid, then start maintenance dose of 25 mg t.i.d. to 100 mg b.i.d.
Children 6 to 10 years: 50 to 150 mg P.O. divided doses q 8 hours.
Preparation for thyroidectomy—
Adults and children: same doses as for hyperthyroidism, then iodine may be added 10 days before surgery.
Thyrotoxic crisis—
Adults and children: same doses as for hyperthyroidism, with concomitant iodine therapy and propranolol.

ADVERSE REACTIONS
Blood: *agranulocytosis,* leukopenia, thrombocytopenia (appear to be dose-related).
CNS: headache, drowsiness, vertigo.
EENT: visual disturbances.
GI: diarrhea, *nausea, vomiting* (may be dose-related).
Hepatic: jaundice, *hepatotoxicity.*
Skin: rash, urticaria, skin discoloration, pruritus.
Other: arthralgia, myalgia, salivary gland enlargement, loss of taste, drug fever, lymphadenopathy, vasculitis.

INTERACTIONS
None significant.

NURSING CONSIDERATIONS
• Use cautiously in pregnancy. Pregnant women may require less drug as pregnancy progresses. Monitor thyroid function studies closely. Thyroid may be added to regimen. Drugs may be stopped during last few weeks of pregnancy.
• Watch for signs of hypothyroidism (mental depression; cold intolerance; hard, nonpitting edema). Dose may

need to be adjusted.
• Monitor CBC periodically to detect impending leukopenia, thrombocytopenia, and agranulocytosis.
• Warn patient to report immediately: fever, sore throat, or mouth sores (possible signs of developing agranulocytosis). Agranulocytosis can develop too rapidly to be detected by periodic blood cell counts. Tell patient to also report skin eruptions (sign of hypersensitivity) immediately.
• Drug should be stopped if severe rash or enlarged cervical lymph nodes develop.
• Tell patient to ask doctor about using iodized salt and eating shellfish during treatment.
• Warn patient against over-the-counter cough medicines; many contain iodine.
• Give with meals to reduce GI side effects.
• Store in light-resistant container.

---

radioactive iodine (sodium iodide) [131]I
Pregnancy Category: X

MECHANISM OF ACTION
Limits thyroid hormone secretion by destroying thyroid tissue. The affinity of thyroid tissue for radioactive iodine facilitates uptake of the drug by cancerous thyroid tissue that has metastasized to other sites in the body.

INDICATIONS & DOSAGE
Hyperthyroidism—
Adults: usual dose is 4 to 10 millicuries P.O. Dose based on estimated weight of thyroid gland and thyroid uptake. Treatment may be repeated after 6 weeks, according to serum thyroxine levels.
Thyroid cancer—
Adults: 50 to 150 millicuries P.O. Dose based on estimated malignant thyroid tissue and metastatic tissue as determined by total body scan. Dose

may be repeated according to clinical status.

ADVERSE REACTIONS
EENT: *feeling of fullness in neck,* metallic taste, "radiation mumps."
Endocrine: hypothyroidism, radiation thyroiditis.
GU: possible increased risk of birth defects in offspring after sufficient ^{131}I dose for thyroid ablation following cancer surgery.
Other: possible increased risk of developing leukemia later in life after sufficient ^{131}I dose for thyroid ablation following cancer surgery.

INTERACTIONS
Lithium carbonate: hypothyroidism may occur. Use with caution.

NURSING CONSIDERATIONS
• Contraindicated in pregnancy and lactation unless used to treat thyroid cancer.
• Stop all antithyroid medications, thyroid preparations, and iodine-containing preparations 1 week before ^{131}I dose. If medications are not stopped, patient may receive thyroid-stimulating hormone for 3 days before ^{131}I dose. When treating women of childbearing age, give dose during menstruation or within 7 days after menstruation.
• Presence of food may delay absorption. Patient should fast overnight before administration.
• After therapy for hyperthyroidism, patient should not resume antithyroid drugs, but should continue propranolol or other drugs used to treat symptoms of hyperthyroidism until onset of full ^{131}I effect (usually 6 weeks).
• Monitor thyroid function with serum thyroxine levels.
• After dose for hyperthyroidism, patient's urine and saliva are slightly radioactive for 24 hours; vomitus is highly radioactive for 6 to 8 hours. Institute full radiation precautions during this time. Instruct patient to use appropriate disposal methods when coughing and expectorating.
• After dose for thyroid cancer, patient's urine, saliva, and perspiration remain radioactive for 3 days. Isolate patient and observe the following precautions: pregnant personnel should not take care of patient; disposable eating utensils and linens should be used; instruct patient to save all urine in lead containers for 24 to 48 hours so amount of radioactive material excreted can be determined. Patient should drink as much fluid as possible for 48 hours after drug administration to facilitate excretion. Limit contact with patient to 30 minutes per shift per person the first day. May increase time to 1 hour second day and longer on third day.
• If patient is discharged less than 7 days after ^{131}I dose for thyroid cancer, warn him to avoid close, prolonged contact with small children (for example, holding children on lap), and instruct him not to sleep in same room with spouse for 7 days after treatment due to increased risk of thyroid cancer in persons exposed to [131]I. Tell patient he may use same bathroom facilities as rest of family.

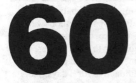

Pituitary hormones

corticotropin (ACTH)
cosyntropin
desmopressin acetate
lypressin
posterior pituitary
somatrem
vasopressin (antidiuretic
   hormone)
vasopressin tannate

COMBINATION PRODUCTS
None.

corticotropin (ACTH)
ACTHAR♦, Duracton♦♦, H.P.
Acthar Gel♦
Pregnancy Category: C

MECHANISM OF ACTION
By replacing the body's own tropic
hormone, stimulates the adrenal cortex to secrete its entire spectrum of
hormones.

INDICATIONS & DOSAGE
*Diagnostic test of adrenocortical func-
tion—*
Adults: up to 80 units I.M. or S.C. in
divided doses; or a single dose of repository form; or 10 to 25 units
(aqueous form) in 500 ml dextrose 5%
in water I.V. over 8 hours, between
blood samplings.
   Individual dosages generally vary
with adrenal glands' sensitivity to
stimulation as well as with specific
disease. Infants and younger children
require larger doses per kilogram than
do older children and adults.
For therapeutic use—

Adults: 40 units S.C. or I.M. in 4 divided doses (aqueous); 40 units q 12
to 24 hours (gel or repository form).

ADVERSE REACTIONS
CNS: *convulsions, dizziness,* papilledema, headache, *euphoria, insomnia,* mood swings, personality
changes, depression, psychosis.
EENT: cataracts, glaucoma.
GI: peptic ulcer with perforation and
hemorrhage, pancreatitis, abdominal
distention, ulcerative esophagitis,
nausea, vomiting.
GU: menstrual irregularities.
Metabolic: *sodium and fluid retention,* calcium and potassium loss, hypokalemic alkalosis, negative nitrogen balance.
Skin: *impaired wound healing,* thin
fragile skin, petechiae, ecchymoses,
facial erythema, increased sweating,
acne, hyperpigmentation, allergic
skin reactions, hirsutism.
Other: muscle weakness, steroid my-
opathy, loss of muscle mass, osteoporosis, vertebral compression fractures, cushingoid state, suppression of
growth in children, *activation of latent diabetes mellitus,* progressive increase in antibodies, loss of ACTH
stimulatory effect, and *hypersensitivity.*

INTERACTIONS
None significant.

NURSING CONSIDERATIONS
• Contraindicated in scleroderma, osteoporosis, systemic fungal infections, ocular herpes simplex, recent

---

Italicized side effects are common or life-threatening.
*Liquid form contains alcohol.   **May contain tartrazine.

surgery, peptic ulcer, congestive heart failure, hypertension, sensitivity to pork and pork products, concomitant smallpox vaccination, adrenocortical hyperfunction or primary insufficiency, or Cushing's syndrome. Use with caution in pregnant women or breast-feeding mothers and in women of childbearing age; patients being immunized; latent tuberculosis or tuberculin reactivity; hypothyroidism; cirrhosis; infection (use anti-infective therapy during and after ACTH treatment); acute gouty arthritis (limit ACTH treatment to a few days, and use conventional therapy during and for several days after ACTH treatment); emotional instability or psychotic tendencies; diabetes; abscess; pyogenic infections; renal insufficiency; myasthenia gravis.

• ACTH treatment should be preceded by verification of adrenal responsiveness and test for hypersensitivity and allergic reactions.

• ACTH should be adjunctive; not sole therapy. Oral agents are preferred for long-term therapy.

• Unusual stress may require additional use of rapidly acting corticosteroids. When possible, gradually reduce ACTH dosage to smallest effective dose to minimize induced adrenocortical insufficiency. Reinstitute therapy if stressful situation (trauma, surgery, severe illness) occurs shortly after stopping drug.

• Watch neonates of ACTH-treated mothers for signs of hypoadrenalism.

• Counteract edema by low-sodium, high-potassium intake; nitrogen loss by high-protein diet; and psychotic changes by reducing ACTH dosage or administering sedatives.

• ACTH may mask signs of chronic disease and decrease host resistance and ability to localize infection.

• Note and record weight changes, fluid exchange, and resting blood pressures until minimal effective dose is achieved.

• Refrigerate reconstituted solution and use within 24 hours.

• If administering gel, warm it to room temperature, draw into large needle, and give slowly deep I.M. with 21G or 22G needle. Warn patient that injection is painful.

cosyntropin
Cortrosyn♦, Synacthen Depot♦♦
Pregnancy Category: C

MECHANISM OF ACTION
By replacing the body's own tropic hormone, stimulates the adrenal cortex to secrete its entire spectrum of hormones.

INDICATIONS & DOSAGE
Diagnostic test of adrenocortical function—
Adults and children: 0.25 to 1 mg I.M. or I.V. (unless label prohibits I.V. administration) between blood samplings.
Children under 2 years: 0.125 mg I.M. or I.V.

ADVERSE REACTIONS
Skin: pruritus.
Other: flushing, hypersensitivity.

INTERACTIONS
None significant.

NURSING CONSIDERATIONS
• Use cautiously in hypersensitivity to natural corticotropin.
• Drug is synthetic duplication of the biologically active part of the ACTH molecule. It is less likely to produce sensitivity than natural ACTH from animal sources.

desmopressin acetate
DDAVP♦, Stimate
Pregnancy Category: B

MECHANISM OF ACTION
Increases the permeability of the renal tubular epithelium to adenosine monophosphate and water; the epithelium promotes reabsorption of water and produces a concentrated urine (antidiuretic hormone effect). Desmopressin also increases Factor VIII activity by releasing endogenous Factor VIII from plasma storage sites.

INDICATIONS & DOSAGE
Nonnephrogenic diabetes insipidus, temporary polyuria and polydipsia associated with pituitary trauma—
Adults: 0.1 to 0.4 ml intranasally daily in 1 to 3 doses. Adjust morning and evening doses separately for adequate diurnal rhythm of water turnover. Alternatively, may administer injectable form in dosage of 0.5 to 1 ml I.V. or S.C. daily, usually in two divided doses.
Children 3 months to 12 years: 0.05 to 0.3 ml intranasally daily in 1 or 2 doses.
Treatment of hemophilia A and von Willebrand's disease—
Adults and children: 0.3 mcg/kg diluted in normal saline and infused I.V. slowly over 15 to 30 minutes. May repeat dose if necessary as indicated by laboratory response and the patient's clinical condition.

ADVERSE REACTIONS
CNS: headache.
CV: slight rise in blood pressure at high dosage.
EENT: nasal congestion, rhinitis.
GI: nausea.
GU: vulval pain.
Other: flushing.

INTERACTIONS
None significant.

NURSING CONSIDERATIONS
• Use with caution in patients with coronary artery insufficiency or hypertensive cardiovascular disease.
• Adjust fluid intake to reduce risk of water intoxication and sodium depletion, especially in very young or old patients.
• Overdose may cause oxytocic or vasopressor activity. Withhold drug until effects subside. Furosemide may be used if fluid retention is excessive.
• Some patients may have difficulty measuring and inhaling drug into nostrils. Teach patient correct method of administration.
• Intranasal use can cause changes in the nasal mucosa resulting in erratic, unreliable absorption. Report any patient's worsening condition to doctor, who may prescribe injectable DDAVP.
• Now indicated for mild-to-moderate hemophilia A and von Willebrand's disease. However, desmopressin injection is *not* indicated in the treatment of hemophilia A with Factor VIII levels of 0% to 5% or in severe cases of von Willebrand's disease.
• In some patients, use of desmopressin may avoid the hazards of contaminated blood products.
• Has been used successfully to reduce blood loss during cardiac surgery.

lypressin
Diapid
Pregnancy Category: B

MECHANISM OF ACTION
Increases the permeability of the renal tubular epithelium to adenosine monophosphate and water; the epithelium promotes reabsorption of water and produces a concentrated urine (antidiuretic hormone effect).

Italicized side effects are common or life-threatening.
*Liquid form contains alcohol.   **May contain tartrazine.

INDICATIONS & DOSAGE
Nonnephrogenic diabetes insipidus—
Adults and children: 1 or 2 sprays (approximately 2 USP posterior pituitary pressor units/spray) in either or both nostrils q.i.d. and an additional dose at bedtime, if needed, to prevent nocturia. If usual dosage is inadequate, increase frequency rather than number of sprays.

ADVERSE REACTIONS
CNS: headache, dizziness.
EENT: nasal congestion or ulceration, irritation, pruritus of nasal passages, rhinorrhea, conjunctivitis.
GI: heartburn due to drip of excess spray into pharynx, abdominal cramps, frequent bowel movements.
GU: possible transient fluid retention due to overdose.
Skin: hypersensitivity reaction.

INTERACTIONS
None significant.

NURSING CONSIDERATIONS
• Use with caution in patients with coronary artery disease.
• Particularly useful if diabetes insipidus is unresponsive to other therapy, or if antidiuretic hormones of animal origin cause adverse reactions.
• Nasal congestion, allergic rhinitis, or upper respiratory infections may diminish drug absorption and require larger dose or adjunctive therapy.
• Instruct patient to clear nasal passage before inhaling drug.
• Inadvertent inhalation of spray may cause tightness in chest, coughing, and transient dyspnea.
• Test patients sensitive to antidiuretic hormone for sensitivity to lypressin.
• To administer a uniform, well-diffused spray, hold bottle upright with patient in vertical position holding head upright.
• Instruct the patient to carry the medication with him at all times because of its fairly short duration.

posterior pituitary
Pituitrin
Pregnancy Category: C

MECHANISM OF ACTION
Provides both oxytocic and vasopressor activity.

INDICATIONS & DOSAGE
To control postoperative ileus; as a surgical aid to achieve hemostasis; treatment of diabetes insipidus—
Adults: 5 to 20 units S.C. or I.M.

ADVERSE REACTIONS
GI: increased gastrointestinal motility.
GU: uterine cramps.
Skin: facial pallor.

INTERACTIONS
Lithium, demeclocycline: reduced antidiuretic activity. Use together cautiously.
Chlorpropamide: increased antidiuretic response. Use together cautiously.

NURSING CONSIDERATIONS
• Contraindicated in toxemia of pregnancy, cardiac disease, hypertension, epilepsy, advanced arteriosclerosis.
• Don't use as an oxytocic. High risk of fetal distress exists.
• Preferred route of administration is I.M.

somatrem
Protropin
Pregnancy Category: C

MECHANISM OF ACTION
Purified growth hormone of recombinant DNA origin that stimulates linear, skeletal muscle, and organ growth.

INDICATIONS & DOSAGE
Long-term treatment of children who have growth failure due to a lack of adequate endogenous growth hormone secretion—
Children (pre-puberty): 0.1 mg/kg I.M. given three times weekly.

ADVERSE REACTIONS
Endocrine: *hypothyroidism, hyperglycemia.*
Other: *antibodies to growth hormone.*

INTERACTIONS
Glucocorticoids: may inhibit growth-promoting action of somatrem. Glucocorticoid dose may need to be adjusted.

NURSING CONSIDERATIONS
• Contraindicated in patients with closed epiphyses, an active underlying intracranial lesion, or known sensitivity to benzyl alcohol.
• Use cautiously in patients whose growth hormone deficiency results from an intracranial lesion. Patient should be examined frequently for progression or recurrence of the underlying disease.
• Observe patient for signs of glucose intolerance and hyperglycemia.
• Monitor periodic thyroid function tests for hypothyroidism, which may require treatment with a thyroid hormone.
• This drug replaces pituitary-derived human growth hormone, which was removed from the market in 1985 because of an association with a rare but fatal virus infection (Jakob-Creutzfeldt disease). Reassure your patient and his family that somatrem is *pure* and that it is *safe.*
• To prepare the solution, inject the bacteriostatic water for injection (which is supplied) into the vial containing the drug. Then swirl the vial with a gentle rotary motion until the contents are completely dissolved.

Don't shake the vial.
• After reconstitution, vial solution should be clear. Don't inject into the patient if the solution is cloudy or contains any particles.
• Store reconstituted vial in refrigerator. Must use within 7 days.
• Be sure to check this product's expiration date.

vasopressin (antidiuretic hormone)
Pitressin Synthetic♦

vasopressin tannate
Pitressin Tannate♦
Pregnancy Category: B

MECHANISM OF ACTION
Increases the permeability of the renal tubular epithelium to adenosine monophosphate and water; the epithelium promotes reabsorption of water and produces a concentrated urine (antidiuretic hormone effect).

INDICATIONS & DOSAGE
Nonnephrogenic, nonpsychogenic diabetes insipidus—
Adults: 5 to 10 units I.M. or S.C. b.i.d. to q.i.d., p.r.n.; or intranasally (spray or cotton balls) in individualized doses, based on response. For chronic therapy, inject 2.5 to 5 units Pitressin Tannate in oil suspension I.M. or S.C. every 2 to 3 days.
Children: 2.5 to 10 units I.M. or S.C. b.i.d. to q.i.d., p.r.n.; or intranasally (spray or cotton balls) in individualized doses. For chronic therapy, inject 1.25 to 2.5 units Pitressin Tannate in oil suspension I.M. or S.C. every 2 to 3 days.
Postoperative abdominal distention—
Adults: 5 units (aqueous) I.M. initially, then q 3 to 4 hours, increasing dose to 10 units, if needed. Reduce dose for children proportionately.
To expel gas before abdominal X-ray—

Italicized side effects are common or life-threatening.
*Liquid form contains alcohol.   **May contain tartrazine.

Adults: inject 10 units S.C. at 2 hours, then again at 30 minutes before X-ray. Enema before first dose may also help to eliminate gas.
Upper GI tract hemorrhage (intraarterial)—
Adults: 0.2 to 0.4 units/minute. Do not use tannate in oil suspension.

ADVERSE REACTIONS
CNS: tremor, dizziness, headache.
CV: *angina in patients with vascular disease,* vasoconstriction. Large doses may cause hypertension, electrocardiographic changes. (With intraarterial infusion: *bradycardia, cardiac arrhythmias, pulmonary edema*.)
GI: abdominal cramps, nausea, vomiting, diarrhea, intestinal hyperactivity.
GU: uterine cramps, anuria.
Skin: circumoral pallor.
Other: water intoxication (drowsiness, listlessness, headache, confusion, weight gain), hypersensitivity reactions (urticaria, angioneurotic edema, bronchoconstriction, fever, rash, wheezing, dyspnea, *anaphylaxis*), sweating.

INTERACTIONS
Lithium, demeclocycline: reduced antidiuretic activity. Use together cautiously.
Chlorpropamide: increased antidiuretic response. Use together cautiously.

NURSING CONSIDERATIONS
• Contraindicated in chronic nephritis with nitrogen retention. Use cautiously in children, elderly persons, pregnant women, and patients with epilepsy, migraine, asthma, cardiovascular disease, or fluid overload.
• Never inject vasopressin tannate in oil I.V.
• Never inject during first stage of labor; may cause ruptured uterus.
• Monitor specific gravity of urine. Monitor intake and output to aid evaluation of drug effectiveness.
• Place tannate in oil in warm water for 10 to 15 minutes. Then shake thoroughly to make suspension uniform before withdrawing I.M. injection dose. Small brown particles must be seen in suspension. Use absolutely dry syringe to avoid dilution.
• Give with 1 to 2 glasses of water to reduce side effects and to improve therapeutic response.
• To prevent possible convulsions, coma, and death, observe patient closely for early signs of water intoxication.
• Overhydration more likely with long-acting tannate oil suspension than with aqueous vasopressin solution.
• Use minimum effective dose to reduce side effects.
• May be used for transient polyuria due to antidiuretic hormone deficiency related to neurosurgery or head injury.
• Synthetic desmopressin is sometimes preferred because of longer duration and less frequent side effects.
• Question the patient with abdominal distention about passage of flatus and stool.
• Monitor blood pressure of patient on vasopressin twice daily. Watch for excessively elevated blood pressure or lack of response to drug, which may be indicated by hypotension. Also monitor fluid intake and output and daily weights.
• A rectal tube will facilitate gas expulsion following vasopressin injection.

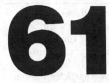

Parathyroid-like agents

calcifediol
calcitonin (human)
calcitonin (Salmon)
calcitriol (1,25-
   dihydroxycholecalciferol)
dihydrotachysterol
etidronate disodium

COMBINATION PRODUCTS
None.

calcifediol
Calderol
Pregnancy Category: A

MECHANISM OF ACTION
Stimulates calcium absorption from
the GI tract and promotes secretion of
calcium from bone to blood.

INDICATIONS & DOSAGE
*Treatment and management of meta-
bolic bone disease associated with
chronic renal failure—*
Adults: initially, 300 to 350 mcg P.O.
weekly, given on a daily or alternate-
day schedule. Dosage may be increased at 4-week intervals. Optimal
dose must be carefully determined for
each patient.

ADVERSE REACTIONS
Vitamin D intoxication associated
with hypercalcemia:
CNS: headache, somnolence.
EENT: conjunctivitis, photophobia,
rhinorrhea.
GI: nausea, vomiting, constipation,
metallic taste, dry mouth, anorexia,
diarrhea.

GU: polyuria.
Other: weakness, bone and muscle
pain.

INTERACTIONS
Cholestyramine: may impair absorption of calcifediol.

NURSING CONSIDERATIONS
• Contraindicated in hypercalcemia
or vitamin D toxicity. Withhold all
preparations containing vitamin D in
patients taking calcifediol. Use cautiously in patients on digitalis because
hypercalcemia may precipitate cardiac arrhythmias.
• Monitor serum calcium; serum calcium times serum phosphate should
not exceed 70. During titration, serum
calcium levels should be determined
at least weekly. If hypercalcemia occurs, calcifediol should be discontinued but resumed after serum calcium
returns to normal.
• Patient should receive adequate
daily intake of calcium—1,000 mg
RDA.
• Advise patient to adhere to diet and
calcium supplementation and to avoid
nonprescription drugs.
• Teach patient to report signs and
symptoms of hypercalcemia.

calcitonin (human)
Cibacalcin
Pregnancy Category: C

MECHANISM OF ACTION
Decreases osteoclastic activity by inhibiting osteocytic osteolysis. Also

decreases mineral release and matrix or collagen breakdown in bone.

INDICATIONS & DOSAGE

Paget's disease (osteitis deformans)—
Adults: 0.5 mg S.C. daily. If patient obtains sufficient improvement, dosage may be reduced to 0.25 mg daily or 2 or 3 times a week. Some patients may need as much as 1 mg daily.

ADVERSE REACTIONS

GI: *nausea, vomiting.*
GU: increased frequency of urination.
Skin: *flushing of face and hands.*
Other: hypocalcemia.

INTERACTIONS

None significant.

NURSING CONSIDERATIONS

• Calcitonin (human) is indicated especially in patients who have developed resistance to calcitonin (Salmon). Calcitonin (human) is associated with risk of diminishing efficacy due to antibody formation or hypersensitivity reactions.
• Administer the drug at bedtime when possible to minimize nausea and vomiting.
• Facial flushing and warmth occur in 20% to 30% of all patients within minutes of injection and usually last about 1 hour. Reassure patient that this effect is transient.
• Observe patient for signs of hypocalcemic tetany during therapy (muscle twitching, tetanic spasms, and convulsions if hypocalcemia is severe).
• Determine serum alkaline phosphatase and urinary hydroxyproline excretion levels before therapy, during the first 3 months, and every 3 to 6 months thereafter during chronic therapy.
• Treatment should continue for at least 6 months. Then, if symptoms have been relieved, it may be discontinued until symptoms or radiologic signs recur.
• Be sure to use the freshly reconstituted solution within 2 hours.

calcitonin (Salmon)
Calcimar♦
Pregnancy Category: B

MECHANISM OF ACTION

Decreases osteoclastic activity by inhibiting osteocytic osteolysis. Also decreases mineral release and matrix or collagen breakdown in bone.

INDICATIONS & DOSAGE

Paget's disease of bone (osteitis deformans)—
Adults: initially, 100 international units daily, S.C. or I.M. Maintenance: 50 to 100 units daily or every other day.
Hypercalcemia—
Adults: 100 to 400 international units I.M. once or twice daily.
Postmenopausal osteoporosis—
Adults: 100 international units S.C. daily.

ADVERSE REACTIONS

CNS: headaches.
GI: transient nausea with or without vomiting, diarrhea, anorexia.
GU: transient diuresis.
Metabolic: hyperglycemia.
Local: inflammation at injection site, skin rashes.
Other: *facial flushing;* hypocalcemia; swelling, tingling, and tenderness of hands; unusual taste sensation; *anaphylaxis.*

INTERACTIONS

None significant.

NURSING CONSIDERATIONS

• Contraindicated in allergy to gelatin diluent used to prepare drug. Not recommended for breast-feeding mothers, or women who are or may become pregnant. Safe use in children not established.

• Periodic serum alkaline phosphatase and 24-hour urine hydroxyproline levels should be determined to evaluate drug effect.

• Skin test is usually done before beginning therapy.

• Systemic allergic reactions possible since hormone is protein. Keep epinephrine handy when administering.

• Patients with good initial clinical response to calcitonin who suffer relapse should be evaluated for antibody formation response to the hormone protein.

• Tell patient in whom calcitonin loses its hypocalcemic activity that further medication or increased dosages will be of no value.

• Facial flushing and warmth occur in 20% to 30% of all patients within minutes of injection; usually last about 1 hour. Reassure patient that this is a transient effect.

• Observe patient for signs of hypocalcemic tetany during therapy (muscle twitching, tetanic spasms, and convulsions if hypocalcemia is severe).

• Monitor calcium levels closely. Watch for signs of hypercalcemic relapse: bone pain, renal calculi, polyuria, anorexia, nausea, vomiting, thirst, constipation, lethargy, bradycardia, muscle hypotonicity, pathologic fracture, psychosis, and coma.

• Periodic examinations of urine sediment advisable.

• Refrigerate solution.

• When administered for postmenopausal osteoporosis, remind patient to take adequate calcium and vitamin D supplementation.

calcitriol (1,25-dihydroxycholecalciferol)
Rocaltrol♦
Pregnancy Category: A (D if used in doses > RDA)

MECHANISM OF ACTION
Stimulates calcium absorption from the GI tract and promotes secretion of calcium from bone to blood.

INDICATIONS & DOSAGE
Management of hypocalcemia in patients undergoing chronic dialysis—
Adults: initially, 0.25 mcg daily. Dosage may be increased by 0.25 mcg daily at 2- to 4-week intervals. Maintenance: 0.25 mcg every other day up to 0.5 to 1.25 mcg daily.
Management of hypoparathyroidism and pseudohypoparathyroidism—
Adults and children over 1 year: initially 0.25 mcg P.O. daily. Dosage may be increased at 2- to 4-week intervals.
Maintenance: 0.25 to 2 mcg daily.

ADVERSE REACTIONS
Vitamin D intoxication associated with hypercalcemia:
CNS: headache, somnolence.
EENT: conjunctivitis, photophobia, rhinorrhea.
GI: nausea, vomiting, constipation, metallic taste, dry mouth, anorexia.
GU: polyuria.
Other: weakness, bone and muscle pain.

INTERACTIONS
None significant.

NURSING CONSIDERATIONS
• Contraindicated in hypercalcemia or vitamin D toxicity. Withhold all preparations containing vitamin D in patients taking calcitriol. Not recommended in breast-feeding mothers. Use cautiously in patients on digitalis; hypercalcemia may precipitate car-

---

Italicized side effects are common or life-threatening.
*Liquid form contains alcohol.   **May contain tartrazine.

diac arrhythmias.
- Monitor serum calcium; serum calcium times serum phosphate should not exceed 70. During titration, determine serum levels twice weekly. If hypercalcemia occurs, discontinue, but resume after serum calcium level returns to normal. Patient should receive adequate daily intake of calcium—1,000 mg RDA.
- Protect from heat and light.
- Instruct patient to adhere to diet and calcium supplementation and to avoid unapproved nonprescription drugs.
- Patients should not use magnesium-containing antacids while taking this drug.
- Patients should report to doctor immediately any of the following symptoms: weakness, nausea, vomiting, dry mouth, constipation, muscle or bone pain, or metallic taste—early symptoms of vitamin D intoxication.
- Tell patient that although this drug is a vitamin, it must not be taken by anyone for whom it was not prescribed due to its potentially serious toxicities.
- Most potent form of vitamin D available.

dihydrotachysterol
DHT Intensol, DHT Oral Solution, Hytakerol♦
Pregnancy Category: A (D if used in doses > RDA)

MECHANISM OF ACTION
Stimulates calcium absorption from the GI tract and promotes secretion of calcium from bone to blood.

INDICATIONS & DOSAGE
Familial hypophosphatemia—
Adults and children: 0.5 to 2 mg P.O. daily. Maintenance: 0.3 to 1.5 mg daily.
Hypocalcemia associated with hypoparathyroidism and pseudohypoparathyroidism—
Adults: initially, 0.8 to 2.4 mg P.O. daily for several days. Maintenance: 0.2 to 2 mg daily, as required for normal serum calcium levels. Average dose 0.6 mg daily.
Children: initially, 1 to 5 mg for several days. Maintenance: 0.2 to 1 mg daily, as required for normal serum calcium levels.
Renal osteodystrophy in chronic uremia—
Adults: 0.1 to 0.6 mg P.O. daily.

ADVERSE REACTIONS
Vitamin D intoxication associated with hypercalcemia:
CNS: headache, somnolence.
EENT: conjunctivitis, photophobia, rhinorrhea.
GI: nausea, vomiting, constipation, metallic taste, dry mouth, anorexia, diarrhea.
GU: polyuria.
Other: weakness, bone and muscle pain.

INTERACTIONS
None significant.

NURSING CONSIDERATIONS
- Contraindicated in hypercalcemia, hypocalcemia associated with renal insufficiency and hyperphosphatemia, renal stones, hypersensitivity to vitamin D, and in breast-feeding mothers.
- Monitor serum and urine calcium levels. Watch for signs of hypercalcemia.
- Adequate dietary calcium intake is necessary; usually supplemented with 10 to 15 g oral calcium lactate or gluconate daily.
- Report hypercalcemia reactions to doctor. Early signs of hypercalcemia include thirst, headache, vertigo, tinnitus, anorexia.
- 1 mg equal to 120,000 units ergocalciferol (vitamin D_2).
- Store in tightly closed, light-resistant containers. Don't refrigerate.

etidronate disodium
Didronel♦
Pregnancy Category: B

MECHANISM OF ACTION
Decreases osteoclastic activity by inhibiting osteocytic osteolysis. Also decreases mineral release and matrix or collagen breakdown in bone.

INDICATIONS & DOSAGE
Symptomatic Paget's disease—
Adults: 5 mg/kg daily P.O. as a single dose 2 hours before a meal with water or juice. Patient should not eat for 2 hours after dose. May give up to 10 mg/kg daily in severe cases. Maximum dose 20 mg/kg daily.
Heterotopic ossification in spinal cord injuries—
Adults: 20 mg/kg daily for 2 weeks, then 10 mg/kg daily for 10 weeks. Total treatment period 12 weeks.
Heterotopic ossification after total hip replacement—
Adults: 20 mg/kg daily for 1 month prior to total hip replacement and for 3 months afterward.

ADVERSE REACTIONS
GI: (seen most frequently at 20 mg/kg daily) diarrhea, increased frequency of bowel movements, nausea.
Other: increased or recurrent bone pain at pagetic sites, pain at previously asymptomatic sites, increased risk of fracture, *elevated serum phosphate*.

INTERACTIONS
None significant.

NURSING CONSIDERATIONS
• Use cautiously in enterocolitis, impaired renal function.
• Therapy should not last more than 6 months. After 3 months, resume if needed. Don't give longer than 3 months at doses above 10 mg/kg daily.
• Don't give drug with food, milk, or antacids; may reduce absorption.
• Monitor renal function before and during therapy.
• Elevated serum phosphate may occur, especially in patients receiving higher doses. However, serum phosphate levels usually return to normal 2 to 4 weeks after drug's discontinued.
• Monitor drug effect by serum alkaline phosphatase and urinary hydroxyproline excretion (both lowered if therapy effective).
• Tell patient that improvement may not occur for up to 3 months but may continue for months after drug is stopped. Stress importance of good nutrition, especially diet high in calcium and vitamin D.

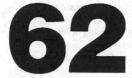

Diuretics

Thiazide diuretics
benzthiazide
chlorothiazide
cyclothiazide
hydrochlorothiazide
methyclothiazide
polythiazide
trichlormethiazide

Thiazide-like diuretics
chlorthalidone
metolazone
quinethazone

Loop diuretics
bumetanide
ethacrynate sodium
ethacrynic acid
furosemide

Carbonic anhydrase inhibitors
acetazolamide
acetazolamide sodium
dichlorphenamide
methazolamide

Miscellaneous diuretics
amiloride hydrochloride
indapamide
mannitol
spironolactone
triamterene
urea (carbamide)

COMBINATION PRODUCTS
ALAZIDE: spironolactone 25 mg and hydrochlorothiazide 25 mg.
ALDACTAZIDE♦: spironolactone 25 mg and hydrochlorothiazide 25 mg.
ALDACTAZIDE 50/50: spironolactone 50 mg and hydrochlorothiazide 50 mg.
ALTEXIDE: spironolactone 25 mg and hydrochlorothiazide 25 mg.
DYAZIDE♦: triamterene 50 mg and hydrochlorothiazide 25 mg.
MAXZIDE: triamterene 75 mg and hydrochlorothiazide 50 mg.
MODURETIC: amiloride hydrochloride 5 mg and hydrochlorothiazide 50 mg.
SPIRONAZIDE: spironolactone 25 mg and hydrochlorothiazide 25 mg.
SPIROZIDE: spironolactone 25 mg and hydrochlorothiazide 25 mg.

acetazolamide
Ak-Zol, Diamox♦, Diamox Sequels♦

acetazolamide sodium
Diamox Parenteral, Diamox Sodium♦♦
Pregnancy Category: C

MECHANISM OF ACTION
By enzymatic blocking, promotes renal excretion of sodium, potassium, bicarbonate, and water. Bicarbonate-ion excretion makes the urine alkaline. Also decreases secretion of aqueous humor in the eye, thereby lowering intraocular pressure. As an anticonvulsant, may inhibit carbonic anhydrase in the central nervous system (CNS) and decrease abnormal paroxysmal or excessive neuronal discharge.

INDICATIONS & DOSAGE
Narrow-angle glaucoma—
Adults: 250 mg q 4 hours; or 250 mg b.i.d. P.O., I.M., or I.V. for short-

term therapy.

Edema, in congestive heart failure—
Adults: 250 to 375 mg P.O., I.M., or I.V. daily in a.m.
Children: 5 mg/kg daily in a.m.
Open-angle glaucoma—
Adults: 250 mg daily to 1 g P.O., I.M., or I.V. divided q.i.d.
Prevention or amelioration of acute mountain sickness—
Adults: 250 mg P.O. q 8 to 12 hours.
Myoclonic seizures, refractory generalized tonic-clonic (grand mal) or absence (petit mal), mixed seizures—
Adults: 375 mg P.O., I.M., or I.V. daily up to 250 mg q.i.d. Or, Diamox Sequels 250 to 500 mg daily or b.i.d. Initial dose when used with other anticonvulsants usually 250 mg daily.
Children: 8 to 30 mg/kg daily, divided t.i.d. or q.i.d. Maximum dose 1.5 g daily, or 300 to 900 mg/m² daily.

ADVERSE REACTIONS
Blood: *aplastic anemia,* hemolytic anemia, leukopenia.
CNS: drowsiness, paresthesias, confusion.
EENT: transient myopia.
GI: nausea, vomiting, anorexia.
GU: crystalluria, renal calculi, hematuria.
Metabolic: *hyperchloremic acidosis,* hypokalemia, asymptomatic hyperuricemia.
Skin: rash.
Local: *pain at injection site,* sterile abscesses.

INTERACTIONS
None significant.

NURSING CONSIDERATIONS
• Contraindicated in long-term therapy for chronic noncongestive narrow-angle glaucoma; also in depressed sodium or potassium serum levels, renal or hepatic disease or dysfunction, adrenal gland failure, and hyperchloremic acidosis. Use cautiously in respiratory acidosis, emphysema, chronic pulmonary disease, or patients receiving other diuretics.
• Monitor intake/output and electrolytes, especially serum potassium. When used in diuretic therapy, consult with doctor and dietitian to provide high-potassium diet.
• Weigh patient daily. Rapid weight loss may cause hypotension.
• Diuretic effect is decreased when acidosis occurs but can be reestablished by withdrawing drug for several days and then restarting, or by using intermittent administration schedules.
• Reconstitute 500-mg vial with at least 5 ml sterile water for injection. Use within 24 hours of reconstitution.
• I.M. injection is painful because of alkalinity of solution. Direct I.V. administration is preferred (100 to 500 mg/minute).
• Elderly patients are especially susceptible to excessive diuresis.
• Sustained-release form available. Permits a reduction in dosage frequency.
• May cause false-positive urine protein tests by alkalinizing the urine.
• Oral liquid: soften 1 tablet in 2 teaspoonfuls of very warm water and add to 2 teaspoonfuls honey or syrup (chocolate, cherry). Don't use fruit juice.

amiloride hydrochloride
Midamor♦
Pregnancy Category: B

MECHANISM OF ACTION
Inhibits sodium reabsorption and potassium excretion by direct action on the distal tubule.

INDICATIONS & DOSAGE
Hypertension; or edema associated with congestive heart failure, usually in patients who are also taking thiazide or other potassium-wasting di-

---

uretics—
Adults: Usual dosage is 5 mg P.O. daily. Dosage may be increased to 10 mg daily, if necessary. As much as 20 mg daily can be given.

ADVERSE REACTIONS
CNS: *headache,* weakness, dizziness.
CV: orthostatic hypotension.
GI: *nausea, anorexia, diarrhea, vomiting,* abdominal pain, constipation.
GU: *impotence.*
Metabolic: *hyperkalemia.*

INTERACTIONS
None significant.

NURSING CONSIDERATIONS
• Contraindicated with elevated serum potassium levels (greater than 5.5 mEq/liter). Don't administer to patients receiving other potassium-sparing diuretics, such as spironolactone and triamterene. Also contraindicated in anuria.
• Use cautiously in patients with renal impairment, because potassium retention is increased.
• Risk of hyperkalemia is greater when a potassium-wasting drug is not taken concurrently. When amiloride is taken this way, be sure to monitor daily potassium levels.
• Discontinue immediately if potassium level exceeds 6.5 mEq/liter.
• Warn patient to avoid excessive ingestion of potassium-rich foods or potassium-containing salt substitutes. Concomitant potassium supplement can lead to serious hyperkalemia.
• Administer amiloride with meals to prevent nausea.

benzthiazide
Aquatag**, Exna**, Hydrex, Marazide, Proaqua
Pregnancy Category: D

MECHANISM OF ACTION
Increases urinary excretion of sodium

and water by inhibiting sodium reabsorption in the cortical diluting site of the nephron.

INDICATIONS & DOSAGE
Edema—
Adults: 50 to 200 mg P.O. daily or in divided doses.
Children: 1 to 4 mg/kg daily in 3 divided doses.
Hypertension—
Adults: 50 mg P.O. daily b.i.d., t.i.d., or q.i.d., adjusted to patient's response.

ADVERSE REACTIONS
Blood: *aplastic anemia, agranulocytosis,* leukopenia, thrombocytopenia.
CV: *volume depletion and dehydration,* orthostatic hypotension.
GI: anorexia, nausea, pancreatitis.
Hepatic: hepatic encephalopathy.
Metabolic: *hypokalemia, asymptomatic hyperuricemia, hyperglycemia and impairment of glucose tolerance,* fluid and electrolyte imbalances including dilutional hyponatremia and hypochloremia, metabolic alkalosis, hypercalcemia, gout.
Skin: dermatitis, photosensitivity, rash.
Other: hypersensitivity reactions, such as pneumonitis and vasculitis.

INTERACTIONS
Cholestyramine, colestipol: intestinal absorption of thiazides decreased. Keep doses as separate as possible.
Diazoxide: increased antihypertensive, hyperglycemic, hyperuricemic effects. Use together cautiously.

NURSING CONSIDERATIONS
• Contraindicated in anuria and in hypersensitivity to other thiazides or other sulfonamide-derived drugs. Use cautiously in severe renal disease, impaired hepatic function.
• Monitor intake/output, weight, and serum electrolytes regularly. Monitor serum potassium levels; consult with

doctor and dietitian to provide high-potassium diet. Watch for signs of hypokalemia (for example, muscle weakness, cramps). Patients on digitalis have an increased risk of digitalis toxicity due to the potassium-depleting side effect of this diuretic. May use with potassium-sparing diuretic to prevent potassium loss.

• Foods rich in potassium include citrus fruits, bananas, tomatoes, dates, and apricots.

• Monitor serum creatinine and BUN levels regularly. Not as effective if these levels are more than twice normal.

• Monitor blood sugar. Check insulin requirements in patients with diabetes. May treat severe hyperglycemia with oral antidiabetic agents.

• Monitor blood uric acid levels, especially in patients with a history of gout.

• Give in a.m. to prevent nocturia.

• Elderly patients are especially susceptible to excessive diuresis.

• In hypertension, therapeutic response may be delayed several days.

• Thiazides and thiazide-like diuretics should be discontinued before tests for parathyroid function are performed.

bumetanide
Bumex
Pregnancy Category: C

MECHANISM OF ACTION
Inhibits reabsorption of sodium and chloride at the proximal portion of the ascending loop of Henle.

INDICATIONS & DOSAGE
Edema (congestive heart failure, hepatic and renal disease)—
Adults: 0.5 to 2 mg P.O. once daily. If diuretic response not adequate, a second or third dose may be given at 4- to 5-hour intervals. Maximum dose is 10 mg/day. May be administered

parenterally when P.O. not feasible. Usual initial dose is 0.5 to 1 mg I.V. or I.M. If response is not adequate, a second or third dose may be given at intervals of 2 to 3 hours. Maximum dose 10 mg/day.

ADVERSE REACTIONS
CNS: dizziness, headache.
CV: *volume depletion and dehydration, orthostatic hypotension,* EKG changes.
EENT: transient deafness.
GI: nausea.
Metabolic: *hypokalemia; hypochloremic alkalosis; asymptomatic hyperuricemia; fluid and electrolyte imbalances, including dilutional hyponatremia, hypocalcemia, hypomagnesemia;* hyperglycemia and impairment of glucose tolerance.
Skin: rash.
Other: muscle pain and tenderness.

INTERACTIONS
Aminoglycoside antibiotics: potentiated ototoxicity. Use together cautiously.
Probenecid, indomethacin: inhibited diuretic response. Use cautiously.

NURSING CONSIDERATIONS
• Contraindicated in anuria, hepatic coma, and in states of severe electrolyte depletion.

• Use cautiously in patients with hepatic cirrhosis and ascites. Supplemental potassium or potassium-sparing diuretics may be used to prevent hypokalemia and metabolic alkalosis in these patients. Use cautiously in patients with depressed renal function.

• Use cautiously in patients allergic to sulfonamides. These patients may show hypersensitivity to bumetanide.

• Potent loop diuretic; can lead to profound water and electrolyte depletion. Monitor blood pressure and pulse rate during rapid diuresis.

• If oliguria or azotemia develops or

Italicized side effects are common or life-threatening.
*Liquid form contains alcohol.   **May contain tartrazine.

increases, may require stopping drug.
• Monitor serum electrolytes, BUN, and CO_2 frequently.
• Monitor serum potassium levels. Watch for signs of hypokalemia (for example, muscle weakness, cramps). Patients also receiving digitalis have an increased risk of digitalis toxicity due to the potassium-depleting effect of this diuretic.
• Consult with doctor and dietitian to provide high-potassium diet.
• Foods rich in potassium include citrus fruits, tomatoes, bananas, dates, and apricots.
• Monitor blood sugar levels in patients with diabetes. May treat severe hyperglycemia with oral antidiabetic agents.
• Monitor blood uric acid levels, especially in patients with a history of gout.
• Give I.V. doses over 1 to 2 minutes.
• Advise patients taking bumetanide to stand up slowly to prevent dizziness and to limit alcohol intake and strenuous exercise in hot weather since these exacerbate orthostatic hypotension.
• Bumetanide can be safely prescribed in patients allergic to furosemide.
• 1 mg of bumetanide is equal to 40 mg of furosemide.
• May be less ototoxic than furosemide, but the clinical relevance of this has not been determined.
• Give in a.m. to prevent nocturia. If second dose is necessary, give in the early afternoon.
• Intermittent dosage given on alternate days, or for 3 to 4 days with 1 or 2 days intervening, is recommended as the safest and most effective dosage schedule for control of edema.

chlorothiazide
Diachlor, Diuril♦, Ro-Chlorozide, SK-Chlorothiazide
Pregnancy Category: D

MECHANISM OF ACTION
Increases urinary excretion of sodium and water by inhibiting sodium reabsorption in the cortical diluting site of the nephron.

INDICATIONS & DOSAGE
Edema, hypertension—
Adults: 500 mg to 2 g P.O. or I.V. daily or in two divided doses.
Diuresis—
Children over 6 months: 20 mg/kg P.O. or I.V. daily in divided doses.
Children under 6 months: may require 30 mg/kg P.O. or I.V. daily in two divided doses.

ADVERSE REACTIONS
Blood: *aplastic anemia, agranulocytosis,* leukopenia, thrombocytopenia.
CV: *volume depletion and dehydration,* orthostatic hypotension.
GI: anorexia, nausea, pancreatitis.
Hepatic: hepatic encephalopathy.
Metabolic: *hypokalemia, asymptomatic hyperuricemia, hyperglycemia and impairment of glucose tolerance,* fluid and electrolyte imbalances including dilutional hyponatremia and hypochloremia, metabolic alkalosis, hypercalcemia, gout.
Skin: dermatitis, photosensitivity, rash.
Other: hypersensitivity reactions such as pneumonitis and vasculitis.

INTERACTIONS
Cholestyramine, colestipol: intestinal absorption of thiazides decreased. Keep doses as separate as possible.
Diazoxide: increased antihypertensive, hyperglycemic, hyperuricemic effects. Use together cautiously.

NURSING CONSIDERATIONS

• Contraindicated in anuria; hypersensitivity to other thiazides or other sulfonamide-derived drugs; impaired hepatic function; progressive hepatic disease. Use cautiously in severe renal disease.

• Monitor intake/output, weight, and serum electrolytes regularly.

• Monitor potassium levels; consult with doctor and dietitian to provide high-potassium diet. Watch for signs of hypokalemia (for example, muscle weakness, cramps). Patients on digitalis have an increased risk of digitalis toxicity due to the potassium-depleting effect of the diuretic. May use with potassium-sparing diuretic to prevent potassium loss.

• Foods rich in potassium include citrus fruits, tomatoes, bananas, dates, and apricots.

• Monitor blood sugar. Check insulin requirements in patients with diabetes. May treat severe hyperglycemia with oral antidiabetic agents.

• Monitor serum creatinine and BUN levels regularly. Not as effective if these levels are more than twice normal.

• Monitor blood uric acid levels, especially in patients with a history of gout.

• Monitor serum calcium levels and for progressive renal impairment.

• Only injectable thiazide. For I.V. use only—not I.M. or subcutaneous. Reconstitute with 18 ml of sterile water for injection/500 mg vial. May store reconstituted solutions at room temperature up to 24 hours. Compatible with intravenous dextrose or sodium chloride solutions.

• Avoid I.V. infiltration; can be very painful.

• Give in a.m. to prevent nocturia.

• In hypertension, therapeutic response may be delayed several days.

• Elderly patients are especially susceptible to excessive diuresis.

• The only thiazide available in liquid form.

• Thiazides and thiazide-like diuretics should be stopped before tests for parathyroid function are performed.

chlorthalidone
Hygroton♦, Novothalidone♦♦, Thalitone, Uridon♦♦
Pregnancy Category: D

MECHANISM OF ACTION
Increases urinary excretion of sodium and water by inhibiting sodium reabsorption in the cortical diluting site of the nephron.

INDICATIONS & DOSAGE
Edema, hypertension—
Adults: 25 to 100 mg P.O. daily, or 100 mg three times weekly or on alternate days.
Children: 2 mg/kg P.O. three times weekly.

ADVERSE REACTIONS
Blood: *aplastic anemia, agranulocytosis,* leukopenia, thrombocytopenia.
CV: *volume depletion and dehydration,* orthostatic hypotension.
GI: anorexia, nausea, pancreatitis.
GU: impotence.
Hepatic: hepatic encephalopathy.
Metabolic: *hypokalemia, asymptomatic hyperuricemia, hyperglycemia and impairment of glucose tolerance,* fluid and electrolyte imbalances including dilutional hyponatremia and hypochloremia, metabolic alkalosis, hypercalcemia, gout.
Skin: dermatitis, photosensitivity, rash.
Other: hypersensitivity reactions, such as pneumonitis and vasculitis.

INTERACTIONS
Cholestyramine, colestipol: intestinal absorption of thiazides decreased. Keep doses as separate as possible.
Diazoxide: increased antihypertensive, hyperglycemic, hyperuricemic

---

effects. Use together cautiously.

NURSING CONSIDERATIONS
• Contraindicated in anuria and in hypersensitivity to thiazides or other sulfonamide-derived drugs. Use cautiously in severe renal disease, progressive hepatic disease, impaired hepatic function.
• Monitor intake/output, weight, and serum electrolytes regularly.
• Monitor serum potassium levels; consult with doctor and dietitian to provide high-potassium diet. Watch for signs of hypokalemia (for example, muscle weakness, cramps). Patients on digitalis have an increased risk of digitalis toxicity due to the potassium-depleting effect of this diuretic. May use with potassium-sparing diuretic to prevent potassium loss.
• Foods rich in potassium include citrus fruits, tomatoes, bananas, dates, and apricots.
• Monitor serum creatinine and BUN levels regularly. Not as effective if these levels are more than twice normal.
• Monitor blood uric acid levels, especially in patients with a history of gout.
• Monitor blood sugar. Check insulin requirements in patients with diabetes. May treat severe hyperglycemia with oral antidiabetic agents.
• In hypertension, therapeutic response may be delayed several days.
• Give in a.m. to prevent nocturia.
• Elderly patients are especially susceptible to excessive diuresis.
• Thiazides and thiazide-like diuretics should be stopped before tests for parathyroid function are performed.

cyclothiazide
Anhydron, Fluidil
Pregnancy Category: D

MECHANISM OF ACTION
Increases urinary excretion of sodium and water by inhibiting sodium reabsorption in the cortical diluting site of the nephron.

INDICATIONS & DOSAGE
Edema—
Adults: 1 to 2 mg P.O. daily. May be used on alternate days as maintenance dose.
Children: 0.02 to 0.04 mg/kg P.O. daily.
Hypertension—
Adults: 2 mg P.O. daily; up to 2 mg b.i.d. or t.i.d.

ADVERSE REACTIONS
Blood: *aplastic anemia, agranulocytosis,* leukopenia, thrombocytopenia.
CV: *volume depletion and dehydration,* orthostatic hypotension.
GI: anorexia, nausea, pancreatitis.
Hepatic: hepatic encephalopathy.
Metabolic: *hypokalemia, asymptomatic hyperuricemia, hyperglycemia and impairment of glucose tolerance,* fluid and electrolyte imbalances including dilutional hyponatremia and hypochloremia, metabolic alkalosis, hypercalcemia, gout.
Skin: dermatitis, photosensitivity, rash.
Other: hypersensitivity reactions, such as pneumonitis and vasculitis.

INTERACTIONS
Cholestyramine, colestipol: intestinal absorption of thiazides decreased. Keep doses as separate as possible.
Diazoxide: increased antihypertensive, hyperglycemic, hyperuricemic effects. Use together cautiously.

NURSING CONSIDERATIONS
• Contraindicated in anuria and in hypersensitivity to other thiazides or other sulfonamide-derived drugs. Use cautiously in severe renal disease, impaired hepatic function, progressive hepatic disease.
• Monitor intake/output, weight, and serum electrolytes regularly.

• Monitor serum potassium levels; consult with doctor and dietitian to provide high-potassium diet. Watch for signs of hypokalemia (for example, muscle weakness, cramps). Patients on digitalis have an increased risk of digitalis toxicity due to the potassium-depleting effect of this diuretic. May use with potassium-sparing diuretic to prevent potassium loss.
• Foods rich in potassium include citrus fruits, tomatoes, bananas, dates, and apricots.
• Monitor blood sugar. Check insulin requirements in patients with diabetes. May treat severe hyperglycemia with oral antidiabetic agents.
• Monitor serum creatinine and BUN levels regularly. Not as effective if these levels are more than twice normal.
• Monitor blood uric acid levels, especially in patients with a history of gout.
• In hypertension, therapeutic response may be delayed several days.
• Give in a.m. to prevent nocturia.
• Elderly patients are especially susceptible to excessive diuresis.
• Thiazides and thiazide-like diuretics should be stopped before tests for parathyroid function are performed.

---

dichlorphenamide
Daranide, Oratrol
Pregnancy Category: C

MECHANISM OF ACTION
Decreases secretion of aqueous humor in the eye, thereby lowering intraocular pressure.

INDICATIONS & DOSAGE
Adjunct in glaucoma—
Adults: initially, 100 to 200 mg P.O., followed by 100 mg q 12 hours until desired response obtained. Maintenance: 25 to 50 mg P.O. daily b.i.d. or t.i.d. Give miotics concomitantly.

ADVERSE REACTIONS
Blood: *aplastic anemia,* hemolytic anemia, leukopenia.
CNS: drowsiness, paresthesias.
EENT: transient myopia.
GI: nausea, vomiting, anorexia.
GU: crystalluria, renal calculi.
Metabolic: *hyperchloremic acidosis,* hypokalemia, asymptomatic hyperuricemia.
Skin: rash.

INTERACTIONS
None significant.

NURSING CONSIDERATIONS
• Contraindicated in hepatic insufficiency, renal failure, adrenocortical insufficiency, hyperchloremic acidosis, depressed sodium or potassium levels, severe pulmonary obstruction with inability to increase alveolar ventilation, Addison's disease. Long-term use contraindicated in severe, absolute, or chronic noncongestive narrow-angle glaucoma. Use cautiously in respiratory acidosis, monitoring blood pH and blood gases.
• Monitor electrolytes, especially serum potassium in initial treatment. Usually no problem in long-term glaucoma therapy unless risk of hypokalemia from other causes; potassium supplements may be necessary.
• May cause false-positive results in urine protein tests.
• Anticipate that drug will be given every day for glaucoma but intermittently for edema.
• Evaluate patient with glaucoma for eye pain to make sure drug is effective in decreasing intraocular pressure.

Italicized side effects are common or life-threatening.
*Liquid form contains alcohol.   **May contain tartrazine.

ethacrynate sodium
Sodium Edecrin

ethacrynic acid
Edecrin♦
Pregnancy Category: D

MECHANISM OF ACTION
Inhibits reabsorption of sodium and chloride at the proximal portion of the ascending loop of Henle.

INDICATIONS & DOSAGE
Acute pulmonary edema—
Adults: 50 to 100 mg of ethacrynate sodium I.V. slowly over several minutes.
Edema—
Adults: 50 to 200 mg P.O. daily. Refractory cases may require up to 200 mg b.i.d.
Children: initial dose 25 mg P.O., cautiously, increased in 25-mg increments daily until desired effect.

ADVERSE REACTIONS
Blood: *agranulocytosis,* neutropenia, thrombocytopenia.
CV: *volume depletion and dehydration, orthostatic hypotension.*
EENT: transient deafness with too-rapid I.V. injection.
GI: abdominal discomfort and pain, diarrhea.
Metabolic: *hypokalemia; hypochloremic alkalosis; asymptomatic hyperuricemia; fluid and electrolyte imbalances including dilutional hyponatremia, hypocalcemia, hypomagnesemia;* hyperglycemia and impairment of glucose tolerance.
Skin: dermatitis.

INTERACTIONS
Aminoglycoside antibiotics: potentiated ototoxic side effects of both ethacrynic acid and aminoglycosides. Use together cautiously.

NURSING CONSIDERATIONS
• Contraindicated in patients with anuria and in infants. Use cautiously in electrolyte abnormalities. If electrolyte imbalance, azotemia, or oliguria develops, may require stopping drug.
• This drug is a very potent diuretic.
• Monitor intake/output, weight, and serum electrolytes regularly.
• Monitor serum potassium levels; consult with doctor and dietitian to provide high-potassium diet. Watch for signs of hypokalemia (e.g., muscle weakness, cramps).
• Foods rich in potassium include citrus fruits, tomatoes, bananas, dates, and apricots.
• Patients also on digitalis have an increased risk of digitalis toxicity due to the potassium-depleting effect.
• I.V. injection painful; may cause thrombophlebitis. Don't give subcutaneously or I.M. Give slowly through tubing of running infusion over several minutes.
• Salt and potassium chloride supplement may be needed during therapy.
• Reconstitute vacuum vial with 50 ml of dextrose 5% injection or NaCl injection. Discard unused solution after 24 hours. Don't use cloudy or opalescent solutions.
• Elderly patients are especially susceptible to excessive diuresis.
• Give P.O. doses in a.m. to prevent nocturia.
• Severe diarrhea may necessitate discontinuing drug.
• Monitor blood uric acid levels, especially in patients with history of gout.
• May potentiate effects of the anticoagulant warfarin; carefully monitor patients receiving both drugs.

---

furosemide

Lasix♦**, Novosemide♦♦, SK-
Furosemide, Uritol♦♦
Pregnancy Category: C

MECHANISM OF ACTION
Inhibits reabsorption of sodium and
chloride at the proximal portion of the
ascending loop of Henle.

INDICATIONS & DOSAGE
Acute pulmonary edema—
Adults: 40 mg I.V. injected slowly;
then 40 mg I.V. in 1 to 1½ hours if
needed.
Edema—
Adults: 20 to 80 mg P.O. daily in
a.m., second dose can be given in 6 to
8 hours; carefully titrated up to 600
mg daily if needed; or 20 to 40 mg
I.M. or I.V. Increase by 20 mg q 2
hours until desired response is
achieved. I.V. dose should be given
slowly over 1 to 2 minutes.
Hypertension—
Adults: 40 mg P.O. b.i.d. Adjust dose
according to response.
Infants and children: 2 mg/kg daily;
dose increased by 1 to 2 mg/kg in 6 to
8 hours if needed; carefully titrated up
to 6 mg/kg daily if needed.
*Hypertensive crisis, acute renal fail-
ure—*
Adults: 100 to 200 mg I.V. over 1 to 2
minutes.
Chronic renal failure—
Adults: initially, 80 mg P.O. daily. Increase by 80 to 120 mg daily until desired response is achieved.

ADVERSE REACTIONS
Blood: *agranulocytosis,* leukopenia,
thrombocytopenia.
CV: *volume depletion and dehydration, orthostatic hypotension.*
EENT: transient deafness with too
rapid I.V. injection.
GI: abdominal discomfort and pain,
diarrhea (with oral solution).
Metabolic: *hypokalemia; hypochlore-*
*mic alkalosis; asymptomatic hyperuri-
cemia, fluid and electrolyte imbalances including dilutional hyponatremia, hypocalcemia, hypomagnesemia;*
hyperglycemia and impairment of
glucose tolerance.
Skin: dermatitis.

INTERACTIONS
Aminoglycoside antibiotics: potentiated ototoxicity. Use together cautiously.
Chloral hydrate: sweating, flushing
with I.V. furosemide.
Clofibrate: enhanced furosemide effects. Use cautiously.
Indomethacin: inhibited diuretic response. Use cautiously.

NURSING CONSIDERATIONS
• Use cautiously in cardiogenic shock
complicated by pulmonary edema,
anuria, hepatic coma, or electrolyte
imbalances. Drug is not routinely administered to women of childbearing
age because its safety in pregnancy
hasn't been established.
• Potent loop diuretic; can lead to
profound water and electrolyte depletion. Monitor blood pressure and
pulse rate during rapid diuresis.
• Sulfonamide-sensitive patients may
have allergic reactions to furosemide.
• If oliguria or azotemia develops or
increases, may require stopping drug.
• Monitor serum electrolytes, BUN,
and CO_2 frequently.
• Monitor serum potassium levels.
Watch for signs of hypokalemia (for
example, muscle weakness, cramps).
Patients also on digitalis have an increased risk of digitalis toxicity due to
the potassium-depleting effect.
• Consult with doctor and dietitian to
provide high-potassium diet.
• Foods rich in potassium include citrus fruits, tomatoes, bananas, dates,
and apricots.
• Monitor blood sugar levels in patients with diabetes. May treat severe
hyperglycemia with oral antidiabetic

Italicized side effects are common or life-threatening.
*Liquid form contains alcohol.   **May contain tartrazine.

agents.
- Monitor blood uric acid levels, especially in patients with a history of gout.
- Give I.V. doses over 1 to 2 minutes.
- Don't use parenteral route in infants and children unless oral dosage form is not practical.
- Give P.O. and I.M. preparations in a.m. to prevent nocturia. Give second doses in early afternoon.
- Elderly patients are especially susceptible to excessive diuresis, with potential for circulatory collapse and thromboembolic complications.
- Store tablets in light-resistant container to prevent discoloration (doesn't affect potency). Don't use discolored (yellow) injectable preparation. Oral furosemide solution should be stored in the refrigerator to ensure stability of the drug.
- Promotes calcium excretion. I.V. furosemide often used to treat hypercalcemia.
- Advise patients taking furosemide to stand slowly to prevent dizziness, and to limit alcohol intake and strenuous exercise in hot weather since these exacerbate orthostatic hypotension.
- Advise patients to report immediately ringing in ears, severe abdominal pain, or sore throat and fever; may indicate furosemide toxicity.
- Discourage patients receiving furosemide therapy at home from storing different types of medication in the same container. This increases the risk of drug errors, especially for patients taking both furosemide and digoxin, since the most popular strengths of these drugs' pills are white tablets approximately equal in size.
- To prepare parenteral furosemide for I.V. infusion, mix drug with dextrose 5% in water, 0.9% sodium chloride solution, or lactated Ringer's solution. Use prepared infusion solution within 24 hours.

hydrochlorothiazide
Chlorzide, Diaqua, Diuchlor H♦♦, Esidrix♦, Hydro DIURIL♦, Hydromal, Hydro-Z-50, Hydrozide♦♦, Hyperetic, Neo-Codema♦♦, Novohydrazide♦♦, Oretic, Ro-Hydrazide, SK-Hydrochlorothiazide, Urozide♦♦
Pregnancy Category: D

MECHANISM OF ACTION
Increases urinary excretion of sodium and water by inhibiting sodium reabsorption in the cortical diluting site of the nephron.

INDICATIONS & DOSAGE
Edema—
Adults: initially, 25 to 100 mg P.O. daily or intermittently for maintenance.
Children over 6 months: 2.2 mg/kg P.O. daily divided b.i.d.
Children under 6 months: up to 3.3 mg/kg P.O. daily divided b.i.d.
Hypertension—
Adults: 25 to 100 mg P.O. daily or divided dosage. Daily dosage increased or decreased according to blood pressure.

ADVERSE REACTIONS
Blood: *aplastic anemia, agranulocytosis,* leukopenia, thrombocytopenia.
CV: *volume depletion and dehydration,* orthostatic hypotension.
GI: anorexia, nausea, pancreatitis.
Hepatic: hepatic encephalopathy.
Metabolic: *hypokalemia, asymptomatic hyperuricemia, hyperglycemia and impairment of glucose tolerance,* fluid and electrolyte imbalances including dilutional hyponatremia and hypochloremia, metabolic alkalosis, hypercalcemia, gout.
Skin: dermatitis, photosensitivity, rash.
Other: hypersensitivity reactions, such as pneumonitis and vasculitis.

INTERACTIONS
Cholestyramine, colestipol: intestinal absorption of thiazides decreased. Keep doses as separate as possible.
Diazoxide: increased antihypertensive, hyperglycemic, hyperuricemic effects. Use together cautiously.

NURSING CONSIDERATIONS
• Contraindicated in anuria and in hypersensitivity to other thiazides or other sulfonamide derivatives. Use cautiously in severe renal disease, impaired hepatic function, progressive hepatic disease.
• Monitor intake/output, weight, and serum electrolytes regularly.
• Monitor serum potassium levels; consult with doctor and dietitian to provide high-potassium diet. Watch for hypokalemia (for example, muscle weakness, cramps). Patients also on digitalis have an increased risk of digitalis toxicity due to the potassium-depleting effect of this diuretic. May use with potassium-sparing diuretic to prevent potassium loss.
• Foods rich in potassium include citrus fruits, tomatoes, bananas, dates, and apricots.
• Monitor serum creatinine and BUN levels regularly. Not as effective if these levels are more than twice normal.
• Monitor blood uric acid levels, especially in patients with a history of gout.
• Check insulin requirements in patients with diabetes. May treat severe hyperglycemia with oral antidiabetic agents.
• In hypertension, therapeutic response may be delayed several days.
• Give in a.m. to prevent nocturia. Studies have shown that the drug is as effective when administered once daily as it is when given more frequently.
• Elderly patients are especially susceptible to excessive diuresis.
• Thiazides and thiazide-like diuret-ics should be stopped before tests for parathyroid function are performed.

indapamide
Lozol
Pregnancy Category: B

MECHANISM OF ACTION
Inhibits sodium reabsorption in the cortical diluting site of the nephron. Also has a direct vasodilating effect that may be a result of calcium channel-blocking action.

INDICATIONS & DOSAGE
Edema, hypertension—
Adults: 2.5 mg P.O. as a single daily dose taken in the morning. Dose may be increased to 5 mg daily.

ADVERSE REACTIONS
CNS: headache, irritability, nervousness.
CV: *volume depletion and dehydration,* orthostatic hypotension.
GI: anorexia, nausea, pancreatitis.
Metabolic: *hypokalemia; asymptomatic hyperuricemia;* fluid and electrolyte imbalances, including dilutional hyponatremia and hypochloremia; metabolic alkalosis; gout.
Skin: dermatitis, photosensitivity, rash.
Other: muscle cramps and spasms.

INTERACTIONS
Diazoxide: increased antihypertensive, hyperglycemic, hyperuricemic effects. Use together cautiously.

NURSING CONSIDERATIONS
• Contraindicated in anuria and hypersensitivity to other sulfonamide-derived drugs.
• Use cautiously in severe renal disease, impaired hepatic function, and progressive hepatic disease.
• Monitor intake/output, weight, and serum electrolytes regularly.
• Monitor serum potassium levels;

Italicized side effects are common or life-threatening.
*Liquid form contains alcohol.   **May contain tartrazine.

consult with doctor and dietitian to provide high-potassium diet. Foods rich in potassium include citrus fruits, tomatoes, bananas, dates, and apricots. Watch for symptoms of hypokalemia (for example, muscle weakness, cramps). May use with potassium-sparing diuretic to prevent potassium loss. Patients also receiving digitalis have an increased risk of digitalis toxicity due to the potassium-depleting effects of this diuretic.

• Monitor serum creatinine and BUN levels regularly. Drug not effective if these levels are more than twice normal.

• Monitor blood uric acid levels, especially in patients with history of gout.

• Check insulin requirements in patients with diabetes. May treat severe hyperglycemia with oral antidiabetic agents.

• Give in a.m. to prevent nocturia.

• In hypertension, therapeutic response may be delayed several days.

• Elderly patients are especially susceptible to excessive diuresis.

• Stop drug before tests for parathyroid function are performed.

mannitol
Osmitrol♦
Pregnancy Category: C

MECHANISM OF ACTION
Increases the osmotic pressure of glomerular filtrate, inhibiting tubular reabsorption of water and electrolytes. Also elevates blood plasma osmolality, resulting in enhanced flow of water into extracellular fluid.

INDICATIONS & DOSAGE
Adults and children over 12 years:
*Test dose for marked oliguria or suspected inadequate renal function—*200 mg/kg or 12.5 g as a 15% or 20% solution I.V. over 3 to 5 minutes. Response adequate if 30 to 50 ml urine/

hour is excreted over 2 to 3 hours.
*Treatment of oliguria—*50 to 100 g I.V. as a 15% to 20% solution over 90 minutes to several hours.
*Prevention of oliguria or acute renal failure—*50 to 100 g I.V. of a concentrated (5% to 25%) solution. Exact concentration is determined by fluid requirements.
*Edema—*100 g as a 10% to 20% solution over 2- to 6-hour period.
*To reduce intraocular pressure or intracranial pressure—*1.5 to 2 g/kg as a 15% to 25% solution I.V. over 30 to 60 minutes.
*To promote diuresis in drug intoxication—*5% to 10% solution continuously up to 200 g I.V., while maintaining 100 to 500 ml urinary output/hour and a positive fluid balance.

ADVERSE REACTIONS
CNS: rebound increase in intracranial pressure 8 to 12 hours after diuresis, headache, confusion.
CV: *transient expansion of plasma volume during infusion causing circulatory overload and pulmonary edema,* tachycardia, angina-like chest pain.
EENT: blurred vision, rhinitis.
GI: thirst, nausea, vomiting.
GU: urinary retention.
Metabolic: *fluid and electrolyte imbalance, water intoxication, cellular dehydration.*

INTERACTIONS
None significant.

NURSING CONSIDERATIONS
• Contraindicated in anuria, severe pulmonary congestion, frank pulmonary edema, severe congestive heart disease, severe dehydration, metabolic edema, progressive renal disease or dysfunction, progressive heart failure during administration, active intracranial bleeding except during craniotomy.
• Monitor vital signs (including CVP)

at least hourly; intake/output hourly (report increasing oliguria). Monitor daily: weight, renal function, fluid balance, serum and urine sodium and potassium levels.
• Solution often crystallizes, especially at low temperatures. To redissolve, warm bottle in hot water bath, shake vigorously. Cool to body temperature before giving. Concentrations greater than 15% have greater tendency to crystallize. Do not use solution with undissolved crystals.
• Infusions should always be given I.V. via an in-line filter.
• Avoid infiltration; observe for inflammation, edema, necrosis.
• For maximum pressure reduction before surgery, give 1 to 1½ hours preoperatively.
• Can be used to measure glomerular filtration rate.
• Give frequent mouth care or fluids as permitted to relieve thirst.
• Urethral catheter is inserted in comatose or incontinent patients because therapy is based on strict evaluation of intake and output. In patients with urethral catheters, use an hourly urometer collection bag to facilitate accurate evaluation of output.

methazolamide
Neptazane♦
Pregnancy Category: C

MECHANISM OF ACTION
Decreases secretion of aqueous humor in the eye, thereby lowering intraocular pressure.

INDICATIONS & DOSAGE
Glaucoma (open-angle, or preoperatively in obstructive or narrow-angle)—
Adults: 50 to 100 mg b.i.d. or t.i.d.

ADVERSE REACTIONS
Blood: *aplastic anemia,* hemolytic anemia, leukopenia.

CNS: drowsiness, paresthesias.
EENT: transient myopia.
GI: nausea, vomiting, anorexia.
GU: crystalluria, renal calculi.
Metabolic: *hyperchloremic acidosis,* hypokalemia, asymptomatic hyperuricemia.
Skin: rash.

INTERACTIONS
None significant.

NURSING CONSIDERATIONS
• Contraindicated in severe or absolute glaucoma; for long-term use in chronic noncongestive narrow-angle glaucoma; in patients with depressed sodium or potassium serum levels, renal or hepatic disease or dysfunction, adrenal gland dysfunction, and hyperchloremic acidosis. Use cautiously in respiratory acidosis, emphysema, chronic pulmonary disease.
• Monitor intake/output, weight, and serum electrolytes frequently.
• May cause false-positive urine protein tests by alkalinizing urine.
• A carbonic anhydrase inhibitor.
• Elderly patients are especially susceptible to excessive diuresis.
• Diuretic effect decreases in acidosis.
• Anticipate that drug will be given every day for glaucoma but intermittently for edema. Caution patient to comply with prescribed dosage and schedule to lessen risk of metabolic acidosis.
• Carefully evaluate the patient with glaucoma for eye pain to make sure drug is effective in decreasing intraocular pressure.

methyclothiazide
Aquatensen, Duretic♦♦, Enduron
Pregnancy Category: D

MECHANISM OF ACTION
Increases urinary excretion of sodium and water by inhibiting sodium reab-

---

Italicized side effects are common or life-threatening.
*Liquid form contains alcohol.   **May contain tartrazine.

sorption in the cortical diluting site of the nephron.

INDICATIONS & DOSAGE
Edema, hypertension—
Adults: 2.5 to 10 mg P.O daily.

ADVERSE REACTIONS
Blood: *aplastic anemia, agranulocytosis,* leukopenia, thrombocytopenia.
CV: *volume depletion and dehydration,* orthostatic hypotension.
GI: anorexia, nausea, pancreatitis.
Hepatic: hepatic encephalopathy.
Metabolic: *hypokalemia, asymptomatic hyperuricemia, hyperglycemia and impairment of glucose tolerance,* fluid and electrolyte imbalances including dilutional hyponatremia and hypochloremia, metabolic alkalosis, hypercalcemia, gout.
Skin: dermatitis, photosensitivity, rash.
Other: hypersensitivity reactions, such as pneumonitis and vasculitis.

INTERACTIONS
Cholestyramine, colestipol: intestinal absorption of thiazides decreased. Keep doses as separate as possible.
Diazoxide: increased antihypertensive, hyperglycemic, hyperuricemic effects. Use together cautiously.

NURSING CONSIDERATIONS
• Contraindicated in renal decompensation; anuria; hypersensitivity to other thiazides or other sulfonamide-derived drugs. Use cautiously in potassium depletion, renal disease or dysfunction, impaired hepatic function, progressive hepatic disease.
• Monitor intake/output, weight, and serum electrolytes regularly.
• Monitor serum potassium levels; consult with doctor and dietitian to provide high-potassium diet. Foods rich in potassium include citrus fruits, tomatoes, bananas, dates, and apricots. Watch for hypokalemia (for example, muscle weakness, cramps).

Patients also on digitalis have an increased risk of digitalis toxicity due to the potassium-depleting effect of this diuretic. May use with potassium-sparing diuretic to prevent potassium loss.
• Check insulin requirements in patients with diabetes. May treat severe hyperglycemia with oral antidiabetic agents.
• Monitor serum creatinine and BUN levels regularly. Not as effective if these levels are more than twice normal.
• Monitor blood uric acid levels, especially in patients with a history of gout.
• In hypertension, therapeutic response may be delayed several days.
• Give in a.m. to prevent nocturia.
• Elderly patients are especially susceptible to excessive diuresis.
• Thiazides and thiazide-like diuretics should be stopped before tests for parathyroid function are performed.

metolazone
Diulo, Zaroxolyn♦**
Pregnancy Category: D

MECHANISM OF ACTION
Increases urinary excretion of sodium and water by inhibiting sodium reabsorption in the cortical diluting site of the ascending loop of Henle.

INDICATIONS & DOSAGE
Edema (heart failure)—
Adults: 5 to 10 mg P.O. daily.
Edema (renal disease)—
Adults: 5 to 20 mg P.O. daily.
Hypertension—
Adults: 2.5 to 5 mg P.O. daily. Maintenance dose determined by patient's blood pressure.

ADVERSE REACTIONS
Blood: *aplastic anemia, agranulocytosis,* leukopenia, thrombocytopenia.
CV: *volume depletion and dehydra-*

tion, orthostatic hypotension.
GI: anorexia, nausea, pancreatitis.
Hepatic: hepatic encephalopathy.
Metabolic: *hypokalemia, asymptomatic hyperuricemia, hyperglycemia and impairment of glucose tolerance,* fluid and electrolyte imbalances including dilutional hyponatremia and hypochloremia, metabolic alkalosis, hypercalcemia, gout.
Skin: dermatitis, photosensitivity, rash.
Other: hypersensitivity reactions, such as pneumonitis and vasculitis.

INTERACTIONS
Cholestyramine, colestipol: intestinal absorption of thiazides decreased. Keep doses as separate as possible.
Diazoxide: increased antihypertensive, hyperglycemic, hyperuricemic effects. Use together cautiously.

NURSING CONSIDERATIONS
• Contraindicated in anuria; hepatic coma or precoma; hypersensitivity to thiazides or other sulfonamide-derived drugs. Use cautiously in hyperuricemia or gout and severely impaired renal function.
• Monitor intake/output, weight, and serum electrolytes regularly.
• Monitor serum potassium levels; consult with doctor and dietitian to provide high-potassium diet. Foods rich in potassium include citrus fruits, tomatoes, bananas, dates, and apricots. Watch for hypokalemia (for example, muscle weakness, cramps). Patients also on digitalis may have an increased risk of digitalis toxicity due to the potassium-depleting effect of this diuretic. May use with potassium-sparing diuretic to prevent potassium loss.
• Check insulin requirements in patients with diabetes. May treat severe hyperglycemia with oral antidiabetic agents.
• Monitor blood uric acid levels, especially in patients with a history of

gout.
• In hypertension, therapeutic response may be delayed several days.
• Give in a.m. to prevent nocturia.
• Elderly patients are especially susceptible to excessive diuresis.
• A thiazide-related diuretic. However, unlike thiazide diuretics, metolazone is effective in patients with decreased renal function.
• Used as an adjunct in furosemide-resistant edema.
• Thiazides and thiazide-like diuretics should be stopped before tests for parathyroid function are performed.

---

polythiazide
Renese
Pregnancy Category: D

MECHANISM OF ACTION
Increases urinary excretion of sodium and water by inhibiting sodium reabsorption in the cortical diluting site of the nephron.

INDICATIONS & DOSAGE
Hypertension—
Adults: 2 to 4 mg P.O. daily.
Edema (heart failure, renal failure)—
Adults: 1 to 4 mg P.O. daily.

ADVERSE REACTIONS
Blood: *aplastic anemia, agranulocytosis,* leukopenia, thrombocytopenia.
CV: *volume depletion and dehydration,* orthostatic hypotension.
GI: anorexia, nausea, pancreatitis.
Hepatic: hepatic encephalopathy.
Metabolic: *hypokalemia, asymptomatic hyperuricemia, hyperglycemia and impairment of glucose tolerance,* fluid and electrolyte imbalances including dilutional hyponatremia and hypochloremia, metabolic alkalosis, hypercalcemia, gout.
Skin: dermatitis, photosensitivity, rash.
Other: hypersensitivity reactions, such as pneumonitis and vasculitis.

INTERACTIONS
Cholestyramine, colestipol: intestinal absorption of thiazides decreased. Keep doses as separate as possible.
Diazoxide: increased antihypertensive, hyperglycemic, hyperuricemic effects. Use together cautiously.

NURSING CONSIDERATIONS
• Contraindicated in anuria and in hypersensitivity to other thiazides or other sulfonamide-derived drugs. Use cautiously in severe renal disease, impaired hepatic function, allergies.
• Monitor intake/output, weight, and serum electrolytes regularly.
• Monitor serum potassium levels; consult with doctor and dietitian to provide high-potassium diet. Foods rich in potassium include citrus fruits, tomatoes, bananas, dates, and apricots. Watch for hypokalemia (for example, muscle weakness, cramps). Patients also on digitalis may have an increased risk of digitalis toxicity due to the potassium-depleting effect of this diuretic. May use with potassium-sparing diuretic to prevent potassium loss.
• Monitor blood uric acid levels, especially in patients with a history of gout.
• Check insulin requirements in patients with diabetes. May treat severe hyperglycemia with oral antidiabetic agents.
• In hypertension, therapeutic response may be delayed several days.
• Give in a.m. to prevent nocturia.
• Elderly patients are especially susceptible to excessive diuresis.
• Thiazides and thiazide-like diuretics should be stopped before tests for parathyroid function are performed.

quinethazone
Aquamox♦♦, Hydromox
Pregnancy Category: D

MECHANISM OF ACTION
Increases urinary excretion of sodium and water by inhibiting sodium reabsorption in the cortical diluting site of the nephron.

INDICATIONS & DOSAGE
Edema—
Adults: 50 to 100 mg P.O. daily or 50 mg P.O. b.i.d. Occasionally, up to 150 to 200 mg P.O. daily may be needed.

ADVERSE REACTIONS
Blood: *aplastic anemia, agranulocytosis,* leukopenia, thrombocytopenia.
CV: *volume depletion and dehydration,* orthostatic hypotension.
GI: anorexia, nausea, pancreatitis.
Hepatic: *hepatic encephalopathy.*
Metabolic: *hypokalemia, asymptomatic hyperuricemia, hyperglycemia and impairment of glucose tolerance,* fluid and electrolyte imbalances including dilutional hyponatremia and hypochloremia, metabolic alkalosis, hypercalcemia, gout.
Skin: dermatitis, photosensitivity, rash.
Other: hypersensitivity reactions, such as pneumonitis and vasculitis.

INTERACTIONS
Cholestyramine, colestipol: intestinal absorption of thiazides decreased. Keep doses as separate as possible.
Diazoxide: increased antihypertensive, hyperglycemic, hyperuricemic effects. Use together cautiously.

NURSING CONSIDERATIONS
• Contraindicated in anuria and in hypersensitivity to quinethazones, thiazides, or other sulfonamide-derived drugs. Use cautiously in severe renal disease, impaired hepatic function,

allergies.
• Monitor intake/output, weight, and serum electrolytes regularly.
• Monitor serum potassium levels; consult with doctor and dietitian to provide high-potassium diet. Foods rich in potassium include citrus fruits, tomatoes, bananas, dates, and apricots. Watch for hypokalemia (for example, muscle weakness, cramps). Patients also on digitalis have an increased risk of digitalis toxicity due to the potassium-depleting effect of this diuretic. May use with potassium-sparing diuretic to prevent potassium loss.
• Monitor serum creatinine and BUN levels regularly.
• Check insulin requirements in patients with diabetes. May treat severe hyperglycemia with oral hypoglycemics.
• Monitor blood uric acid levels, especially in patients with a history of gout.
• In hypertension, therapeutic response may be delayed several days.
• Give in a.m. to prevent nocturia.
• Elderly patients are especially susceptible to excessive diuresis.
• Thiazides and thiazide-like diuretics should be stopped before tests for parathyroid function are performed.

---

spironolactone
Aldactone♦
Pregnancy Category: D

MECHANISM OF ACTION
Antagonizes aldosterone in the distal tubule, increasing excretion of sodium and water but sparing potassium.

INDICATIONS & DOSAGE
Edema—
Adults: 25 to 200 mg P.O. daily in divided doses.
Children: initially, 3.3 mg/kg P.O. daily in divided doses.
Hypertension—

Adults: 50 to 100 mg P.O. daily in divided doses.
Treatment of diuretic-induced hypokalemia—
Adults: 25 to 100 mg P.O. daily when oral potassium supplements are considered inappropriate.
Detection of primary hyperaldosteronism—
Adults: 400 mg P.O. daily for 4 days (short test) or for 3 to 4 weeks (long test). If hypokalemia and hypertension are corrected, a presumptive diagnosis of primary hyperaldosteronism is made.

ADVERSE REACTIONS
CNS: headache.
GI: anorexia, nausea, diarrhea.
Metabolic: *hyperkalemia,* dehydration, hyponatremia, transient rise in BUN, acidosis.
Skin: urticaria.
Other: gynecomastia in males, breast soreness and menstrual disturbances in females.

INTERACTIONS
Aspirin: possible blocked spironolactone effect. Watch for diminished spironolactone response.

NURSING CONSIDERATIONS
• Contraindicated in anuria, acute or progressive renal insufficiency, hyperkalemia. Use cautiously in fluid or electrolyte imbalances, impaired renal function, and hepatic disease.
• A mild acidosis may occur during therapy. This may be dangerous in patients with hepatic cirrhosis.
• Monitor serum potassium levels, electrolytes, intake/output, weight, and blood pressure regularly.
• Potassium-sparing diuretic; useful as an adjunct to other diuretic therapy. Less potent diuretic than thiazide and loop types. Diuretic effect delayed 2 to 3 days when used alone.
• Maximum antihypertensive response may be delayed up to 2 weeks.

Italicized side effects are common or life-threatening.
*Liquid form contains alcohol.   **May contain tartrazine.

- Warn patient to avoid excessive ingestion of potassium-rich foods or potassium-containing salt substitutes. Concomitant potassium supplement can lead to serious hyperkalemia.
- Elderly patients are more susceptible to excessive diuresis.
- Protect drug from light.
- Breast cancer reported in some patients taking spironolactone, but cause-and-effect relationship not confirmed. Warn against taking drug indiscriminately.
- Give with meals to enhance absorption.
- Because of its antiandrogenic properties, spironolactone has been prescribed to treat hirsutism. The dose for this indication is 200 mg daily.

triamterene
Dyrenium♦
Pregnancy Category: D

MECHANISM OF ACTION
Inhibits sodium reabsorption and potassium excretion by direct action on the distal tubule.

INDICATIONS & DOSAGE
Diuresis—
Adults: initially, 100 mg P.O. b.i.d. after meals. Total daily dosage should not exceed 300 mg.

ADVERSE REACTIONS
Blood: megaloblastic anemia related to low folic acid levels.
CNS: dizziness.
CV: hypotension.
EENT: sore throat.
GI: dry mouth, nausea, vomiting.
Metabolic: *hyperkalemia,* dehydration, hyponatremia, transient rise in BUN, acidosis.
Skin: photosensitivity, rash.
Other: *anaphylaxis,* muscle cramps.

INTERACTIONS
None significant.

NURSING CONSIDERATIONS
- Contraindicated in anuria, severe or progressive renal disease or dysfunction, severe hepatic disease, hyperkalemia. Use cautiously in impaired hepatic function, diabetes mellitus, pregnancy, or lactation.
- Watch for blood dyscrasias.
- Monitor BUN and serum potassium, electrolytes.
- A potassium-sparing diuretic, useful as an adjunct to other diuretic therapy. Less potent than thiazides and loop diuretics. Full diuretic effect delayed 2 to 3 days.
- Warn patients to avoid excessive ingestion of potassium-rich foods or potassium-containing salt substitutes. Concomitant potassium supplement can lead to serious hyperkalemia.
- Give medication after meals to prevent nausea.
- Withdraw gradually to prevent excessive rebound potassium excretion.

trichlormethiazide
Diurese, Metahydrin**, Naqua, Trichlorex
Pregnancy Category: D

MECHANISM OF ACTION
Increases urinary excretion of sodium and water by inhibiting sodium reabsorption in the cortical diluting site of the nephron.

INDICATIONS & DOSAGE
Edema—
Adults: 1 to 4 mg P.O. daily or in two divided doses.
Hypertension—
Adults: 2 to 4 mg P.O. daily.

ADVERSE REACTIONS
Blood: *aplastic anemia, agranulocytosis,* leukopenia, thrombocytopenia.
CV: *volume depletion and dehydration,* orthostatic hypotension.
GI: anorexia, nausea, pancreatitis.
Hepatic: hepatic encephalopathy.

Unmarked trade names available in the United States only.
♦ Also available in Canada.   ♦♦ Available in Canada only.

Metabolic: *hypokalemia, asymptomatic hyperuricemia, hyperglycemia and impairment of glucose tolerance,* fluid and electrolyte imbalances including dilutional hyponatremia and hypochloremia, metabolic alkalosis, hypercalcemia, gout.
Skin: dermatitis, photosensitivity, rash.
Other: hypersensitivity reactions, such as pneumonitis and vasculitis.

INTERACTIONS
Cholestyramine, colestipol: intestinal absorption of thiazides decreased. Keep doses as separate as possible.
Diazoxide: increased antihypertensive, hyperglycemic, hyperuricemic effects. Use together cautiously.

NURSING CONSIDERATIONS
• Contraindicated in anuria and in hypersensitivity to other thiazides or other sulfonamide-derived drugs. Use cautiously in severe renal disease, impaired hepatic function.
• Monitor intake/output, weight, and electrolytes regularly.
• Monitor serum potassium levels; consult with doctor and dietitian to provide high-potassium diet. Foods rich in potassium include citrus fruits, tomatoes, bananas, dates, and apricots. Watch for hypokalemia (for example, muscle weakness, cramps). Patients also on digitalis have an increased risk of digitalis toxicity due to the potassium-depleting effect of this diuretic. May use with potassium-sparing diuretic to prevent hypokalemia.
• Monitor serum creatinine and BUN levels regularly. Not as effective if these levels are more than twice normal.
• Check insulin requirements in patients with diabetes. May treat severe hyperglycemia with oral antidiabetic agents. Monitor blood sugar.
• Monitor blood uric acid levels, especially in patients with a history of

gout.
• In hypertension, therapeutic response may be delayed several days.
• Give in a.m. to prevent nocturia.
• Elderly patients are especially susceptible to excessive diuresis.
• Thiazides and thiazide-like diuretics should be stopped before tests for parathyroid function are performed.

urea (carbamide)
Ureaphil, Carbamex♦♦
Pregnancy Category: C

MECHANISM OF ACTION
Increases the osmotic pressure of glomerular filtrate, inhibiting tubular reabsorption of water and electrolytes. Also elevates blood plasma osmolality, resulting in enhanced flow of water into extracellular fluid.

INDICATIONS & DOSAGE
Intracranial or intraocular pressure—
Adults: 1 to 1.5 g/kg as a 30% solution by slow I.V. infusion over 1 to 2.5 hours.
Children over 2 years: 0.5 to 1.5 g/kg slow I.V. infusion.
Children under 2 years: as little as 0.1 g/kg slow I.V. infusion. Maximum 4 ml/minute.
  Maximum adult daily dose 120 g. To prepare 135 ml 30% solution, mix contents of 40-g vial of urea with 105 ml dextrose 5% or 10% in water or 10% invert sugar in water. Each ml of 30% solution provides 300 mg urea.

ADVERSE REACTIONS
CNS: *headache.*
CV: tachycardia, congestive heart failure, *pulmonary edema.*
GI: *nausea, vomiting.*
Metabolic: sodium and potassium depletion.
Local: irritation or necrotic sloughing may occur with extravasation.

Italicized side effects are common or life-threatening.
*Liquid form contains alcohol.   **May contain tartrazine.

INTERACTIONS
None significant.

NURSING CONSIDERATIONS
• Contraindicated in severely impaired renal function, marked dehydration, frank hepatic failure, active intracranial bleeding. Use cautiously in pregnancy, lactation, cardiac disease, hepatic impairment, or sickle cell damage with CNS involvement.
• Avoid rapid I.V. infusion; may cause hemolysis or increased capillary bleeding. Avoid extravasation; may cause reactions ranging from mild irritation to necrosis.
• Don't administer through the same infusion as blood.
• Don't infuse into leg veins; may cause phlebitis or thrombosis, especially in the elderly.
• Watch for hyponatremia or hypokalemia (muscle weakness, lethargy); may indicate electrolyte depletion before serum levels are reduced.
• Maintain adequate hydration; monitor fluid and electrolyte balance.
• In renal disease, monitor BUN frequently.
• Indwelling urethral catheter should be used in comatose patients to assure bladder emptying. Use an hourly urometer collection bag to facilitate accurate evaluation of diuresis.
• If satisfactory diuresis does not occur in 6 to 12 hours, urea should be discontinued and renal function reevaluated.
• Use freshly reconstituted urea only for I.V. infusion; solution becomes ammonia upon standing.
• Use within minutes of reconstitution.

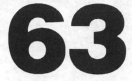

63

Electrolytes and replacement solutions

calcium chloride
calcium gluceptate
calcium gluconate
calcium lactate
dextrans (low molecular weight)
dextrans (high molecular weight)
hetastarch
magnesium sulfate
potassium acetate
potassium bicarbonate
potassium chloride
potassium gluconate
potassium phosphate
Ringer's injection
Ringer's injection, lactated
sodium chloride

COMBINATION PRODUCTS
CALCIUM-SANDOZ FORTE♦♦: calcium lactate-gluconate 2.94 g, calcium carbonate 0.3 g, elemental sodium 275.8 mg; provides 500 mg elemental calcium.
GRAMCAL♦♦: calcium lactate-gluconate 3,080 mg, calcium carbonate 1,500 mg, and potassium 390 mg; provides 1,000 mg of elemental calcium.
KAOCHLOR-EFF: 20 mEq potassium, 20 mEq chloride (from potassium chloride, potassium citrate, potassium bicarbonate, and betaine hydrochloride).
KLORVESS*: 20 mEq each potassium and chloride (from potassium chloride, potassium bicarbonate, and l-lysine monohydrochloride).
KOLYUM: 20 mEq potassium, 3.4 mEq chloride (from potassium gluconate and potassium chloride).
NEUTRA-PHOS: phosphorus 250 mg,

sodium 164 mg, potassium 278 mg (from dibasic and monobasic sodium and potassium phosphate).
POTASSIUM-SANDOZ♦♦: potassium chloride 600 mg and potassium bicarbonate 400 mg (provides 12 mEq potassium and 8 mEq chloride).
TWIN-K-CL: 15 ml supplies 15 mEq of potassium ions as a combination of potassium gluconate, potassium citrate, and ammonium chloride.

---

calcium chloride

calcium gluceptate

calcium gluconate

calcium lactate
Pregnancy Category: C

MECHANISM OF ACTION
Replaces and maintains calcium levels.

INDICATIONS & DOSAGE
Hypocalcemia, hypocalcemic tetany, hypocalcemia during exchange transfusions, cardiac resuscitation for inotropic effect when epinephrine has failed; magnesium intoxication; hypoparathyroidism—
Adults and children: initially 500 mg to 1 g calcium salt I.V., with further dosage based on serum calcium determinations.

Dosage with calcium chloride (1 g [10 ml] yields 13.5 mEq Ca^{++}):
Magnesium intoxication—
Adults and children: initially 500 mg

I.V., with further doses based on calcium and magnesium determination.
Cardiac arrest—
0.5 to 1 g I.V., not to exceed 1 ml/minute; or 200 to 800 mg into the ventricular cavity.
Hypocalcemia—
500 mg to 1 g I.V. at intervals of 1 to 3 days, determined by serum calcium levels.

Dosage with calcium gluconate (1 g [10 ml] yields 4.5 mEq Ca^{++}):
Hypocalcemia—
Adults: 500 mg to 1 g I.V., repeated q 1 to 3 days p.r.n. as determined by serum calcium levels. Further doses depend on serum calcium determination.
Children: 500 mg/kg I.V. daily. Rate of infusion should not exceed 0.5 ml/minute.

Dosage with calcium gluceptate (1.1 g [5 ml] yields 4.5 mEq Ca^{++}) and calcium salts (18 mg [1 ml] yields 0.898 mEq Ca^{++}):
Hypocalcemia—
Adults: initially 5 to 20 ml I.V., with further doses based on serum calcium determinations. If I.V. injection is impossible, 2 to 5 ml I.M. Average adult oral dose, 1 to 2 g elemental calcium daily P.O. in divided doses, t.i.d. or q.i.d. Average oral dose for children, 45 to 65 mg/kg P.O. daily, in divided doses, t.i.d. or q.i.d.
During exchange transfusions—
Adults and children: 0.5 ml I.V. after each 100 ml blood exchanged.

ADVERSE REACTIONS

CNS: from I.V. use, tingling sensations, sense of oppression or heat waves; with rapid I.V. injection, syncope.
CV: mild fall in blood pressure; with rapid I.V. injection, vasodilation, *bradycardia, cardiac arrhythmias, and cardiac arrest.*
GI: with oral ingestion, irritation, hemorrhage, *constipation;* with I.V. administration, chalky taste; with oral

calcium chloride, gastrointestinal hemorrhage, nausea, vomiting, thirst, abdominal pain.
GU: hypercalcemia, polyuria, renal calculi.
Skin: local reaction if calcium salts given I.M.: burning, necrosis, sloughing of tissue, cellulitis, soft-tissue calcification.
Local: with S.C. injection, pain and irritation; *with I.V., venous irritation.*

INTERACTIONS

Cardiac glycosides: increased digitalis toxicity; administer calcium very cautiously (if at all) to digitalized patients.

NURSING CONSIDERATIONS

• Contraindicated in ventricular fibrillation, hypercalcemia, renal calculi. Use cautiously in patients with sarcoidosis and renal or cardiac disease, and in digitalized patients. Use calcium chloride cautiously in cor pulmonale, respiratory acidosis, or respiratory failure.
• Monitor EKG when giving calcium I.V. Such injections should not exceed 0.7 to 1.5 mEq/minute. Stop if patient complains of discomfort. Following I.V. injection, patient should remain recumbent for a short while.
• I.M. injection should be given in the gluteal region in adults; lateral thigh in infants. I.M. route used only in emergencies when no I.V. route available.
• Monitor blood calcium levels frequently. Report abnormalities.
• Hypercalcemia may result after large doses in chronic renal failure.
• If possible, administer I.V. into a large vein.
• I.V. route generally recommended in children, but not by scalp vein (can cause tissue necrosis).
• Solutions should be warmed to body temperature before administration.

• Calcium chloride should be given I.V. only. When adding to parenteral solutions that contain other additives, observe closely for precipitate.
• Severe necrosis and sloughing of tissues follow extravasation. Calcium gluconate is less irritating to veins and tissues than calcium chloride.
• Following injection, patient should be recumbent for 15 minutes.
• If gastrointestinal upset occurs, give oral calcium products 1 to 1½ hours after meals.
• Oxalic acid (found in rhubarb and spinach), phytic acid (in bran and whole cereals), and phosphorus (in milk and dairy products) may interfere with absorption of calcium.
• Crash carts usually contain both gluconate and chloride. Make sure doctor specifies form he wants administered.

dextrans (low molecular weight)
Dextran 40♦, Gentran 40♦, Rheomacrodex♦
Pregnancy Category: C

MECHANISM OF ACTION
Expands plasma volume and provides fluid replacement.

INDICATIONS & DOSAGE
Plasma volume expansion—
Dosage of 10% solution by I.V. infusion depends on amount of fluid loss.

First 500 ml of Dextran 40 may be infused rapidly with central venous pressure monitoring. Infuse remaining dose slowly. Total daily dose not to exceed 2 g/kg body weight. If therapy continued past 24 hours, do not exceed 1 g/kg daily. Continue for no longer than 5 days.
Reduction of blood sludging—
500 ml of 10% solution by I.V. infusion.

ADVERSE REACTIONS
Blood: *decreased level of hemoglobin and hematocrit;* with higher doses, increased bleeding time.
GI: nausea, vomiting.
GU: tubular stasis and blocking, increased viscosity of urine.
Hepatic: increased SGPT and SGOT levels.
Skin: hypersensitivity reaction, urticaria.
Other: *anaphylaxis.*

INTERACTIONS
None significant.

NURSING CONSIDERATIONS
• Contraindicated in marked hemostatic defects; marked cardiac decompensation or pulmonary edema; renal disease with severe oliguria or anuria; or extreme dehydration. Use cautiously in active hemorrhage; may cause additional blood loss. Evaluate patient's hydration status before administration.
• Doctor may order dextran 1 (Promit) to protect against dextran-induced anaphylaxis. Administer Promit, 20 ml I.V. over 60 seconds, 1 to 2 minutes before the I.V. infusion of dextran 40.
• Hazardous when given to patients with heart failure, especially if in saline solution. Use dextrose solution instead.
• Works as plasma expander via colloidal osmotic effect, thereby drawing fluid from interstitial to intravascular space. Provides plasma expansion slightly greater than volume infused. Watch for circulatory overload, rise in central venous pressure readings.
• Monitor urine flow rate during administration. If oliguria or anuria occurs or is not relieved by infusion, stop dextran and give loop diuretic.
• Hydration should be assessed before starting therapy; otherwise, use urine or serum osmolarity because urine specific gravity is affected by

urine dextran concentration.
- Check hemoglobin and hematocrit; don't allow to fall below 30% by volume.
- Observe patient closely during early phase of infusion: most anaphylactoid reactions occur during this time.
- May interfere with analysis of blood grouping, crossmatching, bilirubin, blood glucose, and protein.
- Store at constant 25° C. (77° F.). May precipitate in storage, but can be heated to dissolve if necessary.

dextrans
(high molecular weight)
Dextran 70♦, Dextran 75♦, Gentran 75♦, Macrodex♦
Pregnancy Category: C

MECHANISM OF ACTION
Expands plasma volume and provides fluid replacement.

INDICATIONS & DOSAGE
Plasma expander—
Adults: usual dose 30 g (500 ml of 6% solution) I.V. In emergency situations, may be administered at rate of 1.2 to 2.4 g (20 to 40 ml) per minute. In normovolemic or nearly normovolemic patients, rate of infusion should not exceed 240 mg (4 ml)/minute.

Total dose during first 24 hours not to exceed 1.2 g/kg; actual dose depends on amount of fluid loss and resultant hemoconcentration, and must be determined for each patient.

ADVERSE REACTIONS
Blood: *decreased level of hemoglobin and hematocrit;* with doses of 15 ml/kg body weight, prolonged bleeding time and significant suppression of platelet function.
GI: nausea, vomiting.
GU: increased specific gravity and viscosity of urine, tubular stasis and blocking.
Hepatic: increased SGPT and SGOT

levels.
Skin: hypersensitivity reaction, urticaria.
Other: fever, arthralgia, nasal congestion, *anaphylaxis.*

INTERACTIONS
None significant.

NURSING CONSIDERATIONS
- Contraindicated in marked hemostatic defects; marked cardiac decompensation or pulmonary edema; renal disease with severe oliguria or anuria; and extreme dehydration. Use cautiously in active hemorrhage; may cause additional blood loss.
- Doctor may order dextran 1 (Promit) to protect against dextran-induced anaphylaxis. Administer Promit, 20 ml I.V. over 60 seconds, 1 to 2 minutes before the I.V. infusion of dextran 70.
- Hazardous when given to patients with heart failure, especially if in saline solution. Use dextrose solution instead.
- Works as plasma expander via colloidal osmotic effect, thereby drawing fluid from interstitial to intravascular space. Provides plasma expansion slightly greater than volume infused. Watch for circulatory overload.
- Monitor urine flow rate during administration. If oliguria or anuria occurs or is not relieved by infusion, stop dextran and give loop diuretic.
- Hydration should be assessed before starting therapy; otherwise, use urine or serum osmolarity because urine specific gravity is affected by the urine dextran concentration.
- Check hemoglobin and hematocrit; don't allow to fall below 30% by volume.
- Draw blood samples *before* starting infusion.
- Observe patient closely during early phase of infusion: most anaphylactoid reactions occur during this time.
- May interfere with analysis of

blood grouping, crossmatching, bilirubin, blood glucose, and protein.
• May precipitate in storage, but can be heated to dissolve if necessary.

blood or plasma.
• Available in 500-ml I.V. infusion bottles.
• Discard partially used bottles.

hetastarch
Hespan
Pregnancy Category: C

MECHANISM OF ACTION
Expands plasma volume and provides fluid replacement.

INDICATIONS & DOSAGE
Plasma expander—
Adults: 500 to 1,000 ml I.V. dependent on amount of blood lost and resultant hemoconcentration. Total dosage usually not to exceed 1,500 ml/day. Up to 20 ml/kg hourly may be used in hemorrhagic shock.

ADVERSE REACTIONS
CNS: headaches.
CV: peripheral edema of lower extremities.
EENT: periorbital edema.
GI: nausea, vomiting.
Skin: urticaria.
Other: wheezing, mild fever.

INTERACTIONS
None significant.

NURSING CONSIDERATIONS
• Contraindicated in severe bleeding disorders or with severe congestive heart failure and renal failure with oliguria and anuria.
• To avoid circulatory overload, monitor patients with impaired renal function carefully.
• Discontinue if allergic or sensitivity reactions occur. If necessary, administer an antihistamine.
• When used in continuous-flow centrifugation, leukapheresis ratio is usually 1 part to 8 parts venous whole blood.
• Hetastarch is *not* a substitute for

magnesium sulfate
Pregnancy Category: B

MECHANISM OF ACTION
Replaces and maintains magnesium levels. As an anticonvulsant, reduces muscle contractions by interfering with the release of acetylcholine at the myoneural junction.

INDICATIONS & DOSAGE
Hypomagnesemia—
Adults: 1 g, or 8.12 mEq, of 50% solution (2 ml) I.M. q 6 hours for 4 doses, depending on serum magnesium level.
Severe hypomagnesemia (serum magnesium 0.8 mEq/liter or less, with symptoms)—
6 g, or 50 mEq, of 50% solution I.V. in 1 liter of solution over 4 hours. Subsequent doses depend on serum magnesium levels.
Magnesium supplementation in hyperalimentation—
Adults: 8 to 24 mEq daily added to hyperalimentation solution.
Children over 6 years: 2 to 10 mEq daily added to hyperalimentation solution.
Each 2 ml of 50% solution contains 1 g, or 8.12 mEq, magnesium sulfate.
Acute treatment of preeclampsia and eclampsia—
Adults: loading dose: 2 to 4 g (4 to 8 ml of 50% solution) given by slow I.V. bolus (over 5 minutes).
Maintenance: 1 to 2 g hourly as a constant infusion. Prepare by adding 8 ml of 50% solution to 230 ml dextrose 5% in water.
Hypomagnesemic seizures—
Adults: 1 to 2 g (as 10% solution) I.V. over 15 minutes, then 1 g I.M. q 4 to 6 hours, based on patient's response

---

Italicized side effects are common or life-threatening.
*Liquid form contains alcohol.   **May contain tartrazine.

and magnesium blood levels.
Seizures secondary to hypomagnesemia in acute nephritis—
Adults: 0.2 ml/kg of 50% solution I.M. q 4 to 6 hours, p.r.n. or 100 mg/kg of 10% solution I.V. very slowly. Titrate dosage according to magnesium blood levels and seizure response.

ADVERSE REACTIONS

CNS: toxicity: *weak or absent deep-tendon reflexes,* flaccid paralysis, hypothermia, drowsiness, hypocalcemia (perioral paresthesias, twitching carpopedal spasm, tetany, and seizures).
CV: slow, weak pulse; cardiac arrhythmias (hypocalcemia); *hypotension.*
Skin: flushing, sweating.
Other: *respiratory paralysis,* hypocalcemia.

INTERACTIONS

Neuromuscular blocking agents: may cause increased neuromuscular blockage. Use cautiously.

NURSING CONSIDERATIONS

• Contraindicated in impaired renal function, myocardial damage, heart block, and in actively progressing labor. Use parenteral magnesium with extreme caution in patients receiving digitalis preparations. Treating magnesium toxicity with calcium in such patients could cause serious alterations in cardiac conduction; heart block may result.
• I.V. bolus dose *must* be injected slowly in order to avoid respiratory or cardiac arrest.
• If available, use a constant infusion pump when administering infusion.
• Maximum infusion rate 150 mg/minute. Rapid drip causes feeling of heat.
• Keep I.V. calcium available to reverse magnesium intoxication.
• Monitor vital signs every 15 minutes when giving I.V. for severe hypomagnesemia. Watch for respiratory depression and signs of heart block. Respirations should be more than 16/minute before dose is given.
• Monitor intake/output. Output should be 100 ml or more during 4-hour period before dose.
• Test knee jerk and patellar reflexes before each additional dose. If absent, give no more magnesium until reflexes return; otherwise, patient may develop temporary respiratory failure and need cardiopulmonary resuscitation or I.V. administration of calcium.
• Check magnesium levels after repeated doses.
• After giving to toxemic mothers within 24 hours before delivery, watch newborn for signs of magnesium toxicity, including neuromuscular and respiratory depression.

potassium acetate
Pregnancy Category: C

MECHANISM OF ACTION
Replaces and maintains potassium levels.

INDICATIONS & DOSAGE
Potassium replacement—
I.V. should be used for life-threatening hypokalemia or when oral replacement not feasible. Give no more than 20 mEq hourly in concentration of 40 mEq/liter or less. Total 24-hour dose should not exceed 150 mEq (3 mEq/kg in children). Potassium replacement should be done with EKG monitoring and frequent serum K^+ determinations.
Prevention of hypokalemia—
Adults and children: 20 mEq P.O. daily, in divided doses b.i.d., t.i.d., or q.i.d.
Potassium depletion—
Adults and children: usual dose 40 to 100 mEq P.O. daily, in divided doses b.i.d., t.i.d., or q.i.d.

ADVERSE REACTIONS

Signs of hyperkalemia:

CNS: paresthesias of the extremities, listlessness, mental confusion, weakness or heaviness of legs, flaccid paralysis.

CV: *peripheral vascular collapse with fall in blood pressure, cardiac arrhythmias,* heart block, possible cardiac arrest, EKG changes (prolonged P-R intervals; wide QRS; ST segment depression; tall, tented T waves).

GI: nausea, vomiting, abdominal pain, diarrhea, bowel ulceration.

GU: oliguria.

Skin: cold skin, gray pallor.

INTERACTIONS

None significant.

NURSING CONSIDERATIONS

• Contraindicated in severe renal impairment with oliguria, anuria, azotemia, and untreated Addison's disease; acute dehydration, hyperkalemia, hyperkalemic form of familial periodic paralysis, and conditions associated with extensive tissue breakdown. Use cautiously in patients with cardiac disease, patients receiving potassium-sparing diuretics, and those with renal impairment.

• During therapy, monitor EKG, serum potassium level, renal function, BUN, serum creatinine, and intake/output. Never give potassium postoperatively until urine flow is established.

• Give slowly as diluted solution; potentially fatal hyperkalemia may result from too rapid infusion.

• Parenteral potassium given by infusion only; never I.V. push or I.M.

• Observe for pain and redness at infusion site. Large-bore needle reduces local irritation.

• Watch for signs of GI ulceration: obstruction, hemorrhage, pain, distention, severe vomiting, bleeding.

• Reconstitute potassium acetate powder with liquids; give after meals with a full glass of water or fruit juice to minimize GI irritation.

• To prevent serious hyperkalemia, potassium deficits must be replaced gradually.

potassium bicarbonate

K-Lyte, K-Lyte DS
Pregnancy Category: A

MECHANISM OF ACTION

Replaces and maintains potassium levels.

INDICATIONS & DOSAGE

Hypokalemia—
25 mEq or 50 mEq tablet dissolved in water 1 to 4 times a day.

ADVERSE REACTIONS

CNS: paresthesias of the extremities, listlessness, mental confusion, weakness or heaviness of legs, flaccid paralysis.

CV: *cardiac arrhythmias,* EKG changes (prolonged P-R interval; wide QRS; ST segment depression; tall, tented T waves).

GI: *nausea, vomiting, abdominal pain,* diarrhea, ulcerations, hemorrhage, obstruction, perforation.

INTERACTIONS

None significant.

NURSING CONSIDERATIONS

• Contraindicated in severe renal impairment with oliguria, anuria, azotemia, and untreated Addison's disease; also in acute dehydration, hyperkalemia, hyperkalemic familial periodic paralysis, and conditions associated with extensive tissue breakdown. Use with caution in cardiac disease and patients receiving potassium-sparing diuretics.

• Monitor serum potassium level, BUN, serum creatinine, and intake/output.

• Never switch potassium products

without a doctor's order.
• Dissolve potassium bicarbonate tablets in 6 to 8 ounces of cold water. Dissolve completely to minimize GI irritation.
• Have patient take with meals and sip slowly over a 5- to 10-minute period.
• Potassium bicarbonate cannot be given instead of potassium chloride.
• Potassium bicarbonate does not correct hypochloremic alkalosis.
• Available in lime and orange flavors. Check for patient's flavor preference.

potassium chloride

K-Lor, K-Lyte/Cl♦, Kaochlor 10%♦*, Kaochlor S-F 10%*, Kaon-Cl, Kaon-Cl 20%*, Kato Powder, Kay Ciel♦*, Klor-10%*, Klor-Con, Kloride* **, Klorvess, Klotrix, K-Tab, Micro-K Extencaps♦, SK-Potassium Chloride, Slow-K♦, Ten-K, Twin-K-Cl
Pregnancy Category: A

MECHANISM OF ACTION
Replaces and maintains potassium levels.

INDICATIONS & DOSAGE
Hypokalemia—
40 to 100 mEq P.O. divided into 3 to 4 doses daily for treatment; 20 mEq for prevention. Further dose based on serum potassium determinations. I.V. route when oral replacement not feasible or when hypokalemia life-threatening. Usual dose 20 mEq hourly in concentration of 40 mEq/liter or less. Total daily dose not to exceed 150 mEq (3 mEq/kg in children). Potassium replacement should be done only with EKG monitoring and frequent serum K^+ determinations.

ADVERSE REACTIONS
Signs of hyperkalemia:
CNS: paresthesias of the extremities, listlessness, mental confusion, weakness or heaviness of limbs, flaccid paralysis.
CV: *peripheral vascular collapse with fall in blood pressure, cardiac arrhythmias, heart block, possible cardiac arrest, EKG changes (prolonged P-R interval; wide QRS; ST segment depression; tall, tented T waves).*
GI: *nausea, vomiting, abdominal pain,* diarrhea, GI ulcerations (possible stenosis, hemorrhage, obstruction, perforation).
GU: oliguria.
Skin: cold skin, gray pallor.
Local: *postinfusion phlebitis.*

INTERACTIONS
None significant.

NURSING CONSIDERATIONS
• Contraindicated in severe renal impairment with oliguria, anuria, azotemia, and untreated Addison's disease; also in acute dehydration, hyperkalemia, hyperkalemic form of familial periodic paralysis, conditions associated with extensive tissue breakdown. Use with caution in cardiac disease, patients receiving potassium-sparing diuretics.
• Potassium should not be given during immediate postoperative period until urine flow is established.
• Parenteral potassium given by infusion only; never I.V. push or I.M.
• Small amounts of lidocaine injection (1 to 3 ml of the 1% strength) may be added directly to the potassium chloride solution. This will help reverse postinfusion phlebitis.
• Give slowly as dilute solution; potentially fatal hyperkalemia may result from too rapid infusion.
• Give oral potassium supplements with extreme caution because its many forms deliver varying amounts of potassium. Never switch products without a doctor's order. Tell the doctor if patient tolerates one product better than another.

- Sugar-free liquid available (Ka-ochlor S-F 10%).
- Use a liquid preparation for potassium supplementation if tablet or capsule passage is likely to be delayed, such as in GI obstruction.
- Have patient sip liquid potassium slowly to minimize GI irritation.
- Give with or after meals with full glass of water or fruit juice to lessen GI distress.
- Make sure powders are completely dissolved before giving.
- Enteric-coated tablets not recommended due to potential GI bleeding and small-bowel ulcerations.
- Tablets in wax matrix sometimes lodge in esophagus and cause ulceration in cardiac patients who have esophageal compression due to enlarged left atrium. In such patients and in those with esophageal stasis or obstruction, use liquid form.
- Microencapsulated form (Micro-K) has been shown in one study to cause less GI bleeding than the wax matrix tablets. However, this hasn't been completely confirmed.
- Often used orally with diuretics that cause potassium excretion. Potassium chloride most useful since diuretics waste chloride ion. Hypokalemic alkalosis treated best with potassium chloride.
- Monitor EKG, serum potassium levels, and other electrolytes during therapy.
- Don't crush sustained-release potassium products.

potassium gluconate
Kaon Liquid*, Kaon Tablets♦,
Potassium Rougier♦♦
Pregnancy Category: A

MECHANISM OF ACTION
Replaces and maintains potassium levels.

INDICATIONS & DOSAGE
Hypokalemia—
40 to 100 mEq P.O. divided into 3 to 4 doses daily for treatment; 20 mEq daily for prevention. Further dose based on serum potassium determinations.

ADVERSE REACTIONS
CNS: paresthesias of the extremities, listlessness, mental confusion, weakness or heaviness of legs, flaccid paralysis.
CV: cardiac arrhythmias, EKG changes (prolonged P-R interval; wide QRS; ST segment depression; tall, tented T waves).
GI: *nausea, vomiting, abdominal pain,* diarrhea, GI ulcerations with oral products (especially enteric-coated tablets); ulcerations may be accompanied by stenosis, hemorrhage, obstruction, perforation.

INTERACTIONS
None significant.

NURSING CONSIDERATIONS
- Contraindicated in severe renal impairment with oliguria, anuria, azotemia, and untreated Addison's disease; also in acute dehydration, hyperkalemia, hyperkalemic form of familial periodic paralysis, and conditions associated with extensive tissue breakdown. Use with caution in patients with cardiac disease, and in those receiving potassium-sparing diuretics.
- Monitor serum potassium level, BUN, serum creatinine, and intake/output.
- Give oral potassium supplements with extreme caution because their many forms deliver varying amounts of potassium. Never switch products without doctor's order. If one product is tolerated better than another, tell doctor so brand and dosage can be changed.
- Have patient sip liquid potassium

Italicized side effects are common or life-threatening.
*Liquid form contains alcohol.   **May contain tartrazine.

slowly to minimize GI irritation.
• Give with or after meals with full glass of water or fruit juice to lessen GI distress.
• Potassium gluconate does not correct hypokalemic hypochloremic alkalosis.
• Enteric-coated tablets not recommended due to potential for GI bleeding and small-bowel ulcerations.
• Monitor EKG, serum potassium, and other electrolytes during therapy.

potassium phosphate
Pregnancy Category: C

MECHANISM OF ACTION
Replaces and maintains potassium levels.

INDICATIONS & DOSAGE
Hypokalemia—
I.V. should be used when oral replacement not feasible or when hypokalemia life-threatening. Dosage up to 20 mEq hourly in concentration of 60 mEq/liter or less. Total daily dose not to exceed 150 mEq. Should be done only with EKG monitoring and frequent serum K⁺ determinations. Average P.O. dose: 40 to 100 mEq.
Hypophosphatemia—
0.32 to 0.45 mM/kg of phosphate administered I.V. over 12 hours after diluting in a larger volume of fluid. Dosage is adjusted according to individual needs of patient.

ADVERSE REACTIONS
Signs of hyperkalemia:
CNS: paresthesias of the extremities, listlessness, mental confusion, weakness or heaviness of legs, flaccid paralysis; hypocalcemia—perioral paresthesias, twitching, carpopedal spasm, tetany, and seizures.
CV: *peripheral vascular collapse with fall in blood pressure, cardiac arrhythmias, heart block, possible cardiac arrest,* EKG changes (prolonged

P-R interval; wide QRS; ST segment depression; tall, tented T waves).
GI: nausea, vomiting, abdominal pain, diarrhea.
GU: oliguria.
Skin: cold skin, gray pallor.
Other: soft-tissue calcification.

INTERACTIONS
None significant.

NURSING CONSIDERATIONS
• Contraindicated in severe renal impairment with oliguria, anuria, azotemia, and untreated Addison's disease; also in acute dehydration, hyperkalemia, hyperkalemic form of familial periodic paralysis, extensive tissue damage, and hypocalcemia. Use with caution in patients with cardiac disease, and in those receiving potassium-sparing diuretics.
• Never give potassium postoperatively until urine flow is established.
• Monitor EKG for indications of tissue potassium levels; plasma potassium and calcium levels as well as BUN and creatinine for renal function; inorganic phosphorus levels; intake/output.
• Give slowly as dilute solution; potentially fatal hyperkalemia may result from too rapid an infusion.
• Parenteral potassium given by infusion only; never I.V. push or I.M.
• Reconstitute powder in juice. Give after meals.

Ringer's injection
Pregnancy Category: NR

MECHANISM OF ACTION
Replaces fluids and electrolytes.

INDICATIONS & DOSAGE
Fluid and electrolyte replacement—
Adults and children: dose highly individualized, but generally 1.5 to 3 liters (2% to 6% body weight) infused I.V. over 18 to 24 hours.

ADVERSE REACTIONS
CV: fluid overload.

INTERACTIONS
None significant.

NURSING CONSIDERATIONS
• Contraindicated in renal failure, except as emergency volume expander. Use cautiously in congestive heart failure, circulatory insufficiency, renal dysfunction, hypoproteinemia, or pulmonary edema.
• Ringer's injection contains sodium, 147 mEq/liter; potassium, 4 mEq/liter; calcium, 4.5 mEq/liter; and chloride, 155.5 mEq/liter. This electrolyte content is insufficient for treating severe electrolyte deficiencies, although it does provide electrolytes in levels approximately equal to those of the blood.

Ringer's injection, lactated
(Hartmann's solution, Ringer's lactate solution)
Pregnancy Category: NR

MECHANISM OF ACTION
Replaces fluids and electrolytes.

INDICATIONS & DOSAGE
Fluid and electrolyte replacement—
Adults and children: dose highly individualized, but generally 1.5 to 3 liters (2% to 6% body weight) infused I.V. over 18 to 24 hours.

ADVERSE REACTIONS
CV: fluid overload.

INTERACTIONS
None significant.

NURSING CONSIDERATIONS
• Contraindicated in renal failure, except as emergency volume expander. Use cautiously in congestive heart failure, circulatory insufficiency, renal dysfunction, hypoproteinemia,

and pulmonary edema.
• Ringer's injection, lactated, contains sodium, 130 mEq/liter; potassium, 4 mEq/liter; calcium, 3 mEq/liter; chloride, 109.7 mEq/liter; and lactate, 28 mEq/liter.
• Approximates more closely the electrolyte concentration in blood plasma than Ringer's injection.

---

sodium chloride
Pregnancy Category: C

MECHANISM OF ACTION
Replaces and maintains sodium and chloride levels.

INDICATIONS & DOSAGE
Highly individualized fluid and electrolyte replacement in hyponatremia due to electrolyte loss or in severe salt depletion—
400 ml of 3% or 5% solutions only with frequent electrolyte determination and only if given slow I.V.; *with 0.45% solution:* 3% to 8% of body weight, according to deficiencies, over 18 to 24 hours; *with 0.9% solution:* 2% to 6% of body weight, according to deficiencies, over 18 to 24 hours.
Management of "heat cramp" due to excessive perspiration—
Adults: 1 g P.O. with every glass of water.

ADVERSE REACTIONS
CV: aggravation of congestive heart failure; edema and pulmonary edema if too much given or given too rapidly.
Metabolic: hypernatremia and aggravation of existing acidosis with excessive infusion; serious electrolyte disturbance, loss of potassium.

INTERACTIONS
None significant.

NURSING CONSIDERATIONS
• Use with caution in congestive

---

heart failure, circulatory insufficiency, renal dysfunction, hypoproteinemia.
• Infuse 3% and 5% solutions very slowly and with caution to avoid pulmonary edema. Use only for critical situations. Observe patient constantly.
• Concentrates available for addition to parenteral nutrient solutions. Don't confuse these small volumes of parenterals with sodium chloride injection isotonic 0.9%. *Read label carefully*.
• Monitor serum electrolytes.

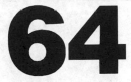

Potassium-removing resin

sodium polystyrene sulfonate

COMBINATION PRODUCTS
None.

sodium polystyrene sulfonate
Kayexalate♦, SPS
Pregnancy Category: C

MECHANISM OF ACTION
The potassium-removing resin exchanges sodium ions for potassium ions in the intestine: 1 g of sodium polystyrene sulfonate is exchanged for 0.5 to 1 mEq of potassium. The resin is then eliminated. Much of the exchange capacity is used for cations other than potassium (calcium and magnesium) and possibly for fats and proteins.

INDICATIONS & DOSAGE
Hyperkalemia—
Adults: 15 g daily to q.i.d. in water or sorbitol (3 to 4 ml/g of resin).
Children: 1 g of resin for each mEq of potassium to be removed.

Oral administration preferred since drug should remain in intestine for at least 6 hours; otherwise, consider nasogastric administration.
Nasogastric administration: mix dose with appropriate medium: aqueous suspension or diet appropriate for renal failure; instill in plastic tube.
Rectal administration:
Adults: 30 to 50 g/100 ml of sorbitol q 6 hours as warm emulsion deep into sigmoid colon (20 cm). In persistent vomiting or paralytic ileus, high retention enema of sodium polystyrene sulfonate (30 g) suspended in 200 ml of 10% methylcellulose, 10% dextrose, or 25% sorbitol solution.

ADVERSE REACTIONS
GI: *constipation,* fecal impaction (in elderly), anorexia, gastric irritation, nausea, vomiting, *diarrhea (with sorbitol emulsions).*
Other: *hypokalemia,* hypocalcemia, hypomagnesemia, sodium retention.

INTERACTIONS
Antacids and laxatives (nonabsorbable cation-donating type, including magnesium hydroxide): systemic alkalosis, reduced potassium exchange capability. Don't use together.

NURSING CONSIDERATIONS
• Use with caution in elderly patients and those on digitalis therapy, with severe congestive heart failure, severe hypertension, and marked edema.
• Treatment may result in potassium deficiency. Monitor serum potassium at least once daily. Usually stopped when potassium level is reduced to 4 or 5 mEq/liter. Watch for other signs of hypokalemia: irritability, confusion, cardiac arrhythmias, EKG changes, severe muscle weakness and sometimes paralysis, and digitalis toxicity in digitalized patients.
• Monitor for symptoms of other electrolyte deficiencies (magnesium, calcium) since drug is nonselective. Monitor serum calcium determination in patients receiving sodium polysty-

---

Italicized side effects are common or life-threatening.
*Liquid form contains alcohol.   **May contain tartrazine.

rene therapy for more than 3 days. Supplementary calcium may be needed.

• Watch for sodium overload. About ⅓ of resin's sodium is retained.

• Premixed forms are available (SPS and others).

• Do not heat resin. This will impair effectiveness of drug. Mix resin only with water or sorbitol for P.O. administration. Above all, *never* mix with orange juice (high K^+ content) to disguise taste.

• Chill oral suspension for greater palatability.

• If sorbitol is given, it may be mixed with resin suspension.

• Consider solid form. Resin cookie and candy recipes are available; perhaps pharmacist or dietitian can supply.

• Watch for constipation in oral or nasogastric administration. Use sorbitol (10 to 20 ml of 70% syrup every 2 hours as needed) to produce one or two watery stools daily.

• If preparing manually, mix polystyrene resin only with water and sorbitol for rectal use. Do not use other vehicles (that is, mineral oil) for rectal administration to prevent impactions. Ion exchange requires aqueous medium. Sorbitol content prevents impaction.

• Prevent fecal impaction in elderly by administering resin rectally. Give cleansing enema before rectal administration. Explain necessity of retaining enema to patient. Retention for 6 to 10 hours is ideal, but 30 to 60 minutes is acceptable.

• Prepare rectal dose at room temperature. Stir emulsion gently during administration.

• Use #28 French rubber tube for rectal dose; insert 20 cm into sigmoid colon. Tape tube in place. Alternatively, consider a Foley catheter with a 30-ml balloon inflated distal to anal sphincter to aid in retention. This is especially helpful for patients with poor sphincter control (for example, after cerebrovascular accident). Use gravity flow. Drain returns constantly through Y-tube connection. When giving rectally, place patient in knee-chest position or with hips on pillow for a while if back-leakage occurs.

• After rectal administration, flush tubing with 50 to 100 ml of nonsodium fluid to ensure delivery of all medication.

• Flush rectum to remove the resin.

• If hyperkalemia is severe, more drastic modalities should be added; for example, dextrose 50% with regular insulin I.V. push. Do not depend solely on polystyrene resin to lower serum potassium levels in severe hyperkalemia.

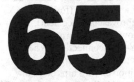

Hematinics

ferrous fumarate
ferrous gluconate
ferrous sulfate
iron dextran

COMBINATION PRODUCTS

FERMALOX: ferrous sulfate 200 mg, and magnesium hydroxide and dried aluminum hydroxide gel 200 mg.
FEROCYL: iron (as fumarate) 50 mg and docusate sodium 100 mg.
FER-REGULES: iron (as fumarate) 150 mg and docusate sodium 100 mg.
FERRO-SEQUELS: iron (as fumarate) 50 mg and docusate sodium 100 mg.
SIMRON: iron (as gluconate) 10 mg and polysorbate 20, 400 mg.

---

ferrous fumarate

Eldofe, F&B Caps, Farbegen, Feco-T, Feostat, Ferranol, Fersamal♦♦, Fumasorb, Fumerin, Hemocyte, Ircon♦, Laud-Iron, Maniron, Novofumar♦♦, Palafer♦♦, Palmiron, Span-FF

Pregnancy Category: A

MECHANISM OF ACTION

Replaces iron, an essential component in the formation of hemoglobin.

INDICATIONS & DOSAGE

Iron deficiency states—
Adults: 200 mg P.O. daily t.i.d. or q.i.d.

ADVERSE REACTIONS

GI: *nausea*, vomiting, *constipation*, *black stools*.
Other: elixir may stain teeth.

INTERACTIONS

Antacids, cholestyramine resin, pancreatic extracts, vitamin E: decreased iron absorption. Separate doses if possible.
Chloramphenicol: watch for delayed response to iron therapy.
Vitamin C: may increase iron absorption. Beneficial drug interaction.

NURSING CONSIDERATIONS

• Contraindicated in hemosiderosis and hemochromatosis. Use cautiously in peptic ulcer, regional enteritis, and ulcerative colitis. Also use cautiously on long-term basis.
• GI upset related to dose. Between-meal dosing preferable, but can be given with some foods although absorption may be decreased. Enteric-coated products reduce GI upset but also reduce amount of iron absorbed.
• Iron is toxic; parents should be aware of iron poisoning in children.
• Tablets may be given with juice or water, but not in milk or antacids. Give with orange juice to promote iron absorption.
• To avoid staining teeth, give elixir iron preparations with glass straw.
• Check for constipation; record color and amount of stool. Teach dietary measures for preventing constipation.
• Oral iron may turn stools black. This is unabsorbed iron and is harmless.
• Monitor hemoglobin and reticulocyte counts during therapy.
• Combination products—Simron, Ferro-Sequels, Ferocyl, Fer-Re-

---

Italicized side effects are common or life-threatening.
*Liquid form contains alcohol.   **May contain tartrazine.

gules—contain stool softeners to help prevent constipation. Fermalox contains antacids to help relieve GI upset, if present; don't use this product unless absolutely necessary because of decreased iron absorption. Generally, combination iron products should be avoided.

ferrous gluconate
Fergon♦*, Ferralet, Fertinic♦♦, Novoferrogluc♦♦
Pregnancy Category: A

MECHANISM OF ACTION
Replaces iron, an essential component in the formation of hemoglobin.

INDICATIONS & DOSAGE
Iron deficiency—
Adults: 200 to 600 mg P.O., t.i.d.
Children 6 to 12 years: 300 to 900 mg P.O. daily.
Children under 6 years: 100 to 300 mg P.O. daily.
1 tablet contains 320 mg ferrous gluconate (37 mg elemental iron).
5 ml of elixir contains 300 mg ferrous gluconate (35 mg elemental iron).

ADVERSE REACTIONS
GI: *nausea,* vomiting, *constipation, black stools.*
Other: elixir may stain teeth.

INTERACTIONS
Antacids, cholestyramine resin, pancreatic extracts, vitamin E: decreased iron absorption. Separate doses if possible.
Chloramphenicol: watch for delayed response to iron therapy.
Vitamin C: may increase iron absorption. Beneficial drug interaction.

NURSING CONSIDERATIONS
• Contraindicated in peptic ulcer, regional enteritis, ulcerative colitis, hemosiderosis, and hemochromatosis. Use cautiously on long-term basis and in patients with anemia.
• GI upset related to dose. Between-meal dosing preferable, but can be given with some foods although absorption may be decreased. Enteric-coated products reduce GI upset but also reduce amount of iron absorbed.
• Tell patient to continue regular dosing schedule if he misses a dose. Patient shouldn't double the dose.
• Iron is toxic; parents should be aware of iron poisoning in children.
• Dilute liquid preparations in juice (preferably orange juice) or water, but not in milk or antacids. Give tablets with orange juice to promote absorption.
• To avoid staining teeth, give elixir iron preparations with glass straw.
• Check for constipation; record color and amount of stool. Teach dietary measures for preventing constipation.
• Oral iron may turn stools black. This is unabsorbed iron and is harmless.
• Monitor hemoglobin and reticulocyte counts during therapy.

ferrous sulfate
Arne Modified Caps, Feosol*, Fer-In-Sol♦*, Fero-Grad♦♦, Fero-Gradumet, Ferolix, Ferospace, Ferralyn, Fesofor♦♦, Irospan, Mol-Iron*, Novoferrosulfa♦♦, Slow-Fe♦, Telefon
Pregnancy Category: A

MECHANISM OF ACTION
Replaces iron, an essential component in the formation of hemoglobin.

INDICATIONS & DOSAGE
Iron deficiency—
Adults: 750 mg to 1.5 g P.O. daily divided t.i.d.; or 225 to 525 mg P.O. sustained-release preparations once daily or q 12 hours.
Children 6 to 12 years: 600 mg P.O. daily in divided doses.

Prophylaxis for iron deficiency anemia—
Pregnant women: 300 to 600 mg P.O. daily in divided doses.
Premature or undernourished infants: 3 to 6 mg/kg P.O. daily in divided doses.

ADVERSE REACTIONS
GI: *nausea*, vomiting, *constipation, black stools.*
Other: elixir may stain teeth.

INTERACTIONS
Antacids, cholestyramine resin, pancreatic extracts, vitamin E: decreased iron absorption. Separate doses if possible.
Chloramphenicol: watch for delayed response to iron therapy.
Vitamin C: may increase iron absorption. Beneficial drug interaction.

NURSING CONSIDERATIONS
• Contraindicated in hemosiderosis and hemochromatosis. Use cautiously in peptic ulcer, ulcerative colitis, and regional enteritis. Also use cautiously on long-term basis.
• GI upset related to dose. Between-meal dosing preferable, but can be given with some foods although absorption may be decreased. Enteric-coated products reduce GI upset but also reduce amount of iron absorbed.
• Tell patient to continue regular dosing schedule if he misses a dose. Patient shouldn't double the dose.
• Iron is toxic; parents should be aware of iron poisoning in children.
• Dilute liquid preparations in juice or water, but not in milk or antacids. Dilute liquids in orange juice; give tablets with orange juice to promote iron absorption.
• To avoid staining teeth, give elixir iron preparations with glass straw.
• Check for constipation; record color and amount of stool. Teach dietary measures for preventing constipation.

• Oral iron may turn stools black. This unabsorbed iron is harmless.
• Monitor hemoglobin and reticulocyte counts during therapy.

iron dextran
Hematran, Hydextran, Imferon♦, K-FeRON
Pregnancy Category: C

MECHANISM OF ACTION
Replaces iron, an essential component in the formation of hemoglobin.

INDICATIONS & DOSAGE
Iron deficiency anemia—
Adults: I.M. or I.V. injections of iron are advisable only for patients for whom oral administration is impossible or ineffective. Test dose (0.5 ml) required before administration.
I.M. (by Z-track): inject 0.5 ml test dose. If no reactions, next daily dose should ordinarily not exceed 0.5 ml (25 mg) for infants under 5 kg; 1 ml (50 mg) for children under 9 kg; 2 ml (100 mg) for patients under 50 kg; 5 ml (250 mg) for patients over 50 kg.
I.V. push: inject 0.5 ml test dose. If no reactions, within 2 to 3 days the dosage may be raised to 2 ml daily I.V., 1 ml/minute undiluted and infused slowly until total dose is achieved. No single dose should exceed 100 mg.
I.V. infusion: dosages are expressed in terms of elemental iron. Dilute in 250 to 1,000 ml of normal saline solution; dextrose increases local vein irritation. Infuse test dose of 25 mg slowly over 5 minutes. If no reaction occurs in 5 minutes, infusion may be started. Infuse total dose slowly over approximately 6 to 12 hours. 1 ml iron dextran = 50 mg elemental iron.

ADVERSE REACTIONS
CNS: headache, transitory paresthesias, arthralgia, myalgia, dizziness, malaise, syncope.
CV: *hypotensive reaction, peripheral*

vascular flushing with overly rapid I.V. administration, tachycardia.
GI: nausea, vomiting, metallic taste, transient loss of taste perception.
Local: *soreness and inflammation at injection site (I.M.); brown skin discoloration at injection site (I.M.); local phlebitis at injection site (I.V.).*
Skin: rash, urticaria.
Other: *anaphylaxis.*

INTERACTIONS
None significant.

NURSING CONSIDERATIONS
• Contraindicated in all anemias other than iron deficiency anemia. Use with extreme caution in patients with impaired hepatic function and rheumatoid arthritis.
• Monitor vital signs for drug reaction. Reactions are varied, ranging from pain, inflammation, and myalgia to hypotension, shock, and death.
• Inject deeply into upper outer quadrant of buttock—never into arm or other exposed area—with a 2- to 3-inch, 19G or 20G needle. Use Z-track technique to avoid leakage into subcutaneous tissue and tattooing of skin.
• Skin staining may be minimized by using a separate needle to withdraw the drug from its container.
• Monitor hemoglobin concentration, hematocrit, and reticulocyte count.
• Use I.V. in these situations: insufficient muscle mass for deep intramuscular injection; impaired absorption from muscle due to stasis or edema; possibility of uncontrolled intramuscular bleeding from trauma (as may occur in hemophilia); and with massive and prolonged parenteral therapy (as may be necessary in cases of chronic substantial blood loss).
• Upon completion of I.V. iron dextran infusion, flush the vein with 10 ml of 0.9% sodium chloride injection.
• Patient should rest 15 to 30 minutes after I.V. administration.
• Check hospital policy before administering I.V. Some do not permit infusion method as its safety is controversial.
• Not removed by hemodialysis.

Anticoagulants and heparin antagonist

dicumarol
dihydroergotamine mesylate/
   heparin sodium
heparin calcium
heparin sodium
phenprocoumon
protamine sulfate
warfarin sodium

COMBINATION PRODUCTS
None.

---

dicumarol
Dicumarol Pulvules
Pregnancy Category: D

MECHANISM OF ACTION
Inhibits vitamin K-dependent activation of clotting factors II, VII, IX, and X, which are formed in the liver.

INDICATIONS & DOSAGE
Treatment of pulmonary emboli; prevention and treatment of deep vein thrombosis, myocardial infarction, rheumatic heart disease with heart valve damage, atrial arrhythmias—
Adults: 200 to 300 mg P.O. on first day, 25 to 200 mg P.O. daily thereafter, based on prothrombin times.

ADVERSE REACTIONS
Blood: *hemorrhage with excessive dosage,* leukopenia, *agranulocytosis.*
GI: anorexia, nausea, vomiting, cramps, *diarrhea,* mouth ulcers.
GU: hematuria.
Skin: dermatitis, urticaria, alopecia, *rash.*
Other: *fever.*

INTERACTIONS
Allopurinol, amiodarone, chloramphenicol, clofibrate, diflunisal, thyroid drugs, heparin, anabolic steroids, cimetidine, disulfiram, glucagon, inhalation anesthetics, metronidazole, quinidine, influenza vaccine, sulindac, sulfinpyrazone, sulfonamides, tricyclic antidepressants: increased prothrombin time. Monitor patient carefully for bleeding. Consider anticoagulant dose reduction.
Ethacrynic acid, indomethacin, mefenamic acid, oxyphenbutazone, phenylbutazone, salicylates: increased prothrombin time; ulcerogenic effects. Don't use together.
Acetaminophen: increased bleeding possible with chronic (greater than 2 weeks) therapy with acetaminophen. Monitor very carefully.
Griseofulvin, haloperidol, ethchlorvynol, carbamazepine, rifampin: decreased prothrombin time with reduced anticoagulant effect. Monitor patient carefully.
Glutethimide, chloral hydrate, sulfinpyrazone, triclofos sodium: increased or decreased prothrombin time. Avoid use if possible, or monitor patient carefully.
Barbiturates: inhibition of hypoprothrombinemic effect of anticoagulants. If barbiturates are withdrawn, reduce anticoagulant dose; inhibition may last weeks after barbiturate is withdrawn, but fatal hemorrhage can occur when inhibiting effect disappears.
Cholestyramine: decreased response when administered too close together.

Italicized side effects are common or life-threatening.
*Liquid form contains alcohol.   **May contain tartrazine.

Administer 6 hours after oral anticoagulants.

NURSING CONSIDERATIONS
• Contraindicated in hemophilia,
thrombocytopenic purpura, leukemia
with pronounced bleeding tendency,
open wounds or ulcers, impaired hepatic or renal function, severe hypertension, acute nephritis, subacute
bacterial endocarditis. Use cautiously
during menses, during use of any
drainage tube, and in any patient in
whom slight bleeding is dangerous.
Use with extreme caution (if at all) in
psychiatric patients, debilitated patients, or cachectic patients.
• Use caution when adding or stopping any drug for patient receiving anticoagulants. May change the clotting
status and result in hemorrhage.
• Fever and skin rash signal severe
complications.
• Give drug at same time daily. Stress
importance of complying with recommended dosage and keeping follow-up
appointments. Patient should carry a
card that identifies him as a potential
bleeder.
• Regularly inspect patient for bleeding gums, bruises on arms or legs, petechiae, nosebleeds, melena, tarry
stools, hematuria, hematemesis. Tell
patient and family to watch for these
signs and notify doctor immediately.
• Warn patient to avoid over-the-
counter products containing aspirin,
other salicylates, or drugs that may
interact with dicumarol.
• Because onset of action is delayed,
heparin sodium is often given during
first few days of treatment. When
heparin is being given simultaneously, don't draw blood for prothrombin time within 5 hours of intermittent I.V. heparin administration.
However, prothrombin time may be
drawn at any time during continuous
heparin infusion.
• Dose given depends on prothrombin
time (PT). Doctors usually try to

maintain PT at 1.5 to 2 times normal.
PT values depend on procedure and
reagents used in individual laboratory.
• Tell patient to notify doctor if menses is heavier than usual.
• Tell patient to use electric razor
when shaving to avoid scratching skin
and to brush teeth with a soft toothbrush.
• May turn alkaline urine red-orange.
• Duration of action 2 to 6 days.
• Light-to-moderate alcohol intake
does not significantly affect prothrombin times.
• Tell patient to eat a consistent
amount of leafy green vegetables every day. These contain vitamin K, and
eating different amounts daily may alter anticoagulant effect.

dihydroergotamine mesylate/heparin sodium
Embolex
Pregnancy Category: X

MECHANISM OF ACTION
Heparin accelerates formation of an
antithrombin III–thrombin complex.
It inactivates thrombin and prevents
conversion of fibrinogen to fibrin. Dihydroergotamine accelerates venous
return and therefore inhibits veno-
stasis.

INDICATIONS & DOSAGE
*Prevention of postoperative deep ve-
nous thrombosis and pulmonary embolism in patients undergoing major
abdominal, thoracic, or pelvic surgery—*
Administer one ampul of Embolex
(dihydroergotamine, 0.5 mg, and heparin, 2500 or 5000 units) S.C. 2 hours
before surgery. Then, as ordered, administer q 12 hours thereafter for 5 to
7 days.

ADVERSE REACTIONS
Blood: *hemorrhage with excessive*

dosage, overly prolonged clotting time.
CV: transient tachycardia and brady-
cardia.
GI: nausea, vomiting.
Local: irritation, mild pain, itching.
Other: numbing and tingling of fin-
gers and toes, muscle pain, leg weak-
ness.

INTERACTIONS
Salicylates, oral anticoagulants: additive bleeding risk. Don't use together.

NURSING CONSIDERATIONS
• Contraindicated in patients with
known peripheral vascular disease,
coronary insufficiency, angina, severe
hypertension, impaired renal or hepatic function, sepsis, severe thrombocytopenia, or in patients receiving
oral anticoagulants.
• Don't administer to patients with
uncontrollable active bleeding.
• Embolex also contains lidocaine,
which is added to act as a local anesthetic at the injection site against pain
and irritation. Before administering,
check for allergy to lidocaine.
• Dihydroergotamine may act as an
oxytocic; don't administer to pregnant
patients.
• Use cautiously in patients with hypertension. Monitor BP regularly.
• Periodically monitor platelet
counts, hematocrit, and tests for occult blood in stool. If any sign of
bleeding occurs, notify doctor.
• Embolex may cause vasospastic reactions due to its dihydroergotamine
content. Patient will show signs and
symptoms of peripheral vascular ischemia, such as muscle pain, numbness, and coldness and pallor of the
fingers. Notify doctor if these symptoms develop.
• Administer by deep subcutaneous
injection into a fold in the anterior abdominal wall above the iliac crest.
Don't administer I.M. to avoid hematoma at the injection site.
• Embolex is more effective than the

same dose of heparin alone in preventing deep vein thrombosis.

heparin calcium
Calcilean♦♦, Calciparine♦

heparin sodium
Hepalean♦♦, Heparin Lock Flush
Solution (Tubex), Hep Lock,
Liquaemin Sodium
Pregnancy Category: C

MECHANISM OF ACTION
Accelerates formation of an antithrombin III–thrombin complex. It inactivates thrombin and prevents conversion of fibrinogen to fibrin.

INDICATIONS & DOSAGE
*Treatment of deep vein thrombosis,
myocardial infarction—*
Adults: initially, 5,000 to 7,500 units
I.V. push, then adjust dose according
to PTT results and give dose I.V. q 4
hours (usually 4,000 to 5,000 units);
or 5,000 to 7,500 units I.V. bolus,
then 1,000 units/hour by I.V. infusion
pump. Wait 8 hours following bolus
dose, and adjust hourly rate according
to PTT.
Treatment of pulmonary embolism—
Adults: initially, 7,500 to 10,000
units I.V. push, then adjust dose according to PTT results and give dose
I.V. q 4 hours (usually 4,000 to 5,000
units); or 7,500 to 10,000 units I.V.
bolus, then 1,000 units hourly by I.V.
infusion pump. Wait 8 hours following bolus dose, and adjust hourly rate
according to PTT.
Prophylaxis of embolism—
Adults: 5,000 units S.C. q 12 hours.
Open heart surgery—
Adults: (total body perfusion) 150 to
300 units/kg continuous I.V infusion.
*Treatment of pulmonary emboli; pre-
vention and treatment of deep vein
thrombosis—*
Children: initially, 50 units/kg I.V.
drip. Maintenance dose 100 units/kg

I.V. drip q 4 hours. Constant infusion: 20,000 units/m² daily. Dosages adjusted according to PTT.

As an I.V. flush to maintain patency of I.V. indwelling catheters—
10 to 100 units as an I.V. flush. Not intended for therapeutic use.

Heparin dosing is highly individualized, depending upon disease state, age, renal and hepatic status.

ADVERSE REACTIONS
Blood: *hemorrhage with excessive dosage, overly prolonged clotting time, thrombocytopenia.*
Local: irritation, mild pain.
Other: *"white clot" syndrome,* hypersensitivity reactions including chills, fever, pruritus, rhinitis, burning of feet, conjunctivitis, lacrimation, arthralgia, urticaria.

INTERACTIONS
Salicylates: increased anticoagulant effect. Don't use together.
Anticoagulants, oral: additive anticoagulation. Monitor prothrombin time and partial thromboplastin time.

NURSING CONSIDERATIONS
• Conditionally contraindicated in active bleeding; blood dyscrasias; or bleeding tendencies such as hemophilia, thrombocytopenia, or hepatic disease with hypoprothrombinemia; suspected intracranial hemorrhage; suppurative thrombophlebitis; inaccessible ulcerative lesions (especially of GI tract); open ulcerative wounds; extensive denudation of skin; ascorbic acid deficiency and other conditions causing increased capillary permeability; during or after brain, eye, or spinal cord surgery; during continuous tube drainage of stomach or small intestine; in subacute bacterial endocarditis; shock; advanced renal disease; threatened abortion; severe hypertension. Although the use of heparin is clearly hazardous in these conditions, a decision to use it depends on the comparative risk in failure to treat the coexisting thromboembolic disorder.
• Use cautiously during menses; in mild hepatic or renal disease; alcoholism; in patients in occupations with the risk of physical injury; immediately postpartum; and in patients with history of allergies, asthma, or GI ulcers.
• Monitor platelet counts regularly. Thrombocytopenia caused by heparin may be associated with a type of arterial thrombosis known as "white clot" syndrome.
• Measure partial thromboplastin time (PTT) carefully and regularly. Anticoagulation present when PTT values are 1.5 to 2 times control values.
• Drug requirements are higher in early phases of thrombogenic diseases and febrile states; lower when patient becomes stabilized.
• Regularly inspect patient for bleeding gums, bruises on arms or legs, petechiae, nosebleeds, melena, tarry stools, hematuria, hematemesis. Tell patient and family to watch for these signs and notify doctor immediately.
• Tell patient to avoid over-the-counter medications containing aspirin, other salicylates, or drugs that may interact with heparin.
• Heparin comes in various concentrations. Check order and vial carefully.
• Low-dose injections given sequentially between iliac crests in lower abdomen deep into subcutaneous fat. Inject drug slowly subcutaneously into fat pad. Leave needle in place for 10 seconds after injection; then withdraw needle. Alternate site every 12 hours—right for a.m., left for p.m.
• Don't massage after subcutaneous injection. Watch for signs of bleeding at injection site. Rotate sites and keep accurate record.
• Check constant I.V. infusions regularly, even when pumps are in good

working order, to prevent overdosage or underdosage.
- I.M. administration not recommended.
- I.V. administration preferred because of long-term effect and irregular absorption when given subcutaneously. Whenever possible, administer I.V. heparin using infusion pump to provide maximum safety.
- Concentrated heparin solutions (greater than 100 units/ml) can irritate blood vessels.
- Place notice above patient's bed to inform I.V. team or lab personnel to apply pressure dressings after taking blood.
- Avoid excessive I.M. injections of other drugs to prevent or minimize hematomas. If possible, don't give I.M. injections at all.
- Elderly patients should usually start at lower doses.
- When intermittent I.V. therapy is utilized, always draw blood ½ hour before next scheduled dose to avoid falsely elevated PTT.
- Blood for PTT can be drawn any time after 8 hours of initiation of continuous I.V. heparin therapy. Never draw blood for PTT from the I.V. tubing of the heparin infusion, or from vein of infusion. Falsely elevated PTT will result. Always draw blood from opposite arm.
- Give on time; try not to skip a dose or "catch up" with an I.V. containing heparin. If I.V. is out, get it restarted as soon as possible, and reschedule bolus dose immediately.
- Never piggyback other drugs into an infusion line while heparin infusion is running. Many antibiotics and other drugs inactivate heparin. Never mix any drug with heparin in syringe when bolus therapy is used.
- Abrupt withdrawal may cause increased coagulability. Usually, heparin therapy is followed by oral anticoagulants for prophylaxis.

phenprocoumon
Liquamar
Pregnancy Category: D

MECHANISM OF ACTION
Inhibits vitamin K–dependent activation of clotting factors II, VII, IX, and X, which are formed in the liver.

INDICATIONS & DOSAGE
Treatment of pulmonary emboli; prevention and treatment of deep vein thrombosis, myocardial infarction, rheumatic heart disease with heart valve damage, atrial arrhythmias—
Adults: initially, 24 mg P.O. Maintenance dose: 0.75 to 6 mg daily, based on prothrombin time.

ADVERSE REACTIONS
Blood: *hemorrhage with excessive dosage, agranulocytosis,* leukopenia.
GI: paralytic ileus and intestinal obstruction (both resulting from hemorrhage), nausea, vomiting, cramps, diarrhea, mouth ulcers.
GU: nephropathy, hematuria.
Skin: *rash,* alopecia, necrosis.
Other: *fever.*

INTERACTIONS
Allopurinol, amiodarone, chloramphenicol, clofibrate, thyroid drugs, heparin, anabolic steroids, disulfiram, glucagon, inhalation anesthetics, metronidazole, quinidine, influenza vaccine, sulindac, sulfonamides, tricyclic antidepressants: increased prothrombin time. Monitor patient carefully for bleeding. Consider anticoagulant dose reduction.
Ethacrynic acid, indomethacin, mefenamic acid, oxyphenbutazone, phenylbutazone, salicylates: increased prothrombin time; ulcerogenic effects. Don't use together.
Acetaminophen: increased bleeding possible with chronic (greater than 2 weeks) therapy with acetaminophen. Monitor very carefully.

Italicized side effects are common or life-threatening.
*Liquid form contains alcohol.   **May contain tartrazine.

Griseofulvin, haloperidol, ethchlorvynol, carbamazepine, rifampin: decreased prothrombin time with reduced anticoagulant effect. Monitor patient carefully.

Glutethimide, chloral hydrate, triclofos sodium: increased or decreased prothrombin time. Avoid use if possible, or monitor patient carefully.

Barbiturates: inhibition of hypoprothrombinemic effect of anticoagulants. If barbiturates are withdrawn, reduce anticoagulant dose; inhibition may last weeks after barbiturate is withdrawn, but fatal hemorrhage can occur when inhibiting effect disappears.

Cholestyramine: decreased response when administered too close together. Administer 6 hours after oral anticoagulants.

NURSING CONSIDERATIONS

• Contraindicated in hemophilia, thrombocytopenic purpura, leukemia with pronounced bleeding tendency, open wounds or ulcers, impaired hepatic or renal function, severe hypertension, acute nephritis, and subacute bacterial endocarditis. Use cautiously in pregnancy or lactation, during menses, during use of any drainage tube in any orifice, and in any patient in whom slight bleeding is dangerous. Use with extreme caution (if at all) in psychiatric, debilitated, or cachectic patients.

• Use caution when adding or stopping any drug for patient receiving anticoagulants. May change the clotting status and result in hemorrhage.

• Fever and skin rash signal severe complications.

• Give drug at same time daily. Stress importance of complying with recommended dosage and keeping follow-up appointments. Patient should carry a card that identifies him as a potential bleeder.

• Regularly inspect patient for bleeding gums, bruises on arms or legs, petechiae, nosebleeds, melena, tarry stools, hematuria, hematemesis. Tell patient and family to watch for these signs and notify doctor immediately.

• Warn patient to avoid over-the-counter products containing aspirin, other salicylates, or drugs that may interact with phenprocoumon.

• Because onset of action is delayed, heparin sodium is often given during first few days of treatment. When heparin is being given simultaneously, don't draw blood for prothrombin time within 5 hours of I.V. heparin administration.

• Dose given depends on prothrombin time (PT). Doctors usually try to maintain PT at 1.5 to 2 times normal. Numerical PT values depend on procedure and reagents used in individual laboratory.

• Tell patient to notify doctor if menses is heavier than usual. May require adjusting dose.

• Tell patient to use electric razor when shaving to avoid scratching skin and to brush teeth with a soft toothbrush.

• Warn patient that alkaline urine may turn orange-red.

• A coumarin derivative.

• Duration of action is 7 to 14 days.

• Light-to-moderate alcohol intake does not significantly affect prothrombin times.

• Tell patient to eat a consistent amount of leafy green vegetables every day. These contain vitamin K, and eating different amounts daily may alter anticoagulant effect.

protamine sulfate
Pregnancy Category: C

MECHANISM OF ACTION
Forms a physiologically inert complex with heparin sodium.

INDICATIONS & DOSAGE
Heparin overdose—

Adults: dosage based on venous blood coagulation studies, generally 1 mg for each 78 to 95 units of heparin. Give diluted to 1% (10 mg/ml) slow I.V. injection over 1 to 3 minutes. Maximum 50 mg/10 minutes.

ADVERSE REACTIONS
CV: fall in blood pressure, bradycardia.
Other: transitory flushing, feeling of warmth, dyspnea.

INTERACTIONS
None significant.

NURSING CONSIDERATIONS
• Use cautiously after cardiac surgery.
• Doctor gives this drug. Should be given slowly to reduce adverse reactions. Have equipment available to treat shock.
• Monitor patient continually. Check vital signs frequently.
• Watch for spontaneous bleeding (heparin "rebound"), especially in patients undergoing dialysis and those who have had cardiac surgery.
• Protamine sulfate may act as anticoagulant in very high doses.
• 1 mg of protamine neutralizes 78 to 95 units of heparin.
• Heparin antagonist.

warfarin sodium
Coufarin, Coumadin♦, Panwarfin, Warfilone Sodium♦♦, Warnerin♦♦
Pregnancy Category: D

MECHANISM OF ACTION
Inhibits vitamin K–dependent activation of clotting factors II, VII, IX, and X, which are formed in the liver.

INDICATIONS & DOSAGE
Treatment of pulmonary emboli; prevention and treatment of deep vein thrombosis, myocardial infarction, rheumatic heart disease with heart valve damage, atrial arrhythmias—
Adults: 10 to 15 mg P.O. for 3 days, then dosage based on daily prothrombin times (PT). Usual maintenance dose 2 to 10 mg P.O. daily. Alternate regimen: initially, 40 to 60 mg P.O. daily; then 2 to 10 mg daily based on PT determinations.
   Warfarin sodium also available for I.V. use (50 mg/vial). Reconstitute with sterile water for injection. I.V. form rarely used and may be in periodic short supply.

ADVERSE REACTIONS
Blood: *hemorrhage with excessive dosage,* leukopenia.
GI: paralytic ileus, intestinal obstruction (both resulting from hemorrhage), diarrhea, vomiting, cramps, nausea.
GU: excessive uterine bleeding.
Skin: dermatitis, urticaria, *rash,* necrosis, alopecia.
Other: *fever.*

INTERACTIONS
Amiodarone, chloramphenicol, clofibrate, diflunisal, thyroid drugs, heparin, anabolic steroids, cimetidine, disulfiram, glucagon, inhalation anesthetics, metronidazole, quinidine, influenza vaccine, sulindac, sulfinpyrazone, sulfonamides: increased prothrombin time. Monitor patient carefully for bleeding. Consider anticoagulant dose reduction.
Ethacrynic acid, indomethacin, mefenamic acid, oxyphenbutazone, phenylbutazone, salicylates: increased prothrombin time; ulcerogenic effects. Don't use together.
Acetaminophen: increased bleeding possible with chronic (greater than 2 weeks) therapy with acetaminophen. Monitor very carefully.
Griseofulvin, haloperidol, ethchlorvynol, carbamazepine, paraldehyde, rifampin: decreased prothrombin time with reduced anticoagulant effect. Monitor patient carefully.

Italicized side effects are common or life-threatening.
*Liquid form contains alcohol.   **May contain tartrazine.

Glutethimide, chloral hydrate, triclofos sodium: increased or decreased prothrombin time. Avoid use if possible, or monitor patient carefully.
Barbiturates: inhibition of hypoprothrombinemic effect of anticoagulants. If barbiturates are withdrawn, reduce anticoagulant dose; inhibition may last weeks after barbiturate is withdrawn, but fatal hemorrhage can occur when inhibiting effect disappears.
Cholestyramine: decreased response when administered too close together. Administer 6 hours after oral anticoagulants.

NURSING CONSIDERATIONS
• Contraindicated in bleeding or hemorrhagic tendencies resulting from open wounds, visceral cancer, GI ulcers, severe hepatic or renal disease, severe uncontrolled hypertension, subacute bacterial endocarditis, vitamin K deficiency; after recent operations in eye, brain, or spinal cord. Use cautiously in diverticulitis, colitis, mild or moderate hypertension, mild or moderate hepatic or renal disease, lactation; in presence of drainage tubes in any orifice; with regional or lumbar block anesthesia; or in any condition increasing risk of hemorrhage.
• Observe nursing infants of mothers on drug for unexpected bleeding.
• PT determinations essential for proper control. High incidence of bleeding when PT exceeds 2.5 times control values. Doctors usually try to maintain PT at 1.5 to 2 times normal.
• Give at same time daily. Stress importance of complying with recommended dosage and keeping follow-up appointments. Patient should carry a card that identifies him as a potential bleeder.
• Elderly patients and patients with renal or hepatic failure are especially sensitive to warfarin effect.
• Half-life of warfarin is 36 to 44

hours.
• Warfarin effect can be neutralized by vitamin K injections.
• Regularly inspect patient for bleeding gums, bruises on arms or legs, petechiae, nosebleeds, melena, tarry stools, hematuria, hematemesis. Tell patient and family to watch for these signs and notify doctor immediately.
• Warn patient to avoid over-the-counter products containing aspirin, other salicylates, or drugs that may interact with warfarin sodium.
• Food and enteral feedings that contain vitamin K may cause inadequate anticoagulation. Warn patient to read labels.
• Because onset of action is delayed, heparin sodium is often given during first few days of treatment. When heparin is being given simultaneously, don't draw blood for prothrombin time within 5 hours of intermittent I.V. heparin administration. However, blood for prothrombin time may be drawn at any time during continuous heparin infusion.
• Fever and skin rash signal severe complications.
• Tell patient to notify doctor if menses is heavier than usual. May require adjusting dose.
• Tell patient to use electric razor when shaving to avoid scratching skin and to brush teeth with a soft toothbrush.
• Best oral anticoagulant when patient must receive antacids or phenytoin.
• Light-to-moderate alcohol intake does not significantly affect prothrombin time.
• Possibly effective in treatment of transient cerebral ischemic attacks.
• Tell patient to eat a consistent amount of leafy green vegetables every day. These contain vitamin K, and eating different amounts daily may alter anticoagulant effects.

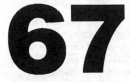

Hemostatics

absorbable gelatin sponge
aminocaproic acid
antihemophilic factor (AHF)
Factor IX complex
microfibrillar collagen hemostat
negatol
oxidized cellulose
thrombin

COMBINATION PRODUCTS
None.

absorbable gelatin sponge
Gelfoam
Pregnancy Category: NR

MECHANISM OF ACTION
Absorbs and holds many times its weight in blood. Also provides a framework for growth of granulation tissue.

INDICATIONS & DOSAGE
Adults:
Decubitus ulcers—place aseptically deep into ulcer. Don't disturb or remove; may add extra p.r.n.
To provide hemostasis in surgery (adjunct)—apply saturated with isotonic NaCl injection or thrombin solution. Hold in place for 10 to 15 seconds. When oozing is controlled, allow material to remain in place.

ADVERSE REACTIONS
None reported.

INTERACTIONS
None significant.

NURSING CONSIDERATIONS
• Contraindicated in frank infection, as sole hemostatic agent in abnormal bleeding, or in postpartum bleeding or hemorrhage.
• Avoid overpacking when placed into body cavities or closed tissue spaces.
• Systemically absorbed within 4 to 6 weeks; no need to remove.

aminocaproic acid
Amicar♦
Pregnancy Category: C

MECHANISM OF ACTION
Inhibits plasminogen activator substances. To a lesser degree, it blocks antiplasmin activity by inhibiting fibrinolysis.

INDICATIONS & DOSAGE
Excessive bleeding resulting from hyperfibrinolysis—
Adults: initially, 5 g P.O. or slow I.V. infusion, followed by 1 to 1.25 g hourly until bleeding is controlled. Maximum dose 30 g daily.

ADVERSE REACTIONS
Blood: generalized thrombosis.
CNS: dizziness, malaise, headache.
CV: hypotension, bradycardia, arrhythmia (with rapid I.V. infusion).
EENT: tinnitus, nasal stuffiness, conjunctival suffusion.
GI: nausea, cramps, diarrhea.
Skin: rash.
Other: malaise.

Italicized side effects are common or life-threatening.
*Liquid form contains alcohol.   **May contain tartrazine.

INTERACTIONS
Oral contraceptives, estrogens: increased probability of hypercoagulability. Use together cautiously.

NURSING CONSIDERATIONS
• Contraindicated in active intravascular clotting. Use cautiously in thrombophlebitis and cardiac, hepatic, or renal disease.
• Monitor coagulation studies, heart rhythm, and blood pressure. Notify doctor of any change immediately.
• Also used as antidote for streptokinase or urokinase toxicity; not beneficial in the treatment of thrombocytopenia.
• Dilute solution with sterile water for injection, normal saline injection, dextrose 5% in water, or Ringer's injection.
• Available in liquid form.
• Drug is sometimes helpful as an adjunct in treating hemophilia.

antihemophilic factor (AHF)
Antihemophilic Globulin (AHG)♦,
Hemofil, Hemofil T, Humafac,
Koate, Profilate
Pregnancy Category: C

MECHANISM OF ACTION
Directly replaces deficient clotting factor.

INDICATIONS & DOSAGE
Hemophilia A (Factor VIII deficiency)—
Adults and children: 10 to 20 units/kg I.V. push or infusion q 8 to 24 hours. Maintenance doses may be less. Infusion rate usually 10 to 20 ml reconstituted solution per 3 minutes. Dosage varies with individual needs.

ADVERSE REACTIONS
CNS: headache, paresthesia, clouding or loss of consciousness.
CV: tachycardia, hypotension, possible intravascular hemolysis in patients with blood type A, B, or AB.
EENT: disturbed vision.
GI: nausea, vomiting.
Skin: erythema, *urticaria.*
Other: chills, *fever, backache, flushing,* constriction in chest; hypersensitivity.

INTERACTIONS
None significant.

NURSING CONSIDERATIONS
• Use cautiously in neonates, infants, and patients with hepatic disease because of susceptibility to hepatitis, which may be transmitted in antihemophilic factor.
• Monitor vital signs regularly. Take baseline pulse rate before I.V. administration. If pulse rate increases significantly, flow rate should be reduced or administration stopped.
• Monitor patient for allergic reactions.
• For I.V. use only. Use plastic syringe; drug may interact with glass syringe, causing binding of ground-glass surface.
• Refrigerate concentrate until ready to use, but not after reconstituted. Refrigeration after reconstitution may cause the active ingredient to precipitate. Before reconstituting, concentrate and diluent bottles should be warmed to room temperature. To mix drug, gently roll vial between your hands. Reconstituted solution unstable; use within 3 hours. Store away from heat. Don't shake or mix with other I.V. solutions.
• As ordered, administer Hepatitis B vaccine before administering antihemophilic factor.
• Monitor coagulation studies before and during therapy.

Unmarked trade names available in the United States only.
♦Also available in Canada.   ♦♦Available in Canada only.

Factor IX complex
Konyne, Profilnine, Proplex
Pregnancy Category: C

MECHANISM OF ACTION
Directly replaces deficient clotting
factors.

INDICATIONS & DOSAGE
*Factor IX deficiency (hemophilia B or
Christmas disease), anticoagulant
overdosage—*
Adults and children: units required
equal 0.8 to 1 × body weight in kg ×
percentage of desired increase of Factor IX level, by slow I.V. infusion or
I.V. push. Dosage is highly individualized, depending on degree of deficiency, level of Factor IX desired,
weight of patient, and severity of
bleeding.

ADVERSE REACTIONS
CNS: headache.
CV: *thromboembolic reactions,* possible intravascular hemolysis in patients
with blood types A, B, AB.
Other: *transient fever, chills, flushing, tingling,* hypersensitivity.

INTERACTIONS
None significant.

NURSING CONSIDERATIONS
• Contraindicated in hepatic disease,
intravascular coagulation, or fibrinolysis. Use cautiously in neonates and
infants because of susceptibility to
hepatitis, which may be transmitted
with Factor IX complex.
• Observe patient for allergic reactions, and monitor vital signs regularly.
• As ordered, administer Hepatitis B
vaccine before administering Factor
IX complex.
• Avoid rapid infusion. If tingling
sensation, fever, chills, or headache
develops during I.V. infusion, decrease flow rate and notify the doctor.

• Reconstitute with 20 ml sterile water for injection for each vial of lyophilized drug. Keep refrigerated until
ready to use; warm to room temperature before reconstituting. Use within
3 hours of reconstitution. Unstable in
solution. Don't shake, refrigerate, or
mix reconstituted solution with other
I.V. solutions. Store away from heat.

microfibrillar collagen hemostat
Avitene
Pregnancy Category: C

MECHANISM OF ACTION
Attracts and aggregates platelets.

INDICATIONS & DOSAGE
*To provide hemostasis in surgery (ad-
junct)—*
Adults and children: amount depends on severity of bleeding. Compress area with dry sponges. Apply
drug directly to bleeding site for 1 to 5
minutes. Gently remove excess. Reapply if needed.

ADVERSE REACTIONS
Blood: hematoma.
Local: exacerbation of wound dehis-
cence, abscess formation, foreign
body reaction, adhesion formation.
Other: enhanced infection in contaminated wounds, mediastinitis, hypersensitivity.

INTERACTIONS
None significant.

NURSING CONSIDERATIONS
• Contraindicated in closure of skin
incisions; it may interfere with heal-
ing.
• Not for injection.
• Don't spill on nonbleeding surfaces.
• Don't dilute. Always apply dry.
• Adheres to wet gloves, instruments,
or tissue surfaces. Handle and apply
with smooth, dry forceps. Apply di-

rectly to source of bleeding.

negatol
Negatan
Pregnancy Category: NR

MECHANISM OF ACTION
An astringent and protein denaturant.

INDICATIONS & DOSAGE
Cervical bleeding—
Women: apply 1-inch gauze dipped in 1:10 dilution of drug; insert in cervical canal. If tolerated, may increase to full-strength solution. Remove pack after 24 hours; give 2-quart douche of dilute negatol or vinegar.
Oral ulcers—
Adults and children: apply to dried lesion with applicator, leave for 1 minute, then neutralize with large amounts of water.

ADVERSE REACTIONS
Local: *burning sensation.*
Skin: erythema, superficial desquamation when applied to skin.

INTERACTIONS
None significant.

NURSING CONSIDERATIONS
• Vaginal membrane turns grayish after vaginal use.
• When used in vagina, patient should wear a perineal pad to prevent soiling of clothing.
• When used for oral ulcers, may apply topical anesthetic first to prevent burning sensation.
• Always clean and dry area to be treated.
• Astringent, styptic, and protein denaturant; highly acidic.

oxidized cellulose
Oxycel♦, Surgicel♦
Pregnancy Category: NR

MECHANISM OF ACTION
Absorbs and holds many times its weight in blood.

INDICATIONS & DOSAGE
To provide hemostasis in surgery (adjunct); external bleeding at tumor sites—
Adults and children: apply with sterile technique, p.r.n. Remove after hemostasis, if possible, with dry sterile forceps. Leave in place if necessary.

ADVERSE REACTIONS
CNS: headache when used as packing for epistaxis, or after rhinologic procedures or application to surface wounds.
EENT: sneezing, epistaxis, stinging, or burning when used as packing for rhinologic procedures; nasal membrane necrosis or septal perforation.
Local: encapsulation of fluid, foreign body reaction, burning or stinging after application to surface wounds.
Other: possible prolongation of drainage in cholecystectomies.

INTERACTIONS
Thrombin: may decrease blood clotting effectiveness.

NURSING CONSIDERATIONS
• Contraindicated in controlling hemorrhage from large arteries; in nonhemorrhagic, serous, oozing surfaces; in implantation in bone defects.
• Don't pack or wad unless it will be removed after hemostasis. Don't apply too tightly when used as wrap sheet in vascular surgery. Apply loosely against bleeding surface.
• Always remove after hemostasis when used in laminectomies or near optic nerve chain.
• Don't autoclave this product.

- Use only amount needed to produce hemostasis. Remove excess before surgical closure.
- Use minimal amounts in urologic procedures.
- In large wounds, don't overlap skin edges.
- Use sterile technique to remove from open wounds after hemostasis. Don't remove without irrigating material first; otherwise, fresh bleeding may occur.
- Don't moisten. Hemostatic effect is greater when applied dry.
- Should not be used for permanent packing in fractures because it may result in cyst formation.

---

thrombin
Fibrindex, Thrombinar♦
Pregnancy Category: C

MECHANISM OF ACTION
Clots to form fibrin in the presence of fibrinogen.

INDICATIONS & DOSAGE
Bleeding from parenchymatous tissue, cancellous bone, dental sockets, nasal and laryngeal surgery, and in plastic surgery and skin-grafting procedures—
Adults: apply 100 units per ml of sterile isotonic NaCl solution or sterile distilled water to area where clotting needed (or may apply dry powder in bone surgery); in major bleeding, apply 1,000 to 2,000 units/ml sterile isotonic NaCl solution. Sponge blood from area before application, but avoid sponging area after application.
GI hemorrhage—
Adults: give 2 oz of milk, followed by 2 oz of milk containing 10,000 to 20,000 units thrombin. Repeat t.i.d. for 4 to 5 days or until bleeding is controlled.

ADVERSE REACTIONS
Systemic: hypersensitivity and fever.

INTERACTIONS
None significant.

NURSING CONSIDERATIONS
- Contraindicated in hypersensitivity to thrombin or bovine products.
- Obtain patient history of reactions to thrombin or bovine products.
- Observe patient for allergic reactions, and monitor vital signs regularly.
- Have blood typed and crossmatched to treat possible hemorrhage.
- Don't inject topical thrombin or allow it to enter large blood vessels. I.V. injection may cause death because of severe intravascular clotting.
- May be used with absorbable gelatin sponge but not with oxidized cellulose. Check sponge labeling before use.
- Neutralize stomach acids before oral use in GI hemorrhage.
- Keep refrigerated, preferably frozen, until ready to use. Unstable in solution. Use within 24 hours of reconstitution; discard after 48 hours. Store away from heat.
- Broken down by diluted acid, alkali, and salts of heavy metals.

Italicized side effects are common or life-threatening.
*Liquid form contains alcohol.   **May contain tartrazine.

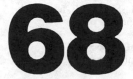

Blood derivatives

normal serum albumin 5%, 25% plasma protein fraction

COMBINATION PRODUCTS
None.

---

normal serum albumin 5%
Albuminar 5%, Albutein 5%, Buminate 5%, Plasbumin 5%

normal serum albumin 25%
Albuminar 25%, Albumisol 25%, Buminate 25%, Plasbumin 25%
Pregnancy Category: C

MECHANISM OF ACTION
Normal serum albumin 25% provides intravascular oncotic pressure in a 5:1 ratio, which causes a shift of fluid from interstitial spaces to the circulation and slightly increases plasma protein concentration. Normal serum albumin 5% supplies colloid to the blood and expands plasma volume.

INDICATIONS & DOSAGE
Shock—
Adults: initially, 500 ml (5% solution) by I.V. infusion, repeat q 30 minutes, p.r.n. Dose varies with patient's condition and response.
Children: 25% to 50% adult dose in nonemergency.
Hypoproteinemia—
Adults: 1,000 to 1,500 ml 5% solution by I.V. infusion daily, maximum rate 5 to 10 ml/minute; or 25 to 100 g 25% solution by I.V. infusion daily, maximum rate 3 ml/minute. Dose varies with patient's condition and re-

sponse.
*Burns—*dosage varies according to extent of burn and patient's condition. Generally maintain plasma albumin at 2 to 3 g/100 ml.
Hyperbilirubinemia—
Infants: 1 g albumin (4 ml 25%)/kg before transfusion.

ADVERSE REACTIONS
CV: *vascular overload after rapid infusion,* hypotension, altered pulse rate.
GI: increased salivation, nausea, vomiting.
Skin: urticaria.
Other: chills, fever, altered respiration.

INTERACTIONS
None significant.

NURSING CONSIDERATIONS
• Contraindicated in severe anemia and heart failure. Use cautiously in low cardiac reserve, absence of albumin deficiency, and restricted salt intake.
• Do not give more than 250 g in 48 hours.
• Watch for hemorrhage or shock if used after surgery or injury.
• Monitor vital signs carefully.
• Watch for signs of vascular overload (heart failure or pulmonary edema).
• Patient should be properly hydrated before infusion of solution.
• Avoid rapid I.V. infusion. Specific rate is individualized according to patient's age, condition, diagnosis.

Unmarked trade names available in the United States only.
♦Also available in Canada.   ♦♦Available in Canada only.

• Dilute with sterile water for injection, 0.9% NaCl solution, or dextrose 5% injection. Use solution promptly; contains no preservatives. Discard unused solution.

• Don't use cloudy solutions or those containing sediment. Solution should be clear amber color.

• Freezing may cause bottle to break. Follow storage instructions on bottle.

• One volume of 25% albumin is equivalent to five volumes of 5% albumin in producing hemodilution and relative anemia.

• This product is very expensive, and random supply shortages occur often.

• Monitor intake and output, hemoglobin, hematocrit, and serum protein and electrolytes during therapy.

---

plasma protein fraction
Plasmanate, Plasma Plex, Plasmatein, Protenate
Pregnancy Category: C

MECHANISM OF ACTION
Supplies colloid to the blood and expands plasma volume.

INDICATIONS & DOSAGE
Shock—
Adults: varies with patient's condition and response, but usual dose is 250 to 500 ml (12.5 to 25 g protein), usually not faster than 10 ml/minute.
Children: 22 to 33 ml/kg I.V. infused at rate of 5 to 10 ml/minute.
Hypoproteinemia—
Adults: 1,000 to 1,500 ml I.V. daily. Maximum infusion rate 8 ml/minute.

ADVERSE REACTIONS
CNS: headache.
CV: variable effects on blood pressure after rapid infusion or intraarterial administration; *vascular overload after rapid infusion.*
GI: nausea, vomiting, hypersalivation.
Skin: erythema, urticaria.

Other: flushing, chills, fever, back pain, dyspnea.

INTERACTIONS
None significant.

NURSING CONSIDERATIONS
• Contraindicated in patients with severe anemia or heart failure, and in patients undergoing cardiac bypass. Use cautiously in hepatic or renal failure, low cardiac reserve, restricted salt intake.

• Monitor blood pressure. Infusion should be slowed or stopped if hypotension suddenly occurs.

• Vital signs should return to normal gradually; monitor hourly.

• Watch for signs of vascular overload (heart failure or pulmonary edema).

• Monitor intake and output. Watch for decreased urinary output.

• Check expiration date on container before using. Discard solutions in containers that have been opened for more than 4 hours. Solution contains no preservatives.

• Don't use solutions that are cloudy, contain sediment, or have been frozen.

• If patient is dehydrated, give additional fluids either P.O. or I.V.

• Do not give more than 250 g (5,000 ml 5%) in 48 hours.

• Contains 130 to 160 mEq sodium/ liter.

Italicized side effects are common or life-threatening.
*Liquid form contains alcohol.   **May contain tartrazine.

Thrombolytic enzymes

streptokinase
urokinase

COMBINATION PRODUCTS
None.

---

streptokinase
Kabikinase, Streptase♦
Pregnancy Category: C

MECHANISM OF ACTION
Activates plasminogen in two steps. Plasminogen and streptokinase form a complex that exposes the plasminogen-activating site. Plasminogen is converted to plasmin by cleavage of the peptide bond.

INDICATIONS & DOSAGE
Arteriovenous cannula occlusion—
Adults: 250,000 IU in 2 ml I.V. solution by I.V. pump infusion into each occluded limb of the cannula over 25 to 35 minutes. Clamp off cannula for 2 hours. Then aspirate contents of cannula; flush with saline solution and reconnect.
Venous thrombosis, pulmonary embolism, and arterial thrombosis and embolism—
Adults: loading dose: 250,000 IU I.V. infusion over 30 minutes. Sustaining dose: 100,000 IU/hour I.V. infusion for 72 hours for deep vein thrombosis and 100,000 IU/hour over 24 to 72 hours by I.V. infusion pump for pulmonary embolism.
Lysis of coronary artery thrombi following acute myocardial infarction—
Adults: loading dose: 20,000 IU via

coronary catheter, followed by a maintenance dose. Maintenance dose: 2,000 IU/minute for 60 minutes as an infusion.

ADVERSE REACTIONS
Blood: *bleeding, low hematocrit.*
CV: transient lowering or elevation of blood pressure.
EENT: periorbital edema.
Local: *phlebitis at injection site.*
Skin: urticaria.
Other: *hypersensitivity to drug, fever, anaphylaxis,* musculoskeletal pain, minor breathing difficulty, bronchospasms, angioneurotic edema.

INTERACTIONS
Anticoagulants: concurrent use of anticoagulants with streptokinase is not recommended. Reversing the effects of oral anticoagulants must be considered before beginning therapy, and heparin must be stopped and its effect allowed to diminish.
Aspirin, indomethacin, phenylbutazone, drugs affecting platelet activity: increased risk of bleeding. Do not use together.

NURSING CONSIDERATIONS
• Contraindicated in ulcerative wounds, active internal bleeding, and recent cerebrovascular accident; recent trauma with possible internal injuries; visceral or intracranial malignancy; ulcerative colitis; diverticulitis; severe hypertension; acute or chronic hepatic or renal insufficiency; uncontrolled hypocoagulation; chronic pulmonary disease with cavi-

---

tation; subacute bacterial endocarditis or rheumatic valvular disease; recent cerebral embolism, thrombosis, or hemorrhage. Also contraindicated within 10 days after intraarterial diagnostic procedure or any surgery, including liver or kidney biopsy, lumbar puncture, thoracentesis, paracentesis, or extensive or multiple cutdowns.

• Use cautiously when treating arterial emboli that originate from left side of heart because of danger of cerebral infarction.

• I.M. injections contraindicated during streptokinase therapy.

• Before initiating therapy, draw blood to determine PTT and PT. Rate of I.V. infusion depends on thrombin time and streptokinase resistance.

• If the patient has had either a recent streptococcal infection or recent treatment with streptokinase, a higher loading dose may be necessary.

• Preparation of I.V. solution: reconstitute each vial with 5 ml sodium chloride for injection. Further dilute to 45 ml. Don't shake; roll gently to mix. Use within 24 hours. Store at room temperature in powder form; refrigerate after reconstitution.

• Monitor patient for excessive bleeding every 15 minutes for the first hour; every 30 minutes for the second through eighth hours; then once every shift. If bleeding is evident, stop therapy. Pretreatment with heparin or drugs affecting platelets causes high risk of bleeding.

• Monitor pulses, color, and sensitivities of extremities every hour.

• Have typed and crossmatched packed red cells and whole blood ready to treat possible hemorrhage.

• Keep aminocaproic acid available to treat bleeding. Corticosteroids are used to treat allergic reactions.

• Before using streptokinase to clear an occluded arteriovenous cannula, try flushing with heparinized saline.

• Bruising more likely during therapy; avoid unnecessary handling of patient. Side rails should be padded.

• Maintain the involved extremity in straight alignment to prevent bleeding from the infusion site.

• Keep venipuncture sites to a minimum; use pressure dressing on puncture sites for at least 15 minutes.

• Keep a laboratory flow sheet on patient's chart to monitor partial thromboplastin time, prothrombin time, hemoglobin, and hematocrit.

• Monitor vital signs frequently.

• Watch for signs of hypersensitivity. Notify doctor immediately.

• Heparin by continuous infusion is usually started within an hour after stopping streptokinase. Use infusion pump to administer heparin.

• Should be used only by doctors with wide experience in thrombotic disease management where clinical and laboratory monitoring can be performed.

• In the treatment of acute MI, streptokinase prevents primary or secondary thrombus formation in the microcirculation surrounding the necrotic area.

urokinase
Abbokinase, Win-Kinase
Pregnancy Category: B

MECHANISM OF ACTION
Activates plasminogen by directly cleaving peptide bonds at two different sites.

INDICATIONS & DOSAGE
Lysis of acute massive pulmonary emboli and lysis of pulmonary emboli accompanied by unstable hemodynamics—

Adults: for I.V. infusion only by constant infusion pump that will deliver a total volume of 195 ml.

Priming dose: 4,400 IU/kg of urokinase-normal saline solution admixture given over 10 minutes. Follow with 4,400 IU/kg hourly for 12 to 24 hours. Total volume should not exceed

200 ml. Follow therapy with continuous I.V. infusion of heparin, then oral anticoagulants.

Coronary artery thrombosis—
Adults: Following a bolus dose of heparin ranging from 2,500 to 10,000 units, infuse 6,000 IU/minute of urokinase into the occluded artery for up to 2 hours. Average total dose is 500,000 IU.

Venous catheter occlusion—
Instill 5,000 IU into occluded line, wait 5 minutes, then aspirate. Repeat aspiration attempts q 5 minutes for 30 minutes. If not patent after 30 minutes, cap line and let urokinase work for 30 to 60 minutes before aspirating. May require second instillation.

ADVERSE REACTIONS
Blood: *bleeding, low hematocrit.*
Local: *phlebitis at injection site.*
Other: hypersensitivity (not as frequent as streptokinase), musculoskeletal pain, bronchospasm, *anaphylaxis.*

INTERACTIONS
Anticoagulants: concurrent use of anticoagulants with urokinase is not recommended. Reversing the effects of oral anticoagulants must be considered before beginning therapy, and heparin must be stopped and its effect allowed to diminish.

Aspirin, indomethacin, phenylbutazone, other drugs affecting platelet activity: increased risk of bleeding. Do not use together.

NURSING CONSIDERATIONS
• Contraindicated in ulcerative wounds, active internal bleeding, and cerebrovascular accident; recent trauma with possible internal injuries; visceral or intracranial malignancy; pregnancy and first 10 days postpartum; ulcerative colitis; diverticulitis; severe hypertension; acute or chronic hepatic or renal insufficiency; uncontrolled hypocoagulation; chronic pulmonary disease with cavitation; subacute bacterial endocarditis or rheumatic valvular disease; and recent cerebral embolism, thrombosis, or hemorrhage. Also contraindicated within 10 days after intraarterial diagnostic procedure or any surgery, including liver or kidney biopsy, lumbar puncture, thoracentesis, paracentesis, or extensive or multiple cutdowns.

• I.M. injections are contraindicated during urokinase therapy.

• Maintain the involved extremity in straight alignment to prevent bleeding from the infusion site.

• Preparation of I.V. solution: add 5.2 ml sterile water for injection to vial. Dilute further with 0.9% saline solution before infusion. Don't use bacteriostatic water for injection to reconstitute; it contains preservatives.

• Monitor patient for bleeding every 15 minutes for the first hour; every 30 minutes for the second through eighth hours; then once every shift. Pretreatment with drugs affecting platelets places patient at high risk of bleeding.

• Monitor pulses, color, and sensitivities of extremities every hour.

• Have typed and crossmatched red cells and whole blood available to treat possible hemorrhage.

• Keep a laboratory flow sheet on patient's chart to monitor partial thromboplastin time, prothrombin time, hemoglobin, and hematocrit.

• Keep aminocaproic acid available to treat bleeding. Corticosteroids are used to treat allergic reactions.

• Watch for signs of hypersensitivity.

• Monitor vital signs.

• Keep venipuncture sites to a minimum; use pressure dressing on puncture sites for at least 15 minutes.

• Heparin by continuous infusion usually started within an hour after urokinase has been stopped.

• Bruising more likely during therapy; avoid unnecessary handling of patient. Side rails should be padded.

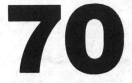

Alkylating agents

busulfan
carmustine (BCNU)
chlorambucil
cisplatin (cis-platinum)
cyclophosphamide
dacarbazine (DTIC)
lomustine (CCNU)
mechlorethamine hydrochloride
  (nitrogen mustard)
melphalan
streptozocin
thiotepa
uracil mustard

COMBINATION PRODUCTS
None.

busulfan
Myleran♦
Pregnancy Category: D

MECHANISM OF ACTION
Cross-links strands of cellular DNA, causing an imbalance of growth that leads to cell death.

INDICATIONS & DOSAGE
Chronic myelocytic (granulocytic) leukemia—
Adults: 4 to 6 mg P.O. daily up to 8 mg P.O. daily until WBC falls to 10,000/mm³; stop drug until WBC rises to 50,000/mm³, then resume treatment as before; or 4 to 8 mg P.O. daily until WBC falls to 10,000 to 20,000/mm³, then reduce daily dose as needed to maintain WBC at this level (usually 2 mg daily).
Children: 0.06 to 0.12 mg/kg or 2.3 to 4.6 mg/m²/day P.O.; adjust dose to maintain WBC at 20,000/mm³, but never less than 10,000/mm³.
Preparation for bone marrow transplantation—
Adults and children: 4 mg/kg/day for 4 days.

ADVERSE REACTIONS
Blood: WBC falling after about 10 days and continuing to fall for 2 weeks after stopping drug; *thrombocytopenia,* leukopenia, anemia.
GI: nausea, vomiting, diarrhea, cheilosis, glossitis.
GU: amenorrhea, testicular atrophy, impotence.
Metabolic: Addison-like wasting syndrome, profound hyperuricemia due to increased cell lysis.
Skin: transient hyperpigmentation, anhidrosis.
Other: gynecomastia; alopecia; *irreversible pulmonary fibrosis, commonly termed "busulfan lung."*

INTERACTIONS
None significant.

NURSING CONSIDERATIONS
• Use cautiously in patients recently given other myelosuppressive drugs or radiation treatment, and in those with depressed neutrophil or platelet count.
• Watch for signs of infection (fever, sore throat).
• Pulmonary fibrosis may be delayed for at least 4 to 6 months.
• Persistent cough and progressive dyspnea with alveolar exudate may result from drug toxicity, not pneu-

---

Italicized side effects are common or life-threatening.
*Liquid form contains alcohol.   **May contain tartrazine.

monia. Instruct patient to report symptoms so dose adjustments can be made.

• Monitor uric acid and CBC.

• Patient response usually begins within 1 to 2 weeks (increased appetite, sense of well-being, decreased total leukocyte count, reduction in size of spleen).

• Anticoagulants and aspirin products should be used cautiously. Watch closely for signs of bleeding. Instruct patient to avoid any OTC product containing aspirin.

• Avoid all I.M. injections when platelets are below 100,000/mm³.

---

carmustine (BCNU)
BiCNU♦
Pregnancy Category: D

MECHANISM OF ACTION
Cross-links strands of cellular DNA, causing an imbalance of growth that leads to cell death.

INDICATIONS & DOSAGE
Brain, colon, and stomach cancer; Hodgkin's disease; non-Hodgkin's lymphomas; melanomas; multiple myeloma; and hepatoma—
Adults: 100 mg/m² I.V. by slow infusion daily for 2 days; repeat q 6 weeks if platelets are above 100,000/mm³ and WBC is above 4,000/mm³. Dose is reduced 50% when WBC less than 2,000/mm³ and platelets less than 25,000/mm³.
Alternate therapy: 200 mg/m² I.V. slow infusion as a single dose, repeated q 6 to 8 weeks; or 40 mg/m² I.V. slow infusion for 5 consecutive days, repeated q 6 weeks.

ADVERSE REACTIONS
Blood: *cumulative bone marrow depression, delayed 4 to 6 weeks, lasting 1 to 2 weeks; leukopenia; thrombocytopenia.*
GI: *nausea, which lasts 2 to 6 hours*
after giving (can be severe); vomiting.
GU: nephrotoxicity.
Hepatic: hepatotoxicity.
Metabolic: possible hyperuricemia in lymphoma patients when rapid cell lysis occurs.
Local: *intense pain at infusion site.*
Other: *pulmonary fibrosis.*

INTERACTIONS
Cimetidine: may increase carmustine's bone marrow toxicity. Avoid combination if possible.

NURSING CONSIDERATIONS
• To reduce pain on infusion, dilute further or slow infusion rate.

• Warn patient to watch for signs of infection and bone marrow toxicity (fever, sore throat, anemia, fatigue, easy bruising, nose or gum bleeds, melena). Take temperature daily.

• Monitor CBC.

• To reduce nausea, give antiemetic before administering.

• Don't mix with other drugs during administration.

• To reconstitute, dissolve 100 mg carmustine in 3 ml absolute alcohol. Dilute solution with 17 ml sterile water for injection. Resultant solution contains 5 mg carmustine/ml in 10% alcohol. Dilute in normal saline solution or dextrose 5% in water for I.V. infusion. Give at least 250 ml over 1 to 2 hours.

• May store reconstituted solution in refrigerator for 24 hours.

• May decompose at temperatures above 80° F. (26.6° C.).

• Solution is unstable in plastic I.V. bags. Administer only in glass containers.

• If powder liquefies or appears oily, it is a sign of decomposition. Discard.

• To prevent hyperuricemia with resultant uric acid nephropathy, allopurinol may be used with adequate hydration. Monitor uric acid.

• Avoid contact with skin, as carmustine will cause a brown stain. If drug

comes into contact with skin, wash off thoroughly.
• Anticoagulants and aspirin products should be used cautiously. Watch closely for signs of bleeding. Instruct patient to avoid any OTC product containing aspirin.
• Avoid all I.M. injections when platelets are below 100,000/mm³.
• Since carmustine crosses the blood-brain barrier, it may be used to treat primary brain tumors.

chlorambucil
Leukeran♦
Pregnancy Category: D

MECHANISM OF ACTION
Cross-links strands of cellular DNA, causing an imbalance of growth that leads to cell death.

INDICATIONS & DOSAGE
Chronic lymphocytic leukemia, diffuse lymphocytic lymphoma, nodular lymphocytic lymphoma, Hodgkin's disease, ovarian carcinoma, mycosis fungoides—
Adults: 0.1 to 0.2 mg/kg P.O. daily for 3 to 6 weeks, then adjust for maintenance (usually 2 mg daily).
Children: 0.1 to 0.2 mg/kg daily or 4.5 mg/m²/day P.O. as single dose or in divided doses.

ADVERSE REACTIONS
Blood: leukopenia, delayed up to 3 weeks, lasting up to 10 days after last dose; thrombocytopenia; anemia; myelosuppression (usually moderate, gradual, and rapidly reversible).
GI: *nausea, vomiting.*
Metabolic: hyperuricemia.
Skin: *exfoliative dermatitis*, rashes.
Other: allergic febrile reactions.

INTERACTIONS
None significant.

NURSING CONSIDERATIONS
• Severe neutropenia reversible up to cumulative dose of 6.5 mg/kg in a single course.
• Monitor CBC.
• To prevent hyperuricemia with resulting uric acid nephropathy, allopurinol may be used with adequate hydration. Monitor uric acid.
• Avoid all I.M. injections when platelets are below 100,000/mm³.
• Anticoagulants and aspirin products should be used cautiously. Watch closely for signs of bleeding. Instruct patient to avoid OTC products containing aspirin.

cisplatin (cis-platinum)
Platinol♦
Pregnancy Category: D

MECHANISM OF ACTION
Cross-links strands of cellular DNA, causing an imbalance of growth that leads to cell death.

INDICATIONS & DOSAGE
Adjunctive therapy in metastatic testicular cancer—
Adults: 20 mg/m² I.V. daily for 5 days. Repeat every 3 weeks for 3 cycles or longer.
Adjunctive therapy in metastatic ovarian cancer—
100 mg/m² I.V. Repeat every 4 weeks; or 50 mg/m² I.V. every 3 weeks with concurrent doxorubicin HCl therapy. Give as I.V. infusion in 2 liters normal saline solution with 37.5 g mannitol over 6 to 8 hours.
Treatment of advanced bladder cancer—
Adults: 50 to 70 mg/m² I.V. once every 3 to 4 weeks. Patients who have received other antineoplastics or radiation therapy should receive 50 mg/m² every 4 weeks.
Note: Prehydration and mannitol diuresis may reduce renal toxicity and ototoxicity significantly.

Italicized side effects are common or life-threatening.
*Liquid form contains alcohol.   **May contain tartrazine.

ADVERSE REACTIONS
Blood: *mild myelosuppression in 25% to 30% of patients, leukopenia, thrombocytopenia,* anemia; nadirs in circulating platelets and leukocytes on days 18 to 23, with recovery by day 39.
CNS: peripheral neuritis, loss of taste, seizures.
EENT: *tinnitus, hearing loss.*
GI: *nausea, vomiting, beginning 1 to 4 hours after dose and lasting 24 hours; diarrhea;* metallic taste.
GU: *more prolonged and severe renal toxicity with repeated courses of therapy.*
Other: *anaphylactoid reaction.*

INTERACTIONS
Aminoglycoside antibiotics: additive nephrotoxicity. Monitor renal function studies very carefully.

NURSING CONSIDERATIONS
• Dose modification may be required in preexisting renal impairment, myelosuppression, or hearing impairment.
• Hydrate patient with normal saline solution before giving drug. Maintain urine output of 100 ml/hour for 4 consecutive hours before therapy and for 24 hours after therapy.
• Mannitol may be given as 12.5 g I.V. bolus before starting cisplatin infusion. Follow, if ordered, by infusion of mannitol at rate of up to 10 g/hour p.r.n. to maintain urine output during and 6 to 24 hours after cisplatin infusion.
• Do not repeat dose unless platelets are over 100,000/mm³, WBC is over 4,000/mm³, creatinine is under 1.5 mg%, or BUN is under 25 mg%.
• Monitor CBC, platelets, and renal function studies before initial and subsequent doses.
• Tell patient to report tinnitus immediately to prevent permanent hearing loss. Do audiometry prior to initial dose and subsequent courses.

• Nausea and vomiting may be severe and protracted (up to 24 hours). Antiemetics can be started 24 hours before therapy. Monitor intake and output. Continue I.V. hydration until patient can tolerate adequate oral intake.
• Delayed-onset vomiting (3 to 5 days after treatment) has been reported. Patients may need prolonged antiemetic coverage.
• Reconstitute with sterile water for injection. Stable for 24 hours in normal saline solution at room temperature. Don't refrigerate.
• Infusions are most stable in chloride-containing solutions (i.e., normal saline, 0.5 normal saline, 0.25 normal saline).
• Given with bleomycin and vinblastine for testicular cancer and with doxorubicin HCl for ovarian cancer.
• Renal toxicity is cumulative. Renal function must return to normal before next dose can be given.
• Avoid all I.M. injections when platelets are below 100,000/mm³.
• Metoclopramide has been used very effectively to treat and prevent nausea and vomiting.
• Anaphylactoid reaction usually responds to immediate treatment with epinephrine, corticosteroids, or antihistamines.

cyclophosphamide
Cytoxan♦**, Neosar, Procytox♦♦
Pregnancy Category: D

MECHANISM OF ACTION
Cross-links strands of cellular DNA, causing an imbalance of growth that leads to cell death.

INDICATIONS & DOSAGE
Breast, head, neck, lung, and ovarian; Hodgkin's disease; chronic lymphocytic leukemia; chronic myelocytic leukemia; acute lymphoblastic leukemia; neuroblastoma; retinoblastoma; non-Hodgkin's lymphomas; multiple

myeloma; mycosis fungoides; sarco mas—
Adults: 40 to 50 mg/kg P.O. or I.V. in single dose or in 2 to 5 daily doses, then adjust for maintenance; or 2 to 4 mg/kg P.O. daily for 10 days, then adjust for maintenance. Maintenance dose 1.5 to 3 mg/kg daily P.O.; or 10 to 15 mg/kg q 7 to 10 days I.V.; or 3 to 5 mg/kg twice weekly I.V.
Children: 2 to 8 mg/kg daily or 60 to 250 mg/m² daily P.O. or I.V. for 6 days (dose depends on susceptibility of neoplasm); divide oral dosages; give I.V. dosages once weekly. Maintenance dose 2 to 5 mg/kg or 50 to 150 mg/m² twice weekly P.O.

ADVERSE REACTIONS
Blood: *leukopenia,* nadir between days 8 to 15, recovery in 17 to 28 days; thrombocytopenia; anemia.
CV: *cardiotoxicity* (with very high doses and in combination with doxorubicin).
GI: anorexia; *nausea and vomiting beginning within 6 hours, lasting 4 hours;* stomatitis; mucositis.
GU: gonadal suppression (may be irreversible), *hemorrhagic cystitis,* bladder fibrosis, nephrotoxicity.
Metabolic: hyperuricemia; syndrome of inappropriate ADH secretion (with high doses).
Other: *reversible alopecia in 50% of patients, especially with high doses;* secondary malignancies, *pulmonary fibrosis (high doses).*

INTERACTIONS
Corticosteroids, chloramphenicol: reduced activity of cyclophosphamide. Use cautiously.
Succinylcholine: may cause apnea. Don't use together.

NURSING CONSIDERATIONS
• Dose modification may be required in severe leukopenia, thrombocytopenia, malignant cell infiltration of bone marrow, recent radiation therapy

or chemotherapy, or hepatic or renal disease.
• Advise both male and female patients to practice contraception while taking this drug and for 4 months after; drug is potentially teratogenic.
• Monitor CBC, renal, and hepatic functions.
• Push fluid (3 liters daily) to prevent hemorrhagic cystitis. Don't give drug at bedtime, since voiding is too infrequent to avoid cystitis. If hemorrhagic cystitis occurs, drug is stopped. Cystitis can occur months after therapy has been stopped.
• Encourage patients to void every 1 to 2 hours while awake to minimize risk of hemorrhagic cystitis.
• Lyophilized preparation is much easier to reconstitute. Request this form from the pharmacy when preparing I.V.
• Reconstituted solution is stable 6 days refrigerated or 24 hours at room temperature.
• Avoid all I.M. injections when platelets are below 100,000/mm³.
• Can be given by direct I.V. push into a running I.V. line or by infusion in normal saline solution or dextrose 5% in water.
• To prevent hyperuricemia with resulting uric acid nephropathy, keep patient well hydrated. Monitor uric acid.
• Warn patient that alopecia is likely to occur, but that it is reversible.
• Monitor for cyclophosphamide toxicity if patient's corticosteroid therapy is discontinued.
• Has been used successfully to treat many nonmalignant conditions.

dacarbazine (DTIC)
DTIC♦
Pregnancy Category: C

MECHANISM OF ACTION
Cross-links strands of cellular DNA, causing an imbalance of growth that

leads to cell death.

INDICATIONS & DOSAGE
Hodgkin's disease, metastatic malignant melanoma, neuroblastoma, sarcomas—
Adults: 2 to 4.5 mg/kg or 70 to 160 mg/m² I.V. daily for 10 days, then repeat q 4 weeks as tolerated; or 250 mg/m² I.V. daily for 5 days, repeated at 3-week intervals.

ADVERSE REACTIONS
Blood: *leukopenia and thrombocytopenia,* nadir between 3 and 4 weeks.
GI: *severe nausea and vomiting begin within 1 to 3 hours in 90% of patients, last 1 to 12 hours; anorexia.*
Local: severe pain if I.V. infiltrates or if solution is too concentrated; tissue damage.
Skin: phototoxicity.
Other: *flu-like syndrome* (fever, malaise, myalgia beginning 7 days after treatment stopped and possibly lasting 7 to 21 days), alopecia.

INTERACTIONS
None significant.

NURSING CONSIDERATIONS
• Use lower dose if renal function or bone marrow is impaired. Stop drug if WBC falls to 3,000/mm³ or platelets drop to 100,000/mm³. Monitor CBC.
• Take temperature daily. Observe for signs of infection.
• Monitor uric acid.
• Discard refrigerated solution after 72 hours, room temperature solution after 8 hours.
• Avoid all I.M. injections when platelets are below 100,000/mm³.
• Give I.V. infusion in 50 to 100 ml dextrose 5% in water over 30 minutes. May dilute further or slow infusion to decrease pain at infusion site. Make sure drug does not infiltrate.
• If I.V. infiltrates, discontinue immediately and apply ice to area for 24 to 48 hours.

• During infusion, protect bag from direct sunlight to avoid possible drug breakdown.
• For Hodgkin's disease, usually given with bleomycin, vinblastine, doxorubicin.
• Advise patient to avoid sunlight and sunlamps for first 2 days after treatment.
• Anticoagulants and aspirin products should be used cautiously. Watch closely for signs of bleeding. Instruct patient to avoid OTC products containing aspirin.
• Administering antiemetics before giving dacarbazine may help decrease nausea. Nausea and vomiting may sometimes subside after several doses.
• Reassure patient that flulike syndrome may be treated with mild antipyretics such as acetaminophen.

lomustine (CCNU)
CeeNU♦
Pregnancy Category: D

MECHANISM OF ACTION
Cross-links strands of cellular DNA, causing an imbalance of growth that leads to cell death.

INDICATIONS & DOSAGE
Brain, colon, lung, and renal cell cancer; Hodgkin's disease; lymphomas; melanomas; multiple myeloma—
Adults and children: 130 mg/m² P.O. as single dose q 6 weeks. Reduce dose according to bone marrow depression. Repeat doses should not be given until WBC is more than 4,000/mm³ and platelet count is more than 100,000/ mm³.

ADVERSE REACTIONS
Blood: *leukopenia, delayed up to 6 weeks, lasting 1 to 2 weeks; thrombocytopenia, delayed up to 4 weeks, lasting 1 to 2 weeks.*
GI: *nausea and vomiting beginning*

within 4 to 5 hours, lasting 24 hours; stomatitis.
GU: nephrotoxicity, progressive azotemia.

INTERACTIONS
None significant.

NURSING CONSIDERATIONS
• Dose modification may be required in patients with decreased platelets, leukocytes, or erythrocytes.
• Give 2 to 4 hours after meals. Lomustine will be more completely absorbed if taken when the stomach is empty. To avoid nausea, give antiemetic before administering.
• May be useful in cancer involving CNS, since CSF level equals 30% to 50% of plasma level 1 hour after administration.
• Monitor CBC weekly. Usually not administered more often than every 6 weeks; bone marrow toxicity is cumulative and delayed.
• Monitor uric acid.
• Avoid all I.M. injections when platelets are below 100,000/mm³.
• Anticoagulants and aspirin products should be used cautiously. Watch closely for signs of bleeding. Instruct patient to avoid OTC products containing aspirin.
• Since lomustine crosses the blood-brain barrier, it may be used to treat primary brain tumors.

---

mechlorethamine hydrochloride (nitrogen mustard)
Mustargen♦
Pregnancy Category: D

MECHANISM OF ACTION
Cross-links strands of cellular DNA, causing an imbalance of growth that leads to cell death.

INDICATIONS & DOSAGE
Breast, lung, and ovarian cancer;

Hodgkin's disease; non-Hodgkin's lymphomas; diffuse lymphocytic lymphoma—
Adults: 0.4 mg/kg or 10 mg/m² I.V. as single or divided dose q 3 to 6 weeks. Give through running I.V. infusion. Dose reduced in prior radiation or chemotherapy to 0.2 to 0.4 mg/kg. Dose based on ideal or actual body weight, whichever is less.
Neoplastic effusions—
Adults: 10 to 20 mg intracavitarily.

ADVERSE REACTIONS
Blood: *nadir of myelosuppression occurring by days 4 to 10, lasting 10 to 21 days;* mild anemia begins in 2 to 3 weeks, possibly lasting 7 weeks.
EENT: tinnitus; *metallic taste* (immediately after dose); deafness in high doses.
GI: *nausea, vomiting, and anorexia* begin within minutes, last 8 to 24 hours.
Metabolic: hyperuricemia.
Local: *thrombophlebitis, sloughing, severe irritation if drug extravasates or touches skin.*
Other: *alopecia*, may precipitate herpes zoster.

INTERACTIONS
None significant.

NURSING CONSIDERATIONS
• Dose modification may be required in severe anemia, depressed neutrophil or platelet count, or patients recently treated with radiation or chemotherapy. Monitor CBC.
• Avoid contact with skin or mucous membranes. Wear gloves when preparing solution to prevent accidental skin contact. If contact occurs, wash with copious amounts of water.
• Be sure I.V. doesn't infiltrate. If drug extravasates, apply cold compresses and infiltrate the area with isotonic sodium thiosulfate.
• When given intracavitarily for sclerosing effect, turn patient from side to

side every 15 minutes to 1 hour to distribute drug.
• Very unstable solution. Prepare immediately before infusion. Use within 15 minutes. Discard unused solution.
• To prevent hyperuricemia with resulting uric acid nephropathy, allopurinol may be given; keep patient well hydrated. Monitor uric acid.
• Avoid all I.M. injections when platelets are below 100,000/mm³.
• Anticoagulants and aspirin products should be used cautiously. Watch closely for signs of bleeding. Instruct patient to avoid OTC products containing aspirin.

melphalan
Alkeran♦
Pregnancy Category: D

MECHANISM OF ACTION
Cross-links strands of cellular DNA, causing an imbalance of growth that leads to cell death.

INDICATIONS & DOSAGE
Multiple myeloma, malignant melanoma, testicular seminoma, reticulum cell sarcoma, osteogenic sarcoma, breast cancer—
Adults: 6 mg P.O. daily for 2 to 3 weeks, then stop drug for up to 4 weeks or until WBC and platelets stop dropping and begin to rise again; resume with maintenance dose of 2 to 4 mg daily. Stop drug if WBC below 3,000/mm³ or platelets below 100,000/mm³. Alternate therapy: 0.15 mg/kg daily P.O. for 7 days, wait for WBC and platelets to recover, then resume with 0.05 mg/kg daily P.O.
Nonresectable advanced ovarian cancer—
Adults: 0.2 mg/kg daily, P.O. in divided doses, for 5 days. Repeat every 4 weeks, depending on bone marrow recovery.

ADVERSE REACTIONS
Blood: *thrombocytopenia, leukopenia, agranulocytosis.*
Other: *pneumonitis and pulmonary fibrosis.*

INTERACTIONS
None significant.

NURSING CONSIDERATIONS
• Not recommended in severe leukopenia, thrombocytopenia, or anemia; or in chronic lymphocytic leukemia.
• Monitor uric acid, CBC.
• Avoid all I.M. injections when platelets are below 100,000/mm³.
• May need dose reduction in renal impairment.
• Drug of choice in multiple myeloma in combination with prednisone.
• Anticoagulants and aspirin products should be used cautiously. Watch closely for signs of bleeding. Instruct patient to avoid OTC products containing aspirin.
• Administer on empty stomach, because absorption is decreased by food.

streptozocin
Zanosar♦
Pregnancy Category: C

MECHANISM OF ACTION
Cross-links strands of cellular DNA, causing an imbalance of growth that leads to cell death.

INDICATIONS & DOSAGE
Treatment of metastatic islet cell carcinoma of the pancreas; colon cancer; exocrine pancreatic tumors; and carcinoid tumors—
Adults and children: 500 mg/m² I.V. for 5 consecutive days every 6 weeks until maximum benefit or until toxicity is observed. Alternatively, 1,000 mg/m² at weekly intervals for the first 2 weeks. Don't exceed a single dose of 1,500 mg/m².

ADVERSE REACTIONS
Blood: *leukopenia, thrombocytopenia.*
GI: *nausea, vomiting,* diarrhea.
Hepatic: elevated liver enzymes.
Metabolic: hyperglycemia and hypoglycemia.
Renal: *renal toxicity (evidenced by azotemia, glycosuria, and renal tubular acidosis),* mild proteinuria.

INTERACTIONS
Other potentially nephrotoxic drugs such as aminoglycosides: increased risk of renal toxicity. Use cautiously.
Phenytoin: may decrease the effects of streptozocin. Monitor carefully.

NURSING CONSIDERATIONS
• Dose modification may be required in patients with preexisting renal or hepatic disease.
• Renal toxicity resulting from streptozocin therapy is dose-related and cumulative. Monitor renal function before and after each course of therapy. Urinalysis, BUN, creatinine, serum electrolytes and creatinine clearance should be obtained before, and at least weekly during, drug administration. Weekly monitoring should continue for 4 weeks after each course.
• Mild proteinuria is one of the first signs of renal toxicity. Make sure doctor is aware if and when this occurs. The dose of the drug may have to be reduced.
• Test urine for protein and glucose each nursing shift.
• Monitor CBC and liver function studies at least weekly.
• Nausea and vomiting occurs in almost *all* patients. Make sure patient is being treated with an antiemetic.
• Reconstitute the streptozocin powder with 0.9% sodium chloride injection. This will produce a pale gold solution.
• Best to use within 12 hours of reconstitution. However, drug will remain stable for at least 48 hours, especially if kept refrigerated.
• The product contains no preservatives and is not intended as a multiple-dose vial.
• When preparing the solution, wear gloves to protect the skin from contact.
• Unopened and unreconstituted vials of streptozocin should be stored in the refrigerator.

---

thiotepa
Thiotepa♦
Pregnancy Category: D

MECHANISM OF ACTION
Cross-links strands of cellular DNA, causing an imbalance of growth that leads to cell death.

INDICATIONS & DOSAGE
Adults and children over 12 years:
Breast, lung, and ovarian cancer; Hodgkin's disease; lymphomas—
0.2 mg/kg I.V. daily for 5 days; then maintenance dose of 0.2 mg/kg I.V. q 1 to 3 weeks.
Bladder tumor—
60 mg in 60 ml water instilled in bladder once weekly for 4 weeks.
Neoplastic effusions—
10 to 15 mg intracavitarily, p.r.n. Stop drug or decrease dosage if WBC below 4,000/mm^3 or if platelets below 150,000/mm^3.

ADVERSE REACTIONS
Blood: *leukopenia begins within 5 to 30 days; thrombocytopenia; neutropenia.*
GI: *nausea, vomiting.*
GU: amenorrhea, decreased spermatogenesis.
Metabolic: hyperuricemia.
Skin: hives, rash.
Local: intense pain at administration site.
Other: headache, fever, tightness of throat, dizziness.

Italicized side effects are common or life-threatening.
*Liquid form contains alcohol.   **May contain tartrazine.

INTERACTIONS
None significant.

NURSING CONSIDERATIONS
• Use cautiously in bone marrow depression and renal or hepatic dysfunction.
• Monitor CBC weekly for at least 3 weeks after last dose. Warn patient to report even mild infections.
• GU adverse reactions reversible in 6 to 8 months.
• May require use of local anesthetic at injection site if intense pain occurs.
• For bladder instillation: dehydrate patient 8 to 10 hours before therapy. Instill drug into bladder by catheter; ask patient to retain solution for 2 hours. Volume may be reduced to 30 ml if discomfort is too great with 60 ml. Reposition patient every 15 minutes for maximum area contact.
• Toxicity delayed and prolonged because drug binds to tissues and stays in body several hours.
• Refrigerate dry powder; protect from light.
• Use only sterile water for injection to reconstitute. Refrigerated solution stable 5 days.
• To prevent hyperuricemia with resulting uric acid nephropathy, allopurinol may be given; keep patient well hydrated. Monitor uric acid.
• Avoid all I.M. injections when platelets are below 100,000/mm³.
• Can be given by all parenteral routes, including direct injection into the tumor.
• Anticoagulants and aspirin products should be used cautiously. Watch closely for signs of bleeding. Instruct patient to avoid OTC products containing aspirin.

uracil mustard
Pregnancy Category: X

MECHANISM OF ACTION
Cross-links strands of cellular DNA, causing an imbalance of growth that leads to cell death.

INDICATIONS & DOSAGE
Chronic lymphocytic and myelocytic leukemia; Hodgkin's disease; non-Hodgkin's lymphomas of the histiocytic and lymphocytic types; reticulum cell sarcoma; lymphomas; mycosis fungoides; polycythemia vera; cancer of ovaries, cervix, and lungs—
Adults: 1 to 2 mg P.O. daily for 3 months or until desired response or toxicity; maintenance 1 mg daily for 3 out of 4 weeks until optimum response or relapse; or 3 to 5 mg P.O. for 7 days not to exceed total dose of 0.5 mg/kg, then 1 mg daily until response, then 1 mg daily 3 out of 4 weeks.

ADVERSE REACTIONS
Blood: bone marrow depression, delayed 2 to 4 weeks; *thrombocytopenia; leukopenia;* anemia.
CNS: irritability, nervousness, mental cloudiness, and depression.
GI: *nausea, vomiting, diarrhea, epigastric distress,* abdominal pain, anorexia.
Metabolic: hyperuricemia.
Skin: pruritus, dermatitis, hyperpigmentation, alopecia.

INTERACTIONS
None significant.

NURSING CONSIDERATIONS
• Dose modification may be required in severe thrombocytopenia, aplastic anemia or leukopenia, or acute leukemia.
• Give at bedtime to reduce nausea.
• Watch for signs of ecchymoses, easy bruising, petechiae.
• Monitor regular platelet count. Do CBC one to two times weekly for 4 weeks; then 4 weeks after stopping drug.
• To prevent hyperuricemia and resulting uric acid nephropathy, allopu-

rinol can be given; keep patient hydrated. Monitor uric acid.
• Avoid all I.M. injections when platelets are below 100,000/mm³.
• Anticoagulants and aspirin products should be used cautiously. Watch closely for signs of bleeding. Instruct patient to avoid OTC products containing aspirin.

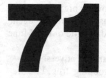

Antimetabolites

cytarabine (ARA-C, cytosine arabinoside)
floxuridine
fluorouracil (5-fluorouracil)
hydroxyurea
mercaptopurine (6-MP)
methotrexate
methotrexate sodium
thioguanine (6-TG)

COMBINATION PRODUCTS
None.

cytarabine (ARA-C, cytosine arabinoside)
Cytosar-U♦
Pregnancy Category: D

MECHANISM OF ACTION
Inhibits pyrimidine synthesis.

INDICATIONS & DOSAGE
Acute myelocytic and other acute leukemias—
Adults and children: 200 mg/m^2 daily by continuous I.V. infusion for 5 days; or 10 to 30 mg/m^2 intrathecally, up to 3 times weekly.

ADVERSE REACTIONS
CNS: neurotoxicity with high doses.
Blood: WBC nadir 5 to 7 days after drug stopped; *leukopenia,* anemia, *thrombocytopenia,* reticulocytopenia; platelet nadir occurring on day 10; *megaloblastosis.*
GI: *nausea, vomiting,* diarrhea, dysphagia; reddened area at juncture of lips, followed by sore mouth, oral ulcers in 5 to 10 days; high dose given via rapid I.V. may cause projectile vomiting.
EENT: *keratitis.*
Hepatic: hepatotoxicity (usually mild and reversible).
Metabolic: hyperuricemia.
Skin: rash.
Other: flulike syndrome.

INTERACTIONS
None significant.

NURSING CONSIDERATIONS
• Dose modification may be required in thrombocytopenia, leukopenia, renal or hepatic disease, and after other chemotherapy or radiation therapy.
• Watch for signs of infection (cough, fever, sore throat). Monitor CBC.
• Excellent mouth care can help prevent oral adverse reactions.
• Nausea and vomiting more frequent when large doses are administered rapidly by I.V. push. These reactions are less frequent with infusion. To reduce nausea, give antiemetic before administering.
• Steroid eye drops are prescribed to prevent drug-induced keratitis.
• Monitor intake/output carefully. Maintain high fluid intake and give allopurinol, if ordered, to avoid urate nephropathy in leukemia induction therapy. Monitor uric acid.
• Monitor hepatic function.
• Use preservative-free normal saline or Elliot's B solution for intrathecal use.
• Optimum schedule is continuous infusion.

- Reconstituted solution is stable for 48 hours. Discard cloudy reconstituted solution.
- Avoid I.M. injections of any drugs in patients with severely depressed platelet count (thrombocytopenia) to prevent bleeding.
- Modify or discontinue therapy if polymorphonuclear granulocyte count is 1,000/mm³ or if platelet count is 50,000/mm³.
- Assess patients receiving high doses for cerebellar dysfunction.

floxuridine
FUDR
Pregnancy Category: D

MECHANISM OF ACTION
Inhibits pyrimidine synthesis.

INDICATIONS & DOSAGE
Brain, breast, head, neck, liver, gallbladder, and bile duct cancer—
Adults: 0.1 to 0.6 mg/kg daily by intraarterial infusion (use pump for continuous, uniform rate); or 0.4 to 0.6 mg/kg daily into hepatic artery.

ADVERSE REACTIONS
Blood: *leukopenia, anemia,* thrombocytopenia.
CNS: cerebellar ataxia, vertigo, nystagmus, convulsions, depression, hemiplegia, hiccups, lethargy.
EENT: blurred vision.
GI: *stomatitis, cramps, nausea, vomiting, diarrhea, bleeding, enteritis.*
Hepatic: cholangitis, jaundice, elevated liver enzymes.
Skin: *erythema,* dermatitis, pruritus, rash.

INTERACTIONS
None significant.

NURSING CONSIDERATIONS
- Dose modification may be required in poor nutritional state, bone marrow depression, or serious infection. Use

cautiously following high-dose pelvic irradiation or use of alkylating agent, and in impaired hepatic or renal function.
- Severe skin and GI adverse reactions require stopping drug. Use of antacid eases but probably won't prevent GI distress.
- Excellent mouth care can help prevent oral adverse reactions.
- Monitor intake/output, CBC, and renal and hepatic function.
- Discontinue if WBC falls below 3,500/mm³ or if platelet count below 100,000/mm³.
- Therapeutic effect may be delayed 1 to 6 weeks. Make sure patient is aware of time it may take for improvement to be noted.
- Reconstitute with sterile water for injection. Dilute further in dextrose 5% in water or normal saline solution for actual infusion.
- Avoid I.M. injections of any drugs in patients with thrombocytopenia to prevent bleeding.
- Refrigerated solution stable no more than 2 weeks.
- Observe arterial perfused area. Check line for bleeding, blockage, displacement, or leakage.
- Often administered via hepatic arterial infusion in treatment of hepatic metastases.

fluorouracil (5-fluorouracil)
Adrucil♦, 5-FU
Pregnancy Category: D

MECHANISM OF ACTION
Inhibits pyrimidine synthesis.

INDICATIONS & DOSAGE
Colon, rectal, breast, ovarian, cervical, bladder, liver, and pancreatic cancer—
Adults: 12.5 mg/kg I.V. daily for 3 to 5 days q 4 weeks; or 15 mg/kg weekly for 6 weeks. (Doses recommended

---

Italicized side effects are common or life-threatening.
*Liquid form contains alcohol.   **May contain tartrazine.

based on lean body weight.) Maximum single recommended dose is 800 mg, although higher single doses (up to 1.5 g) have been used. The injectable form has been given orally but is not recommended.

ADVERSE REACTIONS
CNS: acute cerebellar syndrome.
Blood: *leukopenia,* thrombocytopenia, anemia. WBC nadir 9 to 14 days after first dose; platelet nadir in 7 to 14 days.
GI: *stomatitis, GI ulcer may precede leukopenia, nausea, vomiting in 30% to 50% of patients; diarrhea.*
Skin: *dermatitis,* hyperpigmentation (especially in blacks), nail changes, pigmented palmar creases.
Other: *reversible alopecia in 5% to 20% of patients, weakness, malaise.*

INTERACTIONS
None significant.

NURSING CONSIDERATIONS
• Use cautiously following major surgery; when patient is in poor nutritional state; or with serious infections and bone marrow depression. Use cautiously following high-dose pelvic irradiation or use of alkylating agents, in impaired hepatic or renal function, or in widespread neoplastic infiltration of bone marrow.
• Watch for stomatitis or diarrhea (signs of toxicity). May use topical oral anesthetic to soothe lesions. Discontinue if diarrhea occurs.
• Encourage good and frequent oral hygiene to prevent superinfection of denuded mucosa.
• Give antiemetic before administering to reduce nausea.
• Do WBC and platelet counts daily. Drug should be stopped when WBC is less than 3,500/mm³. Watch for ecchymoses, petechiae, easy bruising, and anemia. Drug should be stopped if platelet count is less than 100,000/mm³.

• Dermatologic side effects reversible when drug is stopped. Patient should use highly protective sun blockers to avoid inflammatory erythematous dermatitis.
• Therapeutic concentrations don't reach cerebrospinal fluid.
• Slowing infusion rate so it takes from 2 to 8 hours lessens toxicity.
• Monitor intake/output, CBC, and renal and hepatic functions.
• Don't refrigerate fluorouracil.
• Don't use cloudy solution. If crystals form, redissolve by warming.
• Solution is more stable in plastic I.V. bags than in glass bottles. Use plastic I.V. containers for administering continuous infusions.
• Sometimes ordered as 5-FU. The numeral 5 is part of the drug name and should not be confused with dosage units.
• Sometimes administered via hepatic arterial infusion in treatment of hepatic metastases.
• Warn patient that alopecia may occur but is reversible.
• To prevent bleeding, avoid I.M. injections of any drugs in patients with thrombocytopenia.
• Fluorouracil toxicity may be delayed for 1 to 3 weeks.

hydroxyurea
Hydrea**♦
Pregnancy Category: D

MECHANISM OF ACTION
Inhibits ribonucleotide reductase.

INDICATIONS & DOSAGE
Melanoma; resistant chronic myelocytic leukemia; recurrent, metastatic, or inoperable ovarian cancer—
Adults: 80 mg/kg P.O. as single dose q 3 days; or 20 to 30 mg/kg P.O. daily.

ADVERSE REACTIONS
Blood: *leukopenia,* thrombocytopenia, anemia, *megaloblastosis; dose-*

limiting and dose-related bone marrow depression, with rapid recovery.
CNS: drowsiness, hallucinations.
GI: *anorexia, nausea, vomiting, diarrhea,* stomatitis.
GU: increased BUN, serum creatinine levels.
Metabolic: hyperuricemia.
Skin: rash, pruritus.

INTERACTIONS
None significant.

NURSING CONSIDERATIONS
• Dose modification may be required following other chemotherapy or radiation therapy.
• Use with caution in renal dysfunction. Discontinue if WBC is less than 2,500/mm³ or if platelet count is less than 100,000/mm³.
• If patient can't swallow capsule, he may empty contents into water and take immediately.
• Monitor intake/output; keep patient hydrated.
• Routinely measure BUN, uric acid, serum creatinine.
• Drug crosses blood-brain barrier.
• Auditory and visual hallucinations and blood toxicity increase when decreased renal function exists.
• May exacerbate postirradiation erythema.
• Avoid all I.M. injections when platelets are below 100,000/mm³.

mercaptopurine (6-MP)
Purinethol♦
Pregnancy Category: D

MECHANISM OF ACTION
Inhibits purine synthesis.

INDICATIONS & DOSAGE
Acute lymphoblastic leukemia (in children), acute myeloblastic leukemia, chronic myelocytic leukemia—
Adults: 80 to 100 mg/m² P.O. daily as a single dose up to 5 mg/kg daily.

Children: 70 mg/m² P.O. daily.
Usual maintenance for adults and children: 1.5 to 2.5 mg/kg daily.

ADVERSE REACTIONS
Blood: *decreased RBC; leukopenia, thrombocytopenia, and anemia; all may persist several days after drug is stopped.*
GI: *nausea, vomiting, and anorexia in 25% of patients;* painful oral ulcers.
Hepatic: *jaundice, hepatic necrosis.*
Metabolic: hyperuricemia.

INTERACTIONS
Allopurinol: slowed inactivation of mercaptopurine. Decrease mercaptopurine to ¼ or ⅓ normal dose.

NURSING CONSIDERATIONS
• Dose modifications may be required following chemotherapy or radiation therapy, in depressed neutrophil or platelet count, and in impaired hepatic or renal function.
• Observe for signs of bleeding and infection.
• Hepatic dysfunction reversible when drug is stopped. Watch for jaundice, clay-colored stools, frothy dark urine. Drug should be stopped if hepatic tenderness occurs.
• Do weekly blood counts; watch for precipitous fall.
• Monitor intake/output. Push fluids (3 liters daily).
• Sometimes ordered as 6-mercaptopurine or 6-MP. The numeral 6 is part of drug name and does not signify number of dosage units.
• Warn patient that improvement may take 2 to 4 weeks or longer.
• GI adverse reactions less common in children than in adults.
• Avoid all I.M. injections when platelets are below 100,000/mm³.
• Monitor serum uric acid. If allopurinol is necessary, use very cautiously.

Italicized side effects are common or life-threatening.
*Liquid form contains alcohol.   **May contain tartrazine.

methotrexate

methotrexate sodium

Folex, Mexate
Pregnancy Category: D

MECHANISM OF ACTION
Prevents reduction of folic acid to tetrahydrofolate by binding to dihydrofolate reductase.

INDICATIONS & DOSAGE
Trophoblastic tumors (choriocarcinoma, hydatidiform mole)—
Adults: 15 to 30 mg P.O. or I.M. daily for 5 days. Repeat after 1 or more weeks, according to response or toxicity.
Acute lymphoblastic and lymphatic leukemia—
Adults and children: 3.3 mg/m^2 P.O., I.M., or I.V. daily for 4 to 6 weeks or until remission occurs; then 20 to 30 mg/m^2 P.O. or I.M. twice weekly.
Meningeal leukemia—
Adults and children: 10 to 15 mg/m^2 intrathecally q 2 to 5 days until cerebrospinal fluid is normal. Use only 20-, 50-, or 100-mg vials of powder with no preservatives; dilute using 0.9% NaCl injection *without* preservatives or Elliot's B solution. Use only new vials of drug and diluent. Use immediately.
Burkitt's lymphoma (Stage I or Stage II)—
Adults: 10 to 25 mg P.O. daily for 4 to 8 days with 1-week rest intervals.
Lymphosarcoma (Stage III)—
Adults: 0.625 to 2.5 mg/kg daily P.O., I.M., or I.V.
Mycosis fungoides—
Adults: 2.5 to 10 mg P.O. daily or 50 mg I.M. weekly; or 25 mg I.M. twice weekly.
Psoriasis—
Adults: 10 to 25 mg P.O., I.M., or I.V. as single weekly dose.

ADVERSE REACTIONS
Blood: WBC and platelet nadir occurring on day 7; anemia, *leukopenia, thrombocytopenia* (all dose-related).
CNS: *arachnoiditis within hours of intrathecal use;* subacute neurotoxicity which may begin a few weeks later; necrotizing demyelinating leukoencephalopathy a few years later.
GI: *stomatitis; diarrhea leading to hemorrhagic enteritis and intestinal perforation; nausea; vomiting.*
GU: *tubular necrosis.*
Hepatic: hepatic dysfunction leading to cirrhosis or hepatic fibrosis.
Metabolic: hyperuricemia.
Skin: exposure to sun may aggravate psoriatic lesions, rash, photosensitivity.
Other: alopecia; *pulmonary interstitial infiltrates;* long-term use in children may cause osteoporosis.

INTERACTIONS
Probenecid, phenylbutazone, salicylates, sulfonamides: increased methotrexate toxicity; don't use together if possible.

NURSING CONSIDERATIONS
• Dose modification may be required in impaired hepatic or renal function, bone marrow depression, aplasia, leukopenia, thrombocytopenia, or anemia. Use cautiously in infection, peptic ulcer, ulcerative colitis, and in very young, old, or debilitated patients.
• Warn patient to avoid conception during and immediately after therapy because of possible abortion or congenital anomalies.
• GI adverse reactions may require stopping drug.
• Rash, redness, or ulcerations in mouth or pulmonary adverse reactions may signal serious complications.
• Monitor uric acid.
• Monitor intake/output daily. Force fluids (2 to 3 liters daily).

• Alkalinize urine by giving NaHCO₃ tablets to prevent precipitation of drug, especially with high doses. Maintain urine pH at more than 6.5. Reduce dose if BUN 20 to 30 mg% or creatinine 1.2 to 2 mg%. Stop drug if BUN more than 30 mg% or creatinine more than 2 mg%.
• Watch for increases in SGOT, SGPT, alkaline phosphatase; may signal hepatic dysfunction.
• Watch for bleeding (especially GI) and infection.
• Warn patient to use highly protective sun screening agent when exposed to sunlight.
• Take temperature daily, and watch for cough, dyspnea, and cyanosis.
• Leucovorin rescue is necessary with high dose protocols (greater than 100-mg doses). Don't confuse with folic acid. This rescue technique is effective against systemic toxicity but does not interfere with the tumor cells' absorption of the methotrexate.
• Avoid all I.M. injections in patients with thrombocytopenia.
• Teach patient good oral care to prevent superinfection of oral cavity.
• Has been used investigationally to treat rheumatoid arthritis that is refractory to other therapy.

thioguanine (6-TG)
Lanvis♦♦
Pregnancy Category: D

MECHANISM OF ACTION
Inhibits purine synthesis.

INDICATIONS & DOSAGE
Acute leukemia, chronic granulocytic leukemia—
Adults and children: initially, 2 mg/kg daily P.O. (usually calculated to nearest 20 mg); then increased gradually to 3 mg/kg daily if no toxic effects occur.

ADVERSE REACTIONS
Blood: *leukopenia,* anemia, *thrombocytopenia* (occurs slowly over 2 to 4 weeks).
GI: nausea, vomiting, stomatitis, diarrhea, anorexia.
Hepatic: hepatotoxicity, jaundice.
Metabolic: hyperuricemia.

INTERACTIONS
None significant.

NURSING CONSIDERATIONS
• Dose modification may be required in renal or hepatic dysfunction.
• Stop drug if hepatotoxicity or hepatic tenderness occurs. Watch for jaundice; may reverse if drug stopped promptly.
• Do CBC during induction, then weekly during maintenance therapy.
• Monitor serum uric acid.
• Sometimes ordered as 6-thioguanine. The numeral 6 is part of drug name and does not signify dosage units.
• Avoid all I.M. injections when platelets are below 100,000/mm³.

Italicized side effects are common or life-threatening.
*Liquid form contains alcohol.   **May contain tartrazine.

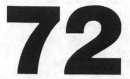

Antibiotic antineoplastic agents

bleomycin sulfate
dactinomycin (actinomycin D)
daunorubicin hydrochloride
doxorubicin hydrochloride
mitomycin
plicamycin (mithramycin)
procarbazine hydrochloride

COMBINATION PRODUCTS
None.

---

bleomycin sulfate
Blenoxane♦
Pregnancy Category: D

MECHANISM OF ACTION
Inhibits deoxyribonucleic acid (DNA) synthesis and causes scission of single- and double-stranded DNA.

INDICATIONS & DOSAGE
Dosage and indications may vary. Check patient's protocol with doctor.
Cervical, esophageal, head, neck, and testicular cancer—
Adults: 10 to 20 units/m² I.V., I.M., or S.C. 1 or 2 times weekly to total 300 to 400 units.
Hodgkin's disease—
Adults: 10 to 20 units/m² I.V., I.M., or S.C. 1 or 2 times weekly. After 50% response, maintenance 1 unit I.M. or I.V. daily or 5 units I.M. or I.V. weekly.
Lymphomas—
Adults: first 2 doses should be 5 units or less, and patient should be monitored for any allergic reaction. If no reaction occurs, then follow above dosing schedule.

ADVERSE REACTIONS
CNS: hyperesthesia of scalp and fingers, headache.
GI: *stomatitis, prolonged anorexia in 13% of patients, nausea, vomiting,* diarrhea.
Skin: *erythema, vesiculation, and hardening and discoloration of palmar and plantar skin in 8% of patients;* desquamation of hands, feet, and pressure areas; *hyperpigmentation; acne.*
Other: *reversible alopecia,* swelling of interphalangeal joints, *pulmonary fibrosis in 10% of patients, pulmonary adverse reactions (fine rales, fever, dyspnea), leukocytosis and nonproductive cough, allergic reaction (fever up to 106° F. [41.1° C.] with chills up to 5 hours after injection; anaphylaxis in 1% to 6% of patients).*

INTERACTIONS
None significant.

NURSING CONSIDERATIONS
• Use cautiously in renal or pulmonary impairment.
• Drug concentrates in keratin of squamous epithelium. To prevent linear streaking, don't use adhesive dressings on skin.
• Allergic reactions may be delayed for several hours, especially in lymphoma.
• Monitor chest X-ray and listen to lungs.
• Pulmonary function tests should be performed to establish baseline. Drug should be stopped if pulmonary function test shows a marked decline.

• Pulmonary adverse reactions common in patients over age 70. Fatal pulmonary fibrosis occurs in 1% of patients, especially when cumulative dose exceeds 400 units.
• Advise patient that alopecia may occur, but that it is usually reversible.
• Refrigerated, reconstituted solution stable 4 weeks; at room temperature, stable 2 weeks.
• Bleomycin-induced fever is common and may be treated with antipyretics. This reaction usually occurs within 3 to 6 hours of administration.
• Refrigerate unopened vials containing dry powder.

dactinomycin (actinomycin D)

Cosmegen♦
Pregnancy Category: C

MECHANISM OF ACTION
Interferes with DNA-dependent ribonucleic acid (RNA) synthesis by intercalation.

INDICATIONS & DOSAGE
Dosage and indications may vary. Check patient's protocol with doctor.
Melanomas, sarcomas, trophoblastic tumors in women, testicular cancer—
Adults: 500 mcg I.V. daily for 5 days; wait 2 to 4 weeks and repeat; or 2 mg I.V. single weekly dose for 3 weeks; wait for bone marrow recovery, then repeat in 3 to 4 weeks.
Wilms' tumor, rhabdomyosarcoma, Ewing's sarcoma—
Children: 15 mcg/kg I.V. daily for 5 days. Maximum dose 500 mcg daily. Wait for marrow recovery.

ADVERSE REACTIONS
Blood: anemia, *leukopenia, thrombocytopenia, pancytopenia.*
GI: *anorexia, nausea, vomiting,* abdominal pain, diarrhea, *stomatitis.*
Skin: *erythema;* desquamation; *hyperpigmentation of skin, especially in previously irradiated areas; acne-like eruptions (reversible).*
Local: phlebitis, severe damage to soft tissue.
Other: reversible alopecia.

INTERACTIONS
None significant.

NURSING CONSIDERATIONS
• Contraindicated in renal, hepatic, or bone marrow impairment.
• Stomatitis, diarrhea, leukopenia, thrombocytopenia may require modifying dosage and schedule.
• Give antiemetic before administering to reduce nausea.
• Monitor renal, hepatic functions.
• Monitor CBC daily and platelet counts frequently.
• Observe for signs of bleeding.
• Warn patient that alopecia may occur but is usually reversible.
• Use only sterile water (without preservatives) as diluent for injection.
• Administer through a running I.V. with good blood return. If infiltration occurs, apply cold compresses to area.

daunorubicin hydrochloride

Cerubidine♦
Pregnancy Category: D

MECHANISM OF ACTION
Interferes with DNA-dependent ribonucleic acid (RNA) synthesis by intercalation.

INDICATIONS & DOSAGE
Dosage and indications may vary. Check patient's protocol with doctor.
Remission induction in acute nonlymphocytic leukemia (myelogenous, monocytic, erythroid) in adults—
As a single agent: 60 mg/m^2 daily I.V. on days 1, 2, and 3 q 3 to 4 weeks.
In combination: 45 mg/m^2 daily I.V. on days 1, 2, and 3 of the first course and on days 1 and 2 of subsequent

courses with cytosine arabinoside infusions.
Note: Dose should be reduced if hepatic function is impaired.

ADVERSE REACTIONS
Blood: *bone marrow depression* (lowest blood counts 10 to 14 days after administration).
CV: *irreversible cardiomyopathy (dose-related), EKG changes, arrhythmias,* pericarditis, myocarditis.
GI: *nausea, vomiting, stomatitis, esophagitis,* anorexia, diarrhea.
GU: nephrotoxicity, transient red urine.
Hepatic: hepatotoxicity.
Skin: rash.
Local: *severe cellulitis or tissue slough if drug extravasates.*
Other: *generalized alopecia,* fever, chills.

INTERACTIONS
Heparin: don't mix. May form a precipitate.

NURSING CONSIDERATIONS
• Use cautiously in myelosuppression, impaired cardiac, renal, and liver function.
• Stop drug immediately in signs of congestive heart failure or cardiomyopathy. Prevent by limiting cumulative dose to 550 mg/m²; 450 mg/m² when patient has been receiving radiation therapy that encompasses the heart or any other cardiotoxic agent, such as cyclophosphamide.
• Monitor EKG before treatment, monthly during therapy.
• Note if resting pulse rate is high (a sign of cardiac adverse reactions).
• *Avoid extravasation;* inject into tubing of freely flowing I.V. *Never* give I.M. or subcutaneously. If extravasation occurs, discontinue I.V. immediately and apply ice to area for 24 to 48 hours.
• Monitor CBC and hepatic function.
• Warn patient that urine may be red

for 1 to 2 days and that it's a normal side effect, not hematuria.
• Advise patient that alopecia may occur, but that it's usually reversible.
• Nausea and vomiting may be very severe and last 24 to 48 hours.
• Reconstituted solution is stable for 24 hours at room temperature or 48 hours refrigerated. Optimally, use within 8 hours of preparation.
• Reddish color looks very similar to doxorubicin (Adriamycin). *Do not confuse the two drugs.*

doxorubicin hydrochloride
Adriamycin♦
Pregnancy Category: D

MECHANISM OF ACTION
Interferes with DNA-dependent ribonucleic acid (RNA) synthesis by intercalation.

INDICATIONS & DOSAGE
Dosage and indications may vary. Check patient's protocol with doctor.
Bladder, breast, cervical, head, neck, liver, lung, ovarian, prostatic, stomach, testicular, and thyroid cancer; Hodgkin's disease; acute lymphoblastic and myeloblastic leukemia; Wilms' tumor; neuroblastomas; lymphomas; sarcomas—
Adults: 60 to 75 mg/m² I.V. as single dose q 3 weeks; or 30 mg/m² I.V. in single daily dose, days 1 to 3 of 4-week cycle. Alternatively, 20 mg/m² I.V. once weekly or 30 mg/m² I.V. on 3 successive days, repeated every 4 weeks. Maximum cumulative dose 550 mg/m².

ADVERSE REACTIONS
Blood: *leukopenia, especially agranulocytosis, during days 10 to 15, with recovery by day 21; thrombocytopenia.*
CV: *cardiac depression, seen in such EKG changes as sinus tachycardia, T-wave flattening, ST segment depres-*

sion, voltage reduction; arrhythmias in 11% of patients; irreversible cardiomyopathy (sometimes with pulmonary edema) with mortality of 30% to 75%.

GI: *nausea, vomiting,* diarrhea, *stomatitis,* esophagitis.

GU: enhancement of cyclophosphamide-induced bladder injury, transient red urine.

Skin: *hyperpigmentation of skin, especially in previously irradiated areas.*

Local: *severe cellulitis or tissue slough if drug extravasates.*

Other: hyperpigmentation of nails and dermal creases, *complete alopecia within 3 to 4 weeks;* hair may regrow 2 to 5 months after drug is stopped.

INTERACTIONS

Streptozocin: increased and prolonged blood levels. Dose may have to be adjusted.

Heparin: don't mix. May form a precipitate.

NURSING CONSIDERATIONS

• Dose modification may be required in myelosuppression and in impaired cardiac or hepatic function.

• Stop drug or slow rate of infusion if tachycardia develops.

• Stop drug immediately in signs of congestive heart failure. Prevent by limiting cumulative dose to 550 mg/m²; 450 mg/m² when patient is also receiving cyclophosphamide or irradiation to cardiac area.

• Monitor EKG before treatment, monthly during therapy.

• *Avoid extravasation;* inject into tubing of freely flowing I.V. *Never give* I.M. or S.C. If extravasation occurs, discontinue I.V. immediately and apply ice to area for 24 to 48 hours.

• If vein streaking occurs, slow administration rate. However, if welts occur, stop administration and report to doctor.

• Monitor CBC and hepatic function.

• Warn patient urine will be red for 1 to 2 days.

• Dose should be reduced in hepatic dysfunction.

• Warn patient that alopecia will occur. A scalp tourniquet or application of ice may decrease alopecia. However, *do not* use if treating leukemias or other neoplasms where tumor stem cells may be present in scalp.

• Refrigerated, reconstituted solution stable 48 hours; at room temperature, stable 24 hours.

• If cumulative dose exceeds 550 mg/m² body surface area, 30% of patients develop cardiac adverse reactions, which begin 2 weeks to 6 months after stopping drug.

• The alternative dosage schedule (once-weekly dosing) has been found to cause a lower incidence of cardiomyopathy.

• Decrease dose if serum bilirubin is increased: 50% dose when bilirubin is 1.2 to 3 mg/100 ml; 25% dose when bilirubin is greater than 3 mg/100 ml.

• Esophagitis very common in patients who have also received radiation therapy.

• Premedicate with antiemetic to reduce nausea.

• Reddish color looks very similar to daunorubicin. *Do not confuse the two drugs.*

---

mitomycin
Mutamycin♦
Pregnancy Category: D

MECHANISM OF ACTION

Acts like an alkylating agent, cross-linking strands of DNA. This causes an imbalance of cell growth, leading to cell death.

INDICATIONS & DOSAGE

Dosage and indications may vary. Check patient's protocol with doctor. *Breast, colon, head, neck, lung, pancreatic, and stomach cancer; malig-*

Italicized side effects are common or life-threatening.
*Liquid form contains alcohol.   **May contain tartrazine.

nant melanoma—
Adults: 2 mg/m² I.V. daily for 5 days. Stop drug for 2 days, then repeat dose for 5 more days; or 20 mg/m² as a single dose. Repeat cycle 6 to 8 weeks. Stop drug if WBC less than 4,000/mm³ or platelets less than 75,000/mm³.

ADVERSE REACTIONS
Blood: *thrombocytopenia, leukopenia (may be delayed up to 8 weeks and may be cumulative with successive doses).*
CNS: paresthesias.
GI: *nausea, vomiting,* anorexia, stomatitis.
Local: desquamation, induration, pruritus, *pain at site of injection.* Extravasation causes cellulitis, ulceration, sloughing.
Other: *reversible alopecia; purple coloration of nail beds;* fever; *microangiopathic hemolytic anemia, syndrome characterized by thrombocytopenia, renal failure, and hypertension; interstitial pneumonitis.*

INTERACTIONS
None significant.

NURSING CONSIDERATIONS
• Dose modification is required when platelet count is below 75,000/mm³, WBC is less than 4,000/mm³; in coagulation or bleeding disorders, serious infections, impaired renal function.
• Continue CBC and blood studies at least 7 weeks after therapy is stopped. Observe for signs of bleeding.
• Advise patient that alopecia may occur, but that it's usually reversible.
• Reconstituted solution stable 1 week at room temperature, 2 weeks refrigerated.
• Has been administered topically by bladder instillation and has been given intraarterially through the hepatic artery.

plicamycin (mithramycin)
Mithracin
Pregnancy Category: C

MECHANISM OF ACTION
Forms a complex with DNA, thus inhibiting RNA synthesis. Also inhibits osteocytic activity, blocking calcium and phosphorus resorption from bone.

INDICATIONS & DOSAGE
Dosage and indications may vary. Check patient's protocol with doctor.
Hypercalcemia—
Adults: 25 mcg/kg I.V. daily for 1 to 4 days.
Testicular cancer—
Adults: 25 to 30 mcg/kg I.V. daily for up to 10 days (based on ideal body weight or actual weight, whichever is less).

ADVERSE REACTIONS
Blood: *thrombocytopenia; bleeding syndrome, from epistaxis to generalized hemorrhage; facial flushing.*
GI: *nausea, vomiting,* anorexia, diarrhea, stomatitis, metallic taste.
GU: proteinuria; increased BUN, serum creatinine.
Metabolic: *decreased serum calcium,* potassium, and phosphorus.
Skin: periorbital pallor, usually the day before toxic symptoms occur.
Local: extravasation causes irritation, cellulitis.

INTERACTIONS
None significant.

NURSING CONSIDERATIONS
• Contraindicated in thrombocytopenia and in coagulation and bleeding disorders. Dose modification may be required in renal, hepatic, or bone marrow impairment.
• Slow infusion reduces nausea that develops with I.V. push.
• Monitor LDH, SGOT, SGPT, alkaline phosphatase, BUN, creatinine,

potassium, calcium, phosphorus.
• Monitor platelet count and prothrombin time before and during therapy.
• Observe for signs of bleeding. Facial flushing early indicator of bleeding.
• Give antiemetic before administering to reduce nausea.
• Avoid extravasation. If I.V. infiltrates, stop immediately; use ice
packs. Restart I.V.
• Avoid contact with skin or mucous
membranes.
• Therapeutic effect in hypercalcemia
may not be seen for 24 to 48 hours;
may last 3 to 15 days.
• Precipitous drop in calcium possible. Monitor patient for tetany, carpopedal spasm, Chvostek's sign, muscle
cramps; check serum calcium levels.
• Store lyophilized powder in refrigerator. Remains stable after reconstitution for 24 hours; 48 hours in refrigerator.

procarbazine hydrochloride
Matulane, Natulan♦♦
Pregnancy Category: D

MECHANISM OF ACTION
Inhibits DNA, RNA, and protein synthesis.

INDICATIONS & DOSAGE
Dosage and indications may vary.
Check patient's protocol with doctor.
*Hodgkin's disease, lymphomas, brain
and lung cancer—*
Adults: 100 to 150 mg/m² P.O. for 10
days until WBC falls below 4,000/
mm³ or platelets fall below 100,000/
mm³. After bone marrow recovers,
resume maintenance dose 50 to 100
mg P.O. daily.
Children: 50 mg P.O. daily for first
week, then 100 mg/m² until response
or toxicity occurs. Maintenance dose
is 50 mg P.O. daily after bone marrow
recovery.

ADVERSE REACTIONS
Blood: bleeding tendency, *thrombocytopenia, leukopenia,* anemia.
CNS: nervousness, depression, insomnia, nightmares, *hallucinations,*
confusion.
EENT: retinal hemorrhage, nystagmus, photophobia.
GI: *nausea, vomiting, anorexia,* stomatitis, dry mouth, dysphagia, diarrhea, constipation.
Skin: dermatitis.
Other: reversible alopecia, pleural effusion.

INTERACTIONS
Alcohol: mild disulfiram (Antabuse)-
like reaction. Warn patient not to
drink alcohol.
Meperidine: may cause severe hypotension and possible death. Don't give
together.

NURSING CONSIDERATIONS
• Use cautiously in inadequate bone
marrow reserve, leukopenia, thrombocytopenia, anemia, impaired hepatic or renal function.
• Observe for signs of bleeding.
• Nausea and vomiting may be decreased if taken at bedtime and in divided doses.
• Warn patient not to drink alcoholic
beverages while taking this drug.
• Procarbazine inhibits monoamine
oxidase (MAO) and can cause disulfiram-like reaction if taken with other
MAO inhibitors, tricyclic antidepressants, or foods with a large tyramine
content.
• Instruct patient to stop medication
and check with doctor immediately if
disulfiram-like reaction occurs (chest
pains, rapid or irregular heartbeat, severe headache, stiff neck).

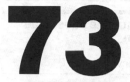

Antineoplastics altering hormone balance

aminoglutethimide
dromostanolone propionate
estramustine phosphate sodium
leuprolide acetate
megestrol acetate
mitotane
tamoxifen citrate
testolactone
trilostane

COMBINATION PRODUCTS
None.

---

aminoglutethimide
Cytadren♦
Pregnancy Category: D

MECHANISM OF ACTION
Blocks conversion of cholesterol to delta-5-pregnenolone in the adrenal cortex, inhibiting the synthesis of glucocorticoids, mineralocorticoids, and other steroids.

INDICATIONS & DOSAGE
Suppression of adrenal function in Cushing's syndrome and adrenal cancer; metastatic breast cancer—
Adults: 250 mg P.O. q.i.d. at 6-hour intervals. Dosage may be increased in increments of 250 mg daily every 1 to 2 weeks to a maximum total daily dose of 2 g.

ADVERSE REACTIONS
Blood: transient leukopenia, *severe pancytopenia.*
CNS: *drowsiness,* headache, dizziness.
CV: hypotension, tachycardia.
Endocrine: adrenal insufficiency, masculinization, hirsutism.
GI: *nausea, anorexia.*
Skin: *morbilliform skin rash,* pruritus, urticaria.
Other: fever, myalgia.

INTERACTIONS
None significant.

NURSING CONSIDERATIONS
• May cause adrenal hypofunction, especially under stressful conditions such as surgery, trauma, or acute illness. Patients may need hydrocortisone and mineralocorticoid supplements in these situations. Monitor such patients carefully.
• Monitor blood pressure frequently. Advise patient to stand up slowly in order to minimize orthostatic hypotension.
• May cause a decrease in thyroid hormone production. Monitor thyroid function studies.
• Perform baseline hematologic studies and monitor CBC periodically.
• Warn patient that drug can cause drowsiness and dizziness. Advise him to avoid activities that require alertness and good psychomotor coordination until response to drug has been determined.
• Tell patient to report if skin rash persists for more than 5 to 8 days. Reassure patient that drowsiness, nausea, and loss of appetite will diminish within 2 weeks after start of aminoglutethimide therapy. However, if these symptoms persist, tell patient to notify doctor.

dromostanolone propionate
Drolban
Pregnancy Category: X

MECHANISM OF ACTION
Changes the tumor's hormonal environment and alters the neoplastic process.

INDICATIONS & DOSAGE
Advanced, inoperable metastatic breast cancer, 1 to 5 years postmenopausal—
Women: 100 mg deep I.M. 3 times weekly.

ADVERSE REACTIONS
GU: clitoral enlargement.
Metabolic: hypercalcemia.
Skin: acne.
Other: *virilism (deepened voice, facial hair growth), which may be intense after long-term treatment;* edema, pain at injection site.

INTERACTIONS
None significant.

NURSING CONSIDERATIONS
• Contraindicated by any route other than I.M.; in male breast cancer; in pregnancy and in premenopausal women. Use cautiously in hepatic disease, cardiac decompensation, nephritis, nephrosis, and prostatic cancer.
• If severe hypercalcemia develops or disease accelerates, drug should be stopped.
• Therapeutic effect may be delayed 8 to 12 weeks. Reassure patient that results are not immediate.
• Do not store in refrigerator; drug precipitates at cold temperatures.
• Explain possible virilizing effects, skin and libido changes to female patients to prevent undue alarm.
• Dromostanolone is an androgen.

estramustine phosphate sodium
Emcyt♦
Pregnancy Category: D

MECHANISM OF ACTION
A combination of estrogen and an alkylating agent; acts by its ability to bind selectively to a protein present in the human prostate.

INDICATIONS & DOSAGE
Palliative treatment of metastatic or progressive cancer of the prostate—
Adults: 10 to 16 mg/kg P.O. in 3 to 4 divided doses. Usual dosage is 14 mg/kg daily. Therapy should continue for up to 3 months and, if successful, be maintained as long as the patient responds.

ADVERSE REACTIONS
Blood: leukopenia, thrombocytopenia.
CV: *myocardial infarction, cerebrovascular accident, edema, pulmonary emboli,* thrombophlebitis, congestive heart failure, hypertension.
GI: *nausea, vomiting,* diarrhea.
Skin: rash, pruritus.
Other: *painful gynecomastia and breast tenderness,* thinning of hair, hyperglycemia.

INTERACTIONS
None significant.

NURSING CONSIDERATIONS
• Contraindicated in patients hypersensitive to estradiol and nitrogen mustard. Also contraindicated in active thrombophlebitis or thromboembolic disorders, except in those cases where the actual tumor mass is the cause of the thromboembolic phenomenon.
• Use cautiously in patients with history of thrombophlebitis or thromboembolic disorders, cerebrovascular and coronary artery disease.

Italicized side effects are common or life-threatening.
*Liquid form contains alcohol.   **May contain tartrazine.

- Estramustine may exaggerate pre-existing peripheral edema or congestive heart failure. Weight gain should be monitored regularly in these patients.
- Monitor blood pressure and glucose tolerance periodically throughout therapy.
- Because of the possibility of mutagenic effects, advise patient and spouse to use contraceptive measures if woman is of childbearing age.
- Estramustine is a combination of the estrogen estradiol and a nitrogen mustard. Shown to be effective in patients refractory to estrogen therapy alone.
- Patient may continue estramustine as long as he's responding favorably. Some patients have taken the drug for more than 3 years.
- Store capsules in refrigerator.

leuprolide acetate
Lupron
Pregnancy Category: NR

MECHANISM OF ACTION
Initially stimulates but then inhibits the release of follicle-stimulating and luteinizing hormone. This results in testosterone suppression.

INDICATIONS & DOSAGE
Management of advanced prostate cancer—
Adults: 1 mg S.C. daily.

ADVERSE REACTIONS
Endocrine: *hot flashes.*
GI: nausea, vomiting.
Local: skin reactions at injection site.
Other: pulmonary embolus, peripheral edema, decrease in libido, transient bone pain during first week of treatment.

INTERACTIONS
None significant.

NURSING CONSIDERATIONS
- Be sure to administer S.C. Don't give I.M. or I.V.
- Leuprolide is a nonsurgical alternative to orchiectomy for prostate cancer.
- Studies show leuprolide is therapeutically equivalent to diethylstilbestrol in "medical castration" palliation treatment but has significantly milder and fewer adverse reactions.
- Reassure your patient who has had undesirable effects from other endocrine therapies that leuprolide is much easier to tolerate.
- Reassure patient that bone pain is transient and will disappear after about 1 week.
- Patients may be maintained on this drug for long-term treatment.

megestrol acetate
Megace♦**
Pregnancy Category: X

MECHANISM OF ACTION
Changes the tumor's hormonal environment and alters the neoplastic process.

INDICATIONS & DOSAGE
Breast cancer—
Women: 40 mg P.O. q.i.d.
Endometrial cancer—
Women: 40 to 320 mg P.O. daily in divided doses.

ADVERSE REACTIONS
GU: dysfunctional uterine bleeding when drug is discontinued.
Other: carpal tunnel syndrome, thrombophlebitis, alopecia.

INTERACTIONS
None significant.

NURSING CONSIDERATIONS
- Use cautiously in patients with history of thrombophlebitis.
- Adequate trial is 2 months. Reas-

sure patient that therapeutic response isn't immediate.

mitotane
Lysodren♦
Pregnancy Category: C

MECHANISM OF ACTION
Selectively destroys adrenocortical tissue and hinders extraadrenal metabolism of cortisol.

INDICATIONS & DOSAGE
Inoperable adrenocortical cancer—
Adults: 9 to 10 g P.O. daily, divided t.i.d. or q.i.d. If severe adverse reactions appear, reduce dose until maximum tolerated dose is achieved (varies from 2 to 16 g daily but is usually 8 to 10 g daily).

ADVERSE REACTIONS
CNS: *depression, somnolence, vertigo;* brain damage and dysfunction in long-term, high-dose therapy.
GI: *severe nausea, vomiting,* diarrhea, anorexia.
Metabolic: adrenal insufficiency.
Skin: dermatitis.

INTERACTIONS
None significant.

NURSING CONSIDERATIONS
• Dose modification may be required in hepatic disease.
• Drug should not be used in a patient with shock or trauma. Use of corticosteroids may avoid acute adrenocorticoid insufficiency.
• Assess and record behavioral and neurologic signs for baseline data daily throughout therapy.
• Give antiemetic before administering to reduce nausea.
• Dosage may be reduced if GI or skin adverse reactions are severe.
• Obese patients may need higher dosage and may have longer-lasting adverse reactions, since drug distributes mostly to body fat.
• Warn ambulatory patient of CNS adverse reactions; advise him to avoid hazardous tasks requiring mental alertness or physical coordination.
• Monitor effectiveness by reduction in pain, weakness, anorexia.
• Adequate trial is at least 3 months, but therapy can continue if clinical benefits are observed.

tamoxifen citrate
Nolvadex♦
Pregnancy Category: C

MECHANISM OF ACTION
Acts as an estrogen antagonist.

INDICATIONS & DOSAGE
Advanced premenopausal and postmenopausal breast cancer—
Women: 10 to 20 mg P.O. b.i.d.

ADVERSE REACTIONS
Blood: transient fall in WBC or platelets.
GI: nausea in 10% of patients, vomiting, anorexia.
GU: vaginal discharge and bleeding.
Metabolic: hypercalcemia.
Skin: rash.
Other: temporary bone or tumor pain, hot flashes in 7% of patients. Brief exacerbation of pain from osseous metastases.

INTERACTIONS
None significant.

NURSING CONSIDERATIONS
• Monitor CBC closely in patients with preexisting leukopenia or thrombocytopenia.
• Acts as an "antiestrogen." Best results in patients with positive estrogen receptors.
• Adverse reactions are usually minor and well tolerated.
• Reassure patient that acute exacerbation of bone pain during tamoxifen

---

Italicized side effects are common or life-threatening.
*Liquid form contains alcohol.   **May contain tartrazine.

therapy usually indicates drug will produce good response. Use analgesic to relieve pain.
• Short-term therapy induces ovulation in premenopausal women. *Mechanical* contraception recommended.
• Monitor serum calcium. Drug may compound hypercalcemia related to bone metastases.
• Also used to treat breast cancer in males and advanced ovarian cancer in women.

testolactone
Teslac
Pregnancy Category: C

MECHANISM OF ACTION
Changes the tumor's hormonal environment and alters the neoplastic process.

INDICATIONS & DOSAGE
Advanced postmenopausal breast cancer—
Women: 100 mg deep I.M. 3 times weekly; or 250 mg P.O. q.i.d.

ADVERSE REACTIONS
Local: pain, inflammation at injection site.
Metabolic: hypercalcemia.

INTERACTIONS
None significant.

NURSING CONSIDERATIONS
• Contraindicated in male breast cancer and not recommended for premenopausal females.
• Adequate trial is 3 months. Reassure patient that therapeutic response isn't immediate.
• Monitor fluids and electrolytes, especially calcium levels.
• Immobilized patients are prone to hypercalcemia. Exercise may prevent it. Force fluids to aid calcium excretion.

• Shake vial vigorously before drawing up injection. Do not refrigerate.
• Use 1½″ needle and inject into upper outer quadrant of gluteal region. Rotate injection sites.
• Advantage over testosterone is less virilization.
• Higher-than-recommended doses do not increase incidence of remission.
• Testolactone is an androgen.

trilostane
Modrastane
Pregnancy Category: X

MECHANISM OF ACTION
Reversibly lowers elevated circulating levels of glucocorticoids by inhibiting the enzyme system essential for their production in the adrenal gland.

INDICATIONS & DOSAGE
Adrenal cortical hyperfunction in Cushing's syndrome—
Adults: 30 mg P.O. q.i.d. initially. May be increased at intervals of 3 to 4 days to maximum of 480 mg daily.

ADVERSE REACTIONS
CNS: headache.
CV: *orthostatic hypotension.*
EENT: burning of oral and nasal membranes.
GI: *diarrhea, upset stomach,* nausea, flatulence, bloating.
Metabolic: hyperkalemia.
Skin: flushing, rash.
Other: fever, fatigue.

INTERACTIONS
Aminoglutethimide, mitotane: may cause severe adrenocortical hypofunction.

NURSING CONSIDERATIONS
• Contraindicated in patients with adrenal insufficiency and in those with severe renal or hepatic disease.
• Use cautiously in patients who are

receiving other drugs that suppress adrenal function.

• Trilostane may prevent the body from responding to a stress situation. Therefore, patients who develop a severe illness or need surgery may need to have this drug temporarily discontinued.

• Because the drug may cause orthostatic hypotension by suppressing aldosterone production, monitor blood pressure regularly in all patients.

• Patient should show therapeutic response within 2 weeks. If no response has occurred, the doctor may discontinue the drug.

• Most patients show a therapeutic response at doses below 360 mg per day.

• Trilostane is prescribed when surgery or pituitary radiation is inappropriate or must be delayed. Explain to your patient that the drug does not cure the underlying disease.

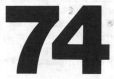

Miscellaneous antineoplastic agents

asparaginase (L-asparaginase)
etoposide (VP-16)
interferon alfa-2a/2b
vinblastine sulfate (VLB)
vincristine sulfate
vindesine sulfate

COMBINATION PRODUCTS
None.

asparaginase (L-asparaginase)
Elspar, Kidrolase♦♦
Pregnancy Category: C

MECHANISM OF ACTION
Destroys the amino acid asparagine, which is needed for protein synthesis in acute lymphocytic leukemia. This leads to death of the leukemic cell.

INDICATIONS & DOSAGE
Acute lymphocytic leukemia (when used along with other drugs)—
Adults and children: 1,000 international units (IU)/kg I.V. daily for 10 days, injected over 30 minutes or by slow I.V. push; or 6,000 IU/m² I.M. at intervals specified in protocol.
Sole induction agent—200 IU/kg I.V. daily for 28 days.

ADVERSE REACTIONS
Blood: *hypofibrinogenemia* and depression of other clotting factors, thrombocytopenia, *leukopenia,* depression of serum albumin.
CNS: lethargy, somnolence.
GI: *vomiting (may last up to 24 hours), anorexia, nausea, cramps,* weight loss.
GU: *azotemia,* renal failure, uric acid nephropathy, glycosuria, polyuria.
Hepatic: elevated SGOT, SGPT; *hepatotoxicity.*
Metabolic: elevated alkaline phosphatase and bilirubin (direct and indirect); increase or decrease in total lipids; *hyperglycemia; increased blood ammonia.*
Skin: *rash, urticaria.*
Other: *hemorrhagic pancreatitis, anaphylaxis (relatively common).*

INTERACTIONS
None significant.

NURSING CONSIDERATIONS
• Contraindicated in pancreatitis, previous hypersensitivity unless desensitized. Use cautiously in preexisting hepatic dysfunction.
• Should be administered in hospital setting with close supervision.
• Don't use as sole agent to induce remission unless combination therapy is inappropriate. Not recommended for maintenance therapy.
• Risk of hypersensitivity increases with repeated doses. Patient may be desensitized, but this doesn't rule out risk of allergic reactions. Routine administration of 2-unit I.V. test dose may identify high-risk patients.
• Intravenous administration of asparaginase with or immediately before vincristine or prednisone may increase toxicity reactions.
• Give I.V. injection over 30-minute period through a running infusion of sodium chloride injection or dextrose

5% injection.
• For I.M. injection, limit dose at single injection site to 2 ml.
• Because of vomiting, patient may need parenteral fluids for 24 hours or until oral fluids are tolerated.
• Monitor CBC and bone marrow function. Bone marrow regeneration may take 5 to 6 weeks.
• Obtain frequent serum amylase determinations to check pancreatic status. If elevated, asparaginase should be discontinued.
• Tumor lysis can result in uric acid nephropathy. Prevent occurrence by increasing fluid intake. Allopurinol should be started before therapy begins.
• Watch for signs of bleeding, such as petechiae and melena.
• Monitor blood sugar and test urine for sugar before and during therapy. Watch for signs of hyperglycemia, such as glycosuria and polyuria.
• Reconstitute with either 2 to 5 ml sterile water for injection or sodium chloride injection.
• Don't shake vial. May cause loss of potency. Don't use cloudy solutions.
• Refrigerate unopened dry powder. Reconstituted solution stable 6 hours at room temperature, 24 hours refrigerated.
• Keep epinephrine, diphenhydramine, and I.V. corticosteroids available for treatment of anaphylaxis.

---

etoposide (VP-16)
VePesid♦
Pregnancy Category: D

MECHANISM OF ACTION
A semi-synthetic derivative of podophyllotoxin that arrests cell mitosis.

INDICATIONS & DOSAGE
Small-cell carcinoma of the lung, acute nonlymphocytic leukemia, lymphosarcoma, Hodgkin's disease, testicular carcinoma—

Adults: 45 to 75 mg/m² daily I.V. or P.O. for 3 to 5 days repeated q 3 to 5 weeks; or 200 to 250 mg/m² I.V. or P.O. weekly; or 125 to 140 mg/m² daily I.V. or P.O. three times a week q 5 weeks.

ADVERSE REACTIONS
Blood: *myelosuppression (dose-limiting), leukopenia,* thrombocytopenia.
CV: hypotension from rapid infusion.
GI: nausea and vomiting.
Local: infrequent phlebitis.
Other: occasional headache and fever, *reversible alopecia, anaphylaxis* (rare).

INTERACTIONS
None significant.

NURSING CONSIDERATIONS
• Intrapleural and intrathecal administration of this drug is contraindicated.
• Give drug by slow I.V. infusion (over at least 30 minutes) to prevent severe hypotension.
• The oral form is now available. It is especially convenient for home care.
• Blood pressure should be monitored before infusion and at 30-minute intervals during infusion. If systolic blood pressure falls below 90 mm Hg, infusion should be stopped and doctor notified.
• Have diphenhydramine, hydrocortisone, epinephrine, and airway available in case of an anaphylactic reaction.
• Monitor CBC. Observe patient for signs of bone marrow depression.
• The drug may be diluted for infusion in either dextrose 5% in water or normal saline solution to a final concentration of 0.2 or 0.4 mg/ml. Higher concentrations may crystalize.
• Solutions diluted to 0.2 mg/ml are stable for 96 hours at room temperature in plastic or glass unprotected from light; solutions diluted to 0.4 mg/ml are stable for 48 hours under

---

Italicized side effects are common or life-threatening.
*Liquid form contains alcohol.   **May contain tartrazine.

the same conditions.
- Do not administer through membrane-type inline filters because the diluent may dissolve the filter.
- Etoposide has produced complete remissions in small-cell lung cancer and testicular cancer. One of the most promising new agents available.

interferon alfa-2a
Roferon-a

interferon alfa-2b
Intron a
Pregnancy Category: C

MECHANISM OF ACTION
Interferons bind to specific membrane receptors on the cell surface. Then, interferon initiates a complex sequence of immunologic events that inhibit virus replication and suppress cell proliferation.

INDICATIONS & DOSAGE
Treatment of hairy cell leukemia—
For alfa-2a:
Adults: for induction, give 3 million units S.C. or I.M. daily for 16 to 24 weeks. For maintenance, 3 million units S.C. or I.M. three times a week.
For alfa-2b:
Adults: 2 million units/m² I.M. or S.C. three times a week (for both induction and maintenance).

ADVERSE REACTIONS
Blood: *leukemia.*
CNS: *fatigue,* headache, *dizziness, confusion,* nervousness, depression, paresthesias.
CV: hypotension, edema, palpitations.
GI: nausea, vomiting, diarrhea, *anorexia.*
Skin: *rash, dry or inflamed oropharynx, dry skin, pruritus,* alopecia.
Other: *flulike symptoms (fever, myalgias, chills).*

INTERACTIONS
None reported.

NURSING CONSIDERATIONS
- Dose modification may be required in patients with cardiac disease or history of cardiac illness; in patients with severe renal or hepatic disease, seizure disorders, or compromised CNS function; and in patients with bone marrow suppression.
- Monitor for CNS adverse reactions, such as decreased mental status and dizziness. Periodic neuropsychiatric monitoring is recommended.
- If patient does not respond within 6 weeks, treatment should be discontinued for reevaluation of therapy.
- Almost all patients experience flulike symptoms at the beginning of therapy. These effects tend to diminish with continued therapy.
- Analgesics and antipyretics such as acetaminophen may help to relieve these symptoms. Bedtime administration may also help to lessen these effects.
- Warn patients against changing brands of interferon. The 2a and 2b forms have different dosages.
- Teach patients correct home administration technique. Advise them to read enclosed patient package insert carefully.
- Patients should be well hydrated during treatment. Encourage adequate fluid intake.
- Subcutaneous administration route should be used in patients whose platelets are below 50,000/mm³.

vinblastine sulfate (VLB)
Velban, Velbe♦♦
Pregnancy Category: D

MECHANISM OF ACTION
Arrests mitosis in metaphase, blocking cell division.

INDICATIONS & DOSAGE

Breast or testicular cancer, Hodgkin's and non-Hodgkin's lymphomas, choriocarcinoma, lymphosarcoma, neuroblastoma, mycosis fungoides, histiocytosis—
Adults and children: 0.1 mg/kg or 3.7 mg/m^2 I.V. weekly or q 2 weeks. May be increased to maximum dose (adults) of 0.5 mg/kg or 18.5 mg/m^2 I.V. weekly according to response. Dose should not be repeated if WBC less than 4,000/mm^3.

ADVERSE REACTIONS

Blood: *leukopenia* (nadir days 4 to 10 and lasts another 7 to 14 days), *thrombocytopenia.*
CNS: depression, *paresthesias, peripheral neuropathy and neuritis, numbness, loss of deep tendon reflexes, muscle pain and weakness.*
EENT: pharyngitis.
GI: *nausea, vomiting, stomatitis,* ulcer and bleeding, *constipation, ileus, anorexia, weight loss,* abdominal pain.
GU: oligospermia, aspermia, urinary retention.
Skin: dermatitis, vesiculation.
Local: *irritation, phlebitis,* cellulitis, necrosis if I.V. extravasates.
Other: *acute bronchospasm;* reversible alopecia in 5% to 10% of patients; *pain in tumor site,* low fever.

INTERACTIONS
None significant.

NURSING CONSIDERATIONS
• Contraindicated in severe leukopenia, bacterial infection. Use cautiously in jaundice or hepatic dysfunction.
• After administering, monitor for life-threatening acute bronchospasm reaction. If this occurs, notify doctor immediately. Reaction most likely to occur in patient who is also receiving mitomycin.
• Give antiemetic before administer-

ing to reduce nausea.
• Drug should be stopped if stomatitis occurs.
• Assess bowel activity. Give laxatives as needed. May use stool softeners prophylactically.
• Don't repeat dose more frequently than every 7 days or severe leukopenia will develop.
• Less neurotoxic than vincristine.
• Assess for numbness and tingling in hands and feet. Assess gait for early evidence of foot drop.
• Should be injected directly into vein or tubing of running I.V. over 1 minute. May also be given in a 50-ml dextrose in water or normal saline solution and infused over 15 minutes. If extravasation occurs, stop infusion. Apply ice packs on and off every 2 hours for 24 hours.
• Warn patient that alopecia may occur but is usually reversible.
• Adequate trial 12 weeks; reassure patient that therapeutic response isn't immediate.
• Reconstitute 10-mg vial with 10 ml of sodium chloride injection or sterile water. This yields 1 mg/ml.
• Refrigerate reconstituted solution. Discard after 30 days.
• Don't confuse vinblastine with vincristine or the investigational agent vindesine.

vincristine sulfate
Oncovin♦
Pregnancy Category: D

MECHANISM OF ACTION
Arrests mitosis in metaphase, blocking cell division.

INDICATIONS & DOSAGE
Acute lymphoblastic and other leukemias, Hodgkin's disease, lymphosarcoma, reticulum cell sarcoma, neuroblastoma, rhabdomyosarcoma, Wilms' tumor, osteogenic and other sarcomas, lung and breast cancer—

Adults: 1 to 2 mg/m² I.V. weekly.
Children: 1.5 to 2 mg/m² I.V. weekly.
Maximum single dose (adults and
children) is 2 mg.

ADVERSE REACTIONS
Blood: rapidly reversible mild anemia
and leukopenia.
CNS: *peripheral neuropathy,* sensory
loss, *deep tendon reflex loss, paresthe-*
sias, wristdrop and footdrop, ataxia,
cranial nerve palsies (headache, *jaw*
pain, hoarseness, vocal cord paralysis, visual disturbances), *muscle*
weakness and cramps, depression, agitation, insomnia; some neurotoxici-
ties may be permanent.
EENT: diplopia, optic and extraocu-
lar neuropathy, ptosis.
GI: *constipation, cramps,* ileus that
mimics surgical abdomen, *nausea,*
vomiting, anorexia, *stomatitis,* weight
loss, dysphagia.
GU: urinary retention.
Local: severe local reaction when ex-
travasated, *phlebitis,* cellulitis.
Other: *acute bronchospasm, revers-*
ible alopecia (up to 71% of patients).

INTERACTIONS
None significant.

NURSING CONSIDERATIONS
• Use cautiously in jaundice or hepatic dysfunction, neuromuscular disease, infection, or with other neurotoxic drugs.
• After administering, monitor for
life-threatening acute bronchospasm
reaction. If this occurs, notify doctor
immediately. Reaction most likely to
occur in patient who is also receiving
mitomycin.
• Because of neurotoxicity, don't give
drug more than once a week. Children
more resistant to neurotoxicity than
adults. Neurotoxicity is dose-related
and usually reversible.
• Should be given directly into vein
or tubing of running I.V. slowly over 1
minute. May also be given in a 50-ml

dextrose in water or normal saline solution and infused over 15 minutes. If
drug infiltrates, apply ice packs on
and off every 2 hours for 24 hours.
• Check for depression of Achilles
tendon reflex, numbness, tingling,
footdrop or wristdrop, difficulty in
walking, ataxia, slapping gait. Also
check ability to walk on heels. Support patient when walking.
• Monitor bowel function. Give stool
softener, laxative, or water before
dosing. Constipation may be an early
sign of neurotoxicity.
• Warn patient that alopecia may occur but is usually reversible.
• Be extremely careful about doses.
Don't confuse vincristine with vinblastine or the investigational agent
vindesine.
• 5-mg vials are for multiple-dose use
only. Don't administer entire vial to
one patient as a single dose.
• All vials (1-mg, 2-mg, 5-mg) contain 1 mg/ml solution and should be
refrigerated.

---

vindesine sulfate
DAVA, Eldisine♦
Pregnancy Category: D

MECHANISM OF ACTION
Arrests mitosis in metaphase, blocking cell division.

INDICATIONS & DOSAGE
Acute lymphoblastic leukemia, breast
cancer, malignant melanoma, lym-
phosarcoma, non–small-cell lung car-
cinoma—
Adults: 3 to 4 mg/m² I.V. q 7 to 14
days, or continuous I.V. infusion 1.2
to 1.5 mg/m² daily for 5 days every 3
weeks.

ADVERSE REACTIONS
Blood: *leukopenia, thrombocyto-*
penia.
CNS: *paresthesias, decreased deep*
tendon reflex, muscle weakness.

Unmarked trade names available in the United States only.
♦Also available in Canada.   ♦♦Available in Canada only.

GI: *constipation, abdominal cramping,* nausea, vomiting.
Local: *phlebitis,* necrosis on extravasation.
Other: *acute bronchospasm, reversible alopecia,* jaw pain, fever with continuous infusions.

INTERACTIONS
None significant.

NURSING CONSIDERATIONS
• Do not give as a continuous infusion unless patient has a central I.V. line.
• After administering, monitor for life-threatening acute bronchospasm reaction. If this occurs, notify doctor immediately. Reaction most likely to occur in patient who is also receiving mitomycin.
• To prevent paralytic ileus, encourage patient to force fluids, increase ambulation, and use stool softeners.
• Instruct patient to report any signs of neurotoxicity: numbness and tingling of extremities, jaw pain, constipation (may be early sign of neurotoxicity).
• Assess for depression of Achilles tendon reflex, footdrop or wristdrop, slapping gait (late signs of neurotoxicity).
• Neuropathy may be assessed by recording patient signatures before each course of therapy and observing for deterioration of handwriting.
• Monitor CBC.
• Avoid extravasation. Drug is a painful vesicant. Give 10-ml normal saline solution flush before drug to test vein patency, and 10-ml normal saline solution flush to remove any remaining drug from tubing after drug is given.
• When reconstituted with the 10-ml diluent provided or normal saline solution, the drug is stable for 30 days under refrigeration.
• Do not mix vindesine with other drugs; compatibility with other drugs has not yet been determined.

Italicized side effects are common or life-threatening.
*Liquid form contains alcohol.   **May contain tartrazine.

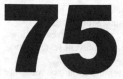

Investigational antineoplastic agents

amsacrine (m-AMSA)
azacytidine (5-azacytidine)
Erwinia asparaginase
hexamethylmelamine (HMM, HXM)
ifosfamide
semustine (methyl CCNU)
teniposide (VM-26)

COMBINATION PRODUCTS
None.

amsacrine (m-AMSA)
Pregnancy Category: C

MECHANISM OF ACTION
Intercalates DNA and inhibits DNA synthesis, producing a cytotoxic effect.

INDICATIONS & DOSAGE
Ovarian carcinoma, lymphomas—
Adults: 30 to 50 mg/m²/day for 3 days, or 90 to 180 mg/m² as a single dose.
Acute myelogenous leukemia—
Adults: 75 to 120 mg/m²/day for 5 days given by I.V. or intraarterial infusion.

ADVERSE REACTIONS
Blood: *leukopenia (usually dose-limiting adverse reaction),* mild thrombocytopenia.
GI: infrequent and mild nausea and vomiting, stomatitis at higher doses.
CNS: *convulsions at doses as low as 40 mg/m²/day.*
CV: rare ventricular arrythmias and cardiac arrests, possibly caused by the diluent.
Other: *local irritation and mild phlebitis,* abnormal liver function tests.

INTERACTIONS
Heparin: don't mix. May form a precipitate.

NURSING CONSIDERATIONS
• Use cautiously in patients with impaired liver function.
• To prepare solution for administration, two sterile liquids are combined. Add 1.5 ml from the amsacrine ampule (50 mg/ml) to the vial containing 13.5 ml of lactic acid. The combined solution will contain 5 mg/ml of amsacrine and is stable for at least 48 hours at room temperature.
• Use glass syringes for combining the amsacrine and lactic acid. The diluent in the amsacrine may dissolve plastic syringes.
• The solution may be further diluted for infusion with dextrose 5% in water (D_5W) to minimize vein irritation. Administer doses of less than 100 mg in at least 100 ml of D_5W, doses from 100 to 199 mg in 250 ml D_5W, and doses 200 mg or greater in a minimum of 500 ml D_5W. Solutions for infusion are stable at least 48 hours at room temperature.
• Solutions should be infused slowly over several hours to minimize vein irritation.
• Do not add amsacrine to normal saline or other chloride-containing solution. Precipitation may occur.
• Do not administer amsacrine through membrane-type inline filters.

The diluent may dissolve the filter.
• Inform the patient that the drug may turn the urine orange.
• Monitor CBC and liver function tests.
• Monitor patient closely for CNS and cardiac toxicity during administration.
• Avoid direct contact of amsacrine with skin due to possible sensitization.

azacytidine (5-azacytidine)
Pregnancy Category: C

MECHANISM OF ACTION
An antimetabolite which disrupts the translation of nucleic acid sequences into protein.

INDICATIONS & DOSAGE
Acute lymphocytic and acute myelogenous leukemia—
Adults and children: 200 to 300 mg/m² I.V. daily for 5 to 10 days. Repeated at 2- to 3-week intervals.

ADVERSE REACTIONS
Blood: *leukopenia (usually dose-limiting adverse reaction), thrombocytopenia.*
CNS: infrequent neurologic toxicities, including generalized muscle pain and weakness.
CV: *Hypotension from rapid infusion.*
GI: *Severe nausea and vomiting, diarrhea.*
Other: rare hepatotoxicity and drug fever.

INTERACTIONS
None significant.

NURSING CONSIDERATIONS
• Contraindicated in patients with liver disease.
• For stability reasons, azacytidine should be infused only in solutions of lactated Ringer's.

• After the drug is diluted for infusion, it is stable for 8 hours.
• The drug should be given by slow I.V. infusion to prevent severe hypotension.
• Blood pressure should be monitored before infusion, at 30-minute intervals during infusion. If systolic blood pressure falls below 90 mm Hg, infusion should be stopped and a doctor notified.
• Nausea and vomiting may be reduced with continuous infusions. Tolerance to nausea and vomiting develops during extended course of treatment.
• Instruct patient to report any signs of neurotoxicity—muscle pain, weakness.
• If necessary, the drug may be given subcutaneously. The drug should be mixed in a smaller quantity of diluent (3 to 5 ml for a 100-mg vial) for subcutaneous administration.
• Monitor temperature, CBC, and liver function tests.

Erwinia asparaginase
Pregnancy Category: C

MECHANISM OF ACTION
Destroys the amino acid asparagine, which is needed for protein synthesis.

INDICATIONS & DOSAGE
Acute lymphocytic leukemia (in combination with other drugs)—
Adults: 5,000 to 10,000 IU/m²/day for 7 days every 3 weeks or 10,000 to 40,000 IU/m² every 2 to 3 weeks.
Doses may be given I.V. over 15 to 30 minutes or by I.M. injection.
Children: 6,000 to 10,000 IU/m² I.V. or I.M. daily for 14 days; or 60,000 IU/m² every other day for a total of 12 doses; or 1,000 IU/kg for 10 days.

ADVERSE REACTIONS
Blood: *hypofibrinogenemia and depression of other clotting factors,* rare

leukopenia, and thrombocytopenia.
CNS: *lethargy,* somnolence.
GI: mild nausea and vomiting, anorexia, weight loss.
GU: rare azotemia and renal failure.
Hepatic: hepatotoxicity, elevated liver function tests, hypoalbuminemia.
Metabolic: *hyperglycemia.*
Skin: rash, urticaria.
Other: *acute pancreatitis, anaphylaxis* (relatively common), *fever.*

INTERACTIONS
None significant.

NURSING CONSIDERATIONS
• Contraindicated in pancreatitis.
• Use cautiously in preexisting hepatic dysfunction.
• Erwinia strain of asparaginase is usually reserved for those patients with previous reactions to *Escherichia coli* asparaginase. The two forms of the drug are not cross-reactive.
• Should be administered in a hospital setting with close supervision.
• Risk of hypersensitivity increases with repeated doses.
• Keep epinephrine, diphenhydramine, and I.V. corticosteroids available for treatment of anaphylaxis.
• Don't use as sole agent to induce remission unless combination therapy is inappropriate. Not recommended for maintenance therapy.
• Give I.V. infusion or I.V. push over 30 minutes through a running infusion of normal saline solution or dextrose 5% in water.
• For I.M. injection, limit dose at single injection site to 2 ml.
• Reconstitute with 2 to 5 ml sterile water for injection or sodium chloride injection. For I.M. use, each 10,000 I.V. vial may be dissolved in 1 ml of diluent.
• Don't shake vial. May cause loss of potency. Don't use cloudy solutions.
• Reconstituted solutions are stable for 3 weeks at either room temperature or refrigerated. Solutions further diluted for infusion are stable at room temperature or refrigerated for at least 4 days.
• The reconstituted solution should be withdrawn from the vial within 15 minutes to minimize protein denaturation resulting from contact with the stopper.
• Monitor CBC and renal and liver function tests.
• Watch for signs of bleeding, such as petechiae and ecchymosis.
• Monitor blood sugar, and test urine for glycosuria before and during therapy.
• Obtain frequent serum amylase and lipase determinations to check pancreatic status. If serum levels are elevated, asparaginase should be discontinued.

hexamethylmelamine (HMM, HXM)
Pregnancy Category: C

MECHANISM OF ACTION
Unknown.

INDICATIONS & DOSAGE
Ovarian carcinoma and lung cancer—
Adults: 4 to 8 mg/kg/day continuously, or 240 to 320 mg/m² daily for 21 days repeated every 6 weeks.

ADVERSE REACTIONS
Blood: *mild leukopenia,* thrombocytopenia.
CNS: *paresthesias, numbness,* sleep disturbances, confusion, hallucinations, seizures, and parkinsonian-like syndrome with ataxia.
GI: *severe GI toxicity including nausea and vomiting, anorexia,* and occasional abdominal cramps and diarrhea.

INTERACTIONS
None significant.

NURSING CONSIDERATIONS
• No special contraindications or cautions.
• GI toxicity may be decreased by giving the daily dose in 4 divided doses. Antiemetics may be useful.
• Neurotoxicity most common in patients receiving continuous daily therapy for longer than 3 months.
• Concomitant administration of pyridoxine 100 mg t.i.d. may decrease neurotoxicity.
• Instruct patient to report any signs of neurotoxicity—CNS or peripheral.
• Monitor CBC.

ifosfamide
Pregnancy Category: NR

MECHANISM OF ACTION
Cross-links strands of cellular DNA, causing an imbalance of growth that leads to cell death.

INDICATIONS & DOSAGE
Lung cancer, Hodgkin's and non-Hodgkin's lymphoma, breast cancer, acute and chronic lymphocytic leukemia, ovarian carcinoma, osteosarcoma—
Adults and children: 1,000 to 1,500 mg/m^2/day × 5 days; or 2,400 mg/m^2/day × 3 days; or up to 5,000 mg/m^2 as a single dose. Regimen usually repeated every 3 weeks.
 The drug may be given by slow I.V. push, intermittent infusion over at least 30 minutes, or by continuous infusion.

ADVERSE REACTIONS
Blood: leukopenia and occasional thrombocytopenia.
CNS: *lethargy and confusion with high doses.*
GI: *nausea, vomiting.*
GU: *hemorrhagic cystitis (dose-limiting adverse reaction occurring in up to 50% of patients),* nephrotoxicity.
Hepatic: elevated liver enzymes.

Other: *alopecia.*

INTERACTIONS
Allopurinol: may produce excessive ifosfamide effect by prolonging half-life. Monitor for enhanced toxicity.
Barbiturates: induce hepatic enzymes, hastening the formation of toxic metabolites. Ifosfamide toxicity may be increased.
Corticosteroids: may inhibit hepatic enzymes, reducing ifosfamide's effect. Monitor for enhanced ifosfamide toxicity if concurrent steroid dose is suddenly reduced or discontinued.

NURSING CONSIDERATIONS
• Use cautiously in patients with renal impairment.
• Push fluids (3 liters daily) to prevent hemorrhagic cystitis. Avoid giving the drug at bedtime, since infrequent voiding during the night may increase the possibility of cystitis. Stop the drug if patient develops cystitis.
• Assess patient for changes in mental status and cerebellar dysfunction. Dose may have to be decreased.
• Bladder irrigation with normal saline solution may decrease the possibility of cystitis.
• Reconstituted solution is stable 2 days at room temperature or 6 weeks refrigerated.
• Infusing each dose over 2 hours or longer will decrease possibility of cystitis.
• Monitor CBC and renal and liver function tests.
• Monitor patient for CNS changes.

semustine (methyl CCNU)
Pregnancy Category: NR

MECHANISM OF ACTION
A nitrosourea compound that probably acts as an alkylating agent. The drug cross-links DNA and also inhib-

---

Italicized side effects are common or life-threatening.
*Liquid form contains alcohol.   **May contain tartrazine.

its several key enzymatic processes.

INDICATIONS & DOSAGE
Advanced GI tumors, brain tumors, Hodgkin's and non-Hodgkin's lymphomas—
Adults: 150 to 200 mg/m² P.O. every 6 to 8 weeks.

ADVERSE REACTIONS
Blood: *delayed thrombocytopenia (about 4 weeks) and leukopenia (about 6 weeks). Myelosuppression may be cumulative.*
GI: *acute nausea and vomiting 2 to 6 hours after administration, anorexia.*
GU: renal toxicity.
Hepatic: elevated liver enzymes.
Other: pulmonary fibrosis with prolonged use.

INTERACTIONS
None significant.

NURSING CONSIDERATIONS
• Use cautiously when other nephrotoxic drugs are also being administered.
• Monitor renal and liver function tests.
• Capsules are usually stored in the refrigerator but are stable for 1 year at room temperature. Avoid storage in high temperatures and excessive moisture.
• The drug should be taken on an empty stomach to assure complete absorption.
• Monitor CBC for delayed myelosuppression, up to 4 weeks for the onset of thrombocytopenia and 6 weeks for leukopenia.

teniposide (VM-26)
Pregnancy Category: NR

MECHANISM OF ACTION
A semi-synthetic derivative of podophyllotoxin that arrests cell mitosis.

INDICATIONS & DOSAGE
Hodgkin's and non-Hodgkin's lymphomas, acute lymphocytic leukemia, bladder carcinoma—
Adults: 50 to 100 mg/m² I.V. once or twice weekly for 4 to 6 weeks, or 40 to 50 mg/m² daily I.V. for 5 days repeated every 3 to 4 weeks.

ADVERSE REACTIONS
Blood: *myelosuppression (dose-limiting), leukopenia, some thrombocytopenia.*
CV: hypotension from rapid infusion.
GI: nausea and vomiting.
Local: *phlebitis, extravasation.*
Other: alopecia (rare), *anaphylaxis (rare).*

INTERACTIONS
None significant.

NURSING CONSIDERATIONS
• May be diluted for infusion in either dextrose 5% in water or normal saline solution, but cloudy solutions should be discarded.
• Infuse over 45 to 90 minutes to prevent hypotension.
• Don't administer through a membrane-type inline filter because the diluent may dissolve the filter.
• Solutions containing 0.5 to 2 mg/ml are stable for 4 hours. Solutions containing 0.1 to 0.2 mg/ml are stable for 6 hours.
• Monitor blood pressure before infusion and at 30-minute intervals during infusion. If systolic blood pressure falls below 90 mm Hg, stop infusion and notify doctor.
• Have diphenhydramine, hydrocortisone, epinephrine, and airway available in case of anaphylaxis.
• Monitor CBC. Observe patient for signs of bone marrow depression.
• Avoid extravasation.
• Drug may be given by local bladder instillation as a treatment for bladder cancer.

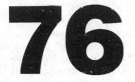

Immunosuppressants

azathioprine
cyclosporine
muromonab-CD3

COMBINATION PRODUCTS
None.

---

azathioprine
Imuran♦
Pregnancy Category: D

MECHANISM OF ACTION
Inhibits purine synthesis.

INDICATIONS & DOSAGE
Immunosuppression in renal transplants—
Adults and children: initially, 3 to 5 mg/kg P.O. daily. Maintain at 1 to 2 mg/kg daily (dose varies considerably according to patient response).
Treatment of severe, refractory rheumatoid arthritis—
Adults: initially, 1 mg/kg taken as a single dose or as 2 doses. If patient response is not satisfactory after 6 to 8 weeks, dosage may be increased by 0.5 mg/kg daily (up to a maximum of 2.5 mg/kg daily) at 4-week intervals.

ADVERSE REACTIONS
Blood: *leukopenia, bone marrow depression,* anemia, pancytopenia, thrombocytopenia.
GI: nausea, vomiting, anorexia, *pancreatitis,* steatorrhea, mouth ulceration, esophagitis.
Hepatic: hepatotoxicity, jaundice.
Skin: rash.
Other: *immunosuppression (possibly profound),* arthralgia, muscle wasting, alopecia.

INTERACTIONS
Allopurinol: impaired inactivation of azathioprine. Decrease azathioprine dose to ¼ or ⅓ normal dose.

NURSING CONSIDERATIONS
• Use cautiously in hepatic or renal dysfunction.
• Watch for clay-colored stools, dark urine, pruritus, and yellow skin and sclera; and for increased alkaline phosphatase, bilirubin, SGOT, and SGPT.
• In renal homotransplants, start drug 1 to 5 days before surgery.
• Hemoglobin, WBC, platelet count should be done at least once monthly; more often at beginning of treatment. Drug should be stopped immediately when WBC is less than 3,000/mm³ to prevent extension to irreversible bone marrow depression.
• This is a potent immunosuppressive. Warn patient to report even mild infections (colds, fever, sore throat, malaise).
• Patient should avoid conception during therapy and up to 4 months after stopping therapy.
• Warn patient that some thinning of hair is possible.
• Avoid I.M. injections of any drugs in patients with severely depressed platelet counts (thrombocytopenia) to prevent bleeding.
• When used for refractory rheumatoid arthritis, inform patient that it may take up to 12 weeks to be effective.

Italicized side effects are common or life-threatening.
*Liquid form contains alcohol.   **May contain tartrazine.

cyclosporine
Sandimmune
Pregnancy Category: C

MECHANISM OF ACTION
Inhibits the action of T lymphocytes.

INDICATIONS & DOSAGE
Prophylaxis of organ rejection in kidney, liver, bone marrow, and heart transplants—
Adults and children: 15 mg/kg P.O. (oral solution) 4 to 12 hours before transplantation. Continue this daily dose postoperatively for 1 to 2 weeks. Then, gradually reduce dosage by 5%/ week to maintenance level of 5 to 10 mg/kg/day. Alternatively, administer I.V. concentrate 4 to 5 mg/kg 4 to 12 hours before transplantation. Postoperatively, repeat this dose daily until patient can tolerate oral solution.

ADVERSE REACTIONS
CNS: *tremor,* headache.
CV: *hypertension.*
GI: *gum hyperplasia,* nausea, vomiting, diarrhea, oral thrush.
GU: *nephrotoxicity.*
Hepatic: hepatotoxicity.
Skin: *hirsutism,* acne.
Other: sinusitis, flushing.

INTERACTIONS
Ketoconazole, amphotericin B, cimetidine: may increase blood levels of cyclosporine. Monitor for increased toxicity.
Phenytoin, rifampin: possible decreased immunosuppressant effect. May need to increase cyclosporine dose.

NURSING CONSIDERATIONS
• Cyclosporine may cause nephrotoxicity. Monitor BUN and serum creatinine levels. Nephrotoxicity may develop as long as 2 to 3 months after transplant surgery. Report these findings to doctor. He may reduce the dose.
• Differentiation between transplanted kidney rejection and cyclosporine-induced nephrotoxicity must be made.
• Monitor liver function tests for hepatotoxicity, which usually occurs during first month post–organ transplant.
• Cyclosporine should always be given concomitantly with adrenal corticosteroids.
• Absorption of cyclosporine oral solution can be erratic. Monitor cyclosporine blood levels at regular intervals.
• Measure oral doses carefully in an oral syringe. To increase palatability, mix with whole milk, chocolate milk, or fruit juice. Use a glass container to minimize adherence to container walls.
• Dose should be given once daily in the morning. Encourage patient to take drug at the same time each day.
• Patient may take with meals if drug causes nausea.
• Stress to patient that therapy should not be stopped without doctor's approval.
• To prevent thrush, patient should swish and swallow nystatin four times daily.
• If hirsutism occurs, tell patient she may use a depilatory.

muromonab-CD3
Orthoclone OKT3
Pregnancy Category: C

MECHANISM OF ACTION
Muromonab-CD3 is an IgG antibody that reacts in the T-lymphocyte membrane with a molecule (CD3) needed for antigen recognition. This drug depletes the blood of CD3-positive T cells, which leads to restoration of allograft function and reversal of rejection.

INDICATIONS & DOSAGE

Treatment of acute allograft rejection in renal transplant patients—
Adults: 5 mg I.V. bolus once daily for 10 to 14 days.
Children: 2.5 mg I.V. bolus once daily for 10 to 14 days.

ADVERSE REACTIONS

CV: *chest pain*.
GI: *nausea, vomiting*, diarrhea.
Other: *severe pulmonary edema, fever, chills, tremors, dyspnea, infection*.

INTERACTIONS

None reported.

NURSING CONSIDERATIONS

• Contraindicated in patients with fluid overload, as evidenced by chest X-ray or a weight gain greater than 3% within the week before treatment.
• Muromonab-CD3 is a monoclonal antibody preparation. Patients develop antibodies to this preparation that can lead to loss of effectiveness and more severe adverse reactions if a second course of therapy is attempted. Therefore, experts believe that this drug should be used for only a single course of treatment.
• Most adverse reactions develop within ½ hour to 6 hours of the first dose.
• Treatment should begin in a facility where the patient can be monitored closely and that is equipped and staffed for cardiopulmonary resuscitation.
• Assess patient for signs of fluid overload before treatment.
• Chest X-ray must be taken within 24 hours before starting drug treatment.
• Inform patient of expected adverse reactions. Reassure him that they will be less severe as treatment progresses.
• Administering an antipyretic before giving the drug may help lower incidence of expected pyrexia and chills.

Corticosteroids may also be administered before first injection to help decrease incidence of adverse reactions.

Italicized side effects are common or life-threatening.
*Liquid form contains alcohol. **May contain tartrazine.

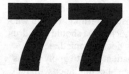

Ophthalmic anti-infectives

bacitracin
boric acid
chloramphenicol
erythromycin
gentamicin sulfate
idoxuridine (IDU)
natamycin
polymyxin B sulfate
silver nitrate 1%
sulfacetamide sodium 10%, 15%, 30%
tetracycline hydrochloride
tobramycin
trifluridine
vidarabine

COMBINATION PRODUCTS

BLEPHAMIDE S.O.P. OPHTHALMIC OINTMENT: sodium sulfacetamide 10% and prednisolone acetate 0.2%.
CETAPRED OINTMENT♦: sodium sulfacetamide 10% and prednisolone acetate 0.25%.
CHLOROMYCETIN HYDROCORTISONE OPHTHALMIC♦: chloramphenicol 1.25% and hydrocortisone acetate 2.5%.
CORTISPORIN OPHTHALMIC OINTMENT♦: polymyxin B sulfate 10,000 units, bacitracin zinc 400 units, neomycin sulfate 0.5%, and hydrocortisone 1%.
CORTISPORIN OPHTHALMIC SUSPENSION♦: polymyxin B sulfate 10,000 units, neomycin sulfate 0.5%, and hydrocortisone 1%.
ISOPTO CETAPRED: sulfacetamide sodium 10% and prednisolone acetate 0.25%.
MAXITROL OPHTHALMIC OINTMENT/ SUSPENSION♦: dexamethasone 0.1%, neomycin sulfate 0.5%, and polymyxin B sulfate 10,000 units.
METIMYD OPHTHALMIC OINTMENT/ SUSPENSION: sodium sulfacetamide 10% and prednisolone acetate 0.5%.
MYCITRACIN OPHTHALMIC: polymyxin B sulfate 5,000 units, neomycin sulfate 3.5 mg, and bacitracin 500 units.
NEODECADRON OPHTHALMIC SOLUTION♦: dexamethasone phosphate 0.1% and neomycin sulfate 0.5%.
NEOSPORIN OPHTHALMIC: polymyxin B sulfate 10,000 units, neomycin sulfate 1.75 mg, and gramicidin 0.025 mg.
NEOSPORIN OPHTHALMIC OINTMENT♦: polymyxin B sulfate 10,000 units, neomycin sulfate 3.5 mg, and bacitracin zinc 400 units/g.
NEOTAL OPHTHALMIC OINTMENT: polymyxin B sulfate 5,000 units, neomycin sulfate 3.5 mg, and bacitracin zinc 400 units.
OPHTHA P/S OPHTHALMIC DROPS: prednisolone acetate 0.5%, sodium sulfacetamide 10%.
OPHTHOCORT OINTMENT: chloramphenicol 1.0%, polymyxin B sulfate 5,000 units, and hydrocortisone acetate 0.5%.
OPTIMYD SOLUTION: prednisolone phosphate 0.5% and sodium sulfacetamide 10%.
POLYSPORIN OPHTHALMIC OINTMENT: polymyxin B sulfate 10,000 units, and bacitracin zinc 500 units.
STATROL OPHTHALMIC SOLUTION: neomycin sulfate 3.5 mg and polymyxin B sulfate 16,250 units.
SULFAPRED OPHTHALMIC SUSPEN-

SION: sodium sulfacetamide 10%, prednisolone acetate 0.25%, and phenylephrine HCl 0.125%.
VASOCIDIN OINTMENT: sodium sulfacetamide 10%, prednisolone acetate 0.2%, and phenylephrine HCl 0.125%.
VASOCIDIN SOLUTION♦: sodium sulfacetamide 10%, prednisolone phosphate 0.2%, and phenylephrine HCl 0.125%.
VASOSULF SOLUTION♦: sodium sulfacetamide 15% and phenylephrine HCl 0.125%.

bacitracin
Pregnancy Category: C

MECHANISM OF ACTION
Inhibits protein synthesis.

INDICATIONS & DOSAGE
Ocular infections—
Adults and children: apply small amount into conjunctival sac several times a day or p.r.n. until favorable response is observed.

ADVERSE REACTIONS
Eye: slowed corneal wound healing, temporary visual haze.
Other: overgrowth of nonsusceptible organisms.

INTERACTIONS
Heavy metals (silver nitrate): inactivate bacitracin. Don't use together.

NURSING CONSIDERATIONS
• Use cautiously in patients with hereditary predisposition to antibiotic hypersensitivity.
• Warn patient to avoid sharing washcloths and towels with family members.
• Always wash hands before and after applying ointment.
• Cleanse eye area of excessive exudate before application.
• Tell patient to watch for signs of

sensitivity, such as itching lids, swelling or constant burning. Patient who develops such signs should stop drug and notify doctor immediately.
• Show patient how to apply. Stress importance of compliance with recommended therapy.
• Warn patient not to touch tip of tube to any part of eye or surrounding tissue.
• Warn patient that ointment may cause blurred vision.
• Solution not commercially available but may be prepared by pharmacy. May be stored up to 3 weeks in refrigerator.
• Bactericidal or bacteriostatic, depending on concentration and infection.
• Store in tightly closed, light-resistant container.
• Tell patient not to share eye medications with family members. If a family member develops the same symptoms, instruct him to contact the doctor.

boric acid
Blinx, Collyrium, Neo-Flo
Pregnancy Category: C

MECHANISM OF ACTION
Unknown. However, drug has fungistatic and bacteriostatic properties.

INDICATIONS & DOSAGE
For irrigation following tonometry, gonioscopy, foreign body removal, or use of fluorescein; used to soothe and cleanse the eye; used in conjunction with contact lens—
Adults: irrigate eye with 2% solution or apply 5% or 10% ointment, p.r.n.

ADVERSE REACTIONS
Note: toxic if absorbed from abraded skin areas, granulating wounds, or ingestion.

Italicized side effects are common or life-threatening.
*Liquid form contains alcohol.   **May contain tartrazine.

INTERACTIONS
Polyvinyl alcohol (Liquifilm): may form insoluble complex. Check with pharmacy on contents in eye drugs and contact lens wetting solutions.

NURSING CONSIDERATIONS
• Contraindicated in eye lacerations.
• Don't apply to abraded cornea or skin.
• Always wash hands before and after instilling solution or ointment.
• Not for use with soft contact lenses.
• Weak bacteriostatic, fungistatic agent.
• Tell patient not to share eye solution with family members.
• Always use sterile solution in the eye.

---

chloramphenicol
Antibiopto, Chloromycetin Ophthalmic♦, Chloroptic♦, Chloroptic S.O.P., Econochlor Ophthalmic, Fenicol♦♦, Isopto Fenicol♦♦, Ophthoclor Ophthalmic, Pentamycetin♦♦
Pregnancy Category: C

MECHANISM OF ACTION
Inhibits protein synthesis.

INDICATIONS & DOSAGE
Surface bacterial infection involving conjunctiva or cornea—
Adults and children: instill 2 drops of solution in eye q hour until condition improves, or instill q.i.d., depending on severity of infection. Apply small amount of ointment to lower conjunctival sac at bedtime as supplement to drops. May use ointment alone by applying a small amount of ointment to lower conjunctival sac q 3 to 6 hours or more frequently, if necessary. Continue until condition improves.

ADVERSE REACTIONS
Note: systemic adverse reactions have not been reported with short-term topical use.
Blood: *bone marrow hypoplasia with prolonged use, aplastic anemia.*
Eye: optic atrophy in children, stinging or burning of eye after instillation.
Other: overgrowth of nonsusceptible organisms; hypersensitivity, including itching and burning eye, dermatitis, angioedema.

INTERACTIONS
None significant.

NURSING CONSIDERATIONS
• Not for long-term use. Notify doctor if no improvement in 3 days.
• If patient has more than a superficial infection, systemic therapy should also be used.
• Apply light finger-pressure on lacrimal sac for 1 minute after drops are instilled.
• One of the safest topical ocular antibiotics, especially for endophthalmitis.
• Warn patient to avoid sharing washcloths and towels with family members.
• Always wash hands before and after applying ointment or solution.
• Cleanse eye area of excessive exudate before application.
• Tell patient to watch for signs of sensitivity, such as itching lids or constant burning. Patient who develops such signs should stop drug and notify doctor immediately.
• Show patient how to instill. Stress importance of compliance with recommended therapy.
• Warn patient not to touch tip of applicator to eye or surrounding tissue.
• If chloramphenicol drops are to be given q 1 hour, then tapered, follow order closely to ensure adequate anterior chamber levels.
• Store in tightly closed, light-resistant container.
• Tell patient not to share eye medications with family members. If a fam-

---

ily member develops the same symptoms, instruct him to contact the doctor.

erythromycin
Ilotycin Ophthalmic♦
Pregnancy Category: NR

MECHANISM OF ACTION
Inhibits protein synthesis.

INDICATIONS & DOSAGE
Acute and chronic conjunctivitis, trachoma, other eye infections—
Adults and children: apply 0.5% ointment 1 or more times daily, depending upon severity of infection.
Prophylaxis of ophthalmia neonatorum—
Neonates: a ribbon of ointment approximately 0.5 to 1 cm long placed in the lower conjunctival sacs shortly after birth.

ADVERSE REACTIONS
Eye: slowed corneal wound healing.
Other: overgrowth of nonsusceptible organisms with long-term use; hypersensitivity, including itching and burning eye, urticaria, dermatitis, angioedema.

INTERACTIONS
None significant.

NURSING CONSIDERATIONS
• Bacteriostatic, but may be bactericidal in high concentrations or against highly susceptible organisms.
• Has a limited antibacterial spectrum. Use only when sensitivity studies show it is effective against infecting organisms. Don't use in infections of unknown etiology.
• For prophylaxis of ophthalmia neonatorum, apply ointment no later than 1 hour after birth.
• Warn patient to avoid sharing washcloths and towels with family members.

• Always wash hands before and after applying ointment.
• Cleanse eye area of excessive exudate before application.
• Tell patient to watch for signs of sensitivity, such as itching lids or constant burning. Patient who develops such signs should stop drug and notify doctor immediately.
• Show patient how to apply. Stress importance of compliance with recommended therapy.
• Warn patient not to touch tube to eye or surrounding tissue.
• Warn patient that ointment may cause blurred vision.
• Store at room temperature in tightly closed, light-resistant container.
• Tell patient not to share eye medications with family members. If a family member develops the same symptoms, instruct him to contact the doctor.

gentamicin sulfate
Garamycin Ophthalmic♦, Genoptic
Pregnancy Category: C

MECHANISM OF ACTION
Inhibits protein synthesis.

INDICATIONS & DOSAGE
External ocular infections (conjunctivitis, keratoconjunctivitis, corneal ulcers, blepharitis, blepharoconjunctivitis, meibomianitis, and dacryocystitis) due to susceptible organisms, especially Pseudomonas aeruginosa, Proteus, Klebsiella pneumoniae, Escherichia coli, *and other gram-negative organisms—*
Adults and children: instill 1 to 2 drops in eye q 4 hours. In severe infections, may use up to 2 drops q 1 hour. Apply ointment to lower conjunctival sac b.i.d. or t.i.d.

ADVERSE REACTIONS
Note: systemic absorption from excessive use may cause systemic toxici-

---

Italicized side effects are common or life-threatening.
*Liquid form contains alcohol.   **May contain tartrazine.

ties.
Eye: burning or stinging with ointment, transient irritation from solution.
Other: hypersensitivity, overgrowth of nonsusceptible organisms with long-term use.

INTERACTIONS
None significant.

NURSING CONSIDERATIONS
• Contraindicated in aminoglycoside hypersensitivity. Use cautiously in impaired renal function.
• Have culture taken before giving drug.
• If topical ocular gentamicin is administered concomitantly with systemic gentamicin, be sure to carefully monitor serum gentamicin levels.
• Stress importance of following recommended therapy. *Pseudomonas* infections can cause complete vision loss within 24 hours if infection is not controlled.
• Warn patient to avoid sharing washcloths and towels with family members.
• Always wash hands before and after applying ointment or solution.
• Cleanse eye area of excessive exudate before application.
• Tell patient to watch for signs of sensitivity, such as itching lids or constant burning. Patient who develops such signs should stop drug and notify doctor immediately.
• Show patient how to instill.
• Apply light finger-pressure on lacrimal sac for 1 minute after drops are instilled.
• Warn patient not to touch tip of tube or dropper to eye or surrounding tissue.
• Store away from heat.
• Tell patient not to share eye medications with family members. If a family member develops the same symptoms, instruct him to contact the doctor.

idoxuridine (IDU)
Herplex♦, Stoxil♦
Pregnancy Category: C

MECHANISM OF ACTION
Interferes with DNA synthesis.

INDICATIONS & DOSAGE
Herpes simplex keratitis—
Adults and children: instill 1 drop of solution into conjunctival sac q 1 hour during day and q 2 hours at night, or apply ointment to conjunctival sac q 4 hours or 5 times daily, with last dose at bedtime. A response should be seen in 7 days; if not, discontinue and begin alternate therapy. Therapy should not be continued longer than 21 days.

ADVERSE REACTIONS
Eye: temporary visual haze; irritation, pain, burning, or inflammation of eye; mild edema of eyelid or cornea; photosensitivity; small punctate defects in corneal epithelium, corneal ulceration; slowed corneal wound healing with ointment.
Other: hypersensitivity.

INTERACTIONS
None significant.

NURSING CONSIDERATIONS
• Contraindicated in deep ulceration.
• Not for long-term use.
• Idoxuridine should not be mixed with other medications.
• Don't use old solution; causes ocular burning and has no antiviral activity.
• Warn patient to avoid sharing washcloths and towels with family members.
• Always wash hands before and after applying ointment or solution.
• Cleanse eye area of excessive exudate before application.
• Tell patient to watch for signs of sensitivity, such as itching lids or constant burning. Patient who develops

such signs should stop drug and notify doctor immediately.
• Show patient how to apply. Stress importance of compliance with recommended therapy.
• Warn patient not to touch tip of tube or dropper to eye or surrounding tissue.
• Refrigerate idoxuridine 0.1% solution. Store in tightly closed, light-resistant container.
• Tell patient not to share eye medications with family members. If a family member develops the same symptoms, instruct him to contact the doctor.
• If sensitivity to light develops, patient should wear sunglasses.

natamycin
Natacyn
Pregnancy Category: C

MECHANISM OF ACTION
Increases fungal cell-membrane permeability.

INDICATIONS & DOSAGE
Treatment of fungal keratitis—
Adults: initial dosage 1 drop instilled in conjunctival sac q 1 to 2 hours. After 3 to 4 days, reduce dosage to 1 drop 6 to 8 times daily.

ADVERSE REACTIONS
Eye: ocular edema, hyperemia.

INTERACTIONS
None significant.

NURSING CONSIDERATIONS
• Only antifungal available as ophthalmic preparation.
• Treatment of choice for fungal keratitis. May also be used to treat fungal blepharitis and conjunctivitis.
• Therapy should be continued for 14 to 21 days, or until active disease subsides.
• Reduce dosage gradually at 4- to 7-

day intervals to assure that organism has been eliminated.
• If infection does not improve with 7 to 10 days of therapy, clinical and laboratory reevaluation is recommended.
• Apply light finger-pressure on lacrimal sac for 1 minute after drops are instilled.
• Warn patient to avoid sharing washcloths and towels with family members.
• Always wash hands before and after applying.
• Cleanse eye area of excessive exudate before application.
• Show patient how to apply. Stress importance of compliance with recommended therapy.
• Warn patient not to touch tip of dropper to eye or surrounding tissue.
• Tell patient not to share eye medications with family members. If a family member develops the same symptoms, instruct him to contact the doctor.
• Shake well before use. May be kept in refrigerator or at room temperature.

polymyxin B sulfate
Pregnancy Category: B

MECHANISM OF ACTION
Inhibits protein synthesis.

INDICATIONS & DOSAGE
Used alone or in combination with other agents for treating corneal ulcers resulting from Pseudomonas *infection or other gram-negative organism infections—*
Adults and children: instill 1 to 3 drops of 0.1% to 0.25% (10,000 to 25,000 units/ml) q 1 hour. Increase interval according to patient response; or up to 10,000 units subconjunctivally daily by doctor.

ADVERSE REACTIONS
Eye: eye irritation, conjunctivitis.

Italicized side effects are common or life-threatening.
*Liquid form contains alcohol.   **May contain tartrazine.

Other: overgrowth of nonsusceptible organisms, hypersensitivity (local burning, itching).

INTERACTIONS
None significant.

NURSING CONSIDERATIONS
• One of the most effective antibiotics against gram-negative organisms, especially *Pseudomonas*.
• Often used in combination with neomycin sulfate.
• In severe, life-threatening *Pseudomonas* infections, polymyxin B may be used as an ocular irrigant.
• Warn patient to avoid sharing washcloths and towels with family members.
• Always wash hands before and after instilling solution.
• Cleanse eye area of excessive exudate before application.
• Tell patient to watch for signs of sensitivity, such as itching lids and lashes or constant burning. Patient who develops such signs should stop drug and notify doctor immediately.
• Show patient how to instill. Stress importance of compliance with recommended therapy.
• Apply light finger-pressure on lacrimal sac for 1 minute after drops are instilled.
• Warn patient not to touch tip of dropper to eye or surrounding tissue.
• Reconstitute carefully to ensure correct drug concentration in solution.
• Tell patient not to share eye medications with family members. If a family member develops the same symptoms, instruct him to contact the doctor.

---

silver nitrate 1%
Pregnancy Category: C

MECHANISM OF ACTION
Causes protein denaturation, which prevents gonorrheal ophthalmia neonatorum.

INDICATIONS & DOSAGE
Prevention of gonorrheal ophthalmia neonatorum—
Neonates: cleanse lids thoroughly; instill 1 drop of 1% solution into each eye.

ADVERSE REACTIONS
Eye: periorbital edema, temporary staining of lids and surrounding tissue, conjunctivitis (with concentrations 1% or greater).

INTERACTIONS
Bacitracin: inactivates silver nitrate. Don't use together.

NURSING CONSIDERATIONS
• Legally required for neonates in most states.
• Don't use repeatedly.
• If 2% solution is accidentally used in eye, prompt irrigation with isotonic sodium chloride is advised to prevent eye irritation.
• Solution may stain skin and utensils. Handle carefully.
• May delay instillation slightly to allow neonate to bond with mother.
• Always wash hands before instilling solution.
• Store wax ampuls away from light and heat.
• Bacteriostatic, germicidal, and astringent.
• Handle solution carefully. May stain skin or utensils.
• Don't irrigate eyes after instillation.

sulfacetamide sodium 10%
Bleph-10 Liquifilm Ophthalmic♦,
Cetamide Ophthalmic♦, Sodium
Sulamyd 10% Ophthalmic♦, Sulf-10
Ophthalmic♦

sulfacetamide sodium 15%
Isopto Cetamide Ophthalmic♦,
Sulfacel-15 Ophthalmic

sulfacetamide sodium 30%
Sodium Sulamyd 30% Ophthalmic♦
Pregnancy Category: C

MECHANISM OF ACTION
Prevents uptake of para-aminobenzoic
acid, a metabolite of bacterial folic-
acid synthesis.

INDICATIONS & DOSAGE
*Inclusion conjunctivitis, corneal ul-
cers, trachoma, prophylaxis to ocular
infection—*
Adults and children: instill 1 to 2
drops of 10% solution into lower conjunctival sac q 2 to 3 hours during
day, less often at night; or instill 1 to 2
drops of 15% solution into lower conjunctival sac q 1 to 2 hours initially,
increasing interval as condition responds; or instill 1 drop of 30% solution into lower conjunctival sac q 2
hours. Instill ½" to 1" of 10% ointment into conjunctival sac q.i.d. and
at bedtime. May use ointment at night
along with drops during the day.

ADVERSE REACTIONS
Eye: slowed corneal wound healing
(ointment), *pain on instilling eye
drop,* headache or browache.
Other: hypersensitivity (including
itching or burning), overgrowth of
nonsusceptible organisms, *Stevens-
Johnson syndrome,* sensitivity to
light.

INTERACTIONS
*Local anesthetics (procaine, tetra-
caine),* p-*aminobenzoic acid deriva-*
tives: decreased sulfacetamide sodium
action. Wait ½ to 1 hour after instilling anesthetic or p-aminobenzoic acid
derivative before instilling sulfacetamide.

NURSING CONSIDERATIONS
• Contraindicated in sulfonamide hypersensitivity.
• Often used with systemic tetracycline in treating trachoma and inclusion conjunctivitis.
• Replaced by antibiotics in treating
major ocular infections; still used in
minor ocular infections.
• Purulent exudate interferes with
sulfacetamide action. Remove as
much exudate as possible from lids
before instilling sulfacetamide.
• Incompatible with silver preparations.
• Warn patient eye drop burns
slightly.
• Warn patient to avoid sharing washcloths and towels with family members.
• Always wash hands before and after
applying ointment or solution.
• Tell patient to watch for signs of
sensitivity, such as itching lids or constant burning. Patient who develops
such signs should stop drug and notify
doctor immediately.
• Show patient how to instill. Stress
importance of compliance with recommended therapy.
• Apply light finger-pressure on lacrimal sac for 1 minute after drops are
instilled.
• Wait at least 5 minutes before administering other eye drops.
• Warn patient not to touch tip of tube
or dropper to eye or surrounding tissue.
• Store in tightly closed, light-resistant container away from heat.
• Don't use discolored (dark brown)
solution.
• Tell patient not to share eye medications with family members. If a family member develops the same symp-

---

toms, instruct him to contact the doctor.

• May minimize sensitivity to bright light by wearing sunglasses.

tetracycline hydrochloride
Achromycin Ophthalmic♦
Pregnancy Category: D

MECHANISM OF ACTION
Inhibits protein synthesis.

INDICATIONS & DOSAGE
Adults and children:
Superficial ocular infections and inclusion conjunctivitis—
instill 1 to 2 drops in eye b.i.d., q.i.d., or more often, depending on severity of infection.
Trachoma—
instill 2 drops in each eye b.i.d., t.i.d., or q.i.d. Continue for 1 to 2 months or longer, or use 1% ointment t.i.d. or q.i.d. for 30 days.
Prophylaxis of ophthalmia neonatorum—
Neonates: 1 to 2 drops into each eye shortly after delivery.

ADVERSE REACTIONS
Eye: itching.
Other: hypersensitivity (eye itching and dermatitis), overgrowth of nonsusceptible organisms with long-term use.

INTERACTIONS
None significant.

NURSING CONSIDERATIONS
• Tell patient or family that trachoma therapy should continue for 1 to 2 months or longer. Trachoma may cause blindness if left untreated or if not treated properly.
• Tell patient that gnats and flies are vectors of the trachoma organism. Warn patient with trachoma not to let them settle around eye area. Also explain that infection is spread by direct contact, so handwashing is essential to prevent spread.
• For prophylaxis of ophthalmia neonatorum, apply ointment no later than 1 hour after birth.
• Apply light finger-pressure on lacrimal sac for 1 minute after drops are instilled.
• Warn patient to avoid sharing washcloths and towels with family members.
• Always wash hands before and after applying solution.
• Cleanse eye area of excessive exudate before application.
• Tell patient to watch for signs of sensitivity, such as itching lids or constant burning. Patient who develops such signs should stop drug and notify doctor immediately.
• Show patient how to instill. Stress importance of compliance with recommended therapy.
• Warn patient not to touch tip of dropper to eye or surrounding tissue.
• Store in tightly closed, light-resistant container.
• Tell patient not to share eye medications with family members. If a family member develops the same symptoms, instruct him to contact the doctor.

tobramycin
Tobrex♦
Pregnancy Category: D

MECHANISM OF ACTION
Inhibits protein synthesis.

INDICATIONS & DOSAGE
Treatment of external ocular infections caused by susceptible gram-negative bacteria—
Adults and children: In mild-to-moderate infections, instill 1 or 2 drops into the affected eye q 4 hours. In severe infections, instill 2 drops into the infected eye hourly.

ADVERSE REACTIONS
Eye: burning or stinging upon instillation, lid itching, lid swelling.
Other: hypersensitivity.

INTERACTIONS
Tetracycline-containing eye preparations: incompatible with tyloxapol, an ingredient in Tobrex. Don't use together.

NURSING CONSIDERATIONS
• Prolonged use may result in overgrowth of nonsusceptible organisms, including fungi.
• If topical ocular tobramycin is administered concomitantly with systemic tobramycin, be sure to carefully monitor serum levels.
• Clinical symptoms of tobramycin overdose include keratitis, erythema, increased lacrimation, edema, and lid itching. Stop drug and notify doctor if any of these occur.
• Always wash hands before and after instilling solution.
• Warn patient to avoid sharing washcloths and towels with family members.
• Tell patient to watch for signs of sensitivity, such as itching lids or constant burning. Patient who develops such signs should discontinue drug and notify doctor immediately.
• Warn patient not to touch tip of dropper to eye or surrounding tissue.
• Show patient how to instill.
• Apply light finger-pressure on lacrimal sac for 1 minute after drops are instilled.
• Often used to combat gram-negative organisms that are resistant to gentamicin.

trifluridine
Viroptic Ophthalmic Solution 1%♦
Pregnancy Category: C

MECHANISM OF ACTION
Interferes with DNA synthesis.

INDICATIONS & DOSAGE
Primary keratoconjunctivitis and recurrent epithelial keratitis due to herpes simplex virus, types I and II—
Adults: 1 drop of solution q 2 hours while patient is awake, to a maximum of 9 drops daily until re-epithelialization of the corneal ulcer occurs; then 1 drop q 4 hours (minimum 5 drops daily) for an additional 7 days.

ADVERSE REACTIONS
Eye: *stinging upon instillation,* edema of eyelids, increased intraocular pressure.

INTERACTIONS
None significant.

NURSING CONSIDERATIONS
• Should be prescribed only for those patients with clinical diagnosis of herpetic keratitis.
• Consider another form of therapy if improvement doesn't occur after 7 days' treatment or complete re-epithelialization after 14 days' treatment. Trifluridine shouldn't be used more than 21 days continuously due to potential ocular toxicity.
• Apply light finger-pressure on lacrimal sac for 1 minute after drops are instilled.
• Reassure patient that mild local irritation of the conjunctiva and cornea that occurs when solution is instilled is usually temporary.
• More effective drug than vidarabine with fewer adverse reactions.
• Warn patient to avoid sharing washcloths and towels with family members.
• Wash hands before and after administration.
• Warn patient not to touch tip of dropper to eye or surrounding tissue.
• Tell patient not to share eye medications with family members. If a family member develops the same disease symptoms, instruct him to contact the doctor.

Italicized side effects are common or life-threatening.
*Liquid form contains alcohol.   **May contain tartrazine.

vidarabine
Vira-A Ophthalmic♦
Pregnancy Category: C

MECHANISM OF ACTION
Interferes with DNA synthesis.

INDICATIONS & DOSAGE
Acute keratoconjunctivitis, superficial keratitis, and recurrent epithelial keratitis resulting from herpes simplex types I and II—
Adults and children: instill ½″ ointment into lower conjunctival sac 5 times daily at 3-hour intervals.

ADVERSE REACTIONS
Eye: temporary visual burning, itching, mild irritation of eye, lacrimation, foreign body sensation, conjunctival injection, superficial punctate keratitis, eye pain, photosensitivity.
Other: hypersensitivity.

INTERACTIONS
None significant.

NURSING CONSIDERATIONS
• Not for long-term use.
• Warn patient not to exceed recommended frequency or duration of dosage.
• Not effective against RNA virus or adenoviral ocular infections, or against bacterial, fungal, or chlamydial infections.
• Warn patient to avoid sharing washcloths and towels with family members.
• Always wash hands before and after applying ointment.
• Tell patient to watch for signs of sensitivity, such as itching lids or constant burning. Patient who develops such signs should stop drug and notify doctor immediately.
• Show patient how to instill.
• Warn patient not to touch tip of tube to eye or surrounding tissue.
• Store in tightly closed, light-resistant container.
• Tell patient not to share eye medications with family members. If a family member develops the same disease symptoms, instruct him to contact the doctor.
• Explain to patient that the ointment may produce a temporary visual haze.
• If sensitivity to light develops, patient should wear sunglasses.

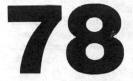

Ophthalmic anti-inflammatory agents

dexamethasone
dexamethasone sodium
   phosphate
fluorometholone
flurbiprofen sodium
medrysone
prednisolone acetate
   (suspension)
prednisolone sodium phosphate
   (solution)

COMBINATION PRODUCTS
Corticosteroids for ophthalmic use
are commonly combined with antibiotics and sulfonamides. See Chapter
77, OPHTHALMIC ANTI-INFECTIVES.

dexamethasone
Maxidex Ophthalmic Suspension♦

dexamethasone sodium phosphate
Decadron Phosphate Ophthalmic♦,
Maxidex Ophthalmic♦
Pregnancy Category: C

MECHANISM OF ACTION
Decreases the infiltration of leukocytes at the site of inflammation.

INDICATIONS & DOSAGE
*Uveitis; iridocyclitis; inflammatory
conditions of eyelids, conjunctiva,
cornea, anterior segment of globe;
corneal injury from chemical or ther-
mal burns, or penetration of foreign
bodies; allergic conjunctivitis—*
Adults and children: instill 1 to 2
drops into conjunctival sac. In severe
disease, drops may be used hourly, tapering to discontinuation as condition
improves. In mild conditions, drops
may be used up to 4 to 6 times daily.
Treatment may extend from a few
days to several weeks.

ADVERSE REACTIONS
Eye: *increased intraocular pressure;*
thinning of cornea, interference with
corneal wound healing, increased susceptibility to viral or fungal corneal
infection, corneal ulceration; with excessive or long-term use, *glaucoma*
exacerbations, *cataracts,* defects in visual acuity and visual field, *optic
nerve damage.*
Other: systemic effects and adrenal
suppression with excessive or long-
term use.

INTERACTIONS
None significant.

NURSING CONSIDERATIONS
• Contraindicated in acute superficial
herpes simplex (dendritic keratitis),
vaccinia, varicella, or other fungal or
viral diseases of cornea and conjunctiva; presence of active diabetes; ocular tuberculosis, or any acute, purulent, untreated infection of the eye.
Use cautiously in corneal abrasions,
since these may be infected (especially with herpes); in patients with
glaucoma (any form), due to possibility of increasing intraocular pressure
(glaucoma medications may need to
be increased to compensate).
• Viral and fungal infections of the
cornea may be exacerbated by the application of steroids.

Italicized side effects are common or life-threatening.
*Liquid form contains alcohol.   **May contain tartrazine.

- Warn patient to call doctor immediately and to stop drug if visual acuity changes or visual field diminishes.
- Not for long-term use.
- May use eye pad with ointment for increased effect.
- Show patient how to instill.
- Apply light finger-pressure on lacrimal sac for 1 minute following instillation.
- Watch for corneal ulceration; may require stopping drug.
- Dexamethasone has greater anti-inflammatory effect than dexamethasone sodium phosphate.
- Warn patient not to use leftover medication for a new eye inflammation; can cause serious problems.
- Tell patient never to share eye medications. If a family member develops similar disease symptoms, instruct him to contact the doctor.

fluorometholone
FML Liquifilm Ophthalmic♦
Pregnancy Category: C

MECHANISM OF ACTION
Decreases the infiltration of leukocytes at the site of inflammation.

INDICATIONS & DOSAGE
Inflammatory and allergic conditions of cornea, conjunctiva, sclera, anterior uvea—
Adults and children: instill 1 to 2 drops in conjunctival sac b.i.d. to q.i.d. May use q hour during first 1 to 2 days if needed.

ADVERSE REACTIONS
Eye: increased intraocular pressure, especially in elderly patients; thinning of cornea, interference with corneal wound healing, corneal ulceration, increased susceptibility to viral or fungal corneal infections; with excessive or long-term use, glaucoma exacerbations, cataracts, decreased visual acuity, diminished visual field, optic

nerve damage.
Other: systemic effects and adrenal suppression in excessive or long-term use.

INTERACTIONS
None significant.

NURSING CONSIDERATIONS
- Contraindicated in vaccinia, varicella, acute superficial herpes simplex (dendritic keratitis), or other fungal or viral eye diseases; ocular tuberculosis; or any acute, purulent, untreated eye infection. Use cautiously in corneal abrasions since they are commonly contaminated (especially with herpes).
- Not for long-term use.
- Less likely to cause increased intraocular pressure with long-term use than other ophthalmic anti-inflammatory drugs (except medrysone).
- Store in tightly covered, light-resistant container.
- Warn patient to call doctor immediately and to stop drug if visual acuity decreases or visual field diminishes.
- Shake well before using.
- Show patient how to instill.
- Apply light finger-pressure on lacrimal sac for 1 minute following instillation.
- Warn patient not to use leftover medication for a new eye inflammation; can cause serious problems.
- Tell patient never to share eye medications. If a family member develops similar disease symptoms, instruct him to contact the doctor.

flurbiprofen sodium
Ocufen
Pregnancy Category: C

MECHANISM OF ACTION
Constricts the iris sphincter, thereby inhibiting miosis. The mechanism is independent of cholinergic action.

INDICATIONS & DOSAGE
Inhibition of intraoperative miosis—
Adults: Instill 1 drop approximately every ½ hour, beginning 2 hours before surgery. Give a total of 4 drops.

ADVERSE REACTIONS
Eye: transient burning and stinging upon instillation, ocular irritation.

INTERACTIONS
None reported.

NURSING CONSIDERATIONS
• Contraindicated in epithelial herpes simplex keratitis.
• This is a nonsteroidal antiinflammatory drug (NSAID). Use cautiously in patients who may be allergic to aspirin and other NSAIDs.
• Use cautiously in patients with bleeding tendencies.
• Wound healing may be delayed.

---

medrysone
HMS Liquifilm Ophthalmic♦
Pregnancy Category: C

MECHANISM OF ACTION
Decreases the infiltration of leukocytes at the site of inflammation.

INDICATIONS & DOSAGE
Allergic conjunctivitis, vernal conjunctivitis, episcleritis, ophthalmic epinephrine sensitivity reaction—
Adults and children: instill 1 drop in conjunctival sac b.i.d. to q.i.d. May use q hour during first 1 to 2 days if needed.

ADVERSE REACTIONS
Eye: thinning of cornea, interference with corneal wound healing, increased susceptibility to viral or fungal corneal infection, corneal ulceration; with excessive or long-term use, glaucoma exacerbations, cataracts, visual acuity and visual field defects, optic nerve damage.

Other: systemic effects and adrenal suppression with excessive or long-term use.

INTERACTIONS
None significant.

NURSING CONSIDERATIONS
• Contraindicated in vaccinia, varicella, acute superficial herpes simplex (dendritic keratitis), viral diseases of conjunctiva and cornea, ocular tuberculosis, fungal or viral eye diseases, iritis, uveitis, or any acute, purulent, untreated eye infection. Use cautiously in corneal abrasions since they are commonly contaminated (especially with herpes).
• Shake well before using. Don't freeze.
• Warn patient not to use leftover medication for a new eye inflammation; can cause serious problems.
• Tell patient never to share eye medications. If a family member develops similar disease symptoms, instruct him to contact the doctor.

---

prednisolone acetate (suspension)
Econopred Ophthalmic,
Econopred Plus Ophthalmic, Pred-Forte♦, Pred Mild Ophthalmic♦,
Predulose Ophthalmic

prednisolone sodium phosphate (solution)
Ak-Pred, Hydeltrasol Ophthalmic,
Inflamase Forte♦, Inflamase Ophthalmic♦, Metreton Ophthalmic
Pregnancy Category: C

MECHANISM OF ACTION
Decreases the infiltration of leukocytes at the site of inflammation.

INDICATIONS & DOSAGE
Inflammation of palpebral and bulbar conjunctiva, cornea, and anterior segment of globe—

Italicized side effects are common or life-threatening.
*Liquid form contains alcohol.   **May contain tartrazine.

Adults and children: instill 1 to 2 drops in eye. In severe conditions, may be used hourly, tapering to discontinuation as inflammation subsides. In mild conditions, may be used up to 4 to 6 times daily.

ADVERSE REACTIONS
Eye: increased intraocular pressure; thinning of cornea, interference with corneal wound healing, increased susceptibility to viral or fungal corneal infection, corneal ulceration; with excessive or long-term use, glaucoma exacerbations, cataracts, visual acuity and visual field defects, optic nerve damage.
Other: systemic effects and adrenal suppression with excessive or long-term use.

INTERACTIONS
None significant.

NURSING CONSIDERATIONS
• Contraindicated in acute untreated purulent ocular infections, acute superficial herpes simplex (dendritic keratitis), vaccinia, varicella, or other viral or fungal eye diseases, ocular tuberculosis. Use cautiously in corneal abrasions since they are commonly contaminated (especially with herpes).
• Tell patient on long-term therapy to have frequent tonometric examinations.
• Shake suspensions before using, and store in tightly covered container.
• Show patient how to instill.
• Apply light finger-pressure on lacrimal sac for 1 minute following instillation.
• Don't stop therapy prematurely.
• Warn patient not to use leftover medication for a new eye inflammation; can cause serious problems.
• Tell patient never to share eye medications. If a family member develops similar disease symptoms, instruct him to contact the doctor.

• Check dosage before administering to ensure using the correct strength.

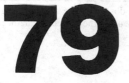

Miotics

acetylcholine chloride
carbachol (intraocular, topical)
echothiophate iodide
pilocarpine hydrochloride
pilocarpine nitrate

COMBINATION PRODUCTS
E-PILO♦: epinephrine bitartrate 1%
and pilocarpine hydrochloride 1%,
2%, 3%, 4%, or 6%.
ISOPTO P-ES: pilocarpine hydrochloride 2% and physostigmine salicylate
0.125%.
P_1E_1, P_2E_1, P_3E_1, P_4E_1, P_6E_1: epinephrine bitartrate 1% and pilocarpine hydrochloride 1%, 2%, 3%, 4%, or 6%.

acetylcholine chloride
Miochol♦
Pregnancy Category: C

MECHANISM OF ACTION
A cholinergic drug that causes contraction of the sphincter muscles of
the iris, resulting in miosis. Also produces ciliary spasm, deepening of the
anterior chamber, and vasodilation of
conjunctival vessels of the outflow
tract.

INDICATIONS & DOSAGE
Anterior segment surgery—
Adults and children: doctor instills
0.5 to 2 ml of 1% solution gently in
anterior chamber of eye.

ADVERSE REACTIONS
None reported with 1% concentration.
Iris atrophy possible with higher concentrations.

INTERACTIONS
None significant.

NURSING CONSIDERATIONS
• Reconstitute immediately before
using.
• Shake vial gently until clear solution is obtained.
• Discard any unused solution.
• Complete miosis within seconds.
• Don't gas-sterilize vial. Ethylene
oxide may produce formic acid.

carbachol (intraocular)
Miostat♦

carbachol (topical)
Carbacel, Isopto Carbachol♦
Pregnancy Category: NR

MECHANISM OF ACTION
A cholinergic drug that causes contraction of the sphincter muscles of
the iris, resulting in miosis. Also produces ciliary spasm, deepening of the
anterior chamber, and vasodilation of
conjunctival vessels of the outflow
tract.

INDICATIONS & DOSAGE
*Ocular surgery (to produce pupillary
miosis)—*
Adults: doctor should gently instill
0.5 ml (intraocular form) into the anterior chamber for production of satisfactory miosis. It may be instilled before or after securing sutures.
Open-angle or narrow-angle glaucoma—
Adults: instill 1 drop (topical form)

Italicized side effects are common or life-threatening.
*Liquid form contains alcohol.   **May contain tartrazine.

into eye daily, b.i.d., t.i.d., or q.i.d.

ADVERSE REACTIONS
CNS: headache.
Eye: accommodative spasm, blurred vision, conjunctival vasodilation, eye and brow pain.
GI: abdominal cramps, diarrhea.
Other: sweating, flushing, asthma.

INTERACTIONS
None significant.

NURSING CONSIDERATIONS
• Contraindicated in acute iritis, corneal abrasion. Use cautiously in acute heart failure, bronchial asthma, peptic ulcer, hyperthyroidism, GI spasm, urinary tract obstruction, Parkinson's disease.
• Used in glaucoma, especially when patient is resistant or allergic to pilocarpine HCl or nitrate.
• Show patient how to instill. Warn him not to exceed recommended dosage.
• Apply light finger-pressure on lacrimal sac for 1 minute following instillation. This minimizes systemic absorption.
• For single-dose intraocular use only. Premixed; discard unused portions.
• Warn patient not to touch tip of dropper to eye or surrounding tissue.
• Tell glaucoma patient that long-term use may be necessary. Stress compliance. Tell him to remain under medical supervision for periodic tonometric readings.
• In case of toxicity, atropine should be given parenterally.
• Caution patient not to drive for 1 or 2 hours after administration.
• Reassure patient that blurred vision usually diminishes with prolonged use.

echothiophate iodide
Phospholine Iodide♦
Pregnancy Category: C

MECHANISM OF ACTION
An anticholinesterase drug that inhibits the enzymatic destruction of acetylcholine by inactivating cholinesterase. This leaves acetylcholine free to act on the effector cells of the iridic sphincter and ciliary muscles, causing pupillary constriction and accommodation spasm.

INDICATIONS & DOSAGE
Open-angle glaucoma, conditions obstructing aqueous outflow, accommodative esotropia—
Adults and children: instill 1 drop 0.03% to 0.125% solution into conjunctival sac daily. Maximum 1 drop b.i.d. Use lowest possible dosage to continuously control intraocular pressure.

ADVERSE REACTIONS
CNS: fatigue, muscle weakness, paresthesias, headache.
CV: bradycardia, hypotension.
Eye: ciliary or accommodative spasm, ciliary or conjunctival injection, nonreversible cataract formation (time- and dose-related), reversible iris cysts, pupillary block, blurred or dimmed vision, eye or brow pain, lid twitching, hyperemia, photosensitivity, lens opacities, lacrimation, retinal detachment.
GI: diarrhea, nausea, vomiting, abdominal pain, intestinal cramps, salivation.
GU: frequent urination.
Other: flushing, sweating, bronchial constriction.

INTERACTIONS
Organophosphorus insecticides (parathion, malathion): may have an additive effect that could cause systemic effects. Warn patient exposed to

insecticides of this danger.
Succinylcholine: respiratory and cardiovascular collapse. Don't use together.
Systemic anticholinesterase for myasthenia gravis: effects may be additive. Monitor patient for signs of toxicity.

NURSING CONSIDERATIONS
• Contraindicated in narrow-angle glaucoma, epilepsy, vasomotor instability, parkinsonism, iodide hypersensitivity, active uveal inflammation, bronchial asthma, spastic GI conditions, urinary tract obstruction, peptic ulcer, severe bradycardia or hypotension, vascular hypertension, myocardial infarction, history of retinal detachment. Use cautiously in patients routinely exposed to organophosphorus insecticides. May cause nausea, vomiting, and diarrhea, progressing to muscle weakness and respiratory difficulty. Use cautiously in patients with myasthenia gravis receiving anticholinesterase therapy.
• Toxicity is cumulative. Toxic systemic symptoms don't appear for weeks or months after initiating therapy.
• Reconstitute powder carefully to avoid contamination. Use only diluent provided. Discard refrigerated, reconstituted solution after 6 months; discard solution at room temperature after 1 month.
• Warn patient that transient browache or dimmed or blurred vision is common at first but usually disappears within 5 to 10 days.
• Instill at bedtime since drug causes transient blurred vision.
• Tell patient to remain under constant medical supervision. Warn him not to exceed recommended dosage.
• Report salivation, diarrhea, profuse sweating, urinary incontinence, or muscle weakness.
• Stop drug at least 2 weeks preoperatively if succinylcholine is to be used in surgery.

• Atropine sulfate (subcutaneous, I.M., or I.V.) is antidote of choice.
• A potent, long-acting, irreversible drug.
• Show patient how to instill. Warn him not to touch tip of dropper to eye or surrounding tissue.
• Apply light finger-pressure on lacrimal sac for 1 minute following instillation. This minimizes systemic absorption.
• Wash hands before and after administering medication.

pilocarpine hydrochloride
Adsorbocarpine, Akarpine, Almocarpine♦, Isopto Carpine♦, Miocarpine♦♦, Ocusert Pilo♦, Pilocar, Pilocel, Pilomiotin♦, Pilopine HS

pilocarpine nitrate
P.V. Carpine Liquifilm♦
Pregnancy Category: C

MECHANISM OF ACTION
A cholinergic drug that causes contraction of the sphincter muscles of the iris, resulting in miosis. Also produces ciliary spasm, deepening of the anterior chamber, and vasodilation of conjunctival vessels of the outflow tract.

INDICATIONS & DOSAGE
Chronic open-angle glaucoma, before, or instead of, emergency surgery in acute narrow-angle glaucoma—
Adults and children: instill 1 to 2 drops in eye daily b.i.d., t.i.d., q.i.d., or as directed by doctor. Or, may apply ointment (Pilopine HS) once daily.
　　Alternatively, apply one Ocusert System (20 or 40 mcg/hour) every 7 days.

ADVERSE REACTIONS
Eye: suborbital headache, *myopia,* ciliary spasm, *blurred vision,* con-

---
Italicized side effects are common or life-threatening.
*Liquid form contains alcohol.　　**May contain tartrazine.

junctival irritation, lacrimation, changes in visual field, *brow pain*.
GI: nausea, vomiting, abdominal cramps, diarrhea, salivation.
Other: bronchiolar spasm, pulmonary edema, hypersensitivity.

INTERACTIONS
Carbachol: additive effect. Don't use together.
Phenylephrine HCl: decreased dilation by phenylephrine HCl. Don't use together.

NURSING CONSIDERATIONS
• Contraindicated in acute iritis, acute inflammatory disease of anterior segment of eye, secondary glaucoma. Use cautiously in bronchial asthma, hypertension.
• Warn patient that vision will be temporarily blurred.
• Transient browache and myopia are common at first; usually disappear in 10 to 14 days.
• Show patient how to instill. Warn him not to touch dropper to eye or surrounding tissue.
• Apply light finger-pressure on lacrimal sac for 1 minute following instillation. This minimizes systemic absorption.
• Widely used drug to treat chronic open-angle glaucoma.
• Used to counteract effects of mydriatics and cycloplegics after surgery or ophthalmoscopic examination.
• May be used alternately with atropine to break adhesions.
• In acute narrow-angle glaucoma before surgery, may be used alone or with mannitol, urea, glycerol, or acetazolamide.
• If the Ocusert System falls out of the eye during sleep, wash hands, rinse the system in cool tap water, and reposition it in the eye.
• If the ointment is prescribed, instruct patient to apply at bedtime, as it will blur vision.
• Because of blurred vision, warn patient to avoid hazardous activities before the drug's effects have been determined.

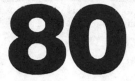

Mydriatics

atropine sulfate
cyclopentolate hydrochloride
epinephrine bitartrate
epinephrine hydrochloride
epinephryl borate
homatropine hydrobromide
phenylephrine hydrochloride
scopolamine hydrobromide
tropicamide

COMBINATION PRODUCTS
MUROCOLL-2: scopolamine HBr
0.3% and phenylephrine HCl 10%.

atropine sulfate
Atropisol, BufOpto Atropine, Isopto
Atropine♦
Pregnancy Category: C

MECHANISM OF ACTION
Anticholinergic action leaves the pupil under unopposed adrenergic influence, causing it to dilate.

INDICATIONS & DOSAGE
Acute iris inflammation (iritis)—
Adults: 1 to 2 drops of 1% solution or small amount of ointment 2 to 3 times daily, b.i.d., or t.i.d.
Children: instill 1 to 2 drops of 0.5% solution daily, b.i.d., or t.i.d.
Cycloplegic refraction—
Adults: instill 1 to 2 drops of 1% solution 1 hour before refracting.
Children: instill 1 to 2 drops of 0.5% solution to each eye b.i.d. for 1 to 3 days before eye examination and 1 hour before refraction, or instill small amount of ointment daily or b.i.d. 2 to 3 days before examination.

ADVERSE REACTIONS
Eye: ocular congestion in long-term use, conjunctivitis, contact dermatitis, edema, *blurred vision,* eye dryness, *photophobia.*
Systemic: flushing, dry skin and mouth, fever, tachycardia, abdominal distention in infants, ataxia, irritability, confusion, somnolence.

INTERACTIONS
None significant.

NURSING CONSIDERATIONS
• Contraindicated in primary glaucoma (narrow-angle). Use cautiously in infants, children, and elderly or debilitated patients.
• Warn patient vision will be temporarily blurred. Dark glasses ease discomfort of photophobia.
• Not for internal use. Treat drops and ointment as poison. Keep physostigmine available as antidote for poisoning. Signs of poisoning are disorientation and confusion.
• Don't touch dropper or tip of tube to eye or surrounding tissue.
• Watch for signs of glaucoma: increased intraocular pressure, ocular pain, headache, progressive blurring of vision.
• Most potent mydriatic and cycloplegic available; long duration.
• Systemic adverse reactions most commonly occur in children and the elderly.
• Warn patient not to operate machinery or drive a car until the temporary visual impairment caused by this drug wears off.

Italicized side effects are common or life-threatening.
*Liquid form contains alcohol.   **May contain tartrazine.

• Show patient how to instill. Wash hands before and after administration.
• Apply light finger-pressure on lacrimal sac for 1 minute following instillation. This minimizes systemic absorption.

cyclopentolate hydrochloride
AK-Pentolate, Cyclogyl♦,
Mydplegic♦♦
Pregnancy Category: C

MECHANISM OF ACTION
Anticholinergic action leaves the pupil under unopposed adrenergic influence, causing it to dilate.

INDICATIONS & DOSAGE
Diagnostic procedures requiring mydriasis and cycloplegia—
Adults: instill 1 drop 1% solution in eye, followed by 1 more drop in 5 minutes. Use 2% solution in heavily pigmented irises.
Children: instill 1 drop of 0.5%, 1%, or 2% solution in each eye, followed in 5 minutes with 1 drop 0.5% or 1% solution, if necessary.

ADVERSE REACTIONS
Eye: burning sensation on instillation, blurred vision, eye dryness, *photophobia*, ocular congestion, contact dermatitis, conjunctivitis.
Systemic: flushing, tachycardia, urinary retention, dry skin, fever, ataxia, irritability, confusion, somnolence, hallucinations, seizures, behavioral disturbances in children.

INTERACTIONS
None significant.

NURSING CONSIDERATIONS
• Contraindicated in narrow-angle glaucoma. Use cautiously in elderly patients.
• Potent drug with mydriatic and cycloplegic effect; superior to homatro-

pine hydrobromide and has shorter duration of action.
• Instruct patient to wear dark glasses to ease discomfort of photophobia.
• Warn patient drug will burn when instilled.
• Warn patient not to operate machinery or drive until the temporary visual impairment caused by this drug has worn off.
• Show patient how to instill.
• Apply light finger-pressure on lacrimal sac for 1 minute following instillation. This minimizes systemic absorption.

epinephrine bitartrate
Epitrate♦, Mytrate

epinephrine hydrochloride
Epifrin♦, Glaucon♦

epinephryl borate
Epinal♦, Eppy♦♦
Pregnancy Category: C

MECHANISM OF ACTION
An adrenergic that dilates the pupil by contracting the dilator muscle.

INDICATIONS & DOSAGE
Adults and children:
Intraocular injection—
0.1 to 0.2 ml of 0.01% or 0.1% epinephrine HCl by doctor.
Open-angle glaucoma—
instill 1 to 2 drops of 1% or 2% bitartrate solution in eye with frequency determined by tonometric readings (once q 2 to 4 days up to q.i.d.), or instill 1 drop 0.5%, 1%, or 2% HCl solution (or 0.5% or 1% epinephryl borate solution) in eye b.i.d.
During surgery—
1 or more drops of 0.1% epinephrine HCl up to 3 times.

ADVERSE REACTIONS
Eye: corneal or conjunctival pigmentation or corneal edema in long-term

use; follicular hypertrophy; chemosis; conjunctivitis; iritis; hyperemic conjunctiva; maculopapular rash; severe stinging, burning, and tearing upon instillation; browache.
Systemic: palpitations, tachycardia.

INTERACTIONS
Cyclopropane or halogenated hydrocarbons: arrhythmias, tachycardia. Use together cautiously, if at all.
Tricyclic antidepressants, antihistamines (diphenhydramine, dexchlorpheniramine): potentiated cardiac effects of epinephrine.

NURSING CONSIDERATIONS
• Contraindicated in shallow anterior chamber or narrow-angle glaucoma.
• Use cautiously in diabetes mellitus, hypertension, Parkinson's disease, hyperthyroidism, aphakia (eye without lens), cardiac disease, or cerebral arteriosclerosis; in elderly patients or pregnant women.
• May stain soft contact lenses.
• Use with pilocarpine: additive effect in lowering intraocular pressure.
• Monitor blood pressure and other systemic effects.
• Don't use darkened solution.
• Also used during surgery to control local bleeding, or injected into the anterior chamber to produce rapid mydriasis during cataract removal.
• Warn patient not to touch dropper to eye or surrounding tissue.
• Show patient how to instill.
• Apply light finger-pressure on lacrimal sac for 1 minute following instillation. This minimizes systemic absorption.
• Epinephrine salts are not interchangeable. Don't substitute one salt if another one is ordered.

homatropine hydrobromide
Homatrocel Ophthalmic, Isopto Homatropine♦
Pregnancy Category: C

MECHANISM OF ACTION
Anticholinergic action leaves the pupil under unopposed adrenergic influence, causing it to dilate.

INDICATIONS & DOSAGE
Adults and children:
Cycloplegic refraction—
instill 1 to 2 drops 2% or 5% solution in eye; repeat in 5 to 10 minutes.
Uveitis—
instill 1 to 2 drops 2% or 5% solution in eye up to every 3 to 4 hours.

ADVERSE REACTIONS
Eye: irritation, *blurred vision, photophobia.*
Systemic: flushing, dry skin and mouth, fever, tachycardia, ataxia, irritability, confusion, somnolence.

INTERACTIONS
None significant.

NURSING CONSIDERATIONS
• Contraindicated in primary glaucoma (narrow-angle). Use cautiously in infants, elderly or debilitated patients, or patients with hypertension, cardiac disease, or increased intraocular pressure.
• Patients who are hypersensitive to atropine will also be hypersensitive to homatropine.
• Warn patient vision will be temporarily blurred after instillation. Tell him not to drive a car or operate machinery until this wears off. Dark glasses should be worn to decrease photophobia.
• May produce symptoms of atropine SO$_4$ poisoning, such as severe dryness of mouth, tachycardia.
• Not for internal use. Treat as poison. Keep physostigmine available as

antidote for poisoning.
- Show patient how to instill.
- Apply light finger-pressure on lacrimal sac for 1 minute following instillation. This minimizes systemic absorption.
- Warn patient not to touch dropper tip to eye or surrounding tissue.
- Similar to atropine SO_4 but weaker, with a shorter duration of action.

phenylephrine hydrochloride
Mydfrin♦, Neo-Synephrine♦
Pregnancy Category: C

MECHANISM OF ACTION
An adrenergic that dilates the pupil by contracting the dilator muscle of the pupil.

INDICATIONS & DOSAGE
Adults and children:
Mydriasis (without cycloplegia)—instill 1 drop 2.5% or 10% solution in eye before examination.
Posterior synechia (adhesion of iris)—instill 1 drop 10% solution in eye.

Do not use 10% concentration in infants; use cautiously in elderly patients.

ADVERSE REACTIONS
Eye: transient burning or stinging on instillation, blurred vision, reactive hyperemia, allergic conjunctivitis, iris floaters, narrow-angle glaucoma, rebound miosis, dermatitis.
CNS: headache, browache.
CV: *hypertension,* tachycardia, palpitations, premature ventricular contractions.
Other: pallor, trembling, sweating.

INTERACTIONS
Guanethidine: increased mydriatic and pressor effects of phenylephrine HCl. Use together cautiously.
Levodopa (systemic): reduced mydriatic effect of phenylephrine HCl. Use

together cautiously.
MAO inhibitors and beta blockers: may cause arrhythmias due to increased pressor effect. Use together cautiously.
Tricyclic antidepressants: potentiated cardiac effects of epinephrine. Use together cautiously.

NURSING CONSIDERATIONS
- Contraindicated in narrow-angle glaucoma, soft contact lens use. Use cautiously in marked hypertension, cardiac disorders, and in children of low body weight.
- Should be avoided in patients with idiopathic orthostatic hypotension. May produce high blood pressure.
- Protect from light and heat.
- Warn patient not to exceed recommended dosage. Systemic effects can result. Monitor blood pressure and pulse rate.
- Warn patient not to touch dropper tip to eye or surrounding tissue.
- Potential for systemic adverse reactions less severe with 2.5% solution. Adverse reactions and toxicity much more likely with 10% solution.
- Show patient how to instill.
- Apply light finger-pressure on lacrimal sac for 1 minute following instillation. This minimizes systemic absorption.
- May cause blurred vision. Warn patient not to drive car or operate machinery until this effect wears off.

scopolamine hydrobromide
Isopto Hyoscine
Pregnancy Category: C

MECHANISM OF ACTION
Anticholinergic action leaves the pupil under unopposed adrenergic influence, causing it to dilate.

INDICATIONS & DOSAGE
Cycloplegic refraction—
Adults: instill 1 to 2 drops 0.25% so-

lution in eye 1 hour before refraction.
Children: instill 1 drop 0.25% solution or ointment b.i.d. for 2 days before refraction.
Iritis, uveitis—
Adults: 1 to 2 drops of 0.25% solution daily, b.i.d., or t.i.d.

ADVERSE REACTIONS
Eye: ocular congestion with prolonged use, conjunctivitis, *blurred vision,* eye dryness, increased intraocular pressure, *photophobia,* contact dermatitis.
Systemic: flushing, fever, dry skin and mouth, tachycardia, hallucinations, ataxia, irritability, confusion, delirium, somnolence, acute psychotic reactions.

INTERACTIONS
None significant.

NURSING CONSIDERATIONS
• Contraindicated in primary glaucoma (shallow anterior chamber or narrow-angle). Use cautiously in cardiac disease, increased intraocular pressure, and in patients over 40 years.
• Observe patient closely for systemic effects (disorientation, delirium).
• Warn patient that vision will be temporarily blurred; tell him not to drive car or operate machinery until this effect wears off.
• Instruct patient to wear dark glasses to ease discomfort of photophobia.
• May be used when patient is sensitive to atropine. Faster acting and has shorter duration of action and fewer adverse reactions.
• Show patient how to instill. Warn him not to touch dropper tip to eye or surrounding tissue. Wash hands before and after administration.
• Apply light finger-pressure on lacrimal sac for 1 minute following instillation. This minimizes systemic absorption.

tropicamide
Mydriacyl♦
Pregnancy Category: C

MECHANISM OF ACTION
Anticholinergic action leaves the pupil under unopposed adrenergic influence, causing it to dilate.

INDICATIONS & DOSAGE
Adults and children:
Cycloplegic refractions—
instill 1 to 2 drops of 1% solution in each eye; repeat in 5 minutes. Additional drop may be instilled in 20 to 30 minutes.
Fundus examinations—
instill 1 to 2 drops 0.5% solution in each eye 15 to 20 minutes before examination.

ADVERSE REACTIONS
Eye: *transient stinging on instillation,* increased intraocular pressure (less than with other mydriatic agents because of shorter duration of action), *blurred vision, photophobia.*
Systemic: flushing, fever, dry skin, dry mouth and throat, ataxia, irritability, confusion, somnolence, hallucinations, behavioral disturbances in children.

INTERACTIONS
None significant.

NURSING CONSIDERATIONS
• Contraindicated in narrow-angle and shallow anterior chamber glaucoma. Use cautiously in elderly.
• Shortest acting cycloplegic, but mydriatic effect greater than cycloplegic effect.
• Causes transient stinging; vision temporarily blurred. Warn patient not to drive car or operate machinery until this effect wears off.
• Instruct patient to wear dark glasses if photosensitivity occurs (lasts about 2 hours).

Italicized side effects are common or life-threatening.
*Liquid form contains alcohol.   **May contain tartrazine.

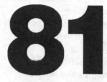

Ophthalmic vasoconstrictors

naphazoline hydrochloride
0.012%, 0.02%, 0.1%
phenylephrine hydrochloride
0.12%, 2.5%, 10%
tetrahydrozoline hydrochloride
zinc sulfate

COMBINATION PRODUCTS
ALBALON-A♦: naphazoline hydrochloride 0.05% and antazoline phosphate 0.5%.
BLEPHAMIDE♦: phenylephrine hydrochloride 0.12%, sulfacetamide sodium 10%, and prednisolone acetate 0.2%.
PHENYLZIN DROPS: zinc sulfate 0.25% and phenylephrine hydrochloride 0.12%.
PREFRIN-A♦: phenylephrine hydrochloride 0.12%, pyrilamine maleate 0.1%, and antipyrine 0.1%.
PREFRIN-Z: phenylephrine hydrochloride 0.12% and zinc sulfate 0.25%.
VASOCIDIN♦: phenylephrine hydrochloride 0.125%, sodium sulfacetamide 10%, and prednisolone sodium phosphate 0.2%.
VASOCON-A♦: naphazoline hydrochloride 0.05% and antazoline phosphate 0.5%.
ZINCFRIN♦: phenylephrine hydrochloride 0.12% and zinc sulfate 0.25%.

naphazoline hydrochloride
0.012%, 0.02%, 0.1%
AK-Con Ophthalmic, Albalon Liquifilm Ophthalmic♦, Clear Eyes, Naphcon, Naphcon Forte Ophthalmic♦, Vasoclear, Vasocon Regular Ophthalmic♦
Pregnancy Category: C

MECHANISM OF ACTION
Produces vasoconstriction by local adrenergic action on the blood vessels of the conjunctiva.

INDICATIONS & DOSAGE
Ocular congestion, irritation, itching—
Adults: instill 1 to 2 drops in eye q 3 to 4 hours.

ADVERSE REACTIONS
Eye: transient stinging, pupillary dilation, irritation.

INTERACTIONS
MAO inhibitors: hypertensive crisis if naphazoline HCl is systemically absorbed. Use together cautiously.

NURSING CONSIDERATIONS
• Contraindicated in narrow-angle glaucoma, hypersensitivity to any ingredients. Use cautiously in patients with hyperthyroidism, cardiac disease, hypertension, and diabetes mellitus, and in elderly patients.
• Can produce marked sedation and coma if ingested by child.
• Advise patient that photophobia may follow pupil dilation if he is sen-

sitive to drug. Tell patient to report this to the doctor if it occurs.
• Warn patient not to exceed recommended dosage. Rebound congestion and conjunctivitis may occur with frequent or prolonged use.
• Notify doctor if blurred vision, pain, or lid edema develops.
• Store in tightly closed container.
• Most widely used ocular decongestant.
• Show patient how to instill. Do not touch tip of dropper to eye or surrounding tissues.

phenylephrine hydrochloride 0.12%, 2.5%, 10%
AK-Dilate, Isopto Frin, Prefrin♦, Tear-Efrin
Pregnancy Category: C

MECHANISM OF ACTION
Produces vasoconstriction by local adrenergic action on the blood vessels of the conjunctiva.

INDICATIONS & DOSAGE
Decongestant, minor eye irritations—
Adults and children: 2 drops of 0.12% in affected eye. May repeat in 3 to 4 hours, p.r.n.

ADVERSE REACTIONS
CNS: headache.
Eye: transient stinging, iris floaters, narrow-angle glaucoma, blurred vision, reactive hyperemia, browache.

INTERACTIONS
MAO inhibitors: may cause hypertensive crisis. Don't use together.

NURSING CONSIDERATIONS
• Contraindicated in narrow-angle glaucoma, in patients taking tricyclic antidepressants or MAO inhibitors, and in hypersensitivity to any ingredient.
• May exacerbate hypertension in hy-

pertensive patients.
• Do not use butacaine drops as local anesthetic, since phenylephrine and butacaine are incompatible.
• Do not exceed prescribed dose.
• Monitor blood pressure and pulse rate; watch for overdosage.
• Do not use if solution is dark brown or contains precipitate.
• Keep container tightly sealed and away from light.
• Do not touch tip of dropper to eye or surrounding tissues.
• Show patient how to instill.
• Caution patient not to share eye medications with others.

tetrahydrozoline hydrochloride
Murine Plus, Optigene, Soothe, Tetrasine, Visine
Pregnancy Category: C

MECHANISM OF ACTION
Produces vasoconstriction by local adrenergic action on the blood vessels of the conjunctiva.

INDICATIONS & DOSAGE
Ocular congestion, irritation, and allergic conditions—
Adults and children over 2 years: instill 1 to 2 drops in eye b.i.d. or t.i.d., or as directed by doctor.

ADVERSE REACTIONS
Eye: transient stinging, pupillary dilation, increased intraocular pressure, irritation, iris floaters in elderly.
Systemic: drowsiness, CNS depression, cardiac irregularities, headache, dizziness, tremors, insomnia.

INTERACTIONS
MAO inhibitors: hypertensive crisis if tetrahydrozoline HCl is systemically absorbed. Don't use together.

NURSING CONSIDERATIONS
• Contraindicated in patients receiv-

Italicized side effects are common or life-threatening.
*Liquid form contains alcohol.   **May contain tartrazine.

ing MAO inhibitors, and in those with hypersensitivity to any ingredients or narrow-angle glaucoma. Use cautiously in patients with hyperthyroidism, heart disease, hypertension, and diabetes mellitus and in the elderly.
• Do not exceed recommended dosage. Rebound congestion may occur with frequent or prolonged use.
• Warn patient to stop drug and notify doctor if relief is not obtained within 48 hours, or if redness or irritation persists or increases.
• Available without prescription.
• Warn patient not to touch dropper tip to eye or surrounding tissues.
• Show patient how to instill.
• Caution patient not to share eye medications with others.

zinc sulfate
Bufopto Zinc Sulfate, Eye-Sed Ophthalmic, Op-Thal-Zin
Pregnancy Category: NR

MECHANISM OF ACTION
Produces astringent action on the conjunctiva.

INDICATIONS & DOSAGE
Ocular congestion, irritation—
Adults and children: solution 0.2%—instill 1 to 2 drops in eye b.i.d. or t.i.d.

ADVERSE REACTIONS
Eye: irritation.

INTERACTIONS
None significant.

NURSING CONSIDERATIONS
• Use cautiously in patients with a shallow anterior chamber, predisposition to narrow-angle glaucoma.
• A decongestant astringent.
• Store in tightly closed container.
• Warn patient not to touch dropper tip to eye or surrounding tissues.

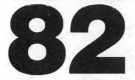

Topical ophthalmic anesthetics

proparacaine hydrochloride
tetracaine hydrochloride

COMBINATION PRODUCTS
None.

proparacaine hydrochloride
Alcaine♦, Ophthaine♦, Ophthetic♦
Pregnancy Category: C

MECHANISM OF ACTION
Produces anesthesia by preventing initiation and transmission of impulses at the nerve-cell membrane.

INDICATIONS & DOSAGE
Anesthesia for tonometry, gonioscopy; suture removal from cornea, removal of corneal foreign bodies—
Adults and children: instill 1 to 2 drops 0.5% solution in eye just before procedure.
Anesthesia for cataract extraction, glaucoma surgery—
Adults and children: instill 1 drop 0.5% solution in eye every 5 to 10 minutes for 5 to 7 doses.

ADVERSE REACTIONS
Eye: occasional conjunctival redness, transient pain.
Other: hypersensitivity.

INTERACTIONS
None significant.

NURSING CONSIDERATIONS
• Use cautiously in patients with cardiac disease and hyperthyroidism.
• *Not* for long-term use; may delay wound healing.
• Warn patient not to rub or touch eye while cornea is anesthetized, since this may cause corneal abrasion and greater discomfort when anesthesia wears off.
• Protective eyepatch recommended following procedure.
• Warn patient that corneal pain is relieved only temporarily in abrasion.
• Systemic reactions unlikely when used in recommended doses.
• Topical ophthalmic anesthetic of choice in diagnostic and minor surgical procedures.
• Don't use discolored solution.
• Store in tightly closed container.
• Ophthaine brand packaged in bottle that looks similar in size and shape to Hemoccult. When taking bottle from shelf, check label carefully.

tetracaine hydrochloride
Anacel, Pontocaine♦
Pregnancy Category: C

MECHANISM OF ACTION
Produces anesthesia by preventing initiation and transmission of impulses at the nerve-cell membrane.

INDICATIONS & DOSAGE
Anesthesia for tonometry, gonioscopy; removal of corneal foreign bodies, suture removal from cornea; other diagnostic and minor surgical procedures—
Adults and children: instill 1 to 2 drops 0.5% solution in eye just before procedure.

Italicized side effects are common or life-threatening.
*Liquid form contains alcohol.   **May contain tartrazine.

ADVERSE REACTIONS
Eye: transient stinging in eye 30 seconds after initial instillation, epithelial damage in excessive or long-term use.
Other: sensitization in repeated use (allergic skin rash, urticaria).

INTERACTIONS
Sulfonamides: interference with sulfonamide antibacterial activity. Wait ½ hour after anesthesia before instilling sulfonamide.

NURSING CONSIDERATIONS
• Systemic absorption unlikely in recommended doses.
• Avoid repeated use.
• Does not dilate the pupil, paralyze accommodation, or increase intraocular pressure.
• Protective eyepatch recommended following procedure.
• Don't use discolored solution. Keep container tightly closed.

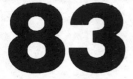

Artificial tears

artificial tears
eye irrigation solutions

COMBINATION PRODUCTS
None.

artificial tears

Adsorbotear♦, Hypotears, Isopto
Alkaline, Isopto Plain, Isopto
Tears♦, Lacril♦, Lacrisert, Liquifilm
Forte, Liquifilm Tears, Lyteers,
Methulose, Neotears, Tearisol,
Tears Naturale♦, Tears Plus, Ultra
Tears, Visculose
Pregnancy Category: NR

MECHANISM OF ACTION
Augments insufficient tear production.

INDICATIONS & DOSAGE
Insufficient tear production—
Adults and children: instill 1 to 2
drops in eye t.i.d., q.i.d., or p.r.n.
Moderate to severe dry eye syndromes,
including keratoconjunctivitis sicca—
Adults: insert 1 Lacrisert rod daily
into inferior cul-de-sac. Some patients may require twice daily use.

ADVERSE REACTIONS
Eye: discomfort; burning, pain on instillation; blurred vision (especially
with Lacrisert); crust formation on
eyelids and eyelashes in products with
high viscosity, such as Adsorbotear,
Isopto Tears, and Tearisol.

INTERACTIONS
Borate external irrigation solutions:

may form gummy deposits on the lid
when used with artificial tear products containing polyvinyl alcohol (Liquifilm Forte, Liquifilm Tears). Keep
patient's eyelids clean.

NURSING CONSIDERATIONS
• Contraindicated in hypersensitivity
to active product or preservatives.
• Show patient how to instill eye
drops.
• To avoid contamination of solution,
warn patient not to touch tip of container to eye, surrounding tissue, or
other surface.
• Instruct patient that product should
be used by one person only.
• Lacrisert rod should be inserted
with special applicator that is included in the package. Familiarize patient with illustrated instructions that
are also included.

eye irrigation solutions

Blinx, Collyrium♦, Dacriose,
EyeStream, I-Lite Eye Drops, Lauro,
Lavoptik Medicinal Eye Wash,
Murine Eye Drops, Neo-Flow,
Sterile Normal Saline (0.9%)
Pregnancy Category: NR

MECHANISM OF ACTION
Cleanse the eye.

INDICATIONS & DOSAGE
Eye irrigation—
Adults and children: flush eye with 1
to 2 drops t.i.d., q.i.d., or p.r.n.

Italicized side effects are common or life-threatening.
*Liquid form contains alcohol.   **May contain tartrazine.

ADVERSE REACTIONS
None reported.

INTERACTIONS
Products containing polyvinyl alcohol: may form gel and gummy deposits on the eye. Keep eyelids clean.

NURSING CONSIDERATIONS
• Contraindicated in hypersensitivity to active ingredient or preservatives.
• To avoid contamination, don't touch tip of container to eye, surrounding tissue, or other surface.
• Check date of expiration to make sure solution is potent.
• Store in tightly closed, light-resistant container.
• Show patient how to instill.
• Should be used by one person only.
• When irrigating, have patient turn his head to side and irrigate from inner to outer canthus. Have tissues handy.

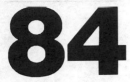

Miscellaneous ophthalmics

betaxolol hydrochloride
cromolyn sodium
dipivefrin
fluorescein sodium
glycerin, anhydrous
isosorbide
levobunolol hydrochloride
sodium chloride, hypertonic
timolol maleate

COMBINATION PRODUCTS
FLURESS: sodium fluorescein 0.25%
and benoxinate HCl 0.4%.

---

betaxolol hydrochloride
Betoptic
Pregnancy Category: C

MECHANISM OF ACTION
Reduces formation and possibly increases outflow of aqueous humor. A
cardioselective beta-blocker.

INDICATIONS & DOSAGE
*Chronic open-angle glaucoma and
ocular hypertension—*
Adults: instill 1 drop in eyes b.i.d.

ADVERSE REACTIONS
CNS: insomnia.
Eye: *stinging upon instillation,* occasional tearing.

INTERACTIONS
None significant.

NURSING CONSIDERATIONS
• Contraindicated in sinus bradycardia, greater than first-degree AV
block, cardiogenic shock, or patients
with overt heart failure.
• Use cautiously in patients with a
history of heart failure; patients with
restricted pulmonary function; patients with diabetes mellitus.
• Betaxolol differs from timolol and levobunolol in that it is a cardioselective
beta-adrenergic blocker. Therefore, this
drug does not significantly affect the
heart rate. Its pulmonary systemic effects are considerably milder than those
of timolol and levobunolol.
• Betaxolol is intended for twice-daily dosage. Encourage your patient
to comply with this regimen.
• In some patients, a few weeks'
treatment may be required to stabilize
pressure-lowering response. Determine intraocular pressure after 4
weeks of treatment.
• Warn patient not to touch dropper
to eye or surrounding tissue.
• Show patient how to instill. Teach
patient to lightly press lacrimal sac
with finger for 1 minute after drug administration to decrease chance of
systemic absorption.

---

cromolyn sodium
Opticrom 4% ophthalmic solution
Pregnancy Category: B

MECHANISM OF ACTION
Inhibits degranulation of sensitized
mast cells that follows exposure to
specific antigens. Also inhibits release of histamine and slow-reacting
substance of anaphylaxis (SRS-A).

Italicized side effects are common or life-threatening.
*Liquid form contains alcohol.   **May contain tartrazine.

INDICATIONS & DOSAGE

Treatment and prevention of allergic ocular disorders such as vernal kerato-conjunctivitis and conjunctivitis, giant papillary conjunctivitis, vernal keratitis, and allergic keratoconjunctivitis—
Adults and children: 1 to 2 drops in each eye 4 to 6 times a day at regular intervals.

ADVERSE REACTIONS

Eye: transient stinging or burning upon instillation.

INTERACTIONS

None significant.

NURSING CONSIDERATIONS

• Because preparation contains ben-zalkonium chloride as a preservative, advise patient not to wear soft contact lenses during treatment period. Patient may resume wearing them a few hours after the drug's discontinued.
• Advise patient to instill medication at regular intervals.
• Tell patient that relief of symptoms may take several days to a week.
• Cromolyn is a safe treatment for some types of allergic conjunctivitis and keratitis and may be as effective as steroids.

dipivefrin
Propine♦
Pregnancy Category: B

MECHANISM OF ACTION

A prodrug of epinephrine (in the eye, dipivefrin is converted to epineph-rine). The liberated epinephrine appears to decrease aqueous production and increase aqueous outflow.

INDICATIONS & DOSAGE

To reduce intraocular pressure in chronic open-angle glaucoma—
Adults: for initial glaucoma therapy, 1 drop in eye q 12 hours.

ADVERSE REACTIONS

Eye: burning, stinging.
CV: tachycardia, hypertension.

INTERACTIONS

None significant.

NURSING CONSIDERATIONS

• Contraindicated in narrow-angle glaucoma.
• Use cautiously in patients with aphakia.
• Dipivefrin is a prodrug of epineph-rine: it's converted to epinephrine when it enters the eye.
• May have fewer adverse reactions than conventional epinephrine therapy.
• Often used concomitantly with other antiglaucoma drugs.
• Available as a 0.1% solution in 5-, 10-, and 15-ml dropper bottles.
• Teach patient how to instill.
• Wash hands before and after administration.
• Don't touch dropper to eye or surrounding tissue.

fluorescein sodium
Fluorescite, Fluor-I-Strip, Fluor-I-Strip A.T.♦, Ful-Glo♦, Funduscein Injections♦
Pregnancy Category: C

MECHANISM OF ACTION

Produces an intense green fluorescence in alkaline solution (pH 5.0 or less) or a bright yellow if viewed under cobalt blue illumination.

INDICATIONS & DOSAGE

Diagnostic in corneal abrasions and foreign bodies; fitting hard contact lenses; lacrimal patency; fundus photography; applanation tonometry—
Topical solution: instill 1 drop of 2% solution followed by irrigation, or moisten strip with sterile water. Touch conjunctiva or fornix with moistened tip. Flush eye with irrigat-

ing solution. Patient should blink several times after application.
Indicated in retinal angiography—
Intravenous:
Adults: 5 ml of 10% solution (500 mg) or 3 ml of 25% solution (750 mg) injected rapidly into antecubital vein, by doctor or a specially trained nurse.
Children: 0.077 ml of 10% solution (7.7 mg/kg body weight) or 0.044 ml of 25% solution (11 mg/kg body weight) injected rapidly into antecubital vein by doctor.

ADVERSE REACTIONS
Topical use:
Eye: stinging, burning, yellow streaks from tears.
Intravenous use:
CNS: headache persisting for 24 to 36 hours.
GI: nausea, vomiting.
GU: bright yellow urine (persists for 24 to 36 hours).
Skin: yellow skin discoloration (fades in 6 to 12 hours).
Local: extravasation at injection site, thrombophlebitis.
Other: hypersensitivity, including urticaria and *anaphylaxis.*

INTERACTIONS
None significant.

NURSING CONSIDERATIONS
• Use with caution in patients with history of allergy or bronchial asthma.
• Never instill while patient is wearing soft contact lens. Drug will ruin it.
• Use topical anesthetic before instilling to partially relieve burning and irritation.
• Always use aseptic technique. Easily contaminated by *Pseudomonas.*
• Yellow skin discoloration may persist 6 to 12 hours.
• Warn patient that urine will be bright yellow after I.V. injection.
• Routine urinalysis will be abnormal within 1 hour after I.V. injection.

• A water-soluble dye.
• Don't freeze; store below 80° F. (26.7° C.).
• Defects appear green under normal light, or bright yellow under cobalt blue illumination. Foreign bodies are surrounded by a green ring. Similar lesions of the conjunctiva are delineated in orange-yellow.
• Always keep an emergency tray with antihistamine, epinephrine, and oxygen available when giving parenterally.

---

glycerin, anhydrous
Ophthalgan
Pregnancy Category: C

MECHANISM OF ACTION
Removes excess fluid from the cornea.

INDICATIONS & DOSAGE
Corneal edema before ophthalmoscopy or gonioscopy in acute glaucoma and bullous keratitis—
Adults and children: instill 1 to 2 drops glycerin, anhydrous after instilling a local anesthetic.

ADVERSE REACTIONS
Eye: pain if instilled without topical anesthetic.

INTERACTIONS
None significant.

NURSING CONSIDERATIONS
• Use topical tetracaine HCl or proparacaine HCl before instilling to prevent discomfort.
• Don't touch tip of dropper to eye, surrounding tissues, or tear-film; glycerin will absorb moisture.
• Used to temporarily restore corneal transparency when cornea is too edematous to permit diagnosis.
• Store in tightly closed container.

Italicized side effects are common or life-threatening.
*Liquid form contains alcohol.   **May contain tartrazine.

isosorbide
Ismotic
Pregnancy Category: C

MECHANISM OF ACTION
Acts as an osmotic agent by promoting redistribution of water and thereby producing diuresis.

INDICATIONS & DOSAGE
Short-term reduction of intraocular pressure due to glaucoma—
Adults: initially, 1.5 g/kg P.O. Usual dosage range is 1 to 3 g/kg.

ADVERSE REACTIONS
CNS: vertigo, light-headedness, lethargy.
GI: gastric discomfort, diarrhea, anorexia.
Metabolic: hypernatremia, hyperosmolality.

INTERACTIONS
None significant.

NURSING CONSIDERATIONS
• Contraindicated in anuria due to severe renal disease, severe dehydration, frank or impending acute pulmonary edema, and hemorrhagic glaucoma.
• Repetitive doses should be used cautiously in patients with diseases associated with salt retention, such as congestive heart failure.
• Pour over cracked ice, and tell patient to sip the medication. This procedure improves palatability.
• Especially useful when a rapid reduction in intraocular pressure is desired.
• As an expected effect of the drug, the patient may become thirsty.

levobunolol hydrochloride
Betagan
Pregnancy Category: C

MECHANISM OF ACTION
Reduces formation and possibly increases outflow of aqueous humor. A nonselective beta-blocker.

INDICATIONS & DOSAGE
Chronic open-angle glaucoma and ocular hypertension—
Adults: instill 1 drop in eyes once or twice daily.

ADVERSE REACTIONS
CNS: headache, dizziness, depression.
CV: slight reduction in resting heart rate.
Eye: *transient stinging and burning.* Long-term use may decrease corneal sensitivity.
GI: nausea.
Skin: urticaria.
Other: evidence of beta blockade and systemic absorption *(hypotension, bradycardia, syncope, exacerbation of asthma,* and *congestive heart failure).*

INTERACTIONS
Propranolol, metoprolol and other oral beta-adrenergic blocking agents: increased ocular and systemic effect. Use together cautiously.

NURSING CONSIDERATIONS
• Contraindicated in bronchial asthma, a history of bronchial asthma or severe chronic obstructive pulmonary disease; sinus bradycardia; second-degree and third-degree AV block; cardiac failure; cardiogenic shock.
• Use cautiously in patients with chronic bronchitis and emphysema, diabetes mellitus, and hyperthyroidism.
• Levobunolol is faster acting than timolol. The onset of action occurs

within 1 hour; maximum effect is between 2 and 6 hours.
• Warn patient not to touch dropper to eye or surrounding tissue.
• Show patient how to instill. Teach patient to lightly press lacrimal sac with finger for 1 minute after drug administration to decrease chance of systemic absorption.

sodium chloride, hypertonic
Adsorbonac Ophthalmic Solution, Muro Ointment, Sodium Chloride Ointment 5%
Pregnancy Category: C

MECHANISM OF ACTION
Removes excess fluid from the cornea.

INDICATIONS & DOSAGE
Corneal edema (postoperative) after cataract extraction or corneal transplantation; also in trauma or bullous keratopathy—
Adults and children: instill 1 to 2 drops q 3 to 4 hours, or apply ointment at bedtime.

ADVERSE REACTIONS
Eye: slight stinging.
Other: hypersensitivity.

INTERACTIONS
None significant.

NURSING CONSIDERATIONS
• An osmotic agent used to reduce corneal edema when repeated instillation is indicated.
• May use a few drops of sterile irrigation solution inside bottle cap to prevent caking on dropper bottle tip.
• Store in tightly closed container.
• Ointment may cause blurred vision.
• Don't touch tip of dropper or tube to eye or surrounding tissue.

timolol maleate
Timoptic Solution
Pregnancy Category: C

MECHANISM OF ACTION
Reduces aqueous formation and possibly increases aqueous outflow. A beta-blocker.

INDICATIONS & DOSAGE
Chronic open-angle glaucoma, secondary glaucoma, aphakic glaucoma, ocular hypertension—
Adults: initially, instill 1 drop 0.25% solution in each eye b.i.d.; reduce to 1 drop daily for maintenance. If patient doesn't respond, instill 1 drop 0.5% solution in each eye b.i.d. If intraocular pressure is controlled, dosage may be reduced to 1 drop in each eye daily.

ADVERSE REACTIONS
CNS: headache, depression, fatigue.
CV: slight reduction in resting heart rate.
Eye: minor irritation. Long-term use may decrease corneal sensitivity.
GI: anorexia.
Other: apnea in infants, *evidence of beta blockade and systemic absorption (hypotension, bradycardia, syncope, exacerbation of asthma, and congestive heart failure).*

INTERACTIONS
Propranolol HCl, metoprolol tartrate, other oral beta-adrenergic blocking agents: increased ocular and systemic effect. Use together cautiously.

NURSING CONSIDERATIONS
• Use cautiously in bronchial asthma, sinus bradycardia, second- and third-degree heart block, cardiogenic shock, right ventricular failure resulting from pulmonary hypertension, congestive heart failure, severe cardiac disease, and in infants with congenital glaucoma.
• In some patients, a few weeks may

Italicized side effects are common or life-threatening.
*Liquid form contains alcohol.   **May contain tartrazine.

be required to stabilize pressure-lowering response. Determine intraocular
pressure after 4 weeks of treatment.
• Warn patient not to touch dropper
to eye or surrounding tissue.
• Can be used safely in patients with
glaucoma who wear conventional
(PMMA) hard contact lenses.
• Show patient how to instill. Teach
patient to lightly press lacrimal sac
with finger after administration to decrease systemic absorption.

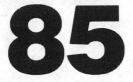

acetic acid
benzocaine
boric acid
carbamide peroxide
chloramphenicol
hydrocortisone
hydrocortisone acetate
methylprednisolone disodium
    phosphate
neomycin sulfate
triethanolamine polypeptide
    oleate-condensate

COMBINATION PRODUCTS

COLY-MYCIN S OTIC: Each ml contains neomycin SO₄ 3.3 mg, colistin SO₄ 3 mg, hydrocortisone acetate 10 mg, and thonzonium bromide 0.05%.
CORTISPORIN OTIC♦: Each ml contains neomycin SO₄ 5 mg, polymyxin.

---

acetic acid

Domeboro Otic♦, VoSol Otic♦
Pregnancy Category: C

MECHANISM OF ACTION

Inhibits or destroys bacteria present in the ear canal.

INDICATIONS & DOSAGE

External ear canal infection—
Adults and children: 4 to 6 drops into ear canal t.i.d. or q.i.d., or insert saturated wick for first 24 hours, then continue with instillations.
Prophylaxis of swimmer's ear—
Adults and children: 2 drops in each ear b.i.d.

ADVERSE REACTIONS

Ear: irritation or itching.
Skin: urticaria.
Other: overgrowth of nonsusceptible organisms.

INTERACTIONS

None significant.

NURSING CONSIDERATIONS

• Use cautiously in perforated eardrum.
• Has anti-infective, anti-inflammatory, and antipruritic effects.
• *Pseudomonas aeruginosa* particularly sensitive to drug.
• Reculture persistent drainage.

---

benzocaine

Americaine-Otic♦, Auralgan♦, Eardro, Myringacaine, Tympagesic
Pregnancy Category: C

MECHANISM OF ACTION

Produces analgesic effects. A local anesthetic.

INDICATIONS & DOSAGE

Cerumen removal—
Adults and children: fill ear canal t.i.d. for 2 days.
Pain from otitis media—
Adults and children: fill ear canal with solution and plug with cotton. May repeat q 1 to 2 hours, p.r.n.

ADVERSE REACTIONS

Ear: irritation or itching.
Skin: urticaria.
Other: edema.

Italicized side effects are common or life-threatening.
*Liquid form contains alcohol.   **May contain tartrazine.

INTERACTIONS
None significant.

NURSING CONSIDERATIONS
• Contraindicated in perforated eardrum.
• Local anesthetic effect only.
• Use with antibiotic to treat underlying cause of pain, because use alone may mask more serious condition.
• Tell patient to call doctor if pain lasts longer than 48 hours.
• Avoid touching ear with dropper. Do not rinse dropper.
• Irrigate ear gently to remove impacted cerumen.
• Keep in dark, tightly closed container, away from moisture and light.

boric acid
Ear-Dry, Swim-Ear
Pregnancy Category: C

MECHANISM OF ACTION
Inhibits or destroys bacteria present in the ear canal.

INDICATIONS & DOSAGE
External ear canal infection—
Adults and children: fill ear canal with solution and plug with cotton. Repeat t.i.d. or q.i.d.

ADVERSE REACTIONS
Ear: irritation or itching.
Skin: urticaria.
Other: overgrowth of nonsusceptible organisms.

INTERACTIONS
None significant.

NURSING CONSIDERATIONS
• Contraindicated in perforated eardrum or excoriated membranes in ear.
• Watch for signs of superinfection (continual pain, inflammation, fever).
• Weak bacteriostatic action; also fungistatic agent.
• If cotton plug used, always moisten

with medication.
• Avoid touching ear with dropper.

carbamide peroxide
Debrox
Pregnancy Category: C

MECHANISM OF ACTION
Emulsifies and disperses accumulated cerumen. A ceruminolytic.

INDICATIONS & DOSAGE
Impacted cerumen—
Adults and children: 5 to 10 drops into ear canal b.i.d. for 3 to 4 days.

ADVERSE REACTIONS
None reported.

INTERACTIONS
None significant.

NURSING CONSIDERATIONS
• Contraindicated in perforated eardrum.
• Tell patient to call doctor if redness, pain, or swelling persists.
• Irrigation of ear may be necessary to aid in removal of cerumen.
• Tip of dropper should not touch ear or ear canal.

chloramphenicol
Chloromycetin Otic♦,
Sopamycetin♦♦
Pregnancy Category: C

MECHANISM OF ACTION
Inhibits or destroys bacteria present in the ear canal.

INDICATIONS & DOSAGE
External ear canal infection—
Adults and children: 2 to 3 drops into ear canal t.i.d. or q.i.d.

ADVERSE REACTIONS
Ear: itching or burning.
Local: pruritus, burning, urticaria,

vesicular or maculopapular dermatitis.
Systemic: sore throat, angioedema.
Other: overgrowth of nonsusceptible organisms.

INTERACTIONS
None significant.

NURSING CONSIDERATIONS
• Avoid prolonged use.
• Obtain history of use and reaction to drug.
• Watch for signs of superinfection (continued pain, inflammation, fever).
• Reculture persistent drainage.
• Watch for signs of sore throat (early sign of toxicity).
• Avoid touching ear with dropper.

hydrocortisone

hydrocortisone acetate
Cortamed♦♦
Pregnancy Category: C

MECHANISM OF ACTION
Controls inflammation, edema, and pruritus.

INDICATIONS & DOSAGE
Inflammation of external ear canal—
Adults and children: 3 to 5 drops into ear canal t.i.d. or q.i.d.
   Available in 0.25%, 0.5%, and 1% concentrations.

ADVERSE REACTIONS
Systemic: adrenal suppression with long-term use.
Other: may mask or exacerbate underlying infection.

INTERACTIONS
None reported.

NURSING CONSIDERATIONS
• Contraindicated in perforated eardrum, fungal infections, herpes or

other viral infections.
• Use with antibiotic to treat inflammation caused by infection.
• Use alone in allergic otitis externa.
• Avoid touching ear with dropper.

methylprednisolone disodium phosphate
Medrol♦♦
Pregnancy Category: C

MECHANISM OF ACTION
Controls inflammation, edema, and pruritus.

INDICATIONS & DOSAGE
Inflammation of external ear canal—
Adults and children: 2 to 3 drops into ear canal t.i.d. or q.i.d.

ADVERSE REACTIONS
Systemic: adrenal suppression with long-term use.
Other: may mask or exacerbate underlying infection.

INTERACTIONS
None significant.

NURSING CONSIDERATIONS
• Contraindicated in perforated eardrum, fungal infection, herpes, or other viral infections.
• Use with antibiotic to treat inflammation caused by infection.
• Use alone to treat seborrheic, contact, or uninfected eczematoid dermatitis.
• Avoid touching ear with dropper.

neomycin sulfate
Otobiotic
Pregnancy Category: C

MECHANISM OF ACTION
Inhibits or destroys bacteria present in the ear canal.

INDICATIONS & DOSAGE
External ear canal infection—
Adults and children: 2 to 5 drops into ear canal t.i.d. or q.i.d.

ADVERSE REACTIONS
Ear: ototoxicity (in patients undergoing tympanoplasty).
Local: burning, erythema, vesicular dermatitis, urticaria.
Other: overgrowth of nonsusceptible organisms.

INTERACTIONS
None significant.

NURSING CONSIDERATIONS
• Contraindicated in perforated eardrum.
• Obtain history of use and reaction to neomycin.
• Observe for signs of hearing loss.
• Watch for signs of superinfection (continued pain, inflammation, fever).
• Reculture persistent drainage.
• Best used in combination with other antibiotics.
• Avoid touching ear with dropper.

---

triethanolamine polypeptide oleate-condensate
Cerumenex♦
Pregnancy Category: C

MECHANISM OF ACTION
Emulsifies and disperses accumulated cerumen. A ceruminolytic.

INDICATIONS & DOSAGE
Impacted cerumen—
Adults and children: fill ear canal with solution and insert cotton plug. After 15 to 30 minutes, flush ear with warm water.

ADVERSE REACTIONS
Ear: erythema, pruritus.
Skin: severe eczema.

INTERACTIONS
None significant.

NURSING CONSIDERATIONS
• Contraindicated in perforated eardrum, otitis media, and allergies. Do patch test by placing 1 drop of drug on inner forearm; cover with small bandage. Read in 24 hours. If any reaction (redness, swelling) occurs, don't use drug.
• Tell patient not to use drops more often than prescribed. Flush ear gently with warm water, using soft rubber bulb ear syringe, within 30 minutes after instillation.
• Moisten cotton plug with medication before insertion.
• Keep container tightly closed and away from moisture.
• Avoid touching ear with dropper.

Nasal agents

beclomethasone dipropionate
dexamethasone sodium
  phosphate
ephedrine sulfate
epinephrine hydrochloride
flunisolide
naphazoline hydrochloride
oxymetazoline hydrochloride
phenylephrine hydrochloride
tetrahydrozoline hydrochloride
xylometazoline hydrochloride

COMBINATION PRODUCTS
4-WAY NASAL SPRAY: phenylephrine hydrochloride 0.5%, naphazoline hydrochloride 0.05%, and pyrilamine maleate 0.2%.

---

beclomethasone dipropionate
Beconase Nasal Inhaler♦,
Vancenase Nasal Inhaler♦
Pregnancy Category: C

MECHANISM OF ACTION
Unknown.

INDICATIONS & DOSAGE
Relief of symptoms of seasonal or perennial rhinitis; prevention of recurrence of nasal polyps after surgical removal—
Adults and children over 12 years:
Usual dosage is one spray (42 mcg) in each nostril 2 to 4 times daily (total dosage 168 to 336 mcg daily). Most patients require one spray in each nostril t.i.d. (252 mcg daily).
Not recommended for children under age 12.

ADVERSE REACTIONS
CNS: headache.
EENT: *mild transient nasal burning and stinging,* nasal congestion, sneezing, epistaxis, watery eyes.
GI: nausea and vomiting.
Other: development of local fungal infections.

INTERACTIONS
None reported.

NURSING CONSIDERATIONS
• Use cautiously, if at all, in patients with active or quiescent respiratory tract tubercular infections or in untreated fungal, bacterial, or systemic viral or ocular herpes simplex infections.
• Use cautiously in patients who have recently had nasal septal ulcers or nasal surgery or trauma.
• Recommended dosages will not suppress hypothalamic-pituitary-adrenal (HPA) function. Warn patient not to exceed this dosage.
• Indicated when conventional treatment (antihistamines, decongestants) fails.
• Beclomethasone is not effective for active exacerbations. Nasal decongestants or oral antihistamines may be needed instead.
• Advise patients to use drug regularly, as prescribed; its effectiveness depends on regular use.
• Explain that the therapeutic effects of this corticosteroid, unlike those of decongestants, are not immediate. Most patients achieve benefit within a few days, but some may need 2 to 3

Italicized side effects are common or life-threatening.
*Liquid form contains alcohol.   **May contain tartrazine.

weeks for maximum benefit.
- If symptoms don't improve within 3 weeks or if nasal irritation persists, patient should stop drug and notify doctor.
- Observe for fungal infections.

dexamethasone sodium phosphate
Decadron Phosphate♦, Turbinaire
Pregnancy Category: C

MECHANISM OF ACTION
Unknown.

INDICATIONS & DOSAGE
Allergic or inflammatory conditions, nasal polyps—
Adults: 2 sprays in each nostril b.i.d. or t.i.d. Maximum 12 sprays daily.
Children 6 to 12 years: 1 or 2 sprays in each nostril b.i.d. Maximum 8 sprays daily.
   Each spray delivers 0.1 mg dexamethasone sodium phosphate equal to 0.084 mg dexamethasone.

ADVERSE REACTIONS
EENT: nasal irritation, dryness, rebound nasal congestion.
Other: hypersensitivity, systemic side effects with prolonged use (pituitary-adrenal suppression, sodium retention, congestive heart failure, hypertension, hypokalemia, headaches, convulsions, peptic ulcer, ecchymoses, petechiae, masking of secondary infection).

INTERACTIONS
None significant.

NURSING CONSIDERATIONS
- Contraindicated in cutaneous tuberculosis, fungal and herpetic lesions. Use cautiously in diabetes mellitus, peptic ulcer, or tuberculosis, as systemic absorption can activate disease.
- Mothers should not breast-feed, as systemic absorption can occur.

- Control underlying bacterial infection with anti-infectives.
- Irritation or sensitivity may require stopping drug.
- Don't break, incinerate, or store in extreme heat; contents under pressure.
- Gradually reduce dose as nasal condition improves.
- Fluid retention can occur as a result of systemic absorption.
- Show patient how to apply. Only one person should use nasal spray.
- Hypertension and hypokalemia can occur with systemic absorption. Monitor blood pressure, serum potassium frequently.
- Should not be used for prolonged periods.

ephedrine sulfate
Efedron Nasal Jelly, Vatronol Nose Drops
Pregnancy Category: C

MECHANISM OF ACTION
Produces local vasoconstriction of dilated arterioles to reduce blood flow and nasal congestion.

INDICATIONS & DOSAGE
Nasal congestion—
Adults and children: apply 3 to 4 drops 0.5% solution or apply a small amount of jelly to nasal mucosa. Use no more frequently than q 4 hours.

ADVERSE REACTIONS
CNS: nervousness, excitation.
CV: *tachycardia.*
EENT: rebound nasal congestion with long-term or excessive use.
Local: mucosal irritation.

INTERACTIONS
MAO inhibitors: hypertensive crisis if ephedrine is absorbed. Don't use together.

NURSING CONSIDERATIONS
• Use cautiously in hyperthyroidism, coronary artery disease, hypertension, or diabetes mellitus, as systemic absorption can occur.
• Tell patient not to exceed recommended dose. Use only when needed.
• Show patient how to apply. Only one person should use dropper bottle or nasal spray.

epinephrine hydrochloride
Adrenalin Chloride♦
Pregnancy Category: C

MECHANISM OF ACTION
Produces local vasoconstriction of dilated arterioles to reduce blood flow and nasal congestion.

INDICATIONS & DOSAGE
Nasal congestion, local superficial bleeding—
Adults and children: apply 0.1% solution to oral or nasal mucosa.

ADVERSE REACTIONS
CNS: nervousness, excitation.
CV: *tachycardia.*
EENT: rebound nasal congestion, slight sting upon application.

INTERACTIONS
None significant.

NURSING CONSIDERATIONS
• Use cautiously in hyperthyroidism, coronary artery disease, hypertension, or diabetes mellitus, as systemic absorption can occur.
• Tell patient not to exceed recommended dose. Use only when needed.
• Show patient how to apply. Only one person should use dropper bottle or nasal spray.

flunisolide
Nasalide Spray
Pregnancy Category: C

MECHANISM OF ACTION
Unknown.

INDICATIONS & DOSAGE
Relief of symptoms of seasonal or perennial rhinitis—
Adults: Starting dose is 2 sprays (50 mcg) in each nostril b.i.d. Total daily dose is 200 mcg. If necessary, dose may be increased to 2 sprays in each nostril t.i.d. Maximum total daily dosage is 8 sprays in each nostril (400 mcg daily).
Children 6 to 14 years: Starting dose is 1 spray (25 mcg) in each nostril t.i.d. or 2 sprays (50 mcg) in each nostril b.i.d. Total daily dose is 150 to 200 mcg. Maximum total daily dose is 4 sprays in each nostril (200 mcg daily).
Not recommended for children under age 6.

ADVERSE REACTIONS
CNS: headache.
EENT: *mild, transient nasal burning and stinging,* nasal congestion, sneezing, epistaxis, watery eyes.
GI: nausea, vomiting.
Other: development of local fungal infections.

INTERACTIONS
None reported.

NURSING CONSIDERATIONS
• Use cautiously, if at all, in patients with active or quiescent respiratory tract tubercular infections or in untreated fungal, bacterial, or systemic viral or ocular herpes simplex infections.
• Use cautiously in patients who have recently had nasal septal ulcers or nasal surgery or trauma.
• Recommended dosages will not

suppress hypothalamic-pituitary-adrenal (HPA) function. Warn patient not to exceed this dosage.
• Indicated when conventional treatment (antihistamines, decongestants) fails.
• Flunisolide is not effective for acute exacerbations. Nasal decongestants or oral antihistamines may be needed instead.
• Advise patient to use drug regularly, as prescribed; its effectiveness depends on regular use.
• Explain that the therapeutic effects of this corticosteroid, unlike those of decongestants, are not immediate. Most patients achieve benefit within a few days, but some may need 2 to 3 weeks for maximum benefit.
• Patients with dryness and crusting of the nasal mucosa may prefer the liquid spray of flunisolide to the aerosolized powder of beclomethasone.
• If symptoms don't improve within 3 weeks or if nasal irritation persists, patient should stop drug and notify doctor.

naphazoline hydrochloride
Privine♦
Pregnancy Category: C

MECHANISM OF ACTION
Produces local vasoconstriction of dilated arterioles to reduce blood flow and nasal congestion.

INDICATIONS & DOSAGE
Nasal congestion—
Adults: apply 2 drops or sprays of 0.05% solution to nasal mucosa q 3 to 4 hours.
Children 6 to 12 years: 1 to 2 drops or sprays of 0.05% solution. Repeat q 3 to 6 hours, p.r.n. Use no longer than 3 to 5 days.

ADVERSE REACTIONS
EENT: rebound nasal congestion with excessive or long-term use,

sneezing, stinging, dryness of mucosa.
Other: systemic side effects in children after excessive or long-term use; marked sedation.

INTERACTIONS
None significant.

NURSING CONSIDERATIONS
• Contraindicated in narrow-angle glaucoma. Use cautiously in hyperthyroidism, heart disease, hypertension, or diabetes mellitus, as systemic absorption can occur.
• Warn patient not to exceed recommended dosage.
• Tell patient to notify doctor if nasal congestion persists after 5 days.
• Show patient how to apply. Hold container upright. Only one person should use dropper bottle or nasal spray.
• Do not shake container.

oxymetazoline hydrochloride
Afrin, Duration
Pregnancy Category: C

MECHANISM OF ACTION
Produces local vasoconstriction of dilated arterioles to reduce blood flow and nasal congestion.

INDICATIONS & DOSAGE
Nasal congestion—
Adults and children over 6 years: apply 2 to 4 drops or sprays 0.05% solution to nasal mucosa b.i.d.
Children 2 to 6 years: apply 2 to 3 drops 0.025% solution to nasal mucosa b.i.d. Use no longer than 3 to 5 days. Dosage for younger children has not been established.

ADVERSE REACTIONS
CNS: headache, drowsiness, dizziness, insomnia.
CV: palpitations, *hypotension with*

cardiovascular collapse, hypertension.

EENT: rebound nasal congestion or irritation with excessive or long-term use, dryness of nose and throat, increased nasal discharge, stinging, sneezing.

Other: systemic side effects in children with excessive or long-term use; possible sedation.

INTERACTIONS
None significant.

NURSING CONSIDERATIONS
• Use cautiously in hyperthyroidism, cardiac disease, hypertension, or diabetes mellitus, as systemic absorption can occur.
• Tell patient not to exceed recommended dose. Use only when needed.
• Warn patient that excessive use may cause bradycardia, hypotension, dizziness, and weakness.
• Show patient how to apply. Have patient bend head forward and sniff spray briskly. Only one person should use dropper bottle or nasal spray.

**phenylephrine
hydrochloride**
Alconefrin, Coricidin Nasal Mist,
Coryzine, Ephrine, Neo-
Synephrine♦, Sinarest Nasal Spray,
Sinophen Intranasal, SuperAnahist
Nasal Spray, Vacon
Pregnancy Category: C

MECHANISM OF ACTION
Produces local vasoconstriction of dilated arterioles to reduce blood flow and nasal congestion.

INDICATIONS & DOSAGE
Nasal congestion—
Adults: 2 to 3 drops or sprays of 0.25% to 1% solution; apply jelly or spray to nasal mucosa.
Children 6 to 12 years: apply 2 to 3 drops or sprays of 0.25% solution.

Children under 6 years: apply 2 to 3 drops or sprays of 0.125% solution.
Drops, spray, or jelly can be given q 4 hours, p.r.n.

ADVERSE REACTIONS
CNS: headache, tremors, dizziness, nervousness.
CV: *palpitations, tachycardia,* premature ventricular contractions, hypertension, pallor.
EENT: transient burning, stinging; dryness of nasal mucosa; rebound nasal congestion may occur with continued use.
GI: nausea.

INTERACTIONS
None significant.

NURSING CONSIDERATIONS
• Contraindicated in narrow-angle glaucoma. Use cautiously in hyperthyroidism, hypertension, diabetes mellitus, or ischemic cardiac disease, as systemic absorption may occur.
• Tell patient not to exceed recommended dose. Use only when needed.
• Show patient how to apply: keep head erect to minimize swallowing of medication. Only one person should use dropper bottle or nasal spray.

**tetrahydrozoline
hydrochloride**
Tyzine HCl, Tyzine Pediatric
Pregnancy Category: C

MECHANISM OF ACTION
Produces local vasoconstriction of dilated arterioles to reduce blood flow and nasal congestion.

INDICATIONS & DOSAGE
Nasal congestion—
Adults and children over 6 years: apply 2 to 4 drops 0.1% solution or spray to nasal mucosa q 4 to 6 hours, p.r.n.
Children 2 to 6 years: apply 2 to 3

Italicized side effects are common or life-threatening.
*Liquid form contains alcohol.   **May contain tartrazine.

drops 0.05% solution to nasal mucosa
q 4 to 6 hours, p.r.n.

ADVERSE REACTIONS
EENT: transient burning, stinging;
sneezing, rebound nasal congestion in
excessive or long-term use.

INTERACTIONS
None significant.

NURSING CONSIDERATIONS
• Contraindicated in narrow-angle
glaucoma. Use cautiously in hyperthyroidism, hypertension, diabetes
mellitus.
• Don't use 0.1% solution in children
under 6 years.
• Tell patient not to exceed recommended dose. Use only as needed.
• Show patient how to apply. Only
one person should use dropper or nasal spray.

xylometazoline hydrochloride
4-Way Long Acting, Neo-
Synephrine II, Otrivin♦, Sine-Off
Nasal Spray, Sinex-L.A.
Pregnancy Category: C

MECHANISM OF ACTION
Produces local vasoconstriction of dilated arterioles to reduce blood flow
and nasal congestion.

INDICATIONS & DOSAGE
Nasal congestion—
Adults and children over 12 years:
apply 2 to 3 drops or 2 sprays of 0.1%
solution to nasal mucosa q 8 to 10
hours.
Children under 12 years: apply 2 to
3 drops or 1 spray of 0.05% solution
to nasal mucosa q 8 to 10 hours.

ADVERSE REACTIONS
EENT: rebound nasal congestion or
irritation with excessive or long-term
use; transient burning, stinging; dry-

ness or ulceration of nasal mucosa;
sneezing.

INTERACTIONS
None significant.

NURSING CONSIDERATIONS
• Contraindicated in narrow-angle
glaucoma. Use cautiously in hyperthyroidism, cardiac disease, hypertension, diabetes mellitus, and advanced arteriosclerosis, as systemic
absorption can occur.
• Tell patient not to exceed recommended dose.
• Show patient how to apply. Only
one person should use dropper bottle
or nasal spray.

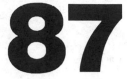

Local anti-infectives

acyclovir
amphotericin B
bacitracin
butoconazole nitrate
carbol-fuchsin solution
chloramphenicol
chlortetracycline hydrochloride
ciclopirox olamine
clotrimazole
econazole nitrate
erythromycin
gentamicin sulfate
gentian violet (methylrosaniline chloride)
haloprogin
iodochlorhydroxyquin (clioquinol)
ketoconazole
mafenide acetate
miconazole nitrate 2%
neomycin sulfate
nitrofurazone
nystatin
silver sulfadiazine
tetracycline hydrochloride
tolnaftate
undecylenic acid (zinc undecylenate)

COMBINATION PRODUCTS

CORDRAN-N CREAM, OINTMENT: flurandrenolide 0.05% and neomycin sulfate 0.5%.
LOTRISONE CREAM: clotrimazole 1% and betamethasone dipropionate 0.05%.
MYCITRACIN OINTMENT: polymyxin B sulfate 5,000 units, bacitracin 500 units, and neomycin sulfate 3.5 mg/g.
MYCOLOG CREAM, OINTMENT: gramicidin 0.25 mg, neomycin sulfate 0.25%, triamcinolone acetonide 0.1%, and nystatin 100,000 units/g.
MYCOLOG CREAM, OINTMENT: triamcinolone acetonide 0.1%, gramicidin 0.25 mg, nystatin 100,000 units, and neomycin sulfate 0.25%.
NEO-CORTEF OINTMENT♦: hydrocortisone acetate 1% and neomycin sulfate 0.5%.
NEODECADRON CREAM: dexamethasone phosphate 0.1% and neomycin sulfate 0.5%.
NEO-POLYCON OINTMENT: polymyxin B sulfate 5,000 units, neomycin sulfate 5 mg, and zinc bacitracin 400 units/g.
NEOSPORIN CREAM♦♦: polymyxin B sulfate 10,000 units, neomycin sulfate 5 mg, and gramicidin 0.25 mg/g.
NEOSPORIN-G CREAM: polymyxin B sulfate 10,000 units, neomycin sulfate 5 mg, and gramicidin 0.25 mg/g.
POLYSPORIN OINTMENT♦: polymyxin B sulfate 10,000 units and zinc bacitracin 500 units/g.

---

acyclovir
Zovirax♦
Pregnancy Category: C

MECHANISM OF ACTION
Inhibits herpes virus DNA synthesis by interfering with the action of viral DNA polymerase.

INDICATIONS & DOSAGE
Initial herpes genitalis; limited, non–life-threatening mucocutaneous herpes simplex virus infections in immunocompromised patients—

Adults and children: Apply sufficient quantity to adequately cover all
lesions every 3 hours six times a day
for 7 days.

ADVERSE REACTIONS
Skin: transient burning and stinging,
rash, pruritus.

INTERACTIONS
None reported.

NURSING CONSIDERATIONS
• For cutaneous use only. Don't apply
to the eye.
• Although the dose size for each application will vary depending upon
the total lesion area, use approximately a ½″ ribbon of ointment on
each 4 in^2 of surface area.
• Ointment must thoroughly cover all
lesions.
• Apply with a finger cot or rubber
glove to prevent autoinoculation of
other body sites and transmission of
infection to other persons.
• Therapy should be initiated as early
as possible following onset of signs
and symptoms of herpes.
• Most studies show that acyclovir is
not effective when used to treat *recurrent* genital herpes.

amphotericin B
Fungizone Cream, Lotion, Ointment
(3% amphotericin B)♦
Pregnancy Category: B

MECHANISM OF ACTION
Alters the permeability of the cell
membrane of fungi.

INDICATIONS & DOSAGE
*Cutaneous or mucocutaneous candi-
dal infections—*
Adults and children: apply liberally
b.i.d., t.i.d., or q.i.d. for 1 to 3
weeks; up to several months for interdigital lesions and paronychias.

ADVERSE REACTIONS
Skin: possible drying, contact sensitivity, erythema, burning, pruritus.

INTERACTIONS
None significant.

NURSING CONSIDERATIONS
• Cream or lotion preferred for such
areas as folds of groin, armpit, and
neck creases.
• Cream discolors skin slightly when
rubbed in; lotion or ointment doesn't.
Lotion may stain nail lesions.
• Watch for and report signs of local
irritation.
• Avoid occlusive dressings.
• Store at room temperature; avoid
freezing.
• Well tolerated, even by infants, for
long periods.
• A fungistatic agent.
• Tell patient to continue using medi-
cation for full time prescribed, even if
condition has improved.

bacitracin
Baciguent♦, Bacitin♦♦
Pregnancy Category: C

MECHANISM OF ACTION
Inhibits bacterial cell-wall synthesis.

INDICATIONS & DOSAGE
*Topical infections, impetigo, abra-
sions, cuts, and minor wounds—*
Adults and children: apply thin film
b.i.d. or t.i.d. or more often, depending on severity of condition.

ADVERSE REACTIONS
Skin: stinging, rashes and other allergic reactions; itching, burning,
swelling of lips or face.
Other: *possible systemic side effects
when used over large areas for prolonged periods: potentially nephrotoxic and ototoxic; allergic reactions;*
tightness in chest, hypotension.

INTERACTIONS
None significant.

NURSING CONSIDERATIONS
• Contraindicated for application in the external ear canal if the eardrum is perforated.
• Patients allergic to neomycin may also be allergic to bacitracin.
• If used on burns that cover more than 20% of body surface, and especially if patient suffers impaired renal function, consider alternative treatment.
• If no improvement or if condition worsens, stop using and notify doctor.
• Prolonged use may result in overgrowth of nonsusceptible organisms.

butoconazole nitrate
Femstat
Pregnancy Category: C

MECHANISM OF ACTION
Controls or destroys fungus by disrupting cell membrane permeability and reducing osmotic resistance.

INDICATIONS & DOSAGE
Local treatment of vulvovaginal mycotic infections caused by Candida *species—*
Adults (nonpregnant): one applicatorful intravaginally at bedtime for 3 days.
Adults (pregnant): one applicatorful intravaginally at bedtime for 6 days. Use only during 2nd and 3rd trimester.

ADVERSE REACTIONS
Skin: vulvar itching, soreness, and swelling; itching of the fingers.

INTERACTIONS
None significant.

NURSING CONSIDERATIONS
• Caution your patient not to use during first trimester of pregnancy.

• Butoconazole may be used with oral contraceptive and antibiotic therapy.
• Diagnosis of *Candida* vulvovaginal infection should be confirmed by smears or cultures.
• Symptom resolution comparable to 7-day miconazole cream therapy. Antifungal effect of butoconazole therapy is apparent after only 3 days of therapy.
• Tell patient not to use tampons during treatment.
• The patient's sexual partner should wear a condom during intercourse. He should consult his doctor if he experiences penile itching, redness, or discomfort.
• Advise patient to do the following to prevent reinfection: keep cool and dry, wear loose-fitting cotton clothing, avoid feminine hygiene sprays, wash daily with unscented soap, dry thoroughly with clean towel, and maintain proper bowel hygiene by wiping from front to back.

carbol-fuchsin solution
Carfusin, Castaderm, Castellani's Paint
Pregnancy Category: C

MECHANISM OF ACTION
Disrupts protein synthesis.

INDICATIONS & DOSAGE
Tinea, dermatophytosis, skin infections—
Adults and children: apply liberally one or two times daily.

ADVERSE REACTIONS
Blood: possibility of bone marrow hypoplasia with use over long periods or at frequent intervals.
Skin: *contact dermatitis.*

INTERACTIONS
None significant.

Italicized side effects are common or life-threatening.
*Liquid form contains alcohol.   **May contain tartrazine.

NURSING CONSIDERATIONS
• Warn patient to expect a stinging sensation.
• A small, initial test application over a small area is recommended. If contact dermatitis or sensitivity occurs, discontinue use.
• Discontinue use after 1 week if no improvement shown; consult doctor. Toxicities may develop in long-term use.
• Poisonous; warn against swallowing. Store in tight, light-resistant container.
• A fungicidal and bactericidal agent.
• Instruct patient to continue using for full treatment period prescribed, even if condition has improved.
• Don't apply to eroded skin or over extensive areas.
• Will stain clothing.
• Clean skin with soap and water before application.

chloramphenicol
Chloromycetin♦
(1% chloramphenicol)
Pregnancy Category: C

MECHANISM OF ACTION
Disrupts protein synthesis.

INDICATIONS & DOSAGE
Superficial skin infections caused by susceptible bacteria—
Adults and children: after thorough cleansing, apply t.i.d. or q.i.d.

ADVERSE REACTIONS
Skin: possible contact sensitivity; itching, burning, urticaria, angioneurotic edema in patients hypersensitive to any of the components.
Other: *blood dyscrasias.*

INTERACTIONS
None significant.

NURSING CONSIDERATIONS
• If no improvement or if condition

worsens, stop using and report to doctor.
• Prolonged use may result in overgrowth of nonsusceptible organisms.
• For all but very superficial infections, topical use of this drug should be supplemented by appropriate systemic medication.
• Discontinue if signs of hypersensitivity develop.
• Tell patient to continue using for full treatment period prescribed, even if condition has improved.

chlortetracycline hydrochloride
Aureomycin 3%♦
Pregnancy Category: D

MECHANISM OF ACTION
Disrupts protein synthesis.

INDICATIONS & DOSAGE
Superficial infections of the skin caused by susceptible bacteria—
Adults and children: rub into affected area b.i.d. or t.i.d.

ADVERSE REACTIONS
Skin: *dermatitis,* drying.

INTERACTIONS
None significant.

NURSING CONSIDERATIONS
• Has lanolin base. Don't use in persons allergic to wool.
• Prolonged use may result in overgrowth of nonsusceptible organisms.
• If no improvement or if condition worsens, stop using and report to doctor.
• Treated skin fluouresces under ultraviolet light.

ciclopirox olamine

Loprox♦
Pregnancy Category: B

MECHANISM OF ACTION

Depletes essential intracellular substrates of fungi.

INDICATIONS & DOSAGE

Treatment of tinea pedis, tinea cruris, and tinea corporis; cutaneous candidiasis; tinea versicolor—
Adults and children over 10 years: massage gently into the affected and surrounding areas b.i.d., in the morning and evening.

ADVERSE REACTIONS

Local: pruritus, burning.

INTERACTIONS

None reported.

NURSING CONSIDERATIONS

• If sensitivity or chemical irritation occurs, discontinue treatment.
• Use the drug for the full treatment period even though symptoms may have improved. Notify doctor if there's no improvement after 4 weeks.
• Available as a 1% cream in a water-soluble base.
• Don't use occlusive dressings.
• Hypopigmentation from *tinea versicolor* will not resolve immediately.

clotrimazole

Canesten♦♦, Gyne-Lotrimin,
Lotrimin (1% clotrimazole),
Mycelex, Mycelex-G
Pregnancy Category: B

MECHANISM OF ACTION

Alters fungal cell wall permeability.

INDICATIONS & DOSAGE

Superficial fungal infections (tinea pedis, tinea cruris, tinea versicolor, candidiasis, and tinea corporis)—
Adults and children: apply thinly and massage into affected and surrounding area, morning and evening, 1 to 8 weeks.
Candidal vulvovaginitis—
Adults: insert 1 full applicator or 1 tablet intravaginally daily for 7 to 14 days at bedtime. Alternatively, insert 2 100 mg tablets once daily for 3 consecutive days or one 500 mg tablet one time only at bedtime.
Oropharyngeal candidiasis—
Adults and children: dissolve lozenge in mouth 5 times daily for 14 consecutive days.

ADVERSE REACTIONS

GI: nausea and vomiting (with lozenges).
GU: *with vaginal use: mild vaginal burning, irritation.*
Hepatic: elevated SGOT levels (from lozenges).
Skin: blistering, *erythema*, edema, pruritus, burning, stinging, peeling, urticaria, skin fissures, general irritation.

INTERACTIONS

None significant.

NURSING CONSIDERATIONS

• Not for ophthalmic use.
• Watch for and report irritation or sensitivity. Discontinue use.
• Improvement usually within a week; if no improvement in 4 weeks, diagnosis should be reviewed.
• Warn patients not to use occlusive wrappings or dressings.
• Shortened dosage schedule with tablets may be used when compliance is a problem.
• Lozenges are indicated in treating oral candidiasis.
• Hypopigmentation from *tinea versicolor* won't resolve immediately.

Italicized side effects are common or life-threatening.
*Liquid form contains alcohol.   **May contain tartrazine.

econazole nitrate
Ecostatin♦, Spectazole
Pregnancy Category: C

MECHANISM OF ACTION
Alters fungal cell wall permeability.

INDICATIONS & DOSAGE
Treatment of tinea pedis, tinea cruris, and tinea corporis; cutaneous candidiasis—
Adults and children: apply sufficient quantity to cover affected areas b.i.d. in the morning and evening.
Tinea versicolor—
Adults and children: apply once daily.

ADVERSE REACTIONS
Local: burning, itching, stinging, erythema.

INTERACTIONS
Topical corticosteroids:
may inhibit antifungal effect.

NURSING CONSIDERATIONS
• If condition persists or worsens or if irritation (burning, itching, stinging, redness) occurs, discontinue use and report this to doctor.
• Use medication for entire treatment period, even though symptoms may have improved. Notify doctor if there is no improvement; after 2 weeks (tinea cruris and corporis) or 4 weeks (tinea pedis).
• Cleanse affected area before applying.
• Available as a 1% cream in a water-soluble base.
• Don't use occlusive dressings.

erythromycin
A/T/S, Eryderm, Staticin ♦
Pregnancy Category: B

MECHANISM OF ACTION
Disrupts protein synthesis.

INDICATIONS & DOSAGE
Superficial skin infections due to susceptible organisms, acne vulgaris—
Adults and children: clean affected area; apply t.i.d. or q.i.d.

ADVERSE REACTIONS
Skin: sensitivity reactions, erythema, burning, *dryness, pruritus.*

INTERACTIONS
None significant.

NURSING CONSIDERATIONS
• Prolonged use may result in overgrowth of nonsusceptible organisms.
• If no improvement or if condition worsens, stop using and notify doctor.
• Wash, rinse, and dry affected areas before application.
• Don't use near eyes, nose, mouth or other mucous membranes.

gentamicin sulfate
Garamycin♦
Pregnancy Category: C

MECHANISM OF ACTION
Disrupts protein synthesis.

INDICATIONS & DOSAGE
Primary and secondary bacterial infections, superficial burns, skin ulcers, infected insect bites and stings, infected lacerations and abrasions, wounds from minor surgery—
Adults and children over 1 year: rub in small amount gently t.i.d. or q.i.d., with or without gauze dressing.

ADVERSE REACTIONS
Skin: small percentage of minor skin irritation; possible photosensitivity; allergic contact dermatitis.

INTERACTIONS
None significant.

NURSING CONSIDERATIONS
• If no improvement or if condition

Unmarked trade names available in the United States only.
♦Also available in Canada.   ♦♦Available in Canada only.

worsens, stop using and report to doctor.
• Should be used in selected patients. Widespread use may lead to resistant organisms.
• Avoid use on large skin lesions or over a wide area because of possible systemic toxic effects.
• Prolonged use may result in overgrowth of nonsusceptible organisms.
• May clear bacterial infections that have not responded to other antibacterial agents.
• Store in cool place.
• Remove crusts before application of gentamicin in impetigo contagiosa.

---

gentian violet (methylrosaniline chloride)
Bismuth Violet Solution (1% and 2%), Crystal Violet
Pregnancy Category: C

MECHANISM OF ACTION
Fungistatic and antibacterial activity.

INDICATIONS & DOSAGE
Superficial infections of skin; lesions, except ulcerative lesions of face, particularly Candida albicans—
Adults and children: apply with swab b.i.d. or t.i.d. Keep affected area clean, dry, and exposed to air to prevent spread of infection.

ADVERSE REACTIONS
Skin: *permanent discoloration if applied to granulation tissue;* irritation or ulceration of mucous membranes.

INTERACTIONS
None significant.

NURSING CONSIDERATIONS
• Do not use on ulcerative lesions of the face.
• Apply carefully to avoid undue staining. Will stain skin and clothing.
• Do not use occlusive dressings.
• Tatooing of the skin may occur if applied to granulation tissue.

---

haloprogin
Halotex♦
Pregnancy Category: B

MECHANISM OF ACTION
Fungistatic and fungicidal activity.

INDICATIONS & DOSAGE
Superficial fungal infections (tinea pedis, tinea cruris, tinea corporis, tinea manuum, and tinea versicolor)—
Adults and children: apply liberally b.i.d. for 2 to 3 weeks.

ADVERSE REACTIONS
Skin: burning sensation, irritation, vesicle formation, increased maceration, *pruritus or exacerbation of preexisting lesions.*

INTERACTIONS
None significant.

NURSING CONSIDERATIONS
• Diagnosis should be reconsidered if no improvement in 4 weeks.
• Tell patient to continue using for full treatment period prescribed, even if condition has improved.

---

iodochlorhydroxyquin (Clioquinol)
Gentleline, Quinoform, Vioform♦
Pregnancy Category: C

MECHANISM OF ACTION
Fungistatic and fungicidal activity.

INDICATIONS & DOSAGE
Inflamed skin conditions, including eczema, athlete's foot, and other fungal infections; cutaneous or mucocutaneous mycotic infections caused by Candida *species (Monilia)*—
Adults and children: apply a thin layer b.i.d. or t.i.d., or as directed.

Italicized side effects are common or life-threatening.
*Liquid form contains alcohol.   **May contain tartrazine.

Continue for 1 week after clinical cure.

ADVERSE REACTIONS
Skin: *possible burning, itching, acneiform eruptions,* allergic contact dermatitis.

INTERACTIONS
Systemic corticosteroids: possible increased absorption. Use together cautiously.

NURSING CONSIDERATIONS
• Contraindicated in hypersensitivity to iodine or iodine-containing preparations. Contraindicated in tuberculosis, vaccinia, and varicella.
• Don't use to treat diaper rash.
• Note all side effects and precautions of each component in the combination antifungals.
• Presence in urine may cause false-positive result for phenylketonuria (PKU) or inaccurate thyroid function tests. Discontinue at least 1 month before thyroid function tests.
• Drug will stain fabric and hair.

---

ketoconazole
Nizoral
Pregnancy Category: C

MECHANISM OF ACTION
Inhibits yeast growth by altering the permeability of the cell membrane.

INDICATIONS & DOSAGE
Treatment of tinea corporis, tinea cruris, and tinea versicolor caused by susceptible organisms—
Adults: apply once daily to cover the affected and immediate surrounding area. Apply twice daily, if necessary, in the more resistant cases.

ADVERSE REACTIONS
Skin: severe irritation, pruritus, stinging.
Systemic: allergic reaction.

INTERACTIONS
None reported.

NURSING CONSIDERATIONS
• Discontinue if sensitivity or chemical irritation occurs.
• Most patients show improvement soon after treatment begins. However, treatment of tinea cruris or tinea corporis should continue for at least 2 weeks to reduce the possibility of recurrence.
• Check with doctor if condition worsens. The drug may have to be discontinued and diagnosis redetermined.

---

mafenide acetate
Sulfamylon♦
Pregnancy Category: C

MECHANISM OF ACTION
Interferes with bacterial cellular metabolism.

INDICATIONS & DOSAGE
Adjunctive treatment of second- and third-degree burns—
Adults and children: apply 1/16″ daily or b.i.d. to cleansed, debrided wounds. Reapply as needed to keep burned area covered.

ADVERSE REACTIONS
Blood: eosinophilia.
Skin: pain, *burning sensation,* rash, itching, swelling, hives, blisters, erythema, facial edema.
Other: *metabolic acidosis.*

INTERACTIONS
None significant.

NURSING CONSIDERATIONS
• Use with caution in acute renal failure and in known hypersensitivity to sulfonamides.
• Closely monitor acid-base balance, especially in the presence of pulmonary and renal dysfunction.

• If acidosis occurs, discontinue use for 24 to 48 hours.
• Causes pain at application site. Check for pain and burning; if they occur, notify doctor. Severe and prolonged pain may indicate allergy. If other allergic reactions occur, treatment may have to be temporarily discontinued.
• Sometimes difficult to distinguish between adverse reactions and effects of severe burn.
• Cleanse area before applying. Mafenide washes off with water.
• Keep burn areas medicated at all times.
• Bathe patient daily, if possible.
• For burns, using reverse isolation technique with sterile gloves and instruments to apply cream minimizes risk of further wound contamination.

miconazole nitrate 2%
Micatin, Monistat-Derm Cream and Lotion♦, Monistat 7 Vaginal Cream♦, Monistat 3 Vaginal Suppository, Monistat 7 Vaginal Suppository♦
Pregnancy Category: C

MECHANISM OF ACTION
Controls or destroys fungus by disrupting fungal cell membrane permeability.

INDICATIONS & DOSAGE
Tinea pedis, tinea cruris, tinea corporis, cutaneous candidiasis (moniliasis), infections from common dermatophytes—
Adults and children: apply or spray sparingly b.i.d. for 2 to 4 weeks.
Vulvovaginal candidiasis—
Adults: insert 1 full applicator or suppository (Monistat 7) intravaginally for 7 days at bedtime; repeat course if necessary. Alternatively, insert suppository (Monistat 3) intravaginally for 3 days at bedtime.

ADVERSE REACTIONS
Skin: isolated reports of irritation, burning, maceration.
Other: (with vaginal cream) vulvovaginal burning, itching, or irritation.

INTERACTIONS
None significant.

NURSING CONSIDERATIONS
• For external or intravaginal use only. Keep out of eyes.
• Discontinue if sensitivity or chemical irritation occurs.
• Tell patient to continue using for full treatment period prescribed, even if condition has improved.
• Do not use occlusive dressings.
• When using intravaginal forms, tell patient to cautiously insert high into the vagina with applicator provided.

neomycin sulfate
Mycifradin♦♦, Myciguent♦, Neocin♦♦
Pregnancy Category: C

MECHANISM OF ACTION
Disrupts protein synthesis.

INDICATIONS & DOSAGE
Topical bacterial infections, burns, wounds, skin grafts, following surgical procedure, lesions, pruritus, trophic ulcerations, edema—
Adults and children: rub in small quantity gently b.i.d., t.i.d., or as directed.

ADVERSE REACTIONS
Skin: *rashes, contact dermatitis,* urticaria.
Other: *possible nephrotoxicity, ototoxicity, and neuromuscular blockade; possible systemic absorption when used on extensive areas of the body.*

INTERACTIONS
None significant.

Italicized side effects are common or life-threatening.
*Liquid form contains alcohol.   **May contain tartrazine.

NURSING CONSIDERATIONS

• If no improvement or if condition worsens, stop using and report to doctor.

• Don't use on more than 20% of the body surface and on patient with impaired renal function unless risk/benefit ratio has been assessed.

• Prolonged use may result in overgrowth of nonsusceptible organisms.

• In those combination products that contain corticosteroids, use of occlusive dressings increases corticosteroid absorption and the likelihood of systemic effects.

• Enhanced systemic absorption occurs on denuded or abraded areas.

• Watch for signs of hypersensitivity and contact dermatitis.

• Evaluate patient for signs of ototoxicity with prolonged or extended use.

---

nitrofurazone
Furacin♦
Pregnancy Category: C

MECHANISM OF ACTION
Inhibits bacterial enzymes.

INDICATIONS & DOSAGE
Adjunctive treatment of second- and third-degree burns (especially when resistance to other antibiotics and sulfonamides occurs); skin grafting—
Adults and children: apply directly to lesion daily or every few days, depending on severity of burn.

ADVERSE REACTIONS
GU: possible renal toxicity.
Skin: *erythema, pruritus,* burning, edema, severe reactions (vesiculation, denudation, ulceration), *allergic contact dermatitis.*

INTERACTIONS
None significant.

NURSING CONSIDERATIONS
• Use cautiously in patients with

known or suspected renal impairment. Monitor serum creatinine regularly.

• If irritation, sensitization, or infection occurs, discontinue use.

• When using wet dressing, protect skin around wound with zinc oxide ointment.

• Cleanse wound as indicated by doctor before each dressing change.

• Solution should be stored in tight, light-resistant containers (brown bottles). Avoid exposure of solution at all times to direct light, prolonged heat, and alkaline materials.

• Drug may discolor in light but is still usable because it retains its potency.

• Discard cloudy solutions if warming to 55° to 60° C. (131° to 140° F.) does not restore clarity.

• Use reverse isolation and/or sterile application technique to prevent further wound contamination.

---

nystatin
Mycostatin♦, Nadostine♦♦, Nilstat
Pregnancy Category: B

MECHANISM OF ACTION
Alters the permeability of the cell membrane of fungi.

INDICATIONS & DOSAGE
Infant eczema, pruritus ani and vulvae, localized forms of candidiasis—
Adults and children: apply to affected area b.i.d. for 2 weeks.
Vulvovaginal candidiosis—
Adults: one vaginal tablet daily or b.i.d. for 14 days.

ADVERSE REACTIONS
Skin: occasional contact dermatitis from preservatives present in some formulations.

INTERACTIONS
None significant.

Unmarked trade names available in the United States only.
♦Also available in Canada.   ♦♦Available in Canada only.

NURSING CONSIDERATIONS
• Generally well tolerated by all age-groups, including debilitated infants.
• Preparation does not stain skin or mucous membranes.
• Cream is recommended for intertriginous areas; powder, for very moist areas; ointment, for dry areas.
• Tell patient to continue using for full treatment period prescribed, even if condition has improved. Immunosuppressed patients may use the drug chronically.
• Do not use occlusive dressings.
• Store vaginal tablets in the refrigerator.

• If hepatic or renal dysfunction occurs, consider discontinuing drug.
• Inspect patient's skin daily, and note any changes. Notify doctor if burning or excessive pain develops.
• Use only on affected areas. Keep medicated at all times.
• For patients with extensive burns, monitor serum sulfadiazine concentrations and renal function, and check urine for sulfa crystals.
• Bathe patient daily, if possible.
• Discard darkened cream.
• Reverse isolation and/or sterile application technique recommended to prevent wound contamination.

silver sulfadiazine
Flamazine◆◆, Silvadene
Pregnancy Category: C

MECHANISM OF ACTION
Acts upon cell membrane and cell wall.

INDICATIONS & DOSAGE
Prevention and treatment of wound infection especially for second- and third-degree burns—
Adults and children: apply 1/16″ thickness of ointment to cleansed and debrided burn wound, then apply daily or b.i.d.

ADVERSE REACTIONS
Blood: *neutropenia (in 3% to 5%) of those receiving extensive applications.*
Skin: pain, burning, rashes, itching.

INTERACTIONS
Topical proteolytic enzymes: inactivity of enzymes when used together. Do not use together.

NURSING CONSIDERATIONS
• Contraindicated in premature and newborn infants during first month of life. (Drug may increase possibility of kernicterus.) Use with caution in hypersensitivity to sulfonamides.

tetracycline hydrochloride
Topicycline
Pregnancy Category: D

MECHANISM OF ACTION
Disrupts protein synthesis.

INDICATIONS & DOSAGE
Acne vulgaris—
Adults and children over 12 years: apply generously to affected areas b.i.d. until skin is thoroughly wet.

ADVERSE REACTIONS
Skin: temporary stinging or burning on application, slight yellowing of treated skin, especially in patients with light complexions; severe dermatitis; treated skin areas fluoresce under black lights.

INTERACTIONS
None significant.

NURSING CONSIDERATIONS
• If no improvement or if condition worsens, stop using and notify doctor.
• Prolonged use may result in overgrowth of nonsusceptible organisms.
• Patient may continue normal use of cosmetics.
• Store at room temperature, away from excessive heat.

Italicized side effects are common or life-threatening.
*Liquid form contains alcohol.   **May contain tartrazine.

- Medication to be used by one person only. Tell patient not to share with family members.
- Apply in morning and evening. Warn that drug should be used within 2 months.
- Explain that floating plug in bottle of Topicycline—an inert and harmless result of proper reconstitution of the preparation—shouldn't be removed.
- Serum levels with topical tetracycline HCl are much lower than those for orally administered drug, so significant systemic effects are unlikely.
- To control flow rate of solution, increase or decrease pressure of the applicator against the skin.

---

tolnaftate
Aftate, Pitrex♦♦, Tinactin♦
Pregnancy Category: C

MECHANISM OF ACTION
Fungistatic and fungicidal activity.

INDICATIONS & DOSAGE
Superficial fungal infections of the skin, infections due to common pathogenic fungi, tinea pedis, tinea cruris, tinea corporis, tinea manuum—
Adults and children: ¼″ to ½″ ribbon of cream or 3 drops of lotion to cover area of one hand; same amount of cream or 3 drops of lotion to cover the toes and interdigital webs of one foot. Apply and massage gently into skin b.i.d. for 2 weeks, up to 6 weeks.

ADVERSE REACTIONS
None significant.

INTERACTIONS
None significant.

NURSING CONSIDERATIONS
- Discontinue if condition worsens. Check with doctor.
- Odorless, greaseless. Won't stain or discolor skin, hair, nails, or clothing.
- Only a small quantity of cream or lotion is needed; area should not be wet with solution when application is completed.
- Commonly available product used to treat athlete's foot (tinea pedis). If no improvement after 10 days, consult doctor.
- Tell patient to continue using for full treatment period prescribed, even if condition has improved.
- Don't use as a side agent to treat hair or nail infections. Will not eradicate fungus from these structures.
- Powder may be sprinkled inside socks and shoes.

---

undecylenic acid (zinc undecylenate)
Cruex, Desenex♦, NP-27, Ting, Unde-Jen
Pregnancy Category: C

MECHANISM OF ACTION
Fungistatic and fungicidal activity.

INDICATIONS & DOSAGE
Athlete's foot and ringworm of the body exclusive of nails and hairy areas—
Adults and children: apply b.i.d. to thoroughly cleansed area.

ADVERSE REACTIONS
Skin: possible irritation in hypersensitive person.

INTERACTIONS
None significant.

NURSING CONSIDERATIONS
- Tell patient to continue using for full treatment period prescribed, even if condition has improved.
- Apply for at least 2 weeks to minimize risk of relapse.
- Liquids are preferable for hairy areas while powders are preferable in moist areas, for example, between skin folds.

Unmarked trade names available in the United States only.
♦Also available in Canada.   ♦♦Available in Canada only.

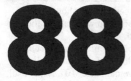

Scabicides and pediculicides

benzyl benzoate lotion
copper oleate solution
  (with tetrahydronaphthalene)
crotamiton
lindane
permethrin
pyrethrins

COMBINATION PRODUCTS
None.

---

benzyl benzoate lotion
Scabanca◆◆
Pregnancy Category: NR

MECHANISM OF ACTION
Unknown.

INDICATIONS & DOSAGE
Parasitic infestation (scabies, Phthirus pubis)—
Adults and children: first, scrub entire body with soap and water. Remove scales or crusts. Then apply the 28% lotion undiluted over entire body, except the face, while still damp. Be sure to apply around nails. Let dry. Apply second coat on the most involved areas. Bathe after 24 to 48 hours. Adults require 30 ml. Children require 20 ml.
Pediculosis capitis—
Adults and children: apply to scalp and leave on overnight; shampoo out in morning. Repeat next night if necessary.

ADVERSE REACTIONS
Skin: *irritation, itching; contact dermatitis with repeated applications.*

INTERACTIONS
None significant.

NURSING CONSIDERATIONS
• Contraindicated when skin is raw or inflamed. Notify doctor immediately if skin irritation or hypersensitivity develops; tell patient to discontinue drug and to wash it off skin.
• If live mites or new lesions occur, retreatment may be indicated in 7 to 10 days.
• Preferred over lindane for treatment of infants, young children, and pregnant or breast-feeding women.
• Do not apply to face, eyes, mucous membranes, or urethral meatus. If accidental contact with eyes does occur, flush with water and notify doctor.
• Instruct patient to change and sterilize (boil, launder, dry clean, or apply very hot iron) all clothing and bed linen after drug is washed off.
• Itching may continue for several weeks; this does not indicate that therapy is ineffective. To prevent acarophobia, reassure patient that itching will cease.
• Topical corticosteroids may be needed if dermatitis develops from scratching.
• Question other family members and sexual contacts about infestation.
• After application for lice infestation, use a fine comb dipped in white vinegar on hair to remove nits from hairy areas.
• Instruct patient to reapply if drug is washed off (hands, for example) during treatment time.
• Don't apply to infant's or small chil-

Italicized side effects are common or life-threatening.
*Liquid form contains alcohol.   **May contain tartrazine.

dren's hands because they will put hands in their mouths.
• Hospitalized patients should be placed in isolation with linen-handling precautions until treatment is completed.
• Store in light-resistant container; avoid exposure to excessive heat.

copper oleate solution (with tetrahydronaphthalene)
Cuprex
Pregnancy Category: NR

MECHANISM OF ACTION
Unknown.

INDICATIONS & DOSAGE
Parasitic infestation (pediculoses capitis and pubis)—
Adults and children: first, scrub entire body with soap and water. Apply gently and sparingly 3 to 4 tablespoonfuls onto affected areas; after 15 minutes wash off with soap and water.

ADVERSE REACTIONS
Skin: *irritation with repeated use, or if used on raw or inflamed skin.*

INTERACTIONS
None significant.

NURSING CONSIDERATIONS
• Contraindicated when skin is raw or inflamed, or when there is a severe infection. Notify doctor immediately if skin irritation or hypersensitivity develops; tell patient to discontinue drug and to wash it off skin.
• Preferred to lindane in treatment of infants, young children, pregnant or breast-feeding women.
• Do not apply more than twice within 48 hours.
• Do not apply to face, eyes, mucous membranes, or urethral meatus. If accidental contact with eyes does occur, flush with water and notify doctor.

• Instruct patient to change and sterilize (boil, launder, dry clean, or apply very hot iron) all clothing and bed linen after application.
• After application, use a fine comb dipped in white vinegar on hair to remove nits.
• Question other family members and sexual contacts about infestation.
• Tendency for overuse of pediculicides. Estimate amount needed.
• Hospitalized patients should be placed in isolation with linen-handling precautions until treatment is completed.
• Solution is flammable. Store away from direct sunlight or open flame.
• If necessary, may retreat in 7 to 10 days.

crotamiton
Eurax♦
Pregnancy Category: C

MECHANISM OF ACTION
Unknown.

INDICATIONS & DOSAGE
Parasitic infestation (scabies)—
Adults and children: scrub entire body with soap and water. Then, apply a thin layer of cream over entire body, from chin down (with special attention to folds, creases, interdigital spaces, and genital area). Apply second coat in 24 hours. Wait additional 48 hours, then wash off.
General itching—
apply locally b.i.d. or t.i.d.

ADVERSE REACTIONS
Skin: *irritation.*

INTERACTIONS
None significant.

NURSING CONSIDERATIONS
• Contraindicated when skin is raw or inflamed. Notify doctor immediately if skin irritation or hypersensitivity

develops; tell patient to discontinue drug and to wash it off skin.
• Do not apply to face, eyes, mucous membranes, or urethral meatus. If accidental contact with eyes does occur, flush with water and notify doctor.
• Instruct patient to change and sterilize (boil, launder, dry clean, or apply very hot iron) all clothing and bed linen after drug is washed off.
• Topical corticosteroids may be needed if dermatitis develops from scratching.
• Tendency to overuse scabicides. Estimate amount needed.
• Question other family members and sexual contacts about infestation.
• Instruct patient to reapply if drug is washed off (hands, for example) during treatment time.
• Hospitalized patients should be placed in isolation with special linen-handling precautions until treatment is completed.

lindane
GBH♦♦, Kwell, Kwellada♦♦, Scabene
Pregnancy Category: C

MECHANISM OF ACTION
Appears to inhibit neuronal membrane function in arthropods.

INDICATIONS & DOSAGE
Parasitic infestation (scabies, pediculosis)—
Adults and children: scrub entire body with soap and water.
Cream or lotion—apply thin layer over entire skin surface (with special attention to folds, creases, interdigital spaces, and genital area) for scabies, or to hairy areas for pediculosis. After 8 to 12 hours, wash off drug. If second application is needed, wait 1 week before repeating, but never more than twice in a week.
Shampoo—apply 30 ml undiluted to affected area and work into lather for

4 to 5 minutes. Rinse thoroughly and rub with dry towel.

ADVERSE REACTIONS
CNS: dizziness, convulsions.
Skin: *irritation with repeated use.*

INTERACTIONS
None significant.

NURSING CONSIDERATIONS
• Contraindicated when skin is raw or inflamed. Notify doctor immediately if skin irritation or hypersensitivity develops; tell patient to discontinue drug and to wash it off skin.
• Use cautiously in infants and young children as there's a greater risk for CNS toxicity in this group.
• Do not apply to open areas or acutely inflamed skin, or to face, eyes, mucous membranes, or urethral meatus. If accidental contact with eyes does occur, flush with water and notify doctor. Avoid inhaling vapors.
• Discourage repeated use, which can lead to skin irritation and systemic toxicity. Repeat use only if live lice or nits are found after 1 week.
• Warn patient that itching may continue for several weeks after effective treatment, especially in scabies.
• Topical corticosteroids or oral antihistamines may be needed for itching.
• Instruct patient to change and sterilize (boil, launder, dry clean, or apply very hot iron) all clothing and bed linen after drug is washed off.
• After application, use a fine comb dipped in white vinegar on hair to remove nits.
• Lindane shampoo can be used to clean combs or brushes; wash them thoroughly afterward. Warn patient not to use routinely.
• Question other family members and sexual contacts about infestation.
• Instruct patient to reapply if drug is washed off (hands, for example) during treatment time.
• Hospitalized patients should be

Italicized side effects are common or life-threatening.
*Liquid form contains alcohol.   **May contain tartrazine.

placed in isolation with special linen-handling precautions until treatment is completed.
• Extremely toxic to CNS if accidentally swallowed.

permethrin
Nix
Pregnancy Category: B

MECHANISM OF ACTION
Acts on the parasites' nerve cells to disrupt the sodium channel current, causing paralysis of the parasite.

INDICATIONS & DOSAGE
Treatment of infestation with Pediculus humanus capitis (head lice) and its nits—
Adults and children: use after hair has been washed with shampoo, rinsed with water, and towel-dried. Apply a sufficient amount (25 to 50 ml) of liquid to saturate the hair and scalp. Allow to remain on hair for 10 minutes before rinsing off with water.

ADVERSE REACTIONS
Skin: itching, burning, stinging, tingling, numbness or scalp discomfort, mild erythema, rash on the scalp.

INTERACTIONS
None reported.

NURSING CONSIDERATIONS
• Contraindicated in patients hypersensitive to pyrethrins or chrysanthemums.
• Don't use in infants because their skin is more permeable than that of children or adults.
• A single treatment is usually all that is necessary. Combing of nits is not required for effectiveness, but drug package supplies a fine-tooth comb for cosmetic use as desired.
• Head lice infestation is frequently accompanied by pruritus, erythema, and edema. Reassure patient that

treatment with permethrin may temporarily worsen these symptoms.
• A second application may be necessary if lice are observed 7 days after the initial application.
• Permethrin has been shown to be at least as effective as lindane (Kwell) in treating head lice.
• Not indicated to treat scabies.

pyrethrins
A-200 Pyrinate, Barc, Pyrin-Aid, Pyrinyl, Rid, TISIT, Triple X
Pregnancy Category: C

MECHANISM OF ACTION
Acts as contact poison that disrupts the parasite's nervous system, causing the parasite's paralysis and death.

INDICATIONS & DOSAGE
Treatment of infestations of head, body, and pubic (crab) lice and their eggs—
Adults and children: apply to hair, scalp, or other infested area until entirely wet. Allow to remain for 10 minutes, but no longer. Wash thoroughly with warm water and soap, or shampoo. Remove dead lice and eggs with fine-toothed comb. Treatment may be repeated, if necessary, but don't exceed two applications within 24 hours. May repeat in 7 to 10 days to kill newly hatched lice.

ADVERSE REACTIONS
Skin: *irritation with repeated use.*

INTERACTIONS
None significant.

NURSING CONSIDERATIONS
• Contraindicated when skin is raw or inflamed. Notify doctor immediately if skin irritation develops; tell patient to discontinue drug and to wash it off skin. Also contraindicated in patients allergic to ragweed. Use cautiously in infants and small children.

• Do not apply to open areas or acutely inflamed skin, or to face, eyes, mucous membranes, or urethral meatus. If accidental contact with eyes does occur, flush with water and notify doctor.

• Discourage repeated use, which can lead to skin irritation and possible systemic toxicity.

• Question other family members and sexual contacts about infestation.

• Topical corticosteroids or oral antihistamines may be needed if dermatitis develops from scratching.

• Instruct patient to change and sterilize (boil, launder, dry clean, or apply very hot iron) all clothing and bed linen after drug is washed off.

• Products containing pyrethrins are available without prescription. Some authorities believe pyrethrins and lindane (Kwell) are equally effective for lice infestation and that pyrethins are less hazardous.

• Not effective against scabies (mites).

Topical corticosteroids

alclometasone dipropionate
amcinonide
betamethasone benzoate
betamethasone dipropionate
betamethasone valerate
clobetasol propionate
clocortolone pivalate
desonide
desoximetasone
dexamethasone
dexamethasone sodium
  phosphate
diflorasone diacetate
fluocinolone acetonide
fluocinonide
flurandrenolide
halcinonide
hydrocortisone
hydrocortisone acetate
hydrocortisone valerate
methylprednisolone acetate
triamcinolone acetonide

COMBINATION PRODUCTS
Corticosteroids for topical use are commonly combined with antibiotics, antifungals, and sulfonamides. (See also Chapter 14, SULFONAMIDES, and Chapter 72, ANTIBIOTIC ANTINEO-PLASTIC AGENTS.)

alclometasone dipropionate
Alclovate
Pregnancy Category: C

MECHANISM OF ACTION
Diffuses across cell membranes to form complexes with specific cytoplasmic receptors.

INDICATIONS & DOSAGE
Inflammation of corticosteroid-responsive dermatoses—
Adults: apply a thin film to affected areas two or three times daily. Gently massage until the medication disappears.

ADVERSE REACTIONS
Skin: burning, itching, irritation, dryness, folliculitis, striae, acneiform eruptions, perioral dermatitis, hypopigmentation, hypertrichosis, allergic contact dermatitis.
With occlusive dressings: *secondary infection, maceration, atrophy, striae, miliaria.*

INTERACTIONS
None significant.

NURSING CONSIDERATIONS
• Use cautiously in viral skin diseases, such as varicella, vaccinia, and herpes simplex; in fungal infections; and in bacterial skin infections.
• Avoid application near eyes or mucous membranes. Do not apply to face, armpits, groin, or under breasts unless specifically ordered.
• Systemic absorption especially likely with occlusive dressings, prolonged treatment, or application to extensive body surface.
• Stop drug and notify doctor if patient develops signs of systemic absorption, skin irritation or ulceration, hypersensitivity, or infection. (If antifungals or antibiotics are being used concurrently, and infection does not respond immediately, corticosteroids

should be discontinued until infection is controlled.)
- Before applying, wash skin gently. To prevent damage to skin, rub medication in gently, leaving a thin coat. When treating hairy sites, part hair and apply directly to lesion.
- Occlusive dressing: apply cream, then cover with a thin, pliable, non-flammable plastic film; seal to adjacent normal skin with hypoallergenic tape. Minimize adverse reactions by using occlusive dressing intermittently. Don't leave in place longer than 16 hours each day.
- Notify doctor and remove occlusive dressing if fever develops.
- Occlusive dressings should not be used in presence of infections or with weeping or exudative lesions.
- Change dressings as ordered by doctor. Inspect skin for infection, striae, and atrophy. Discontinue drug and notify doctor if these occur.
- Treatment should be continued for a few days after clearing of lesions to prevent recurrence.

amcinonide
Cyclocort♦
Pregnancy Category: C

MECHANISM OF ACTION
Diffuses across cell membranes and complexes with specific cytoplasmic receptors.

INDICATIONS & DOSAGE
Inflammation of corticosteroid-responsive dermatoses—
Adults and children: apply a light film to affected areas b.i.d. or t.i.d. Cream should be rubbed in gently and thoroughly until it disappears.

ADVERSE REACTIONS
Skin: burning, itching, irritation, dryness, folliculitis, striae, acneiform eruptions, perioral dermatitis, hypopigmentation, hypertrichosis, allergic

contact dermatitis. *With occlusive dressings: secondary infection, maceration, atrophy, striae, miliaria.*

INTERACTIONS
None significant.

NURSING CONSIDERATIONS
- Use cautiously in viral diseases of skin, such as varicella, vaccinia, herpes simplex; fungal infections; bacterial skin infections.
- Avoid application near eyes or mucous membranes. Do not use on face, armpits, groin, in ear canal, or under breasts unless specifically ordered.
- Systemic absorption especially likely with occlusive dressings, prolonged treatment, or extensive body-surface treatment.
- Stop drug and notify doctor if patient develops signs of systemic absorption, skin irritation or ulceration, hypersensitivity, or infection. (If antifungals or antibiotics are being used with corticosteroids and infection does not respond immediately, corticosteroids should be stopped until infection is controlled.)
- Before applying, gently wash skin. To prevent damage to skin, rub medication in gently, leaving a thin coat. When treating hairy sites, part hair and apply directly to lesion.
- Occlusive dressing: apply cream, then cover with a thin, pliable, non-flammable plastic film; seal to adjacent normal skin with hypoallergenic tape. Minimize adverse reactions by using occlusive dressing intermittently. Don't leave in place longer than 16 hours each day.
- For patient with eczematous dermatitis who may develop irritation with adhesive material, hold dressing in place with gauze, elastic bandages, stockings, or stockinette.
- Notify doctor and remove occlusive dressing if fever develops.
- Occlusive dressings should not be used in presence of infections or with

---

Italicized side effects are common or life-threatening.
*Liquid form contains alcohol.   **May contain tartrazine.

weeping or exudative lesions.
• Change dressings as ordered by doctor. Inspect skin for infection, striae, and atrophy. Discontinue drug and notify doctor if these occur.
• Treatment should be continued for a few days after clearing of lesions to prevent recurrence.

betamethasone benzoate
Beben♦, Benisone, Uticort
Pregnancy Category: C

MECHANISM OF ACTION
Diffuses across cell membranes and complexes with specific cytoplasmic receptors.

INDICATIONS & DOSAGE
Inflammation of corticosteroid-responsive dermatoses—
Adults and children: clean area; apply cream, lotion, or gel sparingly daily to q.i.d.

ADVERSE REACTIONS
Skin: burning, itching, irritation, dryness, folliculitis, striae, acneiform eruptions, perioral dermatitis, hypopigmentation, hypertrichosis, allergic contact dermatitis. *With occlusive dressings: secondary infection, maceration, atrophy, striae, miliaria.*

INTERACTIONS
None significant.

NURSING CONSIDERATIONS
• Use cautiously in viral diseases of skin, such as varicella, vaccinia, herpes simplex; fungal infections; bacterial skin infections.
• Avoid application near eyes, mucous membranes, or in ear canal.
• Due to alcohol content of vehicle, gel preparations may cause mild, transient stinging, especially if used on or near excoriated skin.
• Systemic absorption especially likely with occlusive dressings, pro-

longed treatment, or extensive body-surface treatment.
• Stop drug and notify doctor if patient develops signs of systemic absorption, skin irritation or ulceration, hypersensitivity, or infection. (If antifungals or antibiotics are being used with corticosteroids and infection does not respond immediately, corticosteroids should be stopped until infection is controlled.)
• Before applying, gently wash skin. To prevent damage to skin, rub medication in gently, leaving a thin coat. When treating hairy sites, part hair and apply directly to lesion.
• Occlusive dressing: apply cream, then cover with a thin, pliable, nonflammable plastic film; seal to adjacent normal skin with hypoallergenic tape. Minimize adverse reactions by using occlusive dressing intermittently. Don't leave in place longer than 16 hours each day.
• For patient with eczematous dermatitis who may develop irritation with adhesive material, hold dressing in place with gauze, elastic bandages, stockings, or stockinette.
• Notify doctor and remove occlusive dressing if fever develops.
• Occlusive dressings should not be used in presence of infections or with weeping or exudative lesions.
• Change dressings as ordered by doctor. Inspect skin for infection, striae, and atrophy. Discontinue drug and notify doctor if these occur.
• Treatment should be continued for a few days after clearing of lesions to prevent recurrence.

betamethasone dipropionate
Diprolene, Diprosone♦
Pregnancy Category: C

MECHANISM OF ACTION
Diffuses across cell membranes and complexes with specific cytoplasmic

receptors.

INDICATIONS & DOSAGE
Inflammation of corticosteroid-responsive dermatoses—
Adults and children: clean area; apply cream, lotion, or ointment sparingly b.i.d.
Aerosol—Direct spray onto affected area from a distance of 6″ (15 cm) for only 3 seconds t.i.d. to q.i.d.

ADVERSE REACTIONS
Skin: burning, itching, irritation, dryness, folliculitis, perioral dermatitis, allergic contact dermatitis, hypopigmentation, hypertrichosis, acneiform eruptions. *With occlusive dressings: maceration of skin, secondary infection, atrophy, striae, miliaria.*

INTERACTIONS
None significant.

NURSING CONSIDERATIONS
• Use cautiously in viral diseases of skin, such as varicella, vaccinia, herpes simplex; fungal infections; bacterial skin infections.
• Avoid application near eyes, mucous membranes, or in ear canal.
• Systemic absorption especially likely with occlusive dressings, prolonged treatment, or extensive body-surface treatment.
• Stop drug and notify doctor if patient develops signs of systemic absorption, skin irritation or ulceration, hypersensitivity, or infection. (If antifungals or antibiotics are being used with corticosteroids and infection does not respond immediately, corticosteroids should be stopped until infection is controlled.)
• Before applying, gently wash skin. To prevent damage to skin, rub medication in gently, leaving a thin coat. When treating hairy sites, part hair and apply directly to lesion.
• Aerosol preparation contains alcohol and may produce irritation or

burning in open lesions. When using about the face, cover patient's eyes and warn against inhalation of spray. To avoid freezing tissues, do not spray longer than 3 seconds or closer than 6″ (15 cm).
• For patient with eczematous dermatitis who may develop irritation with adhesive material, hold dressing in place with gauze, elastic bandages, stockings, or stockinette.
• Occlusive dressings should not be used in presence of infection or with weeping or exudative lesions.
• Change dressing as ordered by doctor. Inspect skin for infection, striae, and atrophy. Discontinue drug and notify doctor if these occur.

---

betamethasone valerate
Betnovate♦♦, Betnovate 1/2♦♦, Celestoderm-V♦♦, Celestoderm-V/2♦♦, Valisone♦
Pregnancy Category: C

MECHANISM OF ACTION
Diffuses across cell membranes and complexes with specific cytoplasmic receptors.

INDICATIONS & DOSAGE
Inflammation of corticosteroid-responsive dermatoses—
Adults and children: clean area; apply cream, lotion, ointment, or aerosol sparingly daily to q.i.d.
Betnovate 1/2 and Celestoderm-V/2 contain less betamethasone.

ADVERSE REACTIONS
Skin: burning, itching, irritation, dryness, folliculitis, hypertrichosis, hypopigmentation, acneiform eruptions, perioral dermatitis, allergic contact dermatitis. *With occlusive dressings: maceration of skin, secondary infection, atrophy, striae, miliaria.*

INTERACTIONS
None significant.

Italicized side effects are common or life-threatening.
*Liquid form contains alcohol.   **May contain tartrazine.

NURSING CONSIDERATIONS
• Use cautiously in viral diseases of skin, such as varicella, vaccinia, herpes simplex; fungal infections; bacterial skin infections.
• Avoid application near eyes, mucous membranes, or in ear canal.
• Systemic absorption especially likely with occlusive dressings, prolonged treatment, or extensive body-surface treatment.
• Stop drug and notify doctor if patient develops signs of systemic absorption, skin irritation or ulceration, hypersensitivity, or infection. (If antifungals or antibiotics are being used with corticosteroids and infection does not respond immediately, corticosteroids should be stopped until infection is controlled.)
• Before applying, gently wash skin. To prevent damage to skin, rub medication in gently, leaving a thin coat. When treating hairy sites, part hair and apply directly to lesions.
• Occlusive dressing: apply cream or ointment, then cover with a thin, pliable, nonflammable plastic film; seal to adjacent normal skin with hypoallergenic tape. Minimize adverse reactions by using occlusive dressing intermittently. Don't leave in place longer than 16 hours each day.
• For patient with eczematous dermatitis who may develop irritation with adhesive material, hold dressing in place with gauze, elastic bandages, stockings, or stockinette.
• Notify doctor and remove occlusive dressing if fever develops.
• Occlusive dressings should not be used in presence of infection or with weeping or exudative lesions.
• Change dressing as ordered by doctor. Inspect skin for infection, striae, and atrophy. Discontinue drug and notify doctor if these occur.
• Treatment should be continued for a few days after clearing of lesions to prevent recurrence.

clobetasol propionate
Temovate
Pregnancy Category: C

MECHANISM OF ACTION
Diffuses across cell membranes and forms complexes with specific cytoplasmic receptors.

INDICATIONS & DOSAGE
Inflammation of corticosteroid-responsive dermatoses—
Adults: apply a thin layer to affected skin areas b.i.d., once in the morning and once at night.

ADVERSE REACTIONS
Skin: burning, itching, irritation, dryness, folliculitis, perioral dermatitis, allergic contact dermatitis, hypopigmentation, hypertrichosis, acneiform eruptions.
With occlusive dressings: maceration of skin, secondary infection, atrophy, striae, miliaria.

INTERACTIONS
None significant.

NURSING CONSIDERATIONS
• Use cautiously in viral skin diseases, such as varicella, vaccinia, herpes simplex; fungal infections; bacterial skin infections.
• Clobetasol is a potent, fluoridated corticosteroid. Warn patient not to use for longer than 14 days in a row.
• Avoid application near eyes, mucous membranes, or in ear canal.
• Systemic absorption especially likely with occlusive dressings, prolonged treatment, or extensive body-surface treatment.
• Stop drug and notify doctor if patient develops signs of systemic absorption, skin irritation or ulceration, hypersensitivity, or infection. (If antifungals or antibiotics are being used with corticosteroids and infection does not respond immediately, corti-

costeroids should be stopped until infection is controlled.)
• Before applying, gently wash skin. To prevent damage to skin, rub medication in gently, leaving a thin coat. When treating hairy sites, part hair and apply directly to lesions.
• Occlusive dressings should be applied with extreme caution and only when ordered by the doctor.
• Occlusive dressings: apply cream or ointment, then cover with a thin, pliable, nonflammable plastic film; seal to adjacent normal skin with hypoallergenic tape. Minimize adverse reactions by using occlusive dressing intermittently. Don't leave in place longer than 16 hours each day.
• For patients with eczematous dermatitis who may develop irritation with adhesive material, hold dressing in place with gauze, elastic bandages, stockings, or stockinette.
• Notify doctor and remove occlusive dressing if fever develops.
• Occlusive dressings should not be used in presence of infection or with weeping or exudative lesions.
• Change dressing as ordered by doctor. Inspect skin for infection, striae, and atrophy. Discontinue drug and notify doctor if these occur.

clocortolone pivalate
Cloderm
Pregnancy Category: C

MECHANISM OF ACTION
Diffuses across cell membranes and complexes with specific cytoplasmic receptors.

INDICATIONS & DOSAGE
Inflammation of corticosteroid-responsive dermatoses, such as atopic dermatitis, contact dermatitis, seborrheic dermatitis—
Adults and children: apply cream sparingly to affected areas t.i.d. and rub in gently.

ADVERSE REACTIONS
Skin: burning, itching, irritation, dryness, folliculitis, striae, acneiform eruptions, perioral dermatitis, hypertrichosis, hypopigmentation, allergic contact dermatitis. *With occlusive dressings: secondary infection, maceration, atrophy, striae, miliaria.*

INTERACTIONS
None significant.

NURSING CONSIDERATIONS
• Use cautiously in viral diseases of skin, such as varicella, vaccinia, herpes simplex; fungal infections; bacterial skin infections.
• Avoid application near eyes or mucous membranes.
• Systemic absorption especially likely with occlusive dressings, prolonged treatment, or extensive body-surface treatment.
• Stop drug and notify doctor if patient develops signs of systemic absorption, skin irritation or ulceration, hypersensitivity, or infection. (If antifungals or antibiotics are being used with corticosteroids and infection does not respond immediately, corticosteroids should be stopped until infection is controlled.)
• Before applying, gently wash skin. To prevent damage to skin, rub medication in gently, leaving a thin coat. When treating hairy sites, part hair and apply directly to lesion.
• Occlusive dressing: apply cream, then cover with a thin, pliable, nonflammable plastic film; seal to adjacent normal skin with hypoallergenic tape. Minimize adverse reactions by using occlusive dressing intermittently. Don't leave in place longer than 16 hours each day.
• For patient with eczematous dermatitis who may develop irritation with adhesive material, hold dressing in place with gauze, elastic bandages, or stockings.
• Notify doctor and remove occlusive

Italicized side effects are common or life-threatening.
*Liquid form contains alcohol.   **May contain tartrazine.

dressing if fever develops.
• Occlusive dressings should not be used in presence of infections or with weeping or exudative lesions.
• Change dressings as ordered by doctor. Inspect skin for infection, striae, and atrophy. Discontinue drug and notify doctor if these occur.
• Treatment should be continued for a few days after clearing of lesions to prevent recurrence.

desonide
Tridesilon♦
Pregnancy Category: C

MECHANISM OF ACTION
Diffuses across cell membranes and complexes with specific cytoplasmic receptors.

INDICATIONS & DOSAGE
Adjunctive therapy for inflammation in acute and chronic corticosteroid-responsive dermatoses—
Adults and children: clean area; apply cream, lotion, or gel sparingly b.i.d. or t.i.d.

ADVERSE REACTIONS
Skin: burning, itching, irritation, dryness, folliculitis, perioral dermatitis, allergic contact dermatitis, hypertrichosis, hypopigmentation, acneiform eruptions. *With occlusive dressings: maceration of skin, secondary infection, atrophy, striae, miliaria.*

INTERACTIONS
None significant.

NURSING CONSIDERATIONS
• Use cautiously in viral diseases of skin, such as varicella, vaccinia, herpes simplex; fungal infections; bacterial skin infections.
• Avoid application near eyes, mucous membranes, or in ear canal.
• Systemic absorption especially likely with occlusive dressings, prolonged treatment, or extensive body-surface treatment.
• Stop drug and notify doctor if patient develops signs of systemic absorption, skin irritation or ulceration, hypersensitivity, or infection. (If antifungals or antibiotics are being used with corticosteroids and infection does not respond immediately, corticosteroids should be stopped until infection is controlled.)
• Before applying, gently wash skin. To prevent damage to skin, rub medication in gently, leaving a thin coat. When treating hairy sites, part hair and apply directly to lesion.
• Occlusive dressing: apply cream or ointment, then cover with a thin, pliable, nonflammable plastic film; seal to adjacent normal skin with hypoallergenic tape. Minimize adverse reactions by using occlusive dressing intermittently. Don't leave in place longer than 16 hours each day.
• For patient with eczematous dermatitis who may develop irritation with adhesive material, hold dressing in place with gauze, elastic bandages, stockings, or stockinette.
• Notify doctor and remove occlusive dressing if fever develops.
• Occlusive dressings should not be used in presence of infection or with weeping or exudative lesions.
• Change dressing as ordered by doctor. Inspect skin for infection, striae, and atrophy. Discontinue drug and notify doctor if these occur.
• Treatment should be continued for a few days after clearing of lesions to prevent recurrence.

desoximetasone
Topicort♦
Pregnancy Category: C

MECHANISM OF ACTION
Diffuses across cell membranes and complexes with specific cytoplasmic receptors.

INDICATIONS & DOSAGE
Inflammation of corticosteroid-responsive dermatoses—
Adults and children: clean area; apply cream sparingly b.i.d. to t.i.d.

ADVERSE REACTIONS
Skin: burning, itching, irritation, dryness, folliculitis, hypertrichosis, acneiform eruptions, perioral dermatitis, hypopigmentation, allergic contact dermatitis. *With occlusive dressings: maceration of skin, secondary infection, atrophy, striae, miliaria.*

INTERACTIONS
None significant.

NURSING CONSIDERATIONS
• Use cautiously in viral diseases of skin, such as varicella, vaccinia, herpes simplex; fungal infections; bacterial skin infections.
• Avoid application near eyes, mucous membranes, or in ear canal.
• Systemic absorption especially likely with occlusive dressings, prolonged treatment, or extensive body-surface treatment.
• Stop drug and notify doctor if patient develops signs of systemic absorption, skin irritation or ulceration, hypersensitivity, or infection. (If antifungals or antibiotics are being used with corticosteroids and infection does not respond immediately, corticosteroids should be stopped until infection is controlled.)
• Before applying, gently wash skin. To prevent damage to skin, rub medication in gently, leaving a thin coat. When treating hairy sites, part hair and apply directly to lesions.
• Occlusive dressing: apply cream, then cover with a thin, pliable, nonflammable plastic film; seal to adjacent normal skin with hypoallergenic tape. To minimize adverse reactions, use occlusive dressing intermittently. Don't leave in place longer than 16 hours each day.

• For patient with eczematous dermatitis who may develop irritation with adhesive material, hold dressing in place with gauze, elastic bandages, stockings, or stockinette.
• Notify doctor and remove occlusive dressing if fever develops.
• Occlusive dressings should not be used in presence of infection or with weeping or exudative lesions.
• Change dressing as ordered by doctor. Inspect skin for infection, striae, and atrophy. Discontinue drug and notify doctor if these occur.
• Treatment should be continued for a few days after clearing of lesions to prevent recurrence.

dexamethasone
Aeroseb-Dex, Decaderm, Decaspray
Pregnancy Category: C

MECHANISM OF ACTION
Diffuses across cell membranes and complexes with specific cytoplasmic receptors.

INDICATIONS & DOSAGE
Inflammation of corticosteroid-responsive dermatoses—
Adults and children: clean area; apply gel or aerosol sparingly b.i.d. to q.i.d.
Aerosol use on scalp—shake can well and apply to dry scalp after shampooing. Hold can upright. Slide applicator tube under hair so that it touches scalp. Spray while moving tube to all affected areas, keeping tube under hair and in contact with scalp throughout spraying, which should take about 2 seconds. Inadequately covered areas may be spot sprayed. Slide applicator tube through hair to touch scalp, press and immediately release spray button. Don't massage medication into scalp or spray forehead or eyes.

ADVERSE REACTIONS
Skin: burning, itching, irritation, dryness, folliculitis, hypertrichosis, acneiform eruptions, perioral dermatitis, hypopigmentation, allergic contact dermatitis. *With occlusive dressings: maceration of skin, secondary infection, atrophy, striae, miliaria.*

INTERACTIONS
None significant.

NURSING CONSIDERATIONS
• Use cautiously in viral diseases of skin, such as varicella, vaccinia, herpes simplex; fungal infections; bacterial skin infections.
• Avoid application near eyes, mucous membranes, or in ear canal.
• Systemic absorption especially likely with occlusive dressings, prolonged treatment, or extensive body-surface treatment.
• Stop drug and notify doctor if patient develops signs of systemic absorption, skin irritation or ulceration, hypersensitivity, or infection. (If antifungals or antibiotics are being used with corticosteroids and infection does not respond immediately, corticosteroids should be stopped until infection is controlled.)
• Before applying, gently wash skin. To prevent damage to skin, rub medication in gently, leaving a thin coat. When treating hairy sites, part hair and apply directly to lesions.
• For patient with eczematous dermatitis who may develop irritation with adhesive material, hold dressing in place with gauze, elastic bandages, stockings, or stockinette.
• Notify doctor and remove occlusive dressing if fever develops.
• Change dressing as ordered by doctor. Inspect skin for infection, striae, and atrophy. Discontinue drug and notify doctor if these occur.
• Occlusive dressings should not be used in presence of infection or with weeping or exudative lesions.

• Aerosol preparation contains alcohol and may produce irritation or burning in open lesions. When using about the face, cover patient's eyes and warn against inhalation of the spray. To avoid freezing tissues, do not spray longer than 3 seconds or closer than 6″ (15 cm).
• Treatment should be continued for a few days after clearing of lesions to prevent recurrence.

dexamethasone sodium phosphate
Decadron Phosphate♦
Pregnancy Category: C

MECHANISM OF ACTION
Diffuses across cell membranes and complexes with specific cytoplasmic receptors.

INDICATIONS & DOSAGE
Inflammation of corticosteroid-responsive dermatoses—
Adults and children: clean area; apply cream sparingly b.i.d. or t.i.d.

ADVERSE REACTIONS
Skin: burning, itching, irritation, dryness, folliculitis, hypertrichosis, hypopigmentation, acneiform eruptions, perioral dermatitis, allergic contact dermatitis. *With occlusive dressings: maceration of skin, secondary infection, atrophy, striae, miliaria.*

INTERACTIONS
None significant.

NURSING CONSIDERATIONS
• Use cautiously in viral diseases of skin, such as varicella, vaccinia, herpes simplex; fungal infections; bacterial skin infections.
• Avoid application near eyes, mucous membranes, or in ear canal.
• Systemic absorption especially likely with occlusive dressings, prolonged treatment, or extensive body-

surface treatment.
- Stop drug and notify doctor if patient develops signs of systemic absorption, skin irritation or ulceration, hypersensitivity, or infection. (If antifungals or antibiotics are being used along with corticosteroids and infection does not respond immediately, corticosteroids should be stopped until infection is controlled.)
- Before applying, gently wash skin. To prevent damage to skin, rub medication in gently, leaving a thin coat. When treating hairy sites, part hair and apply directly to lesions.
- Occlusive dressing: apply cream heavily, then cover with a thin, pliable, nonflammable plastic film; seal to adjacent normal skin with hypoallergenic tape. To minimize adverse reactions, use occlusive dressing intermittently. Don't leave in place longer than 16 hours each day. Occlusive dressings should not be used in presence of infection or with weeping or exudative lesions.
- For patient with eczematous dermatitis who may develop irritation with adhesive material, hold dressing in place with gauze, elastic bandages, stockings, or stockinette.
- Notify doctor and remove occlusive dressing if fever develops.
- Change dressing as ordered by doctor. Inspect skin for infection, striae, and atrophy. Discontinue drug and notify doctor if these occur.
- Treatment should be continued for a few days after clearing of lesions to prevent recurrence.

---

diflorasone diacetate
Florone♦, Maxiflor
Pregnancy Category: C

MECHANISM OF ACTION
Diffuses across cell membranes and complexes with specific cytoplasmic receptors.

INDICATIONS & DOSAGE
Inflammation of corticosteroid-responsive dermatoses—
Adults and children: clean area; apply ointment daily to t.i.d.; apply cream b.i.d. to q.i.d. Apply sparingly in a thin film.

ADVERSE REACTIONS
Skin: burning, itching, irritation, dryness, folliculitis, perioral dermatitis, hypertrichosis, hypopigmentation, acneiform eruptions. *With occlusive dressings: maceration, secondary infection, atrophy, striae, miliaria.*

INTERACTIONS
None significant.

NURSING CONSIDERATIONS
- Use cautiously in viral diseases of skin, such as varicella, vaccinia, herpes simplex; fungal infections; bacterial skin infections.
- Use very cautiously in young children. A high-potency corticosteroid.
- Avoid application near eyes, mucous membranes, or in ear canal.
- Systemic absorption especially likely with occlusive dressings, prolonged treatment, or extensive body-surface treatment.
- Stop drug and notify doctor if patient develops signs of systemic absorption, skin irritation or ulceration, hypersensitivity, or infection. (If antifungals or antibiotics are being used concomitantly, corticosteroids should be stopped until infection is controlled.)
- Before applying, gently wash skin. To prevent damage to skin, rub medication in gently, leaving a thin coat. When treating hairy sites, part hair and apply directly to lesion.
- Occlusive dressing: apply cream or ointment, then cover with a thin, pliable, nonflammable plastic film; seal to adjacent normal skin with hypoallergenic tape. Minimize adverse reactions by using occlusive dressing in-

---

termittently. Don't leave in place longer than 16 hours each day. Occlusive dressings should not be used in presence of infection or with weeping or exudative lesions.
• For patient with eczematous dermatitis who may develop irritation with adhesive material, hold dressing in place with gauze, elastic bandages, stockings, or stockinette.
• Notify doctor and remove occlusive dressing if fever develops.
• Change dressing as ordered by doctor. Inspect skin for infection, striae, and atrophy. Discontinue drug and notify doctor if these occur.
• Diflorasone is often effective with once-daily application.

---

fluocinolone acetonide
Fluonid, Synalar♦, Synamol♦, Synemol
Pregnancy Category: C

MECHANISM OF ACTION
Diffuses across cell membranes and complexes with specific cytoplasmic receptors.

INDICATIONS & DOSAGE
Inflammation of corticosteroid-responsive dermatoses—
Adults and children over 2 years: clean area; apply cream, ointment, or solution sparingly b.i.d. to q.i.d. Treat multiple or extensive lesions sequentially, applying to only small areas at any one time.

ADVERSE REACTIONS
Skin: burning, itching, irritation, dryness, folliculitis, hypertrichosis, hypopigmentation, acneiform eruptions, perioral dermatitis, allergic contact dermatitis. *With occlusive dressings: maceration of skin, secondary infection, atrophy, striae, miliaria.*

INTERACTIONS
None significant.

NURSING CONSIDERATIONS
• Use cautiously in viral diseases of skin, such as varicella, vaccinia, herpes simplex; fungal infections; bacterial skin infections.
• Avoid application near eyes, mucous membranes, or in ear canal.
• Systemic absorption especially likely with occlusive dressings, prolonged treatment, or extensive body-surface treatment.
• Stop drug and notify doctor if patient develops signs of systemic absorption, skin irritation or ulceration, hypersensitivity, or infection. (If antifungals or antibiotics are being used with corticosteroids and infection does not respond immediately, corticosteroids should be stopped until infection is controlled.)
• Before applying, gently wash skin. To prevent damage to skin, rub medication in gently, leaving a thin coat. When treating hairy sites, part hair and apply directly to lesion.
• Occlusive dressing: apply gently and sparingly to the lesion until cream disappears. Then reapply, leaving a thin coat. Cover with a thin, pliable, nonflammable plastic film; seal to adjacent normal skin with hypoallergenic tape. To minimize adverse reactions, use occlusive dressing intermittently. Don't leave in place longer than 16 hours each day. Occlusive dressings should not be used in presence of infection or with weeping or exudative lesions.
• For patient with eczematous dermatitis who may develop irritation with adhesive material, hold dressing in place with gauze, elastic bandages, stockings, or stockinette.
• Notify doctor and remove occlusive dressing if fever develops.
• Change dressing as ordered by doctor. Inspect skin for infection, striae, and atrophy. Discontinue drug and notify doctor if these occur.
• Fluonid solution on dry lesions may increase dryness, scaling, or itching;

---

on denuded or fissured areas, may produce burning or stinging. If burning or stinging persists and dermatitis has not improved, solution should be discontinued.

fluocinonide
Lidemol♦♦, Lidex♦, Lidex-E, Topsyn♦
Pregnancy Category: C

MECHANISM OF ACTION
Diffuses across cell membranes and complexes with specific cytoplasmic receptors.

INDICATIONS & DOSAGE
Inflammation of corticosteroid-responsive dermatoses—
Adults and children: clean area; apply cream, ointment, or gel sparingly t.i.d. or q.i.d.

ADVERSE REACTIONS
Skin: burning, itching, irritation, dryness, folliculitis, hypertrichosis, hypopigmentation, acneiform eruptions, perioral dermatitis, allergic contact dermatitis. *With occlusive dressings: maceration of skin, secondary infection, atrophy, striae, miliaria.*

INTERACTIONS
None significant.

NURSING CONSIDERATIONS
• Use cautiously in viral diseases of skin, such as varicella, vaccinia, and herpes simplex; untreated purulent bacterial skin infections; fungal infections; bacterial skin infections.
• Avoid application near eyes, mucous membranes, or in ear canal.
• Systemic absorption especially likely with occlusive dressings, prolonged treatment, or extensive body-surface treatment.
• Stop drug and notify doctor if patient develops signs of systemic absorption, skin irritation or ulceration, hypersensitivity, or infection. (If antifungals or antibiotics are being used with corticosteroids and infection does not respond immediately, corticosteroids should be stopped until infection is controlled.)
• Before applying, gently wash skin. To prevent damage to skin, rub medication in gently, leaving a thin coat. When treating hairy sites, part hair and apply directly to lesion.
• Occlusive dressing: apply cream or ointment heavily, then cover with a thin, pliable, nonflammable plastic film; seal to adjacent normal skin with hypoallergenic tape. To minimize adverse reactions, use occlusive dressing intermittently. Don't leave in place longer than 16 hours each day. Occlusive dressings should not be used in presence of infection or with weeping or exudative lesions.
• For patient with eczematous dermatitis who may develop irritation with adhesive material, hold dressing in place with gauze, elastic bandages, stockings, or stockinette.
• Notify doctor and remove occlusive dressing if fever develops.
• Change dressing as ordered by doctor. Inspect skin for infection, striae, and atrophy. Discontinue drug and notify doctor if these occur.
• Treatment should be continued for a few days after clearing of lesions to prevent recurrence.

flurandrenolide
Cordran, Cordran SP, Cordran Tape, Drenison♦♦, Drenison 1/4♦♦, Drenison Tape♦♦
Pregnancy Category: C

MECHANISM OF ACTION
Diffuses across cell membranes and complexes with specific cytoplasmic receptors.

INDICATIONS & DOSAGE
Inflammation of corticosteroid-

Italicized side effects are common or life-threatening.
*Liquid form contains alcohol.   **May contain tartrazine.

responsive dermatoses—
Adults and children: clean area; apply cream, lotion, or ointment sparingly b.i.d. or t.i.d. Apply tape q 12 to 24 hours. Before applying tape, cleanse skin carefully, removing scales, crust, and dried exudates. Allow skin to dry for 1 hour before applying new tape. Shave or clip hair to allow good contact with skin and comfortable removal. If tape ends loosen prematurely, trim off and replace with fresh tape. Lowest incidence of adverse reactions if tape is replaced q 12 hours, but may be left in place for 24 hours if well tolerated and adheres satisfactorily.
Drenison 1/4—for maintenance therapy of widespread or chronic lesions.

ADVERSE REACTIONS
Skin: burning, itching, irritation, dryness, folliculitis, hypertrichosis, hypopigmentation, acneiform eruptions, allergic contact dermatitis. *With occlusive dressings: maceration of skin, secondary infection, atrophy, striae, miliaria*. With tape: purpura, stripping of epidermis, furunculosis.

INTERACTIONS
None significant.

NURSING CONSIDERATIONS
• Use cautiously in viral diseases of skin, such as varicella, vaccinia, herpes simplex; fungal infections; bacterial skin infections.
• Tape not advised for exudative lesions or those in intertriginous areas.
• Tape should be cut with scissors. Don't tear.
• Avoid application near eyes, mucous membranes, or in ear canal.
• Systemic absorption especially likely with occlusive dressings, prolonged treatment, or extensive body-surface treatment.
• Stop drug and notify doctor if patient develops signs of systemic absorption, skin irritation or ulceration,

hypersensitivity, or infection. (If antifungals or antibiotics are being used with corticosteroids and infection does not respond immediately, corticosteroids should be stopped until infection is controlled.)
• Before applying, gently wash skin. To prevent damage to skin, rub medication in gently, leaving a thin coat. When treating hairy sites, part hair and apply directly to lesion.
• Occlusive dressing: apply cream heavily, then cover with a thin, pliable, nonflammable plastic film; seal to adjacent normal skin with hypoallergenic tape. To minimize adverse reactions, use occlusive dressing intermittently. Don't leave in place longer than 16 hours each day. Occlusive dressings should not be used in presence of infection or with weeping or exudative lesions.
• For patient with eczematous dermatitis who may develop irritation with adhesive material, hold dressing in place with gauze, elastic bandages, stockings, or stockinette.
• Notify doctor and remove occlusive dressing if fever develops.
• Inspect skin for infection, striae, and atrophy. Discontinue drug and notify doctor if these occur.
• Treatment should be continued for a few days after clearing of lesions to prevent recurrence.

---

halcinonide
Halciderm, Halog♦
Pregnancy Category: C

MECHANISM OF ACTION
Diffuses across cell membranes and complexes with specific cytoplasmic receptors.

INDICATIONS & DOSAGE
Inflammation of acute and chronic corticosteroid-responsive dermatoses—
Adults and children: clean area; ap-

ply cream, ointment, or solution sparingly b.i.d. or t.i.d.

ADVERSE REACTIONS
Skin: burning, itching, irritation, dryness, folliculitis, hypertrichosis, hypopigmentation, acneiform eruptions, allergic contact dermatitis. *With occlusive dressings: maceration of skin, secondary infection, atrophy, striae, miliaria.*

INTERACTIONS
None significant.

NURSING CONSIDERATIONS
• Use cautiously in viral diseases of skin, such as varicella, vaccinia, herpes simplex; fungal infections; bacterial skin infections.
• Avoid application near eyes, mucous membranes, or in ear canal.
• Systemic absorption especially likely with occlusive dressings, prolonged treatment, or extensive body-surface treatment.
• Stop drug and notify doctor if patient develops signs of systemic absorption, skin irritation or ulceration, hypersensitivity, or infection. (If antifungals or antibiotics are being used with corticosteroids and infection does not respond immediately, corticosteroids should be stopped until infection is controlled.)
• Before applying, gently wash skin. To prevent damage to skin, rub medication in gently, leaving a thin coat. When treating hairy sites, part hair and apply directly to lesion.
• Occlusive dressing with cream: gently rub small amount into lesion until it disappears. Reapply, leaving a thin coating on lesion, and cover with occlusive dressing. With ointment: apply to lesion and cover with occlusive dressing. Cover with a thin, pliable, nonflammable plastic film; seal to adjacent normal skin with hypoallergenic tape. To minimize adverse reactions, use occlusive dressing inter-

mittently. Don't leave in place longer than 16 hours each day.
• Good results have been obtained by applying occlusive dressings in the evening and removing them in the morning (i.e., 12-hour occlusion). Medication should then be reapplied in the morning, without using the occlusive dressings during the day.
• For patient with eczematous dermatitis who may develop irritation with adhesive material, hold dressing in place with gauze, elastic bandages, stockings, or stockinette.
• Notify doctor and remove occlusive dressing if fever develops.
• Occlusive dressings should not be used in presence of infection or with weeping or exudative lesions.
• Change dressing as ordered by doctor. Inspect skin for infection, striae, and atrophy. Discontinue drug and notify doctor if these occur.
• Treatment should be continued for a few days after clearing of lesions to prevent recurrence.

Italicized side effects are common or life-threatening.
*Liquid form contains alcohol.   **May contain tartrazine.

hydrocortisone
Acticort, Aeroseb-HC♦, Carmol HC, Cetacort, ClearAid, Cort-Dome, Corticreme♦♦, Cortinal, Cortizone 5, Cotacort, Cremesone, Delacort, Dermacort, Dermolate, Durel-Cort, Ecosone, HC Cream, HI-COR-2.5, Hycortole, Hydrocortex, Ivocort, Maso-Cort, Microcort♦, Penetrate, Proctocort, Relecort, Rhus Tox HC, Rocort, Unicort♦

hydrocortisone acetate
Cortaid, Cortamed♦♦, Cortef, Cortifoam, Epifoam, Hydrocortisone Acetate, My-Cort Lotion, Proctofoam-HC

hydrocortisone valerate
Westcort Cream♦
Pregnancy Category: C

MECHANISM OF ACTION
Diffuses across cell membranes and complexes with specific cytoplasmic receptors.

INDICATIONS & DOSAGE
Inflammation of corticosteroid-responsive dermatoses; adjunctive typical management of seborrheic dermatitis of scalp; may be safely used on face, groin, armpits, and under breasts—
Adults and children: clean area; apply cream, lotion, ointment, foam or aerosol sparingly daily to q.i.d. Aerosol—shake can well. Direct spray onto affected area from a distance of 6″ (15 cm). Apply for only 3 seconds (to avoid freezing tissues). Apply to dry scalp after shampooing; no need to massage or rub medication into scalp after spraying. Apply daily until acute phase is controlled, then reduce dosage to 1 to 3 times a week as needed to maintain control.
For rectal administration: shake can well. One applicatorful daily to b.i.d.

for 2 to 3 weeks, then every other day as necessary.

ADVERSE REACTIONS
Skin: burning, itching, irritation, dryness, folliculitis, hypertrichosis, hypopigmentation, acneiform eruptions, allergic contact dermatitis. *With occlusive dressings: maceration of skin, secondary infection, atrophy, striae, miliaria.*

INTERACTIONS
None significant.

NURSING CONSIDERATIONS
• Use cautiously in viral diseases of skin, such as varicella, vaccinia, herpes simplex; fungal infections; bacterial skin infections.
• Avoid application near eyes, mucous membranes, or in ear canal.
• Systemic absorption especially likely with occlusive dressings, prolonged treatment, or extensive body-surface treatment.
• Stop drug and notify doctor if patient develops signs of systemic absorption, skin irritation or ulceration, hypersensitivity, or infection. (If antifungals or antibiotics are being used with corticosteroids and infection does not respond immediately, corticosteroids should be stopped until infection is controlled.)
• Before applying, gently wash skin. To prevent damage to skin, rub medication in gently, leaving a thin coat. When treating hairy sites, part hair and apply directly to lesion.
• Occlusive dressing: apply cream heavily, then cover with a thin, pliable, nonflammable plastic film; seal to adjacent normal skin with hypoallergenic tape. To minimize adverse reactions, use occlusive dressing intermittently. Don't leave in place longer than 16 hours each day. Occlusive dressings should not be used in presence of infection or with weeping or exudative lesions.

Unmarked trade names available in the United States only.
♦Also available in Canada. ♦♦Available in Canada only.

• For patient with eczematous dermatitis who may develop irritation with adhesive material, it may be helpful to hold dressing in place with gauze, elastic bandages, stockings, or stockinette.

• Notify doctor and remove occlusive dressing if fever develops.

• Aerosol preparation contains alcohol and may produce irritation or burning in open lesions. When using about the face, cover patient's eyes and warn against inhalation of the spray. To avoid freezing tissues, do not spray longer than 3 seconds or closer than 6″ (15 cm).

• Change dressing as ordered by doctor. Inspect skin for infection, striae, and atrophy. Discontinue drug and notify doctor if these occur.

• Treatment should be continued for a few days following clearing of lesions to prevent recurrence.

• The 0.5% strength is available without prescription. Urge patients not to self-medicate for longer than 7 days in a row.

---

methylprednisolone acetate
Medrol♦
Pregnancy Category: C

MECHANISM OF ACTION
Diffuses across cell membranes and complexes with specific cytoplasmic receptors.

INDICATIONS & DOSAGE
Inflammation of corticosteroid-responsive dermatoses—
Adults and children: clean area; apply ointment daily to t.i.d.

ADVERSE REACTIONS
Skin: burning, itching, irritation, dryness, folliculitis, hypertrichosis, hypopigmentation, acneiform eruptions, allergic contact dermatitis. *With occlusive dressings: maceration of skin, secondary infection, atrophy, striae, miliaria.*

INTERACTIONS
None significant.

NURSING CONSIDERATIONS
• Use cautiously in viral diseases of skin, such as varicella, vaccinia, herpes simplex; fungal infections; bacterial skin infections.

• Avoid application near eyes, mucous membranes, or in ear canal.

• Systemic absorption especially likely with occlusive dressings, prolonged treatment, or extensive body-surface treatment.

• Stop drug and notify doctor if patient develops signs of systemic absorption, skin irritation or ulceration, hypersensitivity, or infection. (If antifungals or antibiotics are being used with corticosteroids and infection does not respond immediately, corticosteroids should be stopped until infection is controlled.)

• Before applying, gently wash skin. To prevent damage to skin, rub medication in gently, leaving a thin coat. When treating hairy sites, part hair and apply directly to lesion.

• Occlusive dressing: apply ointment heavily, then cover with a thin, pliable, nonflammable plastic film; seal to adjacent normal skin with hypoallergenic tape. To minimize adverse effects, use occlusive dressing intermittently. Don't leave in place longer than 16 hours each day. Occlusive dressings should not be used in presence of infection or with weeping or exudative lesions.

• For patient with eczematous dermatitis who may develop irritation with adhesive material, hold dressing in place with gauze, elastic bandages, stockings, or stockinette.

• Notify doctor and remove occlusive dressing if fever develops.

• Change dressing as ordered by doctor. Inspect skin for infection, striae, and atrophy. Discontinue drug and no-

---

Italicized side effects are common or life-threatening.
*Liquid form contains alcohol.   **May contain tartrazine.

tify doctor if these occur.
• Treatment should be continued for a few days after clearing of lesions to prevent recurrence.

triamcinolone acetonide

Aristocort♦, Aristocort A, Kenalog♦
Pregnancy Category: C

MECHANISM OF ACTION
Diffuses across cell membranes and complexes with specific cytoplasmic receptors.

INDICATIONS & DOSAGE
Inflammation of corticosteroid-responsive dermatoses—
Adults and children: clean area; apply cream, ointment, lotion, foam, or aerosol sparingly b.i.d. to q.i.d. Aerosol: shake can well. Direct spray onto affected area from a distance of approximately 6″ (15 cm) and apply for only 3 seconds.
Paste (for oral lesions): press small amount into lesion without rubbing until thin film develops. Apply after meals and at bedtime.

ADVERSE REACTIONS
Skin: burning, itching, irritation, dryness, folliculitis, hypertrichosis, hypopigmentation, acneiform eruptions, perioral dermatitis, allergic contact dermatitis. *With occlusive dressings: maceration of skin, secondary infection, atrophy, striae, miliaria.*

INTERACTIONS
None significant.

NURSING CONSIDERATIONS
• Use cautiously in viral diseases of skin, such as varicella, vaccinia, herpes simplex; fungal infections; bacterial skin infections.
• Avoid application near eyes, mucous membranes, or in ear canal.
• Systemic absorption especially likely with occlusive dressings, prolonged treatment, or extensive body-surface treatment.
• Stop drug and notify doctor if patient develops signs of systemic absorption, skin irritation or ulceration, hypersensitivity, or infection. (If antifungals or antibiotics are being used with corticosteroids and infection does not respond immediately, corticosteroids should be stopped until infection is controlled.)
• Before applying, gently wash skin. To prevent damage to skin, rub medication in gently, leaving a thin coat. When treating hairy sites, part hair and apply directly to lesion.
• Aerosol preparation contains alcohol and may produce irritation or burning in open lesions. When using about the face, cover patient's eyes and warn against inhalation of the spray. To avoid freezing tissues, do not spray longer than 3 seconds or closer than 6″ (15 cm).
• Occlusive dressing: apply cream or ointment heavily, then cover with a thin, pliable, nonflammable plastic film; seal to adjacent normal skin with hypoallergenic tape. To minimize adverse reactions, use occlusive dressing intermittently. Don't leave in place longer than 16 hours each day.
• Change dressing as ordered by doctor. Inspect skin for infection, striae, and atrophy.
• Treatment should be continued for a few days after clearing of lesions to prevent recurrence.

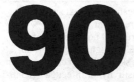

90

Antipruritics and topical anesthetics

benzocaine
carbamide peroxide
dibucaine hydrochloride
dyclonine hydrochloride
ethyl chloride
lidocaine
lidocaine hydrochloride
pramoxine hydrochloride
tetracaine
tetracaine hydrochloride
triamcinolone acetonide

COMBINATION PRODUCTS

BALNETAR♦: water-dispersible emollient tar 2.5% in lanolin fraction, mineral oil, and nonionic emulsifiers.
CARMOL HC: urea 10% and hydrocortisone acetate 1%.
CETACAINE LIQUID: benzocaine 14%, tetracaine HCl 2%, benzalkonium chloride 0.5%, butyl aminobenzoate 2%, and cetyl dimethyl ethyl ammonium bromide in a bland water-soluble base.
DERMOPLAST SPRAY: benzocaine 20% and menthol 0.5%.
ESTAR GEL♦: coal tar 5% and alcohol 29%.
LAVATAR♦: tar distillate 33.3% in water-miscible emulsion base.
MEDICONE DRESSING (CREAM): benzocaine 0.5%, 8-hydroxyquinoline sulfate 0.05%, cod liver oil 12.5%, zinc oxide 12.5%, and menthol 0.18% with petrolatum, lanolin, talcum, and paraffin.
POLYTAR BATH: polytar 25% (juniper, pine, and coal tars, vegetable oil and solubilized crude coal tar) in water-miscible emulsion base.
PRAGMATAR OINTMENT♦: cetyl alcohol-coal tar distillate 4%, precipitated sulfur 3%, and salicylic acid 3% in an oil-in-water emulsion base.
PSORIGEL: coal tar solution 7.5% and alcohol 1%.
SEBUTONE♦: tar (equivalent to 0.5% coal tar) in surface-active soapless cleansers and wetting agents, sulfur 2%, and salicylic acid 2%.
TAR DOAK LOTION♦: tar distillate 5% and nonionic emulsifiers.
ZETAR EMULSION♦: 30% colloidal whole coal tar in polysorbates.
ZETAR SHAMPOO♦: whole coal tar 1% and parachlorometaxylenol 0.5% in foam shampoo base.

---

benzocaine

Americaine♦, Anbesol, Benzocol, Colrex, Dermoplast, Hurricaine♦, Orabase with Benzocaine, Oracin, Ora-Jel, Rhulicream, Solarcaine♦, Spec-T Anesthetic, Trocaine
Pregnancy Category: C

MECHANISM OF ACTION
Blocks conduction of impulses at the sensory nerve endings.

INDICATIONS & DOSAGE
Pain from toothache, cold sore, canker sore, oral irritation, minor sore throat—
Adults and children: apply syrup or jelly to affected area, or suck lozenges.
Local anesthetic for pruritic dermatoses, localized idiopathic pruritus, and sunburn—
Adults and children: apply locally

Italicized side effects are common or life-threatening.
*Liquid form contains alcohol.   **May contain tartrazine.

b.i.d. or t.i.d.
Hemorrhoids or rectal irritation—
Adults and children: apply ointment
b.i.d. or t.i.d.

ADVERSE REACTIONS
Blood: methemoglobinemia (infants).
Local: sensitization, rash.
Other: possible tolerance.

INTERACTIONS
None significant.

NURSING CONSIDERATIONS
• Contraindicated in hypersensitivity
to procaine or other para-aminobenzoic acid (PABA) derivatives (often
used in topical sun-blocking agents).
• Contraindicated in infants under 1
year. Use cautiously in children under
6 years and in severe oral trauma or
sepsis.
• Discontinue if rash or irritation develops.
• Avoid contact with eyes.
• If spray preparation used, hold can
6″ to 12″ (15 to 30 cm) from affected
area and spray liberally. Avoid inhalation.
• If using rectally, cleanse and thoroughly dry rectal area before applying.
• Has a short duration of action.
• Not intended for use in the presence
of infection.
• Obtain history of reactions to local
anesthetics.
• Watch for allergic reactions, such as
reddening or swelling. If condition
persists, drug should be stopped and
doctor notified.
• Show patient how to apply.

carbamide peroxide
Cank-aid, Clear Drops, Gly-Oxide,
Proxigel
Pregnancy Category: C

MECHANISM OF ACTION
Serves as a source of hydrogen peroxide to produce nascent oxygen, which
aids in cleaning and debriding.

INDICATIONS & DOSAGE
*Canker sores, herpetic and other le-
sions, gingivitis, denture irritation,
traumatic or surgical wounds—*
Adults and children over 3 years:
apply, undiluted, to oral mucosa
q.i.d. or p.r.n., leave for several minutes, then expectorate. Don't rinse out
mouth.

ADVERSE REACTIONS
None reported.

INTERACTIONS
None significant.

NURSING CONSIDERATIONS
• Use only as adjunct to regular
professional care.
• Don't dilute. Gently massage affected area with medication. Show
patient how to apply. Tell him not to
drink or rinse his mouth for 5 minutes
after use.
• Warn patient that drug foams in
mouth when mixed with saliva.
• Use after meals and at bedtime for
best results.
• If severe or persistent inflammation
continues, patient should notify doctor or dentist.
• Provides chemomechanical cleansing, debriding action. and has nonselective microbial activity.
• An oxygenating agent.
• Store in cool place.
• Only one person should use dropper
bottle or tube.

dibucaine hydrochloride
D-Caine, Nupercainal Cream♦,
Nupercainal Ointment♦,
Nupercainal Suppositories
Pregnancy Category: C

MECHANISM OF ACTION
Blocks conduction of impulses at the

sensory nerve endings.

INDICATIONS & DOSAGE
Abrasions, sunburn, minor burns, hemorrhoids, and other painful skin conditions—
Adults and children: 0.5% to 1% lotion, cream, or ointment applied locally several times a day.
Suppositories—insert rectally morning, evening, and after every bowel movement.

ADVERSE REACTIONS
Local: sensitization, rash.

INTERACTIONS
None significant.

NURSING CONSIDERATIONS
• Contraindicated in patients allergic to amide-type anesthetics such as lidocaine.
• Avoid contact with eyes.
• Before applying cream or ointment rectally or inserting suppository, cleanse and thoroughly dry rectal area.
• Ointment should be applied rectally using rectal applicator.
• Discontinue use if rash develops.
• Poisoning can occur if these preparations are swallowed. Keep out of reach of children.

---

dyclonine hydrochloride
Dyclone
Pregnancy Category: C

MECHANISM OF ACTION
Blocks conduction of impulses at the sensory nerve endings.

INDICATIONS & DOSAGE
To relieve surface pain and itching caused by minor burns or trauma, surgical wounds, pruritus ani or vulvae, aphthous stomatitis, insect bites, and pruritic dermatoses. Also, to anesthetize mucous membranes before

endoscopic procedures—
Adults and children: 0.5% solution or 1% ointment applied t.i.d. or q.i.d.
Urethral dilation or cystourethroscopy—
Adults: 10 ml of 0.5% solution may be instilled into the urethra.

ADVERSE REACTIONS
Local: *irritation at site of application may occur.*

INTERACTIONS
None significant.

NURSING CONSIDERATIONS
• Avoid prolonged use in patients with chronic conditions.
• May be useful in patients hypersensitive to other local anesthetics because it is a ketone.
• Contraindicated in cystoscopic examinations following an intravenous pyelogram. Iodine-containing contrast material will cause precipitate to form with dyclonine.
• Can be combined with diphenhydramine elixir to provide an effective treatment for stomatitis.
• Avoid accidental contact with drug; it produces temporary numbness.
• Effect lasts 30 to 60 minutes.

---

ethyl chloride
Ethyl Chloride Spray
Pregnancy Category: C

MECHANISM OF ACTION
Produces local anesthesia by producing the sensation of coldness.

INDICATIONS & DOSAGE
For irritation—
Adults and children: hold container about 24" (60 cm) from skin and spray rhythmically to cover area evenly once or twice. Application may be repeated.
As a local anesthetic in minor operative procedures and to relieve pain

---

Italicized side effects are common or life-threatening.
*Liquid form contains alcohol.   **May contain tartrazine.

caused by insect stings and burns and irritation caused by myofascial and visceral pain syndromes—
Adults and children: dosage varies with different procedures. Use smallest dosage needed to produce desired effect. For local anesthesia, hold container about 12″ (30 cm) from area to produce a fine spray.
Infants: hold a cotton ball saturated with ethyl chloride to injection site, and make injection when site dries.

ADVERSE REACTIONS
Skin: sensitization; *frostbite and tissue necrosis may occur with prolonged spraying.*
Other: excessive cooling may increase pain and muscle spasms.

INTERACTIONS
None significant.

NURSING CONSIDERATIONS
• Do not apply to broken skin or mucous membranes.
• Protect skin adjacent to treated area with petrolatum to avoid tissue sloughing.
• Avoid use near eyes.
• Avoid inhalation when spraying.
• Highly flammable; do not use in areas where open flames or sparks are possible.
• Avoid accidental contact with drug; it produces temporary numbness.
• Duration of action is less than 1 minute.

---

lidocaine

lidocaine hydrochloride
Stanacaine, Xylocaine Jelly (2%)♦,
Xylocaine Ointment (5%)♦,
Xylocaine Solution (4%)♦,
Xylocaine Viscous Solution (2%)♦
Pregnancy Category: C

MECHANISM OF ACTION
Blocks conduction of impulses at the sensory nerve endings.

INDICATIONS & DOSAGE
Local anesthesia of skin or mucous membranes, pain from dental extractions, stomatitis—
Adults and children: apply 2% to 5% solution, ointment, or 15 ml of Xylocaine Viscous q 3 to 4 hours to oral or nasal mucosa.
In procedures involving the male or female urethra—
Adults: instill about 15 ml (male) or 3 to 5 ml (female) into urethra.
Pain, burning, or itching caused by burns, sunburn, or skin irritation—
Adults and children: apply liberally.

ADVERSE REACTIONS
Local: sensitization, rash.

INTERACTIONS
None significant.

NURSING CONSIDERATIONS
• Use with caution on severely traumatized mucosa or where sepsis is present or for anesthesia of oropharyngeal mucosa, since gag reflex may be suppressed by lidocaine and aspiration may occur.
• Use cautiously in cardiac disease, hyperthyroidism, or severe oral or nasal trauma or sepsis, as systemic absorption can occur. Don't use in infants.
• The 4% solution can be sprayed or poured onto abrasions to facilitate cleansing and removal of foreign substances (gravel, glass, etc.).
• Discontinue use if rash or irritation develops.
• Apply Xylocaine Ointment carefully to prevent contact with skin in other than the affected area; it produces numbness.
• Duration of action is up to 1 hour. When used for oropharyngeal anesthesia, advise patient to delay eating for 1 hour to avoid aspiration.
• Chronic, prolonged use for oro-

pharynx anesthesia can lead to systemic absorption and toxicity.
• Because of risk of systemic absorption, should be applied to lesions with an oral swab.
• Instruct patient how to use. Xylocaine Viscous should be swished around in mouth. Elderly or debilitated patients shouldn't swallow it.
• Obtain history of reactions to local anesthetics.
• Taste can be improved by adding a drop of oil of peppermint.

pramoxine hydrochloride
Proctofoam, Tronolane, Tronothane♦
Pregnancy Category: C

MECHANISM OF ACTION
Blocks conduction of impulses at the sensory nerve endings.

INDICATIONS & DOSAGE
Pain and itching caused by dermatoses, minor burns, surgical wounds, and insect bites—
Adults and children: apply every 3 to 4 hours.
Hemorrhoids—
Adults: one applicatorful of aerosol foam b.i.d. to t.i.d. and after bowel movements.

ADVERSE REACTIONS
Local: stinging or burning, sensitization.

INTERACTIONS
None significant.

NURSING CONSIDERATIONS
• Can be safely used in those allergic to other local anesthetics.
• May be applied with gauze or sprayed directly on skin. Avoid contact with eyes.
• Cleanse and thoroughly dry rectal area before applying ointment or cream, or inserting suppository.

• Not for prolonged use. Consult doctor after 4 consecutive weeks of use.

tetracaine

tetracaine hydrochloride
Pontocaine♦
Pregnancy Category: C

MECHANISM OF ACTION
Blocks conduction of impulses at the sensory nerve endings.

INDICATIONS & DOSAGE
Pain in hemorrhoids, minor burns, ulcers, sunburn, and poison ivy—
Adults and children: apply 5% ointment or 1% cream—no more than 1 oz for adults or ¼ oz for children daily.

ADVERSE REACTIONS
Local: sensitization, rash.

INTERACTIONS
None significant.

NURSING CONSIDERATIONS
• Contraindicated in hypersensitivity to procaine or other para-aminobenzoic acid (PABA) derivatives.
• Before applying rectally, cleanse and thoroughly dry rectal area.
• Discontinue use if rash develops.

triamcinolone acetonide
Kenalog in Orabase♦
Pregnancy Category: C

MECHANISM OF ACTION
Reduces inflammation and helps heal oral ulcers and lesions by interfering with the protein synthesis of various enzymes.

INDICATIONS & DOSAGE
Stomatitis; erosive lichen planus; traumatic oral lesions, including sore denture spots—

Italicized side effects are common or life-threatening.
*Liquid form contains alcohol.   **May contain tartrazine.

Adults and children: press ¼″ of
0.1% emollient dental paste onto affected area until thin film develops.
Repeat b.i.d. or t.i.d. Don't rub in or
protection of film will be lost.

ADVERSE REACTIONS
Systemic: with prolonged use, adrenal insufficiency, altered glucose metabolism, peptic ulcer activation.

INTERACTIONS
None significant.

NURSING CONSIDERATIONS
• Contraindicated in oral herpetic or
viral lesions. Use cautiously in diabetes mellitus, peptic ulcer, or tuberculosis, as systemic absorption can
occur.
• Apply after meals and at bedtime
for best results.

91

Astringents

acetic acid lotion
aluminum acetate
aluminum sulfate
hamamelis water (witch hazel)

COMBINATION PRODUCTS
ASTRINGENTS WITH ANESTHETICS, for example, Nupercainal Suppositories.
ASTRINGENTS WITH ANTIPRURITIC/ ANTIHISTAMINE, for example, Caladryl, Ziradryl.
ASTRINGENTS WITH ANTIPRURITIC/ ANTIHISTAMINE AND ANESTHETIC, for example, Rhulicream, Rhulihist, Rhulispray.
ASTRINGENTS WITH ANTISEPTICS, for example, Lavoris, Tanac, Tucks Pads.
ASTRINGENTS WITH ANTISEPTICS AND ANESTHETICS, for example, Pazo Hemorrhoid Suppositories and Ointment, Rectal Medicone Suppositories and Unguent, Tanicaine Suppositories and Ointment, Wyanoid Ointment.
ASTRINGENTS WITH DEODORANTS, for example, most antiperspirant/deodorants commonly available.

acetic acid lotion
(0.1% glacial acetic acid in alcohol)
Pregnancy Category: NR

MECHANISM OF ACTION
Precipitates protein, causing tissue to contract.

INDICATIONS & DOSAGE
Superficial fungal or bacterial infection to toughen skin and prevent bedsores—
Adults and children: apply and work into area, p.r.n.

ADVERSE REACTIONS
Skin: burning and irritation of denuded skin and mucous membranes.

INTERACTIONS
Heavy metals: causes precipitation of the metal acetate.

NURSING CONSIDERATIONS
• Contraindicated under occlusive dressings.
• Never confuse acetic acid solutions with *glacial* acetic acid solutions. Glacial form is a concentrate.
• Keep away from eyes and mucous membranes.
• Always apply to freshly cleansed area, free of other medications.
• Especially useful for treating superficial gram-negative infections.

aluminum acetate
(modified Burow's solution or Burow's solution)
Acid Mantle Creme♦, Buro-sol

aluminum sulfate
Bluboro Powder, Domeboro Powder♦ and Tablets♦
Pregnancy Category: C

MECHANISM OF ACTION
Precipitates protein, causing tissue to contract.

INDICATIONS & DOSAGE
Mild skin irritation from exposure to soaps, detergents, chemicals, diaper

---

Italicized side effects are common or life-threatening.
*Liquid form contains alcohol.   **May contain tartrazine.

rash, acne, scaly skin, eczema—
Adults and children: apply p.r.n.
Skin inflammation, insect bites, poison ivy or other contact dermatoses, swelling, athlete's foot—
Adults and children: mix powder or tablet with 1 pint of lukewarm tap water and apply for 15 to 30 minutes every 4 to 8 hours; bandage loosely.

ADVERSE REACTIONS
Skin: irritation; extension of inflammation possible.

INTERACTIONS
None significant.

NURSING CONSIDERATIONS
• Contraindicated under occlusive dressings; use open wet dressings only.
• When solution is prepared, immediately decant clear portion. Discard precipitate. Use only clear solution, *not* precipitate, for soaks. Never strain or filter solutions. Decanted portion may be stored at room temperature for up to 7 days.
• In general, no more than a third of the body should be treated at any one time, since excessive wet dressings may cause chilling and hypothermia.
• Keep away from eyes and mucous membranes.
• Discontinue if irritation develops.
• Prolonged or excessive use may produce necrosis.

hamamelis water (witch hazel)
Mediconet (wipes), Tucks (Cream, Ointment, Pads)
Pregnancy Category: NR

MECHANISM OF ACTION
Precipitates protein, causing tissue to contract.

INDICATIONS & DOSAGE
Anal discomfort, itching, burning, mi-

nor external hemorrhoidal or outer vaginal discomfort, diaper rash—
Adults and children: apply t.i.d. or q.i.d.

ADVERSE REACTIONS
Skin: hypersensitivity.

INTERACTIONS
None significant.

NURSING CONSIDERATIONS
• Discontinue if irritation or itching does not improve.
• Use pads or wipes after or instead of toilet tissue to help prevent pruritus ani or vulvae.
• Cream can be used by breast-feeding mother for nipple care, but wash area clean before breast-feeding baby.

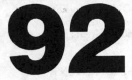

Antiseptics and disinfectants

alcohol, ethyl
alcohol, isopropyl
benzalkonium chloride
boric acid
chlorhexidine gluconate
formaldehyde
hexachlorophene
hydrogen peroxide
iodine
merbromin
potassium permanganate
povidone-iodine
silver protein, mild
sodium hypochlorite
thimerosal

COMBINATION PRODUCTS
ZEASORB POWDER: parachlorometaxylenol 0.5%, aluminum dihydroxy allantoinate 0.2%, and microporous cellulose 45%.

---

alcohol, ethyl
Alcohol, Ethanol
Pregnancy Category: C

MECHANISM OF ACTION
Destroys or inhibits the growth of microorganisms.

INDICATIONS & DOSAGE
To disinfect skin, instruments, and ampuls—
disinfect as needed.

ADVERSE REACTIONS
Skin: dryness, irritation.

INTERACTIONS
None significant.

NURSING CONSIDERATIONS
• Effective as fat-solvent germicidal; ineffective against spore-forming organisms, tubercle bacilli, and viruses.
• Alcohol used as 70% solution known commonly as "rubbing alcohol."
• Should be left on the skin for at least 2 minutes.
• Don't use in an open wound.

---

alcohol, isopropyl
isopropyl alcohol 99%, isopropyl aqueous alcohol 75%, isopropyl rubbing alcohol 70%
Pregnancy Category: C

MECHANISM OF ACTION
Destroys or inhibits the growth of microorganisms.

INDICATIONS & DOSAGE
To disinfect skin, instruments, and ampuls—
disinfect as needed.

ADVERSE REACTIONS
Skin: dryness, irritation.

INTERACTIONS
None significant.

NURSING CONSIDERATIONS
• Isopropyl alcohol is slightly more effective than ethyl alcohol as an antibacterial agent, but it also tends to cause more dryness.
• Should be left on the skin for at least 2 minutes.
• 75% solution for disinfection and

Italicized side effects are common or life-threatening.
*Liquid form contains alcohol.   **May contain tartrazine.

storage of thermometers.
• Not effective against spore-forming organisms, tubercle bacilli, or viruses.
• Combined with formaldehyde, makes effective germicide.
• Don't use in an open wound.

benzalkonium chloride
Benasept, Benzachlor-50♦♦, Benz-All, Ionax Scrub♦♦, Mercurochrome II, Sabol Shampoo♦♦, Zalkon, Zalkonium Chloride, Zephiran♦
Pregnancy Category: C

MECHANISM OF ACTION
Destroys or inhibits the growth of microorganisms.

INDICATIONS & DOSAGE
Preoperative disinfection of unbroken skin—
apply 1:750 to 1:1,000 tincture or spray.
Disinfection of mucous membranes and denuded skin—
apply 1:10,000 to 1:5,000 aqueous solution.
Irrigation of vagina—
instill 1:5,000 to 1:2,000 aqueous solution.
Irrigation of bladder or urethra—
instill 1:20,000 to 1:5,000 aqueous solution.
Irrigation of deep infected wounds—
instill 1:20,000 to 1:3,000 aqueous solution.
Preservation of metallic instruments, ampuls, thermometers, and rubber articles—
wipe with or soak objects in 1:5,000 to 1:750 solution.
Disinfection of operating room equipment—
wipe with 1:5,000 solution.

ADVERSE REACTIONS
Skin: hypersensitivity, allergic contact dermatitis.

INTERACTIONS
Soaps: inactivate benzalkonium chloride. Remove soap traces with alcohol.

NURSING CONSIDERATIONS
• Germicidal for some nonspore-forming organisms and fungi. No effect on tubercle bacilli. Limited viricidal use.
• Used as preservative in some ophthalmic solutions.
• Before applying to skin, remove all traces of soap with water, and apply 70% alcohol.
• Don't store cotton, wool gauze, or sponges in solution. They absorb benzalkonium chloride and reduce the strength of the solution.
• Don't use with occlusive dressings or vaginal packs.
• Store in bottles with screw caps.
• Incompatible with iodine, silver nitrate, fluorescein, nitrates, peroxide, lanolin, potassium permanganate, aluminum, caramel, kaolin, pine oil, zinc sulfate, zinc oxide, and yellow oxide of mercury.
• To prevent rust of metallic instruments stored in benzalkonium chloride, add sodium nitrite to final solution. Change solution weekly.
• Available also as 17% concentrate (Zephiran). Even after dilution, this form of Zephiran should be used only on inanimate objects.
• Mercurochrome II, a brand of benzalkonium chloride, *does not* contain merbromin. Don't confuse with Mercurochrome.

boric acid
Bluboro, boric acid solution 5%, Borofax, Ting
Pregnancy Category: C

MECHANISM OF ACTION
Destroys or inhibits the growth of microorganisms.

INDICATIONS & DOSAGE
Skin conditions (athlete's foot) as a compress, powder, or ointment (2% to 5%)—
Adults and children (not infants): apply as directed.

ADVERSE REACTIONS
Signs of systemic absorption:
CNS: delirium, convulsions, restlessness, headache.
CV: *circulatory collapse,* tachycardia.
GI: irritation, nausea, vomiting, diarrhea.
GU: renal damage.
Other: hypothermia.

INTERACTIONS
None significant.

NURSING CONSIDERATIONS
• Don't use in infants.
• Mild antiseptic and astringent.
• May be significantly absorbed through abraded skin or granulating wounds.
• Avoid long-term use.
• Ingestion of 5 g (infants) or 20 g (adults) may be fatal.

chlorhexidine gluconate
Exidine, Hibiclens Liquid, Hibistat, Peridex
Pregnancy Category: C

MECHANISM OF ACTION
Destroys or inhibits the growth of microorganisms.

INDICATIONS & DOSAGE
Surgical hand scrub, hand wash, hand rinse, skin wound cleanser—
use p.r.n.
Gingivitis—
use 0.12% strength (Peridex oral rinse), p.r.n.

ADVERSE REACTIONS
EENT: irritating to eyes. Causes deafness if instilled into middle ear through perforated eardrum.

INTERACTIONS
None significant.

NURSING CONSIDERATIONS
• Bactericidal; broad spectrum of activity.
• Can be used many times a day without causing excessive irritation or dryness.
• Low potential for producing skin reactions.
• Keep out of eyes and ears.
• Action is residual. Do not cleanse skin with alcohol after application.
• Can be left on skin as an antibacterial lotion.
• Antibacterial effect is not lessened by blood, pus, or soap.
• Action begins 10 seconds after application.

formaldehyde
Formalin (37% solution of formaldehyde)
Pregnancy Category: NR

MECHANISM OF ACTION
Destroys or inhibits the growth of microorganisms.

INDICATIONS & DOSAGE
Cold sterilization of equipment—
disinfect as needed.
Tissue preservative—
cover tissue.

ADVERSE REACTIONS
EENT: fumes cause eye, nose, and throat irritation.
Skin: irritation, allergic contact dermatitis.
Other: pungent odor.

INTERACTIONS
None significant.

Italicized side effects are common or life-threatening.
*Liquid form contains alcohol.   **May contain tartrazine.

NURSING CONSIDERATIONS

• 0.5% solution germicidal against all forms of microorganisms, including spores, in 6 to 12 hours; 10% solution used to disinfect inanimate objects.
• Use the 0.12% strength only as an oral rinse.
• Not affected by organic matter.
• Used with alcohol and sodium nitrite to disinfect instruments and articles that can't tolerate heat (cold sterilization).
• Avoid skin or mucous membrane contact with solutions greater than 0.5%.
• Always dilute 37% solution.

hexachlorophene

Germa-Medica "MG," pHisoHex♦, pHisoScrub, Sept-Soft, WescoHEX♦
Pregnancy Category: C

MECHANISM OF ACTION

Destroys or inhibits the growth of microorganisms.

INDICATIONS & DOSAGE

Surgical scrub, bacteriostatic skin cleanser—
use as directed in 0.25% to 3% concentrations.

ADVERSE REACTIONS

Note: systemic absorption can cause neurotoxic effects, including irritability, generalized clonic muscular contractions, decerebrate rigidity, convulsions, optic atrophy. (Systemic absorption is especially significant when used on mucous membranes and broken skin and burns.)
Skin: dermatitis, mild scaling, dryness (especially when combined with excessive scrubbing).

INTERACTIONS

None significant.

NURSING CONSIDERATIONS

• Don't use in infants (especially premature infants). Use cautiously in burn patients. These patients tend to absorb significant amounts of hexachlorophene through the skin and may develop neurotoxic effects.
• Bacteriostatic agent. Spectrum of activity limited to gram-positive organisms, especially staphylococcus.
• Must be used preoperatively for at least 3 days for maximum effectiveness.
• After cleaning area, rinse thoroughly (especially the scrotum and perineum). Do not apply alcohol or organic solvents to cleansed area.

hydrogen peroxide

3% to 6% solution
Pregnancy Category: NR

MECHANISM OF ACTION

Destroys or inhibits the growth of microorganisms.

INDICATIONS & DOSAGE

Cleansing wound—
use 1.5% to 3% solution.
Mouth wash for necrotizing ulcerative gingivitis—
gargle with 3% solution.
Cleansing douche—
use 2% solution.

ADVERSE REACTIONS

EENT: excessive use as mouthwash may cause "hairy tongue."

INTERACTIONS

None significant.

NURSING CONSIDERATIONS

• Germicidal, particularly against anaerobic organisms.
• Don't inject into closed body cavities or abscesses; generated gas can't escape.
• Useful to remove mucus from inner cannula of tracheostomy tube.

• Store tightly capped in cool, dry place. Protect from light and heat.
• Do not shake bottle. This causes decomposition.
• 6% solution can be used to bleach hair.

iodine

Sepp Antiseptic Applicators (2% mild iodine tincture), solution (2% iodine and 2.4% sodium and iodide in water)♦, strong iodine tincture (7% iodine and 5% potassium iodide in diluted alcohol), tincture (2% iodine and 2.4% sodium iodide in diluted alcohol)
Pregnancy Category: D

MECHANISM OF ACTION
Destroys or inhibits the growth of microorganisms.

INDICATIONS & DOSAGE
Preoperative disinfection of skin (small wounds and abraded areas)—
apply p.r.n.

ADVERSE REACTIONS
Skin: irritation, redness, swelling (sign of hypersensitivity), allergic contact dermatitis.

INTERACTIONS
None significant.

NURSING CONSIDERATIONS
• Microbicidal agent effective against bacteria, fungi, viruses, protozoa, and yeasts.
• If skin reaction develops, remove iodine residue from skin and stop use.
• To prevent skin irritation, do not cover areas treated with iodine.
• Aqueous solution less irritating.
• Sodium thiosulfate renders iodine colorless and is used to remove stains. It is also antidote of choice for accidental ingestion.

merbromin

Mercurochrome (2% aqueous solution)
Pregnancy Category: NR

MECHANISM OF ACTION
Destroys or inhibits the growth of microorganisms.

INDICATIONS & DOSAGE
General antiseptic and first-aid prophylactic—
Adults and children: apply p.r.n. as 1% to 2% solution or tincture.

ADVERSE REACTIONS
Skin: sensitization, allergic contact dermatitis.

INTERACTIONS
None significant.

NURSING CONSIDERATIONS
• Bacteriostatic.
• Don't use on large areas of abraded skin, because mercury may be absorbed and produce systemic toxicity.
• Least effective mercurial antiseptic. Its activity is decreased in presence of organic matter.
• Cleanse injury with soap and water before applying. Let dry.
• Stains may be removed with 2% permanganate solution, followed by 5% oxalic acid solution.
• Never heat solution.
• To prepare 1% solution, dilute with equal parts of water.
• Note that Mercurochrome II does *not* contain merbromin, but contains benzalkonium chloride.

potassium permanganate
Pregnancy Category: C

MECHANISM OF ACTION
Destroys or inhibits the growth of microorganisms.

Italicized side effects are common or life-threatening.
*Liquid form contains alcohol.   **May contain tartrazine.

INDICATIONS & DOSAGE
Topical antiseptic—
apply 1:10,000 to 1:500 solution.
Vaginal douche—
instill 1:5,000 to 1:1,000 solution as directed.

ADVERSE REACTIONS
Skin: solutions greater than 1:5,000 are irritating to skin.

INTERACTIONS
Iodine: precipitates iodine salt. Do not use together.

NURSING CONSIDERATIONS
• Antiseptic astringent with fungicidal properties.
• Germicidal effects reduced by organic matter.
• Stains caused by potassium permanganate removed with dilute acids (lemon juice, oxalic acid, or dilute hydrochloric acid).
• Undissolved crystals may cause chemical burn.
• Never mix with charcoal or give charcoal as antidote. May explode.

---

povidone-iodine
ACU-dyne♦, Aerodine, Betadine♦, Bridine♦♦, Efodine, Final Step, Frepp, Frepp/Sepp, Isodine, Mallisol, Polydine, Proviodine♦♦, Sepp
Pregnancy Category: D

MECHANISM OF ACTION
Destroys or inhibits the growth of microorganisms.

INDICATIONS & DOSAGE
Many uses, including preoperative skin preparation and scrub, germicide for surface wounds, postoperative application to incisions, prophylactic application to urinary meatus of catheterized patients, miscellaneous disinfection—
Adults: apply p.r.n.

ADVERSE REACTIONS
Skin: local hypersensitivity reactions, allergic contact dermatitis.

INTERACTIONS
None significant.

NURSING CONSIDERATIONS
• Should not be used as a vaginal antiseptic during pregnancy.
• Germicidal activity of iodine with minimal irritation to skin and mucous membranes.
• Thought to be superior to soap as a disinfectant; less effective than aqueous or alcoholic solutions of iodine.
• Treated areas may be bandaged or taped.
• Germicidal activity reduced if area cleansed with alcohol or other organic solvents after application of povidone-iodine.
• Prolonged, excessive use may lead to systemic absorption and toxicity.
• Betadine vaginal gel should not be used in patients hypersensitive to iodine.
• Don't combine with alcohol or hydrogen peroxide.

---

silver protein, mild
Argyrol S.S., Silvol, Solargentum
Pregnancy Category: C

MECHANISM OF ACTION
Destroys or inhibits the growth of microorganisms.

INDICATIONS & DOSAGE
Topical application for inflammation of eye, nose, throat—
Adults and children: apply p.r.n. as a 5% to 25% solution.

ADVERSE REACTIONS
Skin: argyria in long-term use.

INTERACTIONS
None significant.

Unmarked trade names available in the United States only.
♦Also available in Canada.   ♦♦Available in Canada only.

NURSING CONSIDERATIONS
• Store in amber glass bottles; protect from light.
• Should not be used chronically.

sodium hypochlorite
0.5% aqueous solution for wounds, Modified Dakin's solution, 5% solution (instruments, swimming pools)
Pregnancy Category: C

MECHANISM OF ACTION
Destroys or inhibits the growth of microorganisms.

INDICATIONS & DOSAGE
Athlete's foot, wound irrigation, disinfection of walls and floors—
apply as directed.

ADVERSE REACTIONS
Skin: irritation, bleeding.

INTERACTIONS
None significant.

NURSING CONSIDERATIONS
• Germicidal and weakly fungicidal.
• Interferes locally with thrombin formation, delaying blood clotting. Dissolves necrotic tissue.
• Unstable in solution. Make fresh solution and use immediately.
• Avoid contact with hair due to its bleaching properties.

thimerosal
Aeroaid Thimerosal, Merthiolate♦
Pregnancy Category: C

MECHANISM OF ACTION
Destroys or inhibits the growth of microorganisms.

INDICATIONS & DOSAGE
Preoperative disinfection of skin; antiseptic for open wounds—
apply or instill to affected area daily, b.i.d., or t.i.d. as a 0.1% solution or tincture.

ADVERSE REACTIONS
Skin: erythematous, vesicular, papular eruptions (indicate hypersensitivity); irritation with tincture; allergic contact dermatitis.

INTERACTIONS
None significant.

NURSING CONSIDERATIONS
• Contraindicated in hypersensitivity to mercury-containing compounds.
• Should not be instilled into external ears. May cause mercury toxicity.
• Do not use when aluminum salts may come in contact with skin.
• Incompatible with permanganate, strong acids, and heavy metals.
• Cleanse wound thoroughly before applying tincture. Allow tincture to dry completely before applying dressing.

Italicized side effects are common or life-threatening.
*Liquid form contains alcohol.   **May contain tartrazine.

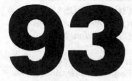

Emollients, demulcents, and protectants

aluminum paste
calamine
collodion, flexible
collodion, USP
compound benzoin tincture
dexpanthenol
glycerin
liquid petrolatum
methyl salicylate
oatmeal
para-aminobenzoic acid
petrolatum
starch
talc (magnesium silicate)
vitamins A and D ointment
zinc gelatin

COMBINATION PRODUCTS
CALADRYL LOTION:diphenhydramine
hydrochloride 1%, calamine, camphor, and alcohol 2%.

aluminum paste
(10% aluminum in zinc oxide
ointment with liquid petrolatum)
Pregnancy Category: C

MECHANISM OF ACTION
Softens dry skin by preventing evaporation of perspiration. Also promotes
healing by reducing irritation and friction.

INDICATIONS & DOSAGE
*Emollient and protectant: colostomy
area or other surgical sites—*
apply p.r.n.

ADVERSE REACTIONS
None.

INTERACTIONS
Topical enzymes: aluminum may inactivate preparations used to debride
wounds. Don't use together.

NURSING CONSIDERATIONS
• Zinc oxide paste can be used as an
alternative.
• Observe for inflammation or infection since protectants are occlusive
layers that retain moisture, exclude
air, and trap cutaneous bacteria.
• Don't use in weeping wounds.
• Skin should be cleaned daily or
more often as needed.
• Emollients and protectants may be
used alone, as vehicles for medications, or with other topical medications. Check with doctor.
• Apply evenly with tongue blade or
finger, and remove with cloth soaked
in mineral or vegetable oil.

calamine
liniment (15% calamine), lotion (8%
calamine), ointment (17%
calamine), Rhulispray (1%
calamine)
Pregnancy Category: C

MECHANISM OF ACTION
Promotes healing by reducing irritation and friction.

INDICATIONS & DOSAGE
*Topical astringent and protectant:
itching, poison ivy and poison oak,
nonpoisonous insect bites, mild sunburn, minor skin irritations—*
apply p.r.n.

Unmarked trade names available in the United States only.
♦Also available in Canada.   ♦♦Available in Canada only.

ADVERSE REACTIONS
Skin: transient, light stinging; irritation; dry skin.

INTERACTIONS
None significant.

NURSING CONSIDERATIONS
• Contraindicated in hypersensitivity to any of the components.
• Watch for sensitivity reactions to calamine. Preparations containing antihistamines can cause sensitivity.
• Always shake well before use.
• Don't use cotton to apply; it will absorb the solute. Use gauze sponge.
• Do not apply to blistered, raw, or oozing areas of the skin.
• Toxic if taken internally.
• Observe for inflammation or infection since protectants are occlusive layers that retain moisture, exclude air, and trap skin bacteria.
• Skin should be cleaned daily or more often as needed.
• Emollients, demulcents, protectants may be used alone, as vehicles for medications, or with other topical medications. Check with doctor.
• May irritate and dry skin.
• Keep away from eyes and mucous membranes.
• Keep container tightly closed so solvent won't evaporate.

---

collodion, flexible
(5% pyroxylin in 1 part alcohol, 3 parts ether plus 20% camphor, 30% castor oil)

collodion, USP
(5% pyroxylin in 1 part alcohol, 3 parts ether)
Pregnancy Category: C

MECHANISM OF ACTION
Promotes healing by reducing irritation and friction.

INDICATIONS & DOSAGE
Protectant; vehicle for other medicinal agents; and sealant for small wounds—
apply to dry skin, p.r.n., or use flexible collodion when a flexible noncontracting film is desired.

ADVERSE REACTIONS
None.

INTERACTIONS
None significant.

NURSING CONSIDERATIONS
• Observe for inflammation or infection since protectants are occlusive layers that retain moisture, exclude air, and trap cutaneous bacteria.
• Skin should be cleaned daily or more often as needed.
• Protectants may be used alone, as vehicles for medications, or with other topical medications. Check with doctor.
• Camphor in flexible collodion is weakly antiseptic and antipruritic; may irritate and dry skin.
• Highly flammable; never use near flame or cigarettes.
• Keep container tightly closed so solvent won't evaporate.
• Toxic if taken internally.
• Avoid excessive inhalation of vapors.

---

compound benzoin tincture
(10% benzoin in alcohol mixed with glycerin and water)
Benzoin Spray♦
Pregnancy Category: C

MECHANISM OF ACTION
Promotes healing by reducing irritation and friction. Also cools and soothes.

INDICATIONS & DOSAGE
Demulcent and protectant: cutaneous ulcers, bedsores, cracked nipples, fis-

---

sures of lips and anus—
apply locally once daily or b.i.d.

ADVERSE REACTIONS
Skin: contact dermatitis

INTERACTIONS
None significant.

NURSING CONSIDERATIONS
• Do not apply to acutely inflamed areas.
• Observe for inflammation or infection since protectants are occlusive layers that retain moisture, exclude air, and trap cutaneous bacteria.
• Skin should be cleaned daily or more often as needed.
• Protectants may be used alone, as vehicles for medications, or with other topical medications.
• For demulcent and expectorant action in laryngitis or croup, use in boiling water and have patient inhale vapors.
• Spray is not intended for use as inhalant.
• Can be mixed with magnesium-aluminum hydroxide and applied on bedsores.

dexpanthenol
Panthoderm♦ (dexpanthenol 2% in a water-miscible cream base)
Pregnancy Category: C

MECHANISM OF ACTION
Softens dry skin by preventing evaporation of perspiration.

INDICATIONS & DOSAGE
Epithelial-bed stimulator in emollient base: itching, wounds, insect bites, poison ivy, poison oak, diaper rash, chafing, mild eczema, decubitus ulcers, dry lesions—
apply topically, p.r.n.

ADVERSE REACTIONS
None.

INTERACTIONS
None significant.

NURSING CONSIDERATIONS
• Contraindicated in wounds of hemophilia patients.
• Before each new application *always* thoroughly cleanse affected area, removing all traces of previously applied medication. Observe for inflammation or infection.
• Dry lesions respond better than oozing lesions.

glycerin
Corn Huskers Lotion (tragacanth 1 g, glycerin 30 ml, propylene glycol 10 ml)
Pregnancy Category: C

MECHANISM OF ACTION
Softens dry skin by preventing evaporation of perspiration.

INDICATIONS & DOSAGE
Emollient and lubricant: rectal tubes and catheters; dry skin, hands—
apply p.r.n.

ADVERSE REACTIONS
None.

INTERACTIONS
None significant.

NURSING CONSIDERATIONS
• Applied undiluted to inflamed, dehydrated skin. Paradoxically, excessive use may dry the skin.
• Diluted with rose water, glycerin is useful for irritated or dry lips.

liquid petrolatum
Light Liquid Petrolatum, NF; Liquid Petrolatum, USP; Mineral Oil
Pregnancy Category: C

MECHANISM OF ACTION
Softens dry skin by preventing evapo-

---

ration of perspiration. Also promotes healing by reducing irritation and friction.

INDICATIONS & DOSAGE
Protectant and emollient— apply locally, full strength, or diluted.

ADVERSE REACTIONS
None.

INTERACTIONS
None significant.

NURSING CONSIDERATIONS
• Occasionally used with other drugs.
• Available in two forms: light mineral oil and heavy mineral oil.
• Heavy mineral oil can be used internally as a laxative. Never use light mineral oil as a laxative. Mineral oil used as nose drops can cause lipid pneumonia.
• Observe for inflammation or infection since protectants are occlusive layers that retain moisture, exclude air, and trap skin bacteria.
• Skin should be cleaned daily or more often as needed.
• Difficult to wash off.
• Emollients and protectants may be used alone, as vehicles for medications, or with other topical medications.

---

methyl salicylate
Banalg, Baumodyne Gel and Ointment, Betula Oil, Gaultheria Oil, Sweet Birch Oil, Wintergreen Oil
Pregnancy Category: NR

MECHANISM OF ACTION
A counterirritant that increases circulation to the area of application.

INDICATIONS & DOSAGE
Counterirritant: minor pains of osteoarthritis, rheumatism, sprains, muscle and tendon soreness and tightness, lumbago, sciatica—

Adults: apply with gentle massage several times daily.
Not recommended for children.

ADVERSE REACTIONS
Skin: rash, irritation, burning, blistering.

INTERACTIONS
None significant.

NURSING CONSIDERATIONS
• Use cautiously in aspirin-allergic patients.
• Never apply directly, undiluted to skin.
• Warning: as little as 4 ml ingested by children can cause fatal toxicity; in adults as little as 30 ml. Since GI absorption may be delayed, treat such ingestion with emetic lavage, then a saline cathartic. Continue lavage until no odor of methyl salicylate can be detected in the washings.
• Absorbed through skin; prolonged increased application can cause toxicity. Toxic effects include hyperpnea leading to respiratory alkalosis, nausea, vomiting, tinnitus, hyperpyrexia, and convulsions.
• Discontinue if rash or redness occurs. Consult doctor if pain or redness persists more than 10 days.
• Avoid getting near eyes, open wounds, or mucous membranes.
• Do not apply to broken or irritated skin.
• Do not wrap or bandage treated area.
• Store in tightly closed container.

---

oatmeal
Aveeno Colloidal♦, Aveeno Oilated Bath (with liquid petrolatum and hypoallergenic lanolin)♦
Pregnancy Category: NR

MECHANISM OF ACTION
Softens dry skin by preventing evaporation of perspiration. Also soothes

---

Italicized side effects are common or life-threatening.
*Liquid form contains alcohol.   **May contain tartrazine.

and cools.

INDICATIONS & DOSAGE
Emollient and demulcent: local irritation—
use as a lotion; 1 level tablespoon to a cup of warm water.
Skin irritation, pruritus, common dermatoses, sunburn, dry skin—
Adults: 1 packet in tub of warm water.
Children: 1 to 2 rounded tablespoons in 3″ to 4″ (8 to 10 cm) of bath water.
Infants: 2 or 3 level teaspoons, depending on size of bath.

ADVERSE REACTIONS
None.

INTERACTIONS
None significant.

NURSING CONSIDERATIONS
• Not to be ingested.
• Instruct patient to exercise caution to avoid slipping in tub.
• Avoid getting in eyes.
• Disperse well by adding to water under running faucet, if possible.

---

para-aminobenzoic acid
PABA♦, Pabagel♦, Pabanol♦, Pre-Sun♦, PreSun Gel♦, RV Paba Lipstick♦
Pregnancy Category: C

MECHANISM OF ACTION
Promotes healing by reducing irritation and friction.

INDICATIONS & DOSAGE
Topical protectant: sunburn protection, sun-sensitive skin, slow tanning—
Adults: apply evenly to skin indoors before exposure to sun. Don't apply to wet skin. Follow directions on various products for number and time of application, which vary from 2 to 6 hours; reapply after swimming.

Not recommended for infants.

ADVERSE REACTIONS
Local: allergic contact dermatitis, irritation, sensitization.
Skin: photocontact dermatitis.

INTERACTIONS
None significant.

NURSING CONSIDERATIONS
• Contraindicated in hypersensitivity to any of the components and for persons with damaged or diseased skin.
• Discontinue if skin rash occurs.
• Encourage slow tanning and short exposure to sun.
• Always apply to thoroughly dried skin. Will not protect if applied to wet skin.
• Avoid contact with eyes and lids.
• Avoid contact with open flame.
• May stain clothing and other fabrics, such as towels and washcloths.
• Follow product directions for correct application.
• Observe for inflammation and infection since protectants produce an occlusive layer that retains perspiration, excludes air, and traps cutaneous bacteria, producing sites for anaerobic infections.

---

petrolatum
Vaseline♦
Pregnancy Category: C

MECHANISM OF ACTION
Promotes healing by reducing irritation and friction. Also softens dry skin by preventing evaporation of perspiration.

INDICATIONS & DOSAGE
Topical protectant and emollient—
use alone or with other drugs, as directed.

ADVERSE REACTIONS
Skin: folliculitis.

Unmarked trade names available in the United States only.
♦Also available in Canada.   ♦♦Available in Canada only.

INTERACTIONS
None significant.

NURSING CONSIDERATIONS
• Stable, does not become rancid.
• Observe for inflammation or infection since protectants are occlusive layers that retain moisture, exclude air, and trap skin bacteria.
• Skin should be cleaned daily or more often as needed.
• Emollients and protectants may be used alone, as vehicles for medications, or with other topical medications.

starch
Pregnancy Category: NR

MECHANISM OF ACTION
Absorbs moisture to relieve dry skin.

INDICATIONS & DOSAGE
Demulcent: minor skin irritations, pruritus associated with common dermatoses—
mix 2 cups of starch with 4 cups of water, add to tub of water, and soak affected area for 30 minutes.

ADVERSE REACTIONS
None.

INTERACTIONS
None significant.

NURSING CONSIDERATIONS
• Instruct patient to exercise caution to avoid slipping in tub.
• Use of cornstarch in intertriginous areas may promote or accelerate a yeast infection since yeast can feed on the sugar.

talc (magnesium silicate)
Pregnancy Category: NR

MECHANISM OF ACTION
Promotes healing by reducing irritation and friction.

INDICATIONS & DOSAGE
Topical lubricant, protectant, drying agent, absorbent dusting powder: irritation, such as intertrigo prickly heat—
sprinkle on affected areas p.r.n. for soothing and lubrication.

ADVERSE REACTIONS
None.

INTERACTIONS
None significant.

NURSING CONSIDERATIONS
• Don't use on surgical gloves; causes granulation and adhesions in open wounds.
• Avoid dust entering eyes or inhalation of talc dust.
• Should not be used on open, weeping surfaces; it cakes and crusts.

vitamins A and D ointment
A&D, Balmex, Caldesene Medicated, Clocream, Comfortine, Desitin, Primaderm
Pregnancy Category: A

MECHANISM OF ACTION
Soothes irritation and cools inflammation. Also softens dry skin by preventing evaporation of perspiration.

INDICATIONS & DOSAGE
Emollient, demulcent, and epithelial-bed stimulant: superficial burns, sunburn, abrasions, slow-healing lesions, chapped skin, diaper rash, skin care of infants or bedridden patients—
apply several times a day, p.r.n.

Italicized side effects are common or life-threatening.
*Liquid form contains alcohol.   **May contain tartrazine.

ADVERSE REACTIONS
Skin: irritation.

INTERACTIONS
None significant.

NURSING CONSIDERATIONS
• Discontinue if skin condition persists or irritation develops.
• Observe for inflammation or infection since emollients and demulcents are occlusive layers that retain moisture, exclude air, and trap cutaneous bacteria.
• Skin should be cleaned daily or more often as needed.
• Emollients and demulcents may be used alone, as vehicles for medications, or with other topical medications. Check with doctor.

zinc gelatin
Dome-Paste, Unna's Boot
Pregnancy Category: C

MECHANISM OF ACTION
Promotes healing by reducing irritation and friction.

INDICATIONS & DOSAGE
Protectant: lesions or injuries of lower legs or arms—
Wrap the wet bandage in place, and retain for about 1 week. Dome-Paste, in 3″ and 4″ (8 to 10 cm) bandages, can be applied directly to arm or leg.

ADVERSE REACTIONS
None.

INTERACTIONS
None significant.

NURSING CONSIDERATIONS
• Observe for inflammation and infection since protectants produce an occlusive layer that retains perspiration, excludes air, and traps cutaneous bacteria, producing sites for anaerobic infections. Before each new application *always* thoroughly cleanse affected area, removing all traces of previously applied medication.
• Don't apply too tightly. Check for vasoconstriction.
• Zinc gelatin boot can be removed by unwinding outer bandage and soaking leg or arm in warm water until dressing floats off. Tell patient not to shower or take tub bath with zinc gelatin boot on leg.
• When applying topical medications to the skin before application of the bandage, apply the medication in the direction of the hair follicle to prevent folliculitis.

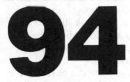

Keratolytics and caustics

podophyllum resin
resorcinol
resorcinol monoacetate
salicylic acid
silver nitrate
sulfur
sulfurated lime solution

COMBINATION PRODUCTS
ACNE-AID CREAM: sulfur 2.5%, resorcinol 1.25%, and parachlorometaxylenol 0.375% in a microporous cellulose base.
ACNOMEL CREAM♦: sulfur 8%, resorcinol 2%, and alcohol 11% in a greaseless base.
CLEARASIL CREAM: benzoyl peroxide 10% and bentonite.
COMPOUND W WART REMOVER: salicylic acid 14%, acetic acid 11%, in castor oil, alcohol, ether, and collodion.

podophyllum resin
Podoben
Pregnancy Category: X

MECHANISM OF ACTION
Inhibits cell division and other cellular processes, leading to the death of the cell.

INDICATIONS & DOSAGE
Venereal warts—
Adults: apply podophyllum resin preparation to the lesion, cover with waxed paper, and bandage. Leave covered for 4 to 6 hours, then wash lesion to remove medication. Repeat at weekly intervals, if indicated.

Multiple superficial epitheliomatoses and keratoses—
Adults: apply daily with applicator and allow to dry. Remove necrotic tissue before each reapplication.

ADVERSE REACTIONS
Blood: thrombocytopenia, leukopenia when systemically absorbed.
Local: irritation of normal skin.
Other: peripheral neuropathy when systemically absorbed.

INTERACTIONS
Other keratolytics: may cause extensive damage to the skin. Do not use together.

NURSING CONSIDERATIONS
• Contraindicated in pregnancy; may be harmful to fetus.
• Resin is irritating and cytotoxic, and should not be applied to normal skin. Petrolatum can be applied to adjacent areas to protect them during treatment.
• Should be applied only by a doctor because of toxicity.
• Do not use on extensive areas or for prolonged therapy; drug is absorbed systemically.
• Warn patient that soreness from local irritation may develop 12 to 48 hours after treatment.
• Should not be used without medical supervision.
• Don't use adjacent to mucous membrane areas.
• Will not remove large venereal warts. Surgery is another option.
• Don't use on recently biopsied

Italicized side effects are common or life-threatening.
*Liquid form contains alcohol.   **May contain tartrazine.

warts.

resorcinol

resorcinol monoacetate
Euresol, Resorcin
Pregnancy Category: C

MECHANISM OF ACTION
Softens keratin and loosens cornified epithelium.

INDICATIONS & DOSAGE
Acute eczema, urticaria, and other inflammatory skin diseases (1% or 2% concentration in alcohol); acne or seborrhea (5% lotion or 10% soap liniment for scalp); chronic eczema, psoriasis (2% to 10% ointment); acne scarring (45% peeling paste)—
Adults and children: apply as directed.

ADVERSE REACTIONS
Skin: irritation, moderate erythema or scaling.
Other: darkening of light hair (resorcinol only).

INTERACTIONS
None significant.

NURSING CONSIDERATIONS
• Do not use preparations on or near eyes.
• Use cautiously on ulcerated surfaces as systemic absorption may occur.
• If skin irritation persists, discontinue medication.
• Apply lotion with cotton ball to affected area.
• When applying the peeling paste, closely observe the patient and site of application until paste is removed.
• Use carefully with topical acne preparations because of local irritation.

salicylic acid
Calicylic, Keralyt♦, Salactic
Liquifilm, Salonil, Tran-Sal
Pregnancy Category: C

MECHANISM OF ACTION
Softens keratin and loosens cornified epithelium.

INDICATIONS & DOSAGE
Superficial fungal infections, acne, psoriasis, seborrheic dermatitis, other scaling dermatoses, hyperkeratosis, calluses, warts—
Adults and children: apply to affected area and place under occlusion at night.

ADVERSE REACTIONS
Skin: irritation, drying.
Other: salicylism with percutaneous absorption.

INTERACTIONS
Iodine, iron salts, and oxidizing substances: incompatible. Don't use together.

NURSING CONSIDERATIONS
• Use with caution in patients with diabetes or peripheral vascular disease. The skin inflammation that may result is difficult to treat. Limit use for children under 12 years. (Do not exceed 1 oz in 24 hours.)
• Avoid contact with eyes and mucous membranes.
• If excessive skin drying or irritation occurs, apply a bland cream or lotion.
• Rinse hands after application (unless they are being treated).
• Transdermal patch (Tran-Sal) now available for removal of warts.
• Skin should be hydrated for at least 5 minutes before treatment and washed the morning after treatment.
• Most preparations are occlusive, which increases percutaneous absorption. Therefore, do not use on large surface areas for prolonged periods.

- Not for use on broken, inflamed, or ulcerated areas.
- Also has bacteristatic and fungistatic properties.

silver nitrate
Pregnancy Category: C

MECHANISM OF ACTION
Denatures protein producing a caustic or corrosive effect.

INDICATIONS & DOSAGE
Cauterization of mucous membranes, fissures, aphthous lesions (5% to 10% solution); cauterization of granulomatous tissues and warts (solid form)—
Adults and children: applied only by doctor at his discretion.

ADVERSE REACTIONS
Local: *argyria (permanent silver discoloration of skin).*

INTERACTIONS
None significant.

NURSING CONSIDERATIONS
- May cause burns. Avoid accidental contact with skin and eyes. If accidental contact with skin occurs, flush with water for at least 15 minutes; accidental contact with eyes, call doctor at once.
- Warn that silver nitrate stains skin and clothing.
- Silver nitrate pencils must be moistened with water before use.
- In low concentrations (0.125% to 0.5%), as a wet dressing, is used as a local anti-infective in treatment of burn patients and in skin wounds or ulcers.
- May be painful in higher concentrations.

sulfur
Acnomead, Bensulfoid, Liquimat, Transact, Xerac
Pregnancy Category: C

MECHANISM OF ACTION
Softens keratin and loosens cornified epithelium.

INDICATIONS & DOSAGE
Acne, ringworm, psoriasis, seborrheic dermatitis, chigger infestation, scabies, favus, staphylococcal folliculitis—
Adults and children: apply preparation to affected areas b.i.d., t.i.d., or as directed.

ADVERSE REACTIONS
Local: excessive drying of skin, blackheads, contact dermatitis.

INTERACTIONS
None significant.

NURSING CONSIDERATIONS
- Prolonged use may cause severe contact dermatitis.
- When initiating therapy, use sparingly for patients with sensitive skin.
- Avoid contact with eyes. If accidental contact occurs, flush with water.
- Wash skin thoroughly before application. Tell patient that tingling sensation may be felt upon application.
- Skin is more reactive to drug in cold, dry climates, so decrease frequency of application. In hot, humid climates, increase frequency of application.
- Do not use on same area with topical acne preparation or preparations containing a peeling agent (for example, benzoyl peroxide); may cause severe irritation.
- The 10% ointment is used for scabies. Don't use on children or infants.
- Do not use on same area with any mercury-containing preparation; may cause a foul odor, irritate the skin, or

---

Italicized side effects are common or life-threatening.
*Liquid form contains alcohol.   **May contain tartrazine.

stain skin black.
• Has antiseptic and parasiticide
properties also.

sulfurated lime solution
Vlemasque, Vlem-Dome,
Vleminckx's solution
Pregnancy Category: C

MECHANISM OF ACTION
Softens keratin and loosens cornified
epithelium.

INDICATIONS & DOSAGE
Acne vulgaris, seborrhea—
Adults and children: dilute 1 packet
in 1 pint hot water and apply as hot
dressing for 15 to 20 minutes daily. Or
apply as a mask to affected, dry areas,
and rinse away with warm water after
15 to 20 minutes once daily.
Generalized furunculosis—
Adults and children: add 30 to 60 ml
solution to bath water.

ADVERSE REACTIONS
Local: may cause excessive drying of
skin.

INTERACTIONS
None significant.

NURSING CONSIDERATIONS
• Discontinue use if excessive drying
or skin irritation develops.
• Avoid contact with jewelry, metallic
objects, or clothing.
• Avoid getting solution in eyes, nose,
or mouth.
• Fumes are irritating and malodo-
rous (rotten eggs). Ventilate adequately. Odors are minimized with
Vlemasque.
• Do not use in same area with topical acne preparations; may cause severe irritation.
• Do not use in same area with
mercury-containing preparations;
may cause a foul odor, irritate skin, or
turn skin black.

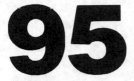

Miscellaneous dermatomucosal agents

anthralin
benzoyl peroxide
collagenase
dextranomer
etretinate
fluorouracil
hydroquinone
isotretinoin
methoxsalen
selenium sulfide
sutilains
tretinoin (vitamin A acid, retinoic
    acid)

COMBINATION PRODUCTS
SULFOXYL REGULAR: benzoyl peroxide 5% and sulfur 2%.
SULFOXYL STRONG: benzoyl peroxide 10% and sulfur 5%.
VANOXIDE♦: benzoyl peroxide 5% and chlorhydroxyquinoline 0.25%.
VANOXIDE-HC♦: benzoyl peroxide 5%, chlorhydroxyquinoline 0.25%, and hydrocortisone 0.5%.

---

anthralin
Anthra-Derm
Pregnancy Category: C

MECHANISM OF ACTION
Acts as a local antieczematous and antipsoriatic agent. Restores normal rate of keratinization and epidermal cell proliferation.

INDICATIONS & DOSAGE
Psoriasis, chronic dermatitis—
Adults and children: apply thinly daily or b.i.d. Concentrations range from 0.1% to 1%; start with lowest

and increase, if necessary.

ADVERSE REACTIONS
GU: possible renal toxicity.
Skin: erythema on healthy skin.

INTERACTIONS
None significant.

NURSING CONSIDERATIONS
• Contraindicated in renal damage. Should not be used on acute or inflammatory eruptions.
• Partial excretion in urine may cause renal irritation, casts, and albuminuria. Check urine weekly.
• Discontinue if allergic reaction, pustular folliculitis, or renal irritation occurs.
• Don't get in eyes. May cause conjunctivitis, keratitis, or corneal opacity.
• Wear plastic gloves to apply anthralin; wash hands thoroughly after using.
• Cover with gauze dressing to protect clothing.
• May cause a temporary yellow-brown discoloration to hair, skin, and alkaline urine. Anthralin stain may be removed from skin by applying 3% to 6% salicylic acid cream or ointment. May stain clothing.
• Avoid applying medication to normal skin by coating the area surrounding the lesion with petrolatum.
• Remove with light application of mineral oil before bathing.

---

benzoyl peroxide

Benoxyl♦, Benzac♦, Benzagel♦,
Clear by Design, Desquam-X♦♦,
Dry and Clear♦, Oxy-5♦, Oxy-10,
OxyCover♦, Panoxyl♦, Persadox
HP, Persa-Gel♦, Xerac BP♦
Pregnancy Category: C

MECHANISM OF ACTION
Has antimicrobial and comedolytic
activity.

INDICATIONS & DOSAGE
Acne—
Adults and children: apply once
daily to q.i.d., depending on tolerance
and effect.

ADVERSE REACTIONS
Skin: transient stinging on application, feeling of warmth, painful irritation, pruritus, vesicles, allergic contact dermatitis.

INTERACTIONS
None significant.

NURSING CONSIDERATIONS
• Contraindicated in sensitivity to
any of the ingredients.
• Don't use near the eyes, on mucous
membranes, or on denuded or highly
inflamed skin.
• Dryness, redness, peeling should
occur 3 to 4 days after starting treatment. If these common reactions
cause considerable discomfort, discontinue temporarily.
• If painful irritation or vesicles develop, discontinue use.
• May cause bleaching of hair or col-
ored fabric.

collagenase

Biozyme-C, Santyl
Pregnancy Category: C

MECHANISM OF ACTION
An enzymatic debriding agent that digests undenatured collagen fibers in
necrotic tissue and removes substrates
for bacterial proliferation.

INDICATIONS & DOSAGE
*Debridement of dermal ulcers and se-
verely burned areas—*
Adults and children: apply ointment
(250 units/g) to lesion daily or every
other day.

ADVERSE REACTIONS
Skin: slight erythema of surrounding
area, especially if ointment is not confined to lesion.
Other: hypersensitivity reactions.

INTERACTIONS
*Detergents; hexachlorophene; antisep-
tics (especially those containing heavy
metal ions, such as mercury or silver);
iodine; soaks or acidic solutions containing metal ions, such as aluminum
acetate (Burow's solution):* decreased
enzymatic activity. Do not use together.

NURSING CONSIDERATIONS
• Use with caution in debilitated patients, since debriding enzymes may
increase risk of bacteremia; watch for
signs of systemic infection.
• Before application, cleanse lesion
with gauze saturated in normal saline
solution, neutral buffer solution, or
hydrogen peroxide; use topical antibacterial agent (such as neomycin-
bacitracin-polymyxin B) if infection
is present. Apply to lesion in powder
form before using collagenase. If infection persists, discontinue collagenase until infection is healed. Confine
collagenase ointment to area of lesion
(Lassar's paste may protect surrounding skin). Apply ointment in thin layers to assure contact with necrotic tissue and complete wound coverage;
apply collagenase ointment with
tongue depressor on deep wounds;
with gauze on shallow wounds. Remove any debris that comes off easily.

Remove excess ointment, and cover wound with sterile gauze pad.
- Discontinue when sufficient debridement has occurred.
- Observe wound to monitor progress of therapy. Appearance of granulation may indicate effectiveness. Notify doctor if inflammation or color of drainage indicates any spread of infection.
- If enzymatic action must be stopped, apply Burow's solution.
- Avoid getting ointment in eyes. If this occurs, flush with water at once.
- Protect drug from heat.

---

dextranomer
Debrisan♦
Pregnancy Category: NR

MECHANISM OF ACTION
A synthetic polymer that aids in granulation by absorbing exudate, bacteria, and contaminants.

INDICATIONS & DOSAGE
To clean secreting wounds, such as venous stasis and decubitus ulcers, infected surgical wounds, and burns—
Adults and children: apply to affected area daily, b.i.d., or more often, p.r.n. Apply to ⅛″ or ¼″ thickness, and cover with sterile gauze.

ADVERSE REACTIONS
Skin: temporary pain.

INTERACTIONS
Ointment bases, such as Vaseline: negates action of dextranomer. Don't mix together.

NURSING CONSIDERATIONS
- Before application, cleanse wound with sterile water, saline solution, or other appropriate solution. Do not dry.
- Don't use in body cavities or deep fistulas.
- Pack cratered wounds with beads,

allowing room for expansion of beads. Cover with dressing to hold beads in place.
- When saturated, medication turns gray-yellow and should be removed.
- To remove, irrigate with sterile water, saline solution, or other cleansing solution.
- Dextranomer beads are not effective in cleaning nonsecreting wounds. When the wound has healed to the point where it is no longer exuding, treatment should be discontinued.
- Dextranomer beads are hydrophilic; each gram of beads can absorb 4 ml of exudate.
- Keep drug away from moisture; store in tightly closed container.
- Avoid contact with eyes.
- Be careful not to spill beads onto floor, as the resultant slipperiness can be a safety hazard.
- Dextranomer reduces tissue edema at site so wound may appear larger after initial use.
- Beads must be thoroughly removed before any surgical procedure.

---

etretinate
Eegison
Pregnancy Category: X

MECHANISM OF ACTION
Unknown.

INDICATIONS & DOSAGE
Treatment of recalcitrant psoriasis, including the erythrodermic and generalized pustular types—
Adults: initially, 0.75 to 1 mg/kg daily in divided doses. Don't exceed maximum initial dose of 1.5 mg/kg daily. After initial response, begin maintenance dose of 0.5 to 0.75 mg/kg daily.

ADVERSE REACTIONS
Blood: *blood dyscrasias,* anemia, altered prothrombin time.
EENT: *eye pain, sore tongue,*

---

chapped lips.
CNS: *benign intracranial hypertension (pseudotumor cerebri), fatigue, headache,* dizziness, lethargy.
CV: thrombosis, edema.
GI: *appetite change, nausea.*
Hepatic: *hepatitis, elevated liver enzymes.*
GU: *white blood cells in urine,* proteinuria, hematuria.
Metabolic: *hypokalemia or hyperkalemia, hyperlipidemia.*
Skin: *skin peeling, itching.*
Other: *bone pain,* dyspnea.

INTERACTIONS
Milk: increases etretinate's absorption. Avoid concomitant consumption of milk.
Vitamin A: additive toxic effects. Avoid concomitant use.

NURSING CONSIDERATIONS
• Etretinate causes severe birth defects if used during pregnancy.
• Contraindicated in women who are pregnant, who intend to become pregnant, or who may not use reliable contraception during treatment. Women of childbearing age must not receive etretinate unless pregnancy is excluded. Perform a pregnancy test within 2 weeks before initiating therapy. Then start therapy on the 2nd or 3rd day of the next normal menstrual period.
• Remind your patient about the importance of using contraception during treatment.
• Monitor liver function tests regularly. They should be performed when therapy begins, at 1- to 2-week intervals for the first 1 to 2 months of therapy, and thereafter at intervals of 1 to 3 months.
• Monitor blood lipids every 1 to 2 weeks during treatment.
• Advise patients not to take vitamin A supplements to avoid possible additive adverse reactions. Etretinate is a vitamin A derivative.

• Reassure patient that transient exacerbation of psoriasis is common during the beginning of therapy.
• Tell patient that he may have difficulty tolerating contact lenses during treatment.
• Advise patient to take this drug with meals, but to avoid taking it with milk or milk products.

fluorouracil
Efudex♦, Fluoroplex♦
Pregnancy Category: D

MECHANISM OF ACTION
Interferes with DNA synthesis by inhibiting thymidylate synthetase.

INDICATIONS & DOSAGE
Multiple actinic or solar keratoses; superficial basal cell carcinoma—
Adults and children: apply cream (5%) or solution (1%, 2%, or 5%) b.i.d.

ADVERSE REACTIONS
Skin: erythema, pain, burning, scaling, pruritus, hyperpigmentation, contact dermatitis, soreness, suppuration, swelling.

INTERACTIONS
None significant.

NURSING CONSIDERATIONS
• Wash hands immediately after handling medication.
• Avoid use with occlusive dressings.
• Patient should avoid prolonged exposure to sunlight or ultraviolet light.
• Apply with caution near eyes, nose, and mouth.
• Warn patient that treated area may be unsightly during therapy and for several weeks after therapy is stopped. Complete healing may not occur until 1 or 2 months after treatment is stopped.
• Ingestion and systemic absorption may cause leukopenia, thrombocyto-

penia, stomatitis, diarrhea; or GI ulceration, bleeding, and hemorrhage.
• Topical application to large ulcerated areas may cause systemic toxicity.
• For superficial basal cell carcinoma confirmed by biopsy, use 5% strength.
• Lesions resistant to fluorouracil shouldn't be retreated; they should be biopsied.
• Use 1% concentration on the face. Reserve higher concentrations for thicker-skinned areas or resistant lesions. Occlusion may be required.

hydroquinone
Artra Skin Tone Cream, Derma-Blanch, Eldopaque♦, Eldopaque-Forte♦, Eldoquin♦, Eldoquin Forte♦, Esoterica Medicated Cream♦, Golden Peacock, HQC Kit, Melanex, Quinnone
Pregnancy Category: C

MECHANISM OF ACTION
Inhibits tyrosinase, preventing the conversion of tyrosine to melanin.

INDICATIONS & DOSAGE
Bleaching of blemished skin, lentigo, chloasma, freckles, old-age spots, and other skin conditions due to increased melanin—
Adults and children 12 years and over: apply 2% to 4% concentration daily or b.i.d.

ADVERSE REACTIONS
Skin: mild irritation, sensitization, rash.

INTERACTIONS
None significant.

NURSING CONSIDERATIONS
• Contraindicated in patients with prickly heat, sunburn, irritated skin; or as depilatory.
• Don't use near eyes.

• If rash or irritation develops, discontinue therapy.
• Sensitivity can be tested by applying a small amount of low-concentration medication on skin before treatment is started. Allergic reactions should appear within 24 hours.
• Doesn't cause permanent depigmentation.
• Advise patient to use opaque sunscreen when outdoors since sun can darken lesions faster than hydroquinone can lighten them.
• Topical steroids can reduce irritation and sensitization.

isotretinoin
Accutane♦
Pregnancy Category: X

MECHANISM OF ACTION
Normalizes keratinization, reversibly decreases the size of sebaceous glands, and alters the composition of sebum to a less viscous form that's less likely to cause follicular plugging.

INDICATIONS & DOSAGE
Severe cystic acne unresponsive to conventional therapy—
Adults and adolescents: 0.5 to 2 mg/kg daily P.O. given in 2 divided doses and continued for 15 to 20 weeks.

ADVERSE REACTIONS
Blood: anemia, elevated platelet count.
CNS: headache, fatigue.
EENT: *conjunctivitis,* corneal deposits, dry eyes.
Endocrine: hyperglycemia.
GI: nonspecific gastrointestinal symptoms, gum bleeding and inflammation.
Hepatic: elevated SGOT, SPGT, alkaline phosphatase.
Skin: *cheilosis (chapped lips), rash, dry skin,* peeling of palms and toes, skin infection, photosensitivity.
Other: *hypertriglyceridemia, muscu-*

loskeletal pain (skeletal hyperostosis), thinning of hair.

INTERACTIONS
Vitamin A and vitamin supplements containing vitamin A: increase in isotretinoin's toxic effects. Don't use together without doctor's permission.

NURSING CONSIDERATIONS
• Isotretinoin shouldn't be used in women of childbearing age unless contraception is used during treatment and for at least 1 month after treatment. *Severe fetal abnormalities may occur if used during pregnancy.*
• Contraindicated in patients hypersensitive to parabens, since parabens are used as a preservative.
• Tell patient to immediately report any bone or skeletal pain.
• Perform blood lipid studies and liver function tests before therapy begins and then at regular intervals until response to drug is established, usually about 4 weeks.
• Monitor blood glucose levels regularly.
• Monitor CPR levels in patients who undergo vigorous physical activity.
• Warn patient that while undergoing isotretinoin therapy, his contact lenses may feel more uncomfortable.
• If a second course of therapy is needed, it shouldn't be started until at least 8 weeks after the completion of the first course because patients may continue to improve after discontinuing the drug.
• Most adverse reactions appear to be dose-related, with most occurring at doses greater than 1 mg/kg daily. They are generally reversible when therapy is discontinued or dose is reduced.
• Advise patient to take with or shortly after meals to insure adequate absorption.

methoxsalen
Oxsoralen♦
Pregnancy Category: C

MECHANISM OF ACTION
A potent photosensitizer of the skin that promotes melanin formation by facilitating the action of ultraviolet light.

INDICATIONS & DOSAGE
Protect against sunburn, enhance pigmentation, and induce repigmentation in vitiligo—
Adults and children over 12 years: for small, well-defined lesions, apply topically weekly or less often and expose to ultraviolet A light gradually, as directed.
Psoriasis—
Adults: oral dosage is based on weight and administered 2 hours before exposure to ultraviolet A light. May repeat 2 to 3 times weekly, at least 48 hours apart.

ADVERSE REACTIONS
CNS: nervousness, insomnia, mental depression.
GI: discomfort, nausea, diarrhea.
Skin: edema, erythema, blistering, burning, peeling, *photosensitivity*.
Other: leg cramps.

INTERACTIONS
Photosensitizing agents: do not use together.

NURSING CONSIDERATIONS
• Contraindicated in hepatic insufficiency, porphyria, acute systemic lupus erythematosus, and hydromorphic, polymorphic light eruptions. Also contraindicated in patients with cataracts or who are aphakic (without lenses). Use with caution in familial history of sunlight allergy, GI diseases, chronic infection, history of basal cell carcinoma.
• Regulate therapy carefully. Overex-

posure to light can cause serious burning or blistering.
- Topical treatment should be directly supervised by a doctor.
- When applied topically to face or hands, patient should protect area from light (except during treatment exposure) for 24 hours before and after therapy.
- Protect eyes and lips during light exposure treatments.
- Significant changes require 6 to 9 months of therapy.
- After oral therapy, patient should wear wrap-around sunglasses with UVA-absorbing properties in daylight during the next 24 hours.

selenium sulfide
Exsel♦, Selsun♦, Sul-Blue
Pregnancy Category: C

MECHANISM OF ACTION
Has irritant, antibacterial, and antifungal properties.

INDICATIONS & DOSAGE
Dandruff, seborrheic scalp dermatitis—
Adults and children: massage 1 to 2 teaspoonfuls into wet scalp. Leave on for 2 to 3 minutes. Rinse thoroughly, and repeat application. Apply twice weekly for 2 weeks, then 2 to 3 times a week, or as often as needed.

ADVERSE REACTIONS
Skin: oily or dry scalp and hair, hair discoloration, hair loss, sensitivity reactions.

INTERACTIONS
None significant.

NURSING CONSIDERATIONS
- Contraindicated in sulfur hypersensitivity.
- Use with caution around areas of acute inflammation or exudation to avoid undue irritation.

- If sensitivity reactions occur, discontinue use.
- Reduce hair discoloration by thorough rinsing after treatment.
- Avoid contact with eyes.
- Highly toxic if ingested.

sutilains
Travase♦
Pregnancy Category: C

MECHANISM OF ACTION
A proteolytic enzyme that selectively digests necrotic tissue.

INDICATIONS & DOSAGE
Debridement of second- and third-degree burns, adjunctive debridement of decubitus ulcers, pyogenic wounds, or ulcers resulting from peripheral vascular disease—
Adults and children: apply thinly to area extending 1/4″ to 1/2″ beyond area to be debrided. Cover with loose, wet dressing t.i.d. or q.i.d.

ADVERSE REACTIONS
CNS: local paresthesias.
Skin: mild pain, bleeding, transient dermatitis.

INTERACTIONS
Detergents, anti-infectives (such as benzalkonium chloride, hexachlorophene, iodine, and nitrofurazone), and compounds containing metallic ions (such as silver nitrate and thimerosal): adversely affects enzymatic activity. Do not use together.

NURSING CONSIDERATIONS
- Contraindicated in wounds involving major body cavities or containing exposed nerves or nerve tissue, fungating neoplastic ulcers, wounds in women of childbearing age, persons having limited cardiac or pulmonary reserves.
- Should be used only on 10% to 15% of the burned area at a time.

- Use cautiously near eyes. If accidental contact occurs, flush eyes repeatedly with large amounts of normal saline solution or sterile water.
- Before application, cleanse and irrigate affected area with normal saline solution or sterile water to remove antibacterial agents.
- May give mild analgesic to reduce painful reactions, but discontinue if pain is severe; also discontinue if bleeding or dermatitis occurs.
- For best response, keep affected area moist.
- In concomitant use of topical antimicrobial agent, apply sutilains first.
- Store at 35.6° to 50° F. (2° to 10° C.). Keep in refrigerator.

tretinoin (vitamin A acid, retinoic acid)
Pregnancy Category: B

MECHANISM OF ACTION
Inhibits comedones by increasing epidermal cell mitosis and epidermal cell turnover.

INDICATIONS & DOSAGE
Acne vulgaris (especially grades I, II, and III)—
Adults and children: cleanse affected area and lightly apply solution once daily at bedtime.

ADVERSE REACTIONS
Skin: *feeling of warmth, slight stinging, local erythema, peeling at site,* chapping and swelling, blistering and crusting, temporary hyperpigmentation or hypopigmentation.

INTERACTIONS
None significant.

NURSING CONSIDERATIONS
- Contraindicated in hypersensitivity to any tretinoin component. Use with caution in eczema.
- If severe local irritation develops,

discontinue temporarily and readjust dosage when application is resumed.
- Some redness and scaling are normal reactions.
- Beneficial effects should be seen within 6 weeks of treatment.
- When treatment is stopped, relapses generally occur within 3 to 6 weeks.
- Patient should wash face with a mild soap no more than two or three times a day. Warn against using strong or medicated cosmetics, soaps, or other skin cleansers.
- Exposure to sunlight or ultraviolet rays should be minimal during treatment. If patient is sunburned, delay therapy until sunburn subsides.
- Patient who can't avoid exposure to sunlight should use a #15 sunscreen and protective clothing.
- Avoid contact with eyes, mouth, and mucous membranes.
- Warn patient not to use topical products containing alcohol, astringents, spices, and lime. These may interfere with action of tretinoin.
- Warn patient to wait until skin is completely dry before applying.

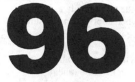

Local anesthetics

**bupivacaine hydrochloride
chloroprocaine hydrochloride
etidocaine hydrochloride
lidocaine hydrochloride
mepivacaine hydrochloride
procaine hydrochloride
tetracaine hydrochloride**

COMBINATION PRODUCTS
None, although epinephrine is added
to some solutions to prolong effect.

---

bupivacaine hydrochloride
Marcaine♦, Sensorcaine
Pregnancy Category: C

MECHANISM OF ACTION
Blocks depolarization by interfering
with sodium-potassium exchange
across the nerve-cell membrane, preventing generation and conduction of
the nerve impulse. When combined
with epinephrine, action is prolonged.

INDICATIONS & DOSAGE
*Available with or without epinephrine.
Dosages given are for drug without
epinephrine.*
Epidural:

Sol.	Vol. (ml)	Dose (mg)
0.50%	10 to 20	50 to 100
0.25%	10 to 20	25 to 50

Caudal:

Sol.	Vol. (ml)	Dose (mg)
0.50%	15 to 30	75 to 150
0.25%	15 to 30	37.5 to 75

Peripheral nerve block:

Sol.	Vol. (ml)	Dose (mg)
0.50%	5 to 80	25 to 400 (max.)

May repeat dose q 3 hours. Dose and
interval may be increased with epinephrine. Maximum 400 mg daily.

ADVERSE REACTIONS
Skin: dermatologic reactions.
Other: edema, status asthmaticus, or
anaphylaxis and anaphylactoid reactions.
Side effects of local anesthetics generally result from high blood levels of
the drug. Examples of these are:
CNS: anxiety, apprehension, nervousness, convulsions followed by
drowsiness, unconsciousness, and *respiratory arrest.*
CV: myocardial depression, *arrhythmias, cardiac arrest.*
EENT: blurred vision, tinnitus.
GI: nausea, vomiting.

INTERACTIONS
*Enflurane, halothane, and related
drugs:* cardiac arrhythmias may occur
when used with bupivacaine *with* epinephrine. Use with extreme caution.
*MAO inhibitors, cyclic antidepres-
sants:* severe, sustained hypertension
may occur when used with bupivacaine *with* epinephrine. Use with extreme caution.
Chloroprocaine: may lessen bupivacaine's action. Don't use both local
anesthetics.

NURSING CONSIDERATIONS
• Contraindicated in children under
12 years and for spinal, paracervical
block, or topical anesthesia. Use cautiously in debilitated, elderly, or
acutely ill patients; and in patients

Italicized side effects are common or life-threatening.
*Liquid form contains alcohol.   **May contain tartrazine.

with severe hepatic disease or drug allergies.
- Although the 0.75% solution is still available, it is not to be used for obstetrical surgery. According to the FDA, lower concentrations are effective and much less hazardous.
- Use solutions with epinephrine cautiously in cardiovascular disorders and in body areas with limited blood supply (ears, nose, fingers, toes).
- Keep resuscitative equipment and drugs available.
- Don't use solution with preservatives for caudal or epidural block.
- Onset in 4 to 17 minutes; duration 3 to 6 hours.
- Discard partially used vials without preservatives.
- Check solution for particles.

---

chloroprocaine hydrochloride
Nesacaine (for infiltration and regional anesthesia), Nesacaine-CE (for caudal and epidural anesthesia)
Pregnancy Category: C

MECHANISM OF ACTION
Blocks depolarization by interfering with sodium-potassium exchange across the nerve-cell membrane, preventing generation and conduction of the nerve impulse.

INDICATIONS & DOSAGE
Available only without epinephrine.
Infiltration and nerve block:

Sol.	Vol. (ml)	Dose (mg)
1%	3 to 20	30 to 200
2%	2 to 40	40 to 800

Caudal and epidural:

Sol.	Vol. (ml)	Dose (mg)
2% to 3%	15 to 25	300 to 750

May repeat with smaller doses q 40 to 50 minutes. Dose and interval may be increased with epinephrine. Maximum adult dose 800 mg, or 1 g when mixed with epinephrine.

ADVERSE REACTIONS
Skin: dermatologic reactions.
Other: edema, status asthmaticus, or *anaphylaxis* and anaphylactoid reactions.
Side effects of local anesthetics generally result from high blood levels of the drug. Examples of these are:
CNS: anxiety, apprehension, nervousness, convulsions followed by drowsiness, unconsciousness, and *respiratory arrest*.
CV: myocardial depression, *arrhythmias, cardiac arrest*.
EENT: blurred vision, tinnitus.
GI: nausea, vomiting.

INTERACTIONS
None significant.

NURSING CONSIDERATIONS
- Contraindicated in hypersensitivity to procaine, tetracaine, or other para-aminobenzoic acid derivatives, and for spinal or topical anesthesia. Epidural and caudal contraindicated in CNS disease. Use cautiously in debilitated, elderly, or acutely ill patients; children; and in patients with drug allergies, paracervical block, or cardiovascular disease.
- With epidural use, a 3-ml test dose should be injected at least 10 minutes before giving total dose to check for intravascular or subarachnoid injection. Motor paralysis and extensive sensory anesthesia indicate subarachnoid injection.
- Repeat the test dose if patient is moved in a way that might displace the epidural catheter.
- At least 5 minutes should elapse after each test before proceeding further.
- Don't use solution with preservatives for caudal or epidural block.
- Don't use discolored solution.
- Keep resuscitative equipment and drugs available.
- Duration is 30 to 60 minutes.
- Discard partially used vials without

preservatives.
• Check solution for particles.

etidocaine hydrochloride
Duranest
Pregnancy Category: B

MECHANISM OF ACTION
Blocks depolarization by interfering with sodium-potassium exchange across the nerve-cell membrane, preventing generation and conduction of the nerve impulse. When combined with epinephrine, action is prolonged.

INDICATIONS & DOSAGE
Available with or without epinephrine. Doses cited are for drug with *epinephrine. Dose and interval may be decreased without epinephrine.*
Peripheral nerve block:

Sol.	Vol. (ml)	Dose (mg)
0.5%	5 to 40	25 to 200
1%	5 to 40	50 to 400

Central neural block:
Lower limbs, cesarean section, lumbar peridural

Sol.	Vol. (ml)	Dose (mg)
1%	10 to 30	100 to 300
1.5%	10 to 20	150 to 300

Vaginal:

Sol.	Vol. (ml)	Dose (mg)
1%	5 to 20	50 to 200

Caudal:

Sol.	Vol. (ml)	Dose (mg)
1%	10 to 30	100 to 300

ADVERSE REACTIONS
Skin: dermatologic reactions.
Other: edema, status asthmaticus, or *anaphylaxis* and anaphylactoid reactions.
Side effects of local anesthetics generally result from high blood levels of the drug. Examples of these are:
CNS: anxiety, apprehension, nervousness, convulsions followed by drowsiness, unconsciousness, and *respiratory arrest.*
CV: myocardial depression, *arrhyth-*

mias, cardiac arrest.
EENT: blurred vision, tinnitus.
GI: nausea, vomiting.

INTERACTIONS
Enflurane, halothane, and related drugs: cardiac arrhythmias may occur when used with etidocaine *with* epinephrine. Use with extreme caution.
MAO inhibitors, cyclic antidepressants, phenothiazines: severe, sustained hypertension or hypotension may occur when used with etidocaine solution *with* epinephrine. Use with extreme caution.

NURSING CONSIDERATIONS
• Contraindicated in inflammation or infection in puncture region, children under 14 years, septicemia, severe hypertension, spinal deformities, neurologic disorders, and spinal block. Use cautiously in debilitated, elderly, or acutely ill patients; severe shock; heart block; epidural block in obstetrics; general drug allergies; hepatic and renal disease.
• Use solutions with epinephrine cautiously in cardiovascular disease and in body areas with limited blood supply (ears, nose, fingers, toes).
• Don't use solution with preservatives for caudal or epidural block.
• Keep resuscitative equipment and drugs available.
• Onset in 2 to 8 minutes; duration, 3 to 6 hours.
• Check solution for particles.

lidocaine hydrochloride
Ardecaine, Dilocaine, Dolicaine, L-Caine, Nervocaine, Norocaine, Rocaine, Stanacaine, Ultracaine, Xylocaine Hydrochloride♦
Pregnancy Category: B

MECHANISM OF ACTION
Blocks depolarization by interfering with sodium-potassium exchange across the nerve-cell membrane, pre-

venting generation and conduction of the nerve impulse. When combined with epinephrine, action is prolonged.

INDICATIONS & DOSAGE
Available with or without epinephrine. Doses cited are for drug without epinephrine except where indicated.
Caudal (obstetrics) *or epidural* (thoracic):

Sol.	Vol. (ml)	Dose (mg)
1%	20 to 30	200 to 300

Caudal (surgery):

Sol.	Vol. (ml)	Dose (mg)
1.5%	15 to 20	225 to 300

Epidural (lumbar anesthesia):

Sol.	Vol. (ml)	Dose (mg)
1.5%	15 to 20	225 to 300
2%	10 to 15	200 to 300

Maximum dose 200 to 300 mg/hour.
For anesthesia other than spinal— maximum single adult dose 4.5 mg/kg or 300 mg.
With epinephrine for anesthesia other than spinal— maximum single adult dose 7 mg/kg or 500 mg. Don't repeat dose more often than q 2 hours.
Spinal surgical anesthesia:

Sol.	Vol. (ml)	Dose (mg)
5% with	1.5 to 2	75 to 100
7.5%		

dextrose
Dose and interval may be increased with epinephrine.

ADVERSE REACTIONS
Skin: dermatologic reactions.
Other: edema, status asthmaticus, or *anaphylaxis* and anaphylactoid reactions.
Side effects of local anesthetics generally result from high blood levels of the drug. Examples of these are:
CNS: anxiety, apprehension, nervousness, convulsions followed by drowsiness, unconsciousness, and *respiratory arrest.*
CV: myocardial depression, *arrhythmias, cardiac arrest.*
EENT: blurred vision, tinnitus.

GI: nausea, vomiting.

INTERACTIONS
Enflurane, halothane, and related drugs: cardiac arrhythmias may occur when used with lidocaine *with* epinephrine. Use with extreme caution.
MAO inhibitors, cyclic antidepressants: severe, sustained hypertension may occur when used with lidocaine *with* epinephrine. Use with extreme caution.

NURSING CONSIDERATIONS
• Contraindicated in inflammation or infection in puncture region, septicemia, severe hypertension, spinal deformities, and neurologic disorders. Use cautiously in debilitated, elderly, or acutely ill patients; severe shock; heart block; obstetrics; general drug allergies; and paracervical block.
• Use solutions with epinephrine cautiously in cardiovascular disorders and in body areas with limited blood supply (ears, nose, fingers, toes).
• Keep resuscitative equipment and drugs available.
• With epidural use, a 2- to 5-ml test dose should be injected at least 5 minutes before giving total dose to check for intravascular or subarachnoid injection. Motor paralysis and extensive sensory anesthesia indicate subarachnoid injection.
• Solutions containing preservatives should not be used for spinal, epidural, or caudal block.
• Discard partially used vials without preservatives.
• Check solution for particles.

mepivacaine hydrochloride
Carbocaine♦, Cavacaine, Isocaine♦
Pregnancy Category: C

MECHANISM OF ACTION
Blocks depolarization by interfering with sodium-potassium exchange

across the nerve-cell membrane, preventing generation and conduction of the nerve impulse. When combined with levonordefrin, action is prolonged.

INDICATIONS & DOSAGE
Available with or without levonordefrin (vasoconstrictor). Doses cited are for drug without levonordefrin.
Nerve block:

Sol.	Vol. (ml)	Dose (mg)
1%	5 to 20	50 to 200
2%	5 to 20	100 to 400

Transvaginal block or infiltration (maximum dose):

Sol.	Vol. (ml)	Dose (mg)
1%	40	400

Paracervical block (obstetrics):

Sol.	Vol. (ml)	Dose (mg)
1%	10	100

Give on each side (200 mg total) per 90-minute period.
Caudal and epidural:

Sol.	Vol. (ml)	Dose (mg)
1%	15 to 30	150 to 300
1.5%	10 to 25	150 to 375
2%	10 to 20	200 to 400

Therapeutic block (pain management):

Sol.	Vol. (ml)	Dose (mg)
1%	1 to 5	10 to 50
2%	1 to 5	20 to 100

Adults: maximum single dose 7 mg/kg up to 550 mg. Don't repeat more often than q 90 minutes. Maximum total dose 1,000 mg daily.
Children: maximum dose 5 to 6 mg/kg. In children under 3 years or weighing less than 14 kg, use 0.5% or 1.5% solution only. Dose and interval may be increased with levonordefrin.

ADVERSE REACTIONS
Skin: dermatologic reactions.
Other: edema, status asthmaticus, or *anaphylaxis* and anaphylactoid reactions.
Side effects of local anesthetics generally result from high blood levels of the drug. Examples of these are:

CNS: anxiety, apprehension, nervousness, convulsions followed by drowsiness, unconsciousness, and *respiratory arrest.*
CV: myocardial depression, *arrhythmias, cardiac arrest.*
EENT: blurred vision, tinnitus.
GI: nausea, vomiting.

INTERACTIONS
Enflurane, halothane, and related drugs: cardiac arrhythmias may occur when used with mepivacaine *with* levonordefrin. Use with extreme caution.
MAO inhibitors, cyclic antidepressants: severe, sustained hypertension may occur when used with mepivacaine *with* levonordefrin. Use with extreme caution.

NURSING CONSIDERATIONS
• Contraindicated in sensitivity to methylparaben, in heart block, or for spinal anesthesia. Use cautiously in debilitated, elderly, or acutely ill patients, or for paracervical block.
• Use solutions with levonordefrin cautiously in cardiovascular disease and in body areas with limited blood supply (nose, ears).
• Monitor fetal heart rate when paracervical block is used in delivery.
• Keep resuscitative equipment and drugs available.
• Don't use solutions with preservatives for caudal or epidural block.
• Onset in 15 minutes; duration, 3 hours.
• Discard partially used vials without preservatives.
• Check solution for particles.

procaine hydrochloride
Novocain♦, Unicaine
Pregnancy Category: C

MECHANISM OF ACTION
Blocks depolarization by interfering with sodium-potassium exchange

---

Italicized side effects are common or life-threatening.
*Liquid form contains alcohol.   **May contain tartrazine.

across the nerve-cell membrane, preventing generation and conduction of
the nerve impulse.

INDICATIONS & DOSAGE
Spinal anesthesia—
before using, dilute 10% solution with
0.9% NaCl injection, sterile distilled
water, or cerebrospinal fluid.
For hyperbaric technique, use dextrose solution.
Perineum: use 0.5 ml 10% solution
and 0.5 ml diluent injected at fourth
lumbar interspace.
Perineum and lower extremities: use 1
ml 10% solution and 1 ml diluent injected at third or fourth lumbar interspace.
Up to costal margin: use 2 ml 10% solution and 1 ml diluent injected at second, third, or fourth lumbar interspace.
Epidural block:

Sol.	Vol. (ml)	Dose (mg)
1.5%	25	375

Peripheral nerve block:

Sol.	Vol. (ml)	Dose (mg)
1%	50	500
2%	25	500

Infiltration: use 250 to 600 mg 0.25%
to 0.5% solution. Maximum initial
dose 1 g. Dose and interval may be increased with epinephrine.

ADVERSE REACTIONS
Skin: dermatologic reactions.
Other: edema, status asthmaticus, or
anaphylaxis and anaphylactoid reactions.
Side effects of local anesthetics generally result from high blood levels of
the drug. Examples of these are:
CNS: anxiety; apprehension; nervousness; convulsions followed by
drowsiness, unconsciousness, and *respiratory arrest.*
CV: myocardial depression, *arrhythmias, cardiac arrest.*
EENT: blurred vision, tinnitus.
GI: nausea, vomiting.

INTERACTIONS
Echothiophate iodide: reduced hydro-
lysis of procaine. Use together cautiously.

NURSING CONSIDERATIONS
• Contraindicated in traumatized urethra and in hypersensitivity to chloroprocaine, tetracaine, or other para-
aminobenzoic acid derivatives. Use
cautiously in hyperexcitable patients
and in patients with CNS diseases, infection at puncture site, shock, profound anemia, cachexia, sepsis, hypertension, hypotension, GI hemorrhage, bowel perforation or strangula-
tion, peritonitis, cardiac decompensation, massive pleural effusions, and
increased intraabdominal pressure.
• Contraindications to obstetric use:
pelvic disporportion, placenta previa,
abruptio placentae, floating fetal
head, intrauterine manipulation.
• Keep resuscitative equipment and
drugs available.
• A 1- to 5-ml test dose should be
given 5 to 15 minutes before total epidural dose. Motor paralysis and extensive sensory anesthesia indicate subarachnoid injection.
• Use solution without preservatives
for epidural block.
• Onset in 2 to 5 minutes; duration 60
minutes.
• Discard partially used vials without
preservatives.
• Check solution for particles.

tetracaine hydrochloride
Pontocaine♦
Pregnancy Category: C

MECHANISM OF ACTION
Blocks depolarization by interfering
with sodium-potassium exchange
across the nerve-cell membrane, preventing generation and conduction of
the nerve impulse.

INDICATIONS & DOSAGE

Low spinal (saddle block) in vaginal delivery—
give 2 to 5 mg as hyperbaric solution (in 10% dextrose). Maximum dose 15 mg.
Perineum and lower extremities: give 5 to 10 mg.
Prolonged spinal anesthesia (2 to 3 hours): dilute 1% solution with equal volume of cerebrospinal fluid, or dissolve 5 mg powdered drug in 1 ml cerebrospinal fluid immediately before giving. Give 1 ml/5 seconds.
Up to costal margin: give 15 to 20 mg.

ADVERSE REACTIONS

Skin: dermatologic reactions.
Other: edema, status asthmaticus, or *anaphylaxis* and anaphylactoid reactions.
Side effects of local anesthetics generally result from high blood levels of the drug. Examples of these are:
CNS: anxiety, apprehension, nervousness, convulsions followed by drowsiness, unconsciousness, and *respiratory arrest.*
CV: myocardial depression, *arrhythmias, cardiac arrest.*
EENT: blurred vision, tinnitus.
GI: nausea, vomiting.

INTERACTIONS

None significant.

NURSING CONSIDERATIONS

• Contraindicated in infection at injection site, serious CNS diseases, and in hypersensitivity to procaine, chloroprocaine, tetracaine, or other para-aminobenzoic acid derivatives. Use cautiously in shock, profound anemia, cachexia, hypertension, hypotension, peritonitis, cardiac decompensation, massive pleural effusion, increased intracranial pressure, infection, and in highly nervous patients.
• Saddle block contraindicated in cephalopelvic disproportion, placenta previa, abruptio placentae, intrauterine manipulation, and floating fetal head.
• Don't use cloudy, discolored, or crystallized solutions.
• Keep resuscitative equipment and drugs available.
• 10 times as strong as procaine HCl.
• Onset in 15 minutes; duration up to 3 hours.
• When cerebrospinal fluid is added to powdered drug or drug solution during spinal anesthesia, solution may be cloudy.
• Protect from light; store in refrigerator.

Italicized side effects are common or life-threatening.
*Liquid form contains alcohol.   **May contain tartrazine.

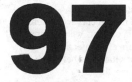

General anesthetics

droperidol
etomidate
fentanyl citrate with droperidol
ketamine hydrochloride
methohexital sodium
thiopental sodium

COMBINATION PRODUCTS
None.

---

droperidol
Inapsine♦
Pregnancy Category: C

MECHANISM OF ACTION
Acts at subcortical levels to produce
sedation.

INDICATIONS & DOSAGE
Premedication—
Adults: 2.5 to 10 mg (1 to 4 ml) I.M.
30 to 60 minutes preoperatively.
Children 2 to 12 years: 1 to 1.5 mg
(0.4 to 0.6 ml) per 20 to 25 lbs of
body weight I.M.
As induction agent—
Adults: 2.5 mg (1 ml) per 20 to 25 lbs
I.V. with analgesic and/or general an-
esthetic.
Children 2 to 12 years: 1 to 1.5 mg
(0.4 to 0.6 ml) per 20 to 25 lbs I.V.
Dose should be titrated.
Elderly, debilitated patients: initial
dose should be decreased.
*Maintenance dose in general anesthe-
sia—*1.25 to 2.5 mg (0.5 to 1 ml) I.V.

ADVERSE REACTIONS
CNS: extrapyramidal reactions (dystonia, akathisia), upward rotation of
eyes and oculogyric crises, extended
neck, flexed arms, fine tremor of
limbs, dizziness, chills or shivering,
facial sweating, restlessness.
CV: hypotension, tachycardia.

INTERACTIONS
None significant.

NURSING CONSIDERATIONS
• Use cautiously in elderly or debilitated patients and in patients with hypotension or other cardiovascular disease, impaired hepatic or renal function, or Parkinson's disease.
• Watch for extrapyramidal reactions.
Call doctor at once if any occur.
• Approved by FDA *only* for use preoperatively and during induction and
maintenance of anesthesia.
• A butyrophenone compound, related to haloperiodol; has greater tendency to cause extrapyramidal reactions than other antipsychotics.
• Keep intravenous fluids and vasopressors handy for hypotension.
• Monitor vital signs frequently; notify doctor of any changes immediately.
• Give intravenous injections slowly.
• Do not place patient in Trendelen-
burg position (that is, shock position);
severe hypotension and deeper anesthesia may result, causing respiratory
arrest.

---

etomidate
Amidate, Hypnomidate
Pregnancy Category: C

MECHANISM OF ACTION
Inhibits the firing rate of neurons within the ascending reticular-activating system.

INDICATIONS & DOSAGE
Induction of general anesthesia—
Adults and children over 10 years:
0.2 to 0.6 mg/kg I.V. over a period of 30 to 60 seconds.

ADVERSE REACTIONS
CNS: *myoclonic movements, averting movements, tonic movements, transient apnea, hyperventilation, hypoventilation.*
CV: hypertension, hypotension, tachycardia, bradycardia.
EENT: *eye movements,* laryngospasms.
Endocrine: inhibition of adrenal steroid production.
GI: nausea or vomiting following induction of anesthesia.
Local: *transient venous pain.*
Other: hiccups, snoring.

INTERACTIONS
None significant.

NURSING CONSIDERATIONS
• Should not be used during labor and delivery, including cesarean sections.
• Smaller increments of I.V. etomidate may be administered to adults during short operations to supplement subpotent anesthetic agents, such as nitrous oxide.
• Other commonly used preanesthesia drugs may be given before etomidate is used.
• Etomidate has a rapid onset of action (about 1 minute). Duration of effect is short (3 to 5 minutes).
• Transient muscle movements can be decreased by first administering 0.1 mg of fentanyl.
• Muscle movements seem more common in patients who feel transient venous pain after injection.
• Monitor vital signs before, during, and after anesthesia.
• Have resuscitative equipment and drugs ready. Maintain airway.
• Corticosteroid supplementation may be ordered to counteract reported inhibition of adrenal steroid production.
• Etomidate has a much lower incidence of cardiovascular and respiratory effects; therefore advantageous for inducing anesthesia in "high risk" surgical patients.

fentanyl citrate with droperidol
Controlled Substance Schedule II
Innovar (Each ml contains [in a 1:50 ratio] fentanyl 0.05 mg as a citrate and droperidol 2.5 mg.)
Pregnancy Category: C

MECHANISM OF ACTION
Acts as a CNS depressant to produce a general calming effect, reduced motor activity, and analgesia.

INDICATIONS & DOSAGE
Doses vary depending on application; use of other agents; and patient's age, body weight, and physical status.
Anesthesia—
Adults:
*Premedication—*0.5 to 2 ml I.M. 45 to 60 minutes before surgery.
*Adjunct to general anesthesia—*Induction: 1 ml/20 to 25 lb body weight by slow I.V. to produce neuroleptanalgesia.
Maintenance: not indicated as sole agent for maintenance of surgical anesthesia. Used in combination with other agents. To prevent excessive accumulation of the relatively long-acting droperidol component, fentanyl alone should be used in increments of

0.025 to 0.05 mg (0.5 to 1 ml) for maintenance of analgesia. However, during prolonged surgery, additional 0.5- to 1-ml amounts of Innovar may be given with caution.

Diagnostic procedures—0.5 to 2 ml I.M. 45 to 60 minutes before procedure. In prolonged procedure, give 0.5 to 1 ml I.V. with caution and without a general anesthetic.

Adjunct in regional anesthesia—1 to 2 ml I.M. or slow I.V.

Children:
Premedication—0.25 ml/20 lb body weight I.M. 45 to 60 minutes before surgery.

Adjunct to general anesthesia—0.5 ml/20 lb body weight (total combined dose for induction and maintenance). Following induction with Innovar, fentanyl alone in a dose of ¼ to ⅓ of adult dose should be used to avoid accumulation of droperidol. However, during prolonged surgery, additional amounts of Innovar may be administered with caution. Safety of use in children under 2 years has not been established.

ADVERSE REACTIONS
CNS: emergence delirium and hallucinations, postoperative drowsiness.
CV: vasodilation, *hypotension,* decreased pulmonary arterial pressure, bradycardia, or tachycardia.
EENT: blurred vision, *laryngospasms.*
GI: *nausea, vomiting.*
Respiratory: *respiratory depression, apnea,* or *arrest.*
Other: drug dependence, muscle rigidity, chills, *shivering,* twitching, diaphoresis.

INTERACTIONS
CNS depressants (such as barbiturates, tranquilizers, narcotics, and general anesthetics): additive or potentiating effect. Dosage should be reduced.
MAO inhibitors: severe and unpredictable potentiation of Innovar. Do not use together or within 2 weeks of MAO inhibitor therapy.

NURSING CONSIDERATIONS
• Contraindicated in intolerance to either component. Use with caution in patients with head injuries and increased intracranial pressure, chronic obstructive pulmonary disease, hepatic and renal dysfunction, bradyarrhythmias, and in elderly or debilitated patients.
• Hypotension is a common side effect. However, if blood pressure drops, also consider hypovolemia as a possible cause. Use appropriate parenteral fluids to help restore blood pressure.
• Vital signs should be monitored frequently.
• Be aware that respiratory depression, rigidity of respiratory muscles, and respiratory arrest can occur. Have narcotic antagonist and CPR equipment on hand.
• Maintain airway.
• Postoperative EEG pattern may return to normal slowly.
• Postoperatively, if narcotic analgesics are required, use initially in reduced doses, as low as ¼ to ⅓ those usually recommended.
• When Innovar is given for anesthesia induction, fentanyl (Sublimaze) should be used for maintenance analgesia during procedure.
• Premedication with Innovar has sometimes been associated with patient agitation and refusal of surgery. Administration of diazepam may relieve this.

---

ketamine hydrochloride
Ketalar♦
Pregnancy Category: C

MECHANISM OF ACTION
Interrupts association pathways in the brain, causing dissociative anesthesia,

a feeling of dissociation from the environment.

INDICATIONS & DOSAGE
Induce anesthesia for procedures, especially short-term diagnostic or surgical, not requiring skeletal muscle relaxation; before giving other general anesthetics or to supplement low-potency agents, such as nitrous oxide—
Adults and children: 1 to 4.5 mg/kg I.V., administered over 60 seconds; or 6.5 to 13 mg/kg I.M. To maintain anesthesia, repeat in increments of half to full initial dose.

ADVERSE REACTIONS
CNS: *tonic and clonic movements resembling convulsions, respiratory depression, apnea when administered too rapidly.*
CV: *increased blood pressure and pulse rate,* hypotension, bradycardia.
EENT: diplopia, nystagmus, slight increase in intraocular pressure, *laryngospasms, salivation.*
GI: mild anorexia, nausea, vomiting.
Skin: transient erythema, measles-like rash.
Other: *dream-like states, hallucinations, confusion, excitement,* irrational behavior, psychic abnormalities.

INTERACTIONS
Thyroid hormones: may elevate blood pressure and cause tachycardia. Give cautiously.

NURSING CONSIDERATIONS
• Contraindicated in patients with history of cerebrovascular accident; patients who would be endangered by a significant rise in blood pressure; and those with severe hypertension; severe cardiac decompensation; surgery of the pharynx, larynx, or bronchial tree (unless used with muscle relaxants). Use with caution in chronic alcoholism, alcohol-intoxicated patients, patients with cerebrospinal fluid pressure elevated before anesthesia.
• Discourage giving anything orally at least 6 hours before elective surgery.
• Because of rapid induction, patient should be physically supported during administration.
• Do not inject barbiturates and ketamine HCl from same syringe, as they are chemically incompatible.
• Monitor vital signs before, during, and after anesthesia.
• Check cardiac function in patients with hypertension or cardiac depression.
• Maintain airway.
• Resuscitation equipment should be available and ready for use.
• Start supportive respiration if respiratory depression occurs. Use mechanical support if possible rather than administering analeptics.
• Keep verbal, tactile, and visual stimulation at a minimum during recovery phase to reduce incidence of emergent reactions.
• Hallucinations and excitement can occur on emergence from anesthesia; they can be abated by administering diazepam.
• A potent hallucinogen that can readily produce dissociative anesthesia (patient feels detached from environment). Dissociative effect and hallucinatory side effects have made this a popular drug of abuse among young people.

---

methohexital sodium
Controlled Substance Schedule IV
Brevital Sodium, Brietal Sodium♦♦
Pregnancy Category: D

MECHANISM OF ACTION
Inhibits the firing rate of neurons within the ascending reticular-activating system.

Italicized side effects are common or life-threatening.
*Liquid form contains alcohol.   **May contain tartrazine.

INDICATIONS & DOSAGE

General anesthetic for short-term procedures (oral surgery, gynecologic and genitourinary examinations); reduction of fractures; before electroconvulsive therapy; for prolonged anesthesia when used with gaseous anesthetics—

Adults and children: 5 to 12 ml 1% solution (50 to 120 mg) I.V. at 1 ml/5 seconds. Dose required for induction may vary from 50 to 120 mg or more; average about 70 mg. Induction dose provides anesthesia for 5 to 7 minutes.

Maintenance—
Intermittent injection: 2 to 4 ml 1% solution (20 to 40 mg) q 4 to 7 minutes.
Continuous I.V. drip: administer 0.2% solution (1 drop/second).

ADVERSE REACTIONS

CNS: *muscular twitching,* headache, emergence delirium.
CV: *temporary hypotension, tachycardia,* circulatory depression, *peripheral vascular collapse.*
GI: excessive salivation, *nausea, vomiting.*
Skin: tissue necrosis with extravasation.
Local: pain at injection site, injury to nerves adjacent to injection site.
Respiratory: *laryngospasm, bronchospasm, respiratory depression, apnea.*
Other: hiccups, coughing, acute allergic reactions, *twitching.* Extended use may cause cumulative effect.

INTERACTIONS
None significant.

NURSING CONSIDERATIONS
• Contraindicated in severe hepatic dysfunction, hypersensitivity to barbiturates, or porphyria; in shock or impending shock; and in patients for whom general anesthetics would be hazardous. Use with caution in debilitated patients; in patients with asthma, respiratory obstruction, severe hypertension or hypotension, myocardial disease, congestive heart failure, severe anemia, or extreme obesity.
• Maintain pulmonary ventilation.
• Avoid extravascular or intraarterial injections.
• Monitor vital signs before, during, and after anesthesia.
• Have resuscitative equipment and drugs ready.
• Reduce postoperative nausea by having patient fast before administration.
• Incompatible with silicone; avoid contact with rubber stoppers or parts of syringes that have been treated with silicone.
• Incompatible with lactated Ringer's solution.
• Do not mix with acid solutions such as atropine sulfate.
• Solvents recommended are 5% glucose solution or isotonic (0.9%) sodium chloride solution instead of distilled water.
• Rate of flow must be individualized for each patient.
• Solutions may be stored and used as long as they remain clear and colorless. Solutions cannot be heated for sterilization.
• Has potential for abuse.

thiopental sodium
Controlled Substance Schedule III
Pentothal Sodium♦
(injection and rectal suspension)
Pregnancy Category: C

MECHANISM OF ACTION
Inhibits the firing rate of neurons within the ascending reticular-activating system.

INDICATIONS & DOSAGE
Induce anesthesia before administering other anesthetics—

210 to 280 mg (3 to 4 ml/kg) usually required for average adult (70 kg).
General anesthetic for short-term procedures—
Adults: 2 to 3 ml 2.5% solution (50 to 75 mg) administered I.V. only at intervals of 20 to 40 seconds, depending on reaction. Dose may be repeated with caution, if necessary.
Convulsive states following anesthesia—
75 to 125 mg (3 to 5 ml of 2.5% solution) immediately.
Psychiatric disorders (narcoanalysis, narcosynthesis)—
100 mg/minute (4 ml/minute 2.5% solution) until confusion occurs and before sleep.
Basal anesthesia by rectal administration—
Adults and children: administer up to 1 g/22.5 kg (50 lb) body weight, or 0.5 ml 10% solution/kg body weight. Maximum 1 to 1.5 g (children weighing 34 kg or more) and 3 to 4 g (adults weighing 91 kg or more).
Note: Thiopental is rarely administered rectally for basal sedation or anesthesia because of variable absorption from the rectum.

ADVERSE REACTIONS
CNS: *prolonged somnolence,* retrograde amnesia.
CV: *myocardial depression, arrhythmias.*
Skin: tissue necrosis with extravasation.
Respiratory: *respiratory depression (momentary apnea following each injection is typical), bronchospasm, laryngospasm.*
Local: pain at injection site.
Other: sneezing, coughing, *shivering.*

INTERACTIONS
None significant.

NURSING CONSIDERATIONS
• Contraindicated in absence of suitable veins for intravenous administra-

tion, hypersensitivity to barbiturates, status asthmaticus, porphyria, respiratory depression or obstruction, decompensated cardiac disease, severe anemia, hepatic cirrhosis, shock, renal dysfunction, myxedema.
• Give test dose (1 to 3 ml 2.5% solution) to assess reaction to drug.
• When used as general anesthetic, give atropine sulfate as premedication to diminish laryngeal reflexes and to prevent laryngeal spasm.
• Have resuscitative equipment and oxygen ready. Maintain airway.
• Avoid extravasation.
• Monitor vital signs before, during, and after anesthesia.
• Solutions of atropine sulfate, *d*-tubocurarine, or succinylcholine may be given concurrently.
• Do not heat solutions for sterilization. Solutions should be used within 24 hours.
• Has potential for abuse.

98

Vitamins and minerals

vitamin A
vitamin B complex
  cyanocobalamin (B_{12})
  folic acid (B_9)
  hydroxocobalamin (B_{12a})
  leucovorin calcium
    (citrovorum factor or
    folinic acid)
  niacin (B_3, nicotinic acid)
  niacinamide (nicotinamide)
  pyridoxine hydrochloride (B_6)
  riboflavin (B_2)
  thiamine hydrochloride (B_1)
vitamin C
  ascorbic acid
vitamin D
  cholecalciferol (D_3)
  ergocalciferol (D_2)
vitamin E
vitamin K analogs
  menadione/menadiol sodium
    diphosphate (K_3)
  phytonadione (K_1)
multivitamins
sodium fluoride
trace elements
  chromium
  copper
  iodine (as iodide)
  manganese
  selenium
  zinc
zinc sulfate

COMBINATION PRODUCTS

B complex vitamins
B complex vitamins with iron
B complex with vitamin C
B vitamin combinations
Calcium and vitamin products
Fluoride with vitamins

Geriatric supplements with multivitamins and minerals
Miscellaneous vitamins and minerals
Multivitamins
Multivitamins and minerals with hormones
Multivitamins with B_{12}
Vitamin A and D combinations

---

vitamin A

Acon, Aquasol A♦, Natola
Pregnancy Category: A (X if >
RDA)

MECHANISM OF ACTION
Coenzyme necessary for retinal function, bone growth, and differentiation of epithelial tissues.

INDICATIONS & DOSAGE
Severe vitamin A deficiency with xerophthalmia—
Adults and children over 8 years:
500,000 IU P.O. daily for 3 days, then 50,000 IU P.O. daily for 14 days, then maintenance with 10,000 to 20,000 IU P.O. daily for 2 months, followed by adequate dietary nutrition and RDA vitamin A supplements.
Severe vitamin A deficiency—
Adults and children over 8 years:
100,000 IU P.O. or I.M. daily for 3 days, then 50,000 IU P.O. or I.M. daily for 14 days, then maintenance with 10,000 to 20,000 IU P.O. daily for 2 months, followed by adequate dietary nutrition and RDA vitamin A supplements.
Children 1 to 8 years: 17,500 to 35,000 IU I.M. daily for 10 days.

Infants under 1 year: 7,500 to 15,000 IU I.M. daily for 10 days.
Maintenance only—
Children 4 to 8 years: 15,000 IU I.M. daily for 2 months, then adequate dietary nutrition and RDA vitamin A supplements.
Children under 4 years: 10,000 IU I.M. daily for 2 months, then adequate dietary nutrition and RDA vitamin A supplements.

ADVERSE REACTIONS
Side effects are usually seen only with toxicity (hypervitaminosis A).
Blood: hypoplastic anemia, leukopenia.
CNS: irritability, headache, increased intracranial pressure, fatigue, lethargy, malaise.
EENT: miosis, papilledema, exophthalmos.
GI: anorexia, epigastric pain, diarrhea.
GU: hypomenorrhea.
Hepatic: jaundice, hepatomegaly.
Skin: alopecia; drying, cracking, scaling of skin; pruritus; lip fissures; massive desquamation; increased pigmentation; night sweating.
Other: skeletal—slow growth, decalcification of bone, fractures, hyperostosis, painful periostitis, premature closure of epiphyses, migratory arthralgia, cortical thickening over the radius and tibia, bulging fontanelles; splenomegaly.

INTERACTIONS
Mineral oil, cholestyramine resin: reduced GI absorption of fat-soluble vitamins. If needed, give mineral oil at bedtime.

NURSING CONSIDERATIONS
• Oral administration contraindicated in presence of malabsorption syndrome; if malabsorption is due to inadequate bile secretion, oral route may be used with concurrent administration of bile salts (dehydrocholic acid). Also contraindicated in hypervitaminosis A. Intravenous administration contraindicated except for special water-miscible forms intended for infusion with large parenteral volumes. Intravenous push of vitamin A of any type is also contraindicated (anaphylaxis or anaphylactoid reactions and death have resulted).
• *Caution:* Evaluate intake from fortified foods, dietary supplements, self-administered drugs, and prescription drug sources.
• In pregnant women, avoid doses exceeding recommended daily allowance (RDA).
• To avoid toxicity, discourage patient self-administration of megavitamin doses without specific indications. Also stress that the patient should not share prescribed vitamins with family or others. If family member feels vitamin therapy may be of value, have him contact his doctor.
• Watch for side effects if dosage is high.
• Acute toxicity has resulted from single doses of 25,000 IU/kg of body weight; 350,000 IU in infants and over 2,000,000 IU in adults have also proved acutely toxic.
• Chronic toxicity in infants (3 to 6 months) has resulted from doses of 18,500 IU daily for 1 to 3 months. In adults, chronic toxicity has resulted from doses of 50,000 IU daily for over 8 months; 500,000 IU daily for 2 months; and 1,000,000 IU daily for 3 days.
• Monitor patient closely during vitamin A therapy for skin disorders since high dosages may induce chronic toxicity.
• Liquid preparations available if nasogastric administration is necessary. May be mixed with cereal or fruit juice.
• Record eating and bowel habits. Report abnormalities to doctor.
• Adequate vitamin A absorption requires suitable protein intake, bile

---

Italicized side effects are common or life-threatening.
*Liquid form contains alcohol.   **May contain tartrazine.

(give supplemental salts if necessary), concurrent RDA doses of vitamin E, and zinc (multivitamins usually supply zinc, but supplements may be necessary in long-term total parenteral nutrition).

• Absorption is fastest and most complete with water-miscible preparations, intermediate with emulsions, and slowest with oil suspensions.

• In severe hepatic dysfunction, diabetes, and hypothyroidism, use vitamin A rather than carotenes for vitamin therapy because the vitamin itself is more easily absorbed and the diseases adversely affect conversion of carotenes into vitamin A. If carotenes are prescribed, dosage should be doubled.

• Because of the potential for additive toxicity, vitamin supplements containing vitamin A should be used cautiously in patients taking isotretinoin (Accutane).

• Protect from light and heat.

cyanocobalamin (vitamin B₁₂)
Anacobin♦♦, Bedoce, Bedoz♦♦, Berubigen, Betalin-12, Crystimin, Cyanabin♦♦, Cyanocobalamin, Cyano-Gel, DBH-B₁₂, Dodex, Kaybovite, Pernavite, Poyamin, Redisol, Rubesol, Rubion♦♦, Rubramin♦, Sigamine, Vibedoz

hydroxocobalamin (vitamin B₁₂ₐ)
Alpha Redisol, Alpha-Ruvite, Codroxomin, Droxomin, Neo-Betalin 12, Rubesol-LA
Pregnancy Category: A (C if > RDA)

MECHANISM OF ACTION
Coenzyme for various metabolic functions. Necessary for cell replication and hematopoiesis.

INDICATIONS & DOSAGE
Vitamin B₁₂ deficiency due to inadequate diet, subtotal gastrectomy, or any other condition, disorder, or disease except malabsorption related to pernicious anemia or other gastrointestinal disease—
Adults: 25 mcg P.O. daily as dietary supplement, or 30 to 100 mcg S.C. or I.M. daily for 5 to 10 days, depending on severity of deficiency. Maintenance dose: 100 to 200 mcg I.M. once monthly. For subsequent prophylaxis, advise adequate nutrition and daily RDA vitamin B₁₂ supplements.
Children: 1 mcg P.O. daily as dietary supplement, or 1 to 30 mcg S.C. or I.M. daily for 5 to 10 days, depending on severity of deficiency. Maintenance: at least 60 mcg/month I.M. or S.C. For subsequent prophylaxis, advise adequate nutrition and daily RDA vitamin B₁₂ supplements.
Pernicious anemia or vitamin B₁₂ malabsorption—
Adults: initially, 100 to 1,000 mcg I.M. daily for 2 weeks, then 100 to 1,000 mcg I.M. once monthly for life. If neurologic complications are present, follow initial therapy with 100 to 1,000 mcg I.M. once every 2 weeks before starting monthly regimen.
Children: 1,000 to 5,000 mcg I.M. or S.C. given over 2 or more weeks in 100-mcg increments; then 60 mcg I.M. or S.C. monthly for life.
Methylmalonic aciduria—
Neonates: 1,000 mcg I.M. daily for 11 days with a protein-restricted diet.
Diagnostic test for vitamin B₁₂ deficiency without concealing folate deficiency in patients with megaloblastic anemias—
Adults and children: 1 mcg I.M. daily for 10 days with diet low in vitamin B₁₂ and folate. Reticulocytosis between days 3 and 10 confirms diagnosis of vitamin B₁₂ deficiency.
Schilling test flushing dose—
Adults and children: 1,000 mcg

I.M. in a single dose.

ADVERSE REACTIONS
CV: peripheral vascular thrombosis.
GI: transient diarrhea.
Skin: itching, transitory exanthema, urticaria.
Local: pain, burning at S.C. or I.M. injection sites.
Other: *anaphylaxis,* anaphylactoid reactions.

INTERACTIONS
Neomycin, colchicine, para-aminosalicylic acid and salts, chloramphenicol: malabsorption of vitamin B_{12}. Don't use together.

NURSING CONSIDERATIONS
• Parenteral administration contraindicated in hypersensitivity to vitamin B_{12} or cobalt. Alternate use of large oral doses of vitamin B_{12} is controversial and should not be considered routine; combined with intrinsic factor increases risk of hypersensitive reactions and should be avoided. Therapeutic dose contraindicated before proper diagnosis; vitamin B_{12} therapy may mask folate deficiency.
• I.V. administration may cause anaphylactic reactions. Use cautiously and only if other routes are ruled out.
• Use cautiously in anemic patients with coexisting cardiac, pulmonary, or hypertensive disease; in patients with early Leber's disease; in patients with severe vitamin B_{12}–dependent deficiencies, especially those receiving cardiotonic glycosides (monitor closely the first 2 to 3 days for hypokalemia, fluid overload, pulmonary edema, congestive heart failure, and hypertension); and in patients with gouty conditions (monitor serum uric acid levels for hyperuricemia).
• Don't mix parenteral liquids in same syringe with other medication.
• Protect from light and heat.
• Infection, tumors, or renal, hepatic, and other debilitating diseases may reduce therapeutic response.
• Deficiencies more common in strict vegetarians and their breast-fed infants.
• Stress need for patients with pernicious anemia to return for monthly injections. Although total body stores may last 3 to 6 years, anemia will recur if not treated monthly.
• May cause false-positive intrinsic factor antibody test.
• Hydroxocobalamin is approved for I.M. use only. Only advantage of hydroxocobalamin over vitamin B_{12} is longer duration.
• 50% to 98% of injected dose may appear in urine within 48 hours. Major portion is excreted within first 8 hours.
• Closely monitor serum potassium levels for first 48 hours. Give potassium if necessary.
• Physically incompatible with dextrose solutions, alkaline or strongly acidic solutions, oxidizing and reducing agents, and many other drugs.

folic acid (vitamin B₉)
Folvite♦, Novofolacid♦♦
Pregnancy Category: A (C if > RDA)

MECHANISM OF ACTION
Necessary for normal erythropoiesis and nucleoprotein synthesis.

INDICATIONS & DOSAGE
Megaloblastic or macrocytic anemia secondary to folic acid or other nutritional deficiency, hepatic disease, alcoholism, intestinal obstruction, excessive hemolysis—
Pregnant and lactating women: 0.8 mg P.O., S.C., or I.M. daily.
Adults and children over 4 years: 1 mg P.O., S.C., or I.M. daily for 4 to 5 days. After anemia secondary to folic acid deficiency is corrected, proper diet and RDA supplements are neces-

---

Italicized side effects are common or life-threatening.
*Liquid form contains alcohol.   **May contain tartrazine.

sary to prevent recurrence.
Children under 4 years: up to 0.3
mg P.O., S.C., or I.M. daily.
Prevention of megaloblastic anemia of pregnancy and fetal damage—
Women: 1 mg P.O., S.C., or I.M. daily throughout pregnancy.
Nutritional supplement—
Adults: 0.1 mg P.O., S.C., or I.M. daily.
Children: 0.05 mg P.O. daily.
Treatment of tropical sprue—
Adults: 3 to 15 mg P.O. daily.
Test of megaloblastic anemia patients to detect folic acid deficiency without masking pernicious anemia—
Adults and children: 0.1 to 0.2 mg P.O. or I.M. for 10 days while maintaining a diet low in folate and vitamin B_{12}.
(Reticulosis, reversion to normoblastic hematopoiesis, and return to normal hemoglobin indicate folic acid deficiency.)

ADVERSE REACTIONS
Skin: allergic reactions (rash, pruritus, erythema).
Other: *allergic bronchospasms*, general malaise.

INTERACTIONS
Chloramphenicol: antagonism of folic acid. Monitor for decreased folic acid effect. Use together cautiously.

NURSING CONSIDERATIONS
• Contraindicated in normocytic, refractory, or aplastic anemias; as sole agent in treatment of pernicious anemia (since it may mask neurologic effects); in treatment of methotrexate, pyrimethamine, or trimethoprim overdose; and in undiagnosed anemia (since it may mask pernicious anemia).
• Patients with small-bowel resections and intestinal malabsorption may require parenteral administration routes.
• Don't mix with other medications

in same syringe for I.M. injections.
• Protect from light and heat.
• May use concurrent folic acid and vitamin B_{12} therapy if supported by diagnosis.
• Proper nutrition is necessary to prevent recurrence of anemia.
• Peak folate activity occurs in the blood in 30 to 60 minutes.
• Patients with pernicious anemia should avoid multivitamins containing folic acid.
• Hematologic response to folic acid in patients receiving chloramphenicol concurrently with folic acid should be carefully monitored.

leucovorin calcium (citrovorum factor or folinic acid)
Calcium Folinate, Wellcovorin
Pregnancy Category: C

MECHANISM OF ACTION
A reduced form of folic acid that is readily converted to other folic acid derivatives.

INDICATIONS & DOSAGE
Overdose of folic acid antagonist—
Adults and children: P.O., I.M., or I.V. dose equivalent to the weight of the antagonist given.
Leucovorin rescue after high methotrexate dose in treatment of malignancy—
Adults and children: dose at doctor's discretion within 6 to 36 hours of last dose of methotrexate.
Toxic effects of methotrexate used to treat severe psoriasis—
Adults and children: 4 to 8 mg I.M. 2 hours after methotrexate dose.
Hematologic toxicity due to pyrimethamine therapy—
Adults and children: 5 mg P.O. or I.M. daily.
Hematologic toxicity due to trimethoprim therapy—
Adults and children: 400 mcg to 5

mg P.O. or I.M. daily.
Megaloblastic anemia due to congenital enzyme deficiency—
Adults and children: 3 to 6 mg I.M. daily, then 1 mg P.O. daily for life.
Folate-deficient megaloblastic anemias—
Adults and children: up to 1 mg of leucovorin I.M daily. Duration of treatment depends on hematologic response.

ADVERSE REACTIONS
Skin: allergic reactions (rash, pruritus, erythema).
Other: *allergic bronchospasms.*

INTERACTIONS
None significant.

NURSING CONSIDERATIONS
• Contraindicated in treatment of undiagnosed anemia, since it may mask pernicious anemia. Use cautiously in pernicious anemia; a hemolytic remission may occur while neurologic manifestations remain progressive.
• Do not confuse leucovorin (folinic acid) with folic acid.
• Follow leucovorin rescue schedule and protocol closely to maximize therapeutic response. Generally, leucovorin should not be administered simultaneously with systemic methotrexate.
• Treat overdosage of folic acid antagonists; administer within 1 hour if possible; usually ineffective after 4-hour delay.
• Protect from light and heat, especially reconstituted parenteral preparations.
• Since allergic reactions have been reported with folic acid, the possibility of allergic reactions to leucovorin should be considered.

niacin
(vitamin B₃, nicotinic acid)
Niac, Nico-400, Nicobid, Nicolar**, Nico-Span

niacinamide (nicotinamide)
Pregnancy Category: A (C if > RDA)

MECHANISM OF ACTION
Necessary for lipid metabolism, tissue respiration, and glycogenolysis. Also (niacin only) decreases synthesis of low-density lipoproteins and inhibits lipolysis in adipose tissue.

INDICATIONS & DOSAGE
Pellagra—
Adults: 10 to 20 mg P.O., S.C., I.M., or I.V. infusion daily, depending on severity of niacin deficiency. Maximum daily dose recommended, 500 mg; should be divided into 10 doses, 50 mg each.
Children: up to 300 mg P.O. or 100 mg I.V. infusion daily, depending on severity of niacin deficiency.
After symptoms subside, advise adequate nutrition and RDA supplements to prevent recurrence.
Peripheral vascular disease and circulatory disorders—
Adults: 250 to 800 mg P.O. daily in divided doses.
Adjunctive treatment of hyperlipidemias, especially associated with hypercholesterolemia—
Adults: 1.5 to 3 g daily in 3 divided doses with or after meals, increased at intervals to 6 g daily.

ADVERSE REACTIONS
Most side effects are dose-dependent.
CNS: dizziness, transient headache.
CV: *excessive peripheral vasodilation (especially niacin).*
GI: *nausea, vomiting, diarrhea,* possible activation of peptic ulcer, epigastric or substernal pain.
Hepatic: hepatic dysfunction.

Italicized side effects are common or life-threatening.
*Liquid form contains alcohol.   **May contain tartrazine.

Metabolic: hyperglycemia, hyperuricemia.
Skin: *flushing,* pruritus, dryness.

INTERACTIONS
Antihypertensive drugs of the sympathetic blocking type: may have an additive vasodilating effect and cause postural hypotension. Use together cautiously. Warn patient about postural hypotension.

NURSING CONSIDERATIONS
• Contraindicated in hepatic dysfunction, active peptic ulcer disease, severe hypotension, arterial hemorrhage. Use with caution in patients with gallbladder disease, diabetes mellitus, or gout.
• Monitor hepatic function and blood glucose early in therapy.
• Give with meals to minimize GI side effects.
• Aspirin may reduce the flushing response to niacin.
• Timed-release niacin or niacinamide may avoid excessive flushing effects with large doses. Give slow I.V. (no faster than 2 mg/minute). Explain harmlessness of flushing syndrome to ease patient's mind.
• Stress that medication used to treat hyperlipoproteinemia or to dilate peripheral vessels is not "just a vitamin." Explain importance of adhering to therapeutic regimen.

---

pyridoxine hydrochloride (vitamin B₆)
Bee six, Hexa-Betalin♦, Hexacrest
Pregnancy Category: A (C if > RDA)

MECHANISM OF ACTION
Acts as coenzyme for various metabolic functions. Required for amino acid metabolism.

INDICATIONS & DOSAGE
Dietary vitamin B₆ deficiency—

Adults: 10 to 20 mg P.O., I.M., or I.V. daily for 3 weeks, then 2 to 5 mg daily as a supplement to a proper diet.
Children: 100 mg P.O., I.M., or I.V. to correct deficiency, then an adequate diet with supplementary RDA doses to prevent recurrence.
Seizures related to vitamin B₆ deficiency or dependency—
Adults and children: 100 mg I.M. or I.V. in single dose.
Vitamin B₆–responsive anemias or dependency syndrome (inborn errors of metabolism)—
Adults: up to 600 mg P.O., I.M., or I.V. daily until symptoms subside, then 50 mg daily for life.
Children: 100 mg I.M. or I.V., then 2 to 10 mg I.M. or 10 to 100 mg P.O. daily.
Prevention of vitamin B₆ deficiency during isoniazid therapy—
Adults: 25 to 50 mg P.O. daily.
Children: at least 0.5 to 1.5 mg daily.
Infants: at least 0.1 to 0.5 mg daily.
If neurologic symptoms develop in pediatric patients, increase dosage as necessary.
Treatment of vitamin B₆ deficiency secondary to isoniazid—
Adults: 100 mg P.O. daily for 3 weeks, then 50 mg daily.
Children: titrate dosages.

ADVERSE REACTIONS
CNS: drowsiness, paresthesias.

INTERACTIONS
None significant.

NURSING CONSIDERATIONS
• Contraindicated in hypersensitivity to parenteral pyridoxine and in doses larger than 5 mg for patients also receiving levodopa. Caution patient to check dosage, especially in multivitamins.
• Protect from light. Do not use injection solution if it contains a precipitate. Slight darkening is acceptable.
• Excessive protein intake increases

daily pyridoxine requirements.
• If sodium bicarbonate is required to control acidosis in isoniazid toxicity, do not mix in same syringe with pyridoxine.
• If prescribed for maintenance therapy to prevent deficiency recurrence, stress importance of compliance and of good nutrition. Explain that pyridoxine in combination therapy with isoniazid has a specific therapeutic purpose and is not "just a vitamin." Emphasize need for adhering to therapeutic regimen.
• Patients receiving levodopa alone (not with carbidopa) shouldn't take pyridoxine.
• Used to treat seizures and coma due to acute isoniazid overdosage. Dosage equal to amount of isoniazid ingested.

riboflavin (vitamin B₂)
Pregnancy Category: A (C if > RDA)

MECHANISM OF ACTION
Converted to two other coenzymes that are necessary for normal tissue respiration.

INDICATIONS & DOSAGE
Riboflavin deficiency or adjunct to thiamine treatment for polyneuritis or cheilosis secondary to pellagra—
Adults and children over 12 years: 5 to 50 mg P.O., S.C., I.M., or I.V. daily, depending on severity.
Children under 12 years: 2 to 10 mg P.O., S.C., I.M., or I.V. daily, depending on severity.
For maintenance, increase nutritional intake and supplement with vitamin B complex.

ADVERSE REACTIONS
GU: high doses make urine bright yellow.

INTERACTIONS
None significant.

NURSING CONSIDERATIONS
• Protect from light.
• Stress proper nutritional habits to prevent recurrence of deficiency.
• Riboflavin deficiency usually accompanies other vitamin B complex deficiencies and may require multivitamin therapy.
• Since food increases absorption of riboflavin, encourage patient to take with meals.

thiamine hydrochloride (vitamin B₁)
Apatate Drops, Betaline S*, Revitonus◆◆, Thia
Pregnancy Category: A (C if > RDA)

MECHANISM OF ACTION
Combines with ATP to form a coenzyme necessary for carbohydrate metabolism.

INDICATIONS & DOSAGE
Beriberi—
Adults: 10 to 500 mg, depending on severity, I.M. t.i.d. for 2 weeks, followed by dietary correction and multivitamin supplement containing 5 to 10 mg thiamine daily for 1 month.
Children: 10 to 50 mg, depending on severity, I.M. daily for several weeks with adequate dietary intake.
Anemia secondary to thiamine deficiency; polyneuritis secondary to alcoholism, pregnancy, or pellagra—
Adults: 100 mg P.O. daily.
Children: 10 to 50 mg P.O. daily in divided doses.
Wernicke's encephalopathy—
Adults: up to 500 mg to 1 g I.V. for crisis therapy, followed by 100 mg b.i.d. for maintenance.
"Wet beriberi," with myocardial failure—
Adults and children: 100 to 500 mg I.V. for emergency treatment.

Italicized side effects are common or life-threatening.
*Liquid form contains alcohol.   **May contain tartrazine.

ADVERSE REACTIONS
CNS: restlessness.
CV: *hypotension after rapid I.V. injection,* angioneurotic edema, cyanosis.
EENT: tightness of throat (allergic reaction).
GI: nausea, hemorrhage, diarrhea.
Skin: feeling of warmth, pruritus, urticaria, sweating.
Other: *anaphylactic reactions,* weakness, pulmonary edema.

INTERACTIONS
None significant.

NURSING CONSIDERATIONS
• Contraindicated in hypersensitivity to thiamine products. I.V. push is contraindicated, except when treating life-threatening myocardial failure in "wet beriberi." Use with caution in I.V. administration of large doses; skin-test patients with history of hypersensitivity before therapy. Have epinephrine on hand to treat anaphylaxis should it occur after a large parenteral dose.
• Thiamine malabsorption is most likely in alcoholism, cirrhosis, or GI disease.
• Use parenteral administration only when P.O. route is not feasible.
• Clinically significant deficiency can occur in approximately 3 weeks of totally thiamine-free diet. Thiamine deficiency usually requires concurrent treatment for multiple deficiencies.
• Doses larger than 30 mg t.i.d. may not be fully utilized. After tissue saturation with thiamine, it is excreted in urine as pyrimidine.
• If beriberi occurs in a breast-fed infant, both mother and child should be treated with thiamine.
• Unstable in alkaline solutions; should not be used with materials that yield alkaline solutions.

ascorbic acid (vitamin C)
Ascorbicap, Ascorbinccd, Best-C, Cecon, Cemill, Cenolate, Cetane, Cevalin, Cevi-Bid, Ce-Vi-Sol♦*, Cevita, C-Long, C-Syrup-500, Redoxon♦♦, Saro-C, Solucap C, Vitacee, Viterra C
Pregnancy Category: A (C if > RDA)

MECHANISM OF ACTION
Necessary for collagen formation and tissue repair; involved in oxidation-reduction reactions throughout the body.

INDICATIONS & DOSAGE
Frank and subclinical scurvy—
Adults: 100 mg to 2 g, depending on severity, P.O., S.C., I.M., or I.V. daily, then at least 50 mg daily for maintenance.
Children: 100 to 300 mg, depending on severity, P.O., S.C., I.M., or I.V. daily, then at least 35 mg daily for maintenance.
Infants: 50 to 100 mg P.O., I.M., I.V., or S.C. daily.
Extensive burns, delayed fracture or wound healing, postoperative wound healing, severe febrile or chronic disease states—
Adults: 200 to 500 mg S.C., I.M., or I.V. daily.
Children: 100 to 200 mg P.O., S.C., I.M., or I.V. daily.
Prevention of vitamin C deficiency in those with poor nutritional habits or increased requirements—
Adults: at least 45 to 50 mg P.O., S.C., I.M., or I.V. daily.
Pregnant and lactating women: at least 60 mg P.O., S.C., I.M., or I.V. daily.
Children: at least 40 mg P.O., S.C., I.M., or I.V. daily.
Infants: at least 35 mg P.O., S.C., I.M., or I.V. daily.
Potentiation of methenamine in urine

acidification—
Adults: 4 to 12 g daily in divided doses.
Before gastrectomy—
Adults: 1 g daily for 4 to 7 days.

ADVERSE REACTIONS
CNS: faintness or dizziness with fast I.V. administration.
GI: diarrhea, epigastric burning.
GU: acid urine, oxaluria, renal calculi, renal failure.
Skin: discomfort at injection site.

INTERACTIONS
None significant.

NURSING CONSIDERATIONS
• Use cautiously in G-6-PD deficiency.
• Administer I.V. infusion cautiously in patients with renal insufficiency.
• Avoid rapid I.V. administration.
• Protect solution from light.

---

vitamin D
(cholecalciferol: vitamin D₃; ergocalciferol: vitamin D₂)
Calciferol♦, Deltalin, Drisdol♦,
Radiostol♦♦, Radiostol Forte♦♦
Pregnancy Category: A (D if >
RDA)

MECHANISM OF ACTION
Promotes absorption and utilization of calcium and phosphate. Helps to regulate calcium concentration.

INDICATIONS & DOSAGE
Rickets and other vitamin D deficiency diseases; renal osteodystrophy—
Adults: 12,000 IU P.O. or I.M. daily initially, increased as indicated by response up to 500,000 IU daily in most cases and up to 800,000 IU daily for vitamin D–resistant rickets.
Children: 1,500 to 5,000 IU P.O. or I.M. daily for 2 to 4 weeks, repeated after 2 weeks, if necessary. Alternatively, a single dose of 600,000 IU.

Monitor serum calcium daily to guide dosage. After correction of deficiency, maintenance includes adequate dietary nutrition and RDA supplements.
Hypoparathyroidism—
Adults and children: 50,000 to 200,000 IU P.O. or I.M. daily, with 4-g calcium supplement.

ADVERSE REACTIONS
Side effects listed are usually seen in vitamin D toxicity only.
CNS: headache, dizziness, ataxia, weakness, somnolence, decreased libido, overt psychosis, convulsions.
CV: calcifications of soft tissues, including the heart.
EENT: dry mouth, metallic taste, rhinorrhea, conjunctivitis (calcific), photophobia, tinnitus.
GI: anorexia, nausea, constipation, diarrhea.
GU: polyuria, albuminuria, hypercalciuria, nocturia, impaired renal function, renal calculi.
Metabolic: hypercalcemia, hyperphosphatemia.
Skin: pruritus.
Other: bone and muscle pain, bone demineralization, weight loss.

INTERACTIONS
Mineral oil, cholestyramine resin: inhibited GI absorption of oral vitamin D. Space doses. Use together cautiously.

NURSING CONSIDERATIONS
• Contraindicated in hypercalcemia, hypervitaminosis A, renal osteodystrophy with hyperphosphatemia.
• If I.V. route is necessary, use only water-miscible solutions intended for dilution in large-volume parenterals. Use cautiously in cardiac patients, especially if they are receiving cardiotonic glycosides.
• Monitor eating and bowel habits; dry mouth, nausea, vomiting, metallic taste, and constipation can be early

---

Italicized side effects are common or life-threatening.
*Liquid form contains alcohol.   **May contain tartrazine.

signs of toxicity.
• Patients with hyperphosphatemia require dietary phosphate restrictions and binding agents to avoid metastatic calcifications and renal calculi.
• When high therapeutic doses are used, frequent serum and urine calcium, potassium, and urea determinations should be made.
• Malabsorption due to inadequate bile or hepatic dysfunction may require addition of exogenous bile salts to oral vitamin D.
• I.M. injection of vitamin D dispersed in oil is preferable in patients who are unable to absorb the oral form.
• This vitamin is fat soluble. Warn patient of the dangers of increasing dosage without consulting the doctor.
• Doses of 60,000 units per day can cause hypercalcemia.
• Patients taking vitamin D should restrict their intake of magnesium-containing antacids.

vitamin E
Aquasol E♦*, D-Alpha-E**, Daltose♦♦, Eprolin, Epsilan-M, Hy-E-Plex, Kell-E, Lethopherol, Maxi-E, Pertropin, Solucap E, Tocopher-Caps
Pregnancy Category: A (C if > RDA)

MECHANISM OF ACTION
Acts as a cofactor and an antioxidant.

INDICATIONS & DOSAGE
Vitamin E deficiency in premature infants and in patients with impaired fat absorption—
Adults: 60 to 75 IU, depending on severity, P.O. or I.M. daily. Maximum 300 IU daily.
Children: 1 mg equivalent/0.6 g of dietary unsaturated fat P.O. or I.M. daily.

ADVERSE REACTIONS
None reported.

INTERACTIONS
Mineral oil, cholestyramine resin: inhibited GI absorption of oral vitamin E. Space doses. Use together cautiously.

NURSING CONSIDERATIONS
• Water-miscible forms more completely absorbed in GI tract than other forms.
• Adequate bile is essential for absorption.
• Requirements increase with rise in dietary polyunsaturated acids.
• May protect other vitamins against oxidation.
• Used for a variety of disorders with mixed successes and failures. Dosages not established.
• Megadoses can cause thrombophlebitis.
• This vitamin is fat soluble. Discourage patient from self-medication with megadoses, as they can cause undesirable side effects.

menadione/menadiol sodium diphosphate (vitamin K₃)
Synkavite♦♦, Synkayvite
Pregnancy Category: C (X near term)

MECHANISM OF ACTION
Promotes hepatic formation of active prothrombin.

INDICATIONS & DOSAGE
Hypoprothrombinemia secondary to vitamin K malabsorption or drug therapy, or when oral administration is desired and bile secretion is inadequate—
Adults: 5 to 15 mg menadiol sodium diphosphate P.O. or parenterally, titrated to patient's requirements.

ADVERSE REACTIONS
CNS: headache, kernicterus.
GI: nausea, vomiting.
Skin: allergic rash, pruritus, urticaria.
Local: pain, hematoma at injection site.

INTERACTIONS
Mineral oil, cholestyramine resin: inhibited GI absorption of oral vitamin K. Space doses. Use together cautiously.

NURSING CONSIDERATIONS
• Contraindicated in treatment of hereditary hypoprothrombinemia (because vitamin K_3 can paradoxically worsen it); in patients with hepatocellular disease, unless it is caused by biliary obstruction; in treatment of heparin-induced bleeding; and during last weeks of pregnancy to avoid toxic reactions in newborns. Use cautiously in G6PD deficiency to avoid hemolysis. In severe bleeding, do not delay other measures, such as giving fresh frozen plasma or whole blood. Use large doses cautiously in severe hepatic disease.
• Failure to respond to vitamin K_3 may indicate coagulation defects.
• Excessive use of vitamin K_3 may temporarily defeat oral anticoagulant therapy. Higher doses of oral anticoagulant or interim use of heparin may be required.
• Protect parenteral products from light.
• When I.V. route must be used, rate shouldn't exceed 1 mg/minute.
• Effects of I.V. injections are more rapid but shorter lived than S.C. or I.M. injections.
• Monitor prothrombin time to determine dosage effectiveness.
• Observe for signs of side effects and report them to doctor.
• Use caution in handling bulk menadione powder. It is irritating to the skin and the respiratory tract.

• Leafy vegetables are high in vitamin K content and may alter warfarin needs.
• This vitamin is fat soluble.

phytonadione (vitamin K₁)
AquaMEPHYTON♦, Konakion♦, Mephyton
Pregnancy Category: C

MECHANISM OF ACTION
Promotes hepatic formation of active prothrombin.

INDICATIONS & DOSAGE
Hypoprothrombinemia secondary to vitamin K malabsorption, drug therapy, or excess vitamin A—
Adults: 2 to 25 mg, depending on severity, P.O. or parenterally, repeated and increased up to 50 mg, if necessary.
Children: 5 to 10 mg P.O. or parenterally.
Infants: 2 mg P.O. or parenterally. I.V. injection rate for children and infants should not exceed 3 mg/m²/minute or a total of 5 mg.
Hypoprothrombinemia secondary to effect of oral anticoagulants—
Adults: 2.5 to 10 mg P.O., S.C., or I.M., based on prothrombin time, repeated, if necessary, 12 to 48 hours after oral dose or 6 to 8 hours after parenteral dose. In emergency, give 10 to 50 mg slow I.V., rate not to exceed 1 mg/minute, repeated q 4 hours, as needed.
Prevention of hemorrhagic disease in neonates—
Neonates: 0.5 to 1 mg S.C. or I.M. immediately after birth, repeated in 6 to 8 hours, if needed, especially if mother received oral anticoagulants or long-term anticonvulsant therapy during pregnancy.
Differentiation between hepatocellular disease or biliary obstruction as source of hypoprothrombinemia—

Adults and children: 10 mg I.M. or S.C.

Prevention of hypoprothrombinemia related to vitamin K deficiency in long-term parenteral nutrition—
Adults: 5 to 10 mg S.C. or I.M. weekly.
Children: 2 to 5 mg S.C. or I.M. weekly.

Prevention of hypoprothrombinemia in infants receiving less than 0.1 mg/liter vitamin K in breast milk or milk substitutes—
Infants: 1 mg S.C. or I.M. monthly.

ADVERSE REACTIONS
CNS: dizziness, convulsive movement.
CV: transient hypotension after I.V. administration, rapid and weak pulse, cardiac irregularities.
GI: nausea, vomiting.
Skin: sweating, flushing, erythema.
Local: pain, swelling, and hematoma at injection site.
Other: bronchospasms, dyspnea, cramp-like pain, *anaphylaxis and anaphylactoid reactions (usually after rapid I.V. administration).*

INTERACTIONS
Mineral oil, cholestyramine resin: inhibited GI absorption of oral vitamin K. Use together cautiously.

NURSING CONSIDERATIONS
• Contraindicated in hereditary hypoprothrombinemia; bleeding secondary to heparin therapy or overdose; hepatocellular disease, unless it is caused by biliary obstruction (vitamin K can paradoxically worsen the hypoprothrombinemia). Oral administration is contraindicated if bile secretion is inadequate, unless supplemented with bile salts. Use cautiously, if at all, during last weeks of pregnancy to avoid toxic reactions in newborns; in G-6-PD deficiency to avoid hemolysis. Use large doses cautiously in severe hepatic disease.

• Failure to respond to vitamin K may indicate coagulation defects.
• In severe bleeding, don't delay other measures such as fresh frozen plasma or whole blood.
• Protect parenteral products from light. Wrap infusion container with aluminum foil.
• Effects of I.V. injections more rapid but shorter lived than S.C. or I.M. injections.
• Monitor prothrombin time to determine dosage effectiveness.
• Observe for signs of side effects and report them to the doctor.
• Phytonadione therapy for hemorrhagic disease in infants causes fewer adverse reactions than do other vitamin K analogs.
• Check brand name labels for administration route restrictions.
• Administer I.V. by slow infusion (over 2 to 3 hours). Mix in normal saline solution, dextrose 5% in water, or dextrose 5% in normal saline solution. Observe patient closely for signs of flushing, weakness, tachycardia, and hypotension; may progress to shock.
• Leafy vegetables are high in vitamin K content and may alter warfarin needs.
• This vitamin is fat soluble.

multivitamins
Available by many brand names.
Contain vitamins A, B complex, C, D, and E in varying amounts.
Pregnancy Category: A

MECHANISM OF ACTION
Source of vitamins.

INDICATIONS & DOSAGE
Prevention of vitamin deficiencies in patients with inadequate diets or increased daily requirements; treatment of multiplevitamin deficiencies and prevention of recurrence; additions to parenteral nutrition solutions to meet

*patient's normal or increased require-
ments—*
Adults and children: dosage depends
on nature and severity of deficiencies
and composition of multivitamin
preparation.

ADVERSE REACTIONS
None reported.

INTERACTIONS
Refer to each component of the multivitamin combination.

NURSING CONSIDERATIONS
• A single discovered vitamin deficiency usually coexists with others.
After initial deficiencies are corrected, stress need for adequate nutrition and multivitamin supplements, if
appropriate.
• Tell patient about possible interactions of vitamins in combinations and
what precautions to take to avoid
problems.
• Stress need to follow doctor's orders regarding daily dosages and follow-up therapy.
• Avoid excessive use of large-volume parenteral solutions of multivitamin supplements containing fat-soluble vitamins to prevent hypervitaminosis. I.V. solutions of water-soluble
multivitamins may be used more
freely.
• Chewable flavored multivitamins
available for children. Prevent use of
these drugs as candy.
• Liquid preparations may contain
varying percentages of alcohol.
Check label; alert patient to content.
• Warn against overdosing. Encourage patient to eat a well-balanced
diet. Stress hazards of self-administered megadoses of vitamins. These
medications are drugs, not just harmless vitamins. Explain possible side
effects.
• Multivitamin preparations with ordinary doses of each component are
usually nontoxic.

• Megavitamin combinations may
promote significant accumulation of
fat-soluble vitamins, with resultant
toxicity.
• Multivitamins containing therapeutic doses of folic acid may mask pernicious anemia. Unless prescribed
otherwise by doctor, patient should
avoid folic acid in undiagnosed but
suspected pernicious anemia.
• Other side effects depend on specific components and concentrations
in each multivitamin preparation.
• Store vitamins in a cool place in
light-resistant containers to limit loss
of potency.

---

sodium fluoride
Fluor-A-Day ♦♦, Fluoritabs, Flura-
Drops, Karidium♦, Luride Lozi-
Tabs, Pediaflor
Pregnancy Category: C

MECHANISM OF ACTION
May catalyze bone remineralization.

INDICATIONS & DOSAGE
Aid in the prevention of dental caries:
Oral—
Children over 3 years: 1 mg daily.
Children under 3 years: 0.5 mg
daily.
Topical—
Adults and children over 12 years:
10 ml of 0.2% solution. Use once
daily after thoroughly brushing teeth
and rinsing mouth. Rinse around and
between teeth for 1 minute, then spit
out.
Children 6 to 12 years: 5 ml of 0.2%
solution.

ADVERSE REACTIONS
CNS: headaches, weakness.
GI: gastric distress.
Skin: hypersensitivity reactions such
as atopic dermatitis, eczema, and ur-
ticaria.

INTERACTIONS
None significant.

NURSING CONSIDERATIONS
• Contraindicated when fluoride intake from drinking water exceeds 0.7 parts/million.
• Chronic toxicity (fluorosis) may result from prolonged use of higher-than-recommended doses.
• Advise patient to notify dentist if tooth mottling occurs.
• Tablets may be dissolved in mouth, chewed, or swallowed whole.
• Drops may be administered orally undiluted or mixed with fluids or food.
• Topical forms (rinses and gels) should not be swallowed. Most effective when used immediately after brushing teeth.
• Tell patient to dilute drops or rinses in plastic containers rather than glass.
• The presence of fluoride in prenatal vitamins has been shown to produce healthier teeth in infants.
• Used investigationally in the treatment of osteoporosis.

trace elements
chromium, copper, iodine (as iodide), manganese, selenium, zinc
Pregnancy Category: C

MECHANISM OF ACTION
Participate in synthesis and stabilization of proteins and nucleic acids in subcellular and membrane transport systems.

INDICATIONS & DOSAGE
Prevention of individual trace element deficiencies in patients receiving long-term total parenteral nutrition—
Chromium—
Adults: 10 to 15 mcg I.V. daily.
Children: 0.14 to 0.20 mcg/kg I.V. daily.
Copper—
Adults: 0.5 to 1.5 mg I.V. daily.

Children: 0.05 to 0.2 mg/kg I.V. daily.
Iodine—
Adults: 1 mcg/kg I.V. daily.
Manganese—
Adults: 1 to 3 mg I.V. daily.
Selenium—
Adults: 40 to 120 mcg/day.
Children: 3 mcg/kg/day.
Zinc—
Adults: 2 to 4 mg I.V. daily.
Children: 0.05 mg/kg I.V. daily.

ADVERSE REACTIONS
None reported.

INTERACTIONS
None significant at recommended dosages.

NURSING CONSIDERATIONS
• Check trace element serum levels of patients who have received total parenteral nutrition for 2 months or longer. Give supplement if ordered. Call doctor's attention to low serum levels of these elements.
• Normal serum levels are 0.07 to 0.15 mg/ml copper; 0.05 to 0.15 mg/100 ml zinc; 4 to 20 mcg/100 ml manganese; selenium 0.1 to 0.19 mcg/ml.
• Solutions of trace elements are compounded by pharmacy for addition to total parenteral nutrition solutions according to various formulas. One common trace element solution is Shil's solution, which contains copper 1 mg/ml, iodide 0.06 mg/ml, manganese 0.4 mg/ml, and zinc 2 mg/ml.
• Trace element solutions are now also commercially available.

zinc sulfate
Orazinc♦
Pregnancy Category: C

MECHANISM OF ACTION
Source of zinc.

INDICATIONS & DOSAGE

Treatment of zinc deficiency or adjunct to treatment of disorders related to low serum zinc levels, including oral and decubitus leg ulcers, acne, granulomata of the ear, rheumatoid arthritis, idiopathic hypogeusia, anosmia; also, as adjunct to vitamin A therapy when patient fails to respond to vitamin A alone and in acrodermatitis enteropathica—

Adults: 200 to 220 mg P.O. t.i.d. (equivalent to 135 to 150 mg elemental zinc daily, 9 times the adult RDA of 15 mg daily).
Children: dosages not established. RDA is 0.3 mg/kg daily.

ADVERSE REACTIONS

GI: distress and irritation, nausea, vomiting with high doses, gastric ulceration.

INTERACTIONS

None significant.

NURSING CONSIDERATIONS

• Beneficial only if patient is zinc-deficient.
• Normal serum levels may not reliably show absence of zinc deficiency.
• Results may not appear for 6 to 8 weeks in zinc-depleted patients.
• Decreasing dosage to 100 mg b.i.d. may ease nausea or other GI side effects; zinc is thought to irritate gastric mucosa.
• Take with meals to prevent possible gastric distress. However, dairy products may hinder zinc absorption.

Calorics

amino acid injection
amino acid solution
corn oil
dextrose (D-glucose)
essential crystalline amino acid solution
fat emulsions
fructose (levulose)
invert sugar
medium-chain triglycerides

COMBINATION PRODUCTS
Various products contain dextrose, fructose, or invert sugar in combination with electrolytes.

---

amino acid injection
FreAmine HBC, HepatAmine
Pregnancy Category: C

MECHANISM OF ACTION
Provides a substrate for protein synthesis or enhances conservation of existing body protein.

INDICATIONS & DOSAGE
Treatment of hepatic encephalopathy in patients with cirrhosis or hepatitis; nutritional support—
Adults: 80 to 120 g of amino acids (12 to 18 g of nitrogen)/day. Typically, 500 ml is mixed with 500 ml dextrose 50% in water and administered over a 24-hour period. Add electrolytes, vitamins, and trace elements needed.

ADVERSE REACTIONS
CNS: mental confusion, unconsciousness, headache, dizziness.

CV: hypervolemia related to congestive heart failure (in susceptible patients), *pulmonary edema,* exacerbation of hypertension (in predisposed patients).
GI: nausea, vomiting.
GU: glycosuria, osmotic diuresis.
Hepatic: fatty liver.
Metabolic: *rebound hypoglycemia* (when long-term infusions are abruptly stopped), *hyperglycemia,* metabolic acidosis, alkalosis, hypophosphatemia, *hyperosmolar syndrome, hyperosmolar hyperglycemic nonketotic syndrome,* hyperammonemia, *electrolyte imbalances,* and dehydration (if hyperosmolar solutions used).
Skin: chills, flushing, feeling of warmth.
Local: tissue sloughing at infusion site due to extravasation, *catheter sepsis, thrombophlebitis,* thrombosis.
Other: allergic reactions.

INTERACTIONS
None significant.

NURSING CONSIDERATIONS
● Contraindicated in patients with anuria and in those with inborn errors of amino acid metabolism, especially involving branched chain amino acid metabolism, such as maple syrup urine disease and isovaleric acidemia.
● Monitor serum electrolytes, magnesium, glucose, BUN, renal and hepatic function.
● Administer very cautiously to diabetic patients. To prevent hyperglycemia, insulin may be required. Admin-

---

ister cautiously to patients with cardiac insufficiency. May cause circulatory overload. Patients with fluid restriction may only tolerate 1 to 2 liters.
- Monitor for extraordinary electrolyte losses that may occur during nasogastric suction, vomiting, or drainage from GI fistula.
- Control infusion rate carefully with infusion pump.
- If infusion rate falls behind, do not attempt to catch up. Notify doctor.
- Check infusion site frequently for erythema, inflammation, irritation, tissue sloughing, necrosis, and phlebitis. Change peripheral I.V. sites routinely to prevent irritation and infection. If a subclavian catheter is used, the solution is administered into the midsuperior vena cava.
- Check fractional urine every 6 hours for glycosuria. Abrupt onset of glycosuria may be an early sign of impending sepsis.
- Assess body temperature every 4 hours; elevation may indicate sepsis or infection.
- If patient has chills, fever, or other signs of sepsis, replace I.V. tubing and bottle, and send them to the laboratory to be cultured.

amino acid solution

(crystalline amino acid solution)
Aminosyn♦, FreAmine III ♦,
Novamine, Travasol♦
Pregnancy Category: C

MECHANISM OF ACTION
Used for protein synthesis of the viscera and skeletal muscles in the protein-depleted patient.

INDICATIONS & DOSAGE
Total, supportive, or supplemental and protein-sparing parenteral nutrition when gastrointestinal system must rest during healing, or when patient can't, shouldn't, or won't eat at all or eat enough to maintain normal nutrition and metabolism—
Adults: 1 to 1.5 g/kg I.V. daily.
Children: 2 to 3 g/kg I.V. daily. Individualize dosage to metabolic and clinical response as determined by nitrogen balance and body weight corrected for fluid balance. Add electrolytes, vitamins, and nonprotein caloric solutions as needed.

ADVERSE REACTIONS
CNS: mental confusion, unconsciousness, headache, dizziness.
CV: hypervolemia related to congestive heart failure (in susceptible patients), *pulmonary edema*, exacerbation of hypertension (in predisposed patients).
GI: nausea, vomiting.
GU: glycosuria, osmotic diuresis.
Hepatic: fatty liver.
Metabolic: *rebound hypoglycemia* (when long-term infusions are abruptly stopped), *hyperglycemia*, metabolic acidosis, alkalosis, hypophosphatemia, *hyperosmolar syndrome, hyperosmolar hyperglycemic nonketotic syndrome,* hyperammonemia, *electrolyte imbalances,* and dehydration (if hyperosmolar solutions used).
Skin: chills, flushing, feeling of warmth.
Local: tissue sloughing at infusion site due to extravasation, *catheter sepsis, thrombophlebitis, thrombosis.*
Other: allergic reactions.

INTERACTIONS
None significant.

NURSING CONSIDERATIONS
- Contraindicated in patients with severe uncorrected electrolyte or acid-base imbalances, in hyperammonemia, and in decreased circulating blood volume. Use cautiously in renal insufficiency or failure, cardiac disease, and hepatic impairment. Long-term use for infants and children must

---

be closely monitored.
• Monitor serum electrolytes, magnesium, glucose, BUN, renal and hepatic function. Check serum calcium levels frequently to avoid bone demineralization in children.
• If long-term therapy is needed, doctor may order trace element and vitamin supplements. Avoid overuse of fat-soluble vitamins A and D—can cause toxic hypervitaminosis.
• Don't mix medications, except electrolytes, vitamins, and trace elements, with total parenteral nutrition solution without first consulting pharmacist.
• Control infusion rate carefully with infusion pump.
• If infusion rate falls behind, do not attempt to "catch up." Notify doctor.
• Check infusion site frequently for erythema, inflammation, irritation, tissue sloughing, necrosis, and phlebitis. Change I.V. sites routinely to prevent irritation and infection. I.V. catheter is usually introduced into subclavian vein.
• Watch closely for signs of fluid overload. Notify doctor promptly.
• Some crystalline amino acid solutions contain large amounts of acetates and lactates; use cautiously in patients with alkalosis or hepatic insufficiency.
• Most side effects are due to mixing amino acids with hypertonic dextrose solutions.
• Check fractional urines every 6 hours for glycosuria (if present, the doctor may order insulin coverage).
• Assess body temperature every 4 hours; elevation may indicate sepsis or infection.
• If patient has chills, fever, or other signs of sepsis, replace I.V. tubing and bottle and send them to the laboratory to be cultured.

corn oil
Lipomul
Pregnancy Category: NR

MECHANISM OF ACTION
Source of calories.

INDICATIONS & DOSAGE
To increase caloric intake—
Adults: 45 ml P.O. b.i.d. to q.i.d. after or between meals, alone or with proteins, milk, or other energy sources.
Children: 30 ml P.O. daily to q.i.d. after or between meals, alone or with proteins, milk, or other energy sources.

ADVERSE REACTIONS
GI: nausea, vomiting, diarrhea.

INTERACTIONS
Griseofulvin: increased GI absorption of griseofulvin. A beneficial interaction.

NURSING CONSIDERATIONS
• Contraindicated in gallbladder calculi or complete GI obstructions. Use cautiously in steatorrhea, partial GI obstruction, enterostomies.
• To minimize nausea, diarrhea, and vomiting, give more frequent, smaller doses with meals or mixed with milk.
• The dosage varies greatly with individual requirements; 30 ml of the emulsion provides 180 calories.

dextrose (D-glucose)
Pregnancy Category: C

MECHANISM OF ACTION
Minimizes glyconeogenesis and promotes anabolism in patients who can't receive sufficient oral caloric intake.

INDICATIONS & DOSAGE
Fluid replacement and caloric supplementation in patient who can't main-

tain adequate oral intake or who is restricted from doing so—

Adults and children: dosage depends on fluid and caloric requirements. Use peripheral I.V. infusion of 2.5%, 5%, or 10% solution, central I.V. infusion of 20% solution for minimal fluid needs. Use 50% solution to treat insulin-induced hypoglycemia. Solutions from 40% to 70% are used diluted in admixtures, normally with amino acid solutions, for total parenteral nutrition given through a central vein.

ADVERSE REACTIONS

CNS: mental confusion, unconsciousness in hyperosmolar syndrome.
CV: (with fluid overload) pulmonary edema, exacerbated hypertension, and congestive heart failure in susceptible patients. *Prolonged or concentrated infusions may cause phlebitis, sclerosis of vein, especially with peripheral route of administration.*
GU: glycosuria, osmotic diuresis.
Metabolic: (with rapid infusion of concentrated solution or prolonged infusion) hyperglycemia, hypervolemia, hyperosmolarity. Rapid termination of long-term infusions may cause hypoglycemia from rebound hyperinsulinemia.
Skin: sloughing and tissue necrosis, if extravasation occurs with concentrated solutions.

INTERACTIONS
None significant.

NURSING CONSIDERATIONS
• Contraindicated in hyperglycemia, diabetic coma, intracranial or intraspinal hemorrhage, and delirium tremens. Use cautiously in cardiac or pulmonary disease, hypertension, renal insufficiency, urinary obstruction, or hypovolemia.
• Control infusion rate carefully. Maximal rate for dextrose infusion is 0.5 g/kg hourly. Use infusion pump when infusing dextrose with amino

acids for total parenteral nutrition.
• Never infuse concentrated solutions rapidly; can cause hyperglycemia, fluid shift.
• Monitor serum glucose carefully. Prolonged therapy with dextrose 5% solution can cause depletion of pancreatic insulin production and secretion.
• Never stop abruptly. If necessary, have dextrose 10% solution available to treat hypoglycemia if rebound hyperinsulinemia occurs.
• Take care to prevent extravasation. Check injection site frequently to prevent irritation, tissue sloughing, necrosis, and phlebitis.
• Watch closely for signs of fluid overload, especially if fluid intake is restricted.
• Monitor intake/output and weight carefully, especially when renal function is impaired.
• Check vital signs frequently. Report side effects promptly.
• Don't give dextrose solutions without saline solution in blood transfusions; may cause clumping of red blood cells. Use central veins to infuse dextrose solutions at concentrations over 10%.

essential crystalline amino acid solution

Aminosyn-RF, Nephramine, Ren-Amine 6.5
Pregnancy Category: C

MECHANISM OF ACTION
Enhances conservation of existing body protein.

INDICATIONS & DOSAGE
Management of potentially reversible renal decompensation—
Adults: 0.3 to 0.5 g/kg I.V., up to 26 g total daily (250 ml with 500 ml dextrose 70% injection), and infuse through central I.V. line at initial rate of 20 to 30 ml/hour, increased in steps

of 10 ml/hour every 24 hours, to a maximum of 60 to 100 ml/hour. Individualize dose and infusion rate to tolerance for glucose, fluid, and nitrogen. Add electrolytes and vitamins as needed.

Children: up to 1 g/kg daily, individualized to patient's tolerance for glucose, fluid, and nitrogen. Add electrolytes, trace elements, and vitamins as needed.

ADVERSE REACTIONS
CNS: mental confusion, dizziness, unconsciousness, headache.
CV: hypervolemia related to congestive heart failure (in susceptible patients), *pulmonary edema,* exacerbation of hypertension (in predisposed patients).
GI: nausea, vomiting.
GU: glycosuria, osmotic diuresis.
Metabolic: *rebound hypoglycemia* (when long-term infusions are abruptly stopped), *hyperglycemia,* metabolic acidosis, alkalosis, hypophosphatemia, hyperosmolar syndrome, *hyperosmolar hyperglycemic nonketotic syndrome,* hyperammonemia, *electrolyte imbalances,* and dehydration (if hyperosmolar solutions used).
Skin: chills, flushing, feeling of warmth.
Local: tissue sloughing at infusion site due to extravasation, *catheter sepsis, thrombophlebitis.*
Other: allergic reactions.

INTERACTIONS
None significant.

NURSING CONSIDERATIONS
• Contraindicated in severe uncorrected electrolyte or acid-base imbalances, hyperammonemia, and decreased circulating blood volume.
• Monitor serum electrolytes, magnesium, glucose, BUN, renal and hepatic function. Check serum calcium levels frequently to avoid bone demineralization in children.
• In long-term therapy, doctor may order trace element and vitamin supplements. Avoid overuse of fat-soluble vitamins.
• Refrigerate solution until ½ hour before it will be infused.
• Don't mix medications, except electrolytes, vitamins, and trace elements with total parenteral nutrition solution without first consulting pharmacist.
• Control infusion rate carefully with infusion pump.
• If infusion rate falls behind, do not attempt to catch up. Notify doctor.
• Check infusion site frequently for erythema, inflammation, irritation, tissue sloughing, necrosis, and phlebitis. Change I.V. sites routinely to prevent irritation. I.V. catheter is usually placed in subclavian vein.
• Watch closely for signs of fluid overload. Notify doctor promptly.
• Essential amino acid solution is used identically to other crystalline amino acid solutions, except that it contains only the essential amino acids. By controlling amino acid content, patients with impaired renal function have decreases in blood urea nitrogen level and minimized deterioration of serum potassium, magnesium, and phosphorus balances. May lead to earlier return of renal function in patients with potentially reversible acute renal failure and may decrease morbidity associated with acute renal failure.
• Most side effects due to mixing essential crystalline amino acid solution with hypertonic dextrose solutions.
• Check blood glucose levels every 6 hours. Doctor may need to order insulin.
• Assess body temperature every 4 hours; elevation may indicate sepsis or infection.
• If patient has chills, fever, or other signs of sepsis, replace I.V. tubing and bottle and send them to the laboratory to be cultured.

fat emulsions

Intralipid 10%♦, Intralipid 20%,
Liposyn 10%, Liposyn 20%,
Liposyn II 10%, Liposyn II 20%,
Soyacal 10%, Soyacal 20%,
Travamulsion 10%, Travamulsion
20%
Pregnancy Category: B for Soyacal
10%; C for all others

MECHANISM OF ACTION

Provides neutral triglycerides, predominantly unsaturated fatty acids.

INDICATIONS & DOSAGE

Intralipid:
*Source of calories adjunctive to total
parenteral nutrition—*
Adults: 1 ml/minute I.V. for 15 to 30
minutes (10% emulsion); 0.5 ml/min-
ute I.V. for 15 to 30 minutes (20%
emulsion). If no adverse reactions, increase rate to deliver 500 ml over 4 to
8 hours. Total daily dose should not
exceed 2.5 g/kg.
Children: 0.1 ml/minute for 10 to 15
minutes (10% emulsion), 0.05 ml/
minute I.V. for 10 to 15 minutes (20%
emulsion). If no adverse reactions, increase rate to deliver 1 g/kg over 4
hours. Daily dose should not exceed 4
g/kg. Equals 60% of daily caloric intake. Protein-carbohydrate total parenteral nutrition should supply remaining 40%.
Fatty acid deficiency—
Adults and children: 8% to 10% of
total caloric intake I.V.
Liposyn:
Prevention of fatty acid deficiency—
Adults: 500 ml (10% emulsion) I.V.
twice weekly. Infuse initially at a rate
of 1 ml/minute for 30 minutes. Rate
may be increased but should not exceed 500 ml over 4 to 6 hours.
Children: 5 to 10 ml/kg (10% emulsion) I.V. daily. Infuse initially at a
rate of 0.1 ml/minute for 30 minutes.
Rate may be increased but should not
exceed 100 ml/hour.

ADVERSE REACTIONS

Early reactions of fat overload:
Blood: hyperlipemia, hypercoagula-
bility, thrombocytopenia (rarely) in
neonates.
CNS: headache, sleepiness, dizzi-
ness.
EENT: pressure over eyes.
GI: nausea, vomiting.
Skin: flushing, diaphoresis.
Local: irritation at infusion site.
Other: fever, dyspnea, chest and back
pains, cyanosis, allergic reactions, de-
position of I.V. fat.
Delayed reactions:
Blood: thrombocytopenia, leuko-
penia, leukocytosis.
CNS: focal seizures.
CV: *shock.*
Hepatic: transient increased liver
function test, hepatomegaly.
Other: fever, splenomegaly, fat accu-
mulation in lungs.

INTERACTIONS

None significant.

NURSING CONSIDERATIONS

• Contraindicated in hyperlipemia,
lipid nephrosis, and acute pancreatitis
accompanied by hyperlipemia. Use
cautiously in severe hepatic disease,
pulmonary disease, anemia, blood coagulation disorders, or patients with
possible danger of fat embolism.
• Lipids support bacterial growth.
Change all I.V. tubing at each infusion.
• Use very cautiously in premature
infants, as they are very susceptible to
I.V. fat overload. Carefully monitor
triglycerides and free fatty acid levels
in these infants.
• Intralipid brand (only) can be mixed
with amino acid solution, dextrose,
electrolytes, and vitamins in the same
I.V. container.
• Do not use an inline filter when administering this drug because the fat
particles are larger than the 0.22-
micron cellulose filter.

Italicized side effects are common or life-threatening.
*Liquid form contains alcohol.   **May contain tartrazine.

- Discard fat emulsion if it separates or becomes oily.
- Refrigeration is not necessary.
- Avoid rapid infusion. Use an infusion pump to regulate rate.
- Check injection site daily. Report signs of inflammation or infection promptly.
- Watch closely for side effects, especially during first half hour of infusion.
- Monitor serum lipids closely when patient is receiving fat emulsion therapy. Lipemia must clear between dosing.
- Check platelet count frequently in neonates receiving fat emulsions I.V.
- Monitor hepatic function carefully in long-term use.
- Intralipid, Travamulsion, and Liposyn differ mainly by their fatty acid components.

fructose (levulose)
Pregnancy Category: C

MECHANISM OF ACTION
Minimizes glyconeogenesis and promotes anabolism in patients who can't receive sufficient oral caloric intake.

INDICATIONS & DOSAGE
Source of carbohydrate calories primarily when fluid replacement is also indicated and as a dextrose substitute for patients with diabetes—
Adults and children: dosage depends on caloric needs. I.V. infusion rate should not exceed 1 g/kg hourly. Single liter 10% solution yields 375 calories.

ADVERSE REACTIONS
CV: increased pulse rate, precipitation or exacerbation of congestive heart failure in susceptible patients, *pulmonary edema*.
Hepatic: hepatomegaly.
Metabolic: metabolic acidosis, hypervolemia.

Local: extravasation at infusion site may cause sloughing of skin, thrombophlebitis.
Other: increased respiratory rate.

INTERACTIONS
None significant.

NURSING CONSIDERATIONS
- Contraindicated in hereditary fructose intolerance, in patients with gout, or in patients receiving therapy for hypoglycemia. Use cautiously in cardiac disease, hypertension, pulmonary disease, hypervolemia, renal insufficiency, or urinary tract obstructions.
- Control infusion rate carefully. Make sure rate does not exceed 1 g/kg hourly in infants.
- Change infusion sites regularly to avoid irritation with prolonged therapy. Take care to avoid extravasation.
- Don't use unless the solution is clear and the seal is intact.
- Watch closely for signs of fluid overload, pulmonary edema, or congestive heart failure.

invert sugar
Travert
Pregnancy Category: C

MECHANISM OF ACTION
Minimizes glyconeogenesis and promotes anabolism in patients who can't receive sufficient oral caloric intake.

INDICATIONS & DOSAGE
Nonelectrolyte fluid replacement and caloric supplementation solution—
Adults and children: dosage depends on patient's age, weight, clinical need. I.V. infusion rate should not exceed 1 g/kg hourly. Single liter 5% invert sugar yields 375 calories.

ADVERSE REACTIONS
CNS: mental confusion.
CV: increased pulse rate, precipita-

tion or exacerbation of congestive heart failure in susceptible patients, *pulmonary edema*, hypertension.
GU: glycosuria, osmotic diuresis.
Metabolic: metabolic acidosis, hypervolemia, hyperglycemia, hypoglycemia.
Local: extravasation at infusion site may cause sloughing of skin, thrombophlebitis.
Other: increased respiratory rate.

INTERACTIONS
None significant.

NURSING CONSIDERATIONS
• Contraindicated in hereditary fructose intolerance, hyperglycemia, diabetic coma, intracranial or intraspinal hemorrhage, or delirium tremens. Use cautiously in cardiac disease, hypertension, pulmonary disease, hypervolemia, renal insufficiency, or urinary tract obstructions.
• Control infusion rate carefully. Make sure rate does not exceed 1 g/kg hourly in infants.
• Change infusion sites regularly to avoid irritation with prolonged therapy. Take care to avoid extravasation.
• Watch closely for signs of fluid overload, pulmonary edema, or congestive heart failure. Monitor blood pressure frequently.
• Monitor serum glucose closely. Prolonged therapy can cause depletion of pancreatic insulin production and secretion.
• Don't stop abruptly. If necessary, have dextrose 10% available to prevent rebound hyperinsulinemia and subsequent hypoglycemia.
• Monitor intake/output and weight closely, especially if renal function is impaired.
• Check vital signs frequently. Tell doctor promptly if side effects develop.

medium-chain triglycerides
M.C.T. Oil♦
Pregnancy Category: C

MECHANISM OF ACTION
Source of rapidly hydrolyzable lipid.

INDICATIONS & DOSAGE
Inadequate digestion or absorption of food fats—
Adults: 15 ml P.O. t.i.d. or q.i.d. Maximum of 100 ml/day.

ADVERSE REACTIONS
CNS: reversible coma and precoma in susceptible patients.
GI: *nausea, vomiting, diarrhea, abdominal distention, cramps.*

INTERACTIONS
None significant.

NURSING CONSIDERATIONS
• Contraindicated in advanced hepatic disease and abetalipoproteinemia. Use cautiously in patients with portacaval shunts.
• To minimize GI side effects, give smaller doses more frequently with meals or mixed with salad dressing or chilled fruit juice.
• More easily absorbed than long-chain fats; not dependent on bile salts for emulsification.
• Rapid metabolism provides quick energy.
• May be useful in lowering cholesterol levels. Also used in patients with short-bowel syndrome.
• Provides 7.7 calories/ml. No essential fatty acids are provided.
• Use metal, glass, or ceramic containers and utensils.

Italicized side effects are common or life-threatening.
*Liquid form contains alcohol.   **May contain tartrazine.

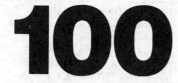

Immune serums

antirabies serum, equine
hepatitis B immune globulin, human
immune globulin
rabies immune globulin, human
Rh₀ (D) immune globulin, human
tetanus immune globulin, human
varicella-zoster immune globulin (VZIG)

COMBINATION PRODUCTS
None.

---

antirabies serum, equine
Pregnancy Category: C

MECHANISM OF ACTION
Provides passive immunity to rabies.

INDICATIONS & DOSAGE
Rabies exposure—
Adults and children: 40 to 55 units/kg at time of first dose of rabies vaccine. Use half dose to infiltrate wound area. Give remainder I.M. Don't give rabies vaccine and antirabies serum in same syringe or at same site.

For wounds including mucous membranes, the entire dose should be administered I.M.

ADVERSE REACTIONS
Local: pain at injection site.
Systemic: within 6 to 12 days serum sickness occurs in 15% to 25% of patients. Symptoms are skin eruptions, arthralgia, pruritus, lymphadenopathy, fever, headache, malaise, abdominal pain, *anaphylaxis.*

INTERACTIONS
Corticosteroids and immunosuppressive agents: interferes with response. Avoid during postexposure immunization period.

NURSING CONSIDERATIONS
• In hypersensitivity to equine serum, use rabies immune globulin, human, instead. If unavailable, desensitize before giving. Consult doctor or pharmacist.
• Do sensitivity test on all patients before giving. Dilute serum 1:100 or 1:1,000 with 0.9% sodium chloride for injection. Inject intradermally on inner forearm. Inject other arm with 0.1 ml of 0.9% sodium chloride for injection intradermally as a control. Read within 20 minutes. Positive reaction: wheal 10 mm or more and erythematous flare 20 × 20 mm.
• Use only when rabies immune globulin, human, is not available.
• Obtain history of animal bite, allergies (especially to equine serum and to eggs), and reaction to immunization.
• Epinephrine solution 1:1,000 should always be available when administering this drug.
• This immune serum provides immediate passive immunity (short-term).
• Do not confuse this drug with rabies vaccine, which is a suspension of attenuated or killed microorganisms used to confer long-term active immunity. These two drugs are often administered together prophylactically after exposure to known or suspected

rabid animals.
• Ask patient when he received last tetanus immunization, since many doctors order a booster at this time.

---

hepatitis B immune globulin, human
H-BIG, Hep-B-Gammagee, HyperHep♦
Pregnancy Category: C

MECHANISM OF ACTION
Provides passive immunity to hepatitis B.

INDICATIONS & DOSAGE
Hepatitis B exposure—
Adults and children: 0.06 ml/kg I.M. within 7 days after exposure. Repeat 28 days after exposure.
Neonates born to HbsAg-positive women—
0.5 ml within 24 hours of birth. Repeat dose at age 3 months and 6 months.

ADVERSE REACTIONS
Systemic: *anaphylaxis.*

INTERACTIONS
None significant.

NURSING CONSIDERATIONS
• Buttocks or deltoid areas are the preferred injection sites.
• Nurse should receive immunization if exposed to hepatitis B (for example, needle-stick, direct contact).
• Obtain history of allergies and reaction to immunization.

---

immune globulin
Gamastan, Gamimune, Gammar, Immuglobin, Sandoglobulin
Pregnancy Category: C

MECHANISM OF ACTION
Provides passive immunity by increasing antibody titer.

INDICATIONS & DOSAGE
Agammaglobulinemia or hypogamma-globulinemia—
Adults: 30 to 50 ml I.M. monthly. Alternatively, administer 100 mg/kg I.V. (Gamimune) once a month. Infuse at 0.01 to 0.02 ml/kg/min for 30 minutes. For Sandoglobulin, administer 200 mg/kg I.V. once a month. Infuse at 0.5 to 1 ml/min. After 15 to 30 minutes, increase infusion rate to 1.5 to 2.5 ml/min.
Children: 20 to 40 ml I.M. monthly.
Hepatitis A exposure—
Adults and children: 0.02 to 0.04 ml/kg I.M. as soon as possible after exposure. Up to 0.1 ml/kg may be given after prolonged or intense exposure.
Serum hepatitis post-transfusion—
Adults and children: 10 ml I.M. within 1 week after transfusion and 10 ml I.M. 1 month later.
Measles exposure—
Adults and children: 0.02 ml/kg within 6 days after exposure.
Modification of measles—
Adults and children: 0.04 ml/kg I.M. within 6 days after exposure.
Measles vaccine complications—
Adults and children: 0.02 to 0.04 ml/kg I.M.
Poliomyelitis exposure—
Adults and children: 0.3 to 0.4 ml/kg I.M. within 7 days after exposure.
Chicken pox exposure—
Adults and children: 0.2 to 1.3 ml/kg I.M. as soon as exposed.
Rubella exposure in first trimester of pregnancy—
Women: 0.2 to 0.4 ml/kg I.M. as soon as exposed.
Prophylaxis in primary immune deficiencies—
Adults and children: 100 mg/kg by I.V. infusion monthly (Gamimune only). Infusion rate is 0.01 to 0.02 ml/kg/minute for 30 minutes. Rate can then be increased to 0.04 ml/minute for remainder of infusion.
Idiopathic thrombocytopenic pur-

Italicized side effects are common or life-threatening.
*Liquid form contains alcohol.   **May contain tartrazine.

pura—
Adults: 0.4 g/kg Sandoglobulin I.V. for 5 consecutive days.

ADVERSE REACTIONS
Skin: urticaria.
Local: pain, erythema, muscle stiffness.
Systemic: angioedema, headache, malaise, fever, nephrotic syndrome, *anaphylaxis.*

INTERACTIONS
Live virus vaccines: don't administer within 3 months after administration of immune globulin.

NURSING CONSIDERATIONS
• Obtain history of allergies and reaction to immunization.
• Have drugs available for anaphylactic reaction.
• Two brands of I.V. immune globulin are now available (Gamimune and Sandoglobulin). They're especially useful in patients with clotting abnormalities or in those with small muscle mass.
• Inject into different sites, preferably buttocks. Do not inject more than 3 ml per injection site.
• Do not give for hepatitis A exposure if 6 weeks or more have elapsed since exposure or after onset of clinical illness.

---

rabies immune globulin, human
Hyperab, Imogam
Pregnancy Category: C

MECHANISM OF ACTION
Provides passive immunity to rabies.

INDICATIONS & DOSAGE
Rabies exposure—
Adults and children: 20 IU/kg at time of first dose of rabies vaccine. Use half dose to infiltrate wound area. Give remainder I.M. Don't give rabies vaccine and rabies immune globulin in same syringe or at same site.

ADVERSE REACTIONS
Local: pain, redness, induration at injection site.
Other: slight fever, *anaphylaxis.*

INTERACTIONS
Corticosteroids and immunosuppressive agents: interferes with response. Avoid during postexposure immunization period.

NURSING CONSIDERATIONS
• Repeated doses contraindicated after rabies vaccine is started.
• Use only with rabies vaccine and immediate local treatment of wound. Give regardless of interval between exposure and initiation of therapy.
• Obtain history of animal bite, allergies, reaction to immunization.
• Don't administer more than 5 ml I.M. at one injection site; divide I.M. doses greater than 5 ml, and administer at different sites.
• This immune serum provides passive immunity.
• Do not confuse this drug with rabies vaccine, which is a suspension of attenuated or killed microorganisms used to confer active immunity. These two drugs are often given together prophylactically after exposure to known or suspected rabid animals.
• Ask the patient when he received his last tetanus immunization, since many doctors order a booster at this time.

Rh₀ (D) immune globulin, human
Gamulin Rh, HypRho-D, MICRhoGAM, Mini-Gamulin Rh, RhoGam♦
Pregnancy Category: C

MECHANISM OF ACTION
Suppresses the active antibody re-

sponse and formation of anti-Rh$_o$(D) in Rh$_o$(D)-negative, D^u-negative individuals, exposed to Rh-positive blood.

INDICATIONS & DOSAGE
Rh exposure—
Women (postabortion, postmiscarriage, ectopic pregnancy, or postpartum): transfusion unit or blood bank determines fetal packed red blood cell volume entering woman's blood, then gives one vial I.M. if fetal packed RBC volume is less than 15 ml. More than one vial I.M. may be required if there is large fetomaternal hemorrhage. Must be given within 72 hours after delivery or miscarriage.
Transfusion accidents—
Adults and children: consult blood bank or transfusion unit at once. Must be given within 72 hours.
Postabortion or postmiscarriage to prevent Rh antibody formation—
Women: consult transfusion unit or blood bank. Ideally should be given within 3 hours, but may be given up to 72 hours after abortion or miscarriage.

ADVERSE REACTIONS
Local: discomfort at injection site.
Other: slight fever.

INTERACTIONS
None significant.

NURSING CONSIDERATIONS
• Contraindicated in Rh$_o$(D)-positive or D^u-positive patients and those previously immunized to Rh$_o$(D) blood factor.
• Immediately after delivery, send a sample of infant's cord blood to laboratory for type and cross match. Confirm mother is Rh$_o$(D)-negative and D^u-negative. Infant must be Rh$_o$(D)-positive or D^u-positive.
• Obtain history of allergies and reaction to immunization.
• MICRhoGAM recommended for

every woman undergoing abortion or miscarriage up to 12 weeks' gestation unless she is Rh$_o$(D)-positive or D^u-positive, has Rh antibodies, or the father and/or fetus is Rh-negative.
• Store at 36° to 46° F. (2° to 8° C.).
• This immune serum provides passive immunity to the woman exposed to Rh$_o$-positive fetal blood during pregnancy. Prevents formation of maternal antibodies (active immunity), which would endanger future Rh$_o$-positive pregnancies.
• Explain to the patient how drug protects future Rh$_o$-positive infants.

tetanus immune globulin, human
Homo-Tet, Hu-Tet, Hyper-Tet♦
Pregnancy Category: C

MECHANISM OF ACTION
Provides passive immunity to tetanus.

INDICATIONS & DOSAGE
Tetanus exposure—
Adults and children: 250 to 500 units I.M.
Tetanus treatment—
Adults and children: single doses of 3,000 to 6,000 units have been used. Optimal dosage schedules not established. Don't give at same site as toxoid.

ADVERSE REACTIONS
Local: pain, stiffness, erythema.
Other: slight fever, allergy, *anaphylaxis.*

INTERACTIONS
None significant.

NURSING CONSIDERATIONS
• Use tetanus immune globulin only if wound is over 24 hours old or patient has had less than two previous tetanus toxoid injections.
• Obtain history of injury, tetanus immunizations, last tetanus toxoid in-

jection, allergies, and reaction to immunization.
• Thoroughly cleanse and remove all foreign matter from wound.
• This immune serum provides passive immunity. Antibodies remain at effective levels for 3 weeks or longer, which is several times the duration of antitoxin-induced antibodies. Protects the patient for the incubation period of most tetanus cases.
• Human globulin is not a substitute for tetanus toxoid, which should be given at the same time to produce active immunization.
• Inject into the deltoid muscle.
• Do not confuse this drug with tetanus toxoid.

varicella-zoster immune globulin (VZIG)
Pregnancy Category: C

MECHANISM OF ACTION
Provides passive immunity to varicella-zoster virus.

INDICATIONS & DOSAGE
Passive immunization of susceptible immunodeficient patients after exposure to varicella (chicken pox or herpes zoster)—
Children to 10 kg: 125 units I.M.
Children 10.1 to 20 kg: 250 units I.M.
Children 20.1 to 30 kg: 375 units I.M.
Children 30.1 to 40 kg: 500 units I.M.
Adults and children over 40 kg: 625 units I.M.

ADVERSE REACTIONS
Local: discomfort at injection site, rash.
Systemic: gastrointestinal distress, malaise, headache, respiratory distress, *anaphylaxis.*

INTERACTIONS
None reported.

NURSING CONSIDERATIONS
• Contraindicated in patients with a history of severe reaction to human immune serum globulin or severe thrombocytopenia.
• For maximum benefit, administer as soon as possible after presumed exposure.
• VZIG is not recommended for non-immunosuppressed patients.
• VZIG should not be administered indiscriminately because supplies are limited.
• Although usually restricted to children under 15 years old, VZIG may be administered to adolescents and adults if necessary.
• Not commercially distributed. Available only from 20 regional distribution centers throughout the United States. These centers will distribute to Canada and overseas. Call the Centers for Disease Control (404-329-3311) for the distribution center in your area.
• Should be administered only by deep I.M. injection. Never administer I.V.
• Store vial in refrigerator.

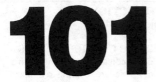

Vaccines and toxoids

COMBINATION PRODUCTS
None.

BCG vaccine
Pregnancy Category: C

MECHANISM OF ACTION
Promotes active immunity to tuberculosis.

INDICATIONS & DOSAGE
Tuberculosis exposure, cancer immunotherapy—
Adults and children: 0.1 ml intradermally.
Newborns: 0.05 ml intradermally.

ADVERSE REACTIONS
Local: lymphangitis, lymph node and skin abscess, ulceration at site of injection (2 to 3 weeks after injection), lupus reaction.
Other: urticaria of trunk and limbs, lymphadenitis, osteomyelitis, *anaphylaxis.*

INTERACTIONS
Isoniazid (INH): inhibited multiplication of BCG. Avoid using together.
Immunosuppressive therapy: may reduce response to BCG vaccine. Avoid if possible.

NURSING CONSIDERATIONS
• Contraindicated in patients with hypogammaglobulinemia, positive tuberculin reaction (when meant for use as immunoprophylactic after exposure to tuberculosis), immunosuppression, fresh smallpox vaccination, and burns

and in patients receiving corticosteroid therapy. Use cautiously in chronic skin disease. Inject in area of healthy skin only.
• Obtain history of allergies and reaction to immunization.
• Vaccine is of no value as immunoprophylactic in patients with positive tuberculin test.
• Keep epinephrine 1:1,000 available to treat anaphylaxis.
• Recommended injection site is over insertion of deltoid muscle.
• Do not shake vial following reconstitution.
• Expected lesion forms in 7 to 10 days.
• Allow an interval of at least 3 weeks between BCG and rubella vaccination.
• Don't administer to children with febrile illness.
• Live vaccine; destroy by autoclaving or formaldehyde solution before disposal.
• Patient should have tuberculin skin test 2 to 3 months after BCG vaccination to determine success of vaccine.
• Use of BCG has shown some value in treatment of various cancers, such as leukemia, some lung cancers, malignant melanoma, multiple myeloma, and some breast tumors. Currently, researchers are trying to find ways of augmenting the immune system's response to cancer. They hope to stimulate the body to destroy tumor cells.

cholera vaccine
Pregnancy Category: C

MECHANISM OF ACTION
Promotes active immunity to cholera.

INDICATIONS & DOSAGE
Primary immunization—
Adults and children over 10 years: 2 doses of 0.5 ml I.M. or 1 ml S.C., 1 week to 1 month apart, before traveling in cholera area. Booster: 0.5 ml q

6 months as long as protection is needed.
Children 5 to 10 years: 0.3 ml I.M. or S.C.
Children 6 months to 4 years: 0.2 ml I.M. or S.C. Boosters of same dose should be given q 6 months as long as protection is needed.

ADVERSE REACTIONS
Systemic: malaise, fever, flushing, urticaria, tachycardia, hypotension, diarrhea, headache, *anaphylaxis.*
Local: erythema, swelling, pain, induration.

INTERACTIONS
None significant.

NURSING CONSIDERATIONS
• Contraindicated in corticosteroid therapy or in immunosuppression. Defer in acute illness.
• Obtain history of allergies and reaction to immunization.
• Keep epinephrine 1:1,000 available.
• May be given intradermally, but I.M. and subcutaneous routes give higher levels of protection.
• Administer I.M. in deltoid muscle in adults and children older than 3 years.

diphtheria and tetanus toxoids, adsorbed
Pregnancy Category: C

MECHANISM OF ACTION
Promotes immunity to diphtheria and tetanus by inducing production of antitoxins.

INDICATIONS & DOSAGE
Primary immunization—
Adults and children over 7 years: use adult strength; 0.5 ml I.M. 4 to 6 weeks apart for 2 doses and a third dose 1 year later. Booster: 0.5 ml I.M. q 10 years.

Infants (6 weeks to 1 year): use pediatric strength. Give three 0.5 ml doses I.M. at least 4 weeks apart. Give booster dose 6 to 12 months after third injection.
Children (1 to 6 years): use pediatric strength. Give two 0.5 ml doses I.M. at least 4 weeks apart. Give booster dose 6 to 12 months after the second injection. If the final immunizing dose is given after the 7th birthday, use the adult strength.

ADVERSE REACTIONS
Systemic: chills, fever, malaise, *anaphylaxis.*
Local: stinging, edema, erythema, pain, induration.

INTERACTIONS
None significant.

NURSING CONSIDERATIONS
• Contraindicated in immunosuppression, radiation, or corticosteroid therapy. Defer in respiratory illness or polio outbreaks, or acute illness except in emergency. Use single antigen during polio risks. In children under 6 years, use only when diphtheria, tetanus, and pertussis toxoid combination is contraindicated because of pertussis component.
• Verify strength (pediatric or adult) of toxoid used.
• Obtain history of allergies and reaction to immunization.
• Keep epinephrine 1:1,000 available.
• Give in site not previously used for vaccines or toxoids.

diphtheria and tetanus toxoids and pertussis vaccine (DPT)
Tri-Immunol
Pregnancy Category: Not applicable

MECHANISM OF ACTION
Promotes active immunity to diphtheria, tetanus, and pertussis by inducing production of antitoxins and antibodies.

INDICATIONS & DOSAGE
Primary immunization—
Children 6 weeks to 6 years: 0.5 ml I.M. 2 months apart for 3 doses and a fourth dose 1 year later. Booster: 0.5 ml I.M. when starting school. Not advised for adults or children over 6 years.

ADVERSE REACTIONS
Systemic: slight fever, chills, malaise, *convulsions, encephalopathy, anaphylaxis.*
Local: *soreness, redness,* expected nodule remaining several weeks.

INTERACTIONS
Immunosuppressive therapy: may reduce response to DPT vaccine. Avoid if possible.

NURSING CONSIDERATIONS
• Contraindicated in corticosteroid therapy, immunosuppression, and history of convulsions. Defer in acute febrile illness.
• Children with preexisting neurologic disorders should not receive pertussis component. Also, children who react to any DPT injection by exhibiting neurologic signs shouldn't receive pertussis component in any succeeding injections. Diphtheria and tetanus toxoids (DT) should be given instead.
• DPT injection may be given at same time as trivalent oral polio vaccine (TOPV).

Italicized side effects are common or life-threatening.
*Liquid form contains alcohol.   **May contain tartrazine.

- Obtain history of allergies and reaction to immunization.
- Keep epinephrine 1:1,000 available.
- Not to be used for active infection.
- Don't give subcutaneously.
- Shake before using. Refrigerate.
- Administer only by deep I.M. injection, preferably in thigh or deltoid.

diphtheria toxoid, adsorbed
Pregnancy Category: Not applicable

MECHANISM OF ACTION
Promotes immunity to diphtheria by inducing production of antitoxin.

INDICATIONS & DOSAGE
Diphtheria immunization—
Children under 6 years: 0.5 ml I.M. 6 to 8 weeks apart for two doses and a third dose 1 year later. Booster: 0.5 ml I.M. at 5- to 10-year intervals. Not advised for adults or for children over 6 years; instead, use adult strength of diphtheria toxoid (usually combined with tetanus toxoid).

ADVERSE REACTIONS
Systemic: fever, malaise, urticaria, tachycardia, flushing, pruritus, hypotension, aches and pains, *anaphylaxis.*
Local: erythema, pain, induration, expected nodule persistent for several weeks.

INTERACTIONS
None significant.

NURSING CONSIDERATIONS
- Contraindicated in immunosuppression, radiation or corticosteroid therapy, children under 12 months with cerebral damage. Defer in acute illness or polio outbreak, except in emergency.
- Obtain history of allergies and reaction to immunization.
- Keep epinephrine 1:1,000 available

to treat anaphylaxis.
- Shake vial well before using. Store in refrigerator.

Haemophilus b polysaccharide vaccine (Hib)
b-Capsa I
Pregnancy Category: Does not apply

MECHANISM OF ACTION
Promotes active immunity to *Haemophilus influenzae* b.

INDICATIONS & DOSAGE
Immunization—
Children 2 to 6 years: 0.5 ml S.C. Single administration only.

ADVERSE REACTIONS
Local: *erythema and pain at injection site.*
Systemic: Fever, *anaphylaxis.*

INTERACTIONS
None significant.

NURSING CONSIDERATIONS
- Contraindicated in immunosuppression. Defer immunization in acute illness.
- Don't administer intradermally or I.V. Must administer S.C.
- All children should receive the vaccine by 24 months of age, but preferably *at* 24 months.
- Not generally recommended for infants younger than 18 months because vaccine will not protect very young children against *H. influenzae* type b. However, vaccine may be given to children 18 to 23 months old if they're at high risk for disease (for example, if attending day-care). Warn parent, however, that vaccine may not be completely effective.
- This vaccine will *not* protect children against any other microorganisms that cause meningitis. Will pro-

tect against *H. influenzae* type b only.
• This vaccine and DPT can be given simultaneously, but should be administered at different sites.
• Don't administer to children with febrile illness.
• Reconstitute vial with diluent provided in package. Inject 6 ml diluent into one vial of vaccine; mix to dissolve contents. The vial will provide 10 doses.
• Record the date of reconstitution on the label of the vaccine vial.
• Store in refrigerator and protect from light. Vaccine is stable for 30 days. Don't freeze.
• Keep epinephrine 1:1,000 available.
• *H. influenzae* type b is an important cause of meningitis in infants and preschool children.

---

hepatitis B vaccine
Heptavax-B♦
Pregnancy Category: C

MECHANISM OF ACTION
Promotes active immunity to hepatitis B.

INDICATIONS & DOSAGE
Immunization against infection caused by all known subtypes of hepatitis B virus. Recommended for immunization of selected populations who are considered to be at increased risk of contracting hepatitis B infection—
Adults and children over 10 years: initial dose 1 ml I.M. followed by another dose of 1 ml 1 month later. This is followed by a third dose of 1 ml 6 months after the first dose.
Children 3 months to 10 years: initial dose 0.5 ml I.M. followed by another dose of 0.5 ml 1 month later. This is followed by a third dose of 0.5 ml 6 months after the first dose.
Dialysis and immunocompromised patients: initial dose 2 ml I.M. followed by another dose of 2 ml 1

month later. This is followed by a third dose of two ml 6 months after the first dose. (The 2-ml doses should be divided into 2 1-ml doses and administered at different sites.)

ADVERSE REACTIONS
Local: discomfort at injection site, local inflammation.
Systemic: slight fever, transient malaise, headache, dizziness, nausea, vomiting.

INTERACTIONS
None reported.

NURSING CONSIDERATIONS
• Use cautiously in patients with any serious, active infection; compromised cardiac or pulmonary status; and in those for whom a febrile or systemic reaction could pose a serious risk.
• Hepatitis B vaccine has *not* been associated with an increased incidence of AIDS (acquired immunodeficiency syndrome).
• The CDC reports that response to hepatitis B vaccine is significantly better when administered in the arm rather than the buttock.
• May be administered S.C., but only to persons, such as hemophiliacs, who are at risk of hemorrhage.
• Although anaphylaxis has not been reported, epinephrine should always be available when administering this drug to counteract any possible reaction.
• The recommended dosage regimen provides immunity for at least 5 years.
• The following persons are at increased risk of infection and should be considered for the vaccine: certain health-care personnel (especially those working with dialysis patients, in blood banks, and in emergency medicine); selected patients and patient contacts; certain endemic populations (Alaskan Eskimos, Indo-

---

Italicized side effects are common or life-threatening.
*Liquid form contains alcohol.   **May contain tartrazine.

Chinese and Haitian refugees); certain military personnel; morticians and embalmers; blood bank employees; sexually active homosexuals; prostitutes; prisoners; and users of illicit, injectable drugs.
• Thoroughly agitate vial just before administration to restore suspension.
• Store both opened and unopened vials in the refrigerator. Don't freeze.

hepatitis B vaccine (recombinant)
Recombivax
Pregnancy Category: C

MECHANISM OF ACTION
Provides active immunity to hepatitis B.

INDICATIONS & DOSAGE
Immunization against infection caused by all known subtypes of hepatitis B virus. Recommended for immunization of selected populations considered at increased risk for hepatitis B infection—
Adults and children over 10 years: initial dose 1 ml I.M., followed by another 1-ml dose 1 month later and a third 1-ml dose 6 months after the first dose.
Children birth to 10 years: initial dose 0.5 ml I.M., followed by another 0.5-ml dose 1 month later and a third 0.5-ml dose 6 months after the first dose.

ADVERSE REACTIONS
Local: discomfort at injection site, local inflammation.
Systemic: fatigue, headache, fever, malaise, nausea, diarrhea, pharyngitis, hypersensitivity.

INTERACTIONS
None reported.

NURSING CONSIDERATIONS
• Don't administer the second or third dose to any patient who develops symptoms of hypersensitivity after the first dose. Ask patients to report any reaction they experience after the first dose.
• Use cautiously in patients with any serious active infection; with compromised cardiac or pulmonary status; and in those for whom a febrile or systemic reaction could pose a serious risk.
• Although anaphylaxis has not been reported, epinephrine should always be available when administering this drug to counteract any possible reaction.
• The Centers for Disease Control reports that response to hepatitis B vaccine is significantly better when vaccine is administered in the arm rather than the buttock.
• May be administered S.C., but only to persons who are at risk for hemorrhage, such as hemophiliacs.
• The following persons are at increased risk for infection and should be considered for the vaccine: certain health care personnel (especially those working with dialysis patients, in blood banks, and in emergency medicine); selected patients and patient contacts; certain endemic populations (Alaskan Eskimos, Indo-Chinese and Haitian refugees); certain military personnel; morticians and embalmers; sexually active homosexuals; prostitutes; prisoners; and users of illicit injectable drugs.
• Thoroughly agitate vial just before administration to restore suspension.
• Store both opened and unopened vials in the refrigerator. Don't freeze.
• Recombivax is manufactured by recombinant DNA technology. It is not a product of human plasma.

influenza virus vaccine, trivalent types A & B (split virus)
Fluogen

influenza virus vaccine, trivalent types A & B (whole virus)
Fluzone-Connaught
Pregnancy Category: C

MECHANISM OF ACTION
Promotes immunity to influenza by inducing production of antibodies.

INDICATIONS & DOSAGE
Chile, Mississippi, Ann Arbor strain influenza prophylaxis—
Adults and children over 12 years: 0.5 ml whole or split virus I.M. Only one dose is required.
Children 3 to 12 years: give 0.5 ml split virus I.M. Repeat dose in 4 weeks unless child received 1978 to 1985 vaccine.
Children 6 to 35 months: 0.25 ml split virus I.M. Repeat dose in 4 weeks unless child received 1978 to 1985 vaccine.
Recommendations are for 1987 only. Must check yearly for new recommendations.

ADVERSE REACTIONS
Systemic: *fever, malaise, myalgia, Guillain-Barré syndrome, anaphylaxis.*
Local: erythema, induration. Side effects occur most often in children and in others not exposed to influenza viruses.

INTERACTIONS
None significant.

NURSING CONSIDERATIONS
• Contraindicated in egg allergy. Defer in acute respiratory or other active infection, or when there is risk of poliomyelitis infection.
• Obtain history of allergies, especially to eggs, and reaction to immunization.
• Give injections in deltoid muscle whenever possible.
• Keep epinephrine 1:1,000 available.
• Recommended for patients with chronic disease, metabolic disorders, and those over age 65.
• Influenza vaccine available as whole virus and split virus preparations. Split virus vaccines cause somewhat fewer side effects than whole virus in children.
• Fever, malaise, and myalgia begin 6 to 12 hours after vaccination and persist 1 to 2 days.
• Allergic reactions, which occur immediately, are extremely rare.
• Paralysis associated with Guillain-Barré syndrome is uncommon. Patient should be made aware of risk as compared with risk of influenza and its complications.
• Pneumococcal vaccine may be given at the same time but at a different injection site.

measles, mumps, and rubella virus vaccine, live
M-M-R-II♦
Pregnancy Category: X

MECHANISM OF ACTION
Promotes immunity to measles, mumps, and rubella virus by inducing production of antibodies.

INDICATIONS & DOSAGE
Immunization—
Children 12 months to puberty: 1 vial (1,000 units) S.C.

ADVERSE REACTIONS
Systemic: fever, rash, regional lymphadenopathy, urticaria, *anaphylaxis.*
Local: erythema.

Italicized side effects are common or life-threatening.
*Liquid form contains alcohol.   **May contain tartrazine.

INTERACTIONS

Immune serum globulin, whole blood, plasma: antibodies in serum may interfere with immune response. Don't use vaccine within 3 months of transfusion.

NURSING CONSIDERATIONS

- Contraindicated in immunosuppression; cancer; blood dyscrasias; corticosteroid or radiation therapy; gamma globulin disorders; fever; active, untreated tuberculosis. Use cautiously in hypersensitivity to neomycin, chickens, ducks, eggs, or feathers. Defer immunization in acute illness.
- Presence of maternal antibodies may prevent response in children under 12 months.
- Treat fever with antipyretics.
- Store in refrigerator; protect from light. Solution may be used if red, pink, or yellow, but must be clear.
- Use only diluent supplied. Discard 8 hours after reconstituting.
- Obtain history of allergies, especially to ducks, rabbits, antibiotics, and reaction to immunization.
- Inject in outer aspect of upper arm. Don't give I.V.
- Keep epinephrine 1:1,000 available.

---

measles (rubeola) and rubella virus vaccine, live attenuated
M-R-Vax-II
Pregnancy Category: X

MECHANISM OF ACTION
Promotes immunity to measles and rubella virus by inducing production of antibodies.

INDICATIONS & DOSAGE
Immunization—
Children 15 months to puberty: 1 vial (1,000 units) S.C.

ADVERSE REACTIONS
Systemic: fever, rash, lymphadenopathy, *anaphylaxis*.

INTERACTIONS
Immune serum globulin, whole blood, plasma: antibodies in serum may interfere with immune response. Don't use vaccine within 3 months of transfusion.
Tuberculin skin test: may temporarily decrease response to test. Defer skin testing.

NURSING CONSIDERATIONS
- Contraindicated in immunosuppression; cancer; blood dyscrasias; corticosteroid or radiation therapy; gamma globulin disorders; fever; active, untreated tuberculosis. Use cautiously in hypersensitivity to neomycin, chickens, ducks, eggs, or feathers; when there is a history of febrile seizures; or in cerebral injury. Defer immunization in acute illness.
- Do not give within 1 month of other live virus vaccines, except oral poliovirus vaccine.
- Allow an interval of at least 3 weeks between BCG and rubella vaccine.
- Store in refrigerator and protect from light. Solution may be used if red, pink, or yellow, but must be clear (with no precipitation).
- Use only diluent supplied. Discard 8 hours after reconstituting.
- Inject in outer aspect of upper arm. Don't inject I.V.
- Keep epinephrine 1:1,000 available.

---

measles (rubeola) virus vaccine, live attenuated
Attenuvax♦
Pregnancy Category: X

MECHANISM OF ACTION
Promotes immunity to measles virus by inducing production of antibodies.

Unmarked trade names available in the United States only.
♦ Also available in Canada.   ♦♦ Available in Canada only.

INDICATIONS & DOSAGE
Immunization—
Adults and children 15 months or over: 0.5 ml (1,000 units) S.C.

ADVERSE REACTIONS
Systemic: fever, rash, lymphadenopathy, *anaphylaxis,* febrile convulsions in susceptible children, anorexia, leukopenia.
Local: erythema, swelling, tenderness.

INTERACTIONS
Immune serum globulin, whole blood, plasma: antibodies in serum may interfere with immune response. Don't use vaccine within 3 months of transfusion.
Tuberculin skin test: may temporarily decrease response to test. Defer skin testing.

NURSING CONSIDERATIONS
• Contraindicated in immunosuppression; cancer; blood dyscrasias; corticosteroid or radiation therapy; gamma globulin disorders; active, untreated tuberculosis; fever. Use with caution in hypersensitivity to neomycin, chickens, eggs, or feathers. Defer in acute illness or after administration of blood or plasma.
• Ideally, should be given during 2nd year of life.
• Warn patient to avoid pregnancy for 3 months after vaccination.
• Do not give I.V.
• Obtain history of allergies, especially to eggs, and reaction to immunization.
• Keep epinephrine 1:1,000 available.
• Store in refrigerator and protect from light. Solution may be used if red, pink, or yellow, but must be clear (with no precipitation).
• Use only diluent supplied. Discard 8 hours after reconstituting.
• May be given with oral poliovirus vaccine.

meningitis vaccines
Menomune-A/C, Menomune-A/C/Y/W-135
Pregnancy Category: C

MECHANISM OF ACTION
Promotes active immunity to meningitis.

INDICATIONS & DOSAGE
Meningococcal meningitis prophylaxis—
Adults and children over 2 years: 0.5 ml S.C.

ADVERSE REACTIONS
Systemic: headache, malaise, chills, fever, cramps, *anaphylaxis.*
Local: pain, erythema, induration.

INTERACTIONS
None significant.

NURSING CONSIDERATIONS
• Contraindicated in immunosuppression. Defer in acute illness.
• Tell patient to avoid pregnancy for 3 months after vaccination.
• Obtain history of allergies and reaction to immunization.
• Do not give I.V.
• Keep epinephrine 1:1,000 available.

mumps virus vaccine, live
Mumpsvax♦
Pregnancy Category: X

MECHANISM OF ACTION
Promotes active immunity to mumps.

INDICATIONS & DOSAGE
Immunization—
Adults and children over 1 year: 1 vial (5,000 units) S.C.

ADVERSE REACTIONS
Systemic: *slight fever,* rash, malaise, mild allergic reactions.

Italicized side effects are common or life-threatening.
*Liquid form contains alcohol.   **May contain tartrazine.

INTERACTIONS
Immune serum globulin, whole blood, plasma: antibodies in serum may interfere with immune response. Don't use vaccine within 3 months of transfusion.
Tuberculin skin test: may temporarily decrease response to test. Defer skin testing.

NURSING CONSIDERATIONS
• Contraindicated in immunosuppression; cancer; blood dyscrasias; corticosteroid or radiation therapy; gamma globulin disorders; active, untreated tuberculosis; pregnancy. Use cautiously in hypersensitivity to neomycin, chickens, ducks, eggs, or feathers. Defer in acute or febrile illness and for 3 months following transfusions or treatment with immune serum globulin.
• Keep epinephrine 1:1,000 available.
• Mumpsvax should not be given less than 1 month before or after immunization with other live virus vaccines, with the exception of Attenuvax, Meruvax, and/or monovalent or trivalent live, oral poliovirus vaccine, which may be administered simultaneously.
• The vaccine will not protect if given after exposure to natural mumps.
• Not recommended for infants younger than 12 months because retained maternal mumps antibodies may interfere with the immune response.
• Stress importance of avoiding pregnancy for 3 months after immunization. If necessary, provide contraceptive information.
• Treat fever with antipyretics.
• Don't give I.V.
• Store in refrigerator and protect from light. Solution may be used if red, pink, or yellow (but must be clear).
• Use only diluent supplied. Discard 8 hours after reconstituting.
• Obtain history of allergies, especially to antibiotics, and reaction to immunization.

plague vaccine
Pregnancy Category: C

MECHANISM OF ACTION
Promotes active immunity to plague.

INDICATIONS & DOSAGE
Primary immunization and booster—
Adults and children over 10 years: 1 ml I.M. followed by 0.2 ml in 4 weeks, then 0.2 ml 6 months after the first dose. Booster: 0.1 to 0.2 ml q 6 months while in plague area.
Children 5 to 10 years: ⅗ adult primary or booster dose.
Children 1 to 4 years: ⅖ adult primary or booster dose.
Children under 1 year: ⅕ adult primary or booster dose.

ADVERSE REACTIONS
Systemic: malaise, headache, slight fever, lymphadenopathy, *anaphylaxis.*
Local: swelling, *induration, erythema.*

INTERACTIONS
None significant.

NURSING CONSIDERATIONS
• Contraindicated in immunosuppression. Defer in respiratory infection.
• Deltoid area is the preferred injection site.
• Obtain history of allergies and reaction to immunization.
• Keep epinephrine 1:1,000 available.

pneumococcal vaccine, polyvalent
Pneumovax-23♦, Pnu-Immune-23
Pregnancy Category: C

MECHANISM OF ACTION
Promotes active immunity to infections caused by *Streptococcus pneu-*

moniae.

INDICATIONS & DOSAGE
Pneumococcal immunization—
Adults and children over 2 years:
0.5 ml I.M. or S.C.
Not recommended for children under
2 years.

ADVERSE REACTIONS
Systemic: *slight fever, anaphylaxis.*
Local: soreness, severe, local reaction
can occur when revaccination takes
place within 3 years.

INTERACTIONS
None significant.

NURSING CONSIDERATIONS
• Check immunization history carefully to avoid revaccination within 3
years.
• Inject in deltoid or midlateral thigh.
Don't inject I.V.
• Keep refrigerated. Reconstitution
or dilution not necessary.
• Treat fever with mild antipyretics.
• Protects against 23 pneumococcal
types, which account for 90% of
pneumococcal disease.
• Also may be administered to children to prevent pneumococcal otitis
media.
• Obtain history of allergies and reaction to immunization.
• Keep epinephrine 1:1,000 available.

poliovirus vaccine, live, oral, trivalent
Orimune
Pregnancy Category: C

MECHANISM OF ACTION
Promotes immunity to poliomyelitis
by inducing humoral antibodies and
antibodies in the lymphatic tissue.

INDICATIONS & DOSAGE
Poliovirus immunization—

**Adults, adolescents (through age
18), and older children:** two 0.5-ml
doses should be administered 8 weeks
apart. Give third 0.5-ml dose 6 to 12
months after second dose. A reinforc-
ing dose of 0.5 ml should be given before entry to school.
Infants: administer 0.5-ml dose at
age 2 months, 4 months, and 18
months. Optional dose may be given
at 6 months.

ADVERSE REACTIONS
Systemic: *paralytic poliomyelitis.*

INTERACTIONS
*Immune serum globulin, whole blood,
plasma:* antibodies in serum may interfere with immune response. Don't
use vaccine within 3 months of transfusion.
Tuberculin skin test: skin test may be
suppressed. Don't test for 6 weeks.

NURSING CONSIDERATIONS
• Contraindicated in immunosuppression, cancer, immunoglobulin abnormalities and in radiation, antimetabolite, alkylating agent, or corticosteroid therapy. Defer in acute illness,
vomiting, or diarrhea.
• Should not be administered to newborns younger than 6 weeks.
• Use with caution in siblings of child
with known immunodeficiency syndrome.
• This vaccine is not effective in
modifying or preventing existing or
incubating poliomyelitis.
• Check the parents' immunization
history when they bring in child for
vaccine; this is an excellent time for
parents to receive booster immunizations.
• Keep frozen until used. Once
thawed, if unopened, may store refrigerated up to 30 days. Opened vials
may be refrigerated up to 7 days.
Thaw before administration.
• Color change from pink to yellow
has no effect on the efficacy of the

vaccine. Yellow color results from vaccine being stored at low temperatures.
• Obtain history of allergies and reaction to immunization.
• Not for parenteral use.

rabies vaccine, human diploid cell (HDCV)
Imovax
Pregnancy Category: C

MECHANISM OF ACTION
Promotes active immunity to rabies.

INDICATIONS & DOSAGE
Postexposure antirabies immunization—
Adults and children: five 1-ml doses of HDCV I.M. (for example, in the deltoid region). Give first dose as soon as possible after exposure; give an additional dose on each of days 3, 7, 14, and 28 after first dose.
Preexposure prophylaxis immunization for persons in high-risk groups—
Adults and children: three 1-ml injections administered I. M. Give first dose on day 0 (the first day of therapy), second dose on day 7, and third dose on either day 21 or 28. Alternatively, give 0.1 ml intradermally on the same dosage schedule.

ADVERSE REACTIONS
Systemic: headache, nausea, abdominal pain, muscle aches, dizziness, fever, diarrhea, *anaphylaxis, serum sickness.*
Local: *pain, erythema, swelling or itching at injection site.*

INTERACTIONS
None significant.

NURSING CONSIDERATIONS
• Stop corticosteroids during immunization period.
• When postexposure immunization is indicated, pregnancy is not a contraindication.
• Persons with a history of hypersensitivity should be given rabies vaccine with caution.
• Some patients who receive booster doses experience serum sickness–like allergic reactions. These reactions usually respond to antihistamines.
• Keep epinephrine 1:1,000 available.
• CDC recommends a booster dose with Imovax for all persons who have been potentially exposed to rabies since October 15, 1984, and who have received postexposure prophylaxis with Wyvac unless acceptable titers were proven.
• The alternative regimen of 0.1-ml doses is only for *preexposure* prophylaxis. For postexposure prophylaxis, only the 1-ml doses should be used.

rubella and mumps virus vaccine, live
Biavax-II
Pregnancy Category: X

MECHANISM OF ACTION
Promotes immunity to rubella and mumps by inducing production of antibodies.

INDICATIONS & DOSAGE
Measles and mumps immunization—
Adults and children over 1 year: 1 vial (1,000 units) S.C.

ADVERSE REACTIONS
Systemic: fever, rash, thrombocytopenic purpura, urticaria, arthritis, arthralgia, polyneuritis, *anaphylaxis.*
Local: pain, erythema, induration, lymphadenopathy.

INTERACTIONS
Immune serum globulin, whole blood, plasma: antibodies in serum may interfere with immune response. Don't give vaccine within 3 months of transfusion.

Tuberculin skin test: may temporarily decrease response to test. Defer skin testing.

NURSING CONSIDERATIONS
• Contraindicated in immunosuppression; cancer; blood dyscrasias; corticosteroid or radiation therapy; gamma globulin disorders; active, untreated tuberculosis; fever; or pregnancy. Use with caution in hypersensitivity to neomycin, chickens, ducks, eggs, or feathers. Defer in acute illness and after administration of immune serum globulin, blood, or plasma.
• Stress importance of avoiding pregnancy for 3 months after immunization. If necessary, provide contraceptive information.
• Store in refrigerator and protect from light. Solution may be used if red, pink, or yellow (but must be clear).
• Use only diluent supplied. Discard 8 hours after reconstituting.
• Obtain history of allergies, especially to ducks, rabbits, and antibiotics, and reaction to immunization.
• Inject into outer aspect of upper arm. Don't inject I.V.
• Keep epinephrine 1:1,000 available.
• Allow an interval of at least 3 weeks between BCG and rubella vaccine.

---

rubella virus vaccine, live attenuated (RA 27/3)
Meruvax II♦
Pregnancy Category: X

MECHANISM OF ACTION
Promotes immunity to rubella by inducing production of antibodies.

INDICATIONS & DOSAGE
Measles immunization—
Adults and children over 1 year: 1 vial (1,000 units) S.C.

ADVERSE REACTIONS
Systemic: *joint pain,* fever, rash, thrombocytopenic purpura, urticaria, arthritis, arthralgia, polyneuritis, *anaphylaxis.*
Local: pain, erythema, induration, lymphadenopathy.

INTERACTIONS
Immune serum globulin, whole blood, plasma: antibodies in serum may interfere with immune response. Don't use vaccine within 3 months of transfusion.
Tuberculin skin test: may temporarily decrease response to test. Defer skin testing.

NURSING CONSIDERATIONS
• Contraindicated in immunosuppression; cancer; blood dyscrasias; corticosteroid or radiation therapy; gamma globulin disorders; active, untreated tuberculosis; fever. Use cautiously in hypersensitivity to neomycin, chickens, ducks, eggs, or feathers. Defer in acute illness and after administration of human immune serum globulin, blood, or plasma.
• Stress importance of avoiding pregnancy for 3 months after immunization. If necessary, provide contraceptive information.
• Store in refrigerator and protect from light. Solution may be used if red, pink, or yellow (but must be clear).
• Use only diluent supplied. Discard 8 hours after reconstituting.
• Obtain history of allergies, especially to ducks and rabbits, and reaction to immunization.
• Inject into outer aspect of upper arm. Don't inject I.V.
• Keep epinephrine 1:1,000 available.
• Allow an interval of at least 3 weeks between BCG and rubella vaccine.

Italicized side effects are common or life-threatening.
*Liquid form contains alcohol.   **May contain tartrazine.

tetanus toxoid, adsorbed

tetanus toxoid fluid
Pregnancy Category: C

MECHANISM OF ACTION
Promotes immunity to tetanus by inducing production of antitoxin.

INDICATIONS & DOSAGE
Primary immunization—
Adults and children: 0.5 ml (adsorbed) I.M. 4 to 6 weeks apart for two doses, then third dose 1 year after the second.
Primary immunization—
Adults and children: 0.5 ml (fluid) I.M. or S.C. 4 to 8 weeks apart, for three doses, then fourth dose of 0.5 ml 6 to 12 months after third dose.
Booster: 0.5 ml I.M. at 10-year intervals.

ADVERSE REACTIONS
Systemic: slight fever, chills, malaise, aches and pains, flushing, urticaria, pruritus, tachycardia, hypotension, *anaphylaxis.*
Local: erythema, induration, nodule.

INTERACTIONS
None significant.

NURSING CONSIDERATIONS
• Contraindicated in immunosuppression and immunoglobulin abnormalities. Defer in acute illness and polio outbreaks, except in emergencies.
• For prevention, not treatment, of tetanus infections.
• Determine date of last tetanus immunization.
• Don't use hot or cold compresses; may increase severity of local reaction.
• Obtain history of allergies and reaction to immunization.
• Keep epinephrine 1:1,000 handy.
• Adsorbed form produces longer duration of immunity. Fluid form provides quicker booster effect in patients actively immunized previously.
• Do not confuse this drug with tetanus immune globulin, human.

typhoid vaccine
Pregnancy Category: C

MECHANISM OF ACTION
Provides active immunity to typhoid fever.

INDICATIONS & DOSAGE
Primary immunization—
Adults and children over 10 years: 0.5 ml S.C.; repeat in 4 weeks. Booster: same dose as primary immunization q 3 years.
Children 6 months to 10 years: 0.25 ml S.C.; repeat in 4 weeks. Booster: same dose as primary immunization q 3 years.

ADVERSE REACTIONS
Systemic: *fever,* malaise, headache, nausea, *anaphylaxis.*
Local: swelling, pain, inflammation.

INTERACTIONS
None significant.

NURSING CONSIDERATIONS
• Contraindicated in corticosteroid therapy. Defer in acute illness.
• Treat fever with antipyretics.
• Do not give intradermally.
• Obtain history of allergies and reaction to immunization.
• Keep epinephrine 1:1,000 available.
• Store at 35.6° to 50° F. (2° to 10° C.).
• Shake thoroughly before withdrawing from vial.

yellow fever vaccine
YF-Vax
Pregnancy Category: D

MECHANISM OF ACTION
Provides active immunity to typhoid
fever.

INDICATIONS & DOSAGE
Primary vaccination—
Adults and children over 6 months:
0.5 ml deep S.C. Booster: repeat 0.5
ml S.C. q 10 years.

ADVERSE REACTIONS
Systemic: fever, malaise, *anaphylaxis.*
Local: mild swelling, pain.

INTERACTIONS
None significant.

NURSING CONSIDERATIONS
• Contraindicated in gamma globulin
deficiency, immunosuppression, cancer, corticosteroid or radiation therapy, allergies to chickens or eggs, and
in pregnancy. Also contraindicated in
infants under 9 months except in
high-risk areas.
• Reconstitute with sodium chloride
injection that contains no preservatives (preservatives decrease potency).
• Must be kept frozen. Don't use unless shipping case contains some dry
ice upon arrival. Avoid vigorous
shaking; carefully swirl mixture until
suspension is uniform. Use within 1
hour after reconstitution. Discard remainder.
• Obtain history of allergies, especially to eggs, and reaction to immunization.
• Don't give within 1 month of other
live virus vaccines.
• Keep epinephrine 1:1,000 available.

Italicized side effects are common or life-threatening.
*Liquid form contains alcohol.   **May contain tartrazine.

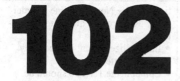

Antitoxins and antivenins

black widow spider antivenin
botulism antitoxin, bivalent
  equine
crotaline antivenin, polyvalent
diphtheria antitoxin, equine
Micrurus fulvius antivenin
tetanus antitoxin (TAT), equine

COMBINATION PRODUCTS
None.

---

black widow spider antivenin
Antivenin *(Latrodectus mactans)*♦
Pregnancy Category: D

MECHANISM OF ACTION
Neutralizes and binds venom.

INDICATIONS & DOSAGE
Black widow spider bite—
Adults and children: 2.5 ml I.M. in deltoid. Second dose may be needed.

ADVERSE REACTIONS
Systemic: hypersensitivity, *anaphylaxis, neurotoxicity*.

INTERACTIONS
None significant.

NURSING CONSIDERATIONS
• If possible, hospitalize patient.
• Immobilize patient; splint the bitten limb to prevent spread of venom.
• Test for sensitivity before giving. Use 0.2 ml of a 1:10 dilution in normal saline solution.
• Epinephrine 1:1,000 should be available in case of adverse reaction.

• Venom is neurotoxic and may cause respiratory paralysis and convulsions. Watch patient carefully for 2 to 3 days.
• Obtain accurate patient history of allergies, especially to horses, and reaction to immunization.
• Earliest possible use of antivenin recommended for best results.
• Antivenin may be given I.V. in severe cases (when patient is in shock), in 10 to 50 ml of saline solution over 15 minutes.

---

botulism antitoxin, bivalent equine
Pregnancy Category: D

MECHANISM OF ACTION
Neutralizes and binds toxin.

INDICATIONS & DOSAGE
Botulism—
Adults and children: 1 vial I.V. stat and q 4 hours, p.r.n., until patient's condition improves. Dilute antitoxin 1:10 in dextrose 5% or 10% in water or normal saline solution before giving. Give first 10 ml of dilution over 5 minutes; after 15 minutes, rate may be increased.

ADVERSE REACTIONS
Systemic: hypersensitivity, *anaphylaxis*, serum sickness (urticaria, pruritus, fever, malaise, arthralgia) may occur in 5 to 13 days.

INTERACTIONS
None significant.

NURSING CONSIDERATIONS
- Test for sensitivity before giving.
- Epinephrine 1:1,000 should be available in case of adverse reaction. Bivalent antitoxin contains antibodies against types A and B *Clostridium botulinum*. Antitoxins against all other types available only from Centers for Disease Control in Atlanta, Georgia (phone 404-329-3311).
- Obtain accurate patient history of allergies, especially to horses, and reaction to immunization.
- Earliest possible use of antitoxin is recommended for best results.

---

crotaline antivenin, polyvalent
Pregnancy Category: D

MECHANISM OF ACTION
Neutralizes and binds venom.

INDICATIONS & DOSAGE
Crotalid (rattlesnake) bites—
Adults and children: initially, 10 to 50 ml or more I.M. or S.C., depending on severity of bite and patient's response. If large amount of venom, 70 to 100 ml I.V. directly into superficial vein. Subsequent doses based on patient's response; may give 10 ml q ½ to 2 hours, p.r.n. If bite is in extremity, inject part of initial dose at various sites around limb above swelling; don't inject in finger or toe. The smaller the patient, the larger the initial dose.

ADVERSE REACTIONS
Systemic: hypersensitivity, *anaphylaxis, neurotoxicity, serum sickness.*

INTERACTIONS
Antihistamines: enhanced toxicity of crotaline venoms. Don't use together.

NURSING CONSIDERATIONS
- Test for sensitivity before giving. Give 0.02 to 0.03 ml of a 1:10 dilu-

tion in 0.9% Normal Saline intradermally. Read results after 5 to 10 minutes.
- Immobilize patient immediately. Splint the bitten extremity.
- Epinephrine 1:1,000 should be available in case of adverse reaction.
- Type and cross match as soon as possible since hemolysis from venom prevents accurate cross matching.
- Early use of antivenin is recommended for best results.
- Watch patient carefully for delayed allergic reaction or relapse.
- Children, who have less resistance and less body fluid to dilute venom, may need twice the adult dose.
- Obtain accurate patient history of allergies, especially to horses, and reaction to immunization.
- Discard unused reconstituted drug.

---

diphtheria antitoxin, equine
Pregnancy Category: D

MECHANISM OF ACTION
Neutralizes and binds toxin.

INDICATIONS & DOSAGE
Diphtheria prevention—
Adults and children: 1,000 to 5,000 units I.M.
Diphtheria treatment—
Adults and children: 20,000 to 80,000 units or more slow I.V. Additional doses may be given in 24 hours. I.M. route may be used in mild cases.

ADVERSE REACTIONS
Systemic: hypersensitivity, *anaphylaxis,* serum sickness (urticaria, pruritus, fever, malaise, arthralgia) may occur in 7 to 12 days.

INTERACTIONS
None significant.

NURSING CONSIDERATIONS
- Test for sensitivity before giving.
- Epinephrine 1:1,000 should be

---

available in case of adverse reaction.
- Obtain accurate patient history of allergies, especially to horses, and reaction to immunization.
- Therapy should be started immediately, without waiting for culture and sensitivity reports, if patient has clinical symptoms of diphtheria (sore throat, fever, tonsillar membrane).
- Refrigerate antitoxin at 35.6° to 50° F. (2° to 10° C.). Warm to 90° to 95° F. (32.2° to 35° C.), never higher.

Micrurus fulvius antivenin
Pregnancy Category: D

MECHANISM OF ACTION
Neutralizes and binds venom.

INDICATIONS & DOSAGE
Eastern and Texas coral snake bite—
Adults and children: 3 to 5 vials slow I.V. through running I.V. of 0.9% normal saline solution. Give first 1 to 2 ml over 3 to 5 minutes, and watch for signs of allergic reaction. If no signs develop, continue injection. Up to 10 vials may be needed. Not effective for Sonoran or Arizona coral snake bites.

ADVERSE REACTIONS
Systemic: hypersensitivity, *anaphylaxis.*

INTERACTIONS
None significant.

NURSING CONSIDERATIONS
- Test for sensitivity before giving.
- Immobilize patient or splint bitten limb to prevent spread of venom.
- If possible, hospitalize patient.
- Early use of antivenin recommended for best results.
- Venom is neurotoxic and may cause respiratory paralysis. Watch patient carefully for 24 hours. Be ready to take supportive measures. Epinephrine 1:1,000 should be available in

case of adverse reaction.
- Obtain accurate patient history of allergies, especially to horses, and reaction to immunization.

tetanus antitoxin (TAT), equine
Pregnancy Category: D

MECHANISM OF ACTION
Neutralizes and binds toxin.

INDICATIONS & DOSAGE
Tetanus prophylaxis—
Patients over 30 kg: 3,000 to 5,000 units I.M. or S.C.
Patients under 30 kg: 1,500 to 3,000 units I.M. or S.C.
Tetanus treatment—
All patients: 10,000 to 20,000 units injected into wound. Give additional 40,000 to 100,000 units I.V. Start tetanus toxoid at same time but at different site and with a different syringe.

ADVERSE REACTIONS
Local: pain, numbness, skin eruptions.
Systemic: joint pain, hypersensitivity, *anaphylaxis, serum sickness.*

INTERACTIONS
None significant.

NURSING CONSIDERATIONS
- Test for sensitivity before giving. Give 0.1 ml as a 1:1,000 dilution in 0.9% Normal Saline intradermally.
- Use only when tetanus immune globulin (human) not available.
- Obtain accurate patient history of allergies, especially to horses, and reaction to immunization. If respiratory difficulty develops, give 0.4 ml of 1:1,000 solution epinephrine HCl.
- Preventive dose should be given to those who have had two or fewer injections of tetanus toxoid and who have tetanus-prone injuries more than 24 hours old.

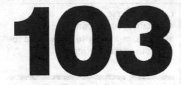

Acidifiers and alkalinizers

Acidifiers
ammonium chloride
dilute hydrochloric acid
Alkalinizers
sodium bicarbonate
sodium lactate
tromethamine

COMBINATION PRODUCTS
None.

ammonium chloride
Pregnancy Category: B

MECHANISM OF ACTION
Increases free hydrogen ion (H^+) concentration. Also acts as an expectorant by causing reflex stimulation of bronchial mucous glands.

INDICATIONS & DOSAGE
Metabolic alkalosis—
Adults and children: Dose is calculated by amount of chloride deficit. Infusion rate: 0.9 to 1.3 ml/minute 2.14% solution. Do not exceed 2 ml/minute. Hypodermoclysis has been used in infants and young children. One half calculated volume should be given, then patient should be reassessed.
As an acidifying agent—
Adults: 4 to 12 g P.O. daily in divided doses.
Children: 75 mg/kg daily P.O. in four divided doses.
As expectorant—
Adults: 250 to 500 mg P.O. q 2 to 4 hours.

ADVERSE REACTIONS
Side effects usually result from ammonia toxicity or too rapid I.V. administration.
CNS: headache, confusion, progressive drowsiness, excitement alternating with coma, hyperventilation, *calcium-deficient tetany, twitching, hyperreflexia, EEG abnormalities.*
CV: bradycardia.
GI: (with oral dose) *gastric irritation, nausea, vomiting,* thirst, anorexia, retching.
GU: glycosuria.
Metabolic: *acidosis, hyperchloremia, hypokalemia,* hyperglycemia.
Skin: rash, pallor.
Local: pain at injection site.
Other: irregular respirations with periods of apnea.

INTERACTIONS
Spironolactone: systemic acidosis. Use together cautiously.

NURSING CONSIDERATIONS
• Contraindicated in severe hepatic or renal dysfunction. Use cautiously in pulmonary insufficiency or cardiac edema and in infants.
• Give after meals to decrease GI side effects. Enteric-coated tablets may also minimize GI symptoms but are absorbed erratically.
• Do not administer drug with milk or other alkaline solutions because they are not compatible.
• Pain of I.V. injection may be lessened by decreasing infusion rate.
• Determine CO_2 combining power and serum electrolytes before and

Italicized side effects are common or life-threatening.
*Liquid form contains alcohol.   **May contain tartrazine.

during therapy to prevent acidosis.
• Monitor urine pH and output. Diuresis is normal for first 2 days.
• Dilute concentrated solutions (21.4%, 26.75%) to 2.14% before giving.
• Monitor rate and depth of respirations frequently.
• Hypodermoclysis should be into lateral aspect of thigh. Stop infusion immediately if pain occurs.
• When using as an expectorant, give with full glass of water.

dilute hydrochloric acid
Pregnancy Category: C

MECHANISM OF ACTION
Increases free hydrogen ion (H^+) concentration.

INDICATIONS & DOSAGE
Metabolic alkalosis—
pharmacy prepares (0.1 normal HCl solution in sterile water) 100 mEq hydrogen and 100 mEq chloride/liter.

ADVERSE REACTIONS
None confirmed.

INTERACTIONS
None significant.

NURSING CONSIDERATIONS
• Not available commercially; prepared in pharmacy.
• Administer I.V. solution slowly through a central venous line.
• Monitor pH, blood gases, and electrolytes at 4- to 6-hour intervals.

sodium bicarbonate
Pregnancy Category: C

MECHANISM OF ACTION
Restores buffering capacity of the body. Also neutralizes excess acid.

INDICATIONS & DOSAGE
Cardiac arrest—
Adults and children: as a 7.5% or 8.4% solution, 1 mEq/kg followed by 0.5 mEq/kg every 10 minutes depending on blood gases. Further doses based on blood gases. If blood gases unavailable, use 0.5 mEq/kg q 10 minutes until spontaneous circulation returns.
Infants up to 2 years: 4.2% solution, I.V. infusion. Rate not to exceed 8 mEq/kg daily.
Metabolic acidosis—
Adults and children: dose depends on blood CO_2 content, pH, and patient's clinical condition. Generally, 2 to 5 mEq/kg I.V. infused over 4- to 8-hour period.
Systemic or urinary alkalinization—
Adults: 325 mg to 2 g P.O. q.i.d.
Children: 12 to 120 mg/kg daily.
Antacid—
Adults: 300 mg to 2 g tablets chewed and taken with glass of water.

ADVERSE REACTIONS
GI: *gastric distention, belching, flatulence.*
GU: renal calculi or crystals.
Metabolic: (with overdose) alkalosis, hypernatremia, hyperkalemia, hyperosmolarity.

INTERACTIONS
None significant.

NURSING CONSIDERATIONS
• No contraindications for use in life-threatening emergencies. Contraindicated in hypertension, in patients with tendency toward edema, in patients who are losing chlorides by vomiting or from continuous GI suction, in patients receiving diuretics known to produce hypochloremic alkalosis, and in patients on salt restriction or with renal disease.
• May be added to other I.V. fluids.
• Because sodium bicarbonate inactivates such catecholamines as norepi-

nephrine and dopamine, do not mix with I.V. solutions of these agents.
• To avoid risk of alkalosis, determine blood pH, PaO_2, $PaCO_2$, and electrolytes. Keep doctor informed of laboratory results.
• Tell patient not to take with milk. May cause hypercalcemia, alkalosis, and possibly renal calculi.
• Discourage use as antacid. Offer nonabsorbable alternative antacid if it is to be used repeatedly.
• May cause enteric-coated drugs to be prematurely released in the stomach.

sodium lactate
Pregnancy Category: C

MECHANISM OF ACTION
Metabolized to sodium bicarbonate. Then produces buffering effect.

INDICATIONS & DOSAGE
Alkalinize urine—
Adults: 30 ml of a $\frac{1}{6}$ molar solution/kg of body weight given in divided doses over 24 hours.
Metabolic acidosis—
Adults: usually given as $\frac{1}{6}$ molar injection (167 mEq lactate/liter). Dosage depends on degree of bicarbonate deficit.

ADVERSE REACTIONS
Metabolic: (with overdose) alkalosis, hypernatremia, hyperosmolarity.

INTERACTIONS
None significant.

NURSING CONSIDERATIONS
• Contraindicated in severe hepatic and renal disease, respiratory alkalosis, and acidosis associated with congenital heart disease with persistent cyanosis.
• Monitor serum electrolytes to avoid alkalosis.

tromethamine
Tham◆
Pregnancy Category: C

MECHANISM OF ACTION
Combines with hydrogen ions and associated acid anions; the resulting salts are excreted.

INDICATIONS & DOSAGE
Metabolic acidosis (associated with cardiac bypass surgery or with cardiac arrest)—
Adults: dose depends on bicarbonate deficit. Calculate as follows: ml of 0.3 M tromethamine solution required = wt in kg × bicarbonate deficit (mEq/liter). Additional therapy based on serial determinations of existing bicarbonate deficit.
Children: calculate dose as above. Give slowly over 3 to 6 hours. Additional therapy based on degree of acidosis. Total 24-hour dose should not exceed 33 to 40 ml/kg.

ADVERSE REACTIONS
CNS: respiratory depression.
Metabolic: hypoglycemia, hyperkalemia (with decreased urinary output).
Local: venospasm; intravenous thrombosis; inflammation, necrosis, and sloughing if extravasation occurs.

INTERACTIONS
None significant.

NURSING CONSIDERATIONS
• Contraindicated in anuria, uremia, chronic respiratory acidosis, pregnancy (except acute, life-threatening situations). Use cautiously in renal disease or poor urinary output. Monitor EKG and serum K^+ in these patients.
• To prevent blood pH from rising above normal, adjust dose carefully.
• Give slowly through large needle (18G to 20G) into largest antecubital vein or by indwelling I.V. catheter.

Italicized side effects are common or life-threatening.
*Liquid form contains alcohol.   **May contain tartrazine.

• Before, during, and after therapy make the following determinations: blood pH; carbon dioxide tension; bicarbonate, glucose, and electrolyte levels.

• Mechanical ventilation should be readily available. Use when giving drug to patient with associated respiratory acidosis.

• Except in life-threatening situations, do not use longer than 1 day.

• If extravasation occurs, infiltrate area with 1% procaine and hyaluronidase 150 units; may reduce vasospasm and dilute remaining drug in local area.

• Concentration of tromethamine should not exceed 0.3 M.

Uricosurics

probenecid
sulfinpyrazone

COMBINATION PRODUCTS
COLBENEMID: probenecid 500 mg
and colchicine 0.5 mg.
PROBEN-C: probenecid 500 mg and
colchicine 0.5 mg.

---

probenecid
Benemid♦, Benn, Benuryl♦♦,
Probalan, Probenimead,
Robenecid
Pregnancy Category: B

MECHANISM OF ACTION
Blocks renal tubular reabsorption of
uric acid, increasing excretion. Also
inhibits active renal tubular secretion
of many weak organic acids (for example, penicillins and cephalosporins).

INDICATIONS & DOSAGE
*Adjunct to penicillin or cephalosporin
therapy—*
Adults and children over 50 kg: 500
mg P.O. q.i.d.
Children 2 to 14 years (under 50 kg):
initially, 25 mg/kg P.O., then 40 mg/
kg divided q.i.d.
Single-dose treatment of gonorrhea—
Adults: 3.5 g ampicillin P.O. with 1 g
probenecid P.O. given together; or 1 g
probenecid P.O. 30 minutes before
dose of 4.8 million units of aqueous
penicillin G procaine I.M., injected at
two different sites.
*Treatment of hyperuricemia of gout,
gouty arthritis—*

Adults: 250 mg P.O. b.i.d. for first
week, then 500 mg b.i.d., to maximum of 2 g daily. Maintenance: 500
mg daily for 6 months.

ADVERSE REACTIONS
Blood: *hemolytic anemia.*
CNS: headache, dizziness.
CV: hypotension.
GI: anorexia, nausea, vomiting, *gas-
tric distress.*
GU: urinary frequency.
Skin: dermatitis, pruritus.
Other: flushing, sore gums, fever.

INTERACTIONS
Salicylates: inhibited uricosuric effect
of probenecid, causing urate retention. Do not use together.

NURSING CONSIDERATIONS
• Contraindicated in blood dyscrasias; acute gout attack; penicillin therapy in presence of known renal impairment; gouty nephropathy; urinary
tract stones or obstruction; azotemia,
hyperuricemia secondary to cancer
chemotherapy, radiation, or myeloproliferative neoplastic diseases. Use
cautiously with peptic ulcer or renal
impairment.
• Usually preferred over sulfinpyrazone because probenecid produces
fewer, less severe GI and hematologic
side effects.
• Contains no analgesic or anti-inflammatory agent, and is of no value
during acute gout attacks. Don't initiate therapy until acute attack subsides.
• Suitable for long-term use; no cu-

---

mulative effects or tolerance.
• Not effective with chronic renal insufficiency (glomerular filtration rate less than 30 ml/minute).
• Periodic BUN and renal function tests recommended in long-term therapy.
• May increase frequency, severity, and length of acute gout attacks during first 6 to 12 months of therapy. Prophylactic colchicine is given during first 3 to 6 months.
• Tell patient to avoid alcohol; it increases urate level.
• Patient should avoid all medications that contain aspirin. These may precipitate gout.
• Force fluids to maintain minimum daily output of 2 to 3 liters. Alkalinize urine with sodium bicarbonate or potassium citrate ordered by doctor. These measures will prevent hematuria, renal colic, urate stone development, and costovertebral pain.
• Give with milk, food, or antacids to minimize GI distress. Continued disturbances might indicate need to lower dose.
• Restrict foods high in purine: anchovies, liver, sardines, kidneys, sweetbreads, peas, lentils.
• Instruct patient and his family that drug must be taken regularly as ordered or gout attacks may result. Tell him to visit doctor regularly so uric acid can be monitored and dosage can be adjusted if necessary. Lifelong therapy may be required in patients with hyperuricemia.
• May produce false-positive glucose tests with Benedict's solution or Clinitest, but not with glucose oxidase method (Clinistix, Diastix, Tes-Tape).
• Decreases urinary excretion of 17-ketosteroids, phenolsulfonphthalein (PSP), Bromsulphalein (BSP), aminohippuric acid, and iodine-related organic acids, interfering with laboratory procedures.

sulfinpyrazone
Anturan◆◆, Anturane
Pregnancy Category: C

MECHANISM OF ACTION
Blocks renal tubular reabsorption of uric acid, increasing excretion. Also inhibits platelet aggregation.

INDICATIONS & DOSAGE
Inhibition of platelet aggregation, increase of platelet survival time in treatment of thromboembolic disorders, angina, myocardial infarction, transient cerebral ischemic attacks, peripheral arterial atherosclerosis—
Adults: 200 mg P.O. q.i.d.
Maintenance therapy for common gout: reduction, prevention of joint changes and tophi formation—
Adults: 100 to 200 mg P.O. b.i.d. first week, then 200 to 400 mg P.O. b.i.d. Maximum 800 mg daily.

ADVERSE REACTIONS
Blood: *agranulocytosis.*
GI: *nausea, dyspepsia,* epigastric pain, blood loss, reactivation of peptic ulcers.
Skin: rash.

INTERACTIONS
Probenecid: inhibited renal excretion of sulfinpyrazone. Use together with caution.
Salicylates: inhibited uricosuric effect of sulfinpyrazone. Do not use together.

NURSING CONSIDERATIONS
• Contraindicated in hypersensitivity to pyrazole derivatives (including oxyphenbutazone, phenylbutazone); active peptic ulcer; gouty nephropathy; urolithiasis or urinary obstruction; bone-marrow depression; azotemia, hyperuricemia secondary to cancer chemotherapy, radiation, or myeloproliferative neoplastic diseases; and during or within 2 weeks

after gout attack. Use cautiously in diminished hepatic or renal function.

• Use in treating thromboembolic conditions is investigational and is most often directed at prevention of recurrent myocardial infarction.

• Recommended for patients unresponsive to probenecid. Suitable for long-term use; no cumulative effects or tolerance.

• Contains no analgesic or anti-inflammatory agent, and is of no value during acute gout attacks.

• Periodic BUN, CBC, and renal function studies advised during long-term use.

• May increase frequency, severity, and length of acute gout attacks during first 6 to 12 months of therapy; prophylactic colchicine is given during first 3 to 6 months.

• Therapy, especially at start, may lead to renal colic and formation of uric acid stones. Until acid levels are normal (about 6 mg/100 ml), monitor intake and output closely.

• Force fluids to maintain minimum daily output of 2 to 3 liters. Alkalinize urine with sodium bicarbonate or other agent ordered by doctor.

• Give with milk, food, or antacids to minimize GI disturbances.

• Restrict foods high in purine: anchovies, liver, sardines, kidneys, sweetbreads, peas, lentils.

• Instruct patient and his family that drug must be taken regularly as ordered or gout attacks may result. Tell him to visit doctor regularly so blood levels can be monitored and dosage adjusted if necessary.

• Lifelong therapy may be required in patients with hyperuricemia.

• Decreases urinary excretion of aminohippuric acid and phenolsulfonphthalein (PSP), interfering with laboratory procedures.

• Alkalinizing agents are used therapeutically to increase sulfinpyrazone activity, preventing urolithiasis.

• Warn patient not to take any aspirin-containing medications.

• Monitor patients taking oral hypoglycemic agents; these drugs' effects may be potentiated by sulfinpyrazone, causing hypoglycemia.

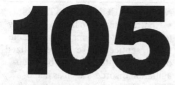

chymopapain
chymotrypsin
fibrinolysin and
   desoxyribonuclease
hyaluronidase

COMBINATION PRODUCTS
CHYMORAL-100: 100,000 units enzymatic activity; trypsin and chymotrypsin in ratio of 6:1.
GRANULEX AEROSOL: trypsin 0.1 mg, balsam Peru 72.5 mg, and castor oil 650 mg/0.82 ml.
ORENZYME BITABS ENTERIC-COATED TABLETS: 100,000 units trypsin and 8,000 units chymotrypsin.

---

chymopapain
Chymodiactin, Discase
Pregnancy Category: C

MECHANISM OF ACTION
Hydrolyzes noncollagenous proteins in the chondromucoprotein of the nucleus pulposus.

INDICATIONS & DOSAGE
Treatment of herniated lumbar intervertebral disk—
Adults: 2,000 to 4,000 units per disk injected intradiskally. Maximum dose in a single patient with multiple disk herniation is 10,000 units. (Should be administered in the hospital by doctors experienced and trained in diagnosis of lumbar disk disease).

ADVERSE REACTIONS
Local: *back pain, stiffness, back spasm.*

Systemic: *anaphylaxis, paraplegia, cerebral hemorrhage, acute transverse myelitis,* nausea, headache, dizziness, leg weakness, paresthesias, numbness of legs and toes.

INTERACTIONS
None significant.

NURSING CONSIDERATIONS
• Contraindicated in patients with history of allergy to papaya or meat tenderizer; patients who have previously received an injection of chymopapain; severe spondylolisthesis plus spinal stenosis; severe progressing paralysis; evidence of spinal cord tumor or a cauda equina lesion.
• Should be used only by doctors qualified by training and experience to perform laminectomy, diskectomy or other spinal procedures, and who have received specialized training in chemonucleolysis. Shouldn't be injected in any region other than the lumbar spine. Chymopapain is extremely toxic if injected into the subarachnoid space.
• A new test (ChymoFAST) can detect allergic sensitivity to chymopapain.
• Monitor very closely for anaphylactic reaction (0.5% of patients). Can be immediate or delayed up to 1 hour after injection and can last for minutes to several hours or longer. Watch for hypotension and bronchospasm. These may lead to laryngeal edema, arrhythmia, cardiac arrest, coma, and death. Other signs of allergic response include erythema, pilomotor

erection, rash, pruritic urticaria, conjunctivitis, vasomotor rhinitis, angioedema, or various GI disturbances.
• Keep an I.V. line open to permit rapid management of anaphylaxis. Keep epinephrine and steroids available.
• Instruct patient to anticipate the possibility of delayed allergic reactions, such as rash, urticaria, or itching, which may occur as late as 15 days after injection. Patient should report these to doctor immediately.
• Patients may experience back pain or involuntary muscle spasm in the lower back for several days after injection. Reassure patient that this is common and will not be chronic.
• Use within 60 minutes after reconstitution. Discard unused drug.

chymotrypsin
Avazyme**
Pregnancy Category: C

MECHANISM OF ACTION
Reverses the decreased tissue permeability that develops with inflammation and edema. Restores flow of blood and other body fluids, and facilitates drainage and tissue repair.

INDICATIONS & DOSAGE
Relief of episiotomy pain—
Women: 20,000 to 40,000 units P.O. q.i.d.

ADVERSE REACTIONS
Blood: increased bleeding tendencies.
GI: nausea, vomiting, diarrhea.
GU: hematuria, albuminuria, menorrhagia.
Other: chills, dizziness, fever, rapid dissolution of animal-origin sutures, *hypersensitivity reactions (rash, urticaria, itching, anaphylaxis)*.

INTERACTIONS
None significant.

NURSING CONSIDERATIONS
• Contraindicated in hypersensitivity to trypsin or to sesame oil (injectable form), septicemia, severe generalized or localized infection, and blood coagulation disorders such as hemophilia. Use with caution in severe hepatic or renal disease.

fibrinolysin and desoxyribonuclease
Elase♦
Pregnancy Category: C

MECHANISM OF ACTION
Desoxyribonuclease attacks DNA and fibrinolysin attacks fibrin of blood clots and fibrinous exudates.

INDICATIONS & DOSAGE
Debridement of inflammatory and infected lesions (surgical wounds, ulcerative lesions, second- and third-degree burns, circumcision, episiotomy, cervicitis, vaginitis, abscesses, fistulas, and sinus tracts)—
Intravaginally—
5 ml ointment may be inserted using applicator supplied, once daily for vaginitis or cervicitis.
Topical use—
apply ointment at intervals as long as enzyme action is desired.
Irrigating agent for infected wounds, empyema cavities, abscesses, otorhinolaryngologic wounds, subcutaneous hematomas—
dilution for irrigation depends on extent and severity of wound.

ADVERSE REACTIONS
Local: hyperemia with high doses, allergic reactions.

INTERACTIONS
None significant.

NURSING CONSIDERATIONS
• Contraindicated for parenteral use.
• Dense, dry eschar must be removed

Italicized side effects are common or life-threatening.
*Liquid form contains alcohol.   **May contain tartrazine.

surgically before enzymatic debridement. Enzyme must be in constant
contact with substrate. Accumulated
necrotic debris must be removed periodically and the enzyme replenished
at least once daily.
• Clean wound with water, normal
saline, or peroxide and dry gently;
cover with thin layer of Elase. Cover
with nonadhering dressing.
• Change dressing at least once a day.
Flush away necrotic debris and reapply ointment.
• Solution as wet to dry dressing: Mix
1 vial of Elase powder with 10 to 50
ml saline solution; saturate strips of
fine gauze with solution. Pack ulcerated area with Elase gauze. Allow
gauze to dry in contact with ulcerated
lesion for about 6 to 8 hours. Remove
dried gauze and repeat 3 to 4 times
daily.
• Solution as irrigating agent: Drain
cavity and replace Elase every 6 to 10
hours to reduce amount of by-product
accumulation and to minimize loss of
enzyme activity. Although parenteral
use is contraindicated, Elase is used
as an irrigating agent in certain specific conditions.
• Prepare solution just before use.
Discard after 24 hours.

hyaluronidase
Wydase♦
Pregnancy Category: C

MECHANISM OF ACTION
Hydrolyzes hyaluronic acid, thereby
promoting diffusion of fluids in the
tissues.

INDICATIONS & DOSAGE
*Adjunct to increase absorption and
dispersion of other injected drugs—*
Adults and children: 150 units to in-
jection medium containing other med-
ication.
Hypodermoclysis—
Adults and children over 3 years:

150 units injected S.C. before clysis
or injected into clysis tubing near needle for each 1,000 ml clysis solution.
Subcutaneous urography—
Adults and children: with patient
prone, give 75 units S.C. over each
scapula, followed by injection of contrast medium at same sites.

ADVERSE REACTIONS
Skin: rash, urticaria.
Local: irritation.

INTERACTIONS
Local anesthetics: increased potential
for toxic local reaction. Use together
cautiously.

NURSING CONSIDERATIONS
• Use with caution in patients with
blood-clotting abnormalities, severe
hepatic or renal disease.
• Do not inject into acutely inflamed
or cancerous areas.
• In hypodermoclysis, adjust dose,
rate of injection, and type of solution
to patient response.
• Administration precautions: Skin-
test for sensitivity. Avoid injecting
into diseased areas (may spread infection). Observe injection site for local
reactions.
• Avoid getting solution in eyes. If solution does get into eyes, flood with
water at once.
• Protect from heat. Do not use
cloudy or discolored solution.
• For children, 15 units are added to
each 100 ml of solution. The drip rate
should not exceed 2 ml/minute.
• Hyaluronidase is incompatible with
epinephrine and heparin. Don't add to
any solutions containing these drugs.

106

Oxytocics

carboprost tromethamine
dinoprostone
dinoprost tromethamine
ergonovine maleate
methylergonovine maleate
oxytocin, synthetic injection
oxytocin, synthetic nasal

COMBINATION PRODUCTS
None.

---

carboprost tromethamine
Prostin/M15
Pregnancy Category: Not
applicable

MECHANISM OF ACTION
Produces strong, prompt contractions
of uterine smooth muscle, possibly-
mediated by calcium and cyclic 3′,5′-
adenosine monophosphate. A prostaglandin.

INDICATIONS & DOSAGE
*Abort pregnancy between 13th and
20th weeks of gestation—*
initially, 250 mcg is administered
deep I.M. Subsequent doses of 250
mcg should be administered at intervals of 1½ to 3½ hours, depending on
uterine response. Increments in dosage may be increased to 500 mcg if
contractility is inadequate after several 250 mcg doses. Total dose should
not exceed 12 mg.
*Postpartum hemorrhage due to uterine
atony which has not responded to conventional management—*
250 mcg by deep I.M. injection. May
administer repeat doses at 15- to 90-

minute intervals. Maximum total dose
is 2 mg.

ADVERSE REACTIONS
GI: *vomiting, diarrhea,* nausea.
Other: *fever,* chills.

INTERACTIONS
None significant.

NURSING CONSIDERATIONS
• Contraindicated in patients with
pelvic inflammatory disease or active
cardiac, pulmonary, renal, or hepatic
disease. Use cautiously in patients
with a history of asthma; hypertension; cardiovascular, renal, or hepatic
disease; anemia; jaundice; diabetes;
epilepsy; previous uterine surgery.
• I.M. injection of this drug is techni-
cally less difficult and poses fewer potential risks than other prostaglandin
abortifacients.
• Carboprost can be used without
concern that expulsion of vaginal suppositories may occur in the presence
of profuse vaginal bleeding.
• Should be used only in a hospital
setting by trained personnel.

---

dinoprostone
Prostin E₂♦
Pregnancy Category: Not
applicable

MECHANISM OF ACTION
Produces strong, prompt contractions
of uterine smooth muscle, possibly
mediated by calcium and cyclic 3′,5′-
adenosine monophosphate. A prosta-

Italicized side effects are common or life-threatening.
*Liquid form contains alcohol.   **May contain tartrazine.

glandin.

INDICATIONS & DOSAGE
*Abort second trimester pregnancy,
evacuate uterus in cases of missed
abortion, intrauterine fetal deaths up
to 28 weeks of gestation, or benign hydatidiform mole—*
insert 20 mg suppository high into
posterior vaginal fornix. Repeat q 3 to
5 hours until abortion is complete.

ADVERSE REACTIONS
CNS: *headache.*
CV: hypotension (in large doses).
GI: *nausea, vomiting, diarrhea.*
GU: vaginal pain, vaginitis.
Other: *fever, shivering, chills, joint
inflammation, nocturnal leg cramps.*

INTERACTIONS
*Alcohol (I.V. infusions of 500 ml of
10% over 1 hour); inhibited uterine
activity.*

NURSING CONSIDERATIONS
• Contraindicated in patients with
pelvic inflammatory disease or history of pelvic surgery, incisions, uterine fibroids, or cervical stenosis. Use
with caution in asthma, epilepsy, anemia, diabetes, hyper- or hypotension,
jaundice, or cardiovascular, renal, or
hepatic disease.
• Just before use, warm dinoprostone
suppositories in their wrapping to
room temperature.
• After administration, patient should
remain supine for 10 minutes.
• Store suppositories in freezer at
temperature of $-20°$ C. ($-4°$ F.).
• Administer only when critical-care
facilities are readily available.
• Dinoprostone-induced fever is self-
limiting and transient, and occurs in
approximately 50% of all patients.
Treat with water or alcohol sponging
and increased fluid intake rather than
with aspirin.
• Check vaginal discharge daily.
• Abortion should be complete within

30 hours.

---

dinoprost tromethamine
Prostin F₂ Alpha
Pregnancy Category: Not
applicable

MECHANISM OF ACTION
Produces strong, prompt contractions
of uterine smooth muscle, possibly
mediated by calcium and cyclic 3′,5′-
adenosine monophosphate. A prostaglandin.

INDICATIONS & DOSAGE
Abort second trimester pregnancy—
1 ml of amniotic fluid is withdrawn by
transabdominal intra-amniotic catheter. If no blood is present in tap, 40
mg of dinoprost is injected directly
into amniotic sac. Initially, 5 mg is
given very slowly (1 mg/minute), and
patient is watched for adverse reactions. Then, remainder is injected. If
abortion not completed in 24 hours,
another 10 to 40 mg may be given.
Uterine activity may continue 10 to
30 minutes after drug is stopped.

ADVERSE REACTIONS
CNS: dizziness, fainting, headache.
CV: bradycardia.
GI: *nausea, vomiting, diarrhea,* ab-
dominal cramps, epigastric pain.
Other: bronchospasm, wheezing,
flushing, hot flashes.

INTERACTIONS
*Alcohol (I.V. infusions of 500 ml of
10% over 1 hour):* inhibited uterine
activity.
I.V. oxytocin: cervical perforation,
especially in primigravida patients or
in those with inadequately dilated cer-
vices. Use with caution.

NURSING CONSIDERATIONS
• Contraindicated in patients with
pelvic inflammatory disease. Use
with caution in cardiovascular, renal,

Unmarked trade names available in the United States only.
♦Also available in Canada.   ♦♦Available in Canada only.

or hypertensive disease; asthma; glaucoma; epilepsy; previous uterine surgery.
• Be aware that inadvertent administration into maternal bloodstream may cause bronchospasm, tetanic contractions, and shock.
• Observe and record character and amount of vaginal bleeding.
• Other measures are required if dinoprost fails to terminate pregnancy completely. Utilization of hypertonic saline solution should be delayed until uterine contractions stop.
• Monitor vital signs. Report rapid fall in blood pressure or hypertonic uterine contractions.
• Instruct patient to empty her bladder before transabdominal tap.
• Instruct patient to remain in prone position.
• After abortion, observe patient frequently for cervical injuries.
• Store at 2° to 8° C. (35.6° to 46.4° F.). Discard 24 months after manufacture date.
• Be aware of late postabortion hemorrhage that can result from retained placental tissue or infection.

---

ergonovine maleate
Ergotrate Maleate♦
Pregnancy Category: Not applicable

MECHANISM OF ACTION
Increases motor activity of the uterus by direct stimulation.

INDICATIONS & DOSAGE
Prevent or treat postpartum and postabortion hemorrhage due to uterine atony or subinvolution—
0.2 mg I.M. q 2 to 4 hours, maximum 5 doses; or 0.2 mg I.V. (only for severe uterine bleeding or other life-threatening emergency) over 1 minute while blood pressure and uterine contractions are monitored. I.V. dose may be diluted to 5 ml with 0.9% sodium

chloride injection. After initial I.M. or I.V. dose, may give 0.2 to 0.4 mg P.O. q 6 to 12 hours for 2 to 7 days. Decrease dose if severe uterine cramping occurs.

ADVERSE REACTIONS
CNS: dizziness, headache.
CV: hypertension, chest pain.
EENT: tinnitus.
GI: *nausea, vomiting.*
GU: uterine cramping.
Other: sweating, dyspnea, hypersensitivity.

INTERACTIONS
Regional anesthetics, dopamine, I.V. oxytocin: excessive vasoconstriction. Use together cautiously.

NURSING CONSIDERATIONS
• Contraindicated for induction or augmentation of labor, before delivery of placenta, in threatened spontaneous abortion, and in patients with allergy or sensitivity to ergot preparations. Use cautiously in hypertension, cardiac disease, venoatrial shunts, mitral valve stenosis, obliterative vascular disease, sepsis, and hepatic or renal impairment.
• Monitor blood pressure, pulse rate, and uterine response. Report sudden changes in vital signs, frequent periods of uterine relaxation, and/or character and amount of vaginal bleeding.
• Hypocalcemia may decrease patient response. If patient is not also taking digitalis, cautious administration of calcium gluconate I.V. may produce desired oxytocic action.
• Contractions begin 5 to 15 minutes after P.O. administration; immediately after I.V. injection. May continue 3 hours or more after P.O. or I.M. administration; 45 minutes after I.V. injection.
• Store in tightly closed, light-resistant container. Discard if discolored.
• Store I.V. solutions below 8° C. (46.4° F.). Daily stock may be kept at

---

cool room temperature for 60 days.
• Keep patient warm.
• Have drug ready for immediate use if it is to be given postpartum.
• I.V. ergonovine is used to diagnose coronary artery spasm (Prinzmetal's angina).

methylergonovine maleate
Methergine
Pregnancy Category: Not applicable

MECHANISM OF ACTION
Increases motor activity of the uterus by direct stimulation.

INDICATIONS & DOSAGE
Prevent and treat postpartum hemorrhage due to uterine atony or subinvolution—
0.2 mg I.M. q 2 to 5 hours for maximum of 5 doses; or I.V. (excessive uterine bleeding or other emergencies) over 1 minute while blood pressure and uterine contractions are monitored. I.V. dose may be diluted to 5 ml with 0.9% sodium chloride injection. Following initial I.M. or I.V. dose, may give 0.2 to 0.4 mg P.O. q 6 to 12 hours for 2 to 7 days. Decrease dose if severe cramping occurs.

ADVERSE REACTIONS
CNS: dizziness, headache.
CV: hypertension, transient chest pain, dyspnea, palpitation.
EENT: tinnitus.
GI: *nausea, vomiting.*
Other: sweating, hypersensitivity.

INTERACTIONS
Regional anesthetics, dopamine, I.V. oxytocin: excessive vasoconstriction.

NURSING CONSIDERATIONS
• Contraindicated for induction of labor; before delivery of placenta; in patients with hypertension, toxemia, or sensitivity to ergot preparations; in threatened spontaneous abortion. Use cautiously in sepsis, obliterative vascular disease, hepatic, renal, and cardiac disease.
• Should not be routinely administered I.V. If must be given by this route, administer slowly over 1 minute with careful blood pressure monitoring.
• Monitor and record blood pressure, pulse rate, uterine response; and report any sudden change in vital signs or frequent periods of uterine relaxation, and character and amount of vaginal bleeding.
• Contractions begin 5 to 15 minutes after P.O. administration; 2 to 5 minutes after I.M. injection; immediately following I.V. injection. Continue 3 hours or more after P.O. or I.M. administration; 45 minutes after I.V.
• Store in tightly closed, light-resistant containers. Discard if discolored.
• Store I.V. solutions below 8° C. (46.4° F.). Daily stock may be kept at room temperature for 60 to 90 days.

oxytocin, synthetic injection
Oxytocin♦, Pitocin♦, Syntocinon♦, Uteracon
Pregnancy Category: Not applicable

MECHANISM OF ACTION
Causes potent and selective stimulation of uterine and mammary gland smooth muscle.

INDICATIONS & DOSAGE
Induction or stimulation of labor—
initially, 1 ml (10 units) ampul in 1,000 ml of dextrose 5% injection or 0.9% sodium chloride solution I.V. infused at 1 to 2 milliunits/minute. Increase rate at 15- to 30-minute intervals until normal contraction pattern is established. Maximum 1 to 2 ml (20 milliunits)/minute. Decrease rate when labor is firmly established.

Reduction of postpartum bleeding after expulsion of placenta—
10 to 40 units added to 1,000 ml of dextrose 5% in water or 0.9% sodium chloride solution infused at rate necessary to control bleeding, usually 20 to 40 milliunits/minute. Also, 1 ml (10 units) can be given I.M. after delivery of the placenta.

Incomplete or inevitable abortion—
I.V. infusion with 10 units of oxytocin in 500 ml of 0.9% sodium chloride solution or dextrose 5% in normal saline solution. Infuse at rate of 20 to 40 milliunits/minute.

ADVERSE REACTIONS
Maternal—
Blood: afibrinogenemia; may be related to increased postpartum bleeding.
CNS: subarachnoid hemorrhage resulting from hypertension; *convulsions or coma resulting from water intoxication*.
CV: hypotension; increased heart rate, systemic venous return, and cardiac output; arrhythmia.
GI: nausea, vomiting.
Other: hypersensitivity, tetanic contractions, abruptio placentae, *impaired uterine blood flow*, and *increased uterine motility*.
Fetal—
Blood: hyperbilirubinemia.
CV: bradycardia, tachycardia, premature ventricular contractions.
Other: *anoxia, asphyxia*.

INTERACTIONS
Cyclopropane anesthetics: less pronounced bradycardia; hypotension.
Thiopental anesthetics: delayed induction reported.
Vasoconstrictors: severe hypertension if oxytocin is given within 3 to 4 hours of vasoconstrictor in patient receiving caudal block anesthetic.

NURSING CONSIDERATIONS
• Contraindicated in cases of cepha-

lopelvic disproportion or where delivery requires conversion, as in transverse lie; fetal distress, when delivery isn't imminent; severe toxemia; and other obstetric emergencies. Use cautiously in history of cervical or uterine surgery, grand multiparity, uterine sepsis, traumatic delivery, or overdistended uterus, and in primipara over 35 years. Use with extreme caution during first and second stages of labor, since cervical laceration, uterine rupture, and maternal and fetal death are reported.
• Don't give by I.V. bolus injection. Must administer by infusion.
• Used to induce or reinforce labor only when pelvis is known to be adequate, when vaginal delivery is indicated, when fetal maturity is assured, and when fetal position is favorable. Should be used only in hospital where critical-care facilities and doctor are immediately available.
• Oxytocin should never be given simultaneously by more than one route.
• Do the following every 15 minutes: monitor and record uterine contractions, heart rate, blood pressure, intrauterine pressure, fetal heart rate, and character of blood loss.
• May produce an antidiuretic effect; monitor fluid intake/output.
• If contractions occur less than 2 minutes apart and if contractions above 50 mm Hg are recorded, or if contractions last 90 seconds or longer, stop infusion, turn patient on her side, and notify doctor.
• Not recommended for routine I.M. use. However, 10 units may be administered I.M. after delivery of the placenta to control postpartum uterine bleeding.
• Should have magnesium sulfate (20% solution) available for relaxation of the myometrium.

Italicized side effects are common or life-threatening.
*Liquid form contains alcohol.   **May contain tartrazine.

oxytocin, synthetic nasal
Pregnancy Category: Not
applicable

MECHANISM OF ACTION
Stimulates impaired milk ejection.

INDICATIONS & DOSAGE
*To promote initial milk ejection; may
relieve postpartum breast engorgement—*
one spray or three drops into one or
both nostrils 2 or 3 minutes before
breast-feeding or pumping breasts.

ADVERSE REACTIONS
None reported.

INTERACTIONS
None significant.

NURSING CONSIDERATIONS
• Instruct patient to clear nasal passages first. With patient's head in vertical position, hold squeeze bottle upright and eject solution into nostril. If
preferred, the solution can be instilled
in drop form by inverting the squeeze
bottle and exerting gentle pressure.

107

Spasmolytics

aminophylline or theophylline ethylenediamine
dyphylline
flavoxate hydrochloride
oxtriphylline
oxybutynin chloride
theophylline
theophylline sodium glycinate

COMBINATION PRODUCTS

BRONCHIAL CAPSULES: 150 mg theophylline and 90 mg guaifenesin.
BRONDECON TABLETS: 200 mg oxtriphylline and 100 mg guaifenesin.
DILOR-G TABLETS: 200 mg dyphylline and 200 mg guaifenesin.
DYFLEX-G TABLETS: 200 mg dyphylline and 200 mg guaifenesin.
DYLINE-GG TABLETS: 200 mg dyphylline and 200 mg guaifenesin.
GLYCERYL-T CAPSULES: 150 mg theophylline and 90 mg guaifenesin.
LANOPHYLLIN-GG CAPSULES: 150 mg theophylline and 90 mg guaifenesin.
NEOTHYLLINE-GG TABLETS: 200 mg dyphylline and 200 mg guaifenesin.
QUIBRON CAPSULES: 150 mg theophylline and 90 mg guaifenesin.
THEOLAIR-PLUS LIQUID: 125 mg theophylline and 100 mg guaifenesin/15 ml.
THEOLAIR-PLUS TABLETS 125: 125 mg theophylline and 100 mg guaifenesin.
THEOLAIR-PLUS TABLETS 250: 250 mg theophylline and 200 mg guaifenesin.

aminophylline or theophylline ethylenediamine

Aminophyllin, Corophyllin♦♦, Phyllocontin, Somophyllin-DF
Pregnancy Category: C

MECHANISM OF ACTION

Inhibits phosphodiesterase, the enzyme that degrades cyclic AMP. Results in relaxation of smooth muscle of the bronchial airways and pulmonary blood vessels.

INDICATIONS & DOSAGE

For treatment of acute and chronic bronchial asthma, bronchospasm; also used for treatment of Cheyne-Stokes respiration—
Oral:
Adults: 500 mg immediately; then 250 to 500 mg q 6 to 8 hours.
Children: 7.5 mg/kg immediately; then 3 to 6 mg/kg q 6 to 8 hours.
I.V.: inject very slowly, minimum time of 4 to 5 minutes; do not exceed 25 mg/minute infusion rate. Loading dose: 5.6 mg/kg over 30 minutes.
Maintenance dose:
Adults: 0.3 to 0.9 mg/kg hourly I.V. by continuous infusion.
Children under 9 years: 1 mg/kg hourly.
Rectal:
Adults: 500 mg suppository or by retention enema q 6 to 8 hours.

ADVERSE REACTIONS

CNS: *restlessness*, *dizziness*, headache, *insomnia*, light-headedness,

Italicized side effects are common or life-threatening.
*Liquid form contains alcohol. **May contain tartrazine.

convulsions, muscle twitching.
CV: *palpitations, sinus tachycardia,* extrasystoles, flushing, marked hypotension, increase in respiratory rate.
GI: *nausea, vomiting, anorexia,* bitter aftertaste, dyspepsia, heavy feeling in stomach, diarrhea.
Skin: urticaria.
Local: *rectal suppositories may cause irritation.*

INTERACTIONS
Alkali-sensitive drugs: reduced activity. Do not add to I.V. fluids containing aminophylline.
Beta-adrenergic blockers: antagonism. Propranolol and nadolol, especially, may cause bronchospasm in sensitive patients. Use together cautiously.
Troleandomycin, erythromycin, cimetidine: decreased hepatic clearance of theophylline; elevated theophylline levels. Monitor for signs of toxicity.
Barbiturates, phenytoin: enhanced metabolism and decreased theophylline blood levels. Monitor for decreased aminophylline effect.

NURSING CONSIDERATIONS
• Contraindicated in hypersensitivity to xanthine compounds (caffeine, theobromine) and in preexisting cardiac arrhythmias, especially tachyarrhythmias. Use cautiously in young children; in elderly patients with congestive heart failure or other cardiac or circulatory impairment, cor pulmonale, or hepatic disease; in patients with active peptic ulcer, since drug may increase volume and acidity of gastric secretions; and in hyperthyroidism or diabetes mellitus.
• Individuals metabolize xanthines at different rates. Adjust dose by monitoring response, tolerance, pulmonary function, and theophylline blood levels: therapeutic level = 10 to 20 mcg/ml; toxicity seen over 20 mcg/ml.
• Plasma clearance may be decreased in patients with congestive heart failure, hepatic dysfunction, or pulmonary edema. Smokers show accelerated clearance. Dose adjustments necessary.
• I.V. drug administration can cause burning; dilute with dextrose in water solution.
• Monitor vital signs; measure and record intake/output. Expected clinical effects include improvement in quality of pulse and respiration.
• Warn elderly patient of dizziness, a common adverse reaction at start of therapy.
• GI symptoms may be relieved by taking oral drug with full glass of water at meals, although food in stomach delays absorption. Enteric-coated tablets may also delay and impair absorption. No evidence that antacids reduce GI adverse reactions.
• Suppositories slowly and erratically absorbed; retention enemas may be absorbed more rapidly. Rectally administered preparations can be given when patient cannot take drug orally. Schedule after evacuation, if possible; may be retained better if given before meal. Advise patient to remain recumbent 15 to 20 minutes after insertion.
• Question patient closely about other drugs used. Warn that over-the-counter remedies may contain ephedrine in combination with theophylline salts; excessive CNS stimulation may result. Tell him to check with doctor or pharmacist before taking *any* other medications.
• Before giving loading dose, check that patient has not had recent theophylline therapy.
• Supply instructions for home care and dosage schedule. Some patients may require round-the-clock dosage schedule.
• Warn patients with allergies that exposure to allergens may exacerbate bronchospasm.

dyphylline

Air-Tabs, Brophylline, Dilin, Dilor,
Dyflex, Dylline, Emfabid, Lufyllin*,
Protophylline♦♦
Pregnancy Category: C

MECHANISM OF ACTION
Inhibits phosphodiesterase, the enzyme that degrades cyclic AMP. Results in relaxation of smooth muscle of the bronchial airways and pulmonary blood vessels.

INDICATIONS & DOSAGE
For relief of acute and chronic bronchial asthma and reversible bronchospasm associated with chronic bronchitis and emphysema—
Adults: 200 to 800 mg P.O. q 6 hours; or 250 to 500 mg I.M. injected slowly at 6-hour intervals.
Children over 6 years: 4 to 7 mg/kg P.O. daily, in divided doses.

ADVERSE REACTIONS
CNS: *restlessness, dizziness,* headache, *insomnia,* light-headedness, *convulsions,* muscle twitching.
CV: *palpitations, sinus tachycardia,* extrasystoles, flushing, marked hypotension, increase in respiratory rate.
GI: *nausea, vomiting, anorexia,* bitter aftertaste, dyspepsia, heavy feeling in stomach.
Skin: urticaria.

INTERACTIONS
Alkali-sensitive drugs: reduced activity. Do not add to I.V. fluids containing aminophylline.
Beta-adrenergic blockers: antagonism. Propanolol and nadolol, especially, may cause bronchospasm in sensitive patients. Use together cautiously.
Troleandomycin, erythromycin, cimetidine: decreased hepatic clearance of theophylline; elevated theophylline levels. Monitor for signs of toxicity.
Barbiturates, phenytoin: enhanced metabolism and decreased theophylline blood levels. Monitor for decreased theophylline effect.

NURSING CONSIDERATIONS
• Contraindicated in hypersensitivity to xanthine compounds (caffeine, theobromine); preexisting cardiac arrhythmias, especially tachycardias. Use cautiously in young children; in elderly patients with congestive heart failure, any impaired cardiac or circulatory function, cor pulmonale, renal or hepatic disease; in patients with peptic ulcer, hyperthyroidism, or diabetes mellitus.
• I.V. use not recommended.
• Dyphylline is metabolized faster than theophylline; dosage intervals may have to be decreased to ensure continual therapeutic effect. Higher daily doses may be needed.
• Dose should be decreased in renal insufficiency.
• Monitor vital signs; measure and record intake/output. Expected clinical effects include improvement in quality of pulse and respiration.
• Warn elderly patient of dizziness, a common adverse reaction.
• Gastric irritation may be relieved by taking oral drug after meals; no evidence that antacids reduce this adverse reaction. May produce less gastric discomfort than theophylline.
• Discard dyphylline ampul if precipitate is present. Protect from light.
• Question patient closely about other drugs used. Warn that over-the-counter remedies may contain ephedrine in combination with theophylline salts; excessive CNS stimulation may result. Tell him to check with doctor or pharmacist before taking *any* other medications.
• Supply instructions for home care and dosage schedule.

Italicized side effects are common or life-threatening.
*Liquid form contains alcohol.   **May contain tartrazine.

flavoxate hydrochloride
Urispas
Pregnancy Category: C

MECHANISM OF ACTION
Has a direct spasmolytic effect on smooth muscles of the urinary tract. It also provides some local anesthesia and analgesia.

INDICATIONS & DOSAGE
Symptomatic relief of dysuria, frequency, urgency, nocturia, incontinence, and suprapubic pain associated with urologic disorders—
Adults and children over 12 years: 100 to 200 mg P.O. q.i.d.

ADVERSE REACTIONS
CNS: *mental confusion* (especially in elderly), nervousness, dizziness, headache, drowsiness, difficulty with concentration.
CV: tachycardia, palpitations.
EENT: *dry mouth and throat, blurred vision,* disturbed eye accommodation.
GI: abdominal pain, constipation (with high doses), nausea, vomiting.
Skin: urticaria, dermatoses.
Other: fever.

INTERACTIONS
None significant.

NURSING CONSIDERATIONS
• Contraindicated in pyloric or duodenal obstruction, obstructive intestinal lesions or ileus, achalasia, GI hemorrhage, obstructive uropathies of lower urinary tract. Use cautiously in patients suspected of having glaucoma.
• Check history for other drug use before giving drugs with anticholinergic side effects.
• Warn about possible drowsiness, mental confusion, and blurred vision.
• Tell the patient to report adverse effects or lack of response to drug.

oxtriphylline
Choledyl♦*, Theophylline Choline
Pregnancy Category: C

MECHANISM OF ACTION
Inhibits phosphodiesterase, the enzyme that degrades cyclic AMP. Results in relaxation of smooth muscle of the bronchial airways and pulmonary blood vessels.

INDICATIONS & DOSAGE
To relieve acute bronchial asthma and reversible bronchospasm associated with chronic bronchitis and emphysema—
Adults and children over 12 years: 200 mg P.O. q 6 hours.
Children 2 to 12 years: 4 mg/kg P.O. q 6 hours. Increase as needed to maintain therapeutic levels of theophylline (10 to 20 mcg/ml).

ADVERSE REACTIONS
CNS: *restlessness, dizziness,* headache, *insomnia,* light-headedness, *convulsions,* muscle twitching.
CV: *palpitations, sinus tachycardia,* extrasystoles, flushing, marked hypotension, increase in respiratory rate.
GI: *nausea, vomiting, anorexia,* bitter aftertaste, dyspepsia, heavy feeling in stomach.
Skin: urticaria.

INTERACTIONS
Erythromycin, troleandomycin, cimetidine: decreased hepatic clearance of theophylline; increased plasma level. Monitor for signs of toxicity.
Barbiturates, phenytoin: enhanced metabolism and decreased theophylline blood levels. Monitor for decreased effect.
Beta-adrenergic blockers: antagonism. Propranolol and nadolol, especially, may cause bronchospasms in sensitive patients. Use together cautiously.

NURSING CONSIDERATIONS

• Contraindicated in hypersensitivity to xanthines (caffeine, theobromine); preexisting cardiac arrhythmias, especially tachyarrhythmias.
• Tell patient to report GI distress, palpitations, irritability, restlessness, nervousness, or insomnia; may indicate excessive CNS stimulation.
• Administer drug after meals and at bedtime.
• Store at 15° to 30° C. (59° to 86° F.). Protect elixir from light, tablets from moisture.
• Equivalent to 64% anhydrous theophylline.
• Monitor therapy carefully.
• Combination products that contain ephedrine not recommended; excessive CNS stimulation may result (nervousness, tremors, akathisia).

oxybutynin chloride
Ditropan♦
Pregnancy Category: C

MECHANISM OF ACTION
Has both a direct spasmolytic effect and an atropine-like effect on urinary tract smooth muscles. It increases urinary bladder capacity and provides some local anesthesia and mild analgesia.

INDICATIONS & DOSAGE
Antispasmodic for neurogenic bladder—
Adults: 5 mg P.O. b.i.d. to t.i.d. to maximum of 5 mg q.i.d.
Children over 5 years: 5 mg P.O. b.i.d. to maximum of 5 mg t.i.d.

ADVERSE REACTIONS
CNS: *drowsiness,* dizziness, insomnia, *dry mouth,* flushing.
CV: *palpitations, tachycardia.*
EENT: *transient blurred vision,* mydriasis, cycloplegia.
GI: nausea, vomiting, *constipation,* bloated feeling.

GU: impotence, *urinary hesitance or retention.*
Skin: urticaria, severe allergic reactions in patients sensitive to anticholinergics.
Other: decreased sweating, fever, suppression of lactation.

INTERACTIONS
None significant.

NURSING CONSIDERATIONS
• Contraindicated in myasthenia gravis, GI obstruction, glaucoma, adynamic ileus, megacolon, severe or ulcerative colitis; in elderly or debilitated patients with intestinal atony; and in patients with obstructive uropathy. Use cautiously in elderly patients; in patients with autonomic neuropathy, reflux esophagitis, or hepatic or renal disease.
• May aggravate symptoms of hyperthyroidism, coronary artery disease, congestive heart failure, cardiac arrhythmias, tachycardia, hypertension, or prostatic hypertrophy.
• Therapy should be stopped periodically to determine whether patient can get along without it. Minimizes tendency toward tolerance.
• Rapid onset of action, peaks at 3 to 4 hours, lasts 6 to 10 hours.
• Neurogenic bladder should be confirmed by cystometry before oxybutynin is given. Evaluate patient response to therapy periodically by cystometry.
• Rule out partial intestinal obstruction in patients with diarrhea, especially those with colostomy or ileostomy, before giving oxybutynin.
• If urinary tract infection is present, patient should receive antibiotics concomitantly.
• Warn patient that drug may impair alertness or vision.
• Since oxybutynin suppresses sweating, its use during very hot weather may precipitate fever or heatstroke.
• Store in tightly closed containers at

Italicized side effects are common or life-threatening.
*Liquid form contains alcohol.   **May contain tartrazine.

59° to 86° F. (15° to 30° C.).

theophylline
(immediate-release tablets and capsules)
Bronkodyl, Elixophyllin, Slo-Phyllin, Somophyllin-T
(immediate-release liquids)
Accurbron*, Aerolate, Aquaphyllin, Asmalix*, Bronkodyl*, Elixicon, Elixomin*, Elixophyllin♦*, Lanophyllin*, Lixolin, Slo-Phyllin, Theolair♦, Theolixir♦*, Theon*, Theophyl*
(timed-release capsules)
Aerolate, Bronkodyl S-R, Elixophyllin SR, Lodrane, Slo-bid, Slow-Phyllin, Somophyllin-CRT, Theo-24, Theobid, Theobid Jr., Theobron SR, Theo-Dur Sprinkle, Theophyl-SR, Theospan-SR, Theovent
(timed-release tablets)
Constant-T, Duraphyl, LABID, Quibron-T/SR, Respbid, Sustaire, Theo-Dur♦, Theolair-SR, Theo-Time, Uniphyl

theophylline sodium glycinate
Acet-Am♦♦, Synophylate
Pregnancy Category: C

MECHANISM OF ACTION
Inhibits phosphodiesterase, the enzyme that degrades cyclic AMP. Results in relaxation of smooth muscle of the bronchial airways and pulmonary blood vessels.

INDICATIONS & DOSAGE
Prophylaxis and symptomatic relief of bronchial asthma, bronchospasm of chronic bronchitis and emphysema—
Adults: 6 mg/kg P.O. followed by 2 to 3 mg/kg q 4 hours for 2 doses. Maintenance—1 to 3 mg/kg q 8 to 12 hours.
Children 9 to 16 years: 6 mg/kg P.O. followed by 3 mg/kg q 4 hours for 3 doses.
Maintenance—3 mg/kg q 6 hours.
Children 6 months to 9 years: 6 mg/kg P.O. followed by 4 mg/kg q 4 hours for 3 doses.
Maintenance—4 mg/kg q 6 hours.
Most oral timed-release forms given q 8 to 12 hours. Several products, however, may be given q 24 hours.
Symptomatic relief of bronchial asthma, pulmonary emphysema, and chronic bronchitis—
Adults: 330 to 660 mg (sodium glycinate) P.O. q 6 to 8 hours, after meals.
Children over 12 years: 220 to 330 mg (sodium glycinate) P.O. q 6 to 8 hours.
Children 6 to 12 years: 330 mg (sodium glycinate) P.O. q 6 to 8 hours.
Children 3 to 6 years: 110 to 165 mg (sodium glycinate) P.O. q 6 to 8 hours.
Children 1 to 3 years: 55 to 110 mg (sodium glycinate) P.O. q 6 to 8 hours.

ADVERSE REACTIONS
CNS: *restlessness, dizziness,* headache, *insomnia,* light-headedness, *convulsions,* muscle twitching.
CV: *palpitations, sinus tachycardia,* extrasystoles, flushing, marked hypotension, increase in respiratory rate.
GI: *nausea, vomiting, anorexia,* bitter aftertaste, dyspepsia, heavy feeling in stomach, diarrhea.
Skin: urticaria.

INTERACTIONS
Erythromycin, troleandomycin, cimetidine: decreased hepatic clearance of theophylline; increased plasma levels. Monitor for signs of toxicity.
Barbiturates, phenytoin: enhanced metabolism and decreased theophylline blood levels. Monitor for decreased effect.
Beta-adrenergic blockers: antagonism. Propranolol and nadolol, especially, may cause bronchospasms in

sensitive patients. Use together cautiously.

NURSING CONSIDERATIONS

• Contraindicated in hypersensitivity to xanthine compounds (caffeine, theobromine); preexisting cardiac arrhythmias, especially tachyarrhythmias. Use cautiously in young children; in elderly patients with congestive heart failure or other circulatory impairment, cor pulmonale, renal or hepatic disease; and in patients with peptic ulcer, hyperthyroidism, or diabetes mellitus.

• Individuals metabolize xanthines at different rates; determine dose by monitoring response, tolerance, pulmonary function, and theophylline plasma levels: therapeutic level = 10 to 20 mcg/ml.

• Monitor vital signs; measure and record intake/output. Expected clinical effects include improvement in quality of pulse and respiration.

• Warn elderly patients of dizziness, a common adverse reaction at start of therapy.

• GI symptoms may be relieved by taking oral drug with full glass of water after meals, although food in stomach delays absorption.

• Question patient closely about other drugs used. Warn that over-the-counter remedies may contain ephedrine in combination with theophylline salts; excessive CNS stimulation may result. Tell him to check with doctor or pharmacist before taking *any* other medications.

• Supply instructions for home care and dosage schedule.

• Daily dosage may need to be decreased in patients with congestive heart failure or hepatic disease, or in elderly patients, since metabolism and excretion may be decreased. Monitor carefully, using blood levels, observation, examination, and interview. Give drug around the clock, using sustained-release product at bedtime.

• Drug dosage may need to be increased in cigarette smokers because smoking causes the drug to be metabolized faster.

• Be careful not to confuse sustained-release dosage forms with standard-release dosage forms.

• Warn patient not to dissolve, crush, or chew slow-release products. Small children unable to swallow these can ingest (without chewing) the contents of bead-filled capsules sprinkled over soft food.

• Warn patients not to exceed prescribed dosages. Patients tend to want to take extra "breathing pills."

• Patients taking Theo-24 brand of theophylline should take it on an empty stomach because food accelerates the drug's absorption.

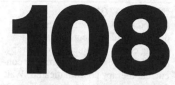

Heavy metal antagonists

deferoxamine mesylate
dimercaprol
edetate calcium disodium
edetate disodium
D-penicillamine
trientine hydrochloride

COMBINATION PRODUCTS
None.

---

deferoxamine mesylate
Desferal♦
Pregnancy Category: C

MECHANISM OF ACTION
Chelates iron by binding ferric ions.

INDICATIONS & DOSAGE
Acute iron intoxication—
Adults and children: 1 g I.M. or I.V. followed by 500 mg I.M. or I.V. for two doses, q 4 hours; then 500 mg I.M. or I.V. q 4 to 12 hours. Infusion rate shouldn't exceed 15 mg/kg hourly. Don't exceed 6 g in 24 hours.
Chronic iron overload resulting from multiple transfusions—
Adults and children: 500 mg to 1 g I.M. daily and 2 g slow I.V. infusion in separate solution along with each unit of blood transfused. Maximum dose 6 g daily. I.V. infusion rate shouldn't exceed 15 mg/kg hourly. S.C.: 1 to 2 g via a subcutaneous infusion pump over 8 to 24 hours.

ADVERSE REACTIONS
Local: pain and induration at injection site.
Other: *After rapid I.V. administra-*
tion: erythema, urticaria, hypotension, shock.
With long term use: sensitivity reaction (cutaneous wheal formation, pruritus, rash, *anaphylaxis), diarrhea, leg cramps, fever, tachycardia, blurred vision, dysuria, abdominal discomfort, cataracts.*

INTERACTIONS
None significant.

NURSING CONSIDERATIONS
• Contraindicated in severe renal disease or anuria. Use cautiously in impaired renal function.
• Monitor intake/output carefully.
• I.M. route preferred.
• Use I.V. only when patient has cardiovascular collapse or shock. For I.V. use, dissolve as for I.M. use; dilute in normal saline, dextrose 5% in water, or lactated Ringer's.
• If giving I.V., change to I.M. as soon as possible.
• For reconstitution, add 2 ml of sterile water for injection to each ampul. Make sure drug is completely dissolved. Reconstituted solution good for 1 week at room temperature. Protect from light.
• Warn patient that urine may be red.
• Have epinephrine 1:1,000 readily available in case of allergic reaction.
• Recommend regular eye exams during long term therapy.

---

dimercaprol
BAL in Oil♦
Pregnancy Category: D

MECHANISM OF ACTION
Forms complexes with heavy metals.

INDICATIONS & DOSAGE
Adults and children:
Severe arsenic or gold poisoning—
3 mg/kg deep I.M. q 4 hours for 2
days, then q.i.d. on 3rd day, then
b.i.d. for 10 days.
Mild arsenic or gold poisoning—
2.5 mg/kg deep I.M. q.i.d. for 2
days, then b.i.d. on 3rd day, then once
daily for 10 days.
Mercury poisoning—
5 mg/kg deep I.M. initially, then 2.5
mg/kg daily or b.i.d. for 10 days.
*Acute lead encephalopathy or lead
level more than 100 mcg/ml—*
4 mg/kg deep I.M. injection, then q 4
hours with edetate calcium disodium
(12.5 mg/kg I.M.). Use separate
sites. Maximum dose 5 mg/kg per
dose.

ADVERSE REACTIONS
CNS: pain or tightness in throat,
chest, or hands; headache; paresthesias; muscle pain or weakness.
CV: *transient increase in blood pressure, returns to normal in 2 hours;
tachycardia.*
EENT: blepharospasm, conjunctivitis, lacrimation, rhinorrhea, excessive
salivation.
GI: *halitosis; nausea; vomiting; burning sensation in lips, mouth, and
throat.*
GU: *renal damage if alkaline urine
not maintained.*
Metabolic: decreased iodine uptake.
Local: sterile abscess, pain at injection site.
Other: *fever (especially in children),*
sweating, pain in teeth.

INTERACTIONS
[131]*I uptake thyroid tests:* decreased;
don't schedule patient for this test
during course of dimercaprol therapy.
Iron: forms toxic metal complex; concurrent therapy contraindicated. Wait
24 hours after last dimercaprol dose.

NURSING CONSIDERATIONS
• Contraindicated in hepatic dysfunction (except postarsenical jaundice),
acute renal insufficiency.
• Should not be used in pregnancy except to treat life-threatening poisoning.
• Don't use for iron, cadmium, or selenium toxicity. Complex formed is
highly toxic, even fatal.
• Ephedrine or antihistamine may
prevent or relieve mild adverse reactions.
• Ineffective in arsine gas poisoning.
• Solution with slight sediment usable.
• Keep urine alkaline to prevent renal
damage. Oral $NaHCO_3$ may be ordered.
• Don't give I.V.; give by deep I.M.
route only. The injection site can be
massaged after drug is given.
• Drug has an unpleasant, garlic-like
odor.
• Be careful when preparing and administering drug not to let drug come
in contact with skin, as it may cause a
skin reaction.

edetate calcium disodium
Calcium Disodium Versenate,
Calcium EDTA
Pregnancy Category: C

MECHANISM OF ACTION
Forms stable, soluble complexes with
metals, particularly lead.

INDICATIONS & DOSAGE
*Lead poisoning (blood levels greater
than 50 mcg/dl)—*
Adults and children: 1 g/m^2 in dex-

---

trose 5% in water or 0.9% normal saline solution I.V. over 1 to 2 hours daily.
Acute lead encephalopathy or lead levels above 100 mcg/dl—
Adults and children: 1.5 g/m² daily for 3 to 5 days, usually in conjunction with dimercaprol. A second course may be administered at least 4 days later, but preferably 2 to 3 weeks should elapse between courses.

ADVERSE REACTIONS
CNS: headache, paresthesias, numbness.
CV: cardiac arrhythmias, hypotension.
GI: anorexia, nausea, vomiting.
GU: *proteinuria, hematuria; nephrotoxicity with renal tubular necrosis leading to fatal nephrosis.*
Other: arthralgia, myalgia, hypercalcemia.
4 to 8 hours after infusion: sudden fever and chills, fatigue, excessive thirst, sneezing, nasal congestion.

INTERACTIONS
None significant.

NURSING CONSIDERATIONS
• Contraindicated in severe renal disease or anuria.
• I.V. use contraindicated in lead encephalopathy; may increase intracranial pressure. Use I.M. route instead.
• Force fluids to facilitate lead excretion in all patients except those with lead encephalopathy.
• Monitor intake/output, urinalysis, BUN, and EKGs.
• To avoid toxicity, use with dimercaprol.
• Procaine HCl may be added to I.M. solutions to minimize pain. Watch for local reactions.
• Avoid rapid I.V. infusions. I.M. route preferred, especially for children.
• Do not confuse this drug with edetate disodium, which is used for the treatment of hypercalcemia.

edetate disodium
Disodium EDTA, Disotate, Endrate
Pregnancy Category: C

MECHANISM OF ACTION
Chelates with metals, such as calcium, to form a stable, soluble complex.

INDICATIONS & DOSAGE
Hypercalcemic crisis—
Adults and children: 15 to 50 mg/kg by slow I.V. infusion. Dilute in 500 ml of dextrose 5% in water or 0.9% normal saline solution. Give over 3 to 4 hours. Maximum adult dose 3 g/day; maximum children's dose 70 mg/kg daily.

ADVERSE REACTIONS
CNS: circumoral paresthesias, numbness, headache, malaise, fatigue, muscle pain or weakness.
CV: hypertension, thrombophlebitis.
GI: nausea, vomiting, diarrhea, anorexia, abdominal cramps.
GU: in excessive doses—nephrotoxicity with urgency, nocturia, dysuria, polyuria, proteinuria, renal insufficiency and failure, tubular necrosis.
Metabolic: *severe hypocalcemia,* decreased magnesium.
Local: pain at site of infusion, erythema, dermatitis.

INTERACTIONS
None significant.

NURSING CONSIDERATIONS
• Contraindicated in anuria, known or suspected hypocalcemia, or significant renal disease; active or healed tubercular lesions; history of seizures or intracranial lesions; generalized arteriosclerosis associated with aging. Use cautiously in limited cardiac reserve, incipient congestive heart failure, hypokalemia, diabetes.

- Avoid rapid I.V. infusion; profound hypocalcemia may occur.
- Monitor EKG, and test renal function frequently.
- Obtain serum calcium levels after each dose.
- Keep I.V. calcium available.
- Monitor blood pressure closely.
- Keep patient in bed for 15 minutes after infusion to avoid postural hypotension.
- Don't use to treat lead toxicity; use edetate calcium disodium instead.
- Record I.V. site used, and try to avoid repeated use of the same site, as this increases likelihood of thrombophlebitis.
- Generalized systemic reactions may occur 4 to 8 hours after drug administration; these include fever, chills, back pain, emesis, muscle cramps, and urinary urgency. Report such reactions to doctor. Treatment is usually supportive. Symptoms generally subside within 12 hours.
- Do not confuse this drug with edetate calcium disodium, which is used to treat lead poisoning.
- Edetate disodium not currently drug of choice for treatment of hypercalcemia; other treatments are safer and more effective.
- EDTA chelation therapy has been inappropriately recommended for treatment of atherosclerosis and related disorders. There's no scientific evidence that the drug is either safe or effective for these indications.

D-penicillamine
Cuprimine♦, Depen♦
Pregnancy Category: D

MECHANISM OF ACTION
Mechanism of action in rheumatoid arthritis is unknown but is probably due to inhibition of collagen formation. Also chelates heavy metals.

INDICATIONS & DOSAGE
Wilson's disease—
Adults: 250 mg P.O. q.i.d. 30 to 60 minutes before meals. Adjust dose to achieve urinary copper excretion of 0.5 to 1 mg daily.
Children: 20 mg/kg daily P.O. divided q.i.d. before meals. Adjust dose to achieve urinary copper excretion of 0.5 to 1 mg daily.
Cystinuria—
Adults: 250 mg P.O. q.i.d. before meals. Adjust dose to achieve urinary cystine excretion of less than 100 mg daily when renal calculi present, or 100 to 200 mg daily when no calculi present. Maximum is 5 g daily.
Children: 30 mg/kg daily P.O. divided q.i.d. before meals. Adjust dose to achieve urinary cystine excretion of less than 100 mg daily when renal calculi present, or 100 to 200 mg daily when no calculi present.
Rheumatoid arthritis—
Adults: 125 to 250 mg P.O. daily initially, with increases of 250 mg q 2 to 3 months if necessary. Maximum dose 1 g daily.

ADVERSE REACTIONS
Blood: *leukopenia, eosinophilia, thrombocytopenia, monocytosis, granulocytopenia,* elevated sedimentation rate, lupus-like syndrome.
EENT: tinnitus.
GU: *nephrotic syndrome, glomerulonephritis, proteinuria.*
Hepatic: hepatotoxicity.
Metabolic: *decreased pyridoxine (may cause optic neuritis),* decreased zinc and mercury.
Skin: friability, especially at pressure spots; wrinkling; erythema; urticaria; ecchymoses.
Other: reversible taste impairment, especially of salts and sweets; hair loss. *About ⅓ of patients develop allergic reactions (rash, pruritus, fever), arthralgia, lymphadenopathy, or pneumonitis.* With long-term use, myasthenia gravis syndrome.

Italicized side effects are common or life-threatening.
*Liquid form contains alcohol.   **May contain tartrazine.

INTERACTIONS
Oral iron: decreased effectiveness of D-penicillamine. If used together, give at least 2 hours apart.

NURSING CONSIDERATIONS
• Contraindicated in pregnant women with cystinuria. Use cautiously in penicillin allergy; cross sensitivity may occur. However, most penicillin-allergic patients can receive penicillamine.
• Report to doctor if fever or other allergic reactions occur.
• Patient should receive pyridoxine daily.
• Handle patient carefully to avoid skin damage.
• Dose should be given on empty stomach to facilitate absorption, preferably 1 hour before or 3 hours after meals.
• Patient should drink large amounts of fluid, especially at night.
• Tell patient that therapeutic effect may be delayed up to 3 months.
• Monitor CBC, and renal and hepatic function regularly throughout therapy (every 2 weeks for the first 6 months, then monthly).
• Monitor urinalysis regularly for protein loss.
• Hold drug and notify doctor if WBC falls below 3,500/mm³ and/or platelet count falls below 100,000/mm³ (these are indications to stop drug). A progressive decline in platelet or WBC in three successive blood tests may necessitate temporary cessation of therapy, even if these counts are within normal limits.
• Advise patient to report fever, sore throat, chills, bruising, increased bleeding time; may be early signs of granulocytopenia.
• Provide appropriate health teaching for patients with Wilson's disease and cystinuria.
• Antihistamines may be tried to manage skin reactions.

trientine hydrochloride
Cuprid
Pregnancy Category: C

MECHANISM OF ACTION
Increases the urinary excretion of copper.

INDICATIONS & DOSAGE
Treatment of Wilson's disease in patients who are intolerant of penicillamine—
Adults: 750 to 2,000 mg in doses divided two, three, or four times daily.
Children: 500 to 1,500 mg in doses divided two, three, or four times daily.
The optimal long-term maintenance dosage should be determined every 6 to 12 months, according to serum copper analysis.

ADVERSE REACTIONS
Blood: iron deficiency anemia.
Skin: rash.
Other: hypersensitivity, fever.

INTERACTIONS
Mineral supplements (including iron): may block trientine absorption. Administer at least 2 hours apart.

NURSING CONSIDERATIONS
• Patients (especially women) should be closely monitored for evidence of iron deficiency anemia throughout therapy.
• Observe patient for signs of hypersensitivity, such as skin rash.
• Tell patient to take trientine on an empty stomach at least 1 hour before meals or 2 hours after meals, and at least 1 hour apart from any other drug, food or milk.
• Capsules should be swallowed whole with water and should not be opened or chewed.
• Exposure to capsule contents may cause contact dermatitis. If capsule is accidentally opened and contents

spilled on the skin, tell patient to wash the site thoroughly.
• Trientine should only be prescribed for patients who cannot tolerate penicillamine, the standard treatment for Wilson's disease.
• Urge your patient to faithfully follow his trientine regimen and low-copper diet as prescribed.

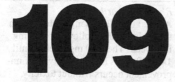

Gold salts

auranofin
aurothioglucose
gold sodium thiomalate

COMBINATION PRODUCTS
None.

---

auranofin
Ridaura
Pregnancy Category: C

MECHANISM OF ACTION
Unknown. Anti-inflammatory effects in rheumatoid arthritis are probably due to inhibition of sulfhydryl systems, which alters cellular metabolism. Auranofin may also alter enzyme function and immune response and suppress phagocytic activity.

INDICATIONS & DOSAGE
Rheumatoid arthritis—
Adults: 6 mg P.O. daily, administered either as 3 mg b.i.d. or 6 mg once daily. After 6 months, may be increased to 9 mg daily.

ADVERSE REACTIONS
Blood: *thrombocytopenia* (with or without purpura), *aplastic anemia, agranulocytosis,* leukopenia, eosinophilia.
GI: *diarrhea, abdominal pain, nausea, vomiting, stomatitis, enterocolitis,* anorexia, metallic taste, dyspepsia, flatulence.
GU: *proteinuria,* hematuria.
Hepatic: jaundice, elevated liver enzymes.
Skin: *rash, pruritus, dermatitis, exfo-*

liative dermatitis.
Other: interstitial pneumonitis.

INTERACTIONS
None significant.

NURSING CONSIDERATIONS
• Contraindicated in patients with history of necrotizing enterocolitis, pulmonary fibrosis, exfoliative dermatitis, bone marrow aplasia, or severe hematologic disorders. Use cautiously with other drugs that cause blood dyscrasias. Use cautiously in patients who have preexisting renal disease, liver disease, inflammatory bowel disease, or skin rash.
• Remind patients to see their doctors on schedule for monthly platelet counts. Auranofin should be stopped if platelet count falls below 100,000 mm^3.
• Reassure patient that beneficial drug effect may be delayed as long as 3 months. However, if response is inadequate after 3 months, doctor will probably discontinue auranofin.
• Encourage patient to take the drug as prescribed and not to alter the dosage schedule.
• Diarrhea is the most common adverse reaction. Tell patient to continue taking this drug if he experiences mild diarrhea; however, if he notes blood in his stool he should contact the doctor immediately.
• Tell patient to continue taking concomitant drug therapy, such as nonsteroidal anti-inflammatory drugs, if prescribed.
• Dermatitis is a common adverse re-

action. Advise patient to report any rashes or other skin problems immediately. Pruritus often precedes dermatitis and should be considered a warning of impending skin reactions. Any pruritic skin eruption while a patient is receiving auranofin should be considered a reaction to this drug until proven otherwise. Therapy is stopped until reaction subsides.

• Stomatitis is another common adverse reaction. Tell patient that stomatitis is often preceded by a metallic taste. Advise him to report this symptom to his doctor immediately.

• Auranofin, like the injectable gold preparations, should be prescribed only for selected rheumatoid arthritis patients. Warn your patient *not* to give the drug to others.

---

aurothioglucose
Solganal

gold sodium thiomalate
Myochrysine♦
Pregnancy Category: C

MECHANISM OF ACTION
Unknown. Anti-inflammatory effects in rheumatoid arthritis are probably due to inhibition of sulfhydryl systems, which alters cellular metabolism. Gold salts may also alter enzyme function and immune response and suppress phagocytic activity.

INDICATIONS & DOSAGE
Rheumatoid arthritis—
Adults: initially, 10 mg (aurothioglucose) I.M., followed by 25 mg for second and third doses at weekly intervals. Then, 50 mg weekly until 1 g has been given. If improvement occurs without toxicity, continue 25 to 50 mg at 3- to 4-week intervals indefinitely as maintenance therapy.
Children 6 to 12 years: ¼ usual adult dose. Alternatively, 1 mg/kg I.M. once weekly for 20 weeks.

Rheumatoid arthritis—
Adults: initially, 10 mg (gold sodium thiomalate) I.M., followed by 25 mg in 1 week. Then, 50 mg weekly until 14 to 20 doses have been given. If improvement occurs without toxicity, continue 50 mg q 2 weeks for 4 doses; then, 50 mg q 3 weeks for 4 doses; then, 50 mg q month indefinitely as maintenance therapy. If relapse occurs during maintenance therapy, resume injections at weekly intervals.
Children: 1 mg/kg weekly I.M. for 20 weeks. If response is good, may be given q 3 to 4 weeks indefinitely.

ADVERSE REACTIONS
Adverse reactions to gold are considered severe and potentially life-threatening. Report any side effect to the doctor at once.
Blood: *thrombocytopenia* (with or without purpura), *aplastic anemia, agranulocytosis,* leukopenia, eosinophilia.
CNS: *dizziness,* syncope, sweating.
CV: bradycardia.
EENT: corneal gold deposition, corneal ulcers.
GI: *metallic taste, stomatitis,* difficulty swallowing, nausea, vomiting.
GU: *albuminuria, proteinuria, nephrotic syndrome,* nephritis, acute tubular necrosis.
Hepatic: hepatitis, jaundice.
Skin: *rash and dermatitis in 20% of patients. (If drug is not stopped, may lead to fatal exfoliative dermatitis.)*
Other: *anaphylaxis,* angioneurotic edema.

INTERACTIONS
None significant.

NURSING CONSIDERATIONS
• Contraindicated in patients with severe uncontrollable diabetes, renal disease, hepatic dysfunction, marked hypertension, heart failure, systemic lupus erythematosus, Sjögren's syndrome, skin rash, and drug allergies

---

Italicized side effects are common or life-threatening.
*Liquid form contains alcohol.   **May contain tartrazine.

or hypersensitivities. Use cautiously with other drugs that cause blood dyscrasias.

• Indicated only in active rheumatoid arthritis that has not responded adequately to salicylates, D-penicillamine, rest, and physical therapy.

• Should be administered only under constant supervision of a doctor who is thoroughly familiar with the drug's toxicities and benefits.

• Most adverse reactions are readily reversible if drug is stopped immediately.

• Administer all gold salts I.M., preferably intragluteally. Color of drug is pale yellow; don't use if it darkens.

• Observe patient for 30 minutes after administration because of possible anaphylactic reaction.

• Inform patient that benefits of therapy may not appear for 6 to 8 weeks or longer.

• Gold therapy may alter liver function studies.

• Aurothioglucose is a suspension. Immerse vial in warm water and shake vigorously before injecting.

• When giving gold sodium thiomalate, advise patient to lie down and to remain recumbent for 10 to 20 minutes after injection.

• Complete blood counts including platelet estimation should be performed before every second injection for the duration of therapy.

• Dermatitis is the most common adverse reaction of these drugs. Advise patient to report any skin rashes or problems immediately. Pruritus often precedes dermatitis and should be considered a warning of impending skin reactions. Any pruritic skin eruption while a patient is receiving gold therapy should be considered a reaction until proven otherwise. Therapy is stopped until reaction subsides.

• Stomatitis is the second most common adverse reaction of gold therapy. Advise patient that stomatitis is often preceded by a metallic taste. This warning should be reported to the doctor immediately.

• Advise patient of the importance of close medical follow-up and the need for frequent blood and urine tests during therapy.

• Urine should be analyzed for protein and sediment changes before each injection.

• Platelet counts should be performed if patient develops purpura or ecchymoses.

• If adverse reactions are mild, some rheumatologists may order resumption of gold therapy after 2 to 3 weeks' rest.

• Dimercaprol should be kept on hand to treat acute toxicity.

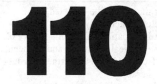

Diagnostic skin tests

coccidioidin
histoplasmin
mumps skin test antigen
**tuberculin purified protein
 derivative (PPD)**
**tuberculosis multiple-puncture
 tests**

COMBINATION PRODUCTS
None.

coccidioidin

Biocox, Spherulin
Pregnancy Category: C

MECHANISM OF ACTION
Causes a cell-mediated immune response.

INDICATIONS & DOSAGE
Suspected coccidioidomycosis; to assess cell-mediated immunity—
Adults and children: 0.1 ml intradermally into the volar surface of the forearm. Use tuberculin syringe with 26G or 27G ⅝″ to ½″ needle.

ADVERSE REACTIONS
Local: hypersensitivity (vesiculation, ulceration, necrosis).
Other: *anaphylaxis,* Arthus reaction.

INTERACTIONS
None significant.

NURSING CONSIDERATIONS
• Test is read at 24 and 48 hours. Induration of 5 mm or more indicates a positive reaction (cell-mediated immune response). Erythema is not considered indicative of a delayed hypersensitivity reaction or positive response.
• Obtain history of allergies and reactions to skin tests. Patients allergic to merthiolate and thimerosol should not receive this skin test.
• Obtain history of any recent residence or travel to endemic areas—southern California, Arizona, New Mexico, and western Texas.
• Keep epinephrine 1:1,000 available.
• Available as either a 1:100 or 1:10 dilution. The more dilute is always tried first. If a patient is suspected of having coccidioidomycosis because of clinical manifestations or X-ray findings and the 1:100 dilution is negative, the 1:10 dilution may be applied.
• Reactivity to this test may be depressed or suppressed for as long as 4 to 6 weeks in individuals who have received concurrent or recent immunization with certain virus vaccines (for example, measles or influenza), in those who are receiving corticosteroid or immunosuppressive agents, and in those who have had viral infections (rubeola, influenza, mumps, and probably others).
• Reaction may be depressed or suppressed in malnourished or immunosuppressed patients.

---

histoplasmin
Histolyn-CYL
Pregnancy Category: NR

MECHANISM OF ACTION
Causes a cell-mediated immune response.

INDICATIONS & DOSAGE
Suspected histoplasmosis; to assess cell-mediated immunity—
Adults and children: 0.1 ml intradermally into the volar surface of the forearm. Use tuberculin syringe with 26G or 27G ⅝″ to ½″ needle.

ADVERSE REACTIONS
Local: urticaria, ulceration or necrosis in highly sensitive patients.
Other: *anaphylaxis.*

INTERACTIONS
None significant.

NURSING CONSIDERATIONS
• Read test at 24 to 48 hours. Induration of 5 mm or more is positive response. In some instances, maximum reactions may not be present until the fourth day.
• Reaction may be depressed in malnourished or immunosuppressed patients.
• A positive reaction may indicate a past infection or a mild subacute or chronic infection with histoplasmosis or such immunologically related organisms as coccidioidomycosis or blastomycosis.
• Obtain history of allergies and reactions to skin tests.
• Histoplasmin should not be administered to known positive reactors because of severity of reaction.
• Cold packs or topical corticosteroids may relieve pain and itching if severe local reaction occurs.
• Serologic titers are often boosted by previous skin test. Draw serologic sample between 48 to 96 hours after skin test administration.
• Tuberculin skin test is advisable concurrently with histoplasmin test.
• Obtain history of any residence or recent travel to endemic areas—central U.S. (Ohio Valley) and eastern U.S.
• Reactivity to this test may be depressed or suppressed for as long as 4 to 6 weeks in individuals who have received concurrent or recent immunization with certain virus vaccines (for example, measles or influenza), in those who are receiving corticosteroid or immunosuppressive agents, and in those who have had viral infections (rubeola, influenza, mumps, and probably others).

mumps skin test antigen
MSTA
Pregnancy Category: NR

MECHANISM OF ACTION
Causes a cell-mediated immune response.

INDICATIONS & DOSAGE
To assess cell-mediated immunity—
Adults and children: 0.1 ml intradermally into the volar surface of the forearm. Use tuberculin syringe with 26G or 27G ⅝″ to ½″ needle.

ADVERSE REACTIONS
Local: hypersensitivity (vesiculation, ulceration).
Other: *anaphylaxis,* Arthus reaction.

INTERACTIONS
None significant.

NURSING CONSIDERATIONS
• Test is read at 48- and 72-hour intervals. A positive reaction (cell-mediated immune response) is 5 mm or more of induration. Erythema is not considered indicative of a delayed hypersensitivity reaction.
• Obtain history of allergies and reac-

tions to skin tests. In patients hypersensitive to eggs, feathers, and chicken, a severe reaction may follow administration.

• Don't administer to patients allergic to thimerosol.

• Keep epinephrine 1:1,000 available.

• Store vials in refrigerator.

• Mumps skin test antigen is *not* used to assess exposure to mumps. This antigen is used in assessing T cell function for immunocompetence.

• Reactivity to this test may be depressed or suppressed for as long as 4 to 6 weeks in individuals who have received concurrent or recent immunization with certain virus vaccines (for example, measles or influenza), in those who are receiving corticosteroid or immunosuppressive agents, and in those who have had viral infections (rubeola, influenza, mumps, and probably others).

• Reaction may be depressed or suppressed in malnourished or immunosuppressed patients.

---

tuberculin purified protein derivative (PPD)

Aplisol, PPD-Stablized Solution (Mantoux), Tubersol
Pregnancy Category: C

MECHANISM OF ACTION

Causes a cell-mediated immune response.

INDICATIONS & DOSAGE

Diagnosis of tuberculosis, evaluation of immunocompetence in patients with cancer, malnutrition—

Adults and children: 5 tuberculin units (0.1 ml) intradermally into volar surface of the forearm. Suspected sensitivity dose use 1 tuberculin unit. First strength equals 1 tuberculin unit/0.1 ml; intermediate strength, 5 tuberculin units/0.1 ml. Second strength equals 250 tuberculin units/

0.1 ml. Use tuberculin syringe with 26G or 27G ⅝″ to ½″ needle.

ADVERSE REACTIONS

Local: pain, pruritus, vesiculation, ulceration, necrosis.
Other: *anaphylaxis,* Arthus reaction.

INTERACTIONS

None significant.

NURSING CONSIDERATIONS

• Contraindicated in known tuberculin-positive reactors; severe reactions may occur.

• Read test in 48 to 72 hours. An induration of 10 mm or greater indicates a significant reaction (formerly called positive reaction). Significance of a reaction is determined not only by the size of the reaction but by circumstances. For example, a reaction of 5 mm or more may be considered significant in a close relative of a person with known tuberculosis. A reaction of 2 mm or more may also be considered significant in infants and children. The amount of induration at the site—not erythema—determines the significance of the reaction.

• Report all known cases of tuberculosis to the appropriate public health agency.

• Obtain history of allergies and reactions to skin tests.

• Reactivity to this test may be depressed or suppressed for as long as 4 to 6 weeks in individuals who have received concurrent or recent immunization with certain virus vaccines (for example, measles or influenza), in those who are receiving corticosteroid or immunosuppressive agents, and in those who have had viral infections (rubeola, influenza, mumps, and probably others).

• Keep epinephrine 1:1,000 available.

• Subcutaneous injection invalidates test results. Bleb (6 to 10 mm in diameter) must form on skin upon intrader-

---

mal injection.
• Cold packs or topical corticosteroids may relieve pain and itching of severe local reaction.
• Never give initial test with second test strength (250 tuberculin units). Use only when a patient has negative response to a 5–tuberculin unit PPD but has the clinical signs and symptoms of tuberculosis.
• Corticosteroids and other immunosuppressives may suppress skin test reaction.

tuberculosis multiple-puncture tests

Aplitest (dried PPD)
Mono-Vacc Test (liquid Old Tuberculin)
Sclavo Test (dried PPD)
Tine Test (dried Old Tuberculin [OT], dried purified protein derivative [PPD])
Pregnancy Category: C

MECHANISM OF ACTION
Causes a cell-mediated immune response.

INDICATIONS & DOSAGE
Screening for tuberculosis—
Adults and children: cleanse skin thoroughly with alcohol; make skin taut on volar surface of forearm and press points firmly into selected site. Hold device at injection site for about 3 seconds. This will assure stabilizing the dried tuberculin B in tissue lymph. All multiple-puncture tests are equivalent to 5 tuberculin units of PPD Mantoux.

ADVERSE REACTIONS
Local: hypersensitivity (vesiculation, ulceration, necrosis).
Other: *anaphylaxis.*

INTERACTIONS
Virus vaccine: TB skin-test reaction may be suppressed if test is given within 4 to 6 weeks after immunization with live or attenuated virus vaccines.

NURSING CONSIDERATIONS
• Contraindicated in known tuberculin-positive reactors.
• False-positive reaction can occur in sensitive patients.
• Reactivity to this test may be depressed or suppressed for as long as 4 to 6 weeks in individuals who have received concurrent or recent immunization with certain virus vaccines (for example, measles or influenza), in those who are receiving corticosteroid or immunosuppressive agents, and in those who have had viral infections (rubeola, influenza, mumps, and probably others).
• Reaction may be depressed in patients with malnutrition, immunosuppression, or miliary tuberculosis.
• Read test in 48 to 72 hours. Questionable or positive reactions to any multiple-puncture test must be verified by the Mantoux test. The amount of induration—not erythema—at the site determines significance of the reaction.
• Induration of 1 to 2 mm is significant.
• If vesiculation is present, the test may be interpreted as positive.
• All tuberculin multiple puncture tests are equivalent to 5 tuberculin units purified protein derivative.
• Obtain history of allergies, especially to acacia (contained in the Tine Test as stabilizer), and reactions to skin tests.
• Keep epinephrine 1:1,000 available.
• Report all known cases of tuberculosis to appropriate public health agency.
• Cold packs or topical corticosteroids may relieve pain and itching if severe local reaction occurs after test.

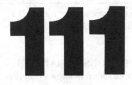

Uncategorized drugs

acetohydroxamic acid
allopurinol
alprostadil
bromocriptine mesylate
clomiphene citrate
colchicine
cromolyn sodium
diazoxide, oral
disulfiram
L-carnitine
levodopa
levodopa-carbidopa
methoxsalen
nicotine resin complex
pentoxifylline
pralidoxime chloride
ritodrine hydrochloride
sodium cellulose phosphate

COMBINATION PRODUCTS
COLBENEMID: probenecid 500 mg
and colchicine 0.5 mg.
PROBENECID WITH COLCHICINE: probenecid 500 mg and colchicine 0.5
mg.

---

acetohydroxamic acid
Lithostat
Pregnancy Category: X

MECHANISM OF ACTION
Prevents formation of renal stones by
inhibiting bacterial urease activity.

INDICATIONS & DOSAGE
*Treatment of infection-related kidney
stones—*
Adults: 250 mg P.O. t.i.d. or q.i.d.
Administer at 6- to 8-hour intervals at
a time when the stomach is empty.

Maximum daily dose is 1.5 g.
Children: 10 mg/kg/day in 2 or 3 divided doses.

ADVERSE REACTIONS
Blood: *hemolytic anemia.*
CNS: *mild headache, depression,*
anxiety, nervousness.
CV: phlebitis.
GI: *nausea, vomiting, anorexia, mal-
aise.*
Skin: *nonpruritic, macular rash in
arms and on face.*
Other: alopecia, deep vein thrombo-
sis.

INTERACTIONS
Oral iron supplements: Reduce absorption of acetohydroxamic acid.
Check with doctor; he may request
iron be administered I.M.

NURSING CONSIDERATIONS
• Contraindicated in patients whose
physical state and disease are amena-
ble to surgery and appropriate antibiotics; in patients whose urine is infected by nonurease-producing organisms in pregnancy; and in patients
with poor renal function.
• Use cautiously in patients predisposed to deep vein thrombosis.
• Coombs'-negative hemolytic anemia has occurred in patients receiving
acetohydroxamic acid.
• Monitor CBC, including a reticulocyte count after 2 weeks of therapy.
Thereafter, monitor at 3-month intervals for the duration of treatment. If
laboratory findings indicate hemolytic
anemia, discontinue drug.

Italicized side effects are common or life-threatening.
*Liquid form contains alcohol.   **May contain tartrazine.

• Skin rash more common during prolonged use and with concomitant use of alcoholic beverages. The rash appears 30 to 45 minutes after ingestion of alcoholic beverages; disappears spontaneously in 30 to 60 minutes. Although skin rash doesn't usually require treatment, advise patient to avoid alcohol.

• Experience with acetohydroxamic acid is limited. About 150 patients have been tested, most for periods of more than 1 year.

allopurinol
Lopurin, Zyloprim♦
Pregnancy Category: C

MECHANISM OF ACTION
Reduces uric-acid production by inhibiting the biochemical reactions preceding its formation.

INDICATIONS & DOSAGE
Gout, primary or secondary to hyperuricemia; secondary to diseases such as acute or chronic leukemia, polycythemia vera, multiple myeloma, and psoriasis—
Dosage varies with severity of disease; can be given as single dose or divided, but doses larger than 300 mg should be divided.
Adults: mild gout, 200 to 300 mg P.O. daily; severe gout with large tophi, 400 to 600 mg P.O. daily. Same dose for maintenance in secondary hyperuricemia.
Hyperuricemia secondary to malignancies—
Children 6 to 10 years: 300 mg P.O. daily.
Children under 6 years: 150 mg P.O. daily.
Impaired renal function—
Adults: 200 mg P.O. daily if creatinine clearance is 10 to 20 ml/minute; 100 mg P.O. daily if creatinine is less than 10 ml/minute; 100 mg P.O. more than 24 hours apart if clearance is less than 3 ml/minute.
To prevent acute gouty attacks—
Adults: 100 mg P.O. daily; increase at weekly intervals by 100 mg without exceeding maximum dose (800 mg), until serum uric acid level falls to 6 mg/100 ml or less.
To prevent uric acid nephropathy during cancer chemotherapy—
Adults: 600 to 800 mg P.O. daily for 2 to 3 days, with high fluid intake.
Recurrent calcium oxalate calculi—
Adults: 200 to 300 mg P.O. daily in single dose or divided doses.

ADVERSE REACTIONS
Blood: *agranulocytosis,* anemia, *aplastic anemia.*
CNS: drowsiness.
EENT: cataracts, retinopathy.
GI: nausea, vomiting, diarrhea, abdominal pain.
Hepatic: altered liver function studies, hepatitis.
Skin: *rash, usually maculopapular;* exfoliative, urticarial, and purpuric lesions; erythema multiforme; severe furunculosis of nose; ichthyosis, *toxic epidermal necrolysis.*

INTERACTIONS
Uricosuric agents: additive effect; may be used to therapeutic advantage.

NURSING CONSIDERATIONS
• Contraindicated in hypersensitivity and in patients with idiopathic hemochromatosis. Use cautiously in patients with cataracts or with hepatic or renal disease.
• Obtain accurate patient history.
• Discontinue at first sign of rash, which may precede severe hypersensitivity reaction or any other adverse reaction. Tell patient to report all adverse reactions immediately. Skin rash is more common in patients taking diuretics and in those with renal disorders.
• Monitor intake/output; daily urinary output of at least 2 liters and

maintenance of neutral or slightly alkaline urine are desirable. Patient should be encouraged to drink plenty of fluids while taking this drug unless otherwise contraindicated.
• If renal insufficiency exists at any time during treatment, allopurinol dose should be reduced.
• Periodically check CBC, hepatic and renal function, especially at start of therapy.
• If patient is taking allopurinol for treatment of recurrent calcium oxalate stones, advise him to also reduce his dietary intake of animal protein, sodium, refined sugars, oxalate-rich foods, and calcium.
• Acute gouty attacks may occur in first 6 weeks of therapy; concurrent use of colchicine may be prescribed prophylactically.
• Minimize GI adverse reactions by administering with meals or immediately after.
• Evaluate effectiveness, using serum uric acid levels.
• Allopurinol may predispose patient to ampicillin-induced rash.
• Allopurinol may cause rash even weeks after discontinuation.
• Since drug may cause drowsiness, advise patient to refrain from driving car or performing tasks requiring mental alertness until CNS response to drug is known.

---

alprostadil
Prostin VR Pediatric♦
Pregnancy Category: Not applicable

MECHANISM OF ACTION
A prostaglandin derivative which relaxes the smooth muscle of the ductus arteriosus.

INDICATIONS & DOSAGE
Palliative therapy for temporary maintenance of patency of ductus arteriosus until surgery can be performed—

Infants: 0.1 mcg/kg/minute by I.V. infusion. When therapeutic response is achieved, reduce infusion rate to give lowest dosage that will maintain response. Maximum dosage is 0.4 mcg/kg/minute. Alternatively, administer through umbilical artery catheter placed at ductal opening.

ADVERSE REACTIONS
Blood: disseminated intravascular coagulation.
CNS: seizures.
CV: *flushing*, bradycardia, hypotension, tachycardia.
GI: diarrhea.
Other: *apnea, fever, sepsis.*

INTERACTIONS
None reported.

NURSING CONSIDERATIONS
• Contraindicated in neonatal respiratory distress syndrome.
• Because drug inhibits platelet aggregation, use cautiously in neonates with bleeding tendencies.
• Monitor arterial pressure by umbilical artery catheter, auscultation, or Doppler transducer. Slow rate of infusion if arterial pressure falls significantly.
• In infants with restricted pulmonary bloodflow, measure drug's effectiveness by monitoring blood oxygenation. In infants with restricted systemic bloodflow, measure drug's effectiveness by monitoring systemic blood pressure and blood pH.
• Drug must be diluted before being administered. Fresh solution must be prepared daily. Discard any solution more than 24 hours old.
• Apnea and bradycardia may reflect drug overdose. If the signs occur, stop infusion immediately.

Italicized side effects are common or life-threatening.
*Liquid form contains alcohol.   **May contain tartrazine.

bromocriptine mesylate
Parlodel♦
Pregnancy Category: C

MECHANISM OF ACTION
Inhibits secretion of prolactin. It acts as a dopamine-receptor agonist by activating postsynaptic dopamine receptors.

INDICATIONS & DOSAGE
To treat amenorrhea and galactorrhea associated with hyperprolactinemia; treatment of female infertility— 2.5 mg P.O. b.i.d. or t.i.d. with meals for 14 days, but for no longer than 6 months.
Prevention of postpartum lactation— 2.5 mg P.O. b.i.d. with meals for 14 days. Treatment may be extended for up to 21 days, if necessary.
Treatment of Parkinson's disease— 1.25 mg P.O. b.i.d. with meals. Dosage may be increased every 14 to 28 days, up to 100 mg daily.
Treatment of acromegaly—
Adults: 1.25 to 2.5 mg P.O. for 3 days. An additional 1.25 to 2.5 mg may be added every 3 to 7 days until patient receives therapeutic benefit.

ADVERSE REACTIONS
CNS: *dizziness, headache,* fatigue, mania, delusions, nervousness, insomnia, depression.
CV: *hypotension,* syncope.
EENT: nasal congestion, tinnitus, blurred vision.
GI: *nausea,* vomiting, *abdominal cramps,* constipation, diarrhea.
GU: urinary retention and frequency.
Other: *pulmonary infiltration and pleural effusion,* coolness and pallor of fingers and toes.

INTERACTIONS
None significant.

NURSING CONSIDERATIONS
• Contraindicated in hypersensitivity to ergot derivatives.
• Use cautiously in patients with pre-existing psychiatric disorders.
• Patient should be examined carefully for pituitary tumor (Forbes-Albright syndrome). Use of Parlodel will not affect tumor size although it may alleviate amenorrhea or galactorrhea.
• May lead to early postpartum conception. Test for pregnancy every 4 weeks or whenever period is missed after menses are reinitiated.
• Advise patient to use contraceptive methods other than oral contraceptives during treatment.
• First-dose phenomenon occurs in 1% of patients. Sensitive patients may collapse for 15 to 60 minutes but can usually tolerate subsequent treatment without ill effects.
• Incidence of adverse effects is high (68%); however, most are mild to moderate, and only 6% of patients discontinue drug for this reason. Nausea is the most common adverse reaction.
• Recurrence rates when used to treat amenorrhea or galactorrhea associated with hyperprolactinemia are high (70% to 80%).
• Advise the patient that it may take 6 to 8 weeks or longer for menses to be reinstated and galactorrhea to be suppressed.
• Should be given with meals.
• When used to treat Parkinson's disease, bromocriptine is usually given in addition to either levodopa alone or levodopa-carbidopa combination (Sinemet).
• Adverse reactions are more frequent when drug is used for Parkinson's disease.
• Also prescribed to treat hyperprolactinemia associated with pituitary adenomas.

---

clomiphene citrate
Clomid♦
Pregnancy Category: X

MECHANISM OF ACTION
Appears to stimulate release of pituitary gonadotropins, follicle-stimulating hormone, and luteinizing hormone. This results in maturation of the ovarian follicle, ovulation, and development of the corpus luteum.

INDICATIONS & DOSAGE
To induce ovulation—
50 to 100 mg P.O. daily for 5 days, starting any time; or 50 to 100 mg P.O. daily starting on day 5 of menstrual cycle (first day of menstrual flow is day 1). Repeat until conception occurs or until 3 courses of therapy are completed.

ADVERSE REACTIONS
CNS: headache, restlessness, insomnia, dizziness, light-headedness, depression, fatigue, tension.
CV: hypertension.
EENT: blurred vision, diplopia, scotoma, photophobia (signs of impending visual toxicity).
GI: nausea, vomiting, bloating, distention, increased appetite, weight gain.
GU: urinary frequency and polyuria; ovarian enlargement and cyst formation, which regress spontaneously when drug is stopped.
Metabolic: hyperglycemia.
Skin: urticaria, rash, dermatitis.
Other: *hot flashes,* reversible alopecia, *breast discomfort.*

INTERACTIONS
None significant.

NURSING CONSIDERATIONS
• Contraindicated in patients who have undiagnosed abnormal genital bleeding, ovarian cyst, or hepatic disease or dysfunction. Use cautiously in hypertension, mental depression, migraines, seizures, diabetes mellitus, or gonadotropin sensitivity. Report development or worsening of these conditions to doctor. May require stopping drug.
• Patient with visual disturbances should report symptoms to doctor immediately.
• Tell patient possibility of multiple births exists with this drug. Risk increases with higher doses.
• Teach patient to take basal body temperature and chart on graph to ascertain whether ovulation has occurred.
• Advise patient to stop drug and contact doctor immediately if abdominal symptoms or pain occurs because these indicate ovarian enlargement or ovarian cyst.
• Reassure patient that response (ovulation) generally occurs after the first course of therapy. If pregnancy does not occur, course of therapy may be repeated twice.
• Since drug may cause dizziness or visual disturbances, caution patient not to perform hazardous tasks until her response to the drug is known.
• Advise patient to stop drug and contact doctor immediately if she suspects she is pregnant (drug may have teratogenic effect).

colchicine
Colchicine♦, Colsalide, Novocolchine
Pregnancy Category: C

MECHANISM OF ACTION
Inhibits migration of granulocytes to an area of inflammation. It decreases lactic acid production associated with phagocytosis and interrupts the cycle of urate crystal deposition and inflammatory response.

INDICATIONS & DOSAGE
To prevent acute attacks of gout as

Italicized side effects are common or life-threatening.
*Liquid form contains alcohol.   **May contain tartrazine.

*prophylactic or maintenance ther-
apy—*
Adults: 0.5 or 0.6 mg P.O. daily; or 1
to 1.8 mg P.O. daily for more severe
cases.
*To prevent attacks of gout in patients
undergoing surgery—*
Adults: 0.5 to 0.6 mg P.O. t.i.d. 3
days before and 3 days after surgery.
*To treat acute gout, acute gouty ar-
thritis—*
Adults: initially, 1 to 1.2 mg P.O.,
then 0.5 or 0.6 mg q hour, or 1 to 1.2
mg q 2 hours until pain is relieved or
until nausea, vomiting, or diarrhea
ensues. Or 2 mg I.V. followed by 2 mg
I.V. in 12 hours if necessary. Total
I.V. dose over 24 hours (one course of
treatment) not to exceed 4 mg.
Note: Give I.V. by slow I.V. push over
2 to 5 minutes. Avoid extravasation.
Don't dilute colchicine injection with
dextrose 5% injection or any other
fluid that might change pH of colchicine solution. If lower concentration
of colchicine injection is needed, dilute with 0.9% sodium chloride or
sterile water for injection. However, if
diluted solution becomes turbid, don't
inject.

ADVERSE REACTIONS
Blood: *aplastic anemia and agranulo-
cytosis with prolonged use;* nonthrom-
bocytopenic purpura.
CNS: peripheral neuritis.
GI: *nausea, vomiting, abdominal
pain, diarrhea.*
Skin: urticaria, dermatitis.
Local: severe local irritation if ex-
travasation occurs.
Other: alopecia.

INTERACTIONS
None significant.

NURSING CONSIDERATIONS
• Use cautiously in hepatic dysfunction, cardiac disease, blood dyscrasias, renal disease, GI disorders, and
in aged or debilitated patients.

• Reduce dosage if weakness, anorexia, nausea, vomiting, or diarrhea
appears. First sign of acute overdosage may be GI symptoms, followed by
vascular damage, muscle weakness,
ascending paralysis. Delirium and
convulsions may occur without the
patient losing consciousness.
• Discontinue drug as soon as gout
pain is relieved or at the first sign of
gastrointestinal symptoms.
• A course of I.V. colchicine should
not be repeated for several weeks to
avoid cumulative toxicity.
• Do not administer I.M. or subcutaneously; severe local irritation occurs.
Administer I.V. over 2 to 5 minutes.
• As maintenance therapy, give with
meals to reduce GI effects. May be
used with uricosuric agents.
• Baseline laboratory studies, including CBC, should precede therapy and
be repeated periodically.
• Monitor fluid intake/output. Keep
output at 2,000 ml daily.
• Store in tightly closed, light-resistant container.
• Change needle before making direct
I.V. injection.
• Has been used effectively to treat
familial Mediterranean fever and hepatic cirrhosis.

cromolyn sodium
Intal♦**, Intal Inhaler, Intal p♦♦,
Nasalcrom, Rynacrom♦♦
Pregnancy Category: B

MECHANISM OF ACTION
Inhibits the degranulation of sensitized mast cells that occurs after a patient's exposure to specific antigens. It
also inhibits release of histamine and
slow-reacting substance of anaphylaxis (SRS-A).

INDICATIONS & DOSAGE
*Adjunct in treatment of severe peren-
nial bronchial asthma—*
Adults and children over 5 years:

contents of 20-mg capsule inhaled q.i.d. at regular intervals. Or, administer two metered sprays using inhaler q.i.d. at regular intervals. Also available as an aqueous solution administered through a nebulizer.

Prevention and treatment of allergic rhinitis—

Adults and children over 5 years: 1 spray in each nostril t.i.d or q.i.d. May give up to 6 times daily.

Prevention of exercise-induced bronchospasm—

Adults and children over 5 years: Inhale contents of one 20-mg capsule or inhale two metered sprays no more than 1 hour before anticipated exercise.

ADVERSE REACTIONS
CNS: dizziness, headache.
EENT: *irritation of the throat and trachea, cough, bronchospasm following inhalation of dry powder; esophagitis;* nasal congestion; pharyngeal irritation; wheezing.
GI: nausea.
GU: dysuria, urinary frequency.
Skin: rash, urticaria.
Other: joint swelling and pain, lacrimation, swollen parotid gland, angioedema, *eosinophilic pneumonia.*

INTERACTIONS
None significant.

NURSING CONSIDERATIONS
• Contraindicated in acute asthma attacks and status asthmaticus.
• Use cautiously in patients with coronary artery disease or history of cardiac arrhythmias.
• Should be discontinued if patient develops eosinophilic pneumonia.
• Capsule not to be swallowed; insert capsule into inhaler provided; follow manufacturer's directions.
• Watch for recurrence of asthmatic symptoms when dosage is decreased, especially when corticosteroids are also used.

• Use only when acute episode has been controlled, airway is cleared, and patient is able to inhale.
• Patient considered for cromolyn therapy should have pulmonary function tests to show significant bronchodilator-reversible component to his airway obstruction.
• Teach correct use of Spinhaler: insert capsule in device properly, exhale completely before placing mouthpiece between lips, then inhale deeply and rapidly with steady, even breath; remove inhaler from mouth, hold breath a few seconds, and exhale. Repeat until all powder has been inhaled.
• Store capsules at room temperature in a tightly closed container; protect from moisture and temperatures higher than 40° C. (104° F.).
• Instruct patient to avoid excessive handling of capsule.
• Esophagitis may be relieved by antacids or a glass of milk.

---

diazoxide, oral
Proglycem
Pregnancy Category: C

MECHANISM OF ACTION
Inhibits the release of insulin from the pancreas and decreases peripheral utilization of glucose.

INDICATIONS & DOSAGE
Management of hypoglycemia due to a variety of conditions resulting in hyperinsulinism—
Adults and children: 3 to 8 mg/kg daily P.O., divided into 3 equal doses q 8 hours.
Infants and newborns: 8 to 15 mg/kg daily P.O., divided into 2 or 3 equal doses q 8 to 12 hours.

ADVERSE REACTIONS
Blood: *leukopenia, thrombocytopenia.*
CV: *cardiac arrhythmias.*
EENT: diplopia.

GI: nausea, vomiting, anorexia, taste alteration.
Metabolic: sodium and fluid retention, ketoacidosis and hyperosmolar nonketotic coma, hyperuricemia.
Other: *severe hypertrichosis (hair growth) in 25% of adults and higher percentage of children.*

INTERACTIONS
Thiazide diuretics: may potentiate hyperglycemic, hyperuricemic, and hypotensive effects. Monitor appropriate laboratory values.

NURSING CONSIDERATIONS
• Contraindicated in thiazide hypersensitivity and functional hypoglycemia.
• Oral diazoxide does not significantly lower blood pressure in dosages used to treat hypoglycemia.
• Most important use is in management of hypoglycemia due to hyperinsulinism in infants and children.
• Monitor urine regularly for glucose and ketones; report any abnormalities to doctor.
• If not effective after 2 or 3 weeks, drug should be stopped.
• Hair growth on arms and forehead is a common adverse reaction that subsides when drug treatment is completed. Reassure patient.
• Available in capsules and oral suspension.

---

disulfiram
Antabuse♦, Cronetal, Ro-Sulfiram
Pregnancy Category: X

MECHANISM OF ACTION
Blocks oxidation of alcohol at the acetaldehyde stage. Excess acetaldehyde produces a highly unpleasant reaction in the presence of even small amounts of alcohol.

INDICATIONS & DOSAGE
Adjunct in management of chronic alcoholism—
Adults: maximum of 500 mg q morning for 1 to 2 weeks. Can be taken in evening if drowsiness occurs. Maintenance: 125 to 500 mg daily (average dose 250 mg) until permanent self-control is established. Treatment may continue for months or years.

ADVERSE REACTIONS
CNS: drowsiness, headache, fatigue, delirium, depression, neuritis.
EENT: optic neuritis.
GI: metallic or garlic-like aftertaste.
GU: impotence.
Skin: acneiform or allergic dermatitis.
Other: disulfiram reaction, which may include flushing, throbbing headache, dyspnea, nausea, copious vomiting, sweating, thirst, chest pain, palpitations, hyperventilation, hypotension, syncope, anxiety, weakness, blurred vision, confusion. In severe reactions, respiratory depression, cardiovascular collapse, arrhythmias, myocardial infarction, acute congestive heart failure, convulsions, unconsciousness, and even death can occur.

INTERACTIONS
Isoniazid (INH): ataxia or marked change in behavior. Avoid use.
Metronidazole: psychotic reaction. Do not use together.
Paraldehyde: toxic levels of the acetaldehyde. Do not use together.
Alcohol: disulfiram reaction.

NURSING CONSIDERATIONS
• Contraindicated in alcohol intoxication, psychoses, myocardial disease, coronary occlusion, or in patients receiving metronidazole, paraldehyde, alcohol, or alcohol-containing preparations; and in pregnancy. Use cautiously in diabetes mellitus, hypothyroidism, epilepsy, cerebral damage, nephritis, hepatic cirrhosis or insufficiency, abnormal EEG, multiple drug dependence.

• Used only under close medical and nursing supervision. Patient should clearly understand consequences of disulfiram therapy and give permission. Drug should be used only in patients who are cooperative, well motivated, and are receiving supportive psychiatric therapy.

• Complete physical examination and laboratory studies, including CBC, SMA-12, and transaminase, should precede therapy and be repeated regularly.

• Warn patient to avoid all sources of alcohol: sauces, cough syrups. Even external application of liniments, shaving lotion, back-rub preparations may precipitate disulfiram reaction. Tell him that alcohol reaction may occur as long as 2 weeks after single dose of disulfiram; the longer patient remains on drug, the more sensitive he will become to alcohol.

• Patient should wear a bracelet or carry a card supplied by drug manufacturer identifying him as disulfiram user.

Note: Mild reactions may occur in sensitive patients with blood alcohol level of 5 to 10 mg/100 ml; symptoms are fully developed at 50 mg/100 ml; unconsciousness usually occurs at 125 to 150 mg/100 ml level. Reaction may last ½ hour to several hours, or as long as alcohol remains in blood.

• Caution patient's family that disulfiram should never be given to the patient without his knowledge; severe reaction or death could result if such a patient then ingested alcohol.

• Reassure patient that disulfiram-induced adverse reactions, such as drowsiness, fatigue, impotence, headache, peripheral neuritis, and metallic- or garlic-like taste, subside after about 2 weeks of therapy.

L-carnitine
Carnitor, Vitacarn
Pregnancy Category: B

MECHANISM OF ACTION
Facilitates the transport of fatty acids into cellular mitochondria. The fatty acids are then used to produce energy.

INDICATIONS & DOSAGE
Primary systemic carnitine deficiency—
Adults: 990 mg (three tablets) P.O. b.i.d. or t.i.d. Alternatively, may give enteral liquid 10 to 30 ml (1 to 3 g) daily.
Children: 50 to 100 mg/kg/day in divided doses of either the tablet or enteral-liquid form.
All doses depend upon the clinical response. Higher doses may be given. However, for children, the maximum dose is 3 g/day.

ADVERSE REACTIONS
GI: *nausea, vomiting, cramps, diarrhea.*
Other: body odor.

INTERACTIONS
D,L carnitive (sold as vitamin B_T in vitamin stores): inhibits L-carnitine and can cause deficiency.

NURSING CONSIDERATIONS
• Monitor patient's tolerance during the 1st week of therapy and after increasing dosage.
• May give enteral liquid alone or dissolved in drinks or liquid food.
• Space doses evenly every 3 to 4 hours if possible. Best to give with or after meals.
• Tell patient to consume enteral liquid slowly to minimize GI distress. If gastrointestinal intolerance persists, dosage may have to be reduced.
• Warn patient to avoid so-called "vitamin B_T" in health food stores. This will interact with the drug and render

it ineffective.
• Caution patient not to share drug with others. Some proponents have used it to improve athletic performance.
• The entire or partial contents of the containers of liquid should be used immediately after opening. Discard any unused contents of opened containers.

levodopa
Dopar, Larodopa♦, Levopa, Parda, Rio-Dopa
Pregnancy Category: C

MECHANISM OF ACTION
Decarboxylated to dopamine, countering the depletion of striatal dopamine in extrapyramidal centers, which is thought to produce parkinsonism.

INDICATIONS & DOSAGE
Treatment of idiopathic parkinsonism, postencephalitic parkinsonism, and symptomatic parkinsonism after carbon monoxide or manganese intoxication; or in association with cerebral arteriosclerosis—
administered orally with food in dosages carefully adjusted to individual requirements, tolerance, response.
Adults: initially, 0.5 to 1 g P.O. daily, given b.i.d., t.i.d., or q.i.d. with food; increase by no more than 0.75 g daily q 3 to 7 days, until usual maximum of 8 g is reached. Larger dose requires close supervision.

ADVERSE REACTIONS
Blood: hemolytic anemia, leukopenia.
CNS: *choreiform, dystonic, dyskinetic movements; involuntary grimacing, head movements, myoclonic body jerks, ataxia, tremors, muscle twitching; bradykinetic episodes; psychiatric disturbances, memory loss, nervousness, anxiety, disturbing dreams,* *euphoria, malaise, fatigue; severe depression, suicidal tendencies, dementia, delirium, hallucinations (may necessitate reduction or withdrawal of drug).*
CV: *orthostatic hypotension,* cardiac irregularities, flushing, hypertension, phlebitis.
EENT: blepharospasm, blurred vision, diplopia, mydriasis or miosis, widening of palpebral fissures, activation of latent Horner's syndrome, oculogyric crises, nasal discharge.
GI: *nausea, vomiting, anorexia;* weight loss may occur at start of therapy; constipation; flatulence; diarrhea; epigastric pain; hiccups; sialorrhea; dry mouth; bitter taste.
GU: urinary frequency, retention, incontinence; darkened urine; excessive and inappropriate sexual behavior; priapism.
Hepatic: hepatotoxicity.
Other: dark perspiration, hyperventilation.

INTERACTIONS
Papaverine, phenothiazines and other antipsychotics, phenytoin: watch for decreased levodopa effect.
Pyridoxine: reduced efficacy of levodopa. Examine vitamin preparations and nutritional supplements for content of vitamin B_6 (pyridoxine).

NURSING CONSIDERATIONS
• Contraindicated in narrow-angle glaucoma, melanoma, or undiagnosed skin lesions. Use cautiously in cardiovascular, renal, hepatic, pulmonary disorders; in patients with peptic ulcer, psychiatric illness, myocardial infarction with residual arrhythmias; and in patients with bronchial asthma, emphysema, and endocrine disease.
• Carefully monitor patients also receiving antihypertensive medication, hypoglycemic agents. Stop MAO inhibitors at least 2 weeks before therapy is begun.
• Adjust dosage according to patient's

responsc and tolerance. Observe and monitor vital signs, especially while adjusting dose. Report significant changes.

• Instruct patient to report adverse reactions and therapeutic effects.

• Warn patient of possible dizziness and orthostatic hypotension, especially at start of therapy. Patient should change position slowly and dangle legs before getting out of bed. Elastic stockings may control this adverse reaction in some patients.

• Muscle twitching and blepharospasm (twitching of eyelids) may be an early sign of drug overdosage; report immediately.

• Patients on long-term use should be tested regularly for diabetes and acromegaly; repeat blood tests, liver and kidney function studies periodically.

• Advise patient and family that multivitamin preparations, fortified cereals, and certain over-the-counter medications may contain pyridoxine (vitamin B₆), which can reverse the effects of levodopa.

• If therapy is interrupted for long period, drug should be adjusted gradually to previous level.

• Therapeutic response usually occurs following each dose and disappears within 5 hours but varies considerably.

• Patient who must undergo surgery should continue levodopa as long as oral intake is permitted, generally 6 to 24 hours before surgery. Drug should be resumed as soon as patient is able to take oral medication.

• Protect from heat, light, moisture. If preparation darkens, it has lost potency and should be discarded.

• Coombs' test occasionally becomes positive during extended use. Expect uric acid elevations with colorimetric method but not with uricase method.

• Alkaline phosphatase, SGOT, SGPT, LDH, bilirubin, BUN, and PBI show transient elevations in patients receiving levodopa; WBC, hemoglobin, and hematocrit show occasional reduction.

• A doctor-supervised period of drug discontinuance (called a drug holiday) may reestablish the effectiveness of a lower dose regimen.

• Combination of levodopa-carbidopa usually reduces amount of levodopa needed by 75%, thereby reducing incidence of adverse reactions.

• Pills may be crushed and mixed with apple sauce or baby food fruits for patients who have difficulty swallowing pills.

• Warn patient and family not to increase drug dose without the doctor's orders (they may be tempted to do this as disease symptoms of parkinsonism progress). Daily dose should not exceed 8 g.

levodopa-carbidopa
(combination)
Sinemet♦
Pregnancy Category: C

MECHANISM OF ACTION
Levodopa is decarboxylated to dopamine, countering the depletion of striatal dopamine in extrapyramidal centers. Carbidopa inhibits the peripheral decarboxylation of levodopa without affecting levodopa's metabolism within the central nervous system. Therefore, more levodopa is available to be decarboxylated to dopamine in the brain.

INDICATIONS & DOSAGE
Treatment of idiopathic Parkinson's disease, postencephalitic parkinsonism, and symptomatic parkinsonism resulting from carbon monoxide or manganese intoxication—
Adults: 3 to 6 tablets of 25 mg carbidopa/250 mg levodopa daily given in divided doses. Do not exceed 8 tablets of 25 mg carbidopa/250 mg levodopa a day. Optimum daily dosage must be determined by careful titration for

---

Italicized side effects are common or life-threatening.
*Liquid form contains alcohol.   **May contain tartrazine.

each patient.

ADVERSE REACTIONS
Blood: hemolytic anemia.
CNS: *choreiform, dystonic, dyskinetic movements; involuntary grimacing, head movements, myoclonic body jerks, ataxia,* tremors, muscle twitching; bradykinetic episodes; psychiatric disturbances, memory loss, nervousness, anxiety, disturbing dreams, euphoria, malaise, fatigue; severe depression, suicidal tendencies, dementia, delirium, hallucinations (may necessitate reduction or withdrawal of drug).
CV: *orthostatic hypotension,* cardiac irregularities, flushing, hypertension, phlebitis.
EENT: blepharospasm, blurred vision, diplopia, mydriasis or miosis, widening of palpebral fissures, activation of latent Horner's syndrome, oculogyric crises, nasal discharge.
GI: nausea, vomiting, anorexia, weight loss may occur at start of therapy; constipation; flatulence; diarrhea; epigastric pain; hiccups; sialorrhea; dry mouth; bitter taste.
GU: urinary frequency, retention, incontinence; darkened urine; excessive and inappropriate sexual behavior; priapism.
Hepatic: hepatotoxicity.
Other: dark perspiration, hyperventilation.

INTERACTIONS
Papaverine, phenothiazines and other antipsychotics, phenytoin: may antagonize anti-Parkinson actions. Use together cautiously.

NURSING CONSIDERATIONS
• Contraindicated in narrow-angle glaucoma, melanoma, or undiagnosed skin lesions. Use cautiously in cardiovascular, renal, hepatic, pulmonary disorders; in history of peptic ulcer, psychiatric illness, myocardial infarction with residual arrhythmias; and in bronchial asthma, emphysema, and endocrine disease.
• Carefully monitor patients also receiving antihypertensive medication, hypoglycemic agents. Discontinue MAO inhibitors at least 2 weeks before therapy is begun.
• Dosage is adjusted according to patient's response and tolerance to drug. Therapeutic and adverse reactions occur more rapidly with levodopa-carbidopa than with levodopa alone. Observe and monitor vital signs, especially while dosage is being adjusted; report significant changes.
• Instruct patient to report adverse reactions and therapeutic effects.
• Warn patient of possible dizziness and orthostatic hypotension, especially at start of therapy. Patient should change position slowly and dangle legs before getting out of bed. Elastic stockings may control this adverse reaction in some patients.
• Muscle twitching and blepharospasm (twitching of eyelids) may be an early sign of drug overdosage; report immediately.
• Patients on long-term therapy should be tested regularly for diabetes and acromegaly; blood tests, liver and kidney function studies should be repeated periodically.
• If patient is being treated with levodopa, discontinue at least 8 hours before starting levodopa-carbidopa.
• This combination drug usually reduces the amount of levodopa needed by 75%, thereby reducing the incidence of adverse reactions.
• Pyridoxine (vitamin B_6) does not reverse the beneficial effects of Sinemet. Multivitamins can be taken without fear of losing control of symptoms.
• If therapy is interrupted temporarily, the usual daily dosage may be given as soon as patient resumes oral medication.
• Available as tablets with carbidopa-levodopa in a 1:10 ratio (Sinemet 10/

100 and Sinemet 25/250); also in a 1:4 ratio (Sinemet 25/100).
• Sinemet 25/100 may reduce many adverse reactions seen with 1:10 ratio strengths.
• Carbidopa (Lodosyn) as a single agent is available from Merck Sharp & Dohme on doctor's request.
• Warn the patient and his family not to increase dose without doctor's order.

methoxsalen
Oxsoralen♦
Pregnancy Category: C

MECHANISM OF ACTION
May enhance melanogenesis, either directly or secondarily, to an inflammatory process.

INDICATIONS & DOSAGE
To induce repigmentation in vitiligo; psoriasis—
Adults and children over 12 years: 20 mg P.O. daily, 2 to 4 hours before carefully timed exposure to ultraviolet light.

ADVERSE REACTIONS
CNS: nervousness, insomnia, depression, vertigo, headache.
GI: *discomfort, nausea, diarrhea.*
Skin: edema, erythema, painful blistering, burning, peeling, pruritus.

INTERACTIONS
Photosensitizing agents: do not use together. May increase toxicity.

NURSING CONSIDERATIONS
• Contraindicated in hepatic insufficiency, porphyria, acute lupus erythematosus, hydromorphic and polymorphic light eruptions. Use with caution in familial history of sunlight allergy, GI diseases, or chronic infection.
• Regulate therapy carefully. Overdosage or overexposure to light can cause serious burning or blistering.
• Drug should be taken orally with meals or milk. Patient should avoid the following foods: limes, figs, parsley, parsnips, mustard, carrots, and celery.
• During light exposure treatments, protect eyes and lips.
• Monthly liver function tests should be done on patients with vitiligo (especially at beginning of therapy).

nicotine resin complex
Nicorette
Pregnancy Category: X

MECHANISM OF ACTION
Stimulates receptors in the central nervous system and causes the release of catecholamines from the adrenal medulla.

INDICATIONS & DOSAGE
Temporary aid to the cigarette smoker seeking to give up smoking while participating in a behavior modification program under medical supervision—
Adults: Chew one piece of gum slowly and intermittently for 30 minutes whenever the urge to smoke occurs. Most patients require approximately 10 pieces of gum per day during the first month. Don't exceed 30 pieces of gum per day.

ADVERSE REACTIONS
CNS: dizziness, light-headedness.
CV: atrial fibrillation.
EENT: throat soreness, jaw muscle ache (from chewing).
GI: nausea, vomiting, indigestion.
Other: hiccups.

INTERACTIONS
None significant.

NURSING CONSIDERATIONS
• Contraindicated in nonsmokers, during the immediate postmyocardial infarction period; in life-threatening

---

Italicized side effects are common or life-threatening.
*Liquid form contains alcohol.   **May contain tartrazine.

arrhythmias, severe or worsening angina pectoris, and active temporomandibular joint disease; and in pregnancy.
• Use cautiously in patients with hyperthyroidism, pheochromocytoma, or insulin-dependent diabetes.
• Nicotine resin complex is the only smoking cessation aid that has been proven safe and effective.
• Smokers most likely to benefit from nicotine gum are those with a high "physical" nicotine dependence. Such smokers show the following characteristics: smoke more than 15 cigarettes daily; prefer brands of cigarettes with high nicotine levels; usually inhale the smoke; smoke the first cigarette within 30 minutes of arising; find the first morning cigarette the hardest to give up; smoke most frequently during the morning; find it difficult to refrain from smoking in places where it's forbidden; or smoke even when they are so ill that they are confined to bed during the day.
• Instruct patient to chew gum slowly and intermittently for about 30 minutes to promote slow and even buccal absorption of nicotine. Fast chewing tends to produce more adverse reactions.
• Successful abstainers will begin gradually withdrawing gum usage after 3 months. Use of the gum for longer than 6 months is not recommended.
• Emphasize the importance of withdrawing the gum gradually.
• The gum is sugar-free and usually doesn't stick to dentures.
• A patient instruction sheet is included in the package dispensed to the patient.

pentoxifylline
Trental
Pregnancy Category: C

MECHANISM OF ACTION
Improves capillary blood flow by increasing erythrocyte flexibility and lowering blood viscosity.

INDICATIONS & DOSAGE
Treatment of intermittent claudication due to chronic occlusive vascular disease—
Adults: 400 mg P.O. t.i.d. with meals.

ADVERSE REACTIONS
CNS: headache, dizziness.
GI: dyspepsia, nausea, vomiting.

INTERACTIONS
None significant.

NURSING CONSIDERATIONS
• Contraindicated in patients who are intolerant to methylxanthines such as caffeine, theophylline, and theobromine.
• Pentoxifylline should be taken for a minimum of 8 weeks to achieve clinical effects. Tell patient not to discontinue the drug during this period unless directed to do so by his doctor.
• Advise patient to take with meals to minimize gastrointestinal upset.
• Patient should report any gastrointestinal or CNS adverse reactions. Doctor may reduce dose.
• Pentoxifylline therapy is useful in patients who are not good surgical candidates.

pralidoxime chloride
Protopam♦
Pregnancy Category: C

MECHANISM OF ACTION
Reactives cholinesterase that has been inactivated by organophosphorus pes-

ticides and related compounds. It permits degradation of accumulated acetylcholine and facilitates normal functioning of neuromuscular junctions.

INDICATIONS & DOSAGE
Antidote for organophosphate poisoning—
Adults: I.V. infusion of 1 to 2 g in 100 ml of saline solution over 15 to 30 minutes. If pulmonary edema is present, give drug by slow I.V. push over 5 minutes. Repeat in 1 hour if muscle weakness persists. Additional doses may be given cautiously. I.M. or S.C. injection can be used if I.V. is not feasible; or 1 to 3 g P.O. q 5 hours.
Children: 20 to 40 mg/kg I.V.
To treat cholinergic crisis in myasthenia gravis—
Adults: 1 to 2 g I.V., followed by increments of 250 mg I.V. q 5 minutes.

ADVERSE REACTIONS
CNS: dizziness, headache, drowsiness, excitement, and manic behavior following recovery of consciousness.
CV: tachycardia.
EENT: blurred vision, diplopia, impaired accommodation, laryngospasm.
GI: nausea.
Other: muscular weakness, muscle rigidity, hyperventilation.

INTERACTIONS
None significant.

NURSING CONSIDERATIONS
• Contraindicated in poisoning with Sevin, a carbamate insecticide, since it increases drug's toxicity. Use with extreme caution in renal insufficiency or myasthenia gravis (overdosage may precipitate myasthenic crisis); also in patients with history of asthma or peptic ulcer.
• Use in hospitalized patients only; have respiratory and other supportive measures available. Obtain accurate medical history and chronology of poisoning if possible. Give as soon as possible after poisoning.
• I.V. preparation should be given slowly, as dilute solution.
• Initial measures should include removal of secretions, maintenance of patent airway, artificial ventilation if needed.
• Drug relieves paralysis of respiratory muscles but is less effective in relieving depression of respiratory center.
• Atropine along with pralidoxime should be given I.V., 2 to 4 mg, if cyanosis is not present. If cyanosis is present, atropine should be given I.M. Give atropine every 5 to 60 minutes until signs of atropine toxicity appear (flushing, tachycardia, dry mouth, blurred vision, excitement, delirium, hallucinations); maintain atropinization for at least 48 hours.
• Dilute with sterile water without preservatives.
• Not effective against poisoning due to phosphorus, inorganic phosphates, or organophosphates with no anticholinesterase activity.
• Difficult to distinguish between toxic effects produced by atropine or by organophosphate compounds and those resulting from pralidoxime. Observe patient for 48 to 72 hours if poison ingested. Delayed absorption may occur from lower bowel.
• Caution patients treated for organophosphate poisoning to avoid contact with insecticides for several weeks.
• Patients with myasthenia gravis treated for overdose of cholinergic drugs should be observed closely for signs of rapid weakening. These patients can pass quickly from a cholinergic crisis to a myasthenic crisis, and require more cholinergic drugs to treat the myasthenia. Keep edrophonium (Tensilon) available in such situations for establishing differential diagnosis.

Italicized side effects are common or life-threatening.
*Liquid form contains alcohol.   **May contain tartrazine.

ritodrine hydrochloride
Yutopar♦
Pregnancy Category: B

MECHANISM OF ACTION
A beta-receptor agonist that stimulates the beta$_2$-adrenergic receptors in uterine smooth muscle, inhibiting contractility.

INDICATIONS & DOSAGE
Management of preterm labor—
I.V. therapy: dilute 150 mg (3 ampuls) in 500 ml of fluid, yielding a final concentration of 0.3 mg/ml. Usual initial dose is 0.1 mg/minute, to be gradually increased according to the results by 0.05 mg/minute q 10 minutes until desired result obtained. Effective dosage range usually lies between 0.15 and 0.35 mg/minute.
Oral maintenance: 1 tablet (10 mg) may be given approximately 30 minutes before termination of I.V. therapy. Usual dosage for first 24 hours of oral maintenance is 10 mg q 2 hours. Thereafter, usual dose is 10 to 20 mg q 4 to 6 hours. Total daily dose should not exceed 120 mg.

ADVERSE REACTIONS
Intravenous
CNS: nervousness, anxiety, headache.
CV: *dose-related alterations in blood pressure, palpitations, pulmonary edema, tachycardia,* EKG changes.
GI: nausea, vomiting.
Metabolic: *hyperglycemia,* hypokalemia.
Other: erythema.
Oral
CNS: tremors, nervousness.
CV: palpitations.
GI: nausea, vomiting.
Skin: rash.

INTERACTIONS
Corticosteroids: may produce pulmonary edema in mother. When these drugs are used concomitantly, monitor closely.
Beta blockers: may inhibit ritodrine's action. Avoid concurrent administration.
Sympathomimetics: additive effects. Use together cautiously.

NURSING CONSIDERATIONS
• Contraindicated before 20th week of pregnancy and in the following conditions: antepartum hemorrhage, eclampsia, intrauterine fetal death, chorioamnionitis, maternal cardiac disease, pulmonary hypertension, maternal hyperthyroidism, uncontrolled maternal diabetes mellitus.
• Because cardiovascular responses are common and more pronounced during I.V. administration, cardiovascular effects—including maternal pulse rate and blood pressure, and fetal heart rate—should be closely monitored. A maternal tachycardia of over 140 or persistent respiratory rate of over 20/minute may be a sign of impending pulmonary edema.
• Monitor blood glucose concentrations during ritodrine infusions, especially in diabetic mothers.
• Discontinue drug if pulmonary edema develops.
• Monitor amount of fluids administered intravenously, to prevent circulatory overload.
• Ritodrine decreases intensity and frequency of uterine contractions.
• Don't use ritodrine I.V. if solution is discolored or contains a precipitate.

sodium cellulose phosphate
Calcibind, Calcisorb♦♦
Pregnancy Category: C

MECHANISM OF ACTION
Binds calcium in the GI tract and decreases the amount absorbed.

INDICATIONS & DOSAGE

Treatment of absorptive hypercalciuria type I with recurrent calcium oxalate or calcium phosphate renal stones—
Adults: 15 g/day (5 g with each meal) in patients with urinary calcium greater than 300 mg/day. When urinary calcium declines to less than 150 mg/day, reduce dosage to 10 g/day (5 g with dinner, 2.5 g with two remaining meals).

ADVERSE REACTIONS

GI: discomfort, *diarrhea,* dyspepsia.
GU: hyperoxaluria, hypomagnesuria.
Other: acute arthralgias.

INTERACTIONS

Magnesium-containing products: May bind drug. Separate doses by at least 1 hour.

NURSING CONSIDERATIONS

• Contraindicated in primary or secondary hyperparathyroidism, including renal hypercalciuria; hypomagnesemic states; bone disease; hypocalcemic states; normal or low intestinal absorption, and renal excretion of calcium; enteric hyperoxaluria.
• Use cautiously in patients with congestive heart failure and ascites.
• Recommended only for the type of absorptive hypercalciuria in which both intestinal calcium absorption and urinary calcium remain abnormally high even with a calcium-restricted diet. When administered inappropriately, it can cause hypocalciuria. This could stimulate parathyroid function and lead to parathyroid bone disease.
• Patient should maintain a calcium-restricted diet and avoid all dairy products.
• Patients taking sodium cellulose phosphate may develop hyperoxaluria and hypomagnesuria, which predispose to stone formation. Therefore, advise patients to restrict dietary intake of oxalate (found in spinach, rhu-barb, chocolate, tea).
• Avoid vitamin C because it can increase urinary oxalate.
• Encourage fluid intake. Urine output should be at least 2 liters/day.
• Patient can mix the powder in fruit juice, water, or a soft drink and take it with meals.
• Encourage a low sodium diet. Tell patient to avoid salty foods and to avoid adding salt at the table.
• Because of the difficulty involved in managing sodium cellulose phosphate therapy, many doctors prefer to treat hypercalciuria with a low calcium diet, high fluid intake, and thiazides, when necessary.

Italicized side effects are common or life-threatening.
*Liquid form contains alcohol.   **May contain tartrazine.

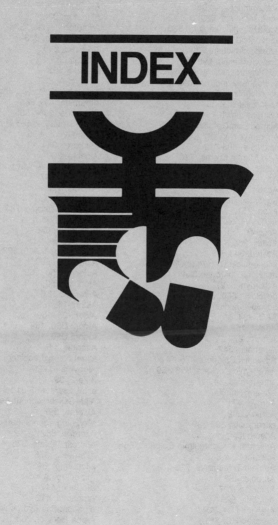

INDEX

Amidrine

A

Ativan, 292
atracurium besylate, **368**
Atromid-S, 200
atropine sulfate, **146, 652**
Atropisol, 652
Atrovent, 339
A/T/S, 685
Attenuvax, 797
Augmentin, 61
Auralgan, 670
auranofin, **837**
Aureomycin 3%, 683
aurothioglucose, **838**
Avazyme, 816
AVC/Dienestrol, 480
Aveeno Colloidal, 732
Aveeno Oilated Bath, 732
Aventyl, 279
Avitene, 582
Avlosulfon, 46
Axotal, 203
Ayercillin, 76
Aygestin, 493
Azactam, 126
azacytidine (5-azacytidine), **626**
5-azacytidine. *See* azacytidine.
azatadine maleate, **377**
azathioprine, **630**
Azlin, 64
azlocillin sodium, **64**
Azmacort, 461
Azo Gantanol, 109, 115
Azo Gantrisin, 109, 115
Azogesic, 210
Azolid, 220
Azo-Mandelamine, 115
Azo-Pyridon, 210
Azo-Standard, 210
aztreonam, **126**
Azulfidine, 112
Azulfidine En-Tabs, 112

B

bacampicillin hydrochloride, **65**
Bacid, 407
Baciguent, 681
Bacitin, 681
bacitracin, **127, 634, 681**
baclofen, **361**
Bactocill, 73
Bactopen, 68
Bactrim, 109
Bactrim DS, 109
Bactrim I.V. Infusion, 109
BAL in Oil, 832
Balmex, 734
Balminil, 390
Balminil DM, 389
Balnetar, 714

Banalg, 732
Bancap HC, 224
Banflex, 367
Banlin, 442
Banthine, 438
Bar, 264
Baramine, 382
Barazole, 113
Barbidonna Elixir, 430
Barbidonna Tablets, 430
Barbidonna #2 Tablets, 430
Barbita, 264
barbiturates. *See* anticonvulsants;
    sedative-hypnotics.
Barc, 695
Baridium, 210
Baritrate, 165
Basaljel, 394, 395
Baumodyne Gel and Ointment, 732
Bax, 382
Bayer Timed-Release, 204
Bayidyl, 386
b-Capsa I, 793
BCG vaccine, **790**
BC Powder, 203
BC Tablets, 203
Beben, 699
beclomethasone dipropionate, **447, 674**
Beclovent, 447
Beconase Nasal Inhaler, 674
Bedoce, 763
Bedoz, 763
Beef Lente Iletin II, 505
Beef NPH Iletin II, 505
Beef Protamine Zinc Iletin II, 505
Beef Regular Iletin II (acid neutral CZI),
    505
Bee six, 767
Belladenal Tablets, 430
belladonna leaf, **432**
Belladonna Tincture USP, 432
Bellafoline, 437
Benachlor, 382
Benadryl, 382
Benahist, 382
Ben-Allergin, 382
Benasept, 723
Benemid, 812
Benisone, 699
Benn, 812
Benoxyl, 741
Bensulfoid, 738
bentiromide, **400**
Bentrac, 382
Bentyl, 434
Bentyl 10 mg with Phenobarbital
    Capsules, 430
Bentyl 20 mg with Phenobarbital
    Tablets, 430
Bentylol, 434

866

E

874

I

M

O

888

Proplex, 582
Pro-Pox 65, 238
propoxyphene hydrochloride, **238**
propoxyphene napsylate, **238**
propranolol hydrochloride, **165**
propylthiouracil (PTU), **519**
Propyl-Thyracil, 519
Prorex, 383
Prosed, 115
Prostaphlin, 73
Prostigmin, 333
Prostigmin Bromide, 333
Prostin E₂, 818
Prostin F₂ Alpha, 819
Prostin/M15, 818
Prostin VR Pediatric, 846
protamine sulfate, **577**
Protamine Zinc Iletin I, 505
protamine zinc insulin suspension (PZI), **505**
Protaphane NPH, 505
protectants, 729-735
Protenate, 586
Proternol (tabs), 349
Protopam, 857
Protophylline, 824
protriptyline hydrochloride, **281**
Protropin, 525
Proval No. 3, 225
Proventil, 344
Proventil Syrup, 344
Provera, 492
Provigan, 383
Proviodine, 727
Proxagesic, 238
Proxigel, 715
pseudoephedrine hydrochloride, **355**
pseudoephedrine sulfate, **355**
psoriGel, 714
PSP-I.V., 458
psychotherapeutics, miscellaneous, 315-316
psyllium, **417**
P-T-T, 165
Purge, 412
Purinethol, 604
P.V. Carpine Liquifilm, 650
PVF K, 77
Pyopen, 66
Pyranistan, 379
pyrantel pamoate, **28**
pyrazinamide, **50**
pyrethrins, **695**
Pyribenzamine, 386
Pyridiate, 210
Pyridium, 210
pyridostigmine bromide, **335**
pyridoxine hydrochloride (vitamin B₆), **767**

pyrimethamine, **41**
Pyrin-Aid, 695
Pyrinyl, 695
pyrvinium pamoate, **28**

Q

Quadrinal, 343
Quarzan, 433
quazepam, **251**
Questran, 199
Quibron Capsules, 824
Quibron Plus, 343
Quibron-T/SR, 829
Quiess, 291
quinacrine hydrochloride, **29**
Quinaglute Dura-Tabs, 155
Quinamm, 42
Quinate, 155
Quinatime, 155
Quine, 155
quinestrol, **489**
quinethazone, **549**
Quinidex Extentabs, 155
quinidine gluconate, **155**
quinidine polygalacturonate, **155**
quinidine sulfate, **155**
quinine sulfate, **42**
Quinnone, 744
Quinoform, 686
Quinora, 155
Quin-Release, 155
Quintrate, 165
Quintrol, 42
Q-Vel, 42

R

rabies immune globulin, human, **787**
rabies vaccine, human diploid cell (HDCV), **801**
radioactive iodine (sodium iodide) ¹³¹I, **520**
Radiostol, 770
Radiostol Forte, 770
Ram, 423
ranitidine, **445**
Rate, 165
Rau, 189
Raudixin, 189
Rauja, 189
Raumason, 189
Rauneed, 189
Raupoid, 189
Rau-Sed, 191
Rausertina, 189
Rautrax, 170
Rautrax-N, 170
Rauval, 189
Rauwoldin, 189

TABLE OF EQUIVALENTS

PENICILLIN UNITS
1 unit = 0.6 mcg penicillin G
1 mg penicillin = 1,667 units

WEIGHTS

APOTHECARY		METRIC	APOTHECARY		METRIC
1 ounce	=	31.1 g	1/150 grain	=	0.4 mg
15.43 grains	=	1 g	1/200 grain	=	0.3 mg
1 grain	=	60 mg	1/250 grain	=	0.25 mg
1/60 grain	=	1.0 mg	1/300 grain	=	0.2 mg
1/80 grain	=	0.8 mg	1/400 grain	=	0.15 mg
1/100 grain	=	0.6 mg	1/500 grain	=	0.12 mg
1/120 grain	=	0.5 mg	1/600 grain	=	0.1 mg

LIQUID MEASURE

HOUSEHOLD		APOTHECARY		APPROXIMATE METRIC
1 teaspoonful	=	1 fluid dram	=	5 ml
1 tablespoonful	=	4 fluid drams	=	15 ml
2 tablespoonfuls	=	1 fluid ounce	=	30 ml
1 measuring cupful	=	8 fluid ounces	=	240 ml
1 pint	=	16 fluid ounces	=	500 ml
1 quart	=	32 fluid ounces	=	1,000 ml

TEMPERATURE

9 C.° = 5 F.° − 160

Centigrade   Fahrenheit
(C.° x 9/5) + 32 = F.°

Fahrenheit   Centigrade
(F.° − 32) x 5/9 = C.°

METRIC WEIGHT EQUIVALENTS
1 kg = 1,000 g
1 g = 1,000 mg
1 mg = 0.001 g
1 mcg or μg = 0.001 mg

CONVERSIONS
1 oz = 30 g
1 lb = 453.6 g
2.2 lb = 1 kg

METRIC VOLUME EQUIVALENTS
1 liter = 1,000 ml
1 deciliter = 100 ml